APA Handbook of

Pediatric Psychology, Developmental-Behavioral Pediatrics, and Developmental Science

APA Handbooks in Psychology® Series

APA Addiction Syndrome Handbook—two volumes
    Howard J. Shaffer, Editor-in-Chief

APA Educational Psychology Handbook—three volumes
    Karen R. Harris, Steve Graham, and Tim Urdan, Editors-in-Chief

APA Handbook of Adolescent and Young Adult Development—one volume
    Lisa J. Crockett, Gustavo Carlo, and John E. Schulenberg, Editors-in-Chief

APA Handbook of Behavior Analysis—two volumes
    Gregory J. Madden, Editor-in-Chief

APA Handbook of Career Intervention—two volumes
    Paul J. Hartung, Mark L. Savickas, and W. Bruce Walsh, Editors-in-Chief

APA Handbook of Clinical Geropsychology—two volumes
    Peter A. Lichtenberg and Benjamin T. Mast, Editors-in-Chief

APA Handbook of Clinical Psychology—five volumes
    John C. Norcross, Gary R. VandenBos, and Donald K. Freedheim, Editors-in-Chief

APA Handbook of Community Psychology—two volumes
    Meg A. Bond, Irma Serrano-García, and Christopher B. Keys, Editors-in-Chief

APA Handbook of Comparative Psychology—two volumes
    Josep Call, Editor-in-Chief

APA Handbook of Consumer Psychology—one volume
    Lynn R. Kahle, Editor-in-Chief

APA Handbook of Contemporary Family Psychology—three volumes
    Barbara H. Fiese, Editor-in-Chief

APA Handbook of Counseling Psychology—two volumes
    Nadya A. Fouad, Editor-in-Chief

APA Handbook of Dementia—one volume
    Glenn E. Smith, Editor-in-Chief

APA Handbook of Ethics in Psychology—two volumes
    Samuel J. Knapp, Editor-in-Chief

APA Handbook of Forensic Neuropsychology—one volume
    Shane S. Bush, Editor-in-Chief

APA Handbook of Forensic Psychology—two volumes
    Brian L. Cutler and Patricia A. Zapf, Editors-in-Chief

APA Handbook of Giftedness and Talent—one volume
    Steven I. Pfeiffer, Editor-in-Chief

APA Handbook of Health Psychology—three volumes
    Neil Schneiderman, Editor-in-Chief

APA Handbook of Human Systems Integration—one volume
    Deborah A. Boehm-Davis, Francis T. Durso, and John D. Lee, Editors-in-Chief

APA Handbook of Industrial and Organizational Psychology—three volumes
    Sheldon Zedeck, Editor-in-Chief

APA Handbook of Intellectual and Developmental Disabilities—two volumes
    Laraine Masters Glidden, Editor-in-Chief

APA Handbook of Men and Masculinities—one volume
    Y. Joel Wong and Stephen R. Wester, Editors-in-Chief

APA Handbook of Multicultural Psychology—two volumes
    Frederick T. L. Leong, Editor-in-Chief
APA Handbook of Neuropsychology—two volumes
    Gregory G. Brown, Bruce Crosson, Kathleen Y. Haaland, and Tricia Z. King, Editors
APA Handbook of Nonverbal Communication—one volume
    David Matsumoto, Hyisung Hwang, and Mark Frank, Editors-in-Chief
APA Handbook of Pediatric Psychology, Developmental-Behavioral Pediatrics, and Developmental Science—two volumes
    Marc H. Bornstein and Prachi E. Shah, Editors-in-Chief
APA Handbook of Personality and Social Psychology—four volumes
    Mario Mikulincer and Phillip R. Shaver, Editors-in-Chief
APA Handbook of Psychology and Juvenile Justice—one volume
    Kirk Heilbrun, Editor-in-Chief
APA Handbook of Psychology, Religion, and Spirituality—two volumes
    Kenneth I. Pargament, Editor-in-Chief
APA Handbook of the Psychology of Women—two volumes
    Cheryl B. Travis and Jacquelyn W. White, Editors-in-Chief
APA Handbook of Psychopathology—two volumes
    James N. Butcher, Editor-in-Chief
APA Handbook of Psychopharmacology—one volume
    Suzette M. Evans, Editor-in-Chief
APA Handbook of Psychotherapy—two volumes
    Frederick T. L. Leong, Editor-in-Chief
APA Handbook of Research Methods in Psychology, Second Edition—three volumes
    Harris Cooper, Editor-in-Chief
APA Handbook of Sexuality and Psychology—two volumes
    Deborah L. Tolman and Lisa M. Diamond, Editors-in-Chief
APA Handbook of Sport and Exercise Psychology—two volumes
    Mark H. Anshel, Editor-in-Chief
APA Handbook of Testing and Assessment in Psychology—three volumes
    Kurt F. Geisinger, Editor-in-Chief
APA Handbook of Trauma Psychology—two volumes
    Steven N. Gold, Editor-in-Chief

APA Handbooks in Psychology

APA Handbook of
Pediatric Psychology, Developmental-Behavioral Pediatrics, and Developmental Science

VOLUME 2

Pediatric Psychology and
Developmental-Behavioral Pediatrics:
Clinical Applications of Developmental Science

Prachi E. Shah and Marc H. Bornstein, *Editors-in-Chief*

AMERICAN PSYCHOLOGICAL ASSOCIATION

Copyright © 2025 by the American Psychological Association. All rights, including for text and data mining, AI training, and similar technologies, are reserved. Except as permitted under the United States Copyright Act of 1976, no part of this publication may be reproduced or distributed in any form or by any means, including, but not limited to, the process of scanning and digitization, or stored in a database or retrieval system, without the prior written permission of the publisher.

The opinions and statements published are those of the Authors, and do not necessarily represent the policies of the American Psychological Association. The information contained in this work does not constitute personalized therapeutic advice. Users seeking medical advice, diagnoses, or treatment should consult a medical professional or health care provider. The Authors have worked to ensure that all information in this book is accurate at the time of publication and consistent with general mental health care standards.

Published by
American Psychological Association
750 First Street, NE
Washington, DC 20002
https://www.apa.org

Order Department
https://www.apa.org/pubs/books
order@apa.org

Typeset in Berkeley by Circle Graphics, Inc., Reisterstown, MD

Printer: Sheridan Books, Chelsea, MI
Cover Designer: Mark Karis

Library of Congress Cataloging-in-Publication Data

Names: Bornstein, Marc H., editor. | Shah, Prachi E. (Prachi Edlagan), editor. |
  American Psychological Association, issuing body.
Title: APA handbook of pediatric psychology, developmental-behavioral pediatrics,
  and developmental science / editors-in-chief, Marc H. Bornstein and Prachi E. Shah.
Other titles: Handbook of pediatric psychology, developmental-behavioral pediatrics,
  and developmental science | APA handbooks in psychology
Description: Washington, DC : American Psychological Association, [2025] |
  Series: APA handbooks in psychology | Includes bibliographical references and index. |
  Contents: v. 1. Developmental science and developmental origins of risk and resilience
  in childhood and adolescence -- v. 2. Pediatric psychology and developmental-behavioral
  pediatrics: clinical applications of developmental science.
Identifiers: LCCN 2024007960 (print) | LCCN 2024007961 (ebook) |
  ISBN 9781433833878 (v. 1 ; hardcover) | ISBN 9781433838774 (v. 2 ; hardcover)
  ISBN 9781433844713 (v. 1 ; ebook) | ISBN 9781433844300 (v. 2 ; ebook)
Subjects: MESH: Psychology, Child | Psychology, Adolescent | Child Development |
  Adolescent Development | Psychology, Developmental | Behavioral Medicine
Classification: LCC RJ499.3 (print) | LCC RJ499.3 (ebook) | NLM WS 105 |
  DDC 618.92/89--dc23/eng/20241107
LC record available at https://lccn.loc.gov/2024007960
LC ebook record available at https://lccn.loc.gov/2024007961

https://doi.org/10.1037/0000414-000

Printed in the United States of America

10 9 8 7 6 5 4 3 2 1

Contents

Volume 2: Pediatric Psychology and Developmental-Behavioral Pediatrics: Clinical Applications of Developmental Science

Editorial Board xi
Contributors xiii

Part I. Family Systems and Ecological Contexts Relevant to Child Health, Development, and Behavior 1

Chapter 1. Family Processes and Child Outcomes in Children With Chronic Health Conditions 3
Thomas G. Power, Wendy M. Gaultney, and Lynnda M. Dahlquist

Chapter 2. Pediatric Treatment Adherence 27
Alexandra M. Psihogios, Annisa M. Ahmed, Christina E. Holbein, and Aimee W. Smith

Chapter 3. Chronic and Recurrent Pain: Considerations for Child Health and Well-Being 49
Tonya M. Palermo and Irina Gorbounova

Chapter 4. Pediatric Medical Traumatic Stress 71
Melissa Carson, Joshua Kallman, and Douglas Vanderbilt

Chapter 5. Pediatric Palliative, End-of-Life, and Bereavement Care 97
Cynthia A. Gerhardt, Anna Olsavsky, Garey Noritz, and Amy E. Baughcum

Part II. Select Child Developmental Contexts, Child Health Conditions, and the Role of Pediatric Psychology 121

Chapter 6. Gender Identity, Gender Dysphoria, and Gender-Affirming Models in Childhood and Adolescence: Clinical and Developmental Science Perspectives 123
Diane Ehrensaft

Chapter 7. Genetic Disorders in Childhood: Chromosome 22q11.2 Deletion Syndrome, Down Syndrome, and Fragile X Syndrome 143
Kathleen Angkustsiri, Angela Thurman, and Randi Hagerman

Chapter 8. Congenital Medical Conditions in Childhood and Adolescence,
  Stigma, and Psychosocial Adjustment 163
    Canice E. Crerand and Jennifer Hansen-Moore
Chapter 9. Pediatric Central Nervous System Disorders: Spina Bifida, Epilepsy,
  and Traumatic Brain Injury...................................... 187
    *Grayson N. Holmbeck, Dhanashree Bahulekar, Olivia E. Clark,
    Julie Doran, Aimee W. Smith, Amery Treble-Barna, and Adrien M. Winning*
Chapter 10. Pediatric Sickle Cell Disease: Implications for Child Health
  and Development 213
    Kemar V. Prussien, Lamia P. Barakat, and Lisa A. Schwartz
Chapter 11. Childhood Cancer: Promoting Health and Well-Being Through
  Pediatric Multidisciplinary Care................................. 235
    *Lisa A. Schwartz, Katie Darabos, Megan N. Perez, Branlyn DeRosa,
    Kemar V. Prussien, Meredith E. MacGregor, and Lamia P. Barakat*
Chapter 12. Pulmonary Disorders: Asthma and Cystic Fibrosis, Considerations
  for Child Health and Well-Being 255
    Emily F. Muther, Courtney Lynn, Emily Skeen, and Monica Federico
Chapter 13. Pediatric and Congenital Heart Disease................. 283
    *Jennifer L. Butcher, Laurel M. Bear, Cheryl L. Brosig Soto,
    Colette Gramszlo, Erica Sood, and Samantha Butler*
Chapter 14. Type 1 and Type 2 Diabetes: Interdisciplinary Management
  in Pediatric Settings... 307
    Luiza Mali, Gabriela Guevara, and Alan M. Delamater
Chapter 15. Pediatric Obesity and Implications for Child Health and Well-Being.... 341
    Bethany J. Gaffka, Susan J. Woolford, Hurley O. Riley, and Alison L. Miller

**Part III. Developmental-Behavioral and Mental Health Conditions
  and the Role of Behavioral Health Providers** 363

Chapter 16. Autism Spectrum Disorder and Disorders of Social Cognition
  Across Childhood and Adolescence 365
    *Christina Toolan, Elaine Clarke, Kathleen Campbell, Paul Carbone,
    and Catherine Lord*
Chapter 17. Preterm Birth: Implications for the Family System and Child and
  Adolescent Health and Well-Being 393
    Maria Spinelli, Julie Poehlmann, and Prachi E. Shah
Chapter 18. Neurosensory Disorders: Hearing, Visual, and Multisensory
  Impairments in Childhood 421
    Desmond Kelly, Anne M. Kinsman, and Erin R. Hahn
Chapter 19. Sleep and Sleep Disorders in Children.................. 445
    Judith A. Owens
Chapter 20. Elimination Disorders in Children and Adolescents 477
    Dawn Dore-Stites and Barbara T. Felt
Chapter 21. Attention and Attention-Deficit/Hyperactivity Disorder
  in Childhood 497
    Tanya E. Froehlich and Stephen P. Becker

Chapter 22. Internalizing and Externalizing Problems in Children and Youth..... 523
    Lana Mahgoub, David Meyer, and Mary Margaret Gleason
Chapter 23. Eating Disorders in Children and Adolescents 551
    Terrill Bravender, Natalie Prohaska, and Jessica Van Huysse
Chapter 24. Suicidal Thinking and Behavior in Youth: Prevention, Intervention,
    and Implications for Child and Adolescent Health. 573
    Cynthia Ewell Foster, Seth Finkelstein, Daniel Epstein, and Cheryl A. King

**Part IV. Multidisciplinary Assessments, Interventions, and Treatments
to Foster Child Health and Well-Being 595**

Chapter 25. Developmental Assessment of Infants and Toddlers: Concepts,
    Psychometric Issues, and Related Brain Development 597
    Glen P. Aylward
Chapter 26. Learning, Cognition, and Intellectual and Learning Disorders—
    Evaluation and Management in Pediatric Settings 615
    Danielle N. Shapiro and Jennifer C. Gidley Larson
Chapter 27. Psychological Consultation in Inpatient Pediatric Medical Settings.... 637
    Cassie N. Ross and Kristin A. Kullgren
Chapter 28. Integrated Behavioral Health in Pediatric Health Care Settings......... 659
    Blake M. Lancaster, Hannah L. Ham, Alexandra Neenan, Eleah Sunde,
    Sharnita D. Harris, Luke K. Turnier, Richard Birnbaum, and
    Alexandros Maragakis
Chapter 29. Relationship-Focused Interventions and Psychotherapy:
    Applications for Child and Adolescent Health and Behavior 681
    Megan M. Julian, Fiona K. Miller, and Jerrica Pitzen

Index.. 707

Editorial Board

EDITORS-IN-CHIEF

Prachi E. Shah, MD, MS, Professor of Pediatrics and Psychiatry, Division of Developmental Behavioral Pediatrics, Department of Pediatrics, and Department of Psychiatry, University of Michigan Medical School, Ann Arbor, MI, United States

Marc H. Bornstein, PhD, holds appointments at the Eunice Kennedy Shriver National Institute of Child Health and Human Development, Bethesda, MD, United States, the Institute for Fiscal Studies, London, United Kingdom of Great Britain and Northern Ireland, and UNICEF, New York, NY, United States

Contributors

Annisa M. Ahmed, BA, Department of Psychological and Brain Sciences, Texas A&M University, College Station, TX, United States

Kathleen Angkustsiri, MD, Department of Pediatrics, University of California, Davis, Davis, CA, and MIND Institute, UC Davis Medical Center, UC Davis Health, Sacramento, CA, United States

Glen P. Aylward, PhD, Professor Emeritus, SIU School of Medicine, Pediatrics, and Psychiatry, Springfield, IL, United States

Dhanashree Bahulekar, MA, Department of Psychological Science, The University of North Carolina at Charlotte, Charlotte, NC, United States

Lamia P. Barakat, PhD, Division of Oncology, Children's Hospital of Philadelphia, and Departments of Pediatrics and Psychiatry, University of Pennsylvania Perelman School of Medicine, Philadelphia, PA, United States

Amy E. Baughcum, PhD, Division of Pediatric Psychology and Neuropsychology, Nationwide Children's Hospital, and Department of Pediatrics, The Ohio State University, Columbus, OH, United States

Laurel M. Bear, MD, Herma Heart Institute, Children's Wisconsin, and Department of Pediatrics, Medical College of Wisconsin, Milwaukee, WI, United States

Stephen P. Becker, PhD, Division of Behavioral Medicine and Clinical Psychology, Cincinnati Children's Hospital Medical Center, and Department of Pediatrics, University of Cincinnati College of Medicine, Cincinnati, OH, United States

Richard Birnbaum, PhD, Division of Pediatric Psychology, Department of Pediatrics, Michigan Medicine, University of Michigan, Ann Arbor, MI, United States

Terrill Bravender, MD, MPH, David S Rosen MD Collegiate Professor of Adolescent Medicine, Division Director of Adolescent Medicine, Professor of Pediatrics and Psychiatry, University of Michigan and C. S. Mott Children's Hospital, Ann Arbor, MI, United States

Cheryl L. Brosig Soto, PhD, Herma Heart Institute, Children's Wisconsin, and Department of Pediatrics, Medical College of Wisconsin, Milwaukee, WI, United States

Jennifer L. Butcher, PhD, Department of Pediatrics, C. S. Mott Children's Hospital, University of Michigan, Ann Arbor, MI, United States

Samantha Butler, PhD, Departments of Psychiatry and Behavioral Sciences, Boston Children's Hospital, and Department of Psychiatry, Harvard Medical School, Boston, MA, United States

Contributors

Kathleen Campbell, MD, MHSc, Division of Developmental and Behavioral Pediatrics, Children's Hospital of Philadelphia, Philadelphia, PA, United States

Paul Carbone, MD, Department of Pediatrics, University of Utah, Salt Lake City, UT, United States

Melissa Carson, PsyD, Division of General Pediatrics, Department of Pediatrics, Children's Hospital Los Angeles, and Keck School of Medicine of the University of Southern California, Los Angeles, CA, United States

Olivia E. Clark, MA, Department of Psychology, Loyola University Chicago, Chicago, IL, United States

Elaine Clarke, MA, Department of Psychiatry and Biobehavioral Sciences, David Geffen School of Medicine, UCLA, Los Angeles, CA, United States

Canice E. Crerand, PhD, Section of Pediatric Psychology and Neuropsychology, Nationwide Children's Hospital; Department of Pediatrics, The Ohio State University College of Medicine; and the Center for Biobehavioral Health, The Abigail Wexner Research Institute at Nationwide Children's Hospital, Columbus, OH, United States

Lynnda M. Dahlquist, PhD, Department of Psychology, University of Maryland Baltimore County, Catonsville, MD, United States

Katie Darabos, PhD, Department of Health Behavior, Society, and Policy, School of Public Health, Rutgers University, New Brunswick, NJ, United States

Alan M. Delamater, PhD, Department of Pediatrics, University of Miami Miller School of Medicine, Miami, FL, United States

Branlyn DeRosa, PhD, Division of Oncology, Children's Hospital of Philadelphia, and Department of Psychiatry, University of Pennsylvania Perelman School of Medicine, Philadelphia, PA, United States

Julie Doran, MS, Department of Psychology, East Carolina University, Greenville, NC, United States

Dawn Dore-Stites, PhD, Pediatric Psychology Clinic, C. S. Mott Children's Hospital, University of Michigan, and Department of Pediatrics, Michigan Medicine, University of Michigan, Ann Arbor, MI, United States

Diane Ehrensaft, PhD, Department of Pediatrics, UCSF Benioff Children's Hospitals, San Francisco, CA, United States

Daniel Epstein, BA, School of Psychology and Counseling, Fairleigh Dickinson University, Teaneck, NJ, United States

Cynthia Ewell Foster, PhD, Department of Psychiatry, Michigan Medicine, and Rackham Graduate School, University of Michigan, Ann Arbor, MI, United States

Monica Federico, University of Colorado School of Medicine, Anschutz Medical Campus, and Children's Hospital Colorado, Aurora, CO, United States

Barbara T. Felt, MD, MS, Division of Developmental Behavioral Pediatrics, Department of Pediatrics, University of Michigan, Ann Arbor, MI, United States

Seth Finkelstein, BA, Department of Psychiatry, Michigan Medicine, University of Michigan, Ann Arbor, MI, United States

Tanya E. Froehlich, MD, MS, FAAP, Division of Developmental and Behavioral Pediatrics, Cincinnati Children's Hospital Medical Center, and Department of Pediatrics, University of Cincinnati College of Medicine, Cincinnati, OH, United States

Bethany J. Gaffka, PhD, Department of Pediatrics, University of Michigan Health, Ann Arbor, MI, United States

Wendy M. Gaultney, PhD, Department of Anesthesiology, University of Colorado Anschutz Medical Campus, Aurora, CO, United States

Cynthia A. Gerhardt, PhD, Center for Biobehavioral Health, The Abigail Wexner Research Institute at Nationwide Children's Hospital, and Departments of Pediatrics and Psychology, The Ohio State University, Columbus, OH, United States

Jennifer C. Gidley Larson, PhD, Department of Physical Medicine and Rehabilitation, Michigan Medicine, University of Michigan, Ann Arbor, MI, United States

Mary Margaret Gleason, MD, Eastern Virginia Medical School and Children's Hospital of the King's Daughters, Norfolk, VA, United States

Irina Gorbounova, MD, Hasbro Children's Hospital, Lifespan Health System, Providence, RI, United States

Colette Gramszlo, PhD, Department of Child and Adolescent Psychiatry and Behavioral Sciences, Children's Hospital of Philadelphia, and Department of Clinical Psychiatry, Perelman School of Medicine, University of Pennsylvania, Philadelphia, PA, United States

Gabriela Guevara, MPH, Department of Pediatrics, University of Miami Miller School of Medicine, Miami, FL, United States

Randi Hagerman, MD, Department of Pediatrics, University of California, Davis, Davis, CA, and MIND Institute, UC Davis Medical Center, UC Davis Health, Sacramento, CA, United States

Erin R. Hahn, PhD, Department of Psychology, Furman University, Greenville, SC, United States

Hannah L. Ham, PhD, Division of Pediatric Psychology, Department of Pediatrics, Michigan Medicine, University of Michigan, Ann Arbor, MI, United States

Jennifer Hansen-Moore, PhD, Section of Pediatric Psychology and Neuropsychology, Nationwide Children's Hospital, and Department of Pediatrics, The Ohio State University College of Medicine, Columbus, OH, United States

Sharnita D. Harris, PhD, College of Medicine, Department of Pediatrics, Ohio State University, Columbus, OH and Department of Psychology and Neuropsychology, Nationwide Children's Hospital, Columbus, OH, United States

Christina E. Holbein, PhD, Department of Child and Adolescent Psychiatry and Behavioral Sciences and the Center for Inflammatory Bowel Disease, Division of Gastroenterology, Hepatology and Nutrition, Children's Hospital of Philadelphia, Philadelphia, PA, United States

Grayson N. Holmbeck, PhD, Department of Psychology, Loyola University Chicago, Chicago, IL, United States

Megan M. Julian, PhD, independent practice, Ann Arbor, MI, United States

Joshua Kallman, MD, Division of Developmental-Behavioral Pediatrics, Department of Pediatrics, Children's Hospital Los Angeles, and Keck School of Medicine of the University of Southern California, Los Angeles, CA, United States

Desmond Kelly, MD, Prisma Health Children's Hospital Developmental Pediatrics—Greenville, and University of South Carolina School of Medicine Greenville, Greenville, SC, United States

Cheryl A. King, PhD, Department of Psychiatry, Michigan Medicine, University of Michigan, Ann Arbor, MI, United States

Anne M. Kinsman, PhD, Prisma Health Pediatric Psychology—Greenville, and University of South Carolina School of Medicine Greenville, Greenville, SC, United States

Kristin A. Kullgren, PhD, Division of Pediatric Psychology, Department of Pediatrics, Michigan Medicine, University of Michigan, Ann Arbor, MI, United States

Blake M. Lancaster, PhD, Division of Pediatric Psychology, Department of Pediatrics, Michigan Medicine, University of Michigan, Ann Arbor, MI, United States

Catherine Lord, PhD, Department of Psychiatry and Biobehavioral Sciences, David Geffen School of Medicine, UCLA, Los Angeles, CA, United States

Courtney Lynn, PhD, School of Education and Human Development, University of Colorado Denver, and Integrated Behavioral Health, Denver, CO, United States

Meredith E. MacGregor, MD, Department of Child and Adolescent Psychiatry and Behavioral Sciences, Children's Hospital of Philadelphia, Philadelphia, PA, United States

Lana Mahgoub, PhD, Eastern Virginia Medical School and Children's Hospital of the King's Daughters, Norfolk, VA, United States

Luiza Mali, PhD, Department of Pediatrics, University of Miami Miller School of Medicine, Miami, FL, United States

Alexandros Maragakis, PhD, School of Graduate and Professional Education, The American College of Greece, Athens, Greece

David Meyer, PhD, Eastern Virginia Medical School and Children's Hospital of the King's Daughters, Norfolk, VA, United States

Alison L. Miller, PhD, Department of Health Behavior and Health Education, University of Michigan School of Public Health, Ann Arbor, MI, United States

Fiona K. Miller, PhD, ABPP, Alba Psychology USA, PLC, Ann Arbor, MI, United States

Emily F. Muther, PhD, University of Colorado School of Medicine, Anschutz Medical Campus, and Children's Hospital Colorado, Aurora, CO, United States

Alexandra Neenan, MS, Department of Psychology, Eastern Michigan University, Ypsilanti, MI, United States

Garey Noritz, MD, Department of Pediatrics, Nationwide Children's Hospital and The Ohio State University School of Medicine, Columbus, OH, United States

Anna Olsavsky, PhD, Center for Biobehavioral Health, The Abigail Wexner Research Institute at Nationwide Children's Hospital, Columbus, OH, United States

Judith A. Owens, MD, MPH, Division of Sleep Medicine, Harvard Medical School, and Center for Pediatric Sleep Disorders, Department of Neurology, Boston Children's Hospital, Boston, MA, United States

Tonya M. Palermo, PhD, Center for Child Health, Behavior and Development, Seattle Children's Research Institute, and Departments of Anesthesiology and Pain Medicine and of Pediatrics, University of Washington, Seattle, WA, United States

Megan N. Perez, PhD, Division of Oncology, Children's Hospital of Philadelphia, Philadelphia, PA, United States

Jerrica Pitzen, PhD, Department of Psychology and Behavioral Science, Rochester Christian University, Rochester Hills, MI, United States

Julie Poehlmann, PhD, Department of Human Development and Family Studies, University of Wisconsin, Madison, WI, United States

Thomas G. Power, PhD, Department of Human Development, Washington State University, Pullman, WA, United States

Natalie Prohaska, MD, Clinical Assistant Professor, Department of Psychiatry and Pediatrics, University of Michigan, Ann Arbor, MI, United States

Kemar V. Prussien, PhD, Divisions of Hematology and Oncology, Department of Child and Adolescent Psychiatry and Behavioral Sciences, Children's Hospital of Philadelphia, Philadelphia, PA, United States

Alexandra M. Psihogios, PhD, Department of Medical Social Sciences, Northwestern University Feinberg School of Medicine, Chicago, IL, United States

Hurley O. Riley, MPH, Department of Health Behavior and Health Education, University of Michigan School of Public Health, Ann Arbor, MI, United States

Cassie N. Ross, PsyD, Division of Pediatric Psychology, Department of Pediatrics, Michigan Medicine, University of Michigan, Ann Arbor, MI, United States

Lisa A. Schwartz, PhD, Division of Oncology, Children's Hospital of Philadelphia, and Department of Pediatrics, University of Pennsylvania Perelman School of Medicine, Philadelphia, PA, United States

Prachi E. Shah, MD, MS, Division of Developmental Behavioral Pediatrics, Department of Pediatrics, and Department of Psychiatry, University of Michigan Medical School, Ann Arbor, MI, United States

Danielle N. Shapiro, PhD, ABPP-CN, Department of Physical Medicine and Rehabilitation, Michigan Medicine, University of Michigan, Ann Arbor, MI, United States

Emily Skeen, MD, University of Colorado School of Medicine, Anschutz Medical Campus, and Children's Hospital Colorado, Aurora, CO, United States

Aimee W. Smith, PhD, Department of Psychological Science, University of North Carolina at Charlotte, Charlotte, NC, United States

Erica Sood, PhD, Nemours Cardiac Center, Nemours Children's Health, Wilmington, DE, and Sidney Kimmel Medical College, Thomas Jefferson University, Philadelphia, PA, United States

Maria Spinelli, PhD, Department of Neurosciences, Imaging and Clinical Sciences, University G. D'Annunzio Chieti-Pescara, Chieti, Italy

Eleah Sunde, PhD, Healthpoint Community Health, Renton, WA, United States

Angela Thurman, PhD, Department of Psychiatry and Behavioral Sciences, University of California, Davis, Davis, CA, and MIND Institute, UC Davis Medical Center, UC Davis Health, Sacramento, CA, United States

Christina Toolan, PhD, Department of Child Development, California State University Dominguez Hills, Carson, CA, United States

Amery Treble-Barna, PhD, School of Medicine, Physical Medicine and Rehabilitation, University of Pittsburgh, Pittsburgh, PA, United States

Luke K. Turnier, PsyD, Division of Pediatric Psychology, Department of Pediatrics, Michigan Medicine, University of Michigan, Ann Arbor, MI, United States

Jessica Van Huysse, PhD, Clinical Assistant Professor, Department of Psychiatry, University of Michigan, Ann Arbor, MI, United States

Douglas Vanderbilt, MD, MS, MBA, Division of Developmental-Behavioral Pediatrics, Department of Pediatrics, Children's Hospital Los Angeles, and Keck School of Medicine of the University of Southern California, Los Angeles, CA, United States

Adrien M. Winning, PhD, The Research Institute at Nationwide Children's Hospital, Center for Biobehavioral Health, Columbus, OH, United States

Susan J. Woolford, MD, MPH, Department of Pediatrics, University of Michigan Health, Ann Arbor, MI, United States

Part I

FAMILY SYSTEMS AND ECOLOGICAL CONTEXTS RELEVANT TO CHILD HEALTH, DEVELOPMENT, AND BEHAVIOR

CHAPTER 1

FAMILY PROCESSES AND CHILD OUTCOMES IN CHILDREN WITH CHRONIC HEALTH CONDITIONS

Thomas G. Power, Wendy M. Gaultney, and Lynnda M. Dahlquist

Chronic health conditions significantly impact family functioning and the physical, cognitive, social, and psychological development of children and adolescents (Pinquart, 2020). Chronic conditions (e.g., asthma, cancer, cystic fibrosis, diabetes, epilepsy, food allergy, juvenile rheumatoid arthritis, kidney disease) typically are of long duration (>12 months), require ongoing medical services, and have functional implications for daily living (van der Lee et al., 2007). Although many children are affected, lack of an approved/widely accepted definition for chronic health conditions leads to prevalence estimates that vary widely. In a review of 64 articles, van der Lee et al. (2007) found prevalence estimates from 0.22% to 44%, with the most frequently cited between 11% and 31%.

Families, especially parents, play an important role in how children address the challenges of chronic health conditions (Crandell et al., 2018; Leeman et al., 2016). In the early 1960s, several historical trends led medical professionals in the United States to focus on families. As a result of environmental changes, higher living standards, improved public health practices, and medical breakthroughs in the 20th century, child mortality rates in the United States had decreased dramatically by mid-century (Field & Behrman, 2003). This led to a new era of pediatrics in the 1960s (Routh, 1975) with a growing need to understand the emotional, psychological, social, and health consequences of children living with chronic health conditions, as well as the role of families in promoting positive child outcomes (Haggerty & Friedman, 2003). Additionally, due to the migration of large numbers of families from small towns to urban/suburban areas (away from extended families), parents increasingly began to rely on medical professionals (particularly pediatricians and family physicians) for guidance in raising their children (Routh, 1975). These developments, along with the growing recognition in the 1960s of the value of collaboration between child psychology and pediatrics (Kagan, 1965), helped contribute to the establishment of the new fields of developmental-behavioral pediatrics and pediatric psychology in the 1960s and 1970s (Haggerty & Friedman, 2003; Routh, 1975).

In this chapter we will integrate findings from pediatric psychology, developmental-behavioral pediatrics, and developmental science to further our understanding of how families contribute to health outcomes in children with chronic health conditions (physical, social, psychological, and emotional health—hereafter referred to as "health outcomes"). Although it is well documented that families play an important role in children's adaptation to such conditions (Crandell et al., 2018; Leeman et al., 2016), most research to date has identified only general

https://doi.org/10.1037/0000414-001
APA Handbook of Pediatric Psychology, Developmental-Behavioral Pediatrics, and Developmental Science: Vol. 2. Pediatric Psychology and Developmental-Behavioral Pediatrics: Clinical Applications of Developmental Science, P. E. Shah and M. H. Bornstein (Editors-in-Chief)
Copyright © 2025 by the American Psychological Association. All rights reserved.

aspects of parenting associated with child health outcomes and provides limited insight into the specific psychological and behavioral processes that account for the associations between these general family factors and child health.

In this chapter, informed by research in developmental science, we will also review the literature on possible mechanisms and explore the implications of these findings for intervention and clinical work with families of children with chronic health conditions. We will selectively review research on conditions diagnosed in the toddler years or later, excluding studies of children with cognitive, sensory, or physical disabilities. First, we will review, from a developmental and ecological perspective, the challenges faced by children with chronic health conditions and examine the impact of these conditions on their health outcomes. Then we will examine the impact of family factors on these outcomes, focusing on specific processes (i.e., parental attitudes and beliefs, parental modeling, family coping, family communication, parental monitoring and shared decision making). Finally, we will examine how these findings inform our understanding of child health disparities, outline directions for future research, and consider implications for clinical practice in pediatric psychology and developmental-behavioral pediatrics.

CHALLENGES FACED BY CHILDREN AND ADOLESCENTS WITH CHRONIC HEALTH CONDITIONS

The impact of chronic conditions on development varies widely by condition. For example,

- children with Type 1 diabetes experience early autonomy demands as they learn to administer insulin and to monitor their diet, blood sugar, and activity levels (Reed-Knight et al., 2014);
- children who experience frequent hospitalizations or who temporarily relocate to a distant location for treatment may experience repeated separations from a parent or siblings (Fluchel et al., 2014);
- children with life-threatening illnesses must cope with emotionally challenging issues rarely addressed by their peers (Bates & Kearney, 2015); and
- children with chronic pain report social isolation and victimization by bullies (Forgeron et al., 2010).

Challenges Across Chronic Health Conditions

Despite differences among various health conditions, reviews of qualitative research have identified similar challenges across conditions. In a review of 18 qualitative studies (including studies of children with cancer, diabetes, arthritis, and asthma), Venning et al. (2008) extracted themes that reflected the views of children (ages 4 to 18 years) living with a chronic health condition. Two themes involved challenges—that is, chronic conditions led to children feeling "uncomfortable in their body and world" (p. 329) and to disruptions to "a normal life" (p. 330). Their review and a review of 55 qualitative studies of children ages 4 to 19 years by Shorey and Ng (2020) described these challenges. Sources of discomfort include

- feeling different from everyone else,
- having concerns about their appearance,
- experiencing pain or fatigue from their condition/treatments,
- feeling that people do not understand what they are going through,
- having concerns about what others think of them,
- receiving unwanted attention, and
- attempting to hide their condition from others.

Factors contributing to disruption include

- the complexities and time-consuming nature of disease management (e.g., treatments, appointments, hospitalizations),
- the restriction of participation in activities (e.g., sports, school, extracurricular activities, social gatherings),
- negative influences on peer relationships (e.g., exclusion, isolation, loss of friendships, victimization by bullies, social anxiety),
- a lack of privacy and autonomy, and
- uncertainty about the present and the future.

Developmental Considerations

Most studies of the challenges associated with chronic conditions do not take a developmental approach; however, the salient challenges likely vary by child age. In the preschool years, when children generally have only a rudimentary understanding of their condition (Myant & Williams, 2005) and parents are primarily responsible for its management (e.g., Reed-Knight et al., 2014), the major challenges likely include pain and discomfort, restrictions on daily activities, and stress from medical procedures. In middle childhood, when children spend more time in school and with peers—contexts that encourage social comparison—they begin to face the challenges of bullying, social exclusion, and concerns about their appearance. Finally, the development of social perspective taking (Van der Graaff et al., 2014), identity (Koepke & Denissen, 2012), and autonomy (Lam et al., 2014) in adolescence may lead to attempts to conceal their condition because they feel different from everyone else, ruminating about what others think, resenting unwanted attention they receive due to their condition, and becoming concerned about privacy. Because friendships, peer acceptance, popularity, and peer group membership in adolescence increasingly depend on social activities outside of the home (e.g., Urberg et al., 2000), adolescents with chronic conditions may be particularly impacted by restrictions on participation in social activities. Finally, due to their developing competence and autonomy, adolescents with certain chronic conditions (e.g., diabetes, asthma, cystic fibrosis) take on greater responsibility for disease management (e.g., Reed-Knight et al., 2014), requiring balancing the management of their condition with the social demands of adolescence.

HEALTH OUTCOMES IN CHILDREN WITH CHRONIC HEALTH CONDITIONS

Quality of Life

Living with chronic health conditions undoubtedly impacts many aspects of children's development. Pinquart (2020) published an analysis of the adjustment of children with chronic health conditions: a meta-analysis of more than 1,200 studies using the Pediatric Quality of Life Inventory (Varni et al., 2001). This widely used child and parent report measure assesses children's quality of life in four domains: physical health, emotional functioning, social functioning, and school functioning. A total score is generated, as well as a psychosocial health score that combines the emotional, social, and school functioning subscales. The meta-analysis examined child health quality of life for children with 29 separate conditions (≥10 effect sizes each) as well as possible moderating variables. Children with chronic conditions showed lower overall health quality of life than healthy children, with significant differences on almost all subscale comparisons. Parents reported lower ratings of children's social and emotional functioning than did children. The largest effect sizes for psychosocial health were for kidney disease, epilepsy, and sickle cell disease; the remaining conditions showed medium effect sizes. Pinquart (2020) speculated that the large effect size for kidney disease may be due to the numerous studies of children on dialysis; the large effect sizes for epilepsy and sickle cell disease may be due to the episodic and unexpected flare-ups associated with these conditions.

Although one might expect that the quality-of-life domains affected by chronic health conditions would vary as a function of the child's developmental level, there were no significant moderating effects of child age in any of the analyses (mean age 11.2 years, $SD = 3.2$, range = 0.4–17 years). This may be due to the limited number of studies of younger children: Only about 2% of the studies included children less than 3 years of age and only about 5% were studies of 3- to 5-year-olds. However, the results revealed that there were no significant differences in the impact of chronic conditions on the children's quality of life across the school years and adolescence, at least on the broad domains assessed by quality-of-life assessments.

Child Behavior Problems

The quality-of-life findings (Pinquart, 2020) extend the findings of an earlier meta-analysis by Pinquart and Shen (2011), who examined child behavior problems (internalizing, externalizing, and total problems) on the Child Behavior Checklist (CBCL; parent report) and the Youth Self-report (YSR; child report), two well-validated measures of children's psychological symptoms (Achenbach, 1991). In this analysis of 569 studies, children with chronic health conditions showed greater internalizing, externalizing, and total symptoms than healthy children (Pinquart & Shen, 2011). As in Pinquart (2020), parents rated their children as having more behavior problems than did children; children with chronic health conditions did not differ from healthy children on self-ratings of externalizing symptoms. Unlike Pinquart (2020), child age was a significant moderator, with differences in psychological symptoms stronger for the older age groups (6–10 and 11–18 years) than for children under age 6. This was true for total problems, internalizing problems, and externalizing problems. Despite being at higher risk for psychological symptoms than healthy children, the vast majority of children with chronic health conditions did not exceed clinical cut-offs on the CBCL or the YSR for psychological symptoms. A significant minority of children, however, showed clinical levels of symptoms. A meta-analysis of 150 studies by Pinquart (2018) showed that 11.5% of children with chronic health conditions met the diagnostic criteria for posttraumatic stress syndrome (PTSS), manifested by subclinical symptoms of posttraumatic stress (e.g., avoidance, irritability, heightened arousal, intrusive thoughts/images), but not the full criteria for a PTSD diagnosis. Children diagnosed with a chronic condition before 6 years of age had lower rates of PTSS than children diagnosed at older ages.

CHILD COPING STRATEGIES ASSOCIATED WITH RESILIENCE

Drawing from research in developmental science, and because of wide individual differences in children's health outcomes, researchers have examined the coping strategies associated with resilience in children and adolescents who experience the challenges of growing up with a chronic health condition. In the reviews of qualitative studies described earlier (Shorey & Ng, 2020; Venning et al., 2008), successful adaptation was facilitated by: (a) gaining information and knowledge about the condition, (b) receiving support from others, (c) accepting the condition and "taking charge," (d) positive thinking, (e) adherence and self-responsibility, and (f) finding balance. These findings are consistent with those from quantitative studies (Compas et al., 2012) in which secondary control coping strategies (e.g., acceptance, positive thinking) showed positive associations with child adjustment, disengagement strategies (e.g., cognitive or behavioral avoidance) showed negative associations, and findings for primary control coping strategies (e.g., problem solving, seeking social support) were mixed.

As noted by Compas et al. (2012), few studies have examined developmental differences in children's coping with chronic health conditions. However, based upon the literature on children's coping with stress (Skinner & Zimmer-Gembeck, 2016), one would expect that the development of cognitive and social skills during middle childhood and adolescence would lead to increases in planful problem solving, cognitive distraction, and self-reliance, and decreases in simple instrumental action, behavioral strategies, and reliance on adults. We would also expect increasing coping flexibility with age and the use of coping strategies in a more discriminating fashion (i.e., using strategies tailored to specific characteristics of the stressful situation).

FAMILY AND PARENTING INFLUENCES ON CHILDREN'S COPING WITH A CHRONIC HEALTH CONDITION: POSSIBLE MECHANISMS

Developmental science has broadened our understanding of how children's biopsychosocial development is shaped by experiences in their family, social, and environmental contexts. This framework is especially helpful in considering the ecological contexts and family processes associated with children's positive adaptation to chronic illness.

Family Ecological Contexts

Meta-analyses of data from the Family Synthesis Project (studies from 2000 to 2014) examined, for multiple chronic conditions, associations between child/adolescent outcomes and measures of family functioning (Leeman et al., 2016) or parenting (Crandell et al., 2018). The family variables showing the most consistent positive associations with child/adolescent adaptation were family cohesion, adaptability, and expressiveness; family conflict was negatively related. Positively associated parenting variables were warmth and autonomy support; rejection and coercion showed negative associations. Unfortunately, the authors were not able to examine whether children's developmental level was a moderating variable in these analyses.

Family Processes Associated With Adaptation

Although these studies help identify some general family functioning and parenting variables associated with adjustment in children with chronic health conditions, a relatively underexplored area centers on the mechanisms by which parents and families promote or interfere with children's adaptation to chronic health conditions. These unanswered questions concern the mechanisms accounting for the associations between child adaptation and such general measures of parenting and family functioning, as well as the larger contextual factors that lead to these patterns of family functioning and parenting in the first place. In the following sections we will examine such mechanisms by selectively reviewing research on (a) parental attitudes and beliefs, (b) family modeling, (c) family stress and coping, (d) family communication, and (e) family monitoring and shared decision making. Because the vast majority of studies in this area have examined parental influences, this review will focus only on parent–child relationships. Although there is extensive literature on siblings of children with chronic health conditions, these studies have focused almost exclusively on the healthy child's adjustment rather than their influence on the adjustment of the child with the chronic condition (Elliott et al., 2020).

Parental attitudes and beliefs. Parental health attitudes and beliefs can play an important role in the outcomes of children with chronic health conditions. According to models of illness representation (Lau & Hartman, 1983), cognitions about several domains of the child's condition are associated with parental adaptation: (a) diagnosis, (b) treatment, (c) causes, (d) consequences/child vulnerability, and (e) controllability. Uncertainty (Szulczewski et al., 2017) and trust in health care providers (Bazargan et al., 2021) are important as well.

Acceptance of diagnosis. Diagnosis is often a complex process, and parents may experience uncertainty (Santacroce, 2001) due to changes in symptoms/diagnoses over time or conflicting information from medical staff, particularly for conditions that are generally hard to diagnose (e.g., chronic pain; Neville et al., 2020) or hard to diagnose in young children (e.g., asthma; Finnvold, 2010).

Parental beliefs and attitudes likely influence parental coping with diagnostic uncertainty. Differences between parents in their attitudes about medical professionals and their understanding of the health care system may lead to different reactions to diagnostic uncertainty. Some parents may actively seek out information (e.g., developing strategies for navigating the health care system, joining support groups, learning to talk with the doctor in ways that yield helpful information; Finnvold, 2010), whereas others may avoid getting new information and even refuse to accept their child's diagnosis (Fawcett, 2019).

Because effective treatment and disease management require parental acceptance of the diagnosis, parental uncertainty may contribute to negative child outcomes. In two studies of children with chronic pain, parents' uncertainty about the pain diagnosis was associated with poorer child-reported outcomes: greater pain intensity and lower health-related quality of life in one study (Neville et al., 2020) and greater pain avoidance in the other (Tanna et al., 2020). These findings suggest that one target for future interventions might be promoting parental acceptance of diagnoses by helping providers understand parents' concerns, clear up misunderstandings, and direct parents toward helpful external resources about the condition. These areas highlight potential clinical opportunities for pediatric psychologists and other behavioral health providers to help support parents' adaptation to their child's chronic illness.

Treatment. Depending on the condition, management and treatment of childhood chronic health conditions are often collaborative processes involving a partnership among the parents, the child, and the health care providers. These partners must coordinate their roles, with parents typically playing the central role in ensuring that management strategies are successfully implemented (Power et al., 2019), including promoting the transition to self-care so that children can eventually manage the condition on their own (Reed-Knight et al., 2014).

Given the substantial parental effort often required in successful disease management, it is likely that parental acceptance of the treatment regimen is an important determinant of child outcomes. If parents are dissatisfied or do not trust their health care provider, the child's health may suffer. Jokinen-Gordon and Quadagno (2013) found that parents who were dissatisfied with their last health care appointment were less likely to have had a preventive care health care visit for their child in the past year and that their child was more likely to have an unmet health care need. In children with asthma, Rotenberg and Petrocchi (2018) found a bidirectional association between mothers' and children's trust beliefs in their physicians over time, but only children's trust beliefs predicted child treatment adherence one year later.

Parents' support of health care treatments is likely influenced by their attitudes toward various medical interventions (e.g., medications, surgery, physical therapy). In studies of children with asthma (Armstrong et al., 2014) and children with celiac disease (Hoffmann et al., 2016), parents' attitudes about medications predicted child treatment adherence.

To promote successful child adaptation, health care providers need to build a therapeutic alliance with families regarding treatment by understanding their concerns, addressing these concerns in language that they can understand, and, when possible, giving them choices in treatment options. One way to promote acceptance is to first recommend less invasive options (e.g., therapy and medication) before recommending more invasive options such as surgery. In multidisciplinary teams, pediatric psychologists can help foster a therapeutic alliance with families and help provide supports and strategies to optimize family adherence to treatment recommendations.

Causes. Parents differ in their beliefs about the causes of child chronic health conditions and may experience significant levels of guilt (Comaroff & Maguire, 1981) about having contributed in some way to their child's condition. Baert et al. (2020), in a study of chronic pain patients, found that children of parents who viewed their child's pain as unjust (including believing that others' negligence may have contributed to the child's suffering) reported greater functional disability and lower health quality of life, even after controlling for parental catastrophizing of the child's pain. Parental emotions such as guilt or anger may contribute to poor child outcomes by interfering with their ability to support their child's coping with the stresses of their condition. Providers might promote successful child outcomes by clarifying parents' misconceptions about the cause of their child's condition and addressing feelings of guilt or anger that may be related to their attributions of their child's diagnosis or condition.

Consequences and parent perceptions of child vulnerability. Parents can overestimate, underestimate, or accurately predict the consequences of their child's condition. Green and Solnit (1964) noted that parents of children who had recovered from life-threatening conditions and were no longer at medical risk still viewed their children as being medically vulnerable. These parents were often "overprotective, overly indulgent, and oversolicitous" (p. 61), and their children were characterized as being "overly dependent, disobedient, irritable, argumentative, and uncooperative" (p. 61). Parents of children with a range of chronic health conditions (e.g., asthma, cancer, Type 1 diabetes, arthritis, cystic fibrosis) are at risk for similar maladaptive patterns, with parent perceptions of child vulnerability being associated with parenting stress, overprotective parenting, and/or child emotional distress, even after controlling for the disease severity (e.g., Mullins et al., 2004). Although maladaptive coping patterns have been observed in parents of children with chronic illness, parents may exhibit a wide range of strategies in the face of their child's chronic medical condition.

Parental catastrophizing. Some parents of children with chronic pain exhibit pain catastrophizing—ruminating about the child's pain, magnifying its severity, and feeling helpless about its control (Goubert et al., 2006). Parental catastrophizing has been associated with more negative child outcomes (e.g., functional disability), even after controlling for the level of child pain (Donnelly et al., 2020). Because such catastrophizing is associated with the modeling and reinforcement of children's illness behaviors (Newton et al., 2019), it may also contribute to children's disability through encouraging illness behaviors such as avoidance of movement and school refusal. Other studies suggest additional paths of influence, with the effects of parent catastrophizing mediated through child catastrophizing (e.g., Feinstein et al., 2018) or playing a moderating role between child catastrophizing and child outcomes (e.g., Sil et al., 2016).

Parental minimizing/dispositional optimism. Much less research has examined parents' minimizing of disease severity. Mack et al. (2007) found that, when disagreements about a child's cancer prognosis occurred, parents typically reported higher levels of optimism than physicians. Sung et al. (2009), in a study of pediatric cancers with poor prognosis, found that this was particularly true if parents showed dispositional optimism—the tendency to hold positive outcome expectancies across multiple situations (Scheier & Carver, 2018). Dispositional optimism is predictive of positive outcomes in adults with numerous health conditions, likely because optimistic individuals use approach-oriented coping styles to address challenges (Scheier & Carver, 2018). As illustrated in a longitudinal study of adolescents with cystic fibrosis or diabetes (D'Angelo et al., 2019), optimistic parents of children may transmit their optimistic viewpoint to their children. In this study, D'Angelo and colleagues found that parental optimism positively predicted adolescent optimism over time whereas the opposite was not true (i.e., adolescent optimism did not predict subsequent parental optimism).

Although parental optimism may promote positive child outcomes, this disposition can also be maladaptive. Parents who minimize the severity of their child's condition may not take the necessary steps to ensure that their child receives the proper treatment or adheres to the management plan. For example, parents' use of avoidant coping strategies (e.g., denial) is associated with poor health quality of life in children with asthma (Sales et al., 2008).

Parental psychological flexibility. An effective way that parents can promote adaptive functioning in children with chronic pain is through psychological flexibility: "being aware of, and open to unwanted and uncontrollable experiences (e.g., seeing your child suffering with chronic pain), while still having the ability to act in line with broader life values (e.g., being an encouraging parent)" (Beeckman et al., 2019, p. 2). After controlling for the level of child pain, greater psychological flexibility (or its subcomponent, parental pain acceptance) was associated with lower child functional disability and/or activity avoidance, with effects mediated through lower parental protectiveness and/or child pain acceptance (Beeckman et al., 2019; Feinstein et al., 2018).

Parental tolerance of uncertainty. Parents of children with chronic health conditions experience high levels of uncertainty that are associated with negative child and parent outcomes (psychological distress and illness-related outcomes;

Szulczewski et al., 2017). However, tolerance of uncertainty may be protective: Higher levels of parental tolerance were associated with less overprotective parenting toward children with life-threatening food allergies (Steiner et al., 2020).

Together, these findings point to the importance of parents having a clear understanding of the severity and consequences of their child's condition and suggest that interventions that help address parental misconceptions about the disease and prognosis may promote positive child outcomes. Interventions that promote psychological flexibility may be particularly effective because they provide parents with a productive approach for addressing the challenges of their child's condition while at the same time promoting a realistic conception of its severity.

Controllability and self-efficacy. Finally, parents' perceptions of control over the consequences of their child's condition and parents' perceptions of self-efficacy are related to more adaptive child outcomes as well. Adolescents with diabetes whose parents believe that they can help prevent further health consequences in their child show better treatment adherence and metabolic control (Prikken et al., 2019). Higher parental self-efficacy is associated with positive child outcomes including greater child self-efficacy (Noser et al., 2017), greater cooperation during medical procedures (Peterson et al., 2014), and better metabolic control (Noser et al., 2017).

In a review of intervention studies for children with chronic health conditions, Mitchell et al. (2020) found that only two of the four studies targeting parent self-efficacy showed significant effects. Because parenting interventions typically increase parent self-efficacy (Wittkowski et al., 2016), future research should examine how programs for parents of children with chronic health conditions can be improved to increase their impact on parent self-efficacy.

Developmental issues. We found no studies that directly examined whether parental attitudes/beliefs associated with child outcomes varied as a function of the child's developmental level. One might expect such differences. For example, as children enter school and spend more time with peers, parents may become more concerned about the impact of the child's condition on school success and peer relations. During the adolescent years, when children take more responsibility for their own care, parents may experience a decreased sense of control over their child's health outcomes. Time since diagnosis may be an important moderator as well. For example, parental attitudes about diagnosis, causes, and treatment may be more important shortly after the diagnosis whereas attitudes about consequences and controllability may become more important once parents have had more experience with the condition. If the developmental level of the child and/or the time since diagnosis play a moderating role, such findings would have important implications for developing interventions targeting parental attitudes and beliefs.

Parent modeling. Children and adolescents mimic the behavior of those around them, and researchers have explored the impact of parental modeling on children's health behaviors. For example, in a study of adolescents with chronic abdominal pain, Stone et al. (2018) found that adolescents who perceived higher levels of pain symptoms in their parents at baseline viewed their own pain as more threatening and later reported greater pain and functional impairment in their own lives.

Modeling also appears to play a role in children's physical activity (Yao & Rhodes, 2015) and healthy eating behaviors (Yee et al., 2017), which have positive effects on many chronic health conditions including diabetes, chronic pain, and arthritis. To experimentally examine the impact of modeling on in-the-moment pain behaviors, Boerner et al. (2017) randomly assigned parents to exaggerate their pain responses, to minimize their responses, or to act naturally during a cold pressor task (submerging their hand into ice water) while their child observed. Children then completed the task themselves. After observing their parents, children of parents in the exaggerated condition reported significantly higher anxiety about the task than children of parents in the minimization condition. Child ratings of their own pain during the task varied by gender. Girls whose parents were in the exaggerated condition reported greater pain intensity than boys; no gender differences were observed in the other conditions.

Various factors, such as parental consistency or developmental level of the child, may moderate the effects of modeling on child outcomes. Parental inconsistency may reduce the impact of parental modeling if, for example, parents with chronic pain model involvement in physical activities in some contexts (e.g., physical therapy) but model pain interference (e.g., not participating in physical activities due to pain) in others. With regard to developmental level, as children enter adolescence, they may become less influenced by parent models and more influenced by peer models as a function of their developing autonomy (Lam et al., 2014).

These studies demonstrate the importance of parents' own illness behavior in children's adaptation, particularly in the area of chronic pain. Children are aware of their parents' responses to pain and may use parental responses in interpreting their own symptoms and guiding their responses to pain. By helping parents become more aware of their own illness behaviors, interventions can help promote child adaptation by preventing the transmission of unwanted messages from parents to their children. Modeling is an understudied topic in the literature on children's health conditions, and future research should examine its role in other domains.

Family stress and coping. The stresses experienced by children with chronic health conditions were described earlier. However, the stress of a child's health condition also impacts other family members, including parents, healthy siblings, and other relatives (Elliott et al., 2020; Power et al., 2019; Ravindran & Rempel, 2011). How well parents cope with such stresses may have an impact on child adaptation. Studies of parents of children with cancer (Sultan et al., 2016) and juvenile rheumatoid arthritis (Hynes et al., 2019) show that parental distress (e.g., parenting stress, depressive symptoms, anxiety, and posttraumatic stress symptoms) is positively associated with child distress (e.g., negative affect, internalizing/externalizing symptoms, posttraumatic stress symptoms, poor health quality of life, and social competence problems).

According to Fisher (2001), parents who successfully cope with the stresses of having a child with a chronic health condition create a "new normal" by managing issues over which they have control, including managing the child's illness and reorganizing family life. Consistent with this conclusion are studies reviewed by Fairfax et al. (2019) which showed that coping flexibility was positively associated with quality of life and that coping strategies characterized by behavioral disengagement and escape/avoidance showed negative associations. Moreover, social support that parents receive is positively associated with caregiver well-being and negatively associated with distress, anxiety, and posttraumatic stress symptoms (Gise & Cohen, 2022).

Parents also play a role in the development of coping strategies in their children by influencing events to which children are exposed and by scaffolding their development of coping skills (Power, 2004). These tasks can be challenging for parents of children with chronic health conditions because of the risks of overprotectiveness and catastrophizing discussed earlier and because of a wide range of nonnormative stressors that children with chronic conditions face during development. Moreover, families must change the way that they adjust to their child's condition over the course of the child's development (Kazak et al., 2017). Finally, parents' distress may interfere with the socialization of effective coping strategies. For example, in a review of the socialization of coping in children with cancer, Koutná and Blatný (2020) argued that the positive association between posttraumatic stress symptoms in mothers and their children may be due to "the parents' reduced ability to provide the appropriate care and support to their child due to their own PTSSs (post-traumatic stress symptoms) and . . . the socialization of maladaptive coping and emotion regulation strategies used by the parents" (p. 8).

Given the numerous stresses experienced by families of children with a chronic health condition and the negative effects on family functioning, programs to promote family coping likely have a positive effect on child outcomes. In a Cochrane meta-analysis, Eccleston et al. (2012) found that problem-solving therapy (PST) interventions show promise for directly improving parental distress associated with parenting a child with chronic illness and that cognitive behavior therapy including parents significantly improved children's immediate posttreatment outcomes in chronic pain conditions. Such programs have good evidence for immediate outcomes posttreatment; however, few studies have examined these outcomes at long-term follow-up, an important area for future research and clinical application.

Family communication. The quality of communication among family members is associated with psychosocial and medical outcomes in children with chronic health conditions. Interactions that are highly critical or negative in tone (DeBoer et al., 2017; Weissberg-Benchell et al., 2009) and those that are unproductive, such as discussions of illness management that do not result in problem resolution, predict poorer adherence (more child resistance and more parental coercion) and poorer health outcomes (Psihogios et al., 2019; Weissberg-Benchell et al., 2009). In contrast, Berg et al. (2017) reported that adolescents were more likely to talk with their parents about diabetes management when they perceived their parents to be accepting and helpful. Taken together, these findings highlight the importance of fostering open adaptive family communication as an intervention target to help support children and families experiencing chronic illness. Pediatric psychologists working in multidisciplinary teams play an important role in supporting family communication and adaptation.

Incorporating both parent and youth reports of family communication is crucial, as parents and children often have different perceptions of family interactions. For example, in families of children with chronic health conditions, parents tend to perceive their communication more favorably than their children do (e.g., DeBoer et al., 2017). Such discrepancies in parent–child report may reflect measurement error, informant bias, or more importantly, the different contexts and experiences of children and parents (Al Ghriwati et al., 2018). Discrepancies in parent versus child reports can serve as markers of family function or predictors of adjustment, with greater discrepancy potentially indicative of less intimate relationships or greater family conflict. Indeed, greater discordance in parent–child reports of family communication is related to family conflict and to poorer metabolic control in adolescents with diabetes (DeBoer et al., 2017) and poorer pulmonary function in adolescents with asthma (Al Ghriwati et al., 2018).

Observational studies suggest additional aspects of family communication processes that contribute to child outcomes (Murphy et al., 2017). For example, when parents of elementary-school-aged children with cystic fibrosis were observed to use praise, reflective statements, and behavioral descriptions rather than verbal disapproval during respiratory treatments, their children demonstrated better cooperation with treatment (Butcher & Nasr, 2015). Similarly, parental verbalizations of praise and prompts to use coping strategies, such as distraction, are associated with less child distress during painful medical procedures whereas parental criticism and reassurance tend to be associated with greater child distress (Caes, 2019).

When direct observation of family communication is not feasible, structured analog observations may shed light on family communication patterns. For example, Chisholm et al. (2014) designed a board game in which 6- to 8-year-old children with diabetes were tasked with "shopping" for food items to serve at a birthday party. Parent–child interactions were coded for positive versus negative content and for positive, neutral, and negative nonverbal affect. More positive dyadic communication correlated with fewer behavior problems, and incongruent communication, in which the nonverbal tone did not match the verbal content, was associated with poorer diet adherence and greater behavior problems.

Communication patterns in families of children with chronic health conditions may differ from patterns seen in families with healthy children (Murphy et al., 2017), suggesting less warmth and structure and more hostile, intrusive, or withdrawn communication. However, the degree to which these patterns reflect adaptive adjustments to the demands of the condition and the associated potential long-term consequences of such communication patterns are difficult to determine from this primarily cross-sectional body of literature. An exception is a longitudinal study by Iskander et al. (2015), who observed communication behaviors as parents and children attempted to achieve a problem solution for a conflictual aspect of diabetes care. Children were observed at 9 to 11 years of age and annually three times thereafter. Baseline levels of positive maternal communication predicted better adherence to blood glucose monitoring three years later.

Together, these studies demonstrate that supportive parent–child communication is associated with positive outcomes for children with chronic health conditions. Communication may be particularly important in these families because management of such conditions often requires a working partnership between children and their parents. The importance of communication may vary with the child's developmental level; however, the meta-analysis by Psihogios et al. (2019) found no moderating effects of child age for the association between family communication and child outcomes. Although the nature of family communication likely changes with development, it may be equally important across ages for child outcomes.

Family monitoring and shared decision making. Greater caregiver involvement in the child's medical care (e.g., providing reminders and monitoring self-management behaviors) is consistently associated with children's better adherence to medical recommendations and better health outcomes (Turner et al., 2021). This is true for both younger and older children, although the nature of parental involvement needs to change as children get older, desire more autonomy, and prepare to assume more responsibility for their own care (Kazak et al., 2017). For example, parents of young children may need to observe the child perform self-care tasks, check for accuracy, or help if the child struggles. For older adolescents, monitoring may simply involve being in the room. Not all parents are in a position to show high levels of involvement. For example, parents who have inflexible work schedules and/or limited access to social support (e.g., single-parent households) may face difficulty providing the support and structure for ongoing management (Gray et al., 2018).

In addition to the amount of parent involvement, the nature of their involvement can help or hinder children's self-management. For example, parental monitoring may be perceived as overly intrusive and/or constraining the child's emerging autonomy (Miller & Jawad, 2019), especially if parents are overly critical or if parents and children disagree about who should assume responsibility for self-management tasks, resulting in more child oppositional behavior (Sweenie et al., 2014). To facilitate the transition from parental responsibility to child responsibility for self-management and minimize such conflicts, Miller and Jawad (2019) argued for decision making that is shared between parents and children throughout the course of the illness and "includes both active participation by the child (e.g., asking parent for advice, expressing an opinion, giving information) and adult attempts to facilitate the child's involvement (e.g., asking for the child's opinion, soliciting questions, sharing information with the child)" (p. 62). Cross-sectional (Turner et al., 2021) and longitudinal (Miller & Jawad, 2019) research shows that shared decision making, particularly child solicitation of information and joint child–parent brainstorming/negotiation processes, predicts better adherence in Type 1 diabetes (Miller & Jawad, 2019) and asthma (Turner et al., 2021).

Given the importance of shared decision making between parents and children in the management of chronic health conditions, health care providers should work closely with both parents and children in the decision-making process. This would best be accomplished by health care providers engaging families in collaborative shared decision-making conversations early and often. In practice, health care providers can facilitate the shift by directly asking children about their opinions, concerns, and questions and ensuring the child's understanding of concepts (Miller, 2018) regardless of who makes the final decision. Parents can also use a similar approach to facilitate shared decision making in daily activities and tasks of condition management. Although these conversations vary substantially according to children's developmental, behavioral, and cultural background and illness state, it is universally recognized as important to engage children early and often (Madrigal & Kelly, 2018).

SUMMARY AND CONCLUSION: THE ROLE OF PARENTING AND FAMILY FUNCTIONING IN CHILDREN'S ADAPTATION TO CHRONIC HEALTH CONDITIONS

Table 1.1 summarizes the family factors positively and negatively associated with children's health outcomes identified in the current review. One of the most important factors associated with health outcomes for children with chronic health conditions is parents' development of a positive collaborative partnership with the child's medical providers. Developing such a partnership shows a high degree of trust in the providers, agreement with the child's diagnosis, comfort with the health care system, and support for the treatment plan, including their own role in disease management. Parents of well-functioning children hold an accurate perception of the severity of the child's condition, are confident in their ability to help their child manage it, and show the tolerance of

TABLE 1.1

Summary of Family Factors Positively and Negatively Associated With Child Health Outcomes

	Positively associated with child health outcomes	Negatively associated with child health outcomes
Family characteristics	Cohesion, adaptability, expressiveness	Conflict
Parenting dimensions	Warmth, autonomy support	Rejection, coercion
Parental attitudes/beliefs		
Regarding diagnosis	Acceptance of diagnosis	Uncertainty about diagnosis
Regarding treatment	Trust in provider, positive attitudes toward treatment	Dissatisfaction with provider, negative attitude toward treatment
Causes	Does not blame self or others	Guilt/anger about cause
Consequences	Accurate perception of condition severity, dispositional optimism, psychological flexibility, tolerance of uncertainty	Uncertainty regarding consequences, catastrophizing, denial
Control	Self-efficacy, feelings of control	Low self-efficacy, helplessness
Parental modeling	Modeling positive coping	Modeling illness behaviors, inconsistent modeling
Family coping	Coping successfully with own stresses, coping flexibility, seeking social support, scaffolding development of children's coping strategies	Poor coping with own stress, disengagement, escape/avoidance, social isolation, overprotectiveness
Family communication	Accepting, helpful, praising, use of reflective statements and behavioral descriptors	Criticism, unproductive discussions, reassurance, incongruent communication
Monitoring	Age-appropriate involvement/monitoring	Intrusive monitoring
Shared decision making	Shared involvement, asking for child's opinions, soliciting questions, sharing information	Lack of involvement, overinvolvement, authoritarian control

Note. Summary of findings described in this chapter; child health outcomes varied by study and included measures of physical, psychological, social, and/or emotional health.

uncertainty and psychological flexibility needed to address the numerous unexpected challenges that arise along the way. These parents acknowledge the challenges of the condition; provide models for coping with those challenges; help the child to cope with the physical, emotional, and social stresses of the condition; create opportunities for the child to have a "normal childhood" despite the challenges of the health condition; and scaffold the development of independent disease management skills with autonomy-supportive parenting practices that promote the gradual transfer of responsibility from parent to child. Families that promote adaptation successfully adjust family roles and responsibilities to meet demands of the child's condition but have the flexibility to change in response to situational and developmental demands. They show responsive respectful patterns of communication and are open and responsive to the input of others. Such parents can effectively cope with the inevitable stresses of caring for a child with a chronic health condition: accepting what they cannot control; actively addressing what that they can control; seeking the emotional support of others; and attending to their own social, emotional, and personal needs.

No family can provide the kinds of support described at all times, but some are in a better position to do so than others. For many families, a wide range of factors (many beyond their control) can work against adopting these supportive behavior patterns: the child's condition may not be easy to diagnose; the course of the condition may be unpredictable; health professionals may offer conflicting diagnoses or treatment plans; or the parent may not have the education, knowledge, skills, or support to understand and/or help manage the child's condition. To further complicate matters, parents may hold a negative view of the medical community (or their particular providers), or the stress of parenting a child with a chronic condition may create high levels of emotional distress. Such parents may ruminate about the child's suffering, magnify its severity, feel that the condition is unjust, blame themselves or others for its occurrence, or feel helpless about its control. Alternatively, parents may deny the seriousness of the condition and not take the appropriate steps necessary to get their child the help needed to effectively manage it. Finally, a range of factors outside of the child's condition (e.g., economic, marital, caregiving, mental health, social network, work-related, neighborhood, public policy, and cultural) may prevent parents from engaging in these practices as well.

Family Factors and Health Disparities: Insights From Developmental Science and Opportunities for Pediatric Psychologists

In the introduction to a special issue of the *Journal of Pediatric Psychology*, Valrie et al. (2020) argued that, although researchers have now documented significant ethnic and socioeconomic health disparities in children's chronic health conditions, limited research has examined the mechanisms contributing to these disparities. Although numerous structural and historical factors play a role (Tourse et al., 2018), family factors often serve as mediators between these more distal factors and child outcomes. For example, a history of structural racism, discrimination, and unethical medical experimentation experienced by members of some ethnic groups (Feagin & Bennefield, 2014), as well as current experiences of discrimination (Bazargan et al., 2021), have contributed to distrust of the health care system by many adults, decreasing the likelihood that some parents can create a working partnership with the child's health care team. Disparities in access to quality health care (Feagin & Bennefield, 2014) likely contribute as well. Given the complexity of many chronic conditions, differences between ethnic groups in educational attainment (U.S. Census Bureau, 2016) put many parents at a disadvantage in understanding the child's disorder and/or treatment.

Ethnic differences in economic hardship (Tourse et al., 2018) and the lack of universal health care in the United States make it difficult for many parents to secure the best treatment for their child. These factors work against many parents having a longterm relationship with a primary care physician who can help with early diagnosis or preventative care; securing referrals to specialists; affording medications and treatments; traveling to regional medical centers for specialty care; getting paid time off from work for doctor's appointments, clinic visits, and hospitalizations; and so on. Moreover, ethnic and socioeconomic differences in residential segregation and rural poverty (Burton et al., 2013; Jargowsky, 2018) can limit the options parents have for high-quality medical care. Provider burnout and turnover in underresourced medical establishments may also reduce the continuity of care, which is important to families to feel supported over time. The stresses resulting from economic hardship, racial discrimination, immigration, neighborhood decay, social isolation, and low-paid employment may lead to parental distress or family conflict that makes it difficult for parents to cope with the demands of their child's condition, to model successful coping for their child, or to successfully scaffold the development of children's self-care skills.

Finally, cultural and language factors (Valrie et al., 2020) and lack of high-quality translation services in medical settings may interfere with parents' ability to understand the child's condition and treatment, to communicate effectively and openly with health care providers, to navigate the complexities of the health care system, to understand the importance of certain interventions, to communicate with teachers and school administrators about the child's condition, and so on.

Primary care providers are sometimes the first to encounter these structural barriers to optimal child outcomes. Some issues can be addressed at the level of the individual provider such as open communication, building trust, cultural sensitivity, providing materials in the patient's primary language, being mindful of the health literacy of the parents, or exploring more affordable treatment options. Telemedicine, mobile medicine, and extended clinic hours can be effective in addressing barriers to care for hard-to-reach populations.

Larger structural changes can help as well. Integrated behavioral health (IBH) approaches (i.e., the provision of behavioral/social/emotional health care in primary care settings; Riley et al., 2022) can help address many of these issues. Asarnow et al. (2015), in a meta-analysis of 31 studies with 13,129 children and adolescents, found a 66% probability that a randomly selected youth who received integrated medical-behavioral health care would have a better outcome (e.g., in terms of anxiety, substance use, and disruptive behaviors) compared with one in usual primary care. Age did not moderate the findings, suggesting that, although the exact behavioral concerns may change with development, access to behavioral health is equally important at all ages. The evidence base for IBH has not yet been evaluated for children with chronic health conditions; however, it likely that, given their demonstrated needs, IBH will show promise in the future for these populations.

These integrated behavioral health care models require attention to equitable access given the increased risk and vulnerability for some families as a result of the inequities discussed earlier. Although outcome studies are limited, culturally and linguistically adapted integrated behavioral health care initiatives have demonstrated improved problem-solving ability and reduced negative affectivity in Spanish-speaking mothers of children with cancer (Sahler et al., 2005) and more sensitive identification of cognitive outcomes in Latino childhood leukemia and lymphoma survivors (Bava et al., 2018).

Methodological Critique and Directions for Future Research

Although the research reviewed in the previous sections provides a rather consistent description of the parenting and family factors associated with children's adaptation to chronic health conditions, the research in this area suffers from a number of shortcomings. First, although many of the models that have been offered for understanding how families promote the well-being of children with chronic health conditions acknowledge how family interactions change with the child's development (e.g., Kazak et al., 2017; Reed-Knight et al., 2014), very few studies have directly examined how the importance of various family processes may vary with the developmental level of the child. Although it is likely that many areas (such as warmth, support, and lack of conflict) may be equally important for children at different developmental levels, we have identified numerous processes in this chapter in which such developmental differences may be present. Second, the research on family effects on child outcomes focuses almost exclusively on parent–child relationships. Although considerable research has been conducted on the adjustment of healthy siblings in such families (Elliott et al., 2020), we have little insight into how healthy siblings influence the adjustment of the child with the chronic health condition. Moreover, we know less about larger family processes such as the impact of the relationship between the caregivers, the role of extended family members, and other family-level variables on child outcomes. Third, the studies in this area are largely cross-sectional. Cross-sectional designs make it impossible to draw even tentative conclusions about the direction of effects—that is, are parents influencing child behavior or is child behavior influencing parenting? Many of the associations described could be explained by "child effects" (e.g., parents may have high levels of self-efficacy because the child's condition is under control). Fourth, many of the studies reviewed here relied on parent and/or child questionnaires to test their hypotheses. Even though researchers often have examined the associations between parent and child questionnaires to eliminate rater effects, self-reports have other problems including "social desirability biases; faulty recall or recall biases; ambiguous, general, or leading questions; limited awareness of one's own behavior; and careless or random responding" (Power et al., 2013, p. S-90).

Examples of more rigorous designs employing multiple methods and innovative measures include the assessment of glycemic control in children with diabetes (e.g., DeBoer et al., 2017; Prikken et al., 2019); the assessment of pulmonary functioning in children with asthma (e.g., Al Ghriwati et al., 2018); behavioral observations of parent–child interactions (e.g., Butcher & Nasr, 2015; Iskander et al., 2015; Peterson et al., 2014); daily records of child pain intensity, activity avoidance, and protective parenting in children with chronic pain (e.g., Beeckman et al., 2019); and the use of mobile technology for tracking contextual variables and diabetes self-management (e.g., Nam et al., 2021).

Although the research to date helps identify important directions for future work in this area, the use of multiple method, longitudinal, and intervention designs would provide considerably more insight into the nature of the associations identified here. Moreover, future studies should consider the following:

- whether the associations between family factors and child outcomes vary with the child's developmental level,
- whether family or parenting variables mediate the associations between distal sociocultural factors and child outcomes,
- whether the impact of parenting or family variables varies as a function of child characteristics (e.g., Slagt et al., 2016), and
- whether the associations between family/parenting variables and child outcomes differ for various ethnic or socioeconomic groups (Davidov, 2021).

Clinical Implications for Pediatric Psychologists and Pediatric Providers

The research reviewed here has implications for the clinical practice of pediatric providers. Along with supporting current best practices in health care (e.g., building trusting collaborative relationships; fostering open communication, cultural respect, and shared decision making), current research points to important modifiable family processes that should be considered in the care of children with chronic health conditions and that can be addressed in a variety of settings in which children with chronic medical conditions and their families are present.

Children with chronic medical conditions may see many providers. It is important for all providers to screen children with chronic health conditions for behavioral and social needs rather than assuming that screening is occurring elsewhere. Integrated behavioral health, characterized by a model of care in which pediatric psychologists are colocated and imbedded in pediatric care settings, is one option for addressing behavioral and social needs efficiently and in a collaborative manner. In addition to offering screening and linkage to needed supports, providers who take the time to hear caregiver and child experiences and to develop relationships with patients and members of their families and communities offer a resource whose value cannot be overstated. The relationship between providers and families is the foundation that allows children with chronic health conditions and their families to succeed in the face of the multiple challenges associated with these chronic conditions.

Given the importance of parents as partners in the management of many conditions, providers should find new ways to help parents effectively carry out these responsibilities and to provide information and support when parents have questions or concerns. The most effective strategies involve modeling, in regular health care visits, a developmentally appropriate transition of responsibility from parent to child. Such efforts should begin early and help parents assess the readiness of their child to take on new responsibilities as they mature (Miller & Jawad, 2019).

Providers also need to be aware of the many challenges facing families of children with chronic conditions and understand how these challenges can influence appraisal of disease severity, feelings of self-efficacy, and the ability to help children cope with the stresses of managing their condition as well as the common daily stressors associated with childhood (e.g., academic and social demands). Although referrals to mental health professionals are important when there are concerns about potential psychopathology, most parents and siblings experience multiple stressors so that standard surveillance of family and child well-being, as well as support in developing strategies for management of conditions, is likely to benefit most families provided that they do not place additional burden on those families.

Integrated behavioral health is gaining support because it can comprehensively meet the complex and intertwined health and behavioral health needs of children and families (Asarnow et al., 2015). Based on their knowledge of what works for other families, behavioral health providers may be particularly helpful in collaborating with parents and health care providers for a range of concerns that may arise given the unpredictable course of many chronic health conditions. If learning or behavior problems are also identified, a referral to a developmental-behavioral pediatrician may also be helpful.

Finally, providers need to be aware of the consequences of overprotectiveness in parents of children with chronic health conditions. Providers need to assess, in a nonjudgmental way, whether parents are being overprotective and give parents strategies, such as those reported in the chronic pain literature (Beeckman et al., 2019), to help them encourage adaptive functioning in their child in a way that is direct yet supportive and respectful of the child's concerns and feelings. Given the range of physical, psychological, and social outcomes observed in children with chronic health conditions and the important role of families in the child's adaptation, the research reviewed here points to many ways that families, children, pediatricians, and mental health professionals can support child development in the face of chronic health conditions.

RESOURCES

For Parents

- American Academy of Pediatrics:

    https://www.healthychildren.org/English/health-issues/conditions/chronic/Pages/default.aspx

    Provides descriptions for parents of a wide range of chronic health conditions affecting children, along with information on symptoms, diagnosis, treatment, care, and effects on the family.

- American Psychological Association: https://www.apa.org/topics/chronic-illness/child

  Provides information for parents on how to cope when their child is diagnosed with a chronic health condition.

- Centers for Disease Control and Prevention: https://www.cdc.gov/healthyschools/chronicconditions.htm

  Provides information for how various health conditions (i.e., asthma, diabetes, epilepsy, obesity, oral behavior) can be successfully managed in the school environment.

- Sileo, F. J., & Potter, C. S. (2021). *When your child has a chronic medical illness: A guide for the parenting journey.* American Psychological Association. https://doi.org/10.1037/0000229-000

  A book written for parents by mental health professionals on how to address the many issues that arise in caring for a child with a chronic health condition. Topics include coping with stress, communicating with your child, working with the school and medical teams, and others.

- Nemours Kids Health: https://kidshealth.org

  Resources for parents for addressing a range of health issues with young children.

- Retrain Pain Foundation: https://www.retrainpain.org

  Resources for applying a science-based approach for coping with pain in adults and children.

For Professionals

- Bogetz, F., Revetter, A., Partin, L., & DeCourcey, D. D. (2022). Relationships and resources supporting children with serious illness and their parents. *Hospital Pediatrics, 12*(9), 832–842. https://doi.org/10.1542/hpeds.2022-006596

  Results of a qualitative, interview study of adolescents and young adults with complex chronic conditions and their parents to inform how to best support children with chronic health conditions and their families.

- Mitchell, A. E., Morawska, A., & Mihelic, M. (2019). A systematic review of parenting interventions for child chronic health conditions. *Journal of Child Health Care, 24*(4), 603–628. https://doi.org/10.1177/1367493519882850

  A review of 10 interventions designed to support parents of children with chronic health conditions with a focus on strategies for increasing parental self-efficacy, parenting behavior, and children's behavior and quality of life.

- Thomas, S., Ryan, N. P., Byrne, L. K., Hendrieckx, C., & White, V. (2023). Unmet supportive care needs of children with chronic illness: A systematic review. *Journal of Clinical Nursing, 32*(19–20), 7101–7124. https://doi.org/10.1111/jocn.16806

  A review of 34 studies designed to identify unmet needs of children with chronic health conditions—primarily studies of children with cancer, but other conditions are considered as well.

- *Standards for Psychosocial Care for Children With Cancer and Their Families*, a special issue of *Pediatric Blood & Cancer, 62*(S5), S419–S895. https://onlinelibrary.wiley.com/toc/15455017/2015/62/S5

  A special issue of the journal *Pediatric Blood & Cancer* with 17 articles written to address various psychosocial issues in caring for children with cancer and their families. Articles cover such topics as psychological assessment, interdisciplinary collaboration, psychoeducation, supporting siblings, and others.

For Parents and Providers

- Meg Foundation for Pain:

  https://www.megfoundationforpain.org

  A source for parents and children to learn scientifically based approaches to managing children's pain.

References

Achenbach, T. M. (1991). *Integrative guide for the 1991 CBCL/4–18, YSR, and TRF profiles*. Department of Psychiatry, University of Vermont.

Al Ghriwati, N., Winter, M. A., Greenlee, J. L., & Thompson, E. L. (2018). Discrepancies between parent and self-reports of adolescent psychosocial symptoms: Associations with family conflict and asthma outcomes. *Journal of Family Psychology, 32*(7), 992–997. https://doi.org/10.1037/fam0000459

Armstrong, M. L., Duncan, C. L., Stokes, J. O., & Pereira, D. (2014). Association of caregiver health beliefs and parenting stress with medication adherence in preschoolers with asthma. *Journal of Asthma, 51*(4), 366–372. https://doi.org/10.3109/02770903.2013.876431

Asarnow, J. R., Rozenman, M., Wiblin, J., & Zeltzer, L. (2015). Integrated medical-behavioral care compared with usual primary care for child and adolescent behavioral health: A meta-analysis. *JAMA Pediatrics, 169*(10), 929–937. https://doi.org/10.1001/jamapediatrics.2015.1141

Baert, F., Miller, M. M., Trost, Z., Hirsh, A. T., McParland, J., De Schryver, M., & Vervoort, T. (2020). Parental injustice appraisals in the context of child pain: Examining the construct and criterion validity of the IEQ-Pc and IEQ-Ps. *The Journal of Pain, 21*(1–2), 195–211. https://doi.org/10.1016/j.jpain.2019.06.012

Bates, A. T., & Kearney, J. A. (2015). Understanding death with limited experience in life: Dying children's and adolescents' understanding of their own terminal illness and death. *Current Opinion in Supportive and Palliative Care, 9*(1), 40–45. https://doi.org/10.1097/SPC.0000000000000118

Bava, L., Johns, A., Kayser, K., & Freyer, D. R. (2018). Cognitive outcomes among Latino survivors of childhood acute lymphoblastic leukemia and lymphoma: A cross-sectional cohort study using culturally competent, performance-based assessment. *Pediatric Blood & Cancer, 65*(2), e26844. https://doi.org/10.1002/pbc.26844

Bazargan, M., Cobb, S., & Assari, S. (2021). Discrimination and medical mistrust in a racially and ethnically diverse sample of California adults. *Annals of Family Medicine, 19*(1), 4–15. https://doi.org/10.1370/afm.2632

Beeckman, M., Simons, L. E., Hughes, S., Loeys, T., & Goubert, L. (2019). Investigating how parental instructions and protective responses mediate the relationship between parental psychological flexibility and pain-related behavior in adolescents with chronic pain: A daily diary study. *Frontiers in Psychology, 10*, 2350. https://doi.org/10.3389/fpsyg.2019.02350

Berg, C. A., Queen, T., Butner, J. E., Turner, S. L., Hughes Lansing, A., Main, A., Anderson, J. H., Thoma, B. C., Winnick, J. B., & Wiebe, D. J. (2017). Adolescent disclosure to parents and daily management of Type 1 diabetes. *Journal of Pediatric Psychology, 42*(1), 75–84. https://doi.org/10.1093/jpepsy/jsw056

Boerner, K. E., Chambers, C. T., McGrath, P. J., LoLordo, V., & Uher, R. (2017). The effect of parental modeling on child pain responses: The role of parent and child sex. *The Journal of Pain, 18*(6), 702–715. https://doi.org/10.1016/j.jpain.2017.01.007

Burton, L. M., Lichter, D. T., Baker, R. S., & Eason, J. S. (2013). Inequality, family processes, and health in the "new" rural America. *American Behavioral Scientist, 57*(8), 1128–1151. https://doi.org/10.1177/0002764213487348

Butcher, J. L., & Nasr, S. Z. (2015). Direct observation of respiratory treatments in cystic fibrosis: Parent–child interactions relate to medical regimen adherence. *Journal of Pediatric Psychology, 40*(1), 8–17. https://doi.org/10.1093/jpepsy/jsu074

Caes, L. (2019). Commentary: Parent–child interactions during painful medical procedures: Recommendations by Blount and colleagues (1991) have not fallen on deaf ears! *Journal of Pediatric Psychology, 44*(7), 794–797. https://doi.org/10.1093/jpepsy/jsz032

Chisholm, V., Atkinson, L., Bayrami, L., Noyes, K., Payne, A., & Kelnar, C. (2014). An exploratory study of positive and incongruent communication in young children with Type 1 diabetes and their mothers. *Child: Care, Health and Development, 40*(1), 85–94. https://doi.org/10.1111/cch.12004

Comaroff, J., & Maguire, P. (1981). Ambiguity and the search for meaning: Childhood leukaemia in the modern clinical context. *Social Science & Medicine, 15B*(2), 115–123.

Compas, B. E., Jaser, S. S., Dunn, M. J., & Rodriguez, E. M. (2012). Coping with chronic illness in childhood and adolescence. *Annual Review of*

Clinical Psychology, 8(1), 455–480. https://doi.org/10.1146/annurev-clinpsy-032511-143108

Crandell, J. L., Sandelowski, M., Leeman, J., Havill, N. L., & Knafl, K. (2018). Parenting behaviors and the well-being of children with a chronic physical condition. *Families, Systems, & Health*, 36(1), 45–61. https://doi.org/10.1037/fsh0000305

D'Angelo, C. M., Mrug, S., Grossoehme, D., Schwebel, D. C., Reynolds, N., & Guion Reynolds, K. (2019). Coping, attributions, and health functioning among adolescents with chronic illness and their parents: Reciprocal relations over time. *Journal of Clinical Psychology in Medical Settings*, 26(4), 495–506. https://doi.org/10.1007/s10880-018-9597-0

Davidov, M. (2021). Cultural moderation of the effects of parenting: Answered and unanswered questions. *Child Development Perspectives*, 15(3), 189–195. https://doi.org/10.1111/cdep.12422

DeBoer, M. D., Valdez, R., Chernavvsky, D. R., Grover, M., Burt Solorzano, C., Herbert, K., & Patek, S. (2017). The impact of frequency and tone of parent–youth communication on Type 1 diabetes management. *Diabetes Therapy* 8(3), 625–636. https://doi.org/10.1007/s13300-017-0259-2

Donnelly, T. J., Palermo, T. M., & Newton-John, T. R. O. (2020). Parent cognitive, behavioural, and affective factors and their relation to child pain and functioning in pediatric chronic pain: A systematic review and meta-analysis. *Pain*, 161(7), 1401–1419. https://doi.org/10.1097/j.pain.0000000000001833

Eccleston, C., Palermo, T. M., Fisher, E., & Law, E. (2012). Psychological interventions for parents of children and adolescents with chronic illness. *Cochrane Database of Systematic Reviews*, 2012(8), CD009660. https://doi.org/10.1002/14651858.CD009660.pub2

Elliott, L., Thompson, K. A., & Fobian, A. D. (2020). A systematic review of somatic symptoms in children with a chronically ill family member. *Psychosomatic Medicine*, 82(4), 366–376. https://doi.org/10.1097/PSY.0000000000000799

Fairfax, A., Brehaut, J., Colman, I., Sikora, L., Kazakova, A., Chakraborty, P., Potter, B. K., & the Canadian Inherited Metabolic Diseases Research Network. (2019). A systematic review of the association between coping strategies and quality of life among caregivers of children with chronic illness and/or disability. *BMC Pediatrics*, 19(1), 215. https://doi.org/10.1186/s12887-019-1587-3

Fawcett, R. (2019). *Experiences of parents and carers managing asthma in children* [Unpublished master's thesis]. University of Adelaide. https://digital.library.adelaide.edu.au/dspace/bitstream/2440/122449/1/Fawcett2019_MClinSc.pdf

Feagin, J., & Bennefield, Z. (2014). Systemic racism and U.S. health care. *Social Science & Medicine*, 103, 7–14. https://doi.org/10.1016/j.socscimed.2013.09.006

Feinstein, A. B., Sturgeon, J. A., Bhandari, R. P., Yoon, I. A., Ross, A. C., Huestis, S. E., Griffin, A. T., & Simons, L. E. (2018). Risk and resilience in pediatric pain: The roles of parent and adolescent catastrophizing and acceptance. *The Clinical Journal of Pain*, 34(12), 1096–1105. https://doi.org/10.1097/AJP.0000000000000639

Field, M. J., & Behrman, R. E. (Eds.). (2003). *When children die: Improving palliative and end-of-live care for children and their families*. National Academies Press. https://doi.org/10.17226/10390

Finnvold, J. E. (2010). In their own words: Early childhood asthma and parents' experiences of the diagnostic process. *Scandinavian Journal of Caring Sciences*, 24(2), 299–306. https://doi.org/10.1111/j.1471-6712.2009.00720.x

Fisher, H. R. (2001). The needs of parents with chronically sick children: A literature review. *Journal of Advanced Nursing*, 36(4), 600–607. https://doi.org/10.1046/j.1365-2648.2001.02013.x

Fluchel, M. N., Kirchhoff, A. C., Bodson, J., Sweeney, C., Edwards, S. L., Ding, Q., Stoddard, G. J., & Kinney, A. Y. (2014). Geography and the burden of care in pediatric cancers. *Pediatric Blood & Cancer*, 61(11), 1918–1924. https://doi.org/10.1002/pbc.25170

Forgeron, P. A., King, S., Stinson, J. N., McGrath, P. J., MacDonald, A. J., & Chambers, C. T. (2010). Social functioning and peer relationships in children and adolescents with chronic pain: A systematic review. *Pain Research & Management*, 15(1), 27–41. https://doi.org/10.1155/2010/820407

Gise, J., & Cohen, L. L. (2022). Social support in parents of children with cancer: A systematic review. *Journal of Pediatric Psychology*, 47(3), 292–305. https://doi.org/10.1093/jpepsy/jsab100

Goubert, L., Eccleston, C., Vervoort, T., Jordan, A., & Crombez, G. (2006). Parental catastrophizing about their child's pain. The parent version of the Pain Catastrophizing Scale (PCS-P): A preliminary validation. *Pain*, 123(3), 254–263. https://doi.org/10.1016/j.pain.2006.02.035

Gray, W. N., Netz, M., McConville, A., Fedele, D., Wagoner, S. T., & Schaefer, M. R. (2018). Medication adherence in pediatric asthma: A systematic review of the literature. *Pediatric Pulmonology*, 53(5), 668–684. https://doi.org/10.1002/ppul.23966

Green, M., & Solnit, A. J. (1964). Reactions to the threatened loss of a child: A vulnerable child syndrome. Pediatric management of the dying child. Part III. *Pediatrics, 34*(1), 58–66. https://doi.org/10.1542/peds.34.1.58

Haggerty, R. J., & Friedman, S. B. (2003). History of developmental-behavioral pediatrics. *Journal of Developmental and Behavioral Pediatrics, 24*(Suppl. 1), S1–S18. https://doi.org/10.1097/00004703-200302001-00001

Hoffmann, M. R., Alzaben, A. S., Enns, S. E., Marcon, M. A., Turner, J., & Mager, D. R. (2016). Parental health beliefs, socio-demographics, and healthcare recommendations influence micronutrient supplementation in youth with celiac disease. *Canadian Journal of Dietetic Practice and Research, 77*(1), 47–53. https://doi.org/10.3148/cjdpr-2015-035

Hynes, L., Saetes, S., McGuire, B., & Caes, L. (2019). Child and family adaptation to juvenile idiopathic arthritis—A systematic review of the role of resilience resources and mechanisms. *Frontiers in Psychology, 10*, 2445. https://doi.org/10.3389/fpsyg.2019.02445

Iskander, J. M., Rohan, J. M., Pendley, J. S., Delamater, A., & Drotar, D. (2015). A 3-year prospective study of parent–child communication in early adolescents with Type 1 diabetes: Relationship to adherence and glycemic control. *Journal of Pediatric Psychology, 40*(1), 109–120. https://doi.org/10.1093/jpepsy/jsu027

Jargowsky, P. A. (2018). The persistence of segregation in the 21st century. *Minnesota Journal of Law and Inequality, 36*(2), 207–230.

Jokinen-Gordon, H., & Quadagno, J. (2013). Variations in parents' perceptions of their children's medical treatment: The effect of dissatisfaction on preventive care and unmet need. In J. J. Kronenfeld (Ed.), *Research in the sociology of health care: Vol. 31. Social determinants, health disparities and linkages to health and health care* (pp. 161–185). https://doi.org/10.1108/S0275-4959(2013)0000031010

Kagan, J. (1965). The new marriage: Pediatrics and psychology. *American Journal of Diseases of Children, 110*(3), 272–278.

Kazak, A. E., Alderfer, M. A., & Reader, S. K. (2017). Families and other systems in pediatric psychology. In M. C. Roberts & R. G. Steele (Eds.), *Handbook of pediatric psychology* (3rd ed., pp. 566–579). Guilford Press.

Koepke, S., & Denissen, J. J. A. (2012). Dynamics of identity development and separation–individuation in parent–child relationships during adolescence and emerging adulthood—A conceptual integration. *Developmental Review, 32*(1), 67–88. https://doi.org/10.1016/j.dr.2012.01.001

Koutná, V., & Blatný, M. (2020). Socialization of coping in pediatric oncology settings: Theoretical consideration on parent–child connections in posttraumatic growth. *Frontiers in Psychology, 11*, 554325. https://doi.org/10.3389/fpsyg.2020.554325

Lam, C. B., McHale, S. M., & Crouter, A. C. (2014). Time with peers from middle childhood to late adolescence: Developmental course and adjustment correlates. *Child Development, 85*(4), 1677–1693. https://doi.org/10.1111/cdev.12235

Lau, R. R., & Hartman, K. A. (1983). Common sense representations of common illnesses. *Health Psychology, 2*(2), 167–185. https://doi.org/10.1037/0278-6133.2.2.167

Leeman, J., Crandell, J. L., Lee, A., Bai, J., Sandelowski, M., & Knafl, K. (2016). Family functioning and the well-being of children with chronic conditions: A meta-analysis. *Research in Nursing & Health, 39*(4), 229–243. https://doi.org/10.1002/nur.21725

Mack, J. W., Cook, E. F., Wolfe, J., Grier, H. E., Cleary, P. D., & Weeks, J. C. (2007). Understanding of prognosis among parents of children with cancer: Parental optimism and the parent–physician interaction. *Journal of Clinical Oncology, 25*(11), 1357–1362. https://doi.org/10.1200/JCO.2006.08.3170

Madrigal, V. N., & Kelly, K. P. (2018). Supporting family decision-making for a child who is seriously ill: Creating synchrony and connection. *Pediatrics, 142*(Suppl. 3), S170–S177. https://doi.org/10.1542/peds.2018-0516H

Miller, V. A. (2018). Involving youth with a chronic illness in decision-making: Highlighting the role of providers. *Pediatrics, 142*(Suppl. 3), S142–S148. https://doi.org/10.1542/peds.2018-0516D

Miller, V. A., & Jawad, A. F. (2019). Decision-making involvement and prediction of adherence in youth with Type 1 diabetes: A cohort sequential study. *Journal of Pediatric Psychology, 44*(1), 61–71. https://doi.org/10.1093/jpepsy/jsy032

Mitchell, A. E., Morawska, A., & Mihelic, M. (2020). A systematic review of parenting interventions for child chronic health conditions. *Journal of Child Health Care, 24*(4), 603–628. https://doi.org/10.1177/1367493519882850

Mullins, L. L., Fuemmeler, B. F., Hoff, A., Chaney, J. H., Van Pelt, J., & Ewing, C. A. (2004). The relationship of parental overprotection and perceived child vulnerability to depressive symptomatology in children with Type 1 diabetes mellitus: The moderating influence of parenting stress. *Children's Health Care, 33*(1), 21–34. https://doi.org/10.1207/s15326888chc3301_2

Murphy, L. K., Murray, C. B., Compas, B. E., & the Guest Editors: Cynthia A. Gerhardt, Cynthia A. Berg, Deborah J. Wiebe, and Grayson N. Holmbeck. (2017). Topical review: Integrating findings on direct observation of family communication in studies comparing pediatric chronic illness and typically developing samples. *Journal of Pediatric Psychology*, 42(1), 85–94. https://doi.org/10.1093/jpepsy/jsw051

Myant, K. A., & Williams, J. M. (2005). Children's concepts of health and illness: Understanding of contagious illnesses, non-contagious illnesses and injuries. *Journal of Health Psychology*, 10(6), 805–819. https://doi.org/10.1177/1359105305057315

Nam, S., Griggs, S., Ash, G. I., Dunton, G. F., Huang, S., Batten, J., Parekh, N., & Whittemore, R. (2021). Ecological momentary assessment for health behaviors and contextual factors in persons with diabetes: A systematic review. *Diabetes Research and Clinical Practice*, 174, 108745. https://doi.org/10.1016/j.diabres.2021.108745

Neville, A., Jordan, A., Pincus, T., Nania, C., Schulte, F., Yeates, K. O., & Noel, M. (2020). Diagnostic uncertainty in pediatric chronic pain: Nature, prevalence, and consequences. *Pain Reports*, 5(6), e871. https://doi.org/10.1097/PR9.0000000000000871

Newton, E., Schosheim, A., Patel, S., Chitkara, D. K., & van Tilburg, M. A. L. (2019). The role of psychological factors in pediatric functional abdominal pain disorders. *Neurogastroenterology and Motility*, 31(6), e13538. https://doi.org/10.1111/nmo.13538

Noser, A. E., Patton, S. R., Van Allen, J., Nelson, M. B., & Clements, M. A. (2017). Evaluating parents' self-efficacy for diabetes management in pediatric Type 1 diabetes. *Journal of Pediatric Psychology*, 42(3), 296–303.

Peterson, A. M., Harper, F. W. K., Albrecht, T. L., Taub, J. W., Orom, H., Phipps, S., & Penner, L. A. (2014). Parent caregiver self-efficacy and child reactions to pediatric cancer treatment procedures. *Journal of Pediatric Oncology Nursing*, 31(1), 18–27. https://doi.org/10.1177/1043454213514792

Pinquart, M. (2018). Posttraumatic stress symptoms and disorders in children and adolescents with chronic physical illnesses: A meta-analysis. *Journal of Child & Adolescent Trauma*, 13(1), 1–10. https://doi.org/10.1007/s40653-018-0222-z

Pinquart, M. (2020). Health-related quality of life of young people with and without chronic conditions. *Journal of Pediatric Psychology*, 45(7), 780–792. https://doi.org/10.1093/jpepsy/jsaa052

Pinquart, M., & Shen, Y. (2011). Behavior problems in children and adolescents with chronic physical illness: A meta-analysis. *Journal of Pediatric Psychology*, 36(9), 1003–1016. https://doi.org/10.1093/jpepsy/jsr042

Power, T. G. (2004). Stress and coping in childhood: The parents' role. *Parenting: Science and Practice*, 4(4), 271–317. https://doi.org/10.1207/s15327922par0404_1

Power, T. G., Dahlquist, L. M., & Pinder, W. (2019). Parenting children with a chronic health condition. In B. H. Bornstein (Ed.), *Handbook of parenting: Vol. 1. Children and parenting* (3rd ed., pp. 597–624). Routledge. https://doi.org/10.4324/9780429440847-18

Power, T. G., Sleddens, E. F. C., Berge, J., Connell, L., Govig, B., Hennessy, E., Liggett, L., Mallan, K., Santa Maria, D., Odoms-Young, A., & St. George, S. M. (2013). Contemporary research on parenting: Conceptual, methodological, and translational issues. *Childhood Obesity*, 9(Suppl. 1), S87–S94. https://doi.org/10.1089/chi.2013.0038

Prikken, S., Raymaekers, K., Oris, L., Rassart, J., Weets, I., Moons, P., & Luyckx, K. (2019). A triadic perspective on control perceptions in youth with Type 1 diabetes and their parents: Associations with treatment adherence and glycemic control. *Diabetes Research and Clinical Practice*, 150, 264–273. https://doi.org/10.1016/j.diabres.2019.03.025

Psihogios, A. M., Fellmeth, H., Schwartz, L. A., & Barakat, L. P. (2019). Family functioning and medical adherence across children and adolescents with chronic health conditions: A meta-analysis. *Journal of Pediatric Psychology*, 44(1), 84–97. https://doi.org/10.1093/jpepsy/jsy044

Ravindran, V. P., & Rempel, G. R. (2011). Grandparents and siblings of children with congenital heart disease. *Journal of Advanced Nursing*, 67(1), 169–175. https://doi.org/10.1111/j.1365-2648.2010.05482.x

Reed-Knight, B., Blount, R. L., & Gilleland, J. (2014). The transition of health care responsibility from parents to youth diagnosed with chronic illness: A developmental systems perspective. *Families, Systems, & Health*, 32(2), 219–234. https://doi.org/10.1037/fsh0000039

Riley, A. R., Walker, B. L., Ramanujam, K., Gualtney, W. M., & Cohen, D. J. (2022). A mixed-method investigation of parent perspectives on early childhood behavioral services in primary care. *The Journal of Behavioral Health Services & Research*, 49(2), 134–148. https://doi.org/10.1007/s11414-021-09772-2

Rotenberg, K. J., & Petrocchi, S. (2018). A longitudinal investigation of trust beliefs in physicians by children with asthma and their mothers: Relations with children's adherence to medical regimes and quality of life. *Child: Care, Health and Development*, 44(6), 879–884. https://doi.org/10.1111/cch.12604

Routh, D. K. (1975). The short history of pediatric psychology. *Journal of Clinical Child Psychology*, 4(3), 6–8. https://doi.org/10.1080/15374417509532658

Sahler, O. J. Z., Fairclough, D. L., Phipps, S., Mulhern, R. K., Dolgin, M. J., Noll, R. B., Katz, E. R., Varni, J. W., Copeland, D. R., & Butler, R. W. (2005). Using problem-solving skills training to reduce negative affectivity in mothers of children with newly diagnosed cancer: Report of a multisite randomized trial. *Journal of Consulting and Clinical Psychology*, 73(2), 272–283. https://doi.org/10.1037/0022-006X.73.2.272

Sales, J., Fivush, R., & Teague, G. W. (2008). The role of parental coping in children with asthma's psychological well-being and asthma-related quality of life. *Journal of Pediatric Psychology*, 33(2), 208–219. https://doi.org/10.1093/jpepsy/jsm068

Santacroce, S. J. (2001). Measuring parental uncertainty during the diagnosis phase of serious illness in a child. *Journal of Pediatric Nursing*, 16(1), 3–12. https://doi.org/10.1053/jpdn.2001.20547

Scheier, M. F., & Carver, C. S. (2018). Dispositional optimism and physical health: A long look back, a quick look forward. *American Psychologist*, 73(9), 1082–1094. https://doi.org/10.1037/amp0000384

Shorey, S., & Ng, E. D. (2020). The lived experience of children and adolescents with non-communicable disease: A systematic review of qualitative studies. *Journal of Pediatric Nursing*, 51, 75–84. https://doi.org/10.1016/j.pedn.2019.12.013

Sil, S., Dampier, C., & Cohen, L. L. (2016). Pediatric sickle cell disease and parent and child catastrophizing. *The Journal of Pain*, 17(9), 963–971. https://doi.org/10.1016/j.jpain.2016.05.008

Skinner, E. A., & Zimmer-Gembeck, M. J. (2016). *The development of coping: Stress, neurophysiology, social relationships, and reliance during childhood and adolescence*. Springer International. https://doi.org/10.1007/978-3-319-41740-0

Slagt, M., Dubas, J. S., Deković, M., & van Aken, M. A. G. (2016). Differences in sensitivity to parenting depending on child temperament: A meta-analysis. *Psychological Bulletin*, 142(10), 1068–1110. https://doi.org/10.1037/bul0000061

Steiner, E. M., Dahlquist, L. M., Power, T. G., & Bollinger, M. E. (2020). Intolerance of uncertainty and protective parenting in mothers of children with food allergy. *Children's Health Care*, 49(2), 184–201. https://doi.org/10.1080/02739615.2019.1650362

Stone, A. L., Bruehl, S., Smith, C. A., Garber, J., & Walker, L. S. (2018). Social learning pathways in the relation between parental chronic pain and daily pain severity and functional impairment in adolescents with functional abdominal pain. *Pain*, 159(2), 298–305. https://doi.org/10.1097/j.pain.0000000000001085

Sultan, S., Leclair, T., Rondeau, É., Burns, W., & Abate, C. (2016). A systematic review on factors and consequences of parental distress as related to childhood cancer. *European Journal of Cancer Care*, 25(4), 616–637. https://doi.org/10.1111/ecc.12361

Sung, L., Klaassen, R. J., Dix, D., Pritchard, S., Yanofsky, R., Ethier, M.-C., & Klassen, A. (2009). Parental optimism in poor prognosis pediatric cancers. *Psycho-Oncology*, 18(7), 783–788. https://doi.org/10.1002/pon.1490

Sweenie, R., Mackey, E. R., & Streisand, R. (2014). Parent–child relationships in Type 1 diabetes: Associations among child behavior, parenting behavior, and pediatric parenting stress. *Families, Systems, & Health*, 32(1), 31–42. https://doi.org/10.1037/fsh0000001

Szulczewski, L., Mullins, L. L., Bidwell, S. L., Eddington, A. R., & Pai, A. L. H. (2017). Meta-analysis: Caregiver and youth uncertainty in pediatric chronic illness. *Journal of Pediatric Psychology*, 42(4), 395–421. https://doi.org/10.1093/jpepsy/jsw097

Tanna, V., Heathcote, L. C., Heirich, M. S., Rush, G., Neville, A., Noel, M., Pate, J. W., & Simons, L. E. (2020). Something else going on? Diagnostic uncertainty in children with chronic pain and their parents. *Children*, 7(10), 165. https://doi.org/10.3390/children7100165

Tourse, R. W. C., Hamilton-Mason, J., & Wewiorski, N. J. (2018). *Systematic racism in the United States: Scaffolding as social construction*. Springer. https://doi.org/10.1007/978-3-319-72233-7

Turner, E. M., Koskela-Staples, N., Voorhees, S., McQuaid, E. L., & Fedele, D. A. (2021). Health-related decision-making in early adolescents with poorly controlled asthma. *Clinical Practice in Pediatric Psychology*, 9(1), 24–34. https://doi.org/10.1037/cpp0000333

Urberg, K. A., Degirmencioglu, S. M., Tolson, J. M., & Halliday-Scher, K. (2000). Adolescent social crowds: Measurement and relationship to friendships. *Journal of Adolescent Research*, 15(4), 427–445. https://doi.org/10.1177/0743558400154001

U.S. Census Bureau. (2016). *Educational attainment in the United States: 2015*. https://www.census.gov/content/dam/Census/library/publications/2016/demo/p20-578.pdf

Valrie, C., Thurston, I., & Santos, M. (2020). Introduction to the special issue: Addressing health disparities in pediatric psychology. *Journal of*

Pediatric Psychology, 45(8), 833–838. https://doi.org/10.1093/jpepsy/jsaa066

Van der Graaff, J., Branje, S., De Wied, M., Hawk, S., Van Lier, P., & Meeus, W. (2014). Perspective taking and empathic concern in adolescence: Gender differences in developmental changes. *Developmental Psychology, 50*(3), 881–888. https://doi.org/10.1037/a0034325

van der Lee, J. H., Mokkink, L. B., Grootenhuis, M. A., Heymans, H. S., & Offringa, M. (2007). Definitions and measurement of chronic health conditions in childhood: A systematic review. *JAMA: Journal of the American Medical Association, 297*(24), 2741–2751. https://doi.org/10.1001/jama.297.24.2741

Varni, J. W., Seid, M., & Kurtin, P. S. (2001). PedsQL 4.0: Reliability and validity of the Pediatric Quality of Life Inventory version 4.0 generic core scales in healthy and patient populations. *Medical Care, 39*(8), 800–812. https://doi.org/10.1097/00005650-200108000-00006

Venning, A., Eliott, J., Wilson, A., & Kettler, L. (2008). Understanding young peoples' experience of chronic illness: A systematic review. *International Journal of Evidence-Based Healthcare, 6*(3), 321–336. https://doi.org/10.1111/j.1744-1609.2008.00107.x

Weissberg-Benchell, J., Nansel, T., Holmbeck, G., Chen, R., Anderson, B., Wysocki, T., Laffel, L., & the Steering Committee of the Family Management of Diabetes Study. (2009). Generic and diabetes-specific parent–child behaviors and quality of life among youth with Type 1 diabetes. *Journal of Pediatric Psychology, 34*(9), 977–988. https://doi.org/10.1093/jpepsy/jsp003

Wittkowski, A., Dowling, H., & Smith, D. M. (2016). Does engaging in a group-based intervention increase parental self-efficacy in parents of preschool children? A systematic review of the current literature. *Journal of Child and Family Studies, 25*(11), 3173–3191. https://doi.org/10.1007/s10826-016-0464-z

Yao, C. A., & Rhodes, R. E. (2015). Parental correlates in child and adolescent physical activity: A meta-analysis. *International Journal of Behavioral Nutrition and Physical Activity, 12*(1), 10. https://doi.org/10.1186/s12966-015-0163-y

Yee, A. Z., Lwin, M. O., & Ho, S. S. (2017). The influence of parental practices on child promotive and preventive food consumption behaviors: A systematic review and meta-analysis. *International Journal of Behavioral Nutrition and Physical Activity, 14*(1), 47. https://doi.org/10.1186/s12966-017-0501-3

CHAPTER 2

PEDIATRIC TREATMENT ADHERENCE

Alexandra M. Psihogios, Annisa M. Ahmed, Christina E. Holbein, and Aimee W. Smith

Among youth with chronic health conditions, a modifiable health behavior has been consistently linked to health outcomes—treatment adherence. The World Health Organization (WHO) defines adherence as "the extent to which a person's behavior—taking medication, following a diet, and/or executing lifestyle changes, corresponds with agreed recommendations from a health care provider" (Sabaté, 2003, pp. 3–4). Thus, adherence is a multifaceted health behavior that can involve a range of treatment tasks (e.g., taking prescribed medications, clinic attendance, and following diet recommendations) that take place across several contexts (e.g., at home, at school, with family and peers). Treatment recommendations are often prescribed by clinicians embedded in multidisciplinary subspecialty clinics (e.g., pediatric hematology clinics), but may be prescribed by pediatricians, as can be the case for common childhood conditions such as asthma and attention-deficit/hyperactivity disorder (ADHD; Drotar, 2013). Suboptimal treatment adherence is highly prevalent among children and adolescents with chronic health conditions. For example, approximately 50% of children and up to 75% of adolescents do not take their medications as prescribed (Rapoff, 2010). Adherence challenges have individual and public health impacts, including increased risks for mortality and secondary morbidities, poorer quality of life, additional health care utilization, and health care spending totaling more than $300 billion (about $920 per person in the United States) per year (McGrady & Hommel, 2016).

Moreover, among various pediatric populations, including cancer (Bhatia et al., 2014), asthma (Lieu et al., 2002), and Type 1 diabetes (Kahkoska et al., 2018), more challenges with adherence have been observed among youth who identify as Black, Hispanic, or a Person of Color. Inequities in managing a complex medical regimen are not caused by biological differences that make certain groups of youth inherently less capable; rather, adherence is influenced by complex interacting socioecological factors at the individual, family, community, and health system level that can shift over the course of child development.

The objective of this chapter is to provide an updated discussion of treatment adherence in pediatrics—including definitions, prevalence, theory, contextual determinants, assessment, interventions, and implications for pediatrics and developmental science. Prior and recent resources on pediatric adherence, including Guilford Press' 2017 *Handbook of Pediatric Psychology* (5th ed.; Roberts & Ric, 2017), similarly discuss these domains but without an integrated focus on the fields of pediatric

https://doi.org/10.1037/0000414-002
APA Handbook of Pediatric Psychology, Developmental-Behavioral Pediatrics, and Developmental Science: Vol. 2. Pediatric Psychology and Developmental-Behavioral Pediatrics: Clinical Applications of Developmental Science, P. E. Shah and M. H. Bornstein (Editors-in-Chief)
Copyright © 2025 by the American Psychological Association. All rights reserved.

psychology, developmental and behavioral pediatrics, and developmental science. Additionally, there has been limited focus on marginalized youth who face barriers to adherence at the systemic level (e.g., access to care). There has been a recent critical examination of racism and other forms of oppression in all parts of society, including developmental and behavioral pediatrics (Spinks-Franklin, 2021) and pediatric psychology (Palermo et al., 2021). Thus, within each subsection of this chapter, we also highlight the strengths and limitations of existing empirical literature for improving adherence and associated health outcomes among marginalized youth.

DEFINING ADHERENCE AND CONTEXTUALIZING ADHERENCE IMPACTS

In this section, we define treatment adherence, then describe prevalence, clinical cut points, and individual and public health impacts of nonadherence.

Defining Treatment Adherence, and the Role of Socioecological Contexts

It is critical to first define treatment adherence and examine those definitions to advance pediatric research and clinical care. As described, WHO's definition of adherence is broadly applicable across developmental stages and diseases, widely accepted across disciplines and provides a cohesive understanding of adherence for research and clinical care. However, this definition also has limitations. It is static, does not capture all medical tasks prescribed to youth with chronic health conditions, does not reflect how treatment recommendations were provided, and orients the construct as a problem that belongs to the patient rather than one that is influenced by socioecological factors (e.g., family medical beliefs, neighborhood access to pharmacies, racism, legislation surrounding medication cost) that pose barriers for equitable disease care. For example, individuals who have experienced discrimination in health care settings may not engage with treatment due to medical mistrust, which is an adaptive functional coping response (Bogart et al., 2021). The WHO definition also focuses on the agreed upon recommendations from clinicians, assuming a shared decision-making framework for health care, which is not always the case.

Limitations to the WHO definition led to development of alternate definitions of adherence. The European Society for Patient Adherence, Compliance and Persistence (ESPA-COMP) developed an empirical taxonomy that conceptualizes adherence as a complex, dynamic, and quantifiable process (Vrijens et al., 2012). This taxonomy comprises three distinct but interrelated phases, including *initiation* (i.e., start of the adherence process), *implementation* (i.e., evaluation of dosing history, including omissions), and *persistence* (i.e., length of time between initiation and treatment abandonment). As compared with other adherence definitions, this approach is based on empirical review and is more clearly operationalized, which can help reduce biased judgments. It also lends itself to developmental cascades (Masten & Cicchetti, 2010; see also Volume 1, Chapter 4, this handbook) present in adherence, as adherence may change over the course of a treatment plan as a result of multiple bidirectional contextual influences. Indeed, the full ESPA-COMP taxonomy integrates with an ecological approach (Bronfenbrenner, 1979) to adherence as it incorporates factors outside of the individual, including health care systems and social networks that assist in managing adherence.

Another important issue is to clarify the distinction between adherence and disease self-management. Self-management encompasses a larger view of what is included in the tasks of disease management and behaviors and is defined as "the interaction of health behaviors and related processes that patients and families engage in to care for a chronic condition" (Modi et al., 2012, p. e474). Therefore, aspects of self-management (e.g., improving knowledge and facilitating social support) can serve as targets for adherence interventions.

Adherence terminology has moved away from characterizing an individual as nonadherent to defining adherence on a continuum that can shift over time and be influenced by socioecological factors. For example, socioecological barriers to adherence can include factors within the individual child or adolescent (e.g., disliking the taste of a medicine limited understanding of the purpose of the medication), family (e.g., caregiver involvement with prompting a child to take a medication), and health system-level factors (e.g., high cost of medication, insufficient clinician communication). Likewise, there has been a movement away from the term "compliance" (implying following orders from an authority figure) to "adherence" (behavior aligned with recommendations that allows the patient more agency).

Adherence is a matter of public health. Based on the abundance of evidence reviewed in the next section on prevalence, adherence challenges are normative and should be expected by clinicians. However, to some extent, the culture of health care systems has not accepted this normative behavior and continues to place the burden of improving adherence on the individual patient or caregiver rather than on any other exosystem (e.g., parent workplace) or macrosystem factors (e.g., cultural values and laws). Indeed, adherence problems disproportionally impact marginalized populations (e.g., Gerber et al., 2010). These disproportionate burdens can lead to increased cumulative health costs over time (e.g., lower quality of life; Wu et al., 2014).

Prevalence and Clinical Cut Points

Approximately 50% of children and up to 75% of adolescents do not take their medications as prescribed (Rapoff, 2010). Rates of medication adherence vary among specific pediatric populations and their recommended treatments, such as clinical samples of youth with chronic illnesses (wide range, averaging 50% adherent; Rapoff, 2010), youth with developmental delay (74.3% adherent; Tan et al., 2015), and youth receiving pediatric primary care (78% adherent; Zweigoron et al., 2012). However, published adherence rates are biased estimates as they include only those who (a) have agreed to participate in research and (b) complete data collection procedures (i.e., have strong adherence to research tasks). Thus, estimates of adherence are likely overestimated in clinical/intervention samples and may be more accurately measured by community-based measurements such as pharmacy refills (e.g., Zweigoron et al., 2012). Moreover, adherence is dynamic and can change rapidly from day to day, a phenomenon not captured by aggregate prevalence scores. Harnessing daily adherence data and advanced statistical techniques (e.g., Modi et al., 2011) may facilitate a richer picture of adherence patterns and allow clinicians to tailor interventions or guide systems-level changes.

There are clinically meaningful thresholds established for some populations (e.g., >95% adherence to oral 6-mercaptopurine to prevent relapse in patients with leukemia; Bhatia et al., 2014). However, for many disease populations, there is not a disease-modifying cut point, and treatment adherence must be examined as a spectrum rather than a dichotomy. Considering adherence as a spectrum (e.g., for diet adherence, the proportion of days in the last week that the diet was followed as prescribed) rather than a cut point (when not clinically indicated) allows more room for patients to succeed and clinicians to note small improvements (e.g., increase in percentage points or fewer missed doses per week). Ideally, the ultimate definition of adherence should correlate with clinical impact and connect with mutually agreed upon health goals (e.g., using shared decision making) to remove unnecessary labeling and marginalization of patients with "good enough" adherence (Pai & Drotar, 2010).

Individual and Public Health Outcomes

Adherence challenges have been associated with a host of negative health outcomes, including preventable disease complications (Walsh et al., 2002), unneeded increases in medications (Carmody et al., 2019), and lower quality of life (Wu et al., 2014). Further, increased urgent health care utilization (emergency department visits, hospitalizations) and decreased outpatient visits are seen in patients with lower adherence (McGrady & Hommel, 2013). Little has been done to examine how the magnitude of adherence problems interacts with ongoing systemic racism and inequitable health care to influence pediatric health. Although research specific to racism and adherence is lacking in children, research on adults has shown that perceived racism negatively impacts adherence (Chakraborty et al., 2011) and engagement in care (Gaston & Alleyne-Green, 2013). Developmental stage also impacts adherence, as adolescents consistently suffer from lower adherence rates than their younger peers (see the section "Patient-Level Factors" later in this chapter; Rapoff, 2010).

On a broader public health level, adherence problems account for up to $300 billion in avoidable health care costs annually, and interventions to improve adherence may lead to lower health care costs (McGrady & Hommel, 2016). Further, there is evidence that imperfect adherence can lead to the development of viruses with increased resistance to treatments (e.g., strains of HIV that are resistant to preferred first-line prescriptions; Wahl & Nowak, 2000), which could increase public health threats. Notably, public health crises such as the COVID-19 pandemic have exacerbated health disparities, including adherence, in marginalized populations through economic hardships, barriers to telemedicine, and reduced community support (Plevinsky et al., 2020).

THEORY AND CONTEXTUAL DETERMINANTS OF ADHERENCE

Here we outline contemporary theoretical models/ frameworks that target pediatric adherence, then discuss socioecological factors that relate to adherence.

Theory and Frameworks

Contemporary models of pediatric treatment adherence and disease self-management are socioecological and include the pediatric self-management model (Modi et al., 2012) and the revised self- and family management framework (Grey et al., 2015). Consistent with ecological systems theory (Bronfenbrenner, 1979), these models describe how treatment adherence can be multiply determined by interconnected contexts at the patient (e.g., internalizing symptoms), family (e.g., caregiver involvement in the regimen), community (e.g., care coordination with schools), and health system levels (e.g., adequate patient–clinician communication; Naar-King et al., 2006). Within these models and the broader pediatric adherence literature, factors that directly influence the child in their immediate environment (e.g., parenting, family functioning) have been the most well studied (i.e., corresponding with Bronfenbrenner's microsystem factors).

Commonly applied frameworks for pediatric adherence also include health behavior change theories that were originally developed for adults (e.g., the COM-B model; McGrady et al., 2015). However, adult-based health behavior change theories are less sensitive to the socioecological contexts that are specifically relevant to youth, including microsystem factors such as the role of families and schools in adherence promotion. Moreover, many adult-based health behavior change theories do not explicitly acknowledge how cultural elements impact health behaviors such as adherence, including systemic racism and economic oppression (i.e., variables that correspond with Bronfenbrenner's macrosystem factors).

The pediatric self-management model possesses multiple strengths; it was developed for pediatric populations, focuses on socioecological determinants of self-management processes (e.g., knowledge of the regimen) that can influence adherence, is generalizable across disease groups, and shows promising predictive utility for the behaviors required to successfully follow a treatment plan (i.e., adherence behaviors; Gray, Netz et al., 2018; Psihogios et al., 2020). This model dichotomizes determinants of self-management into *modifiable* influences (i.e., those that are typically targeted in adherence-promotion interventions such as patient knowledge of the regimen, family functioning, and so on) and *nonmodifiable* influences (i.e., those factors that may be used to tailor interventions to subgroups, such as race, ethnicity, income, and so on). The label of nonmodifiable may shift the focus away from constructs that could be modifiable with structural and systemic changes (e.g., increasing the affordability of health care).

In accordance with the pediatric self-management model, empirical research typically organizes pediatric adherence barriers and facilitators into four levels: patient, family, community, and health system. Thus, in the following, we will similarly describe socioecological determinants of adherence within each of these four levels.

Socioecological Determinants of Adherence

In this section we describe patient, family, community, and health care factors that can influence pediatric treatment adherence.

Patient-level factors. A constellation of patient-level factors has been associated with adherence challenges, including

- adolescent age (e.g., Hilliard et al., 2013);
- neurocognitive status (e.g., more executive function problems, worse impulse control; e.g., Berg et al., 2014; O'Hara & Holmbeck, 2013; Silva & Miller, 2020);
- insufficient disease/treatment knowledge;
- interfering beliefs (e.g., about side effects, doubts about the necessity of treatment; e.g., McQuaid & Landier, 2018); and
- higher levels of depressed mood, worse symptom control, and lower health-related quality of life (e.g., Gray, Netz et al., 2018).

In contrast, adaptive health beliefs such as self-efficacy with the regimen (e.g., Silva & Miller, 2020; Wiebe et al., 2014) have been associated with higher adherence in pediatric populations. Common self-reported barriers to treatment adherence include factors such as forgetting, running out of medications, difficulties with pill swallowing, and taste (Hanghøj & Boisen, 2014). There is evidence that adherence barriers for youth remain stable over time (e.g., Lee et al., 2014; Ramsey et al., 2018), but, as opposed to patient-level barriers, community-level and system-level barriers (e.g., access to pharmacies) are more highly endorsed by Black families than White families (Gutierrez-Colina et al., 2022).

In some pediatric populations (e.g., cancer, asthma, Type 1 diabetes), Youth of Color have demonstrated more challenges with adherence than youth who identify as White (Bhatia et al., 2012; Kahkoska et al., 2018; Lieu et al., 2002; McQuaid et al., 2012; McQuaid & Landier, 2018; Tackett et al., 2021). Although they are often conceptualized as patient-level factors, these differences reflect macro system barriers to adherence, such as explicit (conscious) and implicit (unconscious) bias in health care systems, which can affect patient/family medical trust, communication with clinicians, and how medical resources are provided (Tackett et al., 2021). For example, prior studies have shown that Black youth with asthma were less likely to be seen by a doctor (Mitchell et al., 2016), less likely to receive a written treatment plan (Utidjian et al., 2017), and more likely to have their disease severity underestimated by their doctor (Trivedi et al., 2018). In a study of adolescents and adults with sickle cell disease, patients who reported discrimination in the health care system were less likely to take prescribed medications (Haywood et al., 2014). For youth and families who are not proficient in English, adherence disparities can also reflect lack of access to high-quality medical care in their preferred language (Yun et al., 2019).

Other sociodemographic factors that represent proxies for economic marginalization, including lower income, higher out-of-pocket medical expenses, insurance gaps, housing insecurity, no vehicle access, and longer distance from the hospital, have been associated with lower engagement with pediatric adherence demands (Atkins et al., 2020; Hensley et al., 2018; LePage et al., 2021; McQuaid & Landier, 2018). Financial toxicity, or the negative effects of a disease on one's finances, has emerged as a predictor of adherence in some populations, such as adolescents and young adults with cancer reducing doses of medications or forgoing follow-up care (Salsman et al., 2019). Black community members are at higher risk for financial toxicity because of cancer (Kahkoska et al., 2018), suggesting a likely interplay among race, economic marginalization, and adherence.

Across disease groups, adolescents with chronic health conditions tend to demonstrate more challenges with adherence than younger children (Rapoff, 2010). Aligned with developmental cascade models (Masten & Cicchetti, 2010), a transactional system in which the adolescents and their environment interact over time can influence adherence behaviors and associated health outcomes. Specifically, adolescents with chronic health conditions often gain increased responsibility for managing their medical regimen over time (while parental involvement decreases) and must balance these intensifying self-management demands with their goals, family and peer relationships, self-efficacy with the regimen, social pressures, and transition to adulthood (Palmer et al., 2009; Wiebe et al., 2014). For example, among college-attending adolescents and young adults with ADHD, undergraduates transitioning to college had lower medication adherence (34%) than posttransition undergraduates (68%; Gray, Kavookjian et al., 2018). Neurodevelopmental changes during adolescence, such as developing executive functions, can influence adherence decision making (e.g., based on immediate rather than distal consequences; Steinberg, 2007). Nonetheless, the literature on adolescent adherence has been largely deficit-focused and conceptualized through adolescent stereotypes (e.g., defiant, forgetful) rather than by partnering with adolescents and their communities to understand the complex socioecological contexts that contribute to adherence behaviors—strategies that are important for advancing adolescent-focused antiracist scholarship (Kornbluh et al., 2021).

Family-level factors. For pediatric populations, unlike adult populations, for whom adherence often applies to one primary individual (the patient), caregivers/parents and other family members (e.g., grandparents, siblings) are often intricately involved in managing pediatric adherence demands. Very young children are completely reliant on their caregivers for managing chronic disease demands (Streisand & Monaghan, 2014). In young children, adherence may be challenging for distinct reasons such as lower levels of emotional and behavioral regulation (e.g., in response to disliking the taste of medications, sitting still for injections, following dietary recommendations during mealtimes), thereby requiring considerable parental support to ensure treatment adherence (e.g., Enlow et al., 2020; Spieth et al., 2001). Still, high parental involvement has been observed even among adolescent and young adult patients who must manage complex and intensive treatments for diseases such as cancer (Doshi et al., 2014; Psihogios et al., 2021).

Parental involvement has been shown to positively influence adherence across many pediatric populations, including youth with Type 1 diabetes, sickle cell disease, and epilepsy (Landers et al., 2016; Rhee et al., 2010). Although parental supervision can be adaptive for adherence, it may not be feasible or culturally relevant for all families, and a gradual developmentally appropriate transfer of medical responsibilities from caregivers to adolescents is considered a necessary prerequisite for meeting another self-management milestone—the transfer from pediatric to adult health care settings (Cooley & Sagerman, 2011).

Parental functioning and family functioning as a whole are also important targets for adherence-promoting interventions beyond the individual experiences of the child. For example, among Black mothers of school-aged children in Baltimore, Maryland, and Washington, D.C., mothers with elevated depressive symptoms were five times more likely to report difficulties with using asthma inhalers properly compared with mothers without elevated depressive symptoms (Otsuki et al., 2010). Aspects of the family structure (e.g., married caregiver status, smaller family size) have also been associated with higher adherence (e.g., Hilliard et al., 2016). Family functioning, or the structural and relational aspects of a family environment (e.g., family conflict, cohesion, communication), demonstrated a significant and positive relationship with adherence across several pediatric populations (Psihogios et al., 2019). This finding was significant regardless of child age, adherence assessment features, or study quality, although this meta-analysis did not report or examine other demographic variables beyond child age.

Community-level factors. Compared to patient- and family-level factors, far less research has examined the role of community-level factors such as peers, schools, churches, and neighborhoods, in pediatric adherence. This gap reflects an overarching focus on individual behavior change that neglects the strengths of communities that can be harnessed for adherence as well as the structural change that is needed to ensure equitable access to health (Breland & Stanton, 2022). In the available research, social support for both youth and their family members has been positively associated with adherence (e.g., Janicke et al., 2009). Access to lay community health workers (i.e., trained community members who provide individualized assistance with navigating the health system) and coordination with school nurses may also lead to improvements in pediatric disease management (Raphael et al., 2013; Trivedi et al., 2018).

Health care–level factors. Although relationships between aspects of the health system and adherence are also understudied, communication patterns among patients, caregivers, and pediatric clinicians are particularly salient for pediatric adherence (e.g., establishing a "triadic partnership"; De Civita & Dobkin, 2004). In one meta-analysis, there was a 19% increased risk of adherence challenges among patients whose clinicians communicated poorly compared with patients whose clinicians communicated well (e.g., established rapport, facilitated patient involvement in decision making; Haskard Zolnierek & Dimatteo, 2009). Importantly, this relationship was stronger among pediatricians than among adult clinicians. This relationship has also been observed in community primary care settings. Among youth with ADHD treated in communities, a weaker perceived clinician-family alliance predicted not filling ADHD prescriptions (Kamimura-Nishimura et al., 2019). Clinician communication is particularly salient for marginalized youth given that implicit bias—such as the tendency to prescribe diabetes technologies that improve glycemic outcomes based on insurance type (Addala et al., 2021)— impacts care delivery and quality (Mack et al., 2021; Valenzuela & Smith, 2016).

ASSESSMENT OF TREATMENT ADHERENCE

Previous reviews of adherence assessment omit considerations of language, culture, racism, or other social determinants of health (Al-Hassany et al., 2019; Lehmann & Pietenpol, 2014). Indeed, there are few validated adherence measures in languages other than English (Hsin et al., 2010) or culturally tailored adherence assessments (Plevinsky et al., 2020). From a developmental perspective, adherence assessment must capture a dynamic process, with varying levels of caregiver and child involvement contingent on a range of developmental (e.g., child age, cognitive functioning), family (e.g., caregiver mental health, family stress and resources), and medical factors (e.g., regimen complexity, side effects, shared decision making). Therefore, measures may assess predominantly caregiver behaviors (e.g., in the case of children who are young and/or have developmental delays), child and adolescent behaviors, or some combination of the two that reflects shared responsibilities (Holbein et al., 2019). Adherence assessment is most accurate when a combination of assessment modalities is utilized. It is well established that there is not necessarily a gold standard assessment measure for most treatment regimens and that all methods have specific strengths and weaknesses that must be weighed depending on cultural sensitivity, feasibility, precision, health population, and intended use. As mentioned earlier, patient-focused measures (rather than measures of system-level problems) of adherence can be biased due to the burden placed on the patient.

In the following subsections, we present categories of adherence assessment methods along with racism and diversity considerations and broad strengths and weaknesses.

Subjective Assessment Measures
Subjective assessment measures require the patient or caregiver to provide an estimate of

treatment adherence through an unstructured or structured interview or questionnaire. These methods offer ease of administration, low cost, and standardized formats (Lehmann et al., 2014). Subjective measures may focus on a very specific treatment component (e.g., medication, diet) or multiple treatment regimen tasks. Advances in electronic medical record systems have created opportunities to collect patient-generated data as part of clinical care (Gerhardt et al., 2018).

There are multiple validated self- or caregiver-report adherence questionnaires, including the Medication Adherence Self-report Inventory (Walsh et al., 2002), Medication Adherence Rating Scale (Thompson et al., 2000), and Brief Adherence Rating Scale (Byerly et al., 2008) that are broad in scope and apply to a wide array of pediatric populations required to take medications. Similarly, semi-structured interviews, such as the Medical Adherence Measure (Zelikovsky & Schast, 2008), have been developed to generalize across chronic health conditions that may require medications, therapeutic diets, and consistent clinic visit attendance. Alternatively, condition-specific questionnaires provide comprehensive information about unique treatment regimens and adherence behaviors (Plevinsky et al., 2020); however, they are not available for all pediatric health conditions. For a comprehensive review of validated broad and condition-specific pediatric treatment adherence measures, refer to the recent systematic review by Plevinsky et al. (2020).

Although subjective assessment methods may offer valuable information, they are prone to multiple limitations. General limitations of subjective measures include the potential for inaccuracies associated with retrospective recall and social desirability biases (Lehmann et al., 2014), discrepancies across multiple reporters (Duncan, Mentrikoski, et al., 2014), the requirement of a fairly high degree of health literacy (Basu et al., 2019), and extensive time and resources required for completion that may not be feasible in busy clinic settings (Duncan, Mentrikoski et al., 2014; Ramsey & Holbein, 2020). Clinicians tend to base perceptions of patient or family adherence on observable factors (e.g., race, ethnicity; Lutfey & Ketcham, 2005), and it is well established that clinician perceptions of treatment adherence are biased (Basu et al., 2019; Hall et al., 2015; van Ryn & Burke, 2000). Further, most validated assessment measures have been developed using predominantly White samples to establish normative statistics and psychometric data (Plevinsky et al., 2020). Finally, although standardized assessment measures or questions may help to ensure that treatment adherence is assessed equally across children and families, this does not necessarily ensure an *equitable* assessment.

Traditional Objective Measures

Multiple adherence assessment modalities offer a more objective approach that is less prone to reporting biases and less reliant on idiosyncratic questions, although these measures generally do not allow for identification of day-to-day adherence patterns. Many objective measures assess adherence to medications, thereby limiting opportunities to assess other adherence behaviors, such as diet and physical activity.

Bioassays obtained by bloodwork, urinalysis, and other biospecimen collection (e.g., HIV antiviral loads, hemoglobin A1c) may be part of routine clinical care and can offer insight into medication or dietary adherence based on established values. However, bioassays are influenced by many factors other than adherence, including puberty, pharmacokinetics, and individual differences in drug metabolism (Duncan, Pozehl et al., 2014; Hommel et al., 2017), and they may not be sensitive to infrequent missed doses or occasional deviations from a prescribed diet (Hommel et al., 2008; Lehmann et al., 2014). Inaccuracies may occur if the patient demonstrates stronger adherence shortly before a scheduled clinic visit ("white coat adherence"; Driscoll et al., 2017); this may also complicate validity because many medications for which bioassays are available have short half-lives, thereby limiting efforts to understand long-term adherence outcomes.

Pill counts measure adherence by comparing the number of pills remaining to the expected amount based on prescription dosage and time elapsed (Ramsey & Holbein, 2020). This method assumes that medication has been ingested and does not account for the possibility that medication has been discarded or stored elsewhere. Patients must also have access to pill bottles at the time of assessment. Although this is commonly a barrier in clinic settings, video-based telemedicine may offer opportunities to assess pill counts when children are at home. However, this requires the patient to have reliable internet access, which continues to be a barrier for many youth and families from marginalized groups (Dolcini et al., 2021; McClain et al., 2021).

Adherence may also be measured by analysis of prescription refills through pharmacy records or electronic medical records. Missed doses are captured by prescription refills that are filled later than expected (based on dose and time elapsed) or are not filled at all (Ramsey & Holbein, 2020). Yet prescriptions filled on time, especially in the context of automatic refill programs, do not imply accuracy of medication administration (Duncan, Mentrikoski et al., 2014; Hommel et al., 2017). Many patients may use multiple pharmacies or experience adjustments to their regimens, resulting in inaccurate estimates (Al-Hassany et al., 2019; Hommel et al., 2017).

Technology-Supported Objective Measures

Rapid advances in health care technology have spurred the development of innovative sophisticated assessment methods that harness continuous "real-time" monitoring processes, capture day-to-day assessment data, and identify adherence patterns (Duncan, Mentrikoski et al., 2014; Lehmann et al., 2014; Mulvaney et al., 2013). Although patient monitoring capabilities and prompts may serve as de facto adherence promotion interventions, this effect has not been consistently found (Heron et al., 2017; Mulvaney et al., 2012). Specific to medication, electronic monitors, such as pill containers (e.g., medication event monitoring system [MEMS] TrackCaps) or electronic inhaler caps, have a high degree of accuracy (McGrady et al., 2018). Data imply that a dose was taken at the recorded date and time the monitor was accessed, although they cannot verify that medication has been administered and do not account for deviations when the device is not in use (e.g., when traveling). Further, electronic monitors may not suit all medication dosages or formulations, and they are typically too expensive to integrate into routine clinical practice. There are also multiple electronic methods for assessing adherence behaviors beyond medication, including positive airway pressure devices (Watach et al., 2020), blood glucose meters and insulin pumps (Westen et al., 2019), and Bluetooth-enabled vest therapy (Benoit et al., 2020). As with any technological monitoring system, these adherence measures have unique strengths and limitations depending on their technology platform and the treatment components they assess.

Ecological momentary assessment (EMA) methods offer in-the-moment adherence information in the context of dynamic relationships among behaviors, emotions, physical sensations, and settings (Wen et al., 2017). Patients or caregivers receive prompts via mobile devices to report on their current thoughts, emotions, activities, physical sensations, and adherence behaviors within a limited recall window (Plevinsky et al., 2020). Sensors (e.g., accelerometers, pedometers, smart watches, continuous glucose monitors) that continuously collect adherence outcomes may be used to complement EMA data or provide independent adherence measurement. Despite the rich comprehensive data collected through EMA, mobile devices and wearable technology are expensive. Researchers and clinicians who rely on children and families to provide their own personal devices may exclude economically marginalized youth (McGrady et al., 2018; Patel et al., 2015). Other challenges include deteriorating engagement with surveys, missing data, and difficulties wearing or accessing a device in the context of school or extracurricular activities (Heron et al., 2017; Mulvaney et al., 2013; Patel et al., 2015).

Ingestible sensor systems directly capture medication ingestion by tracking dietary minerals (e.g., copper, magnesium, silicon) or radio frequency identification tags that have been encapsulated within an individual's pill and captured with a wearable sensor patch with wireless data transfer capabilities (Chai et al., 2015; Triplett et al., 2019). Systems may also assess other biometric data (e.g., heart rate, physical activity) and connect to mobile applications. As this technology is new, pill-based sensors have not been widely used or validated with pediatric populations, and the medications eligible for digital encapsulation are still limited (Triplett et al., 2019). However, a study of an ingestible sensor system in youth with solid organ transplant noted difficulties tolerating the sensor patch.

Although technology allows for innovative ways to ameliorate limitations of subjective and traditional objective assessment measures, these methods do not eliminate inequities. Disparities in reliable internet access and connectability, smartphone access, and cellular data connectivity continue to exist, particularly for racially marginalized and low-income youth and families (Dolcini et al., 2021; McClain et al., 2021). Although it is encouraging that some insurance plans have piloted programs to cover or subsidize electronic pill monitors or wearables, there have been no published efforts to expand access to pediatric populations with publicly funded insurance. Beyond technology access, Black and Hispanic adults have reported less confidence than White adults in using their electronic devices independently (McClain et al., 2021). Other broad limitations include technological difficulties (Heron et al., 2017; McGrady et al., 2018) and user concerns about privacy and confidentiality (Triplett et al., 2019).

ADHERENCE INTERVENTIONS

Interventions for promoting adherence are increasingly multicomponent and involve a combination of self-management intervention targets, such as modifying adherence behaviors (e.g., with reminders, feedback, organization strategies, incentives), modifying adherence-related cognitions (e.g., problem solving, coping), or a combination of cognitive behavioral approaches (Pai & McGrady, 2014). In one meta-analysis, medium effect sizes were found for behavioral (mean $d = .54$) and multicomponent adherence-promotion interventions (mean $d = .51$), compared with small effects for education interventions alone (mean $d = .16$; Kahana et al., 2008). However, upon more recent examination, the meta-analytic effect of multicomponent adherence interventions attenuated (mean $d = .20$; Pai & McGrady, 2014), suggesting continual difficulty in identifying the most salient intervention components associated with adherence. Most adherence-promoting interventions target youth and/or their caregivers and have not attempted to intervene upon community or health system factors (Shih & Cohen, 2020).

Patient-Level Interventions

Several interventions have been developed for children and adolescents with chronic health conditions that target their own disease/treatment knowledge, adherence self-monitoring, and self-efficacy (Shih & Cohen, 2020). As an example, one intervention employed the Intensive Training Program (ITP), a mobile health approach that provided educational videos, remote daily monitoring of adherence, and weekly staff feedback to children and adolescents (ages 7 to 18) with sickle cell disease (Anderson et al., 2018). The intervention demonstrated moderate effects, with all participants increasing their medication adherence as measured by pharmacy refill data ($d = .75$). Still, fewer interventions have targeted youth alone than both youth and their families (Pai & McGrady, 2014).

Family-Level Interventions

Interventions that target the family system—typically youth with their caregivers—may be an effective way to improve adherence. For example, behavioral family systems therapy, involving problem solving, communication skills, cognitive modification, and functional-structural family therapy, resulted in improved diabetes adherence (Wysocki et al., 2007). In another study, a family-based teamwork intervention involving parent–youth collaboration and systemic fading of parent supervision with medications improved asthma adherence (Duncan et al., 2013). Bhatia et al. (2020) found that adherence education, daily text message medication reminders to youth, and daily text message prompts to caregivers to supervise medication administration improved adherence among adolescents with leukemia but not in younger children, highlighting the importance of developmental tailoring of interventions.

Limitations of Prior Interventions

There are several criticisms of the existing adherence-promotion intervention literature that may also help to explain the modest effects of prior interventions. First, many interventions have targeted convenience samples of youth who are already engaged in subspecialty care (rather than community samples) and not specifically targeted youth with adherence challenges (Pai & McGrady, 2014). Second, the majority of prior interventions have required additional in-person medical visits, which results in feasibility challenges for families who are already struggling to adhere to existing treatment demands. Third, slightly more than half of existing adherence-promotion interventions have been atheoretical and failed to target multilevel social factors that drive health (McGrady et al., 2015). Fourth, interventions have been developed using top-down strategies based on what clinical researchers expect youth and their families need for adherence, rather than using participatory approaches to co-design interventions with members of the community (Stiles-Shields et al., 2022). Finally, interventions have been one-size-fits-all, rather than providing more personalized support in terms of when, where, and how adherence care is delivered (Harris, 2018).

In the following subsections we will discuss two promising approaches for mitigating these gaps that involve structural changes in where and how adherence care is delivered: multisystemic interventions and digital health approaches.

Multisystemic Interventions

Multisystem interventions are multicomponent, multilevel, and systemic. They target youth and other important individuals who are involved in the youth's medical care, in salient settings such as home, school, and the medical clinic.

Multisystemic therapy. Multisystemic therapy is an intensive home- and community-based treatment adapted for youth with Type 1 diabetes with poor glycemic control. Interventions target the child with diabetes, as well as their family and community (e.g., peers, school, medical team) as needed. Intervention components include home visits, regular phone communication, structural and strategic family therapy interventions, and tailored cognitive behavior therapy based on each family's needs. When compared with a no treatment control group, multisystemic therapy improved the frequency of blood glucose testing and decreased hospital admission rates (Ellis et al., 2005, 2007). These effects were robust, as youth who received multisystemic therapy continued to have fewer hospitalizations for up to 24 months (Ellis et al., 2008).

Novel interventions in children's health care. Another multisystemic approach for promoting adherence among youth with complex health conditions, including youth with Type 1 diabetes who have repeated diabetes ketoacidosis, is Novel Interventions in Children's Healthcare (NICH; Harris et al., 2015). Intervention components include family-based problem solving, skill building, case management, and care coordination. Interventions occur in the youth's natural environment (e.g., home, school, clinic, elsewhere in the community), with interventionists available to families 24 hours per day, 7 days per week (facilitated by telehealth). Although NICH has not yet been tested in a randomized controlled trial, it has been associated with reductions in emergency room visits, improvements in glycemic control, and reductions in yearly health costs among a subgroup of patients who are vulnerable to repeated diabetes ketoacidosis (Harris et al., 2016; Wagner et al., 2017).

Digital Health Interventions

Digital health approaches have proliferated and offer the potential for personalized adherence support in youth's natural environments through technologies that are virtually ubiquitous in society (text messaging, web tools, and mobile applications). Text messaging and mobile application interventions have shown promising feasibility and accessibility among adolescents—a prime population of native smartphone users—with modest efficacy data (Badawy et al., 2017). Similar to traditional face-to-face interventions, digital interventions that incorporate behavioral approaches demonstrated larger effect sizes than those that contained education only (Cushing & Steele, 2010).

Although not yet widely adopted for pediatric digital health, some interventions have begun to adopt human-centered principles to co-design adherence-promotion interventions with (not for) youth (Stiles-Shields et al., 2022). These design approaches may have implications for addressing structural racism and promoting equitable design, as they are participatory and aim to match the technology to the contexts of everyday life (Rubin & Chisnell, 2008). For example, a self-management mobile app called iManage was co-designed with adolescents and young adults with sickle cell disease through surveys about current technology use, interviews about self-management strategies, and cocreation sessions to generate and prioritize design ideas (Crosby et al., 2017). Engagement with the app was positively associated with improvements in self-management skills (Hood et al., 2021), although maintaining engagement was a challenge in this study and a common challenge across digital interventions.

Despite the promise of digital health, these strategies may have unintended consequences that reinforce health inequities. Although smartphone ownership is almost universal in the United States, reliable internet access, sufficient data plans, and adequate digital health literacy are not. Thus, digital health strategies for adherence stand at a critical crossroads for promoting equity, requiring systematic strategies to ensure that health inequities are not replicated onto digital health interventions (Crawford & Serhal, 2020).

IMPLICATIONS FOR PEDIATRICS AND DEVELOPMENTAL SCIENCE

Clinicians, including pediatricians in primary care and developmental-behavioral pediatricians, play an integral role in assessing and promoting adherence. Although the empirical literature has focused on youth with chronic conditions treated in subspecialty clinics, prevalent childhood conditions (e.g., asthma, ADHD) are frequently treated in primary care. As highlighted throughout this chapter, these youth are also at risk for suboptimal adherence, with less access to pediatric psychology services that can help foster adherence in community settings. Moreover, in developmental-behavioral pediatrics clinics, youth and their families may also adhere to a variety of therapies (physical, occupational, and speech and language therapies).

Clinicians who support youth and their families with adherence, regardless of the pediatric care setting, diagnosis, and treatment regimen, may benefit from the following short list of empirically supported core responsibilities in which they play a considerable role:

- joining youth and their families to set and select health goals;
- collecting, processing, and evaluating adherence information (e.g., assessing adherence and adherence barriers routinely);
- engaging in shared treatment decision making with youth and their families;
- supporting youth and families in implementing adherence-related actions such as encouraging open nonjudgmental communication about adherence patterns within families and during clinical visits; and
- monitoring and supporting emotional reactions to the illness and treatment demands (e.g., to prompt discussions of less burdensome treatment options and referrals to mental health support; Drotar, 2013).

When possible, pediatricians and developmental-behavioral pediatricians may also benefit from engaging with social workers, who may play a key role in identifying adherence barriers (e.g., insurance lapses, transportation difficulties, challenges coordinating with school staff) and identifying potential solutions.

Pediatric adherence must be conceptualized within a developmental framework as youth manage long-term conditions that span their childhood, adolescence, and emerging adulthood. As described earlier, many youth gain increasing responsibility for their adherence demands over time while also navigating other developmental factors. As they approach young adulthood, youth must ultimately transfer from family-focused pediatric health care settings to individual-focused adult health settings. At times, caregivers or family members assume that adolescents are responsible for adherence tasks (e.g., taking a daily medication) when in reality the youth still need some level of support (much like the stepwise skill building in driving a car). Still, there are relatively few longitudinal studies of pediatric adherence patterns and predictors over time, including focused study on contextual transactional processes (e.g., how child–parent interactions change over time and influence adherence behaviors). Developmental scientists can substantially contribute to the knowledge base of pediatric treatment adherence through integrative research that harnesses their expertise in development across the lifespan and socioecological factors and processes that influence adherence over time and across contexts. By increasing understanding about the complex dynamic nature of pediatric adherence, more effective tailored interventions can be developed; in fact, such work is critical for improving adherence outcomes for marginalized youth and families at risk for adherence challenges.

CONCLUSION AND FUTURE DIRECTIONS

Pediatric treatment adherence is a complex, dynamic, interdisciplinary, and multilevel behavioral health challenge. Adherence has significant individual and public health implications, including influences on patient morbidity, patient mortality, and health care spending. Socioecological contexts impact pediatric treatment adherence, including individual, family, community, and health system factors, as well as cultural factors such as racism that permeate each of these levels. Moving forward, the field will benefit from an increased focus on research-to-practice translation, such as how evidence-based adherence assessment practices can be successfully implemented on a larger scale in real-world clinic settings (i.e., barriers, facilitators, and implementation strategies). This translation must attend to the systemic challenges that have prevented equitable adherence care and move toward correcting them rather than accepting them or providing temporary solutions that fail to lessen adherence barriers among marginalized youth and their families. Interventions that are multilevel (i.e., those that intervene at the patient, family, community, and/or health system level) and culturally tailored are also needed. One-size-fits-all interventions are likely insufficient for addressing the dynamic contexts that influence pediatric adherence or for advancing health equity. Partnering with and empowering youth, families, and communities to co-design and implement adherence practices is a promising approach for mitigating inequities associated with differential treatment adherence. Finally, advocating for policies that improve equity in pediatric health care access and affordability represents fundamental work to address barriers within the health care system that contribute to suboptimal adherence. Addressing the socioecological factors associated with poor treatment adherence is necessary to promote equitable health and well-being for children and adolescents with chronic health conditions and their families.

RESOURCES

- Cincinnati Children's Medication Adherence Promotion (MAP) Resource:

    https://www.cincinnatichildrens.org/research/divisions/c/adherence/map

- A video by the Alberta Children's Hospital Foundation to aid children in swallowing pills, featuring Bonnie Kaplan:

  https://www.youtube.com/watch?v=MXFMZuNs-Fk

- Marsac, M., & Hogan, M. (2021). *Afraid of the doctor: Every parent's guide to preventing and managing medical trauma*. Rowman and Littlefield. https://www.afraidofthedoctor.com

- Bennett, H. J. (2006). *Lions aren't scared of shots: A story for children about visiting the doctor*. https://www.apa.org/pubs/magination/441A473

- *Supporting Adolescents and Young Adults With Medication Adherence During Cancer Treatment* by Alexandra Psihogios:

  https://www.chop.edu/news/supporting-adolescents-and-young-adults-medication-adherence-during-cancer-treatment

- *Choosing the Right Medication Adherence & Self-Management App: A Guide for Pediatric Psychologists* (created by the Society of Pediatric Psychology Adherence & Self-Management and Digital Health Special Interest Groups):

  https://div54adherencesig.weebly.com/uploads/1/1/0/6/110635105/division_54_a_sm_sig_app_handout.pdf

- *Transitioning Treatment Responsibilities From Caregivers to Adolescents and Young Adults* (created by the Society of Pediatric Psychology Adherence Special Interest Group):

  https://div54adherencesig.weebly.com/uploads/1/1/0/6/110635105/transition_tips_7.19.19.pdf

- Meg Foundation (for procedural-related anxiety adherence challenges):

  https://www.megfoundationforpain.org

References

Addala, A., Hanes, S., Naranjo, D., Maahs, D. M., & Hood, K. K. (2021). Provider implicit bias impacts pediatric Type 1 diabetes technology in the United States: Findings from the Gatekeeper Study. *Journal of Diabetes Science and Technology, 15*(5), 1027–1033. https://doi.org/10.1177/19322968211006476

Al-Hassany, L., Kloosterboer, S. M., Dierckx, B., & Koch, B. C. (2019). Assessing methods of measuring medication adherence in chronically ill children—A narrative review. *Patient Preference and Adherence, 13*, 1175–1189. https://doi.org/10.2147/PPA.S200058

Anderson, L. M., Leonard, S., Jonassaint, J., Lunyera, J., Bonner, M., & Shah, N. (2018). Mobile health intervention for youth with sickle cell disease: Impact on adherence, disease knowledge, and quality of life. *Pediatric Blood & Cancer, 65*(8), e27081. https://doi.org/10.1002/pbc.27081

Atkins, M., Castro, I., Sharifi, M., Perkins, M., O'Connor, G., Sandel, M., Taveras, E. M., & Fiechtner, L. (2020). Unmet social needs and adherence to pediatric weight management interventions: Massachusetts, 2017–2019. *American Journal of Public Health, 110*(S2), S251–S257. https://doi.org/10.2105/AJPH.2020.305772

Badawy, S. M., Barrera, L., Sinno, M. G., Kaviany, S., O'Dwyer, L. C., & Kuhns, L. M. (2017). Text messaging and mobile phone apps as interventions to improve adherence in adolescents with chronic health conditions: A systematic review. *JMIR mHealth and uHealth, 5*(5), e66. https://doi.org/10.2196/mhealth.7798

Basu, S., Berkowitz, S. A., Phillips, R. L., Bitton, A., Landon, B. E., & Phillips, R. S. (2019). Association of primary care physician supply with population mortality in the United States, 2005–2015. *JAMA Internal Medicine, 179*(4), 506–514. https://doi.org/10.1001/jamainternmed.2018.7624

Benoit, C. M., Christensen, E., Nickel, A. J., Shogren, S., Johnson, M., Thompson, E. F., & McNamara, J. (2020). Objective measures of vest therapy adherence among pediatric subjects with cystic fibrosis. *Respiratory Care, 65*(12), 1831–1837. https://doi.org/10.4187/respcare.07421

Berg, C. A., Wiebe, D. J., Suchy, Y., Hughes, A. E., Anderson, J. H., Godbey, E. I., Butner, J., Tucker, C., Franchow, E. I., Pihlaskari, A. K., King, P. S., Murray, M. A., & White, P. C. (2014). Individual differences and day-to-day fluctuations in perceived self-regulation associated with daily adherence in late adolescents with Type 1 diabetes. *Journal of Pediatric Psychology, 39*(9), 1038–1048. https://doi.org/10.1093/jpepsy/jsu051

Bhatia, S., Hageman, L., Chen, Y., Wong, F. L., McQuaid, E. L., Duncan, C., Mascarenhas, L., Freyer, D., Mba, N., Aristizabal, P., Walterhouse, D., Lew, G., Kempert, P. H., Russell, T. B., McNall-Knapp, R. Y., Jacobs, S., Dang, H., Raetz, E., Relling, M. V., &

Landier, W. (2020). Effect of a daily text messaging and directly supervised therapy intervention on oral mercaptopurine adherence in children with acute lymphoblastic leukemia: A randomized clinical trial. *JAMA Network Open, 3*(8), e2014205. https://doi.org/10.1001/jamanetworkopen.2020.14205

Bhatia, S., Landier, W., Hageman, L., Kim, H., Chen, Y., Crews, K. R., Evans, W. E., Bostrom, B., Casillas, J., Dickens, D. S., Maloney, K. W., Neglia, J. P., Ravindranath, Y., Ritchey, A. K., Wong, F. L., & Relling, M. V. (2014). 6MP adherence in a multi-racial cohort of children with acute lymphoblastic leukemia: A Children's Oncology Group study. *Blood, 124*(15), 2345–2353. https://doi.org/10.1182/blood-2014-01-552166

Bhatia, S., Landier, W., Shangguan, M., Hageman, L., Schaible, A. N., Carter, A. R., Hanby, C. L., Leisenring, W., Yasui, Y., Kornegay, N. M., Mascarenhas, L., Ritchey, A. K., Casillas, J. N., Dickens, D. S., Meza, J., Carroll, W. L., Relling, M. V., & Wong, F. L. (2012). Nonadherence to oral mercaptopurine and risk of relapse in Hispanic and non-Hispanic White children with acute lymphoblastic leukemia: A report from the Children's Oncology Group. *Journal of Clinical Oncology, 30*(17), 2094–2101. https://doi.org/10.1200/JCO.2011.38.9924

Bogart, L. M., Takada, S., & Cunningham, W. E. (2021). Medical mistrust, discrimination, and the domestic HIV epidemic. In B. O. Ojikutu & V. E. Stone (Eds.), *HIV in US communities of color* (pp. 207–231). Springer. https://doi.org/10.1007/978-3-030-48744-7_12

Breland, J. Y., & Stanton, M. V. (2022). Anti-Black racism and behavioral medicine: Confronting the past to envision the future. *Translational Behavioral Medicine, 12*(1), ibab090. https://doi.org/10.1093/tbm/ibab090

Bronfenbrenner, U. (1979). *The ecology of human development: Experiments by nature and design*. Harvard University Press.

Byerly, M. J., Nakonezny, P. A., & Rush, A. J. (2008). The Brief Adherence Rating Scale (BARS) validated against electronic monitoring in assessing the antipsychotic medication adherence of outpatients with schizophrenia and schizoaffective disorder. *Schizophrenia Research, 100*(1–3), 60–69. https://doi.org/10.1016/j.schres.2007.12.470

Carmody, J. K., Plevinsky, J., Peugh, J. L., Denson, L. A., Hyams, J. S., Lobato, D., LeLeiko, N. S., & Hommel, K. A. (2019). Longitudinal non-adherence predicts treatment escalation in paediatric ulcerative colitis. *Alimentary Pharmacology & Therapeutics, 50*(8), 911–918. https://doi.org/10.1111/apt.15445

Chai, P. R., Castillo-Mancilla, J., Buffkin, E., Darling, C., Rosen, R. K., Horvath, K. J., Boudreaux, E. D., Robbins, G. K., Hibberd, P. L., & Boyer, E. W. (2015). Utilizing an ingestible biosensor to assess real-time medication adherence. *Journal of Medical Toxicology, 11*(4), 439–444. https://doi.org/10.1007/s13181-015-0494-8

Chakraborty, A., King, M., Leavey, G., & McKenzie, K. (2011). Perceived racism, medication adherence, and hospital admission in African-Caribbean patients with psychosis in the United Kingdom. *Social Psychiatry and Psychiatric Epidemiology, 46*(9), 915–923. https://doi.org/10.1007/s00127-010-0261-8

Cooley, W. C., Sagerman, P. J., American Academy of Pediatrics, American Academy of Family Physicians, & American College of Physicians, Transitions Clinical Report Authoring Group. (2011). Supporting the health care transition from adolescence to adulthood in the medical home. *Pediatrics, 128*(1), 182–200. https://doi.org/10.1542/peds.2011-0969

Crawford, A., & Serhal, E. (2020). Digital health equity and COVID-19: The innovation curve cannot reinforce the gradient of health. *Journal of Medical Internet Research, 22*(6), e19361. https://doi.org/10.2196/19361

Crosby, L. E., Ware, R. E., Goldstein, A., Walton, A., Joffe, N. E., Vogel, C., & Britto, M. T. (2017). Development and evaluation of iManage: A self-management app co-designed by adolescents with sickle cell disease. *Pediatric Blood & Cancer, 64*(1), 139–145. https://doi.org/10.1002/pbc.26177

Cushing, C. C., & Steele, R. G. (2010). A meta-analytic review of eHealth interventions for pediatric health promoting and maintaining behaviors. *Journal of Pediatric Psychology, 35*(9), 937–949. https://doi.org/10.1093/jpepsy/jsq023

De Civita, M., & Dobkin, P. L. (2004). Pediatric adherence as a multidimensional and dynamic construct, involving a triadic partnership. *Journal of Pediatric Psychology, 29*(3), 157–169. https://doi.org/10.1093/jpepsy/jsh018

Dolcini, M. M., Canchola, J. A., Catania, J. A., Song Mayeda, M. M., Dietz, E. L., Cotto-Negrón, C., & Narayanan, V. (2021). National-level disparities in internet access among low-income and Black and Hispanic youth. *Journal of Medical Internet Research, 23*(10), e27723. https://doi.org/10.2196/27723

Doshi, K., Kazak, A. E., Hocking, M. C., DeRosa, B. W., Schwartz, L. A., Hobbie, W. L., Ginsberg, J. P., & Deatrick, J. (2014). Why mothers accompany adolescent and young adult childhood cancer survivors to follow-up clinic visits. *Journal of*

Pediatric Oncology Nursing, 31(1), 51–57. https://doi.org/10.1177/1043454213518111

Driscoll, K. A., Wang, Y., Johnson, S. B., Gill, E., Wright, N., & Deeb, L. C. (2017). White coat adherence occurs in adolescents with Type 1 diabetes receiving intervention to improve insulin pump adherence behaviors. *Journal of Diabetes Science and Technology*, 11(3), 455–460. https://doi.org/10.1177/1932296816672691

Drotar, D. (2013). Strategies of adherence promotion in the management of pediatric chronic conditions. *Journal of Developmental and Behavioral Pediatrics*, 34(9), 716–729. https://doi.org/10.1097/DBP.0b013e31829f6781

Duncan, C. L., Hogan, M. B., Tien, K. J., Graves, M. M., Chorney, J. M., Zettler, M. D., Koven, L., Wilson, N. W., Dinakar, C., & Portnoy, J. (2013). Efficacy of a parent–youth teamwork intervention to promote adherence in pediatric asthma. *Journal of Pediatric Psychology*, 38(6), 617–628. https://doi.org/10.1093/jpepsy/jss123

Duncan, C. L., Mentrikoski, J. M., Wu, Y. P., & Fredericks, E. M. (2014). Practice-based approach to assessing and treating non-adherence in pediatric regimens. *Clinical Practice in Pediatric Psychology*, 2(3), 322–336. https://doi.org/10.1037/cpp0000066

Duncan, K., Pozehl, B., Hertzog, M., & Norman, J. F. (2014). Psychological responses and adherence to exercise in heart failure. *Rehabilitation Nursing*, 39(3), 130–139. https://doi.org/10.1002/rnj.106

Ellis, D. A., Frey, M. A., Naar-King, S., Templin, T., Cunningham, P., & Cakan, N. (2005). Use of multisystemic therapy to improve regimen adherence among adolescents with Type 1 diabetes in chronic poor metabolic control: A randomized controlled trial. *Diabetes Care*, 28(7), 1604–1610. https://doi.org/10.2337/diacare.28.7.1604

Ellis, D. A., Naar-King, S., Templin, T., Frey, M., Cunningham, P., Sheidow, A., Cakan, N., & Idalski, A. (2008). Multisystemic therapy for adolescents with poorly controlled Type 1 diabetes: Reduced diabetic ketoacidosis admissions and related costs over 24 months. *Diabetes Care*, 31(9), 1746–1747. https://doi.org/10.2337/dc07-2094

Ellis, D. A., Templin, T., Naar-King, S., Frey, M. A., Cunningham, P. B., Podolski, C. L., & Cakan, N. (2007). Multisystemic therapy for adolescents with poorly controlled Type I diabetes: Stability of treatment effects in a randomized controlled trial. *Journal of Consulting and Clinical Psychology*, 75(1), 168–174. https://doi.org/10.1037/0022-006X.75.1.168

Enlow, P. T., Wasserman, R., Aroian, K., Lee, J., Wysocki, T., & Pierce, J. (2020). Development and validation of the Parent-Preschoolers Diabetes Adjustment Scale (PP-DAS). *Journal of Pediatric Psychology*, 45(2), 170–180. https://doi.org/10.1093/jpepsy/jsz093

Forsyth, J., Schoenthaler, A., Chaplin, W. F., Ogedegbe, G., & Ravenell, J. (2014). Perceived discrimination and medication adherence in Black hypertensive patients: The role of stress and depression. *Psychosomatic Medicine*, 76(3), 229–236. https://doi.org/10.1097/PSY.0000000000000043

Gaston, G. B., & Alleyne-Green, B. (2013). The impact of African Americans' beliefs about HIV medical care on treatment adherence: A systematic review and recommendations for interventions. *AIDS and Behavior*, 17(1), 31–40. https://doi.org/10.1007/s10461-012-0323-x

Gerber, B. S., Cho, Y. I., Arozullah, A. M., & Lee, S. Y. (2010). Racial differences in medication adherence: A cross-sectional study of Medicare enrollees. *American Journal of Geriatric Pharmacotherapy*, 8(2), 136–145. https://doi.org/10.1016/j.amjopharm.2010.03.002

Gerhardt, W. E., Mara, C. A., Kudel, I., Morgan, E. M., Schoettker, P. J., Napora, J., Britto, M. T., & Alessandrini, E. A. (2018). Systemwide implementation of patient-reported outcomes in routine clinical care at a children's hospital. *Joint Commission Journal on Quality and Patient Safety*, 44(8), 441–453. https://doi.org/10.1016/j.jcjq.2018.01.002

Gray, W. N., Kavookjian, J., Shapiro, S. K., Wagoner, S. T., Schaefer, M. R., Resmini Rawlinson, A., & Hinnant, J. B. (2018). Transition to college and adherence to prescribed attention deficit hyperactivity disorder medication. *Journal of Developmental and Behavioral Pediatrics*, 39(1), 1–9. https://doi.org/10.1097/DBP.0000000000000511

Gray, W. N., Netz, M., McConville, A., Fedele, D., Wagoner, S. T., & Schaefer, M. R. (2018). Medication adherence in pediatric asthma: A systematic review of the literature. *Pediatric Pulmonology*, 53(5), 668–684. https://doi.org/10.1002/ppul.23966

Grey, M., Schulman-Green, D., Knafl, K., & Reynolds, N. R. (2015). A revised self- and family management framework. *Nursing Outlook*, 63(2), 162–170. https://doi.org/10.1016/j.outlook.2014.10.003

Gutierrez-Colina, A. M., Wetter, S. E., Mara, C. A., Guilfoyle, S., & Modi, A. C. (2022). Racial disparities in medication adherence barriers: Pediatric epilepsy as an exemplar. *Journal of Pediatric Psychology*, 47(6), 620–630. https://doi.org/10.1093/jpepsy/jsac001

Hall, W. J., Chapman, M. V., Lee, K. M., Merino, Y. M., Thomas, T. W., Payne, B. K., Eng, E., Day, S. H., &

Coyne-Beasley, T. (2015). Implicit racial/ethnic bias among health care professionals and its influence on health care outcomes: A systematic review. *American Journal of Public Health, 105*(12), e60–e76. https://doi.org/10.2105/AJPH.2015.302903

Hanghøj, S., & Boisen, K. A. (2014). Self-reported barriers to medication adherence among chronically ill adolescents: A systematic review. *Journal of Adolescent Health, 54*(2), 121–138. https://doi.org/10.1016/j.jadohealth.2013.08.009

Harris, M. A. (2018). Your exclusion, my inclusion: Reflections on a career working with the most challenging and vulnerable in. *Diabetes Spectrum, 31*(1), 113–118. https://doi.org/10.2337/ds17-0080

Harris, M. A., Wagner, D. V., & Dukhovny, D. (2016). Commentary: Demon$trating (our) value. *Journal of Pediatric Psychology, 41*(8), 898–901. https://doi.org/10.1093/jpepsy/jsw029

Harris, M. A., Wagner, D. V., Wilson, A. C., Spiro, K., Heywood, M., & Hoehn, D. (2015). Novel interventions in children's healthcare for youth hospitalized for chronic pain. *Clinical Practice in Pediatric Psychology, 3*(1), 48–58. https://doi.org/10.1037/cpp0000088

Haskard Zolnierek, K. B., & Dimatteo, M. R. (2009). Physician communication and patient adherence to treatment: A meta-analysis. *Medical Care, 47*(8), 826–834. https://doi.org/10.1097/MLR.0b013e31819a5acc

Haywood, C., Jr., Lanzkron, S., Bediako, S., Strouse, J. J., Haythornthwaite, J., Carroll, C. P., Diener-West, M., Onojobi, G., Beach, M. C., & the IMPORT Investigators. (2014). Perceived discrimination, patient trust, and adherence to medical recommendations among persons with sickle cell disease. *Journal of General Internal Medicine, 29*(12), 1657–1662. https://doi.org/10.1007/s11606-014-2986-7

Hensley, C., Heaton, P. C., Kahn, R. S., Luder, H. R., Frede, S. M., & Beck, A. F. (2018). Poverty, transportation access, and medication. *Pediatrics, 141*(4), e20173402. https://doi.org/10.1542/peds.2017-3402

Heron, K. E., Everhart, R. S., McHale, S. M., & Smyth, J. M. (2017). Using mobile-technology-based ecological momentary assessment (EMA) methods with youth: Systematic review and recommendations. *Journal of Pediatric Psychology, 42*(10), 1087–1107. https://doi.org/10.1093/jpepsy/jsx078

Hilliard, M. E., Mann, K. A., Peugh, J. L., & Hood, K. K. (2013). How poorer quality of life in adolescence predicts subsequent Type 1 diabetes management and control. *Patient Education and Counseling, 91*(1), 120–125. https://doi.org/10.1016/j.pec.2012.10.014

Hilliard, M. E., Powell, P. W., & Anderson, B. J. (2016). Evidence-based behavioral interventions to promote diabetes management in children, adolescents, and families. *American Psychologist, 71*(7), 590–601. https://doi.org/10.1037/a0040359

Holbein, C. E., Smith, A. W., Peugh, J., & Modi, A. C. (2019). Allocation of treatment responsibility in adolescents with epilepsy: Associations with cognitive skills and medication adherence. *Journal of Pediatric Psychology, 44*(1), 72–83. https://doi.org/10.1093/jpepsy/jsy006

Hommel, K. A., Mackner, L. M., Denson, L. A., & Crandall, W. V. (2008). Treatment regimen adherence in pediatric gastroenterology. *Journal of Pediatric Gastroenterology and Nutrition, 47*(5), 526–543. https://doi.org/10.1097/MPG.0b013e318175dda1

Hommel, K. A., Ramsey, R. R., Rich, K. L., & Ryan, J. L. (2017). *Adherence to pediatric treatment regimens.* Guilford Press.

Hood, A. M., Nwankwo, C., Walton, A., McTate, E., Joffe, N., Quinn, C. T., Britto, M. T., Peugh, J., Mara, C. A., & Crosby, L. E. (2021). Mobile health use predicts self-efficacy and self-management in adolescents with sickle cell disease. *Translational Behavioral Medicine, 11*(10), 1823–1831. https://doi.org/10.1093/tbm/ibab041

Hsin, O., La Greca, A. M., Valenzuela, J., Moine, C. T., & Delamater, A. (2010). Adherence and glycemic control among Hispanic youth with Type 1 diabetes: Role of family involvement and acculturation. *Journal of Pediatric Psychology, 35*(2), 156–166. https://doi.org/10.1093/jpepsy/jsp045

Hughes, K., Bellis, M. A., Hardcastle, K. A., Sethi, D., Butchart, A., Mikton, C., Jones, L., & Dunne, M. P. (2017). The effect of multiple adverse childhood experiences on health: A systematic review and meta-analysis. *The Lancet Public Health, 2*(8), e356–e366. https://doi.org/10.1016/S2468-2667(17)30118-4

Janicke, D. M., Gray, W. N., Kahhan, N. A., Follansbee Junger, K. W., Marciel, K. K., Storch, E. A., & Jolley, C. D. (2009). Brief report: The association between peer victimization, prosocial support, and treatment adherence in children and adolescents with inflammatory bowel disease. *Journal of Pediatric Psychology, 34*(7), 769–773. https://doi.org/10.1093/jpepsy/jsn116

Kahana, S., Drotar, D., & Frazier, T. (2008). Meta-analysis of psychological interventions to promote adherence to treatment in pediatric chronic health conditions. *Journal of Pediatric Psychology, 33*(6), 590–611. https://doi.org/10.1093/jpepsy/jsm128

Kahkoska, A. R., Shay, C. M., Crandell, J., Dabelea, D., Imperatore, G., Lawrence, J. M., Liese, A. D.,

Pihoker, C., Reboussin, B. A., Agarwal, S., Tooze, J. A., Wagenknecht, L. E., Zhong, V. W., & Mayer-Davis, E. J. (2018). Association of race and ethnicity with glycemic control and hemoglobin A$_{1c}$ levels in youth with Type 1 diabetes. *JAMA Network Open*, *1*(5), e181851. https://doi.org/10.1001/jamanetworkopen.2018.1851

Kamimura-Nishimura, K. I., Epstein, J. N., Froehlich, T. E., Peugh, J., Brinkman, W. B., Baum, R., Gardner, W., Langberg, J. M., Lichtenstein, P., Chen, D., & Kelleher, K. J. (2019). Factors associated with attention deficit hyperactivity disorder medication use in community care settings. *The Journal of Pediatrics*, *213*, 155–162.e1. https://doi.org/10.1016/j.jpeds.2019.06.025

Kornbluh, M., Rogers, L. O., & Williams, J. L. (2021). Doing anti-racist scholarship with adolescents: Empirical examples and lessons learned. *Journal of Adolescent Research*, *36*(5), 427–436. https://doi.org/10.1177/07435584211031450

Landers, S. E., Friedrich, E. A., Jawad, A. F., & Miller, V. A. (2016). Examining the interaction of parental involvement and parenting style in predicting adherence in youth with Type 1 diabetes. *Families, Systems, & Health*, *34*(1), 41–50. https://doi.org/10.1037/fsh0000183

Lee, J. L., Eaton, C., Gutiérrez-Colina, A. M., Devine, K., Simons, L. E., Mee, L., & Blount, R. L. (2014). Longitudinal stability of specific barriers to medication adherence. *Journal of Pediatric Psychology*, *39*(7), 667–676. https://doi.org/10.1093/jpepsy/jsu026

Lehmann, A., Aslani, P., Ahmed, R., Celio, J., Gauchet, A., Bedouch, P., Bugnon, O., Allenet, B., & Schneider, M. P. (2014). Assessing medication adherence: Options to consider. *International Journal of Clinical Pharmacy*, *36*(1), 55–69. https://doi.org/10.1007/s11096-013-9865-x

Lehmann, B. D., & Pietenpol, J. A. (2014). Identification and use of biomarkers in treatment strategies for triple-negative breast cancer subtypes. *The Journal of Pathology*, *232*(2), 142–150. https://doi.org/10.1002/path.4280

LePage, A. K., Wise, J. B., Bell, J. J., Tumin, D., & Smith, A. W. (2021). Distance from the endocrinology clinic and diabetes control in a rural pediatric population. *Journal of Pediatric Endocrinology & Metabolism*, *34*(2), 187–193. https://doi.org/10.1515/jpem-2020-0332

Lieu, T. A., Lozano, P., Finkelstein, J. A., Chi, F. W., Jensvold, N. G., Capra, A. M., Quesenberry, C. P., Selby, J. V., & Farber, H. J. (2002). Racial/ethnic variation in asthma status and management practices among children in managed Medicaid. *Pediatrics*, *109*(5), 857–865. https://doi.org/10.1542/peds.109.5.857

Lutfey, K. E., & Ketcham, J. D. (2005). Patient and provider assessments of adherence and the sources of disparities: Evidence from diabetes care. *Health Services Research*, *40*(6 Pt. 1), 1803–1817. https://doi.org/10.1111/j.1475-6773.2005.00433.x

Mack, J. W., Jaung, T., Uno, H., & Brackett, J. (2021). Parent and clinician perspectives on challenging parent–clinician relationships in pediatric oncology. *JAMA Network Open*, *4*(11), e2132138. https://doi.org/10.1001/jamanetworkopen.2021.32138

Masten, A. S., & Cicchetti, D. (2010). Developmental cascades. *Development and Psychopathology*, *22*(3), 491–495. https://doi.org/10.1017/S0954579410000222

McClain, C., Vogels, E. A., Perrin, A., Sechopoulos, S., & Rainie, L. (2021, September 1). *The internet and the pandemic*. Pew Research Center. https://www.pewresearch.org/internet/2021/09/01/the-internet-and-the-pandemic/

McGrady, M. E., Holbein, C. E., Smith, A. W., Morrison, C. F., Hommel, K. A., Modi, A. C., Pai, A. L. H., & Ramsey, R. R. (2018). An independent evaluation of the accuracy and usability of electronic adherence monitoring devices. *Annals of Internal Medicine*, *169*(6), 419–422. https://doi.org/10.7326/M17-3306

McGrady, M. E., & Hommel, K. A. (2013). Medication adherence and health care utilization in pediatric chronic illness: A systematic review. *Pediatrics*, *132*(4), 730–740. https://doi.org/10.1542/peds.2013-1451

McGrady, M. E., & Hommel, K. A. (2016). Targeting health behaviors to reduce health care costs in pediatric psychology: Descriptive review and recommendations. *Journal of Pediatric Psychology*, *41*(8), 835–848. https://doi.org/10.1093/jpepsy/jsv083

McGrady, M. E., Ryan, J. L., Brown, G. A., & Cushing, C. C. (2015). Topical review: Theoretical frameworks in pediatric adherence-promotion interventions: Research findings and methodological implications. *Journal of Pediatric Psychology*, *40*(8), 721–726. https://doi.org/10.1093/jpepsy/jsv025

McQuaid, E. L., Everhart, R. S., Seifer, R., Kopel, S. J., Mitchell, D. K., Klein, R. B., Esteban, C. A., Fritz, G. K., & Canino, G. (2012). Medication adherence among Latino and non-Latino White children with asthma. *Pediatrics*, *129*(6), e1404–e1410. https://doi.org/10.1542/peds.2011-1391

McQuaid, E. L., & Landier, W. (2018). Cultural issues in medication adherence: Disparities and directions. *Journal of General Internal Medicine*, *33*(2), 200–206. https://doi.org/10.1007/s11606-017-4199-3

Mitchell, S. J., Bilderback, A. L., & Okelo, S. O. (2016). Racial disparities in asthma morbidity among pediatric patients seeking asthma specialist care. *Academic Pediatrics, 16*(1), 64–67. https://doi.org/10.1016/j.acap.2015.06.010

Modi, A. C., Pai, A. L., Hommel, K. A., Hood, K. K., Cortina, S., Hilliard, M. E., Guilfoyle, S. M., Gray, W. N., & Drotar, D. (2012). Pediatric self-management: A framework for research, practice, and policy. *Pediatrics, 129*(2), e473–e485. https://doi.org/10.1542/peds.2011-1635

Modi, A. C., Rausch, J. R., & Glauser, T. A. (2011). Patterns of nonadherence to antiepileptic drug therapy in children with newly diagnosed epilepsy. *JAMA: Journal of the American Medical Association, 305*(16), 1669–1676. https://doi.org/10.1001/jama.2011.506

Mulvaney, D., Woodward, B., Datta, S., Harvey, P., Vyas, A., Thakker, B., Farooq, O., & Istepanian, R. (2012). Monitoring heart disease and diabetes with mobile internet communications. *International Journal of Telemedicine and Applications, 2012*, 195970. https://doi.org/10.1155/2012/195970

Mulvaney, S. A., Ho, Y. X., Cala, C. M., Chen, Q., Nian, H., Patterson, B. L., & Johnson, K. B. (2013). Assessing adolescent asthma symptoms and adherence using mobile phones. *Journal of Medical Internet Research, 15*(7), e141. https://doi.org/10.2196/jmir.2413

Naar-King, S., Arfken, C., Frey, M., Harris, M., Secord, E., & Ellis, D. (2006). Psychosocial factors and treatment adherence in paediatric HIV/AIDS. *AIDS Care, 18*(6), 621–628. https://doi.org/10.1080/09540120500471895

O'Hara, L. K., & Holmbeck, G. N. (2013). Executive functions and parenting behaviors in association with medical adherence and autonomy among youth with spina bifida. *Journal of Pediatric Psychology, 38*(6), 675–687. https://doi.org/10.1093/jpepsy/jst007

Otsuki, M., Eakin, M. N., Arceneaux, L. L., Rand, C. S., Butz, A. M., & Riekert, K. A. (2010). Prospective relationship between maternal depressive symptoms and asthma morbidity among inner-city African American children. *Journal of Pediatric Psychology, 35*(7), 758–767. https://doi.org/10.1093/jpepsy/jsp091

Pai, A. L., & McGrady, M. (2014). Systematic review and meta-analysis of psychological interventions to promote treatment adherence in children, adolescents, and young adults with chronic illness. *Journal of Pediatric Psychology, 39*(8), 918–931. https://doi.org/10.1093/jpepsy/jsu038

Pai, A. L. H., & Drotar, D. (2010). Treatment adherence impact: The systematic assessment and quantification of the impact of treatment adherence on pediatric medical and psychological outcomes. *Journal of Pediatric Psychology, 35*(4), 383–393. https://doi.org/10.1093/jpepsy/jsp073

Palermo, T. M., Alderfer, M. A., Boerner, K. E., Hilliard, M. E., Hood, A. M., Modi, A. C., & Wu, Y. P. (2021). Editorial: Diversity, equity, and inclusion: Reporting race and ethnicity in the *Journal of Pediatric Psychology*. *Journal of Pediatric Psychology, 46*(7), 731–733. https://doi.org/10.1093/jpepsy/jsab063

Palmer, D. L., Berg, C. A., Butler, J., Fortenberry, K., Murray, M., Lindsay, R., Donaldson, D., Swinyard, M., Foster, C., & Wiebe, D. J. (2009). Mothers', fathers', and children's perceptions of parental diabetes responsibility in adolescence: Examining the roles of age, pubertal status, and efficacy. *Journal of Pediatric Psychology, 34*(2), 195–204. https://doi.org/10.1093/jpepsy/jsn073

Patel, M. S., Asch, D. A., & Volpp, K. G. (2015). Wearable devices as facilitators, not drivers, of health behavior change. *JAMA: Journal of the American Medical Association, 313*(5), 459–460. https://doi.org/10.1001/jama.2014.14781

Plevinsky, J. M., Young, M. A., Carmody, J. K., Durkin, L. K., Gamwell, K. L., Klages, K. L., Ghosh, S., & Hommel, K. A. (2020). The impact of COVID-19 on pediatric adherence and self-management. *Journal of Pediatric Psychology, 45*(9), 977–982. https://doi.org/10.1093/jpepsy/jsaa079

Psihogios, A. M., Fellmeth, H., Schwartz, L. A., & Barakat, L. P. (2019). Family functioning and medical adherence across children and adolescents with chronic health conditions: A meta-analysis. *Journal of Pediatric Psychology, 44*(1), 84–97. https://doi.org/10.1093/jpepsy/jsy044

Psihogios, A. M., King-Dowling, S., O'Hagan, B., Darabos, K., Maurer, L., Young, J., Fleisher, L., Barakat, L. P., Szalda, D., Hill-Kayser, C. E., & Schwartz, L. A. (2021). Contextual predictors of engagement in a tailored mHealth intervention for adolescent and young adult cancer survivors. *Annals of Behavioral Medicine, 55*(12), 1220–1230. https://doi.org/10.1093/abm/kaab008

Psihogios, A. M., Schwartz, L. A., Ewing, K. B., Czerniecki, B., Kersun, L. S., Pai, A. L. H., Deatrick, J. A., & Barakat, L. P. (2020). Adherence to multiple treatment recommendations in adolescents and young adults with cancer: A mixed methods, multi-informant investigation. *Journal of Adolescent and Young Adult Oncology, 9*(6), 651–661. https://doi.org/10.1089/jayao.2020.0013

Ramsey, R. R., & Holbein, C. E. (2020). Treatment adherence within consultation-liaison services. In B. D. Carter & K. A. Kullgren (Eds.), *Clinical handbook of psychological consultation in pediatric medical settings* (pp. 425–438). Springer. https://doi.org/10.1007/978-3-030-35598-2_32

Ramsey, R. R., Zhang, N., & Modi, A. C. (2018). The stability and influence of barriers to medication adherence on seizure outcomes and adherence in children with epilepsy over 2 years. *Journal of Pediatric Psychology, 43*(2), 122–132. https://doi.org/10.1093/jpepsy/jsx090

Raphael, J. L., Rueda, A., Lion, K. C., & Giordano, T. P. (2013). The role of lay health workers in pediatric chronic disease: A systematic review. *Academic Pediatrics, 13*(5), 408–420. https://doi.org/10.1016/j.acap.2013.04.015

Rapoff, M. A. (2010). *Adherence to pediatric medical regimens* (2nd ed.). Springer. https://doi.org/10.1007/978-1-4419-0570-3

Rhee, H., Belyea, M. J., & Brasch, J. (2010). Family support and asthma outcomes in adolescents: Barriers to adherence as a mediator. *Journal of Adolescent Health, 47*(5), 472–478. https://doi.org/10.1016/j.jadohealth.2010.03.009

Roberts, M. C., & Ric, G. S. (2017). *Handbook of pediatric psychology* (5th ed.). Guilford Press.

Rubin, J., & Chisnell, D. (2008). *Handbook of usability testing: How to plan, design, and conduct effective tests* (2nd ed.). Wiley.

Sabaté, E. (2003). *Adherence to long-term therapies: Evidence for action.* World Health Organization. https://iris.who.int/bitstream/handle/10665/42682/9241545992.pdf

Salsman, J. M., Pustejovsky, J. E., Schueller, S. M., Hernandez, R., Berendsen, M., McLouth, L. E. S., & Moskowitz, J. T. (2019). Psychosocial interventions for cancer survivors: A meta-analysis of effects on positive affect. *Journal of Cancer Survivorship: Research and Practice, 13*(6), 943–955. https://doi.org/10.1007/s11764-019-00811-8

Shih, S., & Cohen, L. L. (2020). A systematic review of medication adherence interventions in pediatric sickle cell disease. *Journal of Pediatric Psychology, 45*(6), 593–606. https://doi.org/10.1093/jpepsy/jsaa031

Silva, K., & Miller, V. A. (2020). Does self-efficacy mediate the link between impulse control and diabetes adherence? *Journal of Pediatric Psychology, 45*(4), 445–453. https://doi.org/10.1093/jpepsy/jsaa007

Spieth, L. E., Stark, L. J., Mitchell, M. J., Schiller, M., Cohen, L. L., Mulvihill, M., & Hovell, M. F. (2001). Observational assessment of family functioning at mealtime in preschool children with cystic fibrosis. *Journal of Pediatric Psychology, 26*(4), 215–224. https://doi.org/10.1093/jpepsy/26.4.215

Spinks-Franklin, A. A. (2021, July 1). How pediatricians can advance equity in care of children with developmental/behavioral concerns. *AAP News.*

Steinberg, L. (2007). Risk taking in adolescence: New perspectives from brain and behavioral science. *Current Directions in Psychological Science, 16*(2), 55–59. https://doi.org/10.1111/j.1467-8721.2007.00475.x

Stiles-Shields, C., Cummings, C., Montague, E., Plevinsky, J. M., Psihogios, A. M., & Williams, K. D. A. (2022). A call to action using and extending human-centered design methodologies to improve mental and behavioral health equity. *Frontiers in Digital Health, 4*, 848052. https://doi.org/10.3389/fdgth.2022.848052

Streisand, R., & Monaghan, M. (2014). Young children with Type 1 diabetes: Challenges, research, and future directions. *Current Diabetes Reports, 14*(9), 520. https://doi.org/10.1007/s11892-014-0520-2

Tackett, A. P., Farrow, M., Kopel, S. J., Coutinho, M. T., Koinis-Mitchell, D., & McQuaid, E. L. (2021). Racial/ethnic differences in pediatric asthma management: The importance of asthma knowledge, symptom assessment, and family-provider collaboration. *Journal of Asthma, 58*(10), 1395–1406. https://doi.org/10.1080/02770903.2020.1784191

Tan, X., Marshall, V. D., Balkrishnan, R., Patel, I., Chang, J., & Erickson, S. R. (2015). Psychotropic medication adherence among community-based individuals with developmental disabilities and mental illness. *Journal of Mental Health Research in Intellectual Disabilities, 8*(1), 1–22. https://doi.org/10.1080/19315864.2014.959216

Thompson, K., Kulkarni, J., & Sergejew, A. A. (2000). Reliability and validity of a new Medication Adherence Rating Scale (MARS) for the psychoses. *Schizophrenia Research, 42*(3), 241–247. https://doi.org/10.1016/S0920-9964(99)00130-9

Triplett, K. N., El-Behadli, A. F., Masood, S. S., Sullivan, S., & Desai, D. M. (2019). Digital medicine program with pediatric solid organ transplant patients: Perceived benefits and challenges. *Pediatric Transplantation, 23*(7), e13555. https://doi.org/10.1111/petr.13555

Trivedi, M., Fung, V., Kharbanda, E. O., Larkin, E. K., Butler, M. G., Horan, K., Lieu, T. A., & Wu, A. C. (2018). Racial disparities in family-provider interactions for pediatric asthma care. *Journal of Asthma, 55*(4), 424–429. https://doi.org/10.1080/02770903.2017.1337790

Utidjian, L. H., Fiks, A. G., Localio, A. R., Song, L., Ramos, M. J., Keren, R., Bell, L. M., & Grundmeier, R. W. (2017). Pediatric asthma hospitalizations among urban minority children and the continuity of primary care. *Journal of Asthma, 54*(10), 1051–1058. https://doi.org/10.1080/02770903.2017.1294695

Valenzuela, J. M., & Smith, L. (2016). Topical review: Provider-patient interactions: An important consideration for racial/ethnic health disparities in youth. *Journal of Pediatric Psychology*, *41*(4), 473–480. https://doi.org/10.1093/jpepsy/jsv086

van Ryn, M., & Burke, J. (2000). The effect of patient race and socio-economic status on physicians' perceptions of patients. *Social Science & Medicine*, *50*(6), 813–828. https://doi.org/10.1016/S0277-9536(99)00338-X

Vrijens, B., De Geest, S., Hughes, D. A., Przemyslaw, K., Demonceau, J., Ruppar, T., Dobbels, F., Fargher, E., Morrison, V., Lewek, P., Matyjaszczyk, M., Mshelia, C., Clyne, W., Aronson, J. K., Urquhart, J., & the ABC Project Team. (2012). A new taxonomy for describing and defining adherence to medications. *British Journal of Clinical Pharmacology*, *73*(5), 691–705. https://doi.org/10.1111/j.1365-2125.2012.04167.x

Wagner, D. V., Barry, S. A., Stoeckel, M., Teplitsky, L., & Harris, M. A. (2017). NICH at its best for diabetes at its worst: Texting teens and their caregivers for better outcomes. *Journal of Diabetes Science and Technology*, *11*(3), 468–475. https://doi.org/10.1177/1932296817695337

Wahl, L. M., & Nowak, M. A. (2000). Adherence and drug resistance: Predictions for therapy outcome. *Proceedings of the Royal Society B: Biological Sciences*, *267*(1445), 835–843. https://doi.org/10.1098/rspb.2000.1079

Walsh, J. C., Mandalia, S., & Gazzard, B. G. (2002). Responses to a 1 month self-report on adherence to antiretroviral therapy are consistent with electronic data and virological treatment outcome. *AIDS*, *16*(2), 269–277. https://doi.org/10.1097/00002030-200201250-00017

Watach, A. J., Xanthopoulos, M. S., Afolabi-Brown, O., Saconi, B., Fox, K. A., Qiu, M., & Sawyer, A. M. (2020). Positive airway pressure adherence in pediatric obstructive sleep apnea: A systematic scoping review. *Sleep Medicine Reviews*, *51*, 101273. https://doi.org/10.1016/j.smrv.2020.101273

Wen, C. K. F., Schneider, S., Stone, A. A., & Spruijt-Metz, D. (2017). Compliance with mobile ecological momentary assessment protocols in children and adolescents: A systematic review and meta-analysis. *Journal of Medical Internet Research*, *19*(4), e132. https://doi.org/10.2196/jmir.6641

Westen, S. C., Warnick, J. L., Albanese-O'Neill, A., Schatz, D. A., Haller, M. J., Entessari, M., & Janicke, D. M. (2019). Objectively measured adherence in adolescents with Type 1 diabetes on multiple daily injections and insulin pump therapy. *Journal of Pediatric Psychology*, *44*(1), 21–31. https://doi.org/10.1093/jpepsy/jsy064

Wiebe, D. J., Chow, C. M., Palmer, D. L., Butner, J., Butler, J. M., Osborn, P., & Berg, C. A. (2014). Developmental processes associated with longitudinal declines in parental responsibility and adherence to Type 1 diabetes management across adolescence. *Journal of Pediatric Psychology*, *39*(5), 532–541. https://doi.org/10.1093/jpepsy/jsu006

Wu, Y. P., Follansbee-Junger, K., Rausch, J., & Modi, A. (2014). Parent and family stress factors predict health-related quality in pediatric patients with new-onset epilepsy. *Epilepsia*, *55*(6), 866–877. https://doi.org/10.1111/epi.12586

Wysocki, T., Harris, M. A., Buckloh, L. M., Mertlich, D., Lochrie, A. S., Mauras, N., & White, N. H. (2007). Randomized trial of behavioral family systems therapy for diabetes: Maintenance of effects on diabetes outcomes in adolescents. *Diabetes Care*, *30*(3), 555–560. https://doi.org/10.2337/dc06-1613

Yun, K., Jenicek, G., & Gerdes, M. (2019). Overcoming language barriers in mental and behavioral health care for children and adolescents—Policies and priorities. *JAMA Pediatrics*, *173*(6), 511–512. https://doi.org/10.1001/jamapediatrics.2019.0400

Zelikovsky, N., & Schast, A. P. (2008). Eliciting accurate reports of adherence in a clinical interview: Development of the Medical Adherence Measure. *Pediatric Nursing*, *34*(2), 141–146.

Zweigoron, R. T., Binns, H. J., & Tanz, R. R. (2012). Unfilled prescriptions in pediatric primary care. *Pediatrics*, *130*(4), 620–626. https://doi.org/10.1542/peds.2011-3480

CHAPTER 3

CHRONIC AND RECURRENT PAIN: CONSIDERATIONS FOR CHILD HEALTH AND WELL-BEING

Tonya M. Palermo and Irina Gorbounova

Many children and adolescents struggle with chronic pain. Chronic pain affects nearly one quarter to one third of children and adolescents in the United States and worldwide (King et al., 2011). Although the prevalence of chronic pain varies among studies, it increases with age, and chronic pain is more common among females. Chronic pain may arise from a chronic health condition, such as inflammatory bowel disease or cancer, or it may be from a primary pain disorder (a chronic pain disorder that cannot be explained by appropriate medical assessment[s] in terms of conventionally defined medical disease). Children with chronic pain experience poor quality of life, disability, school absenteeism, frequent health care utilization, anxiety, and depression. Chronic pain affects children's relationships with peers and family members. Pediatric chronic pain is a risk factor for chronic pain in adulthood and places a significant economic burden on society. There have been substantial advances in our understanding and management of pediatric chronic pain, evidenced by expansion of scientific literature on this subject since the early 2000s.

In this chapter, we provide an overview of current knowledge of pediatric chronic pain, we highlight the multisystemic contexts, informed by developmental science and associated with development and maintenance of chronic pain, and we offer future directions for research and clinical management by subspecialty providers, including developmental-behavioral pediatricians and pediatric psychologists. We begin the chapter by providing the definition and classification of chronic pain. We then discuss the epidemiology and impact of chronic pain at the level of the individual, family, and society. We provide the reader with an overview of conceptual models of chronic pain, with an emphasis on the biopsychosocial model. We describe common types of chronic pain and discuss the approach to assessment and management of chronic pain, highlighting the importance of an interdisciplinary approach. Finally, we discuss the impact of the COVID-19 pandemic on chronic pain and provide resources for patients and providers in understanding and managing chronic pain.

DEFINITION AND CLASSIFICATION OF CHRONIC PAIN

Pain is a complex biopsychosocial phenomenon defined by the International Association for the Study of Pain (IASP) as "an unpleasant sensory and emotional experience associated with, or resembling that associated with, actual or potential tissue damage" (Raja et al., 2020, p. 2). Pain is classified based on timing and duration as acute or chronic. Acute pain is meant to be protective and serve as a warning of threat or

https://doi.org/10.1037/0000414-003
APA Handbook of Pediatric Psychology, Developmental-Behavioral Pediatrics, and Developmental Science: Vol. 2. Pediatric Psychology and Developmental-Behavioral Pediatrics: Clinical Applications of Developmental Science, P. E. Shah and M. H. Bornstein (Editors-in-Chief)
Copyright © 2025 by the American Psychological Association. All rights reserved.

disease. For instance, experiencing pain on touching a hot stove is protective against developing a burn injury. Chronic pain is defined as lasting longer than 3 or 6 months, and it can be either persistent or recurrent (Dinakar & Stillman, 2016; Friedrichsdorf et al., 2016; Manworren & Stinson, 2016; Treede et al., 2015). Unlike acute pain, chronic pain is maladaptive, with the ongoing signal or "warning" no longer serving a protective purpose. For instance, patients who are in remission after undergoing chemotherapy may suffer from chronic pain despite absence of tumor. Chronic pain begins as acute pain, and the transition from acute to chronic pain is an active area of research that has important implications for prevention. Identifying modifiable factors associated with this transition has potential for early intervention to change the trajectory of pain and reduce the development of chronic pain.

Different approaches to classifying chronic pain are based on etiology, location, or whether the pain is related to a disease process. To standardize diagnosis and management of chronic pain, the IASP and World Health Organization proposed inclusion of the diagnosis of chronic pain for the *International Classification of Diseases*, 11th revision (*ICD-11*; Nicholas et al., 2019). Chronic pain was further classified into seven categories: chronic primary pain, chronic cancer-related pain, chronic postsurgical or posttraumatic pain, chronic neuropathic pain, chronic secondary headache or orofacial pain, chronic secondary visceral pain, and chronic secondary musculoskeletal pain (Smith et al., 2019). Billing codes now offer a description of chronic pain, a major advance expected to aid with diagnosis and future research related to chronic pain. In turn, this typology may lead to better treatment options for chronic pain based on etiology. We address comprehensive approaches to understanding pain-related impairment and psychosocial contributors in the section on assessment.

Common Types of Chronic and Recurrent Pain

Chronic pain can occur as a result of a chronic health condition (such as inflammatory bowel disease and sickle cell disease) or it can be a primary pain disorder (functional abdominal pain, primary headaches, or musculoskeletal pain). In some instances, a child can experience multiple types of chronic pain. Primary pain disorders in children and adolescents are common yet they are underdiagnosed and undertreated (Friedrichsdorf et al., 2016). The most common sources of chronic and recurrent pain in children are headaches, abdominal pain, and musculoskeletal pain (King et al., 2011). Although previously viewed as separate entities with different underlying pathophysiologies, chronic primary pain conditions are now viewed as manifestations of the same underlying condition in varying locations, as described in greater detail in the following section.

Pain in children with underlying health conditions. Children diagnosed with chronic illness are at risk for chronic pain. Some of the more common conditions with painful symptoms include inflammatory bowel disease (IBD), sickle cell disease (SCD), and juvenile idiopathic arthritis (JIA). Children with these disorders suffer from inflammation and are at risk for acute flares of pain, such as acute pain crises during a sickle cell episode (Brandow & DeBaun, 2018) and pain in inflammatory bowel disease (Murphy et al., 2021). Typically, these flares or crises are short-lived. However, recurrent acute episodes can be interposed on top of chronic pain, which may be due to changes to the tissue (such as avascular necrosis in patients with SCD; Martí-Carvajal et al., 2019). Chronic pain can also develop despite good control of the primary disease (e.g., functional abdominal pain in a child with well-controlled IBD; Watson et al., 2017). Thus, children with underlying health conditions can suffer from pain as a result of their medical condition, or chronic pain can be a disease on its own.

Primary pain disorder. Primary pain disorder is a chronic pain disorder that cannot be explained by appropriate medical assessment(s) in terms of conventionally defined medical disease, as based on biochemical or structural abnormalities

(Friedrichsdorf et al., 2016), and can be diagnosed across the entire pediatric age range. We discuss some of the more common primary pain disorders in the following subsections.

Primary headache. Primary headaches are typically diagnosed in childhood as migraines or tension-type headaches (Headache Classification Committee, 2013). Primary headaches are more common in females. Migraines are typically subdivided into migraines without aura and migraines with aura (Kelly et al., 2018). An aura is a neurological phenomenon that involves changes in vision (e.g., absence of vision, seeing flashing lights), changes in hearing or sensitivity to sounds, and changes in smell. They can include temporary changes in vision, sensation, speech, or motor function and typically last from several minutes up to 1 hour. Migraines without aura are typically recurrent headaches that last between 4 and 72 hours, afflict one side of the head, are pulsatile in quality, and are aggravated by physical activity. They are frequently accompanied by nausea and/or photophobia and phonophobia. In children and adolescents, migraines with aura are more often bilateral; they become unilateral nearing adult years (Headache Classification Committee, 2013). Migraines with aura are associated with preceding or accompanying neurological symptoms that are fully reversible.

Diagnosis of tension-type headaches can be challenging as there is significant overlap in symptoms with migraines. Tension-type headaches are frequently accompanied by muscular tenderness on palpation of the scalp, are typically bilateral, and have a tight or pressing band-like quality that lasts from 30 minutes to 7 days. The pain does not worsen with physical activity and is not associated with nausea. In some cases, there is presence of either photophobia or phonophobia (but not both). Tension headaches are further subdivided based on frequency and duration (e.g., chronic daily headache).

Functional abdominal pain. Functional abdominal pain disorders (FAPD) consist of four subtypes (Hyams et al., 2016): functional dyspepsia, irritable bowel syndrome (IBS), abdominal migraine, and functional abdominal pain not otherwise specified. An individual patient can suffer from more than one FAPD. In a meta-analysis, Korterink et al. (2015) found that the prevalence of FAPD worldwide was 13.5%, yet it varied widely from 1.6% to 41.2%. This disorder occurs more frequently in girls and is associated with anxiety and depressive disorders as well as stress and traumatic life events. Diagnosis of these disorders requires that, after appropriate evaluation, the abdominal pain cannot be fully explained by another medical condition.

Musculoskeletal and joint pain. The most common forms of musculoskeletal and joint pain are isolated low back pain and diffuse musculoskeletal pain. The prevalence of low back pain in the pediatric population varies among studies. Generally, low back pain increases in adolescence and is more prevalent in girls than boys. Widespread musculoskeletal pain is termed fibromyalgia in adults. However, the diagnosis of juvenile-onset fibromyalgia is controversial. The terminology is not mutually agreed on, and at times the term "widespread musculoskeletal pain" is used as a pediatric equivalent of fibromyalgia in adults. It more commonly affects adolescent girls and is associated with fatigue, poor sleep, other pain conditions, and mood disorders (Kashikar-Zuck & Ting, 2014). In a review of risk factors for onset and persistence of musculoskeletal pain in childhood, Huguet et al. (2016) found that low socioeconomic status, smoking, and negative emotional symptoms are risk factors for onset of musculoskeletal pain.

EPIDEMIOLOGY AND ECONOMIC IMPACT OF CHRONIC PAIN

Prevalence rates of chronic pain in children and adolescents vary across different studies, likely due to a lack of a commonly accepted definition of chronic pain. In a systematic review by King et al. (2011), prevalence rates according to location were found to be 8%–83% for headache, 4%–53% for abdominal pain, 14%–24% for back pain, 4%–40% for musculoskeletal pain, 4%–49% for multiple pains, and 5%–88% for other pains. Girls reported higher prevalence rates than boys, and with the exception of abdominal pain, prevalence rates of chronic pain increased with age, with a peak in prevalence in mid-adolescence. There is very limited data on prevalence rates for chronic pain in young children under age 6, although studies of specific pain types suggest that abdominal pain is diagnosed in 2.25% of children ages 0 to 5 years and musculoskeletal pain in 2.4% to 5.7% of 3-year-old children (Chitkara et al., 2007; De Inocencio, 2004).

Chronic pain leads to frequent health care utilization and high health care costs. Expenditures for pain-related conditions in childhood are higher than those for other common childhood conditions (Groenewald et al., 2014). Approximately 5% of youth have moderate to severe pain with disability (Huguet & Miró, 2008). It has been estimated that in the United States the total costs to society for adolescents with chronic pain amount to $19.5 billion annually (Groenewald et al., 2014). Direct medical costs are the primary contributor to annual costs, followed by productivity losses. These costs are even more striking in considering that they may accumulate from childhood into adulthood. Estimated societal costs for adult chronic pain are $560 to $635 billion annually in the United States, far outpacing other priority health conditions such as obesity, heart disease, and substance abuse (Gaskin & Richard, 2012).

Chronic pain is associated with impairments in physical, psychological, and social health (Bohr et al., 2015; Vinall et al., 2016). Children with chronic pain experience higher rates of school absenteeism than peers without pain (Logan et al., 2008). These children also experience limitations in performing vigorous physical activities and report limitations in a range of activities in their daily lives (Roth-Isigkeit et al., 2005). Adolescents with chronic pain have more physical impairment than healthy adolescents based on subjective measures of physical functioning, as well lower levels of physical activity based on actigraphy monitoring (Wilson & Palermo, 2012).

ECOLOGICAL AND CONTEXTUAL FACTORS: CONSIDERATIONS FROM DEVELOPMENTAL SCIENCE

Pediatric chronic pain is situated in an ecological system in which the child's pain is affected by multiple levels of the surrounding environment (see Bronfenbrenner, 1979). This includes individual factors and parent and family factors, as well as peer, school, and broader societal factors, and is applicable to all types of chronic pain (disease-related and primary pain). These contextual factors may contribute to the development of pain (vulnerability/risk factors) or may serve as maintaining factors, prolonging pain and disability over time.

Individual Factors

Several individual factors have a strong evidence base, including emotional vulnerabilities such as pain catastrophizing and threat appraisal as well as general symptoms of anxiety and depression, demonstrating links with development and maintenance of chronic pain (Palermo, 2020).

Mood disorders. Chronic pain is highly comorbid with mood disorders such as anxiety and depression. In an epidemiological study, affective disorders were found to frequently precede and serve as early risk factors for subsequent development of chronic pain (Tegethoff et al., 2015). A history of chronic pain in adolescence is associated with an approximately 1.3 times higher rate of anxiety and depressive disorders in adulthood (Noel et al., 2016).

Sleep disturbances. Another important individual variable concerns health behavior vulnerabilities such as sleep disturbances. Sleep disturbances often precede the onset of new chronic pain complaints (Afolalu et al., 2018; Finan et al., 2013). Across many different types of chronic pain, children and adolescents experience a high rate of comorbid sleep disturbances, most commonly difficulties with sleep onset and maintenance, and poor quality of sleep. In a systematic review, Valrie et al. (2013) found strong evidence for increased sleep problems across samples of youth with persistent pain in comparison with healthy controls. When compared with healthy teens, adolescents with chronic pain are six times more likely to report symptoms of insomnia and lower sleep quality (Palermo et al., 2011). Adolescents with more severe sleep disturbances experience greater functional disability and reduced social and emotional functioning.

Developmental considerations. The experience and impact of chronic pain varies based on a child's developmental stage as the child's developmental goals change across the preschool, school, and adolescent age range (Palermo et al., 2014). Given the high prevalence of chronic pain in adolescence as compared to other age groups, most of the research on developmental influences has focused on this developmental stage. Adolescents with chronic pain are more likely to experience increased family conflict and to strive for increased autonomy in their health care management; thus, parent–adolescent communication around chronic pain is an important contextual factor shown to be associated with pain-related disability (Palermo et al., 2007).

Parent and Family Factors

At the level of the parent/family, individual behaviors and mental health, pain history, dyadic communication, and overall family environment are all important influences on the child's pain experience (Palermo & Chambers, 2005).

Parent emotional distress. Parents experience high levels of emotional distress and make adaptations in their personal lives in parenting youth with chronic pain (Jastrowski Mano et al., 2011). A subgroup of parents experience clinically significant levels of anxiety and depression (Fussner et al., 2018), which is associated with severity of child pain and extent of pain-related disability (Conte et al., 2003; Harrison et al., 2020). Children's pain behaviors can elicit potentially reinforcing parental behaviors and responses, such as increased attention and sympathy, discouragement of activity, and relief from responsibilities (e.g., chores, going to school). Whitehead et al. suggested that these types of parental responses, also conceptualized as *protectiveness or solicitousness*, reward somatic complaints and increase the probability of future illness behavior by the child (i.e., the child's reaction to somatic sensations such as excessive attention to them, preoccupation or worry, and avoidance of activities; Whitehead et al., 1979, 1982).

Family history of chronic illness. Chronic pain conditions often occur among multiple family members, pointing toward possible genetic predisposition to pain or social learning. For example, offspring of parents with IBS have a three times greater risk of developing functional abdominal pain disorder than offspring of parents without IBS (Saito et al., 2010). Current conceptual models for the transmission of risk for chronic pain from parents to offspring highlight potential mechanisms including genetics, alterations in early neurobiological development, pain-specific social learning, general parenting and family health, and exposure to a stressful environment (Stone & Wilson, 2016). In particular, ample evidence points to solicitous or protective parental reactions to children's expressions of discomfort and maternal modeling of their own illness behavior as major contributors to a greater focus on somatic sensations, leading to illness behaviors in children (Levy et al., 2007).

Parental beliefs. Parental beliefs may explain why some parents are more likely to reinforce child illness behaviors. Parents' catastrophizing (i.e., appraising an event or experience as a threat or as beyond the ability of the individual to cope) about their child's pain has been associated with their emotional and behavioral responses to the child's pain (Caes et al., 2011, 2014; Hechler et al., 2011) as well as increased pain and disability in the child (Hechler et al., 2011; Lynch-Jordan et al., 2010, 2013). Parental catastrophizing may lead parents to interpret child pain as indicating harm or threat to the well-being of the child and thus may increase the likelihood that parents intervene to comfort or help the child, which can lead to increased expressions of pain and disability (Langer et al., 2014). Logan et al. (2012) found that parental pain catastrophizing and solicitous responses independently predicted child school attendance and school functioning, with solicitousness mediating the association between parent catastrophizing and child school functioning.

Social Context

The social context includes the child's peer network; historical, political, and legal structures and processes (e.g., colonialism, migration); and organizations and institutions (e.g., schools, clinics, community). Peer relationships seem to be impacted among youth with chronic pain; these children tend to have fewer friends, are subjected to more peer victimization, and are viewed as less likeable than children without pain (Forgeron et al., 2010).

Social determinants of health and health disparities. Disparities in pain, including inequitable pain treatment and worse pain outcomes, have been identified by sociodemographic characteristics. The highest burden of pain is experienced in ethnic and racial minority groups. In particular, individuals who are Black and Latin American self-report higher prevalence of pain, greater pain severity, and greater functional disability than non-Hispanic White individuals (Evans et al., 2010; Goyal et al., 2020; Miller et al., 2020). Moreover, socioeconomic status, including lower levels of education, low income, and unemployment, is associated with higher rates of chronic pain (Prego-Domínguez et al., 2021). Longitudinal studies demonstrate that poor socioeconomic conditions and housing quality (i.e., material home conditions in regard to type, age, state of repair, and crowding) in childhood are associated with an increased likelihood of chronic pain in adulthood (Muthuri et al., 2018), highlighting the link between childhood experiences and subsequent health in adulthood.

Further inequities have been identified in access to pain care and in pain treatment experienced by ethnic minorities as compared with non-Hispanic Whites (Green et al., 2003). For example, racial disparities in use of analgesia in emergency departments for pain (e.g., resulting from limb fractures, appendicitis) have been previously documented in which Black and Hispanic children are less likely to receive opioids than White children (Goyal et al., 2020; Guedj et al., 2021). Moreover, Black and Hispanic children with limb fractures are less likely to achieve optimal pain reduction (i.e., reduction to mild or no pain; Goyal et al., 2020). Inadequate acute pain management has consequences beyond the immediate perception of pain. Unrelieved acute pain may increase the risk of developing chronic pain (Sinatra, 2010). We need to understand underlying factors resulting in differences of acute pain management and provide equitable analgesic care to reduce consequent disparities that follow inadequate management of pain in acute medical settings. Further research is needed to understand pain care inequities in children. Overall, we know little about how various cultures experience and communicate about pain as the majority of research has involved White middle class subjects, typically in North America or the United Kingdom (Eccleston et al., 2021; Fisher et al., 2022).

With regard to the contextual factors influencing pediatric pain, it is also important to consider intergenerational social mobility including the impact of family socioeconomic position in childhood and into adult life as children grow up. Socioeconomic position in childhood is determined by the parent's socioeconomic position and can not only influence risk for pain and access to medical care but also be affected by child pain and pain treatment costs. Taking care of children with chronic pain comes at a burden of time and cost. According to data gathered by the 2016 National Survey of Children's Health (Datz et al., 2019), the general health status of adolescents with chronic pain and the extent of their health care needs predicted caregiver burden. This burden included direct time spent on the child's health care, reduction of paid work hours, and increased health care expenditures (Datz et al., 2019). Cumulative exposure to a higher socioeconomic position in childhood and adulthood has been associated with a number of positive health outcomes, including higher physical activity level in adulthood (Elhakeem et al., 2017). Thus, a potential outcome of policies and interventions that aim to minimize exposure to socioeconomic adversity may be increased leisure time physical activity among adults, which may be protective against developing chronic pain.

CONCEPTUAL MODELS OF CHRONIC PAIN: PATHOPHYSIOLOGY OF CHRONIC AND RECURRENT PAIN

From a biological standpoint, repetitive episodes of acute pain lead to pain hypersensitivity to help with early detection of pain as a protective mechanism against further injury (Dinakar & Stillman, 2016). Initially, pain is a symptom of possible injury or disease (such as acute inflammation in IBD), but over time it can become a disease in itself. Eventually pain is experienced in the absence of a painful stimulus, or an increased sensation of pain is experienced that is out of proportion to the painful stimulus. This is partially explained by peripheral and central sensitization to pain. Peripheral sensitization occurs when neurotransmitters stimulate the nociceptors and the pain response becomes sustained (Dinakar & Stillman, 2016). Central sensitization occurs on the level of the dorsal horn neurons in the spinal cord due to sustained peripheral inputs over an extended period of time. However, sensitization alone is not enough to explain chronic pain, and a more comprehensive biopsychosocial model that incorporates emotional, cognitive, and behavioral factors that influence the experience of pain is the most successful current approach to understanding pain.

Biopsychosocial Models of Chronic and Recurrent Pain

The biopsychosocial model of chronic pain describes pain as a dynamic interaction among and within the biological, psychological (behavior, emotions, and beliefs), and social factors (cultural norms, socioeconomic position, and social support) personally relevant to the individual. Beliefs, appraisals, mood, and behaviors have been identified as relevant and significant to the pain experience. This model has been used to understand and identify factors that contribute to the development of pain (vulnerability/risk factors) or that prolong pain and disability over time, focusing on individual differences in the overall pain experience to guide assessment and intervention approaches. The biopsychosocial model has helped to disentangle psychosocial factors and has led to targeted psychosocial treatments.

Fear avoidance model. The fear avoidance model of chronic pain describes how individuals experiencing pain may enter a vicious cycle of fear, avoidance, and chronic disability (Crombez et al., 2012). In the fear avoidance model, when pain is perceived as threatening, catastrophic misinterpretation and excessive fear of pain and injury lead to avoidance of physical activity. This circumstance often results in physical deconditioning, decline in mental health, and social isolation that can in turn exacerbate chronic pain (Crombez et al., 2012; Vlaeyen & Linton, 2000). Based on empirical evidence, Asmundson et al. (2012) proposed a pediatric fear avoidance model of chronic pain that acknowledges the interactive effects of child and parental factors in development and maintenance of chronic pain, drawing from other established associations found between parental cognitions and behaviors and child pain experiences (Palermo & Chambers, 2005). This model incorporates the influence of caregiver psychological responses and pain management behaviors in pediatric chronic pain.

Life course model. Developmental or life course models of pain explain factors that contribute to the persistence of pain from childhood to adulthood. Because upwards of 50% of youth will continue to live with chronic pain in adulthood (Kashikar-Zuck et al., 2019; Walker et al., 2010), developmental models play an important role in considering approaches to support pain management across the life course. In a study by Hassett et al. (2013), 17% of adult chronic pain patients reported suffering from chronic pain in childhood or adolescence, with close to 80% indicating that the pain in childhood continued and persisted until adulthood. Several long-term follow-up studies have examined adult outcomes of children with chronic pain, revealing that youth are at high risk for continued chronic pain and adverse developmental and health outcomes, including educational failure, poor vocational functioning, mood disorders, and opioid misuse (Kashikar-Zuck et al., 2014; Murray et al., 2020; Noel et al., 2016). Palermo (2020) proposed a developmental model that links childhood chronic pain to adult chronic pain and adverse adult developmental and health outcomes through effects on emotions (e.g., depression, anxiety), health behaviors (e.g., sleep problems), social and family (e.g., socioeconomic status, parental pain), and neurobiological vulnerabilities. The model is used as an approach to psychosocial prevention and pain management interventions directed at childhood vulnerabilities.

Resilience Factors Associated With Adjustment in Chronic Pain

Resilience to pain is an important factor in adjustment. Resilience mechanisms refer to cognitions, affect, and behaviors used by the individual at the time of the stressor that sustain well-being, aid recovery, and promote new learning/growth. A strengths-based or resiliency approach focuses on both individual cognitive-affective (positive affect, acceptance, and self-efficacy) resources and family and social resources (i.e., social support) that may promote adaptation to pain (Palit et al., 2021).

Cousins et al. (2015) outlined the complex bidirectional interplay of resilience and risk factors in youth with pain: resilience resources, resilience mechanisms, risk factors, and risk mechanisms on the individual and family/social environment level. Resilience resources are relatively stable whereas resilience mechanisms are dynamic and modifiable. Individual resilience mechanisms include pain acceptance (i.e., living life to the fullest according to personal values despite experiencing pain), and social environmental resilience mechanisms include adaptive parent behaviors (i.e., modeling coping behaviors by staying active despite pain). Research is emerging on how to tailor interventions to incorporate resilience-enhancing strategies such as mindfulness, benefit finding, and cultivating strong social support.

ASSESSMENT OF CHRONIC PAIN

Pain assessment is critical in choosing the appropriate treatment and considers the multi-dimensional experience of pain, including its impact on activities of daily life, its emotional impact, and social and contextual factors (e.g., social determinants of health) that affect the child's perception of pain.

Interview and Screening Questions

A comprehensive biopsychosocial assessment of a child with chronic pain consists of a clinical interview with the child and accompanying caregiver and a physical exam and may also include patient-reported measures. Consistent with the biopsychosocial model of pediatric pain, a standard evaluation should include not only the child's medical history and physical examination but also information on the history and functional impact of pain elicited with clinical interview questions and supplemented by questionnaire measures of the child and caregiver as needed. Eccleston et al. (2021) recommended a set of questions for making pain visible and understanding personal impact:

1. What impact does pain have on your life?
2. What is the typical day like for you when you have pain?
3. What would you be doing if your pain was lessened?
4. What are the things you do that make your pain better and the things you do that make your pain worse?
5. What are your concerns and worries about your pain?
6. How would you know that a pain treatment was working for you?
7. What would be a meaningful change for you?

Moreover, the physician should identify and investigate any red flags or clinical indicators of pathologic findings indicative of a specific underlying disease such as JIA or IBD (e.g., bone pain, joint swelling, blood in the stool, weight loss; for further guidance see Liossi & Howard, 2016).

Children who are able to understand and communicate should use an age-appropriate self-report scale to report pain intensity. It is always preferable to use a self-report scale when possible (typically above age 4) as it is considered to be the gold standard given the subjective experience of pain (Eccleston et al., 2021). In a review by Birnie et al. (2019), of 60 available self-report measures of pain intensity, eight were considered of high methodological quality (e.g., validity and reliability) based on the COnsensus based Standards for the selection of health Measurement INstruments (COSMIN) criteria:

- the 11-point Numerical Pain Rating Scale
- the Color Analog Scale
- the Faces Pain Scale–Revised
- the Oucher photographic and numeric scales
- the Pieces of Hurt/Poker Chip Tool
- the Visual Analog Pain Rating Scale
- the Wong-Baker FACES Pain Rating Scale

The evidence for and validity of these scales vary based on a child's age and type of pain. The majority of research on pain scales has been conducted in the context of acute and procedural pain; by contrast, there is a paucity of validation studies of pain scales for evaluation of chronic pain.

Assessment of Pain Interference

Pain interference is a measure of the extent to which pain affects daily activities such as engagement in social, emotional, physical, and recreational activities. There are several well-validated measures of pain interference, including the Functional Disability Inventory (Walker & Greene, 1991), the Child Activity Limitations Interview (Holley et al., 2018; Palermo et al., 2004), and the Patient Reported Outcomes Measurement Information System (PROMIS) Pediatric Pain Interference Scale (Amtmann et al., 2010). They are all brief measures and recommended for assessment of pain interference. For example, the PROMIS Pediatric Pain Interference Scale is an eight-item scale validated for children ages 8 to 17 for self-report and for ages 5 to 17 for parent proxy (Varni et al., 2010). This scale has been validated for evaluating pain interference in multiple chronic conditions (Forrest et al., 2020; Fussner et al., 2019).

Screening for behavioral comorbidities. There is a high concurrence of anxiety and depression in children with chronic pain, and thus it is important to assess these mental health conditions in caring for this patient population. There are multiple measurement tools available to evaluate pediatric anxiety and depressive symptoms, some being multi-item and others single item (Lazor et al., 2017). Some of the more commonly used measures include PROMIS Pediatric Anxiety (Schalet et al., 2016) and Screen for Child Anxiety and Related Emotional Disorders (Birmaher et al., 1997). Some of the commonly used scales for assessing depressive symptoms are Beck Depression Inventory (Beck et al., 1961) and Patient Health Questionnaire-9 (Maurer, 2012).

Screening for sleep disturbances. Children with chronic pain frequently report symptoms of insomnia and lower sleep quality compared with healthy children (Palermo et al., 2011). There are more than 70 tools to evaluate sleep in the pediatric population. The majority of these tools are directed at measuring quality of sleep, identification of sleep pathologies, sleep initiation/maintenance, daytime sleepiness, sleep habits/hygiene, and cognitions/beliefs about sleep (Lewandowski et al., 2011; Sen & Spruyt, 2020). Common measures of sleep disturbances used in children with chronic pain are the Adolescent Sleep Wake Scale (Essner et al., 2015), and the PROMIS Sleep Disturbance Scale (Yu et al., 2012).

Screenings for quality of life. Clinicians may consider multidimensional measures that assess the broad impact of chronic pain on the child, parent, and family. The Bath Adolescent Pain Questionnaire (Eccleston et al., 2005) and Pediatric

Quality of Life Inventory (Varni et al., 1999) are examples. These measures encompass the effect of chronic pain on the child's overall quality of life, as well as the effect of a child's pain on the quality of life of their family members.

Recognizing key outcome domains in chronic pain that are meaningful to children, parents, and providers, the following areas are recommended for assessment following implementation of pain management interventions: pain severity, pain interference, overall well-being, adverse events, mental health, physical functioning, and sleep (Palermo et al., 2021).

CHRONIC PAIN TREATMENT

Families look to their primary care providers to evaluate and treat their child's chronic pain yet providers may feel unsure about how to manage pain and make appropriate referrals (Jandial et al., 2009). In some cases, a clear diagnosis such as JIA or IBD may emerge from the exam and evaluation. However, for the majority of youth, medical evaluation and diagnostic testing can indicate that painful symptoms are not attributed to underlying disease processes, and there may not be a clear next step to assessment or treatment. The lack of clarity around a diagnosis and explanation for their child's pain can create considerable frustration and distress in families, especially if they fear that a medical diagnosis has been missed (diagnostic uncertainty has received some research attention; Neville et al., 2019).

As a result, initial discussions and explanation of chronic pain with the child and their caregiver are critical and should be approached with sensitivity and clarity. The primary care provider plays an important role in educating children and families about the etiology of chronic pain, setting collaborative goals for treatment, and coordinating treatment with an interdisciplinary team of health professionals. An interdisciplinary approach is the reference standard for patients with primary pain disorders as well as chronic pain due to chronic illnesses (Dinakar & Stillman, 2016; Landry et al., 2015). Refer to the section on the role of interdisciplinary pediatric pain clinics for discussion of the role of various providers in caring for children with chronic pain.

In a review of a wide range of pharmacological and nonpharmacological interventions for pediatric chronic pain, Fisher et al. (2022) found that children and adolescents with chronic pain improved in physical functioning with physical and psychological therapies. Although pharmacological therapies such as central and peripheral neuromodulators reduced pain, they did not lead to improved physical functioning (Fisher et al., 2022). Unfortunately, none of the aforementioned therapies improved other core outcome domains such as health-related quality of life, emotional functioning, or sleep. Overall, psychological therapies were found to have the most benefit for children and adolescents with chronic pain; pharmacological and physical therapies were understudied; and pharmaceuticals were overprescribed. More details on specific therapies are provided in the following sections.

Physical Therapy

Physical therapy and exercise play important roles in treatment of children with chronic pain. With physical therapy, the goal is to regain physical functioning despite having pain. As children regain their strength and endurance and become more physically active, they become more functional and start to enjoy activities and lead more meaningful lives. Unfortunately, physical therapy for chronic pain is understudied, with only a few reviews in the literature (Birnie et al., 2020). An evidence-based recommendation for time, intensity, and frequency of physical exercise for patients with chronic pain does not yet exist (Ambrose & Golightly, 2015), but physical exercise is considered a core component of interdisciplinary treatment for pediatric chronic pain.

Other research has examined exercise training within the context of intensive inpatient or outpatient pain treatment programs (Simons et al., 2017). Combined interventions integrating cognitive behavior therapy (CBT) with therapeutic exercise have also shown promising results. For example, a novel pilot intervention integrating CBT and specialized neuromuscular training in adolescents with juvenile fibromyalgia showed enhanced efficacy compared with CBT alone (Kashikar-Zuck et al., 2018).

Psychological Therapies for Chronic Pain: The Role of Pediatric Psychologists

CBT is the most well-studied psychological therapy for chronic pain and has the most evidence showing benefit for children and adolescents (Fisher et al., 2014). Specifically, CBT has been well studied in children with headaches, abdominal pain, mixed chronic pain conditions, and fibromyalgia; benefits have been found for reducing pain frequency and intensity, disability, and anxiety (Fisher et al., 2018). CBT is often implemented by pediatric psychologists with specialized training in pain management, and treatment typically includes multiple components delivered individually to children: pain education, relaxation skills, cognitive strategies, behavioral strategies, and parent training. Parents may be taught strategies for decreasing their own worries, modifying unhelpful beliefs about pain, and encouraging adaptive behaviors (e.g., school attendance) using praise and rewards. (For a detailed CBT protocol for pediatric chronic pain management, see Palermo, 2012.) The goals of CBT are to promote self-efficacy, increase functioning, and reduce maladaptive behavior that may contribute to chronic pain.

A systematic review and meta-analysis of 43 randomized controlled trials examining effects of psychological therapies (delivered face-to-face) for chronic pain management in children (with headache, abdominal pain, neuropathic pain, and musculoskeletal pain) showed that psychological interventions reduced pain symptoms and disability post treatment (Fisher et al., 2018). However, this review found no beneficial effect of psychological therapies on depression and anxiety. This highlights the importance of psychological treatments in overall approach and treatment of children with chronic pain.

There are great disparities in access to pediatric chronic pain treatment based on the family's household income and the limited availability of chronic pain providers, especially in low and middle income countries (Ruhe et al., 2016; Walters et al., 2018). In the United States, families with private insurance are more likely to engage in chronic pain treatment programs (Boppana et al., 2020). Unfortunately there are limited available interdisciplinary pediatric chronic pain programs (about 50 programs exist in the United States), and most families will not have ready access in their own communities. In those communities that have access to chronic pain clinics, children typically experience long wait times during which they feel frustration and anxiety and experience lack of improvement in pain intensity and disability while on the wait-list (Palermo et al., 2019).

Given that specialized face-to-face CBT for chronic pain is not widely available in many communities, internet-based and mobile app programs are being developed to expand access (Palermo et al., 2020). Promising data are emerging on the benefits of internet-delivered family CBT intervention for youth with chronic headache and abdominal and musculoskeletal pain who report greater reduction in pain intensity and increased function compared with youth receiving standard medical care (Palermo et al., 2009, 2016). The evidence base for remotely delivered psychological therapies is rapidly growing for children with chronic pain (Fisher et al., 2019), and future work is needed to make these programs universally available across digital literacy levels, socioeconomic positions, and languages. (See the Resources box for information on available online tools.)

There are other psychological treatments for chronic pain, such as hypnosis, acceptance and commitment therapy, biofeedback, memory reframing, and mindfulness. However, the evidence of their use in children with chronic pain is limited (Eccleston et al., 2021).

Integrative Medicine/Complementary and Alternative Medicine

Integrative medicine (also known as complementary and alternative medicine) modalities such as hypnosis, yoga, acupuncture, and massage are of interest to many patients with chronic pain and have been frequently used clinically as adjunctive interventions (Friedrichsdorf et al., 2016). Some additional mind–body therapies include therapeutic touch, faith healing, aromatherapy, tai chi, and qigong; benefits of these modalities on chronic pain are unclear. The exact mechanisms of how these modalities help with pain are yet to be determined, but they are thought to release endogenous opioids and suppress transmission of pain. Most studies of mind–body therapies have been performed in adults with chronic pain and have shown equivocal findings. The evidence for using these therapies varies across modalities, and more studies with children are needed (Lee et al., 2014) as it is unknown for which pain conditions or ages these modalities may be useful.

Adjunctive Pharmacologic Therapy

In the past, pharmacotherapy was viewed as the primary treatment for chronic pain. This view has fallen out of favor due to low efficacy, limited evidence base, and advancement of the biopsychosocial model of pain. However, pharmacologic treatments remain commonly used for chronic pain despite lack of robust evidence of efficacy (Eccleston et al., 2021; Fisher et al., 2022). There are few randomized controlled trials of pharmacologic treatments in children with chronic pain, and frequently efficacy is extrapolated from adult trials. Pharmaceutical targets for pain management are centrally and peripherally mediated. Some of the commonly used medications include tricyclic antidepressants (amitriptyline and nortriptyline), gabapentinoids (gabapentin and pregabalin), alpha-2 adrenergic receptor agonist (clonidine and dexmedetomidine), selective serotonin reuptake inhibitors, and serotonin and norepinephrine reuptake inhibitors. These drugs have different mechanisms of action and varying targets along the pain pathway. The evidence for using these medications for treatment of pediatric pain is sparse (Friedrichsdorf et al., 2016).

Centers for Disease Control and Prevention guidelines do not discuss whether opioids should be prescribed to children with chronic pain. However, most pain experts recommend that opioids should not be prescribed to children with primary pain disorders. Opioids may provide benefits for some children with chronic pain due to an underlying health condition, but recommendations are to use them in conjunction with nonpharmacologic therapies such as physical therapy, CBT, and so on.

Role of Interdisciplinary Pediatric Pain Clinics, and Developmental Behavioral Pediatrics

Typically housed within tertiary care medical centers, interdisciplinary pediatric pain clinics provide intensive multimodal treatment (e.g., physical, psychological, and complementary and alternative medicine therapies) through outpatient and/or inpatient services. These programs have demonstrated efficacy in improving pain, pain-related disability, and school absenteeism in children with complex and disabling chronic pain (Hechler et al., 2014; Simons et al., 2017) and improving several pediatric chronic pain outcome domains, such as pain intensity, functional disability, school attendance and functioning, and anxiety and depression (Liossi et al., 2019). Unfortunately, dedicated pediatric pain treatment facilities are sparse, with most centers located in major urban cities. For an online international listing of pediatric chronic pain programs, see the Resources at the end of this chapter.

Inpatient interdisciplinary pain rehabilitation is available in only a dozen or so centers in the United States, offering an option for youth who are not benefiting from outpatient treatment or who are severely disabled and unable to participate in outpatient treatment. There is evidence of the efficacy of these programs for improving patient outcomes (Hechler et al., 2015) and for reducing health care utilization and costs. In an analysis performed by Evans et al. (2016), a 3-week inpatient pain rehabilitation program saved approximately $27,119 per family during the year following an inpatient rehabilitation admission based on reduction in self-reported health care utilization and parental missed workdays (Evans et al., 2016). In another study, pain clinic utilization was associated with fewer emergency room visits and hospitalizations and led to hospital savings of $36,228 per patient per year and insurance savings of $11,482 per patient per year (Mahrer et al., 2018).

When an interdisciplinary pain clinic is not available, the developmental behavioral pediatrician can assist in coordination of services with other disciplines in the community (e.g., physical therapy and psychology) and maintain close follow-up with the child and family. In addition, if a child with chronic pain manifests academic or behavioral difficulties, a developmental-behavioral pediatrician can help evaluate for signs of school failure and can help advocate for services on an individualized education plan to provide school-based supports to optimize school functioning.

ROLE OF COVID-19 PANDEMIC ON CHRONIC PAIN

Coronavirus (caused by SARS-CoV-2) spread rapidly around the world in early 2020, resulting in a global COVID-19 pandemic. Clinicians and investigators in the pain community were concerned about the public health impact on individuals with chronic pain (Eccleston et al., 2020). In particular, because health care resources and personnel were redistributed to areas with acute patient care, such as emergency departments and intensive care units, delays of care arose for nonurgent and long-term conditions, including chronic pain (Puntillo et al., 2020). Mobility restrictions due to lockdowns also made health care less accessible.

There is now ample evidence that the COVID-19 pandemic negatively impacted mental health for many people, with epidemiologic studies estimating an additional 53.2 million cases of major depressive disorder and an additional 76.2 million cases of anxiety disorders globally; younger populations were more affected (COVID-19 Mental Disorders Collaborators, 2021). However, less is known about the condition-specific impact for individuals with chronic pain, including the impact on the experience of pain and disability. In pediatric populations with chronic pain, Law et al. (2021) found clinically elevated and persistent anxiety, depression, and insomnia symptoms whereas pain interference remained relatively stable. Minority ethnicity and pandemic-related economic stress were identified as risk factors for poor outcomes.

Positive aspects of the pandemic such as reduced school-related stress and increased family time were also noted by participants. In a community school-age sample in Germany, investigators reported that chronic pain prevalence was lower at the assessment during the COVID-19 pandemic (22.8%) than in the year before the pandemic (29.9%; Rau et al., 2021). Preliminary data from the United States are similar, with reduced rates of chronic pain for children during 2020 across sociodemographic groups (Kapos et al., 2022). Preliminary hypotheses are that reductions in school stress and increased family time may have protective effects, at least initially, and subsequent longitudinal data are needed to understand whether there are rebounds in later years. Despite the aforementioned challenges of the rapidly evolving pandemic that brought unpredictable demands on the health care system, there was a rapid adaptation of telemedicine in efforts to provide medical care, including transformation of virtual pediatric chronic pain clinic care (D'Alessandro et al., 2020). The impact of the pandemic on childhood chronic pain remains unclear, and further studies are needed on access to and efficacy of virtual management of chronic pain conditions.

CONCLUSION

Pediatric chronic pain has immense physical, social, and economic effects on the individual and society. Although we are making strides in understanding chronic pain, significant work remains to be done in uncovering how to prevent and treat chronic pediatric pain effectively. As highlighted by Eccleston et al. (2021), to make an impact on chronic pain in children we must strive toward four transformational goals: to make pain in children matter, to make pain visible, to make pain understood, and to make pain better. Successful pain management requires

(1) an understanding of the multisystemic contexts, informed by developmental science, that are associated with the development and maintenance of chronic pain, and (2) multidisciplinary clinical management by subspecialty providers, including pediatricians, pediatric psychologists, and other health professionals, to help children optimize health and well-being.

RESOURCES

- International Association for the Study of Pain:

    https://www.iasp-pain.org/

    Pain in childhood special interest group website:

    http://childpain.org

    International directory of Pediatric Chronic Pain Programs: This list of dedicated pediatric chronic pain programs in the United States, Canada, and internationally has been developed and maintained since 2012 by Tonya Palermo.

    http://childpain.org/index.php/resources

- WebMAP Mobile: A free app designed to help teens cope with chronic pain; available for download for Apple and Android devices. This app was designed to track pain, provide educational information about chronic pain, and teach relaxation and imagery strategies.

    https://www.seattlechildrens.org/research/centers-programs/child-health-behavior-and-development/labs/pediatric-pain-and-sleep-innovations-lab/resources/

- Comfort Ability:

    https://www.thecomfortability.com

    Program developed by Boston Children's Hospital and Harvard Medical School to help parents and children with chronic or recurrent pain learn strategies to cope with pain and improve their daily functioning.

- Creative Healing for Youth in Pain:

    https://mychyp.org

    Online resource for teens with chronic pain and their parents. Contains educational resources, creative healing experiences, and social support.

- SickKids Online Pediatric Pain Curriculum:

    https://www.sickkids.ca/en/care-services/centres/pain-centre/#oppc

    Aimed at health care professionals and includes a variety of topics, including a section on chronic pain ("Chronic Pain Management: Special Considerations").

- SKIP (Solutions for Kids in Pain):

    https://www.kidsinpain.ca

    Aimed at improving children's pain management in Canada and around the world. See "Pain Management Apps and Online Resources" at

    https://kidsinpain.ca/wp-content/uploads/2021/02/4fdfcf_da931f8a4ad14f2d9591ff41466e0e40-1.pdf

- PROMIS measures website:

    https://www.healthmeasures.net/explore-measurement-systems/promis/obtain-administer-measures

    PROMIS measures are available free and include child self-report (ages 8–17) and parent proxy report (ages 5–17) across multiple domains of functioning relevant to children with chronic pain.

- *The Lancet Child & Adolescent Health* Commission:

    https://www.thelancet.com/commissions/paediatric-pain

References

Afolalu, E. F., Ramlee, F., & Tang, N. K. Y. (2018). Effects of sleep changes on pain-related health outcomes in the general population: A systematic review of longitudinal studies with exploratory meta-analysis. *Sleep Medicine Reviews*, 39, 82–97. https://doi.org/10.1016/j.smrv.2017.08.001

Ambrose, K. R., & Golightly, Y. M. (2015). Physical exercise as non-pharmacological treatment of chronic pain: Why and when. *Best Practice & Research: Clinical Rheumatology, 29*(1), 120–130. https://doi.org/10.1016/j.berh.2015.04.022

Amtmann, D., Cook, K. F., Jensen, M. P., Chen, W. H., Choi, S., Revicki, D., Cella, D., Rothrock, N., Keefe, F., Callahan, L., & Lai, J. S. (2010). Development of a PROMIS item bank to measure pain interference. *Pain, 150*(1), 173–182. https://doi.org/10.1016/j.pain.2010.04.025

Asmundson, G. J., Noel, M., Petter, M., & Parkerson, H. A. (2012). Pediatric fear-avoidance model of chronic pain: Foundation, application and future directions. *Pain Research & Management, 17*(6), 397–405. https://doi.org/10.1155/2012/908061

Beck, A. T., Ward, C. H., Mendelson, M., Mock, J., & Erbaugh, J. (1961). An inventory for measuring depression. *Archives of General Psychiatry, 4*(6), 561–571. https://doi.org/10.1001/archpsyc.1961.01710120031004

Birmaher, B., Khetarpal, S., Brent, D., Cully, M., Balach, L., Kaufman, J., & Neer, S. M. (1997). The Screen for Child Anxiety Related Emotional Disorders (SCARED): Scale construction and psychometric characteristics. *Journal of the American Academy of Child & Adolescent Psychiatry, 36*(4), 545–553. https://doi.org/10.1097/00004583-199704000-00018

Birnie, K. A., Hundert, A. S., Lalloo, C., Nguyen, C., & Stinson, J. N. (2019). Recommendations for selection of self-report pain intensity measures in children and adolescents: A systematic review and quality assessment of measurement properties. *Pain, 160*(1), 5–18. https://doi.org/10.1097/j.pain.0000000000001377

Birnie, K. A., Ouellette, C., Do Amaral, T., & Stinson, J. N. (2020). Mapping the evidence and gaps of interventions for pediatric chronic pain to inform policy, research, and practice: A systematic review and quality assessment of systematic reviews. *Canadian Journal of Pain, 4*(1), 129–148. https://doi.org/10.1080/24740527.2020.1757384

Bohr, A. H., Nielsen, S., Müller, K., Karup Pedersen, F., & Andersen, L. B. (2015). Reduced physical activity in children and adolescents with juvenile idiopathic arthritis despite satisfactory control of inflammation. *Pediatric Rheumatology Online Journal, 13*(1), 57. https://doi.org/10.1186/s12969-015-0053-5

Boppana, S. S., Miller, R., Wrona, A., Tumin, D., Wrona, S., Smith, T. P., Bhalla, T., Kim, S. S., & Tobias, J. D. (2020). Barriers to outpatient pediatric chronic pain clinic participation among referred patients. *Clinical Pediatrics, 59*(9–10), 859–864. https://doi.org/10.1177/0009922820922847

Brandow, A. M., & DeBaun, M. R. (2018). Key components of pain management for children and adults with sickle cell disease. *Hematology/Oncology Clinics of North America, 32*(3), 535–550. https://doi.org/10.1016/j.hoc.2018.01.014

Bronfenbrenner, U. (1979). *The ecology of human development: Experiments by nature and design.* Harvard University Press.

Caes, L., Vervoort, T., Devos, P., Verlooy, J., Benoit, Y., & Goubert, L. (2014). Parental distress and catastrophic thoughts about child pain: Implications for parental protective behavior in the context of child leukemia-related medical procedures. *The Clinical Journal of Pain, 30*(9), 787–799. https://doi.org/10.1097/AJP.0000000000000028

Caes, L., Vervoort, T., Eccleston, C., Vandenhende, M., & Goubert, L. (2011). Parental catastrophizing about child's pain and its relationship with activity restriction: The mediating role of parental distress. *Pain, 152*(1), 212–222. https://doi.org/10.1016/j.pain.2010.10.037

Chitkara, D. K., Talley, N. J., Weaver, A. L., Katusic, S. K., De Schepper, H., Rucker, M. J., & Locke, G. R., III. (2007). Incidence of presentation of common functional gastrointestinal disorders in children from birth to 5 years: A cohort study. *Clinical Gastroenterology and Hepatology, 5*(2), 186–191. https://doi.org/10.1016/j.cgh.2006.06.012

Conte, P. M., Walco, G. A., & Kimura, Y. (2003). Temperament and stress response in children with juvenile primary fibromyalgia syndrome. *Arthritis and Rheumatism, 48*(10), 2923–2930. https://doi.org/10.1002/art.11244

Cousins, L. A., Kalapurakkel, S., Cohen, L. L., & Simons, L. E. (2015). Topical review: Resilience resources and mechanisms in pediatric chronic. *Journal of Pediatric Psychology, 40*(9), 840–845. https://doi.org/10.1093/jpepsy/jsv037

COVID-19 Mental Disorders Collaborators. (2021). Global prevalence and burden of depressive and anxiety disorders in 204 countries and territories in 2020 due to the COVID-19 pandemic. *The Lancet, 398*(10312), 1700–1712. https://doi.org/10.1016/S0140-6736(21)02143-7

Crombez, G., Eccleston, C., Van Damme, S., Vlaeyen, J. W., & Karoly, P. (2012). Fear-avoidance model of chronic pain: The next generation. *The Clinical Journal of Pain, 28*(6), 475–483. https://doi.org/10.1097/AJP.0b013e3182385392

D'Alessandro, L. N., Brown, S. C., Campbell, F., Ruskin, D., Mesaroli, G., Makkar, M., & Stinson, J. N. (2020). Rapid mobilization of a virtual pediatric chronic pain clinic in Canada during the COVID-19 pandemic. *Canadian Journal of Pain, 4*(1), 162–167. https://doi.org/10.1080/24740527.2020.1771688

Datz, H., Tumin, D., Miller, R., Smith, T. P., Bhalla, T., & Tobias, J. D. (2019). Pediatric chronic pain and caregiver burden in a national survey. *Scandinavian Journal of Pain*, 19(1), 109–116. https://doi.org/10.1515/sjpain-2018-0121

De Inocencio, J. (2004). Epidemiology of musculoskeletal pain in primary care. *Archives of Disease in Childhood*, 89(5), 431–434. https://doi.org/10.1136/adc.2003.028860

Dinakar, P., & Stillman, A. M. (2016). Pathogenesis of pain. *Seminars in Pediatric Neurology*, 23(3), 201–208. https://doi.org/10.1016/j.spen.2016.10.003

Eccleston, C., Blyth, F. M., Dear, B. F., Fisher, E. A., Keefe, F. J., Lynch, M. E., Palermo, T. M., Reid, M. C., & Williams, A. C. C. (2020). Managing patients with chronic pain during the COVID-19 outbreak: Considerations for the rapid introduction of remotely supported (eHealth) pain management services. *Pain*, 161(5), 889–893. https://doi.org/10.1097/j.pain.0000000000001885

Eccleston, C., Fisher, E., Howard, R. F., Slater, R., Forgeron, P., Palermo, T. M., Birnie, K. A., Anderson, B. J., Chambers, C. T., Crombez, G., Ljungman, G., Jordan, I., Jordan, Z., Roberts, C., Schechter, N., Sieberg, C. B., Tibboel, D., Walker, S. M., Wilkinson, D., & Wood, C. (2021). Delivering transformative action in paediatric pain: A *Lancet Child & Adolescent Health* Commission. *The Lancet Child & Adolescent Health*, 5(1), 47–87. https://doi.org/10.1016/S2352-4642(20)30277-7

Eccleston, C., Jordan, A., McCracken, L. M., Sleed, M., Connell, H., & Clinch, J. (2005). The Bath Adolescent Pain Questionnaire (BAPQ): Development and preliminary psychometric evaluation of an instrument to assess the impact of chronic pain on adolescents. *Pain*, 118(1–2), 263–270. https://doi.org/10.1016/j.pain.2005.08.025

Elhakeem, A., Hardy, R., Bann, D., Caleyachetty, R., Cosco, T. D., Hayhoe, R. P., Muthuri, S. G., Wilson, R., & Cooper, R. (2017). Intergenerational social mobility and leisure-time physical activity in adulthood: A systematic review. *Journal of Epidemiology and Community Health*, 71(7), 673–680. https://doi.org/10.1136/jech-2016-208052

Essner, B., Noel, M., Myrvik, M., & Palermo, T. (2015). Examination of the factor structure of the Adolescent Sleep-Wake Scale (ASWS). *Behavioral Sleep Medicine*, 13(4), 296–307. https://doi.org/10.1080/15402002.2014.896253

Evans, J. R., Benore, E., & Banez, G. A. (2016). The cost-effectiveness of intensive interdisciplinary pediatric chronic pain rehabilitation. *Journal of Pediatric Psychology*, 41(8), 849–856. https://doi.org/10.1093/jpepsy/jsv100

Evans, S., Taub, R., Tsao, J. C., Meldrum, M., & Zeltzer, L. K. (2010). Sociodemographic factors in a pediatric chronic pain clinic: The roles of age, sex and minority status in pain and health characteristics. *Journal of Pain Management*, 3(3), 273–281. https://www.ncbi.nlm.nih.gov/pubmed/21686073

Finan, P. H., Goodin, B. R., & Smith, M. T. (2013). The association of sleep and pain: An update and a path forward. *The Journal of Pain*, 14(12), 1539–1552. https://doi.org/10.1016/j.jpain.2013.08.007

Fisher, E., Heathcote, L., Palermo, T. M., de C Williams, A. C., Lau, J., & Eccleston, C. (2014). Systematic review and meta-analysis of psychological therapies for children with chronic pain. *Journal of Pediatric Psychology*, 39(8), 763–782. https://doi.org/10.1093/jpepsy/jsu008

Fisher, E., Law, E., Dudeney, J., Eccleston, C., & Palermo, T. M. (2019). Psychological therapies (remotely delivered) for the management of chronic and recurrent pain in children and adolescents. *Cochrane Database of Systematic Reviews*, 2019(4), CD011118. https://doi.org/10.1002/14651858.CD011118.pub3

Fisher, E., Law, E., Dudeney, J., Palermo, T. M., Stewart, G., & Eccleston, C. (2018). Psychological therapies for the management of chronic and recurrent pain in children and adolescents. *Cochrane Database of Systematic Reviews*, 2018(9), CD003968. https://doi.org/10.1002/14651858.CD003968.pub5

Fisher, E., Villanueva, G., Henschke, N., Nevitt, S. J., Zempsky, W., Probyn, K., Buckley, B., Cooper, T. E., Sethna, N., & Eccleston, C. (2022). Efficacy and safety of pharmacological, physical, and psychological interventions for the management of chronic pain in children: A WHO systematic review and meta-analysis. *Pain*, 163(1), e1–e19. https://doi.org/10.1097/j.pain.0000000000002297

Forgeron, P. A., King, S., Stinson, J. N., McGrath, P. J., MacDonald, A. J., & Chambers, C. T. (2010). Social functioning and peer relationships in children and adolescents with chronic pain: A systematic review. *Pain Research & Management*, 15(1), 27–41. https://doi.org/10.1155/2010/820407

Forrest, C. B., Forrest, K. D., Clegg, J. L., de la Motte, A., Amaral, S., Grossman, A. B., & Furth, S. L. (2020). Establishing the content validity of PROMIS pediatric pain interference, fatigue, sleep disturbance, and sleep-related impairment measures in children with chronic kidney disease and Crohn's disease. *Journal of Patient-Reported Outcomes*, 4(1), 11. https://doi.org/10.1186/s41687-020-0178-2

Friedrichsdorf, S. J., Giordano, J., Desai Dakoji, K., Warmuth, A., Daughtry, C., & Schulz, C. A. (2016). Chronic pain in children and adolescents: Diagnosis and treatment of primary pain disorders in head, abdomen, muscles and joints. *Children*, *3*(4), 42. https://doi.org/10.3390/children3040042

Fussner, L. M., Black, W. R., Lynch-Jordan, A., Morgan, E. M., Ting, T. V., & Kashikar-Zuck, S. (2019). Utility of the PROMIS Pediatric Pain Interference Scale in juvenile fibromyalgia. *Journal of Pediatric Psychology*, *44*(4), 436–441. https://doi.org/10.1093/jpepsy/jsy110

Fussner, L. M., Schild, C., Holley, A. L., & Wilson, A. C. (2018). Parent chronic pain and mental health symptoms impact responses to children's pain. *Canadian Journal of Pain*, *2*(1), 258–265. https://doi.org/10.1080/24740527.2018.1518119

Gaskin, D. J., & Richard, P. (2012). The economic costs of pain in the United States. *The Journal of Pain*, *13*(8), 715–724. https://doi.org/10.1016/j.jpain.2012.03.009

Goyal, M. K., Johnson, T. J., Chamberlain, J. M., Cook, L., Webb, M., Drendel, A. L., Alessandrini, E., Bajaj, L., Lorch, S., Grundmeier, R. W., Alpern, E. R., & the Pediatric Emergency Care Applied Research Network (PECARN). (2020). Racial and ethnic differences in emergency department pain management of children with fractures. *Pediatrics*, *145*(5), e20193370. https://doi.org/10.1542/peds.2019-3370

Green, C. R., Anderson, K. O., Baker, T. A., Campbell, L. C., Decker, S., Fillingim, R. B., Kaloukalani, D. A., Lasch, K. E., Myers, C., Tait, R. C., Todd, K. H., & Vallerand, A. H. (2003). The unequal burden of pain: Confronting racial and ethnic disparities in pain. *Pain Medicine*, *4*(3), 277–294. https://doi.org/10.1046/j.1526-4637.2003.03034.x

Groenewald, C. B., Essner, B. S., Wright, D., Fesinmeyer, M. D., & Palermo, T. M. (2014). The economic costs of chronic pain among a cohort of treatment-seeking adolescents in the United States. *The Journal of Pain*, *15*(9), 925–933. https://doi.org/10.1016/j.jpain.2014.06.002

Guedj, R., Marini, M., Kossowsky, J., Berde, C. B., Kimia, A. A., & Fleegler, E. W. (2021). Racial and ethnic disparities in pain management of children with limb fractures or suspected appendicitis: A retrospective cross-sectional study. *Frontiers in Pediatrics*, *9*, 652854. https://doi.org/10.3389/fped.2021.652854

Harrison, L. E., Timmers, I., Heathcote, L. C., Fisher, E., Tanna, V., Duarte Silva Bans, T., & Simons, L. E. (2020). Parent responses to their child's: Systematic review and meta-analysis of measures. *Journal of Pediatric Psychology*, *45*(3), 281–298. https://doi.org/10.1093/jpepsy/jsaa005

Hassett, A. L., Hilliard, P. E., Goesling, J., Clauw, D. J., Harte, S. E., & Brummett, C. M. (2013). Reports of chronic pain in childhood and adolescence among patients at a tertiary care pain clinic. *The Journal of Pain*, *14*(11), 1390–1397. https://doi.org/10.1016/j.jpain.2013.06.010

Headache Classification Committee of the International Headache Society. (2013). The international classification of headache disorders (3rd ed., beta version). *Cephalalgia*, *33*(9), 629–808. https://doi.org/10.1177/0333102413485658

Hechler, T., Kanstrup, M., Holley, A. L., Simons, L. E., Wicksell, R., Hirschfeld, G., & Zernikow, B. (2015). Systematic review on intensive interdisciplinary pain treatment of children with chronic pain. *Pediatrics*, *136*(1), 115–127. https://doi.org/10.1542/peds.2014-3319

Hechler, T., Ruhe, A. K., Schmidt, P., Hirsch, J., Wager, J., Dobe, M., Krummenauer, F., & Zernikow, B. (2014). Inpatient-based intensive interdisciplinary pain treatment for highly impaired children with severe chronic pain: Randomized controlled trial of efficacy and economic effects. *Pain*, *155*(1), 118–128. https://doi.org/10.1016/j.pain.2013.09.015

Hechler, T., Vervoort, T., Hamann, M., Tietze, A. L., Vocks, S., Goubert, L., Hermann, C., Wager, J., Blankenburg, M., Schroeder, S., & Zernikow, B. (2011). Parental catastrophizing about their child's chronic pain: Are mothers and fathers different? *European Journal of Pain*, *15*(5), 515.e1–515.e9. https://doi.org/10.1016/j.ejpain.2010.09.015

Holley, A. L., Zhou, C., Wilson, A. C., Hainsworth, K., & Palermo, T. M. (2018). The CALI-9: A brief measure for assessing activity limitations in children and adolescents with chronic pain. *Pain*, *159*(1), 48–56. https://doi.org/10.1097/j.pain.0000000000001063

Huguet, A., & Miró, J. (2008). The severity of chronic pediatric pain: An epidemiological study. *The Journal of Pain*, *9*(3), 226–236. https://doi.org/10.1016/j.jpain.2007.10.015

Huguet, A., Tougas, M. E., Hayden, J., McGrath, P. J., Stinson, J. N., & Chambers, C. T. (2016). Systematic review with meta-analysis of childhood and adolescent risk and prognostic factors for musculoskeletal pain. *Pain*, *157*(12), 2640–2656. https://doi.org/10.1097/j.pain.0000000000000685

Hyams, J. S., Di Lorenzo, C., Saps, M., Shulman, R. J., Staiano, A., & van Tilburg, M. (2016). Functional disorders: Child/adolescent. *Gastroenterology*, *150*(6), 1456–1468. https://doi.org/10.1053/j.gastro.2016.02.015

Jandial, S., Myers, A., Wise, E., & Foster, H. E. (2009). Doctors likely to encounter children with musculoskeletal complaints have low confidence in their clinical skills. *Journal of Pediatrics*, *154*(2), 267–271. https://doi.org/10.1016/j.jpeds.2008.08.013

Jastrowski Mano, K. E., Khan, K. A., Ladwig, R. J., & Weisman, S. J. (2011). The impact of pediatric chronic pain on parents' health-related quality of life and family functioning: Reliability and validity of the PedsQL 4.0 Family Impact Module. *Journal of Pediatric Psychology*, *36*(5), 517–527. https://doi.org/10.1093/jpepsy/jsp099

Kapos, F. P., Palermo, T. M., & Groenewald, C. B. (2022). Prevalence of chronic pain among school-aged children in the United States during the first year of the COVID-19 pandemic: A nationally representative study. *Journal of Pain*, *23*(5), 51. https://doi.org/10.1016/j.jpain.2022.03.194

Kashikar-Zuck, S., Black, W. R., Pfeiffer, M., Peugh, J., Williams, S. E., Ting, T. V., Thomas, S., Kitchen, K., & Myer, G. D. (2018). Pilot randomized trial of integrated cognitive-behavioral therapy and neuromuscular training for juvenile fibromyalgia: The FIT Teens Program. *The Journal of Pain*, *19*(9), 1049–1062. https://doi.org/10.1016/j.jpain.2018.04.003

Kashikar-Zuck, S., Cunningham, N., Peugh, J., Black, W. R., Nelson, S., Lynch-Jordan, A. M., Pfeiffer, M., Tran, S. T., Ting, T. V., Arnold, L. M., Carle, A., Noll, J., Powers, S. W., & Lovell, D. J. (2019). Long-term outcomes of adolescents with juvenile-onset fibromyalgia into adulthood and impact of depressive symptoms on functioning over time. *Pain*, *160*(2), 433–441. https://doi.org/10.1097/j.pain.0000000000001415

Kashikar-Zuck, S., Cunningham, N., Sil, S., Bromberg, M. H., Lynch-Jordan, A. M., Strotman, D., Peugh, J., Noll, J., Ting, T. V., Powers, S. W., Lovell, D. J., & Arnold, L. M. (2014). Long-term outcomes of adolescents with juvenile-onset fibromyalgia in early adulthood. *Pediatrics*, *133*(3), e592–e600. https://doi.org/10.1542/peds.2013-2220

Kashikar-Zuck, S., & Ting, T. V. (2014). Juvenile fibromyalgia: Current status of research and future developments. *Nature Reviews Rheumatology*, *10*(2), 89–96. https://doi.org/10.1038/nrrheum.2013.177

Kelly, M., Strelzik, J., Langdon, R., & DiSabella, M. (2018). Pediatric headache: Overview. *Current Opinion in Pediatrics*, *30*(6), 748–754. https://doi.org/10.1097/MOP.0000000000000688

King, S., Chambers, C. T., Huguet, A., MacNevin, R. C., McGrath, P. J., Parker, L., & MacDonald, A. J. (2011). The epidemiology of chronic pain in children and adolescents revisited: A systematic review. *Pain*, *152*(12), 2729–2738. https://doi.org/10.1016/j.pain.2011.07.016

Korterink, J. J., Diederen, K., Benninga, M. A., & Tabbers, M. M. (2015). Epidemiology of pediatric functional abdominal pain disorders: A meta-analysis. *PLOS ONE*, *10*(5), e0126982. https://doi.org/10.1371/journal.pone.0126982

Landry, B. W., Fischer, P. R., Driscoll, S. W., Koch, K. M., Harbeck-Weber, C., Mack, K. J., Wilder, R. T., Bauer, B. A., & Brandenburg, J. E. (2015). Managing chronic pain in children and adolescents: A clinical review. *PM&R*, *7*(115, Suppl.), S295–S315. https://doi.org/10.1016/j.pmrj.2015.09.006

Langer, S. L., Romano, J. M., Mancl, L., & Levy, R. L. (2014). Parental catastrophizing partially mediates the association between parent-reported child pain behavior and parental protective responses. *Pain Research and Treatment*, *2014*, 751097. https://doi.org/10.1155/2014/751097

Law, E. F., Zhou, C., Seung, F., Perry, F., & Palermo, T. M. (2021). Longitudinal study of early adaptation to the coronavirus disease pandemic among youth with chronic pain and their parents: Effects of direct exposures and economic stress. *Pain*, *162*(7), 2132–2144. https://doi.org/10.1097/j.pain.0000000000002290

Lazor, T., Tigelaar, L., Pole, J. D., De Souza, C., Tomlinson, D., & Sung, L. (2017). Instruments to measure anxiety in children, adolescents, and young adults with cancer: A systematic review. *Supportive Care in Cancer*, *25*(9), 2921–2931. https://doi.org/10.1007/s00520-017-3743-3

Lee, C., Crawford, C., Hickey, A., & Active Self-Care Therapies for Pain (PACT) Working Group. (2014). Mind-body therapies for the self-management of chronic pain symptoms. *Pain Medicine*, *15*(Suppl. 1), S21–S39. https://doi.org/10.1111/pme.12383

Levy, R. L., Langer, S. L., & Whitehead, W. E. (2007). Social learning contributions to the etiology and treatment of functional abdominal pain and inflammatory bowel disease in children and adults. *World Journal of Gastroenterology*, *13*(17), 2397–2403. https://doi.org/10.3748/wjg.v13.i17.2397

Lewandowski, A. S., Toliver-Sokol, M., & Palermo, T. M. (2011). Evidence-based review of subjective pediatric sleep measures. *Journal of Pediatric Psychology*, *36*(7), 780–793. https://doi.org/10.1093/jpepsy/jsq119

Liossi, C., & Howard, R. F. (2016). Pediatric chronic pain: Biopsychosocial assessment and formulation. *Pediatrics*, *138*(5), e20160331. https://doi.org/10.1542/peds.2016-0331

Liossi, C., Johnstone, L., Lilley, S., Caes, L., Williams, G., & Schoth, D. E. (2019). Effectiveness of interdisciplinary interventions in paediatric chronic pain management: A systematic review and subset meta-analysis. *British Journal of Anaesthesia*, *123*(2), e359–e371. https://doi.org/10.1016/j.bja.2019.01.024

Logan, D. E., Simons, L. E., & Carpino, E. A. (2012). Too sick for school? Parent influences on school functioning among children with chronic pain.

Pain, 153(2), 437–443. https://doi.org/10.1016/j.pain.2011.11.004

Logan, D. E., Simons, L. E., Stein, M. J., & Chastain, L. (2008). School impairment in adolescents with chronic pain. The Journal of Pain, 9(5), 407–416. https://doi.org/10.1016/j.jpain.2007.12.003

Lynch-Jordan, A. M., Kashikar-Zuck, S., & Goldschneider, K. R. (2010). Parent perceptions of adolescent pain expression: The adolescent pain behavior questionnaire. Pain, 151(3), 834–842. https://doi.org/10.1016/j.pain.2010.09.025

Lynch-Jordan, A. M., Kashikar-Zuck, S., Szabova, A., & Goldschneider, K. R. (2013). The interplay of parent and adolescent catastrophizing and its impact on adolescents' pain, functioning, and pain behavior. The Clinical Journal of Pain, 29(8), 681–688. https://doi.org/10.1097/AJP.0b013e3182757720

Mahrer, N. E., Gold, J. I., Luu, M., & Herman, P. M. (2018). A cost-analysis of an interdisciplinary pediatric chronic pain clinic. The Journal of Pain, 19(2), 158–165. https://doi.org/10.1016/j.jpain.2017.09.008

Manworren, R. C., & Stinson, J. (2016). Pediatric pain measurement, assessment, and evaluation. Seminars in Pediatric Neurology, 23(3), 189–200. https://doi.org/10.1016/j.spen.2016.10.001

Martí-Carvajal, A. J., Solà, I., & Agreda-Pérez, L. H. (2019). Treatment for avascular necrosis of bone in people with sickle cell disease. Cochrane Database of Systematic Reviews, 2019(12), CD004344. https://doi.org/10.1002/14651858.CD004344.pub7

Maurer, D. M. (2012). Screening for depression. American Family Physician, 85(2), 139–144. https://www.ncbi.nlm.nih.gov/pubmed/22335214

Miller, M. M., Williams, A. E., Zapolski, T. C. B., Rand, K. L., & Hirsh, A. T. (2020). Assessment and treatment recommendations for pediatric pain: The influence of patient race, patient gender, and provider pain-related attitudes. The Journal of Pain, 21(1–2), 225–237. https://doi.org/10.1016/j.jpain.2019.07.002

Murphy, L. K., de la Vega, R., Kohut, S. A., Kawamura, J. S., Levy, R. L., & Palermo, T. M. (2021). Systematic review: Psychosocial correlates of pain in pediatric inflammatory bowel disease. Inflammatory Bowel Diseases, 27(5), 697–710. https://doi.org/10.1093/ibd/izaa115

Murray, C. B., Groenewald, C. B., de la Vega, R., & Palermo, T. M. (2020). Long-term impact of adolescent chronic pain on young adult educational, vocational, and social outcomes. Pain, 161(2), 439–445. https://doi.org/10.1097/j.pain.0000000000001732

Muthuri, S. G., Kuh, D., & Cooper, R. (2018). Longitudinal profiles of back pain across adulthood and their relationship with childhood factors: Evidence from the 1946 British birth cohort. Pain, 159(4), 764–774. https://doi.org/10.1097/j.pain.0000000000001143

Neville, A., Jordan, A., Beveridge, J. K., Pincus, T., & Noel, M. (2019). Diagnostic uncertainty in youth with chronic pain and their parents. The Journal of Pain, 20(9), 1080–1090. https://doi.org/10.1016/j.jpain.2019.03.004

Nicholas, M., Vlaeyen, J. W. S., Rief, W., Barke, A., Aziz, Q., Benoliel, R., Cohen, M., Evers, S., Giamberardino, M. A., Goebel, A., Korwisi, B., Perrot, S., Svensson, P., Wang, S. J., Treede, R. D., Pain, I. T. C. C., & the IASP Taskforce for the Classification of Chronic Pain. (2019). The IASP classification of chronic pain for ICD-11: Chronic primary pain. Pain, 160(1), 28–37. https://doi.org/10.1097/j.pain.0000000000001390

Noel, M., Groenewald, C. B., Beals-Erickson, S. E., Gebert, J. T., & Palermo, T. M. (2016). Chronic pain in adolescence and internalizing mental health disorders: A nationally representative study. Pain, 157(6), 1333–1338. https://doi.org/10.1097/j.pain.0000000000000522

Palermo, T. M. (2012). Cognitive-behavioral therapy for chronic pain in children and adolescents. Oxford University Press. https://doi.org/10.1093/med:psych/9780199763979.001.0001

Palermo, T. M. (2020). Pain prevention and management must begin in childhood: The key role of psychological interventions. Pain, 161(Suppl. 1), S114–S121. https://doi.org/10.1097/j.pain.0000000000001862

Palermo, T. M., & Chambers, C. T. (2005). Parent and family factors in pediatric chronic pain and disability: An integrative approach. Pain, 119(1–3), 1–4. https://doi.org/10.1016/j.pain.2005.10.027

Palermo, T. M., de la Vega, R., Murray, C., Law, E., & Zhou, C. (2020). A digital health psychological intervention (WebMAP Mobile) for children and adolescents with chronic pain: Results of a hybrid effectiveness-implementation stepped-wedge cluster randomized trial. Pain, 161(12), 2763–2774. https://doi.org/10.1097/j.pain.0000000000001994

Palermo, T. M., Law, E. F., Fales, J., Bromberg, M. H., Jessen-Fiddick, T., & Tai, G. (2016). Internet-delivered cognitive-behavioral treatment for adolescents with chronic pain and their parents: A randomized controlled multicenter trial. Pain, 157(1), 174–185. https://doi.org/10.1097/j.pain.0000000000000348

Palermo, T. M., Putnam, J., Armstrong, G., & Daily, S. (2007). Adolescent autonomy and family functioning are associated with headache-related disability.

The Clinical Journal of Pain, 23(5), 458–465. https://doi.org/10.1097/AJP.0b013e31805f70e2

Palermo, T. M., Slack, M., Zhou, C., Aaron, R., Fisher, E., & Rodriguez, S. (2019). Waiting for a pediatric chronic pain clinic evaluation: A prospective study characterizing wait times and symptom trajectories. *The Journal of Pain*, 20(3), 339–347. https://doi.org/10.1016/j.jpain.2018.09.009

Palermo, T. M., Valrie, C. R., & Karlson, C. W. (2014). Family and parent influences on pediatric chronic pain: A developmental perspective. *American Psychologist*, 69(2), 142–152. https://doi.org/10.1037/a0035216

Palermo, T. M., Walco, G. A., Paladhi, U. R., Birnie, K. A., Crombez, G., de la Vega, R., Eccleston, C., Kashikar-Zuck, S., & Stone, A. L. (2021). Core outcome set for pediatric chronic pain clinical trials: Results from a Delphi poll and consensus meeting. *Pain*, 162(10), 2539–2547. https://doi.org/10.1097/j.pain.0000000000002241

Palermo, T. M., Wilson, A. C., Lewandowski, A. S., Toliver-Sokol, M., & Murray, C. B. (2011). Behavioral and psychosocial factors associated with insomnia in adolescents with chronic pain. *Pain*, 152(1), 89–94. https://doi.org/10.1016/j.pain.2010.09.035

Palermo, T. M., Wilson, A. C., Peters, M., Lewandowski, A., & Somhegyi, H. (2009). Randomized controlled trial of an internet-delivered family cognitive-behavioral therapy intervention for children and adolescents with chronic pain. *Pain*, 146(1), 205–213. https://doi.org/10.1016/j.pain.2009.07.034

Palermo, T. M., Witherspoon, D., Valenzuela, D., & Drotar, D. D. (2004). Development and validation of the Child Activity Limitations Interview: A measure of pain-related functional impairment in school-age children and adolescents. *Pain*, 109(3), 461–470. https://doi.org/10.1016/j.pain.2004.02.023

Palit, S., Palermo, T. M., Fillingim, R. B., & Bartley, E. J. (2021). Topical review: Examining multidomain pain resilience in late adolescents and young adults. *Journal of Pediatric Psychology*, 46(3), 280–285. https://doi.org/10.1093/jpepsy/jsaa108

Prego-Domínguez, J., Khazaeipour, Z., Mallah, N., & Takkouche, B. (2021). Socioeconomic status and occurrence of chronic pain: A meta-analysis. *Rheumatology*, 60(3), 1091–1105. https://doi.org/10.1093/rheumatology/keaa758

Puntillo, F., Giglio, M., Brienza, N., Viswanath, O., Urits, I., Kaye, A. D., Pergolizzi, J., Paladini, A., & Varrassi, G. (2020). Impact of COVID-19 pandemic on chronic pain management: Looking for the best way to deliver care. *Best Practice & Research Clinical Anaesthesiology*, 34(3), 529–537. https://doi.org/10.1016/j.bpa.2020.07.001

Raja, S. N., Carr, D. B., Cohen, M., Finnerup, N. B., Flor, H., Gibson, S., Keefe, F. J., Mogil, J. S., Ringkamp, M., Sluka, K. A., Song, X. J., Stevens, B., Sullivan, M. D., Tutelman, P. R., Ushida, T., & Vader, K. (2020). The revised International Association for the Study of Pain definition of pain: Concepts, challenges, and compromises. *Pain*, 161(9), 1976–1982. https://doi.org/10.1097/j.pain.0000000000001939

Rau, L. M., Grothus, S., Sommer, A., Grochowska, K., Claus, B. B., Zernikow, B., & Wager, J. (2021). Chronic pain in schoolchildren and its association with psychological wellbeing before and during the COVID-19 pandemic. *Journal of Adolescent Health*, 69(5), 721–728. https://doi.org/10.1016/j.jadohealth.2021.07.027

Roth-Isigkeit, A., Thyen, U., Stöven, H., Schwarzenberger, J., & Schmucker, P. (2005). Pain among children and adolescents: Restrictions in daily living and triggering factors. *Pediatrics*, 115(2), e152–e162. https://doi.org/10.1542/peds.2004-0682

Ruhe, A. K., Wager, J., Hirschfeld, G., & Zernikow, B. (2016). Household income determines access to specialized pediatric chronic pain treatment in Germany. *BMC Health Services Research*, 16(1), 140. https://doi.org/10.1186/s12913-016-1403-9

Saito, Y. A., Petersen, G. M., Larson, J. J., Atkinson, E. J., Fridley, B. L., de Andrade, M., Locke, G. R., III, Zimmerman, J. M., Almazar-Elder, A. E., & Talley, N. J. (2010). Familial aggregation of irritable bowel syndrome: A family case-control study. *The American Journal of Gastroenterology*, 105(4), 833–841. https://doi.org/10.1038/ajg.2010.116

Schalet, B. D., Pilkonis, P. A., Yu, L., Dodds, N., Johnston, K. L., Yount, S., Riley, W., & Cella, D. (2016). Clinical validity of PROMIS depression, anxiety, and anger across diverse clinical samples. *Journal of Clinical Epidemiology*, 73, 119–127. https://doi.org/10.1016/j.jclinepi.2015.08.036

Sen, T., & Spruyt, K. (2020). Pediatric sleep tools: An updated literature review. *Frontiers in Psychiatry*, 11, 317. https://doi.org/10.3389/fpsyt.2020.00317

Simons, L. E., Sieberg, C. B., Conroy, C., Randall, E. T., Shulman, J., Borsook, D., Berde, C., Sethna, N. F., & Logan, D. E. (2017). Children with chronic pain: Response trajectories after intensive pain rehabilitation treatment. *The Journal of Pain*, 19(2), 207–218. https://doi.org/10.1016/j.jpain.2017.10.005

Sinatra, R. (2010). Causes and consequences of inadequate management of acute pain. *Pain Medicine*, 11(12), 1859–1871. https://doi.org/10.1111/j.1526-4637.2010.00983.x

Smith, B. H., Fors, E. A., Korwisi, B., Barke, A., Cameron, P., Colvin, L., Richardson, C., Rief, W., Treede, R. D., & the IASP Taskforce for the Classification of Chronic Pain. (2019). The IASP classification of chronic pain for *ICD-11*: Applicability in primary care. *Pain, 160*(1), 83–87. https://doi.org/10.1097/j.pain.0000000000001360

Stone, A. L., & Wilson, A. C. (2016). Transmission of risk from parents with chronic pain to offspring: An integrative conceptual model. *Pain, 157*(12), 2628–2639. https://doi.org/10.1097/j.pain.0000000000000637

Tegethoff, M., Belardi, A., Stalujanis, E., & Meinlschmidt, G. (2015). Comorbidity of mental disorders and chronic pain: Chronology of onset in adolescents of a national representative cohort. *The Journal of Pain, 16*(10), 1054–1064. https://doi.org/10.1016/j.jpain.2015.06.009

Treede, R. D., Rief, W., Barke, A., Aziz, Q., Bennett, M. I., Benoliel, R., Cohen, M., Evers, S., Finnerup, N. B., First, M. B., Giamberardino, M. A., Kaasa, S., Kosek, E., Lavand'homme, P., Nicholas, M., Perrot, S., Scholz, J., Schug, S., Smith, B. H., ... Wang, S. J. (2015). A classification of chronic pain for *ICD-11*. *Pain, 156*(6), 1003–1007. https://doi.org/10.1097/j.pain.0000000000000160

Valrie, C. R., Bromberg, M. H., Palermo, T., & Schanberg, L. E. (2013). A systematic review of sleep in pediatric pain populations. *Journal of Developmental and Behavioral Pediatrics, 34*(2), 120–128. https://doi.org/10.1097/DBP.0b013e31827d5848

Varni, J. W., Seid, M., & Rode, C. A. (1999). The PedsQL: Measurement model for the pediatric quality of life inventory. *Medical Care, 37*(2), 126–139. https://doi.org/10.1097/00005650-199902000-00003

Varni, J. W., Stucky, B. D., Thissen, D., Dewitt, E. M., Irwin, D. E., Lai, J. S., Yeatts, K., & Dewalt, D. A. (2010). PROMIS Pediatric Pain Interference Scale: An item response theory analysis of the pediatric pain item bank. *The Journal of Pain, 11*(11), 1109–1119. https://doi.org/10.1016/j.jpain.2010.02.005

Vinall, J., Pavlova, M., Asmundson, G. J., Rasic, N., & Noel, M. (2016). Mental health comorbidities in pediatric chronic pain: A narrative review of epidemiology, models, neurobiological mechanisms and treatment. *Children, 3*(4), 40. https://doi.org/10.3390/children3040040

Vlaeyen, J. W. S., & Linton, S. J. (2000). Fear-avoidance and its consequences in chronic musculoskeletal pain: A state of the art. *Pain, 85*(3), 317–332. https://doi.org/10.1016/S0304-3959(99)00242-0

Walker, L. S., Dengler-Crish, C. M., Rippel, S., & Bruehl, S. (2010). Functional abdominal pain in childhood and adolescence increases risk for chronic pain in adulthood. *Pain, 150*(3), 568–572. https://doi.org/10.1016/j.pain.2010.06.018

Walker, L. S., & Greene, J. W. (1991). The functional disability inventory: Measuring a neglected dimension of child health status. *Journal of Pediatric Psychology, 16*(1), 39–58. https://doi.org/10.1093/jpepsy/16.1.39

Walters, C. B., Kynes, J. M., Sobey, J., Chimhundu-Sithole, T., & McQueen, K. A. K. (2018). Chronic pediatric pain in low- and middle-income countries. *Children, 5*(9), Article 113. https://doi.org/10.3390/children5090113

Watson, K. L., Jr., Kim, S. C., Boyle, B. M., & Saps, M. (2017). Prevalence and impact of functional abdominal pain in children with inflammatory bowel diseases (IBD-FAPD). *Journal of Pediatric Gastroenterology and Nutrition, 65*(2), 212–217. https://doi.org/10.1097/MPG.0000000000001479

Whitehead, W. E., Fedoravicius, A. S., Blackwell, B., & Wooley, S. (1979). A behavioral conceptualization of psychosomatic illness: Psychosomatic symptoms as learned responses. In J. R. McNamara (Ed.), *Behavioral approaches in medicine: Application and analysis* (pp. 65–99). Plenum. https://doi.org/10.1007/978-1-4615-9122-1_4

Whitehead, W. E., Winget, C., Fedoravicius, A. S., Wooley, S., & Blackwell, B. (1982). Learned illness behavior in patients with irritable bowel syndrome and peptic ulcer. *Digestive Diseases and Sciences, 27*(3), 202–208. https://doi.org/10.1007/BF01296915

Wilson, A. C., & Palermo, T. M. (2012). Physical activity and function in adolescents with chronic pain: A controlled study using actigraphy. *The Journal of Pain, 13*(2), 121–130. https://doi.org/10.1016/j.jpain.2011.08.008

World Health Organization. (2019). *International statistical classification of diseases and related health problems* (11th ed.). https://icd.who.int/

Yu, L., Buysse, D. J., Germain, A., Moul, D. E., Stover, A., Dodds, N. E., Johnston, K. L., & Pilkonis, P. A. (2012). Development of short forms from the PROMIS™ sleep disturbance and sleep-related impairment item banks. *Behavioral Sleep Medicine, 10*(1), 6–24. https://doi.org/10.1080/15402002.2012.636266

PEDIATRIC MEDICAL TRAUMATIC STRESS

Melissa Carson, Joshua Kallman, and Douglas Vanderbilt

Pediatric medical traumatic stress (PMTS) encompasses a host of "psychological and physiological responses of children and their families to pain, injury, serious illness, medical procedures, and invasive or frightening treatment experiences" (National Child Traumatic Stress Network, n.d.-b, para. 1). The consequences of unrecognized and persistent PMTS in the long-term may be widespread and could include avoidance of seeking appropriate medical care to avoid re-experiencing the medical trauma, which may lead to delays in medical care and more significant medical trauma later once care is finally sought (Kazak et al., 2006).

There are a few conceptual models, largely informed by foundational theories in developmental science, that seek to characterize the trajectory of PMTS and identify key risk and protective factors. Central to the understanding of these conceptual models is the idea that medical traumatic events happen to children in the context of a family system and that both child and family characteristics influence one's reaction to a traumatic event. A complex set of factors determines whether a particular illness, injury, or intervention will become traumatic. Some factors relate directly to the objective characteristics of the illness, injury, or medical event, such as the severity and chronicity of the medical condition, the prognosis of the condition, the presence of potentially life-threatening or painful experiences, and the need for invasive procedures (Kazak et al., 2006). Subjective factors, such as one's developmentally based interpretation of the severity of the medical event and the level of child and parental distress, also play a critical role in determining whether the potential traumatic event (PTE) will lead to clinically significant PMTS (Balluffi et al., 2004).

In this chapter, we define and discuss the epidemiology of PMTS, introduce conceptual models for PMTS, describe common clinical conditions associated with PMTS, discuss risks and protective factors, explore common outcomes, and finally, turn to assessment and treatment interventions, with an emphasis on the roles of pediatric psychology and developmental-behavioral pediatrics in the assessment and management of PMTS. Understanding the complex, multilevel factors contributing to the development of PMTS is critical to inform multidisciplinary interventions in both clinical and research settings so that the field can better prevent, recognize, and treat traumatic stress seen in medical environments.

DEFINITION, SYMPTOMS, AND EPIDEMIOLOGY OF PEDIATRIC MEDICAL TRAUMATIC STRESS

It is important to distinguish PMTS from posttraumatic stress symptoms (PTSS), acute stress disorder, and posttraumatic stress disorder (PTSD). PMTS is the overarching term for a wide variety of distressing physiological and psychological responses to a medical event or condition that can occur in the child experiencing the medical trauma or in a family member of the child experiencing the medical trauma (Price et al., 2016). PMTS may or may not result in PTSS, which includes a wide variety of subdiagnostic symptoms of PTSD that are not severe or comprehensive enough to meet the diagnostic criteria for acute stress disorder or PTSD (Price et al., 2016). If it is severe enough, PMTS may also result in acute stress disorder or PTSD, but it does not have to. Acute stress disorder and PTSD are clinical diagnoses based on criteria from the *Diagnostic and Statistical Manual of Mental Disorders*, 5th edition (*DSM-5*; American Psychiatric Association, 2013). While acute stress disorder and PTSD may result from exposure to a wide variety of both medical and nonmedical traumas, PMTS refers specifically to the distressing physiological and psychological responses that may result from exposure to a medical event or treatment of a medical event. Unlike acute stress disorder and PTSD, PMTS does not have specific, agreed-upon diagnostic criteria and can be thought of more as a clinical spectrum of PTSS that may result from acute or chronic medical trauma.

Children frequently undergo intensive and painful medical procedures for a wide variety of illnesses and injuries. There are 5.9 million U.S. pediatric hospital admissions annually (Witt et al., 2014). Rates of pediatric hospitalization in other countries are variable but these admissions are still quite common. Pediatric hospital admission rates among seven European countries ranged from 9.41 admissions per 100 person-years in Spain to 19.59 admissions per 100 person-years in Germany (Adetunji et al., 2020). It is estimated that 1.5% of pediatric hospital admissions include time in an intensive care unit (ICU; Ibiebele et al., 2018). The medical events leading to these hospital admissions and resultant interventions and treatments can lead to PMTS. Since PMTS refers to a spectrum of posttraumatic responses to medical trauma, the true epidemiology of PMTS is unclear. However, there is much data investigating rates of PTSS, acute stress disorder, and PTSD among children who have experienced medical trauma and their families. It has been estimated that about one-fifth to one-third of adolescents hospitalized for physical injuries will go on to develop PTSD (Zatzick et al., 2006). About 10% to 15% of parents of children with a serious childhood injury or illness go on to develop clinically significant levels of PTSS (Muscara et al., 2018).

OBJECTIVE NATURE OF THE TRAUMA, AND RISK FOR THE DEVELOPMENT OF PEDIATRIC MEDICAL TRAUMATIC STRESS

A complex set of factors determines whether a particular illness, injury, or intervention will become traumatic. Some factors relate directly to the objective characteristics of the illness, injury, or medical event, such as the severity and chronicity of the medical condition, the prognosis of the condition, the presence of potentially life-threatening or painful experiences, and the need for invasive procedures (Kazak et al., 2006). The characteristics of an event that are likely to contribute to PTSD are also likely to contribute to PMTS (Kazak et al., 2006). *DSM-5* criteria for PTSD include exposure to actual or threatened death or serious injury (American Psychiatric Association, 2013). Applying this same traumatic stress framework to PMTS, medical conditions or events that pose a high risk of morbidity or mortality would be more likely to contribute to PMTS. For instance, childhood cancers with a poor prognosis would be more likely than cancers with a good prognosis to lead to clinically significant PTSS. Similarly, serious medical complications that pose a high risk of death or severe long-term morbidity would have a high probability of contributing to PMTS (Pinquart, 2020).

In other cases, acute injuries may pose a high risk of death or serious complications such as motor vehicle accidents, traumatic brain injury (TBI), and gunshot wounds (Martin-Herz et al., 2012). These injuries often require immediate surgical intervention that can be quite risky. Certain medical procedures are extremely invasive and pose a high risk of injury, morbidity, or mortality such as intubation and mechanical ventilation, extracorporeal membrane oxygenation (ECMO), and bone marrow transplant (Garcia Guerra et al., 2014; Gavin & Roesler, 1997; Stuber et al., 1991). In some cases, the *nature* of the traumatic event may play a role in the eventual development of PTSS. Those experiencing intentional or violence-related injuries are more likely to develop symptoms of acute stress disorder, and those experiencing assault and penetrating traumatic injuries are more likely to develop PTSD compared to other types of injuries (Holbrook et al., 2005).

Although the objective characteristics of the medical condition or event play a role in the eventual development of PMTS, there is much variability. The same medical condition or event may be traumatogenic for one child or family, but not for another. Thus, these conditions and events are more appropriately referred to as potential traumatic events (PTEs; Kazak et al., 2006). In addition to the objective characteristics of the PTE, subjective factors, such as one's interpretation of the severity of the medical event and level of child and parental distress, also play a critical role in determining whether the PTE will lead to clinically significant PMTS.

RISK AND PROTECTIVE FACTORS ASSOCIATED WITH THE DEVELOPMENT OF PEDIATRIC MEDICAL TRAUMATIC STRESS

In understanding the origination of PMTS, various contextual factors around and within the child and family shape its ultimate expression. These factors will be explored in this section.

Subjective Experience of Potential Traumatic Event

One's subjective experience of a PTE seems to play an integral role in the eventual development of PTSS (Balluffi et al., 2004). A child's or parent's subjective interpretation of medical events, such as perception of life threat, regardless of the severity of the injury, is one of the strongest predictors of PMTS (Holbrook et al., 2001; Price et al., 2016). Subjective experiences vary based on the child's developmental level and temperament of the child, preexisting psychopathology in the child and family, levels of child and parental distress, perceptions of the health care services being provided, and understanding the illness and prognosis (Kazak et al., 2006). Preexisting mental or emotional health problems in the child and/or parent are associated with child or parent PTSS (Daviss et al., 2000). Among childhood cancer survivors, higher baseline levels of child anxiety predict persistent PTSS in children (Stuber et al., 1997). Among hospitalized children, preexisting parental anxiety and depression are associated with the development of parent PTSS (Muscara et al., 2017). Preexisting parent psychopathology also increases the risk of PMTS in the child (Saxe, Miller, et al., 2005).

Level of Parental Distress

A parent's level of distress during their child's treatment is associated with later higher levels of PTSS (Kazak et al., 2006). If the mother of a child who was hospitalized in the neonatal intensive care unit (NICU) has extreme levels of distress at baseline, she is more likely to experience persistently elevated PTSS over time compared to a mother with lower levels; one study showed that at least 65% of mothers with extreme baseline distress had clinically significant PTSS from 2 to 24 months after NICU experience compared to 11% or fewer mothers with low distress (Holditch-Davis et al., 2009). A parental feeling of powerlessness over their child's illness has also been associated with the development of PTSD in both the child and parent (Hofmann et al., 2007). Parents who have a higher degree of worry that their hospitalized child might die have a higher likelihood of developing PTSD, regardless of the objective measures of the severity of the child's illness (Balluffi et al., 2004). Family stressors also play an important role. A larger number of family stressors (i.e., conflict between parents and/or children, financial strain, and caring for an ill relative) is associated with a higher risk of the child developing acute stress disorder (Saxe, Miller, et al., 2005).

Child Psychological and Physiological Response

A child's psychological response to the medically traumatic experience also plays a role in the development of PTSS. Peritraumatic dissociation has been shown to be the strongest predictor in the transition from acute stress disorder to PTSD (Brown et al., 2016). Symptoms of peritraumatic dissociation include a subjective sense of numbing, reduction in awareness, derealization, depersonalization, and dissociative amnesia (Miller et al., 2009). Furthermore, perceiving the injury-related event to have a medium-to-high chance of recurrence is associated with a greater odds ratio of developing PTSD (Holbrook et al., 2001). In addition, the child's physiological response to the medically traumatic experience also plays a role in the eventual development of PMTS. Children who experience higher levels of pain are more likely to develop acute stress disorder in response to a traumatic injury (Saxe, Miller, et al., 2005). Higher levels of physiological arousal in the child (as manifested by heart rate) following the trauma have been associated with an increased risk of developing PTSD (Kassam-Adams et al., 2005).

Sociodemographic Factors

Sociodemographic factors among both the child and their family members have also been associated with the development of PMTS. Among mothers with babies who were admitted to the NICU, mothers who had a lower education level were more likely to have extreme levels of distress and a higher risk of having clinically significant PTSS up to 2 years after NICU discharge (Holditch-Davis et al., 2009). Among adolescents admitted to the hospital with traumatic injuries, female sex predicted risk of the development of acute stress disorder (Holbrook et al., 2005). Females may be at a slightly higher risk than males for PTSS (Brosbe et al., 2011; Cox et al., 2008; Stuber et al., 1997; Taylor et al., 2012). However, a meta-analysis of 26 studies among youth experiencing injury or illness did not find significant gender differences in rates of diagnostic PTSD (Kahana et al., 2006). Younger child age at the time of a PTE is associated with a greater risk of developing clinically significant PMTS and a greater likelihood of developing acute PTSS following pediatric ICU (PICU) admission (Dow et al., 2019). Similarly, among parents of children who were admitted to a hospital with serious illness or injury, younger age of the parent was associated with a higher level of parental acute stress disorder (Muscara et al., 2017).

Developmental Considerations

Constructive cognitive processing of the trauma following a traumatic experience enhances positive outcomes (Cryder et al., 2006). Through a neurodevelopmental lens, children of younger ages have less mature cognitive processing abilities, which impacts their ability to appraise and understand a traumatic experience in the same way that adolescents or adults do (Picoraro et al., 2014). Younger children may be more reliant on their parents' functioning and sense parental distress. Parental PTSS has been found to contribute to PTSS in young children (De Young et al., 2014; Haag & Landolt, 2017). Closely aligned with age, children of lower developmental levels would be at higher risk of developing PTSS in response to traumatic experiences, including medically traumatic experiences. Indeed, children with intellectual disability are more likely to develop PTSD compared to children with normal cognitive abilities (Kremen et al., 2007; Mevissen et al., 2020). This difference underscores the importance of considering the child's developmental level when considering their risk for developing PMTS in response to a medically traumatic event.

Protective Factors

Protective factors also may mitigate the risk of a child or caregiver developing PMTS following a child's PTE. Among young adult childhood cancer survivors, the experience of positive psychological outcomes was significantly more likely among female survivors, survivors of minority ethnicities, survivors who were older at the time of initial diagnosis, survivors with the psychosocial characteristic of optimism, and survivors with social support (Yi et al., 2015). Understanding the protective factors that can mitigate the risk of developing PMTS can help inform the development of interventions to enhance resilience in children at risk for PMTS.

CONCEPTUAL FRAMEWORKS FOR PEDIATRIC MEDICAL TRAUMATIC STRESS: INTEGRATIVE TRAJECTORY MODEL

Risk for the development of PMTS can be depicted in a conceptual framework. Kazak et al. (2006) originally described an integrative model of PMTS that categorized experiences surrounding a PTE into three distinct phases: peritrauma, early/ongoing/evolving responses, and longer-term PMTS. The updated version of the model, the Integrative Trajectory Model of PMTS, has renamed the phases to emphasize the importance of medical events: Phase I: peritrauma, Phase II: acute medical care, and Phase III: ongoing care or discharge from care (Price et al., 2016; see Figure 4.1). The specific time frame of each of these phases varies based on the specific medical issue and the treatments and interventions used. The Integrative Model emphasizes that medical traumatic events are experienced in the context of family systems with child

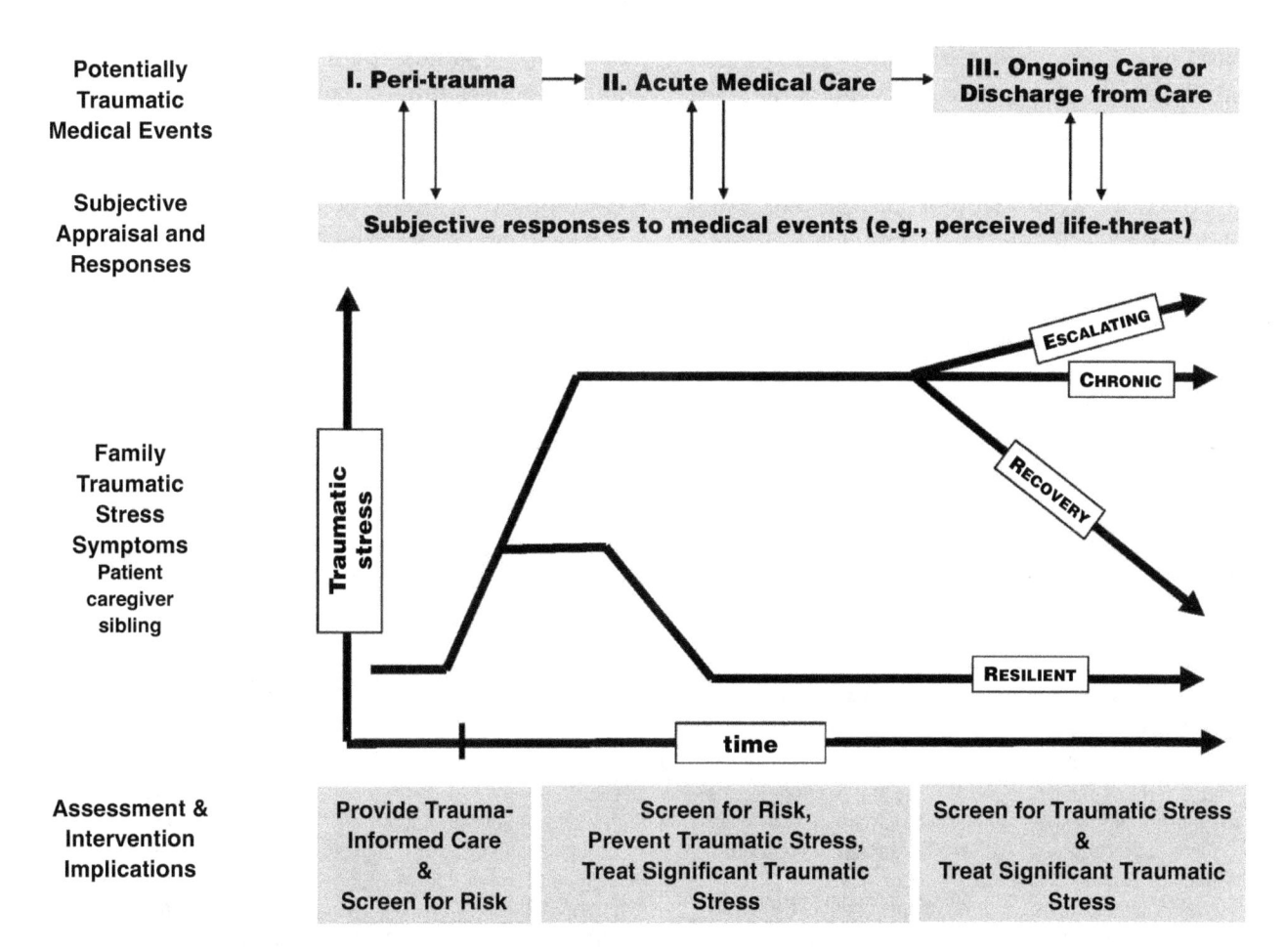

FIGURE 4.1. Integrative Trajectory Model of pediatric medical traumatic stress. A schematic of the model includes medical phases and psychological responses to pediatric injury and illness, as well as important risk factors and indicated psychosocial assessment and intervention practices. From "Systematic Review: A Reevaluation and Update of the Integrative (Trajectory) Model of Pediatric Medical Traumatic Stress," by J. Price, N. Kassam-Adams, M. A. Alderfer, J. Christofferson, and A. E. Kazak, 2016, *Journal of Pediatric Psychology*, 41(1), p. 93 (https://doi.org/10.1093/jpepsy/jsv074). Copyright 2016 by Oxford University Press. Reprinted with permission.

and family characteristics influencing the generation of PTSS.

Peritrauma Phase

The peritrauma phase (Phase I) includes the PTE and the immediate aftermath following the medical event. Examples may include the initial diagnosis of cancer or a chronic medical problem, the experience of a traumatic injury, an emergent surgical procedure, admission for a serious illness, or the need for a medical invasive procedure such as intubation or ECMO. Important factors in the peritrauma phase include the objective characteristics of the medically traumatic event, the preexisting characteristics of the child and parent (including baseline psychopathology, demographic factors, levels of parental distress, baseline cognitive levels, and the presence of family stressors), and the child and parents' immediate psychological and physiological reactions to the PTE and initial interventions (Kazak et al., 2006). Outlined in Table 4.1, these factors play a role in the development of the subjective experience of the PTE, which plays an integral role in the eventual development of PTSS (Balluffi et al., 2004).

Acute Medical Care Phase

The acute medical care phase (Phase II) incorporates early, ongoing, and evolving responses to a PTE following the initial event and immediate medical interventions. Factors in this phase include both the child's and family members' early responses to and appraisals of the PTE, perceived threat to life, and fears about recurrence of the event. Other factors involve the child's experience of pain following the event and during subsequent interventions, and level of parental anxiety surrounding the treatment process and worry that the child may die (Kazak et al., 2006).

Ongoing Care Phase

Finally, ongoing care or discharge from care phase (Phase III) includes the longer-term responses of the child and parent to the medical trauma once the immediate sequelae and interventions have resolved. Factors related to this phase include some of the same child and parental attitudes and responses inherent to Phase II that persist. Long-term consequences of unrecognized and persistent PTSS may include avoidance of seeking appropriate medical care to avoid reexperiencing the medical trauma, which could delay medical care and more significant medical trauma later once care is finally sought (Kazak et al., 2006).

Trajectories of Pediatric Medical Traumatic Stress

The revised Integrative Trajectory Model describes four possible trajectories of PMTS that children

TABLE 4.1

Risk and Protective Factors Associated With the Development of Pediatric Medical Traumatic Stress (PMTS)

Objective nature of the medical trauma	Preexisting demographic characteristics	Response/perceptions about the medical trauma	Protective factors decrease PMTS
■ High risk of death or long-term morbidity ■ High-risk or invasive medical procedures ■ Intentional and violence-related injuries ■ Type of trauma: assault and penetrating trauma	■ Preexisting emotional or behavioral health problems in child/parent ■ Younger age of the child/parent ■ Temperament of the child and family ■ Preexisting family stressors ■ Lower maternal education ■ Lower cognition ■ Parental level of distress	■ Experience of peritraumatic dissociation ■ Higher levels of physiological arousal following trauma ■ Perception of higher trauma recurrence of ■ Parental feeling of powerlessness over child's illness ■ Perceived life threat ■ Child experiencing higher levels of pain ■ Parental worry of child death	■ Female gender (mixed risk/protect evidence) ■ Non-White race ■ Positive processing cognitive/affective of subjective experience ■ Utilizing of "sense making" and "benefit finding" cognitive processing ■ Older age at time of PTE ■ Higher levels of optimism ■ More social supports

Note. PTE = potential traumatic event.

and parents may follow over time, depending on the risk and protective factors previously discussed. The Integrative Trajectory Model of PMTS includes the roles of family and ongoing medical events and is characterized by four trajectories: *resilient*, *recovery*, *chronic*, and *escalating* trajectories, with most families following a Resilient trajectory, that is, experiencing initial distress but adapting over time (Price et al., 2016). The Resilient trajectory is demonstrated by a typical and expected level of distress in response to the medical trauma that tapers off during the acute medical care phase and gradually reaches pretrauma distress levels. A smaller number of children and families follow a Recovery trajectory with persistently elevated levels of PTSS throughout the acute medical care phase, but then have a decline in traumatic stress levels throughout the third phase. Only a small percentage of children and families follow the Chronic trajectory, where elevated levels of PTSS persist into the third phase, or the Escalating trajectory, in which PTSS continues to increase (Price et al., 2016). Although specific predictors for each trajectory have not yet been identified, certain child and family characteristics increase the likelihood of developing PTSS. For instance, preexisting mental health conditions in both the child and caregiver have been shown to be strongly associated with the development of PTSS (Price et al., 2016). Other risk factors are outlined in Table 4.1. Although there have been no specific studies investigating this yet, it would be reasonable to assume that children and families with a higher degree of these risk factors would be more likely to fall into the Chronic or Escalating trajectories. Similarly, children and families with more protective factors (also outlined in Table 4.1) would likely have a higher likelihood of following the Recovery or Resilient trajectories.

Clinical Conditions Associated With Pediatric Medical Traumatic Stress

A variety of medically traumatic experiences may lead to a range of PMTS symptoms depending on the subjective experience of children and caregivers.

Chronic diseases.

Asthma. Asthma is one of the most prevalent pediatric diseases with 6.5% of all children affected; the percentage affected is higher (9.5%) among older teens (Centers for Disease Control and Prevention [CDC], 2023). It is characterized by lung airway inflammation that creates symptoms of wheezing, breathlessness, chest tightness, and coughing (CDC, n.d.-a). It can be exacerbated by the physical environment (allergens and pollution), illnesses (colds), and psychosocial factors such as stress (Barnthouse & Jones, 2019). An asthma exacerbation that causes acute respiratory symptoms may be experienced by the child as "feeling like dying" due to the inability to breathe. PMTS can result from asthma; in one sample of children with asthma from an underserved community, up to one-quarter experienced these breathless episodes as traumatic (Vanderbilt et al., 2008). Asthma exacerbations and subsequent ICU admissions among their children are also traumatic experiences for parents (Boeschoten et al., 2020).

Sickle cell disease. Sickle cell disease is an inherited disorder of red blood cells that causes oxygen-carrying hemoglobin to form a "sickle" shape instead of the normal round shape; this alteration blocks blood flow (National Heart, Lung, and Blood Institute [NHLBI], 2021). Sickle cell disease occurs in 1 out of 365 African American individuals, with the allele for this trait being carried by 1 out of 13 African American children, but can also occur in other races at lower prevalence (CDC, 2021a). Physical symptoms of sickle cell disease and to a lesser degree in those with the sickle cell trait include pain crises, hand and foot swelling, anemia, acute chest syndrome (pain, difficulty breathing, fever), strokes, vision loss, clots, and infections (NHLBI, 2021). These episodic medical complications are experienced by children as life-threatening and can precipitate PMTS, with PTSD prevalence rates reported as 27% in one study of children exposed to at least one hospitalization due to pain crisis and ranging from 7% to 19% in a specialty care sample depending on the child or caregiver reporter (Hofmann et al., 2007; Ingerski et al., 2010). PTSD was also seen in the caregivers of these children with rates ranging from 14% to 40% depending on the severity of physical symptoms in the sample (Hofmann et al., 2007; Ingerski et al., 2010).

Cancer. Cancer is a potent generator of PMTS for children. In 2021, over 15,000 children were diagnosed with cancer in the United States, with over 1,700 of those dying (Siegel et al., 2021). The most common types of pediatric cancer are leukemias, brain and central nervous system (CNS) tumors, and lymphomas with over 450,000 children surviving these diseases (Howlader et al., 2021). Among 254 children with cancer in one study, 54% described the overall cancer experience as the most stressful event they had ever experienced (Sharp et al., 2017). Aspects of cancer that elicited these reactions included: (a) diagnosis and subsequent adjustment, (b) treatment and acute side effects, (c) family/social impact, (d) prediagnosis period of uncertainty, (e) later persistent effects of treatment, and (f) possibility of death (Sharp et al., 2017). In one study of pediatric leukemia survivors and their families, 12.5% of children and up to 40% of their parents experienced severe PTSS (Stuber, 1996). A systematic review noted high rates of PMTS symptoms years after the diagnosis among acute leukemia, solid cancer, and lymphoma survivors ranging from 2% to 20%, with a lifetime prevalence of a diagnosis of PTSD estimated at 20% to 35% (Pelcovitz et al., 1998; Taïeb et al., 2003). In the same review, between 10% and 30% of childhood cancer survivors' parents suffered from PTSS (Taïeb et al., 2003).

Transplants. PMTS occurs at high rates in children requiring a transplant. Common organs that fail and require transplantation include kidney, liver, heart, lung, and intestines. Bone marrow transplantation is also a treatment in the setting of red blood cell disorders such as sickle cell anemia, rare genetic and immunological diseases, and an interventional treatment for some cancers such as leukemia and lymphoma. These children suffer both a life-threatening illness and painful intensive medical interventions with ongoing immunosuppression to prevent rejection of the organ. In a systematic review of pediatric solid organ transplants, 30% of recipients self-reported significant PMTS (Supelana et al., 2016). In a study of bone marrow transplantation, PTSS were seen even 12 months afterward, with more denial and avoidance reported versus children exposed to violent experiences (Stuber et al., 1991). In another study, 40% of caregivers of childhood liver transplant recipients were noted to have above-average distress and a high likelihood of seeking mental health services (Annunziato et al., 2020).

Accidents and burns.

Accidents. More than 7,000 children die annually because of unintentional injuries in the United States, and many more are hospitalized (CDC, 2021b). Childhood unintentional injuries include motor vehicle crashes, suffocation, drowning, poisoning, fires, and falls, all of which can create PMTS (Kassam-Adams, 2006; Stoddard & Saxe, 2001). In one study of children with serious injuries requiring an acute hospital stay, 27.7% met the criteria for acute stress disorder, with predictive risk factors including family and caregiver stress, child pain, and younger age (Saxe, Miller, et al., 2005). In another sample of children hospitalized for serious accidental injury, 12.5% had PTSD, and 16.7% more had subsyndromal PTSD with predictive risk factors of prior psychopathology and trauma, parental distress, and child's acute distress (Daviss et al., 2000). Beyond child symptoms, Kassam-Adams et al. (2015) found PTSS in 5% of parents 5 months after emergency department care for an unintentional injury.

Burns. Burn injuries result in 435 children being seen in emergency departments daily with two children unfortunately dying (CDC, n.d.-b). Burns are the third most frequent cause of injury in children resulting in death behind car accidents and drowning, and they result in a greater length of hospital stay than all other admissions for injuries (Toon et al., 2011). Burn injuries in children are often hot-liquid scald injuries resulting from exploratory behavior, accidental spills, or intentional abuse (Toon et al., 2011). A systematic review of pediatric burn survivors noted that nearly 30% of preschool and school-age victims had an acute stress disorder diagnosis in the first month, with symptoms typically improving postburn but persisting for some children, with PTSD rates of 10%–20% up to 1 year or later, especially with large burns (Bakker et al., 2013; Stoddard et al., 2006). Saxe, Stoddard, and colleagues noted that risk factors for acute stress disorder and later PTSD following the burn included the size of the burn, pain, and high heart rate in the hospital, low body image, parent acute stress disorder symptoms, and child separation anxiety and dissociation (Saxe, Stoddard, Chawla, et al., 2005; Saxe, Stoddard, Hall, et al., 2005). In another study, 10% of young children had PTSD 6 months postinjury and 25% of their parents had acute stress disorder in the first month, which declined to 5% having PTSD by 6 months (De Young et al., 2014). Other studies demonstrated caregivers having significant PTSS reactions, up to 47% at 3 months after the burn (Hall et al., 2006).

Intensive care unit hospitalization impacts on the family system. It has been well recognized that caregiver PMTS is highly prevalent in ICU settings. The NICU experience creates parental distress generating depression, anxiety, stress, feelings of loss of control and uncertainty regarding their caregiving ability (Obeidat et al., 2009). Maternal educational underachievement, stressful life events, postnatal depression, and infant unsettled-irregular behavior all worsen stress symptomatology (Woodward et al., 2014). Gateau et al. (2021) noted 33% positive Postnatal Posttraumatic Stress Questionnaire screens among preterm birth caregivers up to 2 years postpartum. Vanderbilt et al. (2009) found rates of acute stress disorder of 23% in an underserved community sample of NICU-exposed mothers as compared to 3% amongst those in a newborn nursery. Similar rates of parental PMTS have been found at 6 and 18 months as well (Feeley et al., 2011; Pierrehumbert et al., 2003). Among a higher-income sample, Shaw et al. (2009) found rates of 28% for acute stress disorder with increased risk for women, alteration in parental role, family cohesiveness, and emotional restraint and, at 4 months postpartum, rates of PTSD were 33% for fathers and 9% for mothers.

Similar to NICU-exposed populations, studies of the PICU experience on parents and children show high rates of parental PMTS. After a PICU admission, over 75% of parents experienced persistent symptoms of PTSD and 12.6% had diagnosable PTSD at 3 months postdischarge (Bronner et al., 2008). In addition to the parents, children who have experienced PICU hospitalization are at risk for the development of PMTS. A systematic review of five studies of PICU survivors found clinically significant PTSD symptom prevalence ranging from 10% to 28% (Davydow et al., 2010). A study of 50 PICU-admitted school-age children also noted the effects of PICU hospitalization on the family system; 26% of children and 24% of parents developed substantial PTSD symptoms, with early child and parent symptoms in the PICU precipitating later ones (Stowman et al., 2015).

Other acute and chronic conditions. Worldwide, increased PTSD symptoms in children have been noted due to COVID-related disruptions (Ma et al., 2021; Zhang et al., 2021). When considering chronic conditions, children with special health care needs constitute up to 18% of the pediatric population and require more medical exposures, such as hospitalization, medical interventions and procedures, and reliance on technology and/or medication (Cohen et al., 2011). Intensive interventions include dialysis, intubation, and ECMO (Gavin & Roesler, 1997; Neul, 2012; Valentine & Randolph, 2015) and associated pain (Brosbe et al., 2011) that can contribute to PMTS. Just over 50% of children admitted to PICUs have complex chronic conditions (Edwards et al., 2012). Given the intensive needs of this population, children with special health care needs and their caregivers are at higher risk for PMTS compared to the general population (Pinquart, 2020). Additionally, medical complexity is a factor in generating PMTS symptoms in conditions such as craniofacial anomalies, severe infections like meningococcemia, significant inflammatory responses to infections such as multisystem inflammatory syndrome (MIS-C) in the setting of COVID-19, congenital heart disease, or the need for cardiopulmonary resuscitation (Aspesberro et al., 2015; Feragen et al., 2020; Penner et al., 2021; Saxe et al., 2003; Vyse et al., 2013).

Pediatric Medical Traumatic Stress Screening and Assessment

Along with behavioral health providers, such as pediatric psychologists and developmental-behavioral pediatricians, medical providers are in a unique position to screen for PMTS given they are among the first contacts when injury or illness occurs. The importance of early screening around the time of a potentially traumatic medical event is supported by pediatric injury research demonstrating that functioning near the time of the injury predicts later PTSS and PTSD. Guidance has been provided for pediatricians on the importance of trauma screening and assessment as an aspect of trauma-informed care in the context of PMTS (Forkey et al., 2021; Ramsdell et al., 2015). Additionally, the Integrative Trajectory Model recommends screening for the risk of PTSS during all phases of medical care, including peritrauma, acute medical care, and ongoing care or discharge from care (Price et al., 2016).

Screening and assessment tools. There are several empirically validated measures available for the screening or assessment of PTSS, which if unaddressed can lead to acute stress disorder and PTSD. PMTS can be viewed as a set of PTSS that may not meet the criteria for acute stress disorder or PTSD (Kazak et al., 2006). Some of these instruments have been developed to screen youth who have experienced a potentially traumatic medical experience. The Screening Tool for Early Predictors of PTSD (Winston et al., 2003) was developed as a nondiagnostic tool that can be used post injury in acute hospital settings (e.g., inpatient unit, emergency department) to identify patients and families who may benefit from monitoring and additional support (Ward-Begnoche et al., 2006; Winston et al., 2003). The Child Trauma Screening Questionnaire (Kenardy et al., 2006) can screen children ages 7 to 16 at risk of developing PTSD and has been implemented in hospital settings to screen children after injuries.

The Pediatric Emotional Distress Scale (Saylor et al., 1999) can also be used to rapidly screen for symptoms in children 2 to 10 years old following a traumatic event. The UCLA PTSD Reaction Index for *DSM-5* is a developmentally informed tool that assesses trauma exposure, including life-threatening medical illness and accidents, and PTSD symptom frequency in children and adolescents ages 7 to 18 years via semistructured interview (Kaplow et al., 2020; Steinberg et al., 2004). The Trauma Symptom Checklist for Children (Briere, 1996) is a child self-report measure for ages 8 to 16 years, and the Trauma Symptom Checklist for Young Children (Briere, 2005) is a caregiver report measure for children ages 3 to 12 years, both developed to assess trauma-related symptoms in children. In addition to screening for PTSD or PTSS, it is important to assess psychosocial functioning given its importance in PMTS outcomes. The Psychosocial Assessment Tool (Kazak et al., 2001, 2011, 2015) is an evidence-based screener developed for families of pediatric oncology patients, and generalized for use across pediatric illnesses, to screen for risks that indicate the need for a higher level of psychosocial support. The NCTSN website (n.d.-d) also provides information regarding measures for trauma screening and trauma-informed mental health assessments.

IMPACT OF PEDIATRIC MEDICAL TRAUMATIC STRESS ON CHILD WELL-BEING: IMPLICATIONS FOR DEVELOPMENTAL AND BEHAVIORAL HEALTH CARE

Rates of PMTS in children, adolescents, and parents are roughly 30%, including subclinical levels of symptoms and symptoms that decline across time (Price et al., 2016). A developmental lens is essential when considering the impact of trauma (Kazak et al., 2006; Price et al., 2016) and it is important to understand how medical PTEs may impact child and family functioning.

Impact of Pediatric Medical Traumatic Stress on Child and Adolescent Functioning

The severity of PMTS symptoms can impact the short- and long-term functioning of children and adolescents. It is estimated that, "15–25% of children and siblings experience persistent traumatic stress reactions that can impair daily functioning and affect treatment adherence and recovery" (NCTSN, n.d.-c). PMTS and PTSS can impact child and adolescent functioning across several domains including, but not limited to, psychological functioning, academic functioning, health outcomes and quality of life.

Psychological functioning. Children and adolescents impacted by PMTS may experience traumatic stress symptoms, such as reexperiencing, avoidance, and hyperarousal (NCTSN, n.d.-b). In a study of children aged 1 to 6 years, 1 month following a burn, 25% of children met *DSM-5* (American Psychiatric Association, 2013) criteria for PTSD for preschool children with 73% having a comorbid mental health diagnosis such as major depressive disorder, attention-deficit/hyperactivity disorder, oppositional defiant disorder, separation anxiety disorder, or a phobia (De Young et al., 2021). While there has been some concern about possible misdiagnosis by focusing on externalizing symptoms, rather than the underlying trauma, it is believed that updated *DSM-5* criteria may better capture trauma symptoms in young children and prevent potential misdiagnosis (American Psychiatric Association, 2013).

A meta-analysis of studies of youth aged 6 to 19, experiencing injury or illness also found that internalizing symptoms, such as depression and anxiety, were comorbid with PTSD in injured youth; however, Kahana et al. (2006) could not determine if the symptoms developed postinjury or were present prior to the injury, contributing to higher risk for developing PTSD. Similarly, a systematic review of research on PMTS found that preexisting internalizing and externalizing difficulties were risk factors for PMTS (Price et al., 2016). Also, rates of anxiety, depression, and PTSD were found to be greater in pediatric liver transplant patients compared to a control group, with a higher rate of PTSD in pediatric patients who had significant anxiety and depression (Ünay et al., 2020).

Academic/school functioning. Injury or illness may contribute to school absenteeism, which can negatively impact school performance, and the development of PMTS following pediatric illness or injury can further impact school performance. Adolescents with a TBI and higher levels of PTSS at 3 months postinjury had poorer school functioning at 1 year and 2 years postinjury that was unexplained by TBI severity (O'Connor et al., 2012). PTSS includes intrusive thoughts, dissociation, and alterations in arousal and reactivity that can impact concentration and school functioning (American Psychiatric Association, 2013). Any child with a history of PMTS and signs of school failure or deteriorating academic functioning should be referred for further evaluation of learning by a provider with specialized training in assessment (e.g., developmental-behavioral pediatrician, pediatric psychologist, pediatric neuropsychologist).

Health outcomes. The PMTS model was revised to include a new assumption reflecting the impact of PTSS on adherence and health outcomes in families (Price et al., 2016). One study found parental PTSS symptoms did not contribute to worse adherence in a pediatric transplant population, but parental depression was significantly associated with worse adherence, which could contribute to poorer health outcomes (Annunziato et al., 2020). In pediatric liver transplant patients, child PTSD symptoms, especially avoidance of illness reminders, were associated with nonadherence with taking medication (Shemesh et al., 2008). Young adults who were childhood cancer survivors and reported higher levels of PTSS also reported poorer self-efficacy on items related to managing a chronic disease that was associated with their ability to communicate with health care providers or seek appropriate follow-up care (Taylor et al., 2012).

Quality of life. PTSS and PTSD are negatively associated with quality of life in pediatric solid-organ transplant candidates and recipients, including heart, liver, and kidney recipients (Hind et al., 2021; Ünay et al., 2020) and pediatric burn survivors (Landolt et al., 2009). Long-term impact on quality of life has also been found in childhood cancer survivors, who were more likely to have PTSD and a lower health-related quality of life as young adults than healthy peers (Schwartz & Drotar, 2006).

Impact of Pediatric Medical Traumatic Stress on Parents/Caregivers

When combining chronic illness groups, almost 25% of parents of a child with a chronic disease met the criteria for PTSD, with the prevalence being higher in mothers than fathers (Cabizuca et al., 2009). Levels of PTSD symptoms in mothers and fathers have been found to correlate with a family history of anxiety and depression (Lefkowitz et al., 2010). Prior trauma history, acute distress, number of invasive procedures for the child, history of guilt, and child PTSS are additional risk factors for the development of PTSD by mothers (De Young et al., 2014). Other factors, such as a history of trait anxiety, depression, and child behavior problems, have the strongest association with acute parental stress, when compared to demographic factors or illness-related factors (Muscara et al., 2017). For parents of children with a history of hospitalization in the PICU, levels of anxiety and depression 12 months after hospital discharge were double the levels of anxiety and depression in a community sample, indicating that long-term monitoring should continue to assess for PTSS and other emotional symptoms in parents (Colville & Pierce, 2012).

It is also important to consider how parents are coping and functioning in response to a PTE because parental adaptation to a pediatric medical trauma can impact the child's functioning. PTSD severity in mothers has been associated with an increased risk for PTSD in preschool children with cancer (Graf et al., 2013). Initial parental depression has been correlated with child PTSS 2 to 4 weeks and 6 weeks after an emergency department visit for an assault or a motor vehicle accident (Meiser-Stedman et al., 2006). Parental distress has also been correlated with a child's level of PMTS (Ben-Ari et al., 2021), though the directionality of the association is not clear. It may be that the child's reaction to the medical trauma influences the parent's psychological response, because mothers of children who had more avoidance symptoms at 3 months after PICU admission were more likely to endorse PTSS at 1 year postadmission (Colville & Pierce, 2012). Conversely, high levels of PTSS in parents have also been associated with poorer recovery of PTSS in children (Landolt et al., 2012). Although the direction of the relationship is not clear, and the associations are likely transactional (Sameroff, 2009), caregiver and child functioning interactions should be considered across time in PMTS assessment and intervention.

Impact of Pediatric Medical Traumatic Stress on Siblings

Having a sibling diagnosed with a chronic illness impacts household functioning, parent availability, and daily routines. Siblings of children with cancer experience elevated PTSS, negative mood symptoms, and lower quality of life scores (Alderfer et al., 2010). Another study found that 25% of siblings of children with cancer met criteria for PTSD, and 62% reported moderate to severe PTSS (Long et al., 2013). PTSS symptoms improve over time for siblings of children with cancer; however, 10 months after diagnosis, moderate to severe PTSS remained for 20% of siblings; siblings showing less improvement in PTSS had higher levels of anxiety at the beginning of this study (Alderfer et al., 2020). The psychological impact of stem cell transplants on healthy sibling donors and nondonors may include PTSS, anxiety, low self-esteem, and school problems (Packman et al., 2010). Nondonor siblings of bone marrow transplant survivors have higher PTSD scores and lower health-related quality of life scores as compared to a control group of healthy peers (Gizli Çoban et al., 2017). Sibling adjustment is also impacted by the quality of relationship with parents and is negatively impacted by lower parental acceptance and more parental control, leaving less sibling independence (Long et al., 2013). Developmentally appropriate independence may promote positive functioning for a sibling while the family deals with a PTE. Taken together, siblings of children with chronic illness may also benefit from surveillance with a behavioral health specialist to monitor for signs of PTSS and problematic adjustment to their sibling's medical condition.

Impact of Pediatric Medical Traumatic Stress on Family Functioning

Family functioning impacts the rates of PTSS in adolescent cancer survivors, who were five times more likely to exhibit PTSS if their family exhibited poor family functioning (Alderfer et al., 2009). Family functioning also impacts the functioning of siblings of a child who is ill (Long et al., 2013). Caregivers, patients, and siblings of patients identified the following as being PTEs related to a medical event: receiving the child's medical diagnosis; being at the hospital; medical procedures; medical emergencies; experiencing symptoms and physical changes; and communicating with the medical team (Christofferson et al., 2020). Families endorsed common themes in reaction to medical PTE, including strong emotional reactions and distressing thoughts; changes in family routines; increases in family conflict; and feeling different from peers (Christofferson et al., 2020). Because of the impact of chronic illness and PMTS on the family system, and the importance of considering the systems in which the child exists (Price et al., 2016), family-based supports and interventions should be considered when concerns are identified.

Posttraumatic Growth and Resilience Following Pediatric Medical Traumatic Stress

While most research regarding PMTS has identified negative outcomes associated with experiencing medical trauma, there is also evidence that PMTS can contribute to the development of resilience. Children and their parents may also experience posttraumatic growth (PTG) in response to medical trauma, which consists of positive psychological changes over time following medical trauma (Picoraro et al., 2014). Positive outcomes for siblings of children with cancer have also been reported, including resiliency, maturity, and empathy (Alderfer et al., 2010). Similar to the Integrative Trajectory Models for PMTS, there are also three distinct phases associated with the development of PTG: the *Pretraumatic Event*, the *Traumatic Event*, and the *Posttraumatic Event* (Picoraro et al., 2014). Baseline characteristics in the Pretraumatic Event phase associated with better adaptation include the presence of protective factors that mitigate the risk of PTSS, as well as select demographic and psychosocial characteristics including female gender, minority ethnicity, older age at the time of PTE, higher levels of optimism, and more social supports (Yi et al., 2015). In the Traumatic Event phase, the subjective experience of the medically traumatic event and the presence of social supports play an important role in this phase as well (Picoraro et al., 2014). Finally, in the Posttraumatic Event phase, the adoption of two forms of cognitive processing, known as "sense making" and "benefit finding," in the period following the medical trauma has been associated with PTG (Picoraro et al., 2014). PTG has been reported when family members developed positive narratives about the events related to the PTE that resulted in positive outcomes (Christofferson et al., 2020). Taken together, for families experiencing PMTS, interventions to support the development of a positive narrative, and PTG may help to foster adaptation and resilience following a medical trauma.

Pediatric Medical Traumatic Stress Interventions

When considering intervention for PMTS, the Integrative Model proposes goals for intervention for each phase of PMTS, including, "changing the subjective experience of the PTE in Phase I, preventing PTSS in Phase II, and reducing PTS in Phase III" (Price et al., 2016, p. 87). Approaches to intervention, ranging from providing a trauma-informed care approach within a medical setting to more specific, evidence-based interventions based upon presenting symptoms, vary depending on the time period during which intervention is provided related to the medical PTE, as well as based on individual child or family needs.

Trauma-informed care. Approaching all interactions from a trauma-informed care perspective means recognizing and acknowledging the prevalence and impact of trauma for children and families across the systems in which they function, including medical settings. In pediatric care, the steps of trauma-informed care are (1) minimize the traumatic aspects of medical care, (2) provide all pediatric patients and their families with basic support and information, (3) screen to identify those who may need more help, and (4) ensure health care providers remain aware of their own stress (Center for Pediatric Traumatic Stress, n.d.). A trauma-informed care approach asks medical providers to assume that all families have experienced a previous trauma or may experience their child's medical diagnosis and treatment as traumatic (Marsac et al., 2016). Training for health care providers in trauma-informed care is an essential step and resources have been developed to assist providers in minimizing the impact of potentially traumatic medical events on both families and providers. The American Academy of Pediatrics has developed resources for education and implementation of trauma-informed care within pediatric settings including how to recognize trauma symptoms in pediatric patients, recommended screening tools, and interventions to reduce further traumatization for a range of traumatic experiences and reactions, including PMTS (Forkey et al., 2021).

The Pediatric Psychosocial Preventative Health Model (PPPHM) identifies a three-tiered, dose-specific approach (universal, targeted, and clinical) to guide psychosocial support based on the specific family's level of risk factors and needs as they adjust to their child's medical condition (Kazak, 2006). Screening and a thorough history assist in identifying the level of support needed. Universal intervention targets the largest proportion of patients and families that are resilient with adequate-to-strong coping skills but are experiencing understandable distress in response to their child's diagnosis (Kazak et al., 2006). These families may benefit from general support and psychoeducation provided by physicians, nurses, child life specialists, or social workers regarding common reactions to illness or injury and further assessment for additional risk factors (Kazak et al., 2006). Based on screening, a smaller subset of families with preexisting factors that place them at greater risk for difficulty coping with their child's medical condition, may be identified and benefit from targeted intervention, such as focusing on specific emotional symptoms (Kazak et al., 2006). These families may have a history of mental health concerns, substance use, or legal involvement. Intervention can be provided by a range of professionals, including pediatric psychologists or mental health counselors (Kazak et al., 2006). The third tier, indicated for the smallest subset of families, is clinical intervention by a behavioral health specialist (i.e., psychologist, psychiatrist, social worker); these families have risk factors for ongoing distress, such as anxiety, depression, or trauma history (Kazak et al., 2006).

The National Child Traumatic Stress Network (NCTSN) has developed references and training materials on pediatric medical traumatic stress for families and health care providers (see the Resources box at the end of this chapter), such as the *Pediatric Medical Traumatic Stress Toolkit for Health Care Providers* (NCTSN, 2014).

Resources are also available for both medical providers and families through the Health Care Toolbox (Center for Pediatric Traumatic Stress, n.d.; see the Resources box). This resource includes direct materials for family psychoeducation and resources to assist medical professionals when providing universal intervention. One example in this tool kit is the "D-E-F Framework" to guide health care providers in assessing, addressing, and preventing traumatic stress in pediatric patients by assessing the areas of Distress, Emotional Support, and Family. The Health Care Toolbox website also provides information on many common PMTS topics such as typical stress reactions following an illness or injury; how to help a child who is having difficulty sleeping after a hospitalization; how to help a child who is experiencing pain; and when to seek professional intervention (Center for Pediatric Traumatic Stress, n.d.).

Given the impact of pain symptoms in PMTS and in the development of acute stress disorder and PTSD (Saxe, Miller, et al., 2005), effective pain management is an essential area for intervention. Pain management resources, ranging from cancer-related pain to pediatric postsurgery pain, are also available online at the website for It Doesn't Have to Hurt (https://itdoesnthavetohurt.ca/). The link for this organization's website is in the Resources section.

Psychological modalities. Beyond education and resources for parents, children, and health care professionals, interventions have been developed to specifically address PMTS. A review of PMTS interventions found some common factors: the majority of interventions for young children are brief, parent-mediated, and include psychoeducation and cognitive behavior therapy (CBT) skills. Across development, the majority of interventions continue to involve caregivers and utilize CBT (Christian-Brandt et al., 2019; Price et al., 2016). Evidence-based interventions for older children and adolescents who have experienced PMTS draw heavily from CBT approaches. Subjective responses to medical events such as perceived life-threat, rather than objective data, relate to PMTS (Price et al., 2016), thereby, providing a focus for CBT-informed interventions that replace maladaptive, catastrophic thoughts with more realistic, adaptive thoughts.

PMTS impacts the functioning of families; therefore, family interventions are often utilized to improve family functioning and reduce the likelihood of ongoing PTSS or PTSD. The Surviving Cancer Competently Intervention Program (Kazak et al., 1999, 2004) is a time-limited, one-day, four-session, multifamily group intervention to reduce PTSS, based on CBT principles and family therapy approaches. Creating Opportunities for Parent Empowerment (COPE; Melnyk et al., 2004) is also a time-limited intervention developed for parents and children in the PICU, given the high risk of children and parents developing PTSD after a PICU stay. This brief intervention provides psychoeducation about children's reactions to PICU admission, strategies to increase parental involvement in caregiving in the PICU, and activities to help the child and parent express and cope with emotions while developing mastery related to the hospital experience. Melnyk and colleagues (2004) found that mothers who participated in COPE had fewer PTSD symptoms and improved coping; children who received COPE exhibited fewer externalizing behaviors compared to a control group up to 1 year after hospitalization.

De Young and colleagues (2021) introduced a stepped-model-of-care framework of PMTS intervention for young children, aged 0 to 6 years, that incorporates many of the approaches and resources described, applied in a developmentally appropriate manner, varying based on the phase of the trauma and the level of intervention indicated. Their approach is based on the Integrative Trajectory Model of PMTS (Price et al., 2016; see Figure 4.1) and follows the PPPHM (Kazak, 2006) framework, beginning with universal, trauma-informed care for all children and families. The next stage is targeted intervention for children screened at high risk using the 1- to 2-session CARE intervention, based on principles of trauma-focused CBT (TF-CBT; Cohen & Mannarino, 2008), consisting of psychoeducation, developmentally appropriate resources, a trauma narrative, and information on trauma-related parenting behaviors (De Young et al., 2016; Haag et al., 2020). If symptoms persist, De Young and colleagues (2021) recommend clinical intervention using developmentally appropriate, evidence-based interventions, such as child–parent psychotherapy (CPP) or TF-CBT.

CPP is an evidence-based, relationship-focused, dyadic intervention for young children who have experienced trauma, and its effectiveness for abuse, domestic violence, and infants with depressed mothers has been demonstrated through randomized controlled trials (Lieberman et al., 2015). A published case study demonstrated the application of CPP with young children with PMTS and a developmental disability (Harley et al., 2014; Williams et al., 2014). CPP also appears to have promise for families that have an infant in the NICU (Lakatos et al., 2019). The goal of CPP is to restore an optimal developmental trajectory for a parent and a child who have experienced trauma and promote healing by focusing on the parent–child relationship.

TF-CBT is an evidence-based intervention for children who have experienced trauma that provides children and caregivers with coping skills to deal with stressful topics prior to processing the child's traumatic experience (Cohen & Mannarino, 2008). Children should be exhibiting trauma-related symptoms, such as PTSS, but a PTSD diagnosis is not required (Cohen & Mannarino, 2015). The acronym PRACTICE represents TF-CBT interventions: Psychoeducation, Parenting skills, Relaxation skills, Affective modulation skills, Cognitive coping skills, Trauma narrative and cognitive processing of the traumatic event, In vivo mastery of trauma reminders, Conjoint parent sessions, and Enhancing safety and future developmental trajectory (Cohen & Mannarino, 2008). In a small sample, TF-CBT was effective for children and adolescents who experienced an accidental injury and presented with PTSD 2 years following the injury (van Meijel et al., 2019). A NICU group intervention based on TF-CBT principles also found reductions in the levels of anxiety, depression, and PTSS in mothers at 6-week and 6-month follow-up (Simon et al., 2021).

Acceptance and commitment therapy (ACT; Hayes et al., 2012) focuses on increasing psychological flexibility and may have applications in the treatment of PMTS. ACT is effective in improving coping with a broad range of medical conditions perhaps due to promoting resilience and increasing the individual's ability to engage in developmentally expected behavior despite adversity (Ernst & Mellon, 2016).

Some families prefer internet-based interventions (Christian-Brandt et al., 2019; Price et al., 2016), given the distance families may have to travel to their child's hospital setting for periodic mental health appointments and ongoing medical appointments. Additionally, the COVID-19 pandemic necessitated a rapid increase in telehealth for medical and behavioral health appointments. PMTS interventions should utilize technology, when clinically appropriate, for implementation. The interventions described, beginning with the underlying principles of TIC, align well with the goals of the Integrative Model to change the subjective experience of the PTE, prevent PTSS, or reduce PTSS (Price et al., 2016). It is important to implement pediatric medical intervention in a trauma-informed manner across all medical settings to decrease risk for PTSS and provide dose-specific interventions based on the child, adolescent, or family's level of need that may vary across the phases of medical treatment (Price et al., 2016).

Medication modalities. Three medications have shown some evidence in the prevention of PMTS with a few other potentially efficacious prevention options on the horizon. Saxe and Stoddard found that young and older children with burn injuries who had higher cumulative dosages of morphine while in the hospital showed lower rates of PTSD symptoms at 6 months especially in the arousal domain (Saxe et al., 2001; Stoddard et al., 2009). Sertraline may reduce parent-reported but not child-reported PTSD symptoms over 6 months following pediatric burns, but more studies are needed (Stoddard et al., 2011). Some researchers found propranolol efficacious in PTSD prevention in child abuse victims and in physical injuries among girls (Famularo et al., 1988; Nugent et al., 2010), but Rosenberg et al. (2018) failed to find an effect for propranolol in preventing PTSD symptoms in a randomized controlled trial of pediatric burn ICU patients. Few randomized placebo-controlled trials have evaluated the efficacy of medications for pediatric PTSD and none in the setting of PMTS (Strawn et al., 2023). Guanfacine and possibly clonidine, both alpha-2 adrenergic agonists, can reduce intrusive (nightmares) and hyperarousal symptoms in children with PTSD (Connor et al., 2013). These drugs also have a favorable side effect profile, with sedation and gastrointestinal complaints (dry mouth and constipation) being most common (Strawn et al., 2010). Thus, the best evidence and side effect profile suggest that, in addition to adequate pain control, guanfacine and clonidine may be the first-line medications to trial for PTSD symptoms, and prazosin (alpha-1 agonist) may be used with sleep disruption specifically.

Cultural and generational considerations. In trauma-informed care, interventions should be approached from a perspective of cultural humility. Having a trauma-informed system means acknowledging the impact of structural inequity and responding to the needs of diverse communities (NCTSN, n.d.-a). When considering PMTS, the impact of some cultural identity factors, such as ethnicity on PTSS, is inconsistent across the literature, with some studies indicating that minority ethnicity is a protective factor toward PTG (Yi et al., 2015). Another study found that acculturation, assessed by proxy of preferred language spoken, had an inverse relation with PTG and that adolescents and young adults who identified as Latin American and came from English-speaking home had significantly lower PTG than other groups who came from Spanish-speaking homes (Arpawong et al., 2013). More research is needed on the role of cultural factors in PMTS and how health care systems can better promote a family's use of culturally based sources of support in decreasing the impact of PTE and promoting PTG.

Another aspect related to trauma-informed medical care is considering the impact of intergenerational trauma. Infants born to mothers who experienced their own childhood traumas and traumas throughout their life prior to pregnancy have a higher risk of certain health conditions, including bronchiolitis (Adgent et al., 2019), which can lead to childhood asthma, thereby possibly increasing that mother and child's interaction with medical systems and future potentially traumatic medical experiences and PMTS. Thus, asthma can generate intergenerational transmission of maternal traumatic stress through later child asthma attack traumas (Brunst et al., 2017). Mechanisms of the transmission of intergenerational trauma have implications for assessment and intervention. Through a trauma-informed system of care, information can be obtained regarding the family and child's trauma history as well as their protective factors. Protective factors can be supported and promoted by the health care team and, if necessary, referrals provided for evidence-based, early intervention that could improve long-term health and psychological outcomes for the child and family (Amaya-Jackson et al., 2021).

CONCLUSION

PMTS is a frequent psychological response seen in pediatric medical care. Most children and families cope well following PMTS after an initial period of expected stress. It is critical to contextualize and assess the unique risk factors and symptoms to guide early intervention in decreasing the likelihood of negative long-term psychological and health outcomes. Evidence-based interventions are available for those who experience distress and ongoing PMTS symptoms. Medical systems should implement trauma-informed systems of care as a form of prevention and intervention for PMTS. To improve care and guide psychological and medication interventions, more research is needed specifically on PMTS in medical settings. Interdisciplinary care that is attuned to the needs of children and their families who have experienced medical trauma is necessary to mitigate risks associated with PMTS and to support the development of resilience. This can occur through routine psychosocial screenings in clinics that care for children and families with chronic illness and can include referrals to psychologists, neuropsychologists, and developmental-behavioral pediatricians for assessment and interventions when risks and concerns are identified.

RESOURCES

Resources for Providers, Parents, Families, and Youth

Many resources are available for free from the National Child Traumatic Stress Network's website (https://www.nctsn.org). Their medical trauma resources page (https://www.nctsn.org/what-is-child-trauma/trauma-types/medical-trauma/nctsn-resources) includes information for medical providers and families regarding how to support children and adolescents who are experiencing PMTS related to accident, illness, or hospitalization. Resources are available in English and Spanish.

The Health Care Toolbox (https://www.healthcaretoolbox.org/) is another resource that helps families and children cope with illness and injury. The website is presented by the Center for Pediatric Traumatic Stress to provide information and resources related to PMTS. Free information is available for patients, families, and medical professionals. The website contains educational materials about PMTS developed for parents, caregivers, children, and adolescents. The website also contains an overview of screening and assessment tools, interventions, and trauma-informed care.

It Doesn't Have to Hurt: Proven Pain Control for Children (https://itdoesnthavetohurt.ca) contains resources for pain management for children and adolescents, including videos and blog posts. Examples of topics covered include needle pain, pain assessment, and coping strategies for pain. This website brings together researchers, parents, and other stakeholders to address pain management in children.

References

Adetunji, O., Ottino, K., Tucker, A., Al-Attar, G., Abduljabbar, M., & Bishai, D. (2020). Variations in pediatric hospitalization in seven European countries. *Health Policy*, 124(11), 1165–1173. https://doi.org/10.1016/j.healthpol.2020.07.002

Adgent, M. A., Elsayed-Ali, O., Gebretsadik, T., Tylavsky, F. A., Kocak, M., Cormier, S. A., Wright, R. J., & Carroll, K. N. (2019). Maternal childhood and lifetime traumatic life events and infant bronchiolitis. *Paediatric and Perinatal Epidemiology*, 33(4), 262–270. https://doi.org/10.1111/ppe.12559

Alderfer, M. A., Logan, B. A., DiDonato, S., Jackson, L., Hayes, M. J., & Sigmon, S. T. (2020). Change across time in cancer-related traumatic stress symptoms of siblings of children with cancer: A preliminary investigation. *Journal of Clinical Psychology in Medical Settings*, 27(1), 48–53. https://doi.org/10.1007/s10880-019-09618-2

Alderfer, M. A., Long, K. A., Lown, E. A., Marsland, A. L., Ostrowski, N. L., Hock, J. M., & Ewing, L. J. (2010). Psychosocial adjustment of siblings of children with cancer: A systematic review. *Psycho-Oncology*, 19(8), 789–805. https://doi.org/10.1002/pon.1638

Alderfer, M. A., Navsaria, N., & Kazak, A. E. (2009). Family functioning and posttraumatic stress disorder in adolescent survivors of childhood cancer. *Journal of Family Psychology*, 23(5), 717–725. https://doi.org/10.1037/a0015996

Amaya-Jackson, L., Absher, L. E., Gerrity, E. T., Layne, C. M., & Halladay Goldman, J. (2021). *Beyond the ACE Score: Perspectives from the NCTSN on child trauma and adversity screening and impact*. National Center for Child Traumatic Stress.

American Psychiatric Association. (2013). *Diagnostic and statistical manual of mental disorders* (5th ed.). https://doi.org/10.1176/appi.books.9780890425596

Annunziato, R. A., Stuber, M. L., Supelana, C. J., Dunphy, C., Anand, R., Erinjeri, J., Alonso, E. M., Mazariegos, G. V., Venick, R. S., Bucuvalas, J., & Shemesh, E. (2020). The impact of caregiver post-traumatic stress and depressive symptoms on pediatric transplant outcomes. *Pediatric Transplantation*, 24(1), e13642. https://doi.org/10.1111/petr.13642

Arpawong, T. E., Oland, A., Milam, J. E., Ruccione, K., & Meeske, K. A. (2013). Post-traumatic growth among an ethnically diverse sample of adolescent and young adult cancer survivors. *Psycho-Oncology*, 22(10), 2235–2244. https://doi.org/10.1002/pon.3286

Aspesberro, F., Mangione-Smith, R., & Zimmerman, J. J. (2015). Health-related quality of life following pediatric critical illness. *Intensive Care Medicine*, 41(7), 1235–1246. https://doi.org/10.1007/s00134-015-3780-7

Bakker, A., Maertens, K. J., Van Son, M. J., & Van Loey, N. E. (2013). Psychological consequences of pediatric burns from a child and family perspective: A review of the empirical literature. *Clinical Psychology Review*, 33(3), 361–371. https://doi.org/10.1016/j.cpr.2012.12.006

Balluffi, A., Kassam-Adams, N., Kazak, A., Tucker, M., Dominguez, T., & Helfaer, M. (2004). Traumatic stress in parents of children admitted to the pediatric intensive care unit. *Pediatric Critical Care Medicine*, 5(6), 547–553. https://doi.org/10.1097/01.PCC.0000137354.19807.44

Barnthouse, M., & Jones, B. L. (2019). The impact of environmental chronic and toxic stress on asthma. *Clinical Reviews in Allergy & Immunology*, 57(3), 427–438. https://doi.org/10.1007/s12016-019-08736-x

Ben-Ari, A., Aloni, R., Ben-David, S., Benarroch, F., & Margalit, D. (2021). Parental psychological flexibility as a mediating factor of post-traumatic stress disorder in children after hospitalization or surgery. *International Journal of Environmental Research and Public Health*, 18(21), 11699. https://doi.org/10.3390/ijerph182111699

Boeschoten, S. A., Dulfer, K., Boehmer, A. L. M., Merkus, P. J. F. M., van Rosmalen, J., de Jongste, J. C., de Hoog, M., & Buysse, C. M. P. (2020). Quality of life and psychosocial outcomes in children with severe acute asthma and their parents. *Pediatric Pulmonology, 55*(11), 2883–2892. https://doi.org/10.1002/ppul.25034

Briere, J. (1996). *Trauma symptom checklist for children (TSCC), professional manual*. Psychological Assessment Resources.

Briere, J. (2005). *Trauma symptom checklist for young children (TSCYC): Professional manual*. Psychological Assessment Resources.

Bronner, M. B., Knoester, H., Bos, A. P., Last, B. F., & Grootenhuis, M. A. (2008). Follow-up after paediatric intensive care treatment: Parental post-traumatic stress. *Acta Paediatrica, 97*(2), 181–186. https://doi.org/10.1111/j.1651-2227.2007.00600.x

Brosbe, M. S., Hoefling, K., & Faust, J. (2011). Predicting posttraumatic stress following pediatric injury: A systematic review. *Journal of Pediatric Psychology, 36*(6), 718–729. https://doi.org/10.1093/jpepsy/jsq115

Brown, R. C., Nugent, N. R., Hawn, S. E., Koenen, K. C., Miller, A., Amstadter, A. B., & Saxe, G. (2016). Predicting the transition from acute stress disorder to posttraumatic stress disorder in children with severe injuries. *Journal of Pediatric Health Care, 30*(6), 558–568. https://doi.org/10.1016/j.pedhc.2015.11.015

Brunst, K. J., Rosa, M. J., Jara, C., Lipton, L. R., Lee, A., Coull, B. A., & Wright, R. J. (2017). Impact of maternal lifetime interpersonal trauma on children's asthma: Mediation through maternal active asthma during pregnancy. *Psychosomatic Medicine, 79*(1), 91–100. https://doi.org/10.1097/PSY.0000000000000354

Cabizuca, M., Marques-Portella, C., Mendlowicz, M. V., Coutinho, E. S. F., & Figueira, I. (2009). Posttraumatic stress disorder in parents of children with chronic illnesses: A meta-analysis. *Health Psychology, 28*(3), 379–388. https://doi.org/10.1037/a0014512

Centers for Disease Control and Prevention (CDC). (n.d.-a). *Asthma*. Retrieved February 7, 2025, from https://www.cdc.gov/asthma/index.html

Centers for Disease Control and Prevention (CDC). (n.d.-b). *Protect the ones you love: Burns*. Retrieved February 7, 2025, from https://stacks.cdc.gov/view/cdc/12352

Centers for Disease Control and Prevention (CDC). (2021a). *Data & statistics on sickle cell disease*. https://www.cdc.gov/ncbddd/sicklecell/data.html

Centers for Disease Control and Prevention (CDC). (2021b). *Injuries among children and teens*. https://www.cdc.gov/injury/features/child-injury/index.html

Centers for Disease Control and Prevention (CDC). (2023). *Most recent national asthma data*. Retrieved September 19, 2024, from https://www.cdc.gov/asthma/most_recent_national_asthma_data.htm

Center for Pediatric Traumatic Stress. (n.d.). *Providing trauma informed care for children*. Retrieved September 19, 2024, from https://www.healthcaretoolbox.org/trauma-informed-care-the-basics

Christian-Brandt, A. S., Santacrose, D. E., Farnsworth, H. R., & MacDougall, K. A. (2019). When treatment is traumatic: An empirical review of interventions for pediatric medical traumatic stress. *American Journal of Community Psychology, 64*(3–4), 389–404. https://doi.org/10.1002/ajcp.12392

Christofferson, J. L., Okonak, K., Kazak, A. E., Pierce, J., Kelly, C., Schifano, E., Sciolla, J., Deatrick, J. A., & Alderfer, M. A. (2020). Family consequences of potentially traumatic pediatric medical events: Implications for trauma-informed care. *Journal of Family Psychology, 34*(2), 237–246. https://doi.org/10.1037/fam0000597

Cohen, E., Kuo, D. Z., Agrawal, R., Berry, J. G., Bhagat, S. K. M., Simon, T. D., & Srivastava, R. (2011). Children with medical complexity: An emerging population for clinical and research initiatives. *Pediatrics, 127*(3), 529–538. https://doi.org/10.1542/peds.2010-0910

Cohen, J. A., & Mannarino, A. P. (2008). Trauma-focused cognitive behavioural therapy for children and parents. *Child and Adolescent Mental Health, 13*(4), 158–162. https://doi.org/10.1111/j.1475-3588.2008.00502.x

Cohen, J. A., & Mannarino, A. P. (2015). Trauma-focused cognitive behavior therapy for traumatized children and families. *Child and Adolescent Psychiatric Clinics of North America, 24*(3), 557–570. https://doi.org/10.1016/j.chc.2015.02.005

Colville, G., & Pierce, C. (2012). Patterns of post-traumatic stress symptoms in families after paediatric intensive care. *Intensive Care Medicine, 38*(9), 1523–1531. https://doi.org/10.1007/s00134-012-2612-2

Connor, D. F., Grasso, D. J., Slivinsky, M. D., Pearson, G. S., & Banga, A. (2013). An open-label study of guanfacine extended release for traumatic stress related symptoms in children and adolescents. *Journal of Child and Adolescent Psychopharmacology, 23*(4), 244–251. https://doi.org/10.1089/cap.2012.0119

Cox, C. M., Kenardy, J. A., & Hendrikz, J. K. (2008). A meta-analysis of risk factors that predict psychopathology following accidental trauma. *Journal for Specialists in Pediatric Nursing, 13*(2), 98–110. https://doi.org/10.1111/j.1744-6155.2008.00141.x

Cryder, C. H., Kilmer, R. P., Tedeschi, R. G., & Calhoun, L. G. (2006). An exploratory study of posttraumatic growth in children following a natural disaster. *American Journal of Orthopsychiatry*, 76(1), 65–69. https://doi.org/10.1037/0002-9432.76.1.65

Daviss, W. B., Mooney, D., Racusin, R., Ford, J. D., Fleischer, A., & McHugo, G. J. (2000). Predicting posttraumatic stress after hospitalization for pediatric injury. *Journal of the American Academy of Child & Adolescent Psychiatry*, 39(5), 576–583. https://doi.org/10.1097/00004583-200005000-00011

Davydow, D. S., Richardson, L. P., Zatzick, D. F., & Katon, W. J. (2010). Psychiatric morbidity in pediatric critical illness survivors: A comprehensive review of the literature. *Archives of Pediatrics & Adolescent Medicine*, 164(4), 377–385. https://doi.org/10.1001/archpediatrics.2010.10

De Young, A. C., Haag, A., Kenardy, J. A., Kimble, R. M., & Landolt, M. A. (2016). Coping with accident reactions (CARE) early intervention programme for preventing traumatic stress reactions in young injured children: Study protocol for two randomised controlled trials. *Trials*, 17(362). https://doi.org/10.1186/s13063-016-1490-2

De Young, A. C., Hendrikz, J., Kenardy, J. A., Cobham, V. E., & Kimble, R. M. (2014). Prospective evaluation of parent distress following pediatric burns and identification of risk factors for young child and parent posttraumatic stress disorder. *Journal of Child and Adolescent Psychopharmacology*, 24(1), 9–17. https://doi.org/10.1089/cap.2013.0066

De Young, A. C., Paterson, R. S., Brown, E. A., Egberts, M. R., Le Brocque, R. M., Kenardy, J. A., Landolt, M. A., Marsac, M. L., Alisic, E., & Haag, A.-C. (2021). Topical review: Medical trauma during early childhood. *Journal of Pediatric Psychology*, 46(7), 739–746. https://doi.org/10.1093/jpepsy/jsab045

Dow, B. L., Kenardy, J. A., Long, D. A., & Le Brocque, R. M. (2019). Cognitive/affective factors are associated with children's acute posttraumatic stress following pediatric intensive care. *Psychological Trauma*, 11(1), 55–63. https://doi.org/10.1037/tra0000349

Edwards, J. D., Houtrow, A. J., Vasilevskis, E. E., Rehm, R. S., Markovitz, B. P., Graham, R. J., & Dudley, R. A. (2012). Chronic conditions among children admitted to U.S. pediatric intensive care units: Their prevalence and impact on risk for mortality and prolonged length of stay. *Critical Care Medicine*, 40(7), 2196–2203. https://doi.org/10.1097/CCM.0b013e31824e68cf

Ernst, M. M., & Mellon, M. W. (2016). Acceptance and commitment therapy (ACT) to foster resilience in pediatric chronic illness. In C. DeMichelis & M. Ferrari (Eds.), *Child and adolescent resilience within medical contexts: Integrating research and practice* (pp. 193–207). Springer International. https://doi.org/10.1007/978-3-319-32223-0_11

Famularo, R., Kinscherff, R., & Fenton, T. (1988). Propranolol treatment for childhood posttraumatic stress disorder, acute type: A pilot study. *American Journal of Diseases of Children*, 142(11), 1244–1247. https://doi.org/10.1001/archpedi.1988.02150110122036

Feeley, N., Zelkowitz, P., Cormier, C., Charbonneau, L., Lacroix, A., & Papageorgiou, A. (2011). Posttraumatic stress among mothers of very low birthweight infants at 6 months after discharge from the neonatal intensive care unit. *Applied Nursing Research*, 24(2), 114–117. https://doi.org/10.1016/j.apnr.2009.04.004

Feragen, K. B., Stock, N. M., Myhre, A., & Due-Tønnessen, B. J. (2020). Medical stress reactions and personal growth in parents of children with a rare craniofacial condition. *The Cleft Palate Craniofacial Journal*, 57(2), 228–237. https://doi.org/10.1177/1055665619869146

Forkey, H., Szilagyi, M., Kelly, E. T., Duffee, J., & the Council on Foster Care, Adoption, and Kinship Care, Council on Community Pediatrics, Council on Child Abuse and Neglect, Committee on Psychosocial Aspects of Child and Family Health. (2021). Trauma-informed care. *Pediatrics*, 148(2), e2021052580. https://doi.org/10.1542/peds.2021-052580

Garcia Guerra, G., Robertson, C. M. T., Alton, G. Y., Joffe, A. R., Moez, E. K., Dinu, I. A., Ross, D. B., Rebeyka, I. M., Lequier, L., & the Western Canadian Complex Pediatric Therapies Follow-Up Group. (2014). Health-related quality of life in pediatric cardiac extracorporeal life support survivors. *Pediatric Critical Care Medicine*, 15(8), 720–727. https://doi.org/10.1097/PCC.0000000000000212

Gateau, K., Song, A., Vanderbilt, D. L., Gong, C., Friedlich, P., Kipke, M., & Lakshmanan, A. (2021). Maternal post-traumatic stress and depression symptoms and outcomes after NICU discharge in a low-income sample: A cross-sectional study. *BMC Pregnancy and Childbirth*, 21, 48. https://doi.org/10.1186/s12884-020-03536-0

Gavin, L. A., & Roesler, T. A. (1997). Posttraumatic distress in children and families after intubation. *Pediatric Emergency Care*, 13(3), 222–224. https://doi.org/10.1097/00006565-199706000-00013

Gizli Çoban, Ö., Sürer Adanır, A., & Özatalay, E. (2017). Post-traumatic stress disorder and health-related quality of life in the siblings of the pediatric bone marrow transplantation survivors and post-traumatic stress disorder in their mothers. *Pediatric Transplantation, 21*(6), e13003. https://doi.org/10.1111/petr.13003

Graf, A., Bergstraesser, E., & Landolt, M. A. (2013). Posttraumatic stress in infants and preschoolers with cancer. *Psycho-Oncology, 22*(7), 1543–1548. https://doi.org/10.1002/pon.3164

Haag, A. C., & Landolt, M. A. (2017). Young children's acute stress after a burn injury: Disentangling the role of injury severity and parental acute stress. *Journal of Pediatric Psychology, 42*(8), 861–870. https://doi.org/10.1093/jpepsy/jsx059

Haag, A. C., Landolt, M. A., Kenardy, J. A., Schiestl, C. M., Kimble, R. M., & De Young, A. C. (2020). Preventive intervention for trauma reactions in young injured children: Results of a multi-site randomised controlled trial. *Journal of Child Psychology and Psychiatry, 61*(9), 988–997. https://doi.org/10.1111/jcpp.13193

Hall, E., Saxe, G., Stoddard, F., Kaplow, J., Koenen, K., Chawla, N., Lopez, C., King, L., & King, D. (2006). Posttraumatic stress symptoms in parents of children with acute burns. *Journal of Pediatric Psychology, 31*(4), 403–412. https://doi.org/10.1093/jpepsy/jsj016

Harley, E., Williams, M. E., Zamora, I., & Lakatos, P. P. (2014). Trauma treatment in young children with developmental disabilities: Applications of the Child-Parent Psychotherapy model to the cases of "James" and "Juan." *Pragmatic Case Studies in Psychotherapy, 10*(3), 156–195. https://doi.org/10.14713/pcsp.v10i3.1869

Hayes, S. C., Pistorello, J., & Levin, M. E. (2012). Acceptance and commitment therapy as a unified model of behavior change. *The Counseling Psychologist, 40*(7), 976–1002. https://doi.org/10.1177/0011000012460836

Hind, T., Lui, S., Moon, E., Broad, K., Lang, S., Schreiber, R. A., Armstrong, K., & Blydt-Hansen, T. D. (2021). Post-traumatic stress as a determinant of quality of life in pediatric solid-organ transplant recipients. *Pediatric Transplantation, 25*(4), e14005. https://doi.org/10.1111/petr.14005

Hofmann, M., de Montalembert, M., Beauquier-Maccotta, B., de Villartay, P., & Golse, B. (2007). Posttraumatic stress disorder in children affected by sickle-cell disease and their parents. *American Journal of Hematology, 82*(2), 171–172. https://doi.org/10.1002/ajh.20722

Holbrook, T. L., Hoyt, D. B., Coimbra, R., Potenza, B., Sise, M., & Anderson, J. P. (2005). High rates of acute stress disorder impact quality-of-life outcomes in injured adolescents: Mechanism and gender predict acute stress disorder risk. *The Journal of Trauma, 59*(5), 1126–1130. https://doi.org/10.1097/01.ta.0000196433.61423.f2

Holbrook, T. L., Hoyt, D. B., Stein, M. B., & Sieber, W. J. (2001). Perceived threat to life predicts posttraumatic stress disorder after major trauma: Risk factors and functional outcome. *The Journal of Trauma, 51*(2), 287–293. https://doi.org/10.1097/00005373-200108000-00010

Holditch-Davis, D., Miles, M. S., Weaver, M. A., Black, B., Beeber, L., Thoyre, S., & Engelke, S. (2009). Patterns of distress in African-American mothers of preterm infants. *Journal of Developmental and Behavioral Pediatrics, 30*(3), 193–205. https://doi.org/10.1097/DBP.0b013e3181a7ee53

Howlader, N., Noone, A. M., Krapcho, M., Miller, D., Brest, A., Yu, M., Ruhl, J., Tatalovich, Z., Mariotto, A., Lewis, D. R., Chen, H. S., Feuer, E. J., & Cronin, K. A. (Eds.). (2021). *SEER Cancer Statistics Review, 1975–2018*. National Cancer Institute. https://seer.cancer.gov/csr/1975_2018/

Ibiebele, I., Algert, C. S., Bowen, J. R., & Roberts, C. L. (2018). Pediatric admissions that include intensive care: A population-based study. *BMC Health Services Research, 18*(1), 264. https://doi.org/10.1186/s12913-018-3041-x

Ingerski, L. M., Shaw, K., Gray, W. N., & Janicke, D. M. (2010). A pilot study comparing traumatic stress symptoms by child and parent report across pediatric chronic illness groups. *Journal of Developmental and Behavioral Pediatrics, 31*(9), 713–719. https://doi.org/10.1097/DBP.0b013e3181f17c52

Kahana, S. Y., Feeny, N. C., Youngstrom, E. A., & Drotar, D. (2006). Posttraumatic stress in youth experiencing illnesses and injuries: An exploratory meta-analysis. *Traumatology, 12*(2), 148–161. https://doi.org/10.1177/1534765606294562

Kaplow, J. B., Rolon-Arroyo, B., Layne, C. M., Rooney, E., Oosterhoff, B., Hill, R., Steinberg, A. M., Lotterman, J., Gallagher, K. A. S., & Pynoos, R. S. (2020). Validation of the UCLA PTSD reaction index for *DSM-5*: A developmentally informed assessment tool for youth. *Journal of the American Academy of Child & Adolescent Psychiatry, 59*(1), 186–194. https://doi.org/10.1016/j.jaac.2018.10.019

Kassam-Adams, N. (2006). Introduction to the special issue: Posttraumatic stress related to pediatric illness and injury. *Journal of Pediatric Psychology, 31*(4), 337–342. https://doi.org/10.1093/jpepsy/jsj052

Kassam-Adams, N., Bakker, A., Marsac, M. L., Fein, J. A., & Winston, F. K. (2015). Traumatic stress, depression, and recovery: Child and parent responses after emergency medical care for unintentional injury. *Pediatric Emergency*

Care, *31*(11), 737–742. https://doi.org/10.1097/PEC.0000000000000595

Kassam-Adams, N., Garcia-España, J. F., Fein, J. A., & Winston, F. K. (2005). Heart rate and posttraumatic stress in injured children. *Archives of General Psychiatry*, *62*(3), 335–340. https://doi.org/10.1001/archpsyc.62.3.335

Kazak, A. E. (2006). Pediatric psychosocial preventative health model (PPPHM): Research, practice, and collaboration in pediatric family systems medicine. *Families, Systems, & Health*, *24*(4), 381–395. https://doi.org/10.1037/1091-7527.24.4.381

Kazak, A. E., Alderfer, M. A., Streisand, R., Simms, S., Rourke, M. T., Barakat, L. P., Gallagher, P., & Cnaan, A. (2004). Treatment of posttraumatic stress symptoms in adolescent survivors of childhood cancer and their families: A randomized clinical trial. *Journal of Family Psychology*, *18*(3), 493–504. https://doi.org/10.1037/0893-3200.18.3.493

Kazak, A. E., Barakat, L. P., Ditaranto, S., Biros, D., Hwang, W. T., Beele, D., Kersun, L., Alderfer, M. A., Mougianis, I., Hocking, M. C., & Reilly, A. (2011). Screening for psychosocial risk at pediatric cancer diagnosis: The psychosocial assessment tool. *Journal of Pediatric Hematology/Oncology*, *33*(4), 289–294. https://doi.org/10.1097/MPH.0b013e31820c3b52

Kazak, A. E., Kassam-Adams, N., Schneider, S., Zelikovsky, N., Alderfer, M. A., & Rourke, M. (2006). An integrative model of pediatric medical traumatic stress. *Journal of Pediatric Psychology*, *31*(4), 343–355. https://doi.org/10.1093/jpepsy/jsj054

Kazak, A. E., Prusak, A., McSherry, M., Simms, S., Beele, D., Rourke, M., Alderfer, M., & Lange, B. (2001). The Psychosocial Assessment Tool (PAT)©: Pilot data on a brief screening instrument for identifying high risk families in pediatric oncology. *Families, Systems, & Health*, *19*(3), 303–317. https://doi.org/10.1037/h0089454

Kazak, A. E., Schneider, S., Didonato, S., & Pai, A. L. (2015). Family psychosocial risk screening guided by the Pediatric Psychosocial Preventative Health Model (PPPHM) using the Psychosocial Assessment Tool (PAT). *Acta Oncologica*, *54*(5), 574–580. https://doi.org/10.3109/0284186X.2014.995774

Kazak, A. E., Simms, S., Barakat, L., Hobbie, W., Foley, B., Golomb, V., & Best, M. (1999). Surviving cancer competently intervention program (SCCIP): A cognitive-behavioral and family therapy intervention for adolescent survivors of childhood cancer and their families. *Family Process*, *38*(2), 176–191. https://doi.org/10.1111/j.1545-5300.1999.00176.x

Kenardy, J. A., Spence, S. H., & Macleod, A. C. (2006). Screening for posttraumatic stress disorder in children after accidental injury. *Pediatrics*, *118*(3), 1002–1009. https://doi.org/10.1542/peds.2006-0406

Kremen, W. S., Koenen, K. C., Boake, C., Purcell, S., Eisen, S. A., Franz, C. E., Tsuang, M. T., & Lyons, M. J. (2007). Pretrauma cognitive ability and risk for posttraumatic stress disorder: A twin study. *Archives of General Psychiatry*, *64*(3), 361–368. https://doi.org/10.1001/archpsyc.64.3.361

Lakatos, P. P., Matic, T., Carson, M., & Williams, M. E. (2019). Child–parent psychotherapy with infants hospitalized in the neonatal intensive care unit. *Journal of Clinical Psychology in Medical Settings*, *26*(4), 584–596. https://doi.org/10.1007/s10880-019-09614-6

Landolt, M. A., Buehlmann, C., Maag, T., & Schiestl, C. (2009). Brief report: Quality of life is impaired in pediatric burn survivors with posttraumatic stress disorder. *Journal of Pediatric Psychology*, *34*(1), 14–21. https://doi.org/10.1093/jpepsy/jsm088

Landolt, M. A., Ystrom, E., Sennhauser, F. H., Gnehm, H. E., & Vollrath, M. E. (2012). The mutual prospective influence of child and parental posttraumatic stress symptoms in pediatric patients. *Journal of Child Psychology and Psychiatry*, *53*(7), 767–774. https://doi.org/10.1111/j.1469-7610.2011.02520.x

Lefkowitz, D. S., Baxt, C., & Evans, J. R. (2010). Prevalence and correlates of posttraumatic stress and postpartum depression in parents of infants in the neonatal intensive care unit (NICU). *Journal of Clinical Psychology in Medical Settings*, *17*(3), 230–237. https://doi.org/10.1007/s10880-010-9202-7

Lieberman, A. F., Ghosh Ippen, C., & Van Horn, P. (2015). *Don't hit my mommy: A manual for child parent psychotherapy with young witnesses of family violence* (2nd ed.). Zero to Three Press.

Long, K. A., Marsland, A. L., & Alderfer, M. A. (2013). Cumulative family risk predicts sibling adjustment to childhood cancer. *Cancer*, *119*(13), 2503–2510. https://doi.org/10.1002/cncr.28077

Ma, L., Mazidi, M., Li, K., Li, Y., Chen, S., Kirwan, R., Zhou, H., Yan, N., Rahman, A., Wang, W., & Wang, Y. (2021). Prevalence of mental health problems among children and adolescents during the COVID-19 pandemic: A systematic review and meta-analysis. *Journal of Affective Disorders*, *293*, 78–89. https://doi.org/10.1016/j.jad.2021.06.021

Marsac, M. L., Kassam-Adams, N., Hildenbrand, A. K., Nicholls, E., Winston, F. K., Leff, S. S., & Fein, J. (2016). Implementing a trauma-informed approach in pediatric healthcare networks. *JAMA Pediatrics, 170*(1), 70–77. https://doi.org/10.1001/jamapediatrics.2015.2206

Martin-Herz, S. P., Zatzick, D. F., & McMahon, R. J. (2012). Health-related quality of life in children and adolescents following traumatic injury: A review. *Clinical Child and Family Psychology Review, 15*(3), 192–214. https://doi.org/10.1007/s10567-012-0115-x

Meiser-Stedman, R. A., Yule, W., Dalgleish, T., Smith, P., & Glucksman, E. (2006). The role of the family in child and adolescent posttraumatic stress following attendance at an emergency department. *Journal of Pediatric Psychology, 31*(4), 397–402. https://doi.org/10.1093/jpepsy/jsj005

Melnyk, B. M., Alpert-Gillis, L., Feinstein, N. F., Crean, H. F., Johnson, J., Fairbanks, E., Small, L., Rubenstein, J., Slota, M., & Corbo-Richert, B. (2004). Creating opportunities for parent empowerment: Program effects on the mental health/coping outcomes of critically ill young children and their mothers. *Pediatrics, 113*(6), e597–e607. https://doi.org/10.1542/peds.113.6.e597

Mevissen, L., Ooms-Evers, M., Serra, M., de Jongh, A., & Didden, R. (2020). Feasibility and potential effectiveness of an intensive trauma-focused treatment programme for families with PTSD and mild intellectual disability. *European Journal of Psychotraumatology, 11*(1), 1777809. https://doi.org/10.1080/20008198.2020.1777809

Miller, A., Enlow, M. B., Reich, W., & Saxe, G. (2009). A diagnostic interview for acute stress disorder for children and adolescents. *Journal of Traumatic Stress, 22*(6), 549–556. https://doi.org/10.1002/jts.20471

Muscara, F., McCarthy, M. C., Hearps, S. J. C., Nicholson, J. M., Burke, K., Dimovski, A., Darling, S., Rayner, M., & Anderson, V. A. (2018). Trajectories of posttraumatic stress symptoms in parents of children with a serious childhood illness or injury. *Journal of Pediatric Psychology, 43*(10), 1072–1082. https://doi.org/10.1093/jpepsy/jsy035

Muscara, F., McCarthy, M. C., Thompson, E. J., Heaney, C. M., Hearps, S. J. C., Rayner, M., Burke, K., Nicholson, J. M., & Anderson, V. A. (2017). Psychosocial, demographic, and illness-related factors associated with acute traumatic stress responses in parents of children with a serious illness or injury. *Journal of Traumatic Stress, 30*(3), 237–244. https://doi.org/10.1002/jts.22193

National Child Traumatic Stress Network. (n.d.-a). *Creating trauma-informed systems.* https://www.nctsn.org/trauma-informed-care/creating-trauma-informed-systems

National Child Traumatic Stress Network. (n.d.-b). *Medical trauma.* https://www.nctsn.org/what-is-child-trauma/trauma-types/medical-trauma

National Child Traumatic Stress Network. (n.d.-c). *Medical trauma: Effects.* https://www.nctsn.org/what-is-child-trauma/trauma-types/medical-trauma/effects

National Child Traumatic Stress Network. (n.d.-d). *Screening and assessment.* https://www.nctsn.org/treatments-and-practices/screening-and-assessment/

National Child Traumatic Stress Network. (2014). *Pediatric medical traumatic stress toolkit for health care providers.* https://www.nctsn.org/resources/pediatric-medical-traumatic-stress-toolkit-health-care-providers

National Heart, Lung, and Blood Institute. (2021). *What is sickle cell disease?* https://www.nhlbi.nih.gov/health-topics/sickle-cell-disease

Neul, S. K. (2012). Medical traumatic stress symptoms in pediatric patients on dialysis and their caregivers: A pilot study. *Nephrology Nursing Journal, 39*(6), 483–488.

Nugent, N. R., Christopher, N. C., Crow, J. P., Browne, L., Ostrowski, S., & Delahanty, D. L. (2010). The efficacy of early propranolol administration at reducing PTSD symptoms in pediatric injury patients: A pilot study. *Journal of Traumatic Stress, 23*(2), 282–287. https://doi.org/10.1002/jts.20517

O'Connor, S. S., Zatzick, D. F., Wang, J., Temkin, N., Koepsell, T. D., Jaffe, K. M., Durbin, D., Vavilala, M. S., Dorsch, A., & Rivara, F. P. (2012). Association between posttraumatic stress, depression, and functional impairments in adolescents 24 months after traumatic brain injury. *Journal of Traumatic Stress, 25*(3), 264–271. https://doi.org/10.1002/jts.21704

Obeidat, H. M., Bond, E. A., & Callister, L. C. (2009). The parental experience of having an infant in the newborn intensive care unit. *Journal of Perinatal Education, 18*(3), 23–29. https://doi.org/10.1624/105812409X461199

Packman, W., Weber, S., Wallace, J., & Bugescu, N. (2010). Psychological effects of hematopoietic SCT on pediatric patients, siblings and parents: A review. *Bone Marrow Transplantation, 45*(7), 1134–1146. https://doi.org/10.1038/bmt.2010.74

Pelcovitz, D., Libov, B. G., Mandel, F., Kaplan, S., Weinblatt, M., & Septimus, A. (1998). Post-traumatic stress disorder and family functioning in adolescent cancer. *Journal of Traumatic Stress, 11*(2), 205–221. https://doi.org/10.1023/A:1024442802113

Penner, J., Abdel-Mannan, O., Grant, K., Maillard, S., Kucera, F., Hassell, J., Eyre, M., Berger, Z.,

Hacohen, Y., & Moshal, K. (2021). 6-month multidisciplinary follow-up and outcomes of patients with paediatric inflammatory multisystem syndrome (PIMS-TS) at a UK tertiary paediatric hospital: A retrospective cohort study. *The Lancet Child & Adolescent Health*, 5(7), 473–482. https://doi.org/10.1016/S2352-4642(21)00138-3

Picoraro, J. A., Womer, J. W., Kazak, A. E., & Feudtner, C. (2014). Posttraumatic growth in parents and pediatric patients. *Journal of Palliative Medicine*, 17(2), 209–218. https://doi.org/10.1089/jpm.2013.0280

Pierrehumbert, B., Nicole, A., Muller-Nix, C., Forcada-Guex, M., & Ansermet, F. (2003). Parental post-traumatic reactions after premature birth: Implications for sleeping and eating problems in the infant. *Archives of Disease in Childhood. Fetal and Neonatal Edition*, 88(5), F400–F404. https://doi.org/10.1136/fn.88.5.F400

Pinquart, M. (2020). Posttraumatic stress symptoms and disorders in children and adolescents with chronic physical illnesses: A meta-analysis. *Journal of Child & Adolescent Trauma*, 13(1), 1–10. https://doi.org/10.1007/s40653-018-0222-z

Price, J., Kassam-Adams, N., Alderfer, M. A., Christofferson, J., & Kazak, A. E. (2016). Systematic review: A reevaluation and update of the integrative (trajectory) model of pediatric medical traumatic stress. *Journal of Pediatric Psychology*, 41(1), 86–97. https://doi.org/10.1093/jpepsy/jsv074

Ramsdell, K. D., Smith, A. J., Hildenbrand, A. K., & Marsac, M. L. (2015). Posttraumatic stress in school-age children and adolescents: Medical providers' role from diagnosis to optimal management. *Pediatric Health, Medicine and Therapeutics*, 6, 167–180. https://doi.org/10.2147/PHMT.S68984

Rosenberg, L., Rosenberg, M., Sharp, S., Thomas, C. R., Humphries, H. F., Holzer, C. E., III, Herndon, D. N., & Meyer, W. J., III. (2018). Does acute propranolol treatment prevent posttraumatic stress disorder, anxiety, and depression in children with burns? *Journal of Child and Adolescent Psychopharmacology*, 28(2), 117–123. https://doi.org/10.1089/cap.2017.0073

Sameroff, A. (2009). *The transactional model*. American Psychological Association. https://doi.org/10.1037/11877-001

Saxe, G., Chawla, N., Stoddard, F., Kassam-Adams, N., Courtney, D., Cunningham, K., Lopez, C., Hall, E., Sheridan, R., King, D., & King, L. (2003). Child Stress Disorders Checklist: A measure of ASD and PTSD in children. *Journal of the American Academy of Child & Adolescent Psychiatry*, 42(8), 972–978. https://doi.org/10.1097/01.CHI.0000046887.27264.F3

Saxe, G., Stoddard, F., Chawla, N., Lopez, C. G., Hall, E., Sheridan, R., King, D., & King, L. (2005). Risk factors for acute stress disorder in children with burns. *Journal of Trauma & Dissociation*, 6(2), 37–49. https://doi.org/10.1300/J229v06n02_05

Saxe, G., Stoddard, F., Courtney, D., Cunningham, K., Chawla, N., Sheridan, R., King, D., & King, L. (2001). Relationship between acute morphine and the course of PTSD in children with burns. *Journal of the American Academy of Child and Adolescent Psychiatry*, 40(8), 915–921. https://doi.org/10.1097/00004583-200108000-00013

Saxe, G. N., Miller, A., Bartholomew, D., Hall, E., Lopez, C., Kaplow, J., Koenen, K. C., Bosquet, M., Allee, L., Erikson, I., & Moulton, S. (2005). Incidence of and risk factors for acute stress disorder in children with injuries. *The Journal of Trauma*, 59(4), 946–953. https://doi.org/10.1097/01.ta.0000187659.37385.16

Saxe, G. N., Stoddard, F., Hall, E., Chawla, N., Lopez, C., Sheridan, R., King, D., King, L., & Yehuda, R. (2005). Pathways to PTSD, part I: Children with burns. *The American Journal of Psychiatry*, 162(7), 1299–1304. https://doi.org/10.1176/appi.ajp.162.7.1299

Saylor, C. F., Swenson, C. C., Stokes Reynolds, S., & Taylor, M. (1999). The pediatric emotional distress scale: A brief screening measure for young children exposed to traumatic events. *Journal of Clinical Child Psychology*, 28(1), 70–81. https://doi.org/10.1207/s15374424jccp2801_6

Schwartz, L., & Drotar, D. (2006). Posttraumatic stress and related impairment in survivors of childhood cancer in early adulthood compared to healthy peers. *Journal of Pediatric Psychology*, 31(4), 356–366. https://doi.org/10.1093/jpepsy/jsj018

Sharp, K. M. H., Lindwall, J. J., Willard, V. W., Long, A. M., Martin-Elbahesh, K. M., & Phipps, S. (2017). Cancer as a stressful life event: Perceptions of children with cancer and their peers. *Cancer*, 123(17), 3385–3393. https://doi.org/10.1002/cncr.30741

Shaw, R. J., Bernard, R. S., Deblois, T., Ikuta, L. M., Ginzburg, K., & Koopman, C. (2009). The relationship between acute stress disorder and posttraumatic stress disorder in the neonatal intensive care unit. *Psychosomatics*, 50(2), 131–137. https://doi.org/10.1176/appi.psy.50.2.131

Shemesh, E., Annunziato, R. A., Shneider, B. L., Dugan, C. A., Warshaw, J., Kerkar, N., & Emre, S. (2008). Improving adherence to medications in pediatric liver transplant recipients. *Pediatric Transplantation*, 12(3), 316–323. https://doi.org/10.1111/j.1399-3046.2007.00791.x

Siegel, R. L., Miller, K. D., Fuchs, H. E., & Jemal, A. (2021). Cancer statistics, 2021. *CA: A Cancer*

Journal for Clinicians, 71(1), 7–33. https://doi.org/10.3322/caac.21654

Simon, S., Moreyra, A., Wharton, E., Dowtin, L. L., Borkovi, T. C., Armer, E., & Shaw, R. J. (2021). Prevention of posttraumatic stress disorder in mothers of preterm infants using trauma-focused group therapy: Manual development and evaluation. Early Human Development, 154, 105282. https://doi.org/10.1016/j.earlhumdev.2020.105282

Steinberg, A. M., Brymer, M. J., Decker, K. B., & Pynoos, R. S. (2004). The University of California at Los Angeles post-traumatic stress disorder reaction index. Current Psychiatry Reports, 6(2), 96–100. https://doi.org/10.1007/s11920-004-0048-2

Stoddard, F. J., Jr., Luthra, R., Sorrentino, E. A., Saxe, G. N., Drake, J., Chang, Y., Levine, J. B., Chedekel, D. S., & Sheridan, R. L. (2011). A randomized controlled trial of sertraline to prevent posttraumatic stress disorder in burned children. Journal of Child and Adolescent Psychopharmacology, 21(5), 469–477. https://doi.org/10.1089/cap.2010.0133

Stoddard, F. J., & Saxe, G. (2001). Ten-year research review of physical injuries. Journal of the American Academy of Child and Adolescent Psychiatry, 40(10), 1128–1145. https://doi.org/10.1097/00004583-200110000-00007

Stoddard, F. J., Saxe, G., Ronfeldt, H., Drake, J. E., Burns, J., Edgren, C., & Sheridan, R. (2006). Acute stress symptoms in young children with burns. Journal of the American Academy of Child and Adolescent Psychiatry, 45(1), 87–93. https://doi.org/10.1097/01.chi.0000184934.71917.3a

Stoddard, F. J., Jr., Sorrentino, E. A., Ceranoglu, T. A., Saxe, G., Murphy, J. M., Drake, J. E., Ronfeldt, H., White, G. W., Kagan, J., Snidman, N., Sheridan, R. L., & Tompkins, R. G. (2009). Preliminary evidence for the effects of morphine on posttraumatic stress disorder symptoms in one- to four-year-olds with burns. Journal of Burn Care & Research, 30(5), 836–843. https://doi.org/10.1097/BCR.0b013e3181b48102

Stowman, S., Kearney, C. A., & Daphtary, K. (2015). Mediators of initial acute and later posttraumatic stress in youth in a PICU. Pediatric Critical Care Medicine, 16(4), 113. https://doi.org/10.1097/PCC.0b013e31822f1916

Strawn, J. R., Keeshin, B. R., & Cohen, J. A. (2023). Pharmacotherapy for posttraumatic stress disorder in children and adolescents. UpToDate. https://www.uptodate.com/contents/posttraumatic-stress-disorder-in-children-and-adolescents-treatment-overview

Strawn, J. R., Keeshin, B. R., DelBello, M. P., Geracioti, T. D., Jr., & Putnam, F. W. (2010). Psychopharmacologic treatment of posttraumatic stress disorder in children and adolescents: A review. The Journal of Clinical Psychiatry, 71(7), 932–941. https://doi.org/10.4088/JCP.09r05446blu

Stuber, M. L. (1996). Psychiatric sequelae in seriously ill children and their families. Psychiatric Clinics of North America, 19(3), 481–493.

Stuber, M. L., Christakis, D. A., Houskamp, B., & Kazak, A. E. (1996). Posttrauma symptoms in childhood leukemia survivors and their parents. Psychosomatics, 37(3), 254–261. https://doi.org/10.1016/S0033-3182(96)71564-5

Stuber, M. L., Kazak, A. E., Meeske, K., Barakat, L., Guthrie, D., Garnier, H., Pynoos, R., & Meadows, A. (1997). Predictors of posttraumatic stress symptoms in childhood cancer survivors. Pediatrics, 100(6), 958–964. https://doi.org/10.1542/peds.100.6.958

Stuber, M. L., Nader, K., Yasuda, P., Pynoos, R. S., & Cohen, S. (1991). Stress responses after pediatric bone marrow transplantation: Preliminary results of a prospective longitudinal study. Journal of the American Academy of Child and Adolescent Psychiatry, 30(6), 952–957. https://doi.org/10.1097/00004583-199111000-00013

Supelana, C., Annunziato, R. A., Kaplan, D., Helcer, J., Stuber, M. L., & Shemesh, E. (2016). PTSD in solid organ transplant recipients: Current understanding and future implications. Pediatric Transplantation, 20(1), 23–33. https://doi.org/10.1111/petr.12628

Taïeb, O., Moro, M. R., Baubet, T., Revah-Lévy, A., & Flament, M. F. (2003). Posttraumatic stress symptoms after childhood cancer. European Child & Adolescent Psychiatry, 12(6), 255–264. https://doi.org/10.1007/s00787-003-0352-0

Taylor, N., Absolom, K., Snowden, J., Eiser, C., & the Late Effects Group Sheffield. (2012). Need for psychological follow-up among young adult survivors of childhood cancer. European Journal of Cancer Care, 21(1), 52–58. https://doi.org/10.1111/j.1365-2354.2011.01281.x

Toon, M. H., Maybauer, D. M., Arceneaux, L. L., Fraser, J. F., Meyer, W., Runge, A., & Maybauer, M. O. (2011). Children with burn injuries—Assessment of trauma, neglect, violence and abuse. Journal of Injury and Violence Research, 3(2), 99–110. https://doi.org/10.5249/jivr.v3i2.91

Ünay, M., Önder, A., Gizli Çoban, Ö., Atalay, A., Sürer Adanir, A., Artan, R., & Özatalay, E. (2020). Psychopathology, quality of life, and related factors in pediatric liver transplantation candidates and recipients. Pediatric Transplantation, 24(1), e13633. https://doi.org/10.1111/petr.13633

Valentine, S. L., & Randolph, A. G. (2015). Long-term outcomes after mechanical ventilation in children. Pediatric and neonatal mechanical ventilation.

Springer Berlin Heidelberg. https://doi.org/10.1007/978-3-642-01219-8_64

van Meijel, E. P. M., Gigengack, M. R., Verlinden, E., van der Steeg, A. F. W., Goslings, J. C., Bloemers, F. W., Luitse, J. S. K., Boer, F., Grootenhuis, M. A., & Lindauer, R. J. L. (2019). Long-term posttraumatic stress following accidental injury in children and adolescents: Results of a 2–4-year follow-up study. *Journal of Clinical Psychology in Medical Settings*, 26(4), 597–607. https://doi.org/10.1007/s10880-019-09615-5

Vanderbilt, D., Bushley, T., Young, R., & Frank, D. A. (2009). Acute posttraumatic stress symptoms among urban mothers with newborns in the neonatal intensive care unit: A preliminary study. *Journal of Developmental and Behavioral Pediatrics*, 30(1), 50–56. https://doi.org/10.1097/DBP.0b013e318196b0de

Vanderbilt, D., Young, R., MacDonald, H. Z., Grant-Knight, W., Saxe, G., & Zuckerman, B. (2008). Asthma severity and PTSD symptoms among inner city children: A pilot study. *Journal of Trauma & Dissociation*, 9(2), 191–207. https://doi.org/10.1080/15299730802046136

Vyse, A., Anonychuk, A., Jäkel, A., Wieffer, H., & Nadel, S. (2013). The burden and impact of severe and long-term sequelae of meningococcal disease. *Expert Review of Anti-Infective Therapy*, 11(6), 597–604. https://doi.org/10.1586/eri.13.42

Ward-Begnoche, W. L., Aitken, M. E., Liggin, R., Mullins, S. H., Kassam-Adams, N., Marks, A., & Winston, F. K. (2006). Emergency department screening for risk for post-traumatic stress disorder among injured children. *Injury Prevention*, 12(5), 323–326. https://doi.org/10.1136/ip.2006.011965

Williams, M., Carson, M., Zamora, I., Harley, E. K., & Lakatos, P. P. (2014). Child-parent psychotherapy in the context of developmental disability and medical service systems. *Pragmatic Case Studies in Psychotherapy*, 10(3), 212–226. https://doi.org/10.14713/pcsp.v10i3.1871

Winston, F. K., Kassam-Adams, N., Garcia-España, F., Ittenbach, R., & Cnaan, A. (2003). Screening for risk of persistent posttraumatic stress in injured children and their parents. *JAMA: Journal of the American Medical Association*, 290(5), 643–649. https://doi.org/10.1001/jama.290.5.643

Witt, W. P., Weiss, A. J., & Elixhauser, A. (2014). *Overview of hospital stays for children in the United States, 2012. HCUP Statistical Brief #187*. Agency for Healthcare Research and Quality. https://www.hcup-us.ahrq.gov/reports/statbriefs/sb187-Hospital-Stays-Children-2012.pdf

Woodward, L. J., Bora, S., Clark, C. A., Montgomery-Hönger, A., Pritchard, V. E., Spencer, C., & Austin, N. C. (2014). Very preterm birth: Maternal experiences of the neonatal intensive care environment. *Journal of Perinatology*, 34(7), 555–561. https://doi.org/10.1038/jp.2014.43

Yi, J., Zebrack, B., Kim, M. A., & Cousino, M. (2015). Posttraumatic growth outcomes and their correlates among young adult survivors of childhood cancer. *Journal of Pediatric Psychology*, 40(9), 981–991. https://doi.org/10.1093/jpepsy/jsv075

Zatzick, D. F., Grossman, D. C., Russo, J., Pynoos, R., Berliner, L., Jurkovich, G., Sabin, J. A., Katon, W., Ghesquiere, A., McCauley, E., & Rivara, F. P. (2006). Predicting posttraumatic stress symptoms longitudinally in a representative sample of hospitalized injured adolescents. *Journal of the American Academy of Child & Adolescent Psychiatry*, 45(10), 1188–1195. https://doi.org/10.1097/01.chi.0000231975.21096.45

Zhang, H., Xu, H., Huang, L., Wang, Y., Deng, F., Wang, X., Tang, X., Wang, W., Fu, X., Tao, Y., & Yin, L. (2021). Increased occurrence of PTSD symptoms in adolescents with major depressive disorder soon after the start of the COVID-19 outbreak in China: A cross-sectional survey. *BMC Psychiatry*, 21(1), 395. https://doi.org/10.1186/s12888-021-03400-1

CHAPTER 5

PEDIATRIC PALLIATIVE, END-OF-LIFE, AND BEREAVEMENT CARE

Cynthia A. Gerhardt, Anna Olsavsky, Garey Noritz, and Amy E. Baughcum

The death of a child has a profound impact on the family, as well as the providers who care for them. In this chapter, we summarize the current state of research and clinical practice in pediatric palliative, end-of-life, and bereavement care with attention to the characteristics of childhood death in the context of increasing medical advancements, unique trajectories of pediatric life-limiting conditions, and the barriers to quality palliative and end-of-life care. We discuss the importance of effective communication and shared decision making while highlighting interventions to mitigate the psychosocial impact on parents and siblings through family-centered approaches. We consider the impact of death, dying, and grief on the child and family system, and note how these processes vary by the developmental age of the child. We examine the ecological contexts, informed by developmental science, that are associated with more positive adaptation and family resilience. We also summarize the current state of research and clinical practice in pediatric palliative, end-of-life, and bereavement care with consideration for the roles of pediatric psychologists and developmental-behavioral pediatricians as partners in this difficult process.

By way of organization, the chapter begins with an overview and epidemiology of death and dying in childhood; considers a developmental approach to death and dying across the childhood lifespan; and presents clinical models of care for terminally ill children, with a focus on palliative and end-of-life care. We consider the impact of death and dying on the family system and discuss interventions to address grief. Drawing from research in developmental science, we consider factors associated with resilience and more positive family adaptation, and we discuss how pediatric psychologists and developmental-behavioral pediatricians can support families in this process. With an emphasis on developmentally tailored and culturally responsive approaches, attention is paid to the characteristics of childhood death in the context of increasing medical advancements. Lastly, we discuss how, through continued efforts, pediatric providers, researchers, and advocates can play a pivotal role in improving care and promoting resilience among families affected by a child's life-limiting condition and death.

OVERVIEW AND EPIDEMIOLOGY

About 40,000 U.S. children under the age of 20 die each year, resulting in a growing population of grieving parents and siblings (Goldstick et al., 2022; Xu et al., 2022). Despite improvements in prenatal and neonatal care, half of childhood deaths still occur in the first year of life (Xu et al., 2022).

https://doi.org/10.1037/0000414-005
APA Handbook of Pediatric Psychology, Developmental-Behavioral Pediatrics, and Developmental Science: Vol. 2. Pediatric Psychology and Developmental-Behavioral Pediatrics: Clinical Applications of Developmental Science, P. E. Shah and M. H. Bornstein (Editors-in-Chief)
Copyright © 2025 by the American Psychological Association. All rights reserved.

The top five causes of death in infancy include congenital anomalies, prematurity and low birth weight, sudden infant death syndrome, injuries, and complications of pregnancy. In contrast, firearm-related injuries and motor vehicle crashes are the primary causes of death in children aged 1 to 19 years (Goldstick et al., 2022). All injury-related causes (i.e., suicide, homicide, unintentional injuries) now account for 60% of childhood deaths. Cancer remains the leading cause of disease-related death in children at 9%, with congenital anomalies (5%) and heart disease (3%) as close second and third causes. Furthermore, social determinants of health result in significant disparities in mortality rates, as the highest rates of infant and childhood deaths occur in males, Black and Indigenous populations, as well as youth residing in rural areas (Goldstick et al., 2022; Xu et al., 2022). Thus, death in infancy and childhood is often unexpected, but it is also largely preventable.

Current estimates indicate that nearly 700,000 U.S. children have an acute or chronic condition that may shorten life expectancy (Connor et al., 2017). Life-limiting conditions can include (a) conditions with curative treatments that may be unsuccessful (e.g., cancer, organ failure); (b) conditions where treatments can prolong life, but premature death is inevitable (e.g., Duchenne muscular dystrophy, Batten disease); (c) progressive conditions without effective treatment options (e.g., Tay-Sachs disease, Menkes disease); and (d) irreversible but non-progressive conditions causing disability and susceptibility to severe health complications (e.g., cerebral palsy, traumatic brain or spinal cord injury). Children with medical complexity are defined as having conditions that involve multiple organ systems and result in functional limitations, high health care utilization, and/or the use of medical technology (Kuo & Houtrow, 2016). Collectively, this group accounts for only 1% of all children but one-third of all pediatric health care expenditures due to their frequent need for specialty services and higher risk of mortality (Cohen et al., 2012). These children are the highest utilizers of pediatric hospitalization and intensive care services, and they have the highest mortality rate.

DEATH AND DYING: CHILD LIFESPAN CONSIDERATIONS

Death in infancy presents unique challenges for families and health care providers, with 68% of these deaths occurring in the first month of life (Heron, 2018).

End-of-Life Care of Infants in the NICU

When a critically ill infant is admitted to the neonatal intensive care unit (NICU), they are often separated from their parents, who may still be recovering postbirth. This separation adds a level of complexity to the care of critically ill neonates. Symptom management can be difficult, requiring monitoring and interpretation of infant cues, as well as ongoing communication between parents and providers, who may have different perspectives (Cortezzo et al., 2015). In addition, infant physiological or behavioral distress may indicate a variety of symptoms or needs, which may be difficult to interpret. For example, changes in heart rate while crying can signal pain, agitation, a soiled diaper, hunger, or a desire to be held. Infants nearing death experience an average of six symptoms, such as respiratory distress, agitation, pain, and lethargy (Fortney et al., 2022; Shultz et al., 2017), but some infants may be obtunded and unable to mount a physiologic response to pain and other symptoms when death is imminent. Thus, infants in the final stages of life exhibit different symptom profiles and trajectories than older children, requiring unique approaches to care (Bertaud et al., 2023).

Aggressive care often occurs until the day of death in the NICU (Currie et al., 2023; Fortney et al., 2022). While some treatments can exacerbate infant suffering and offer limited benefit, medical interventions that are painful, burdensome, or otherwise compromise current quality of life may be acceptable to the family and providers if there is a reasonable chance that future quality of life could be improved by the treatment. Although most infant deaths occur in the neonatal period within hours or days of birth, lengthy stays in the NICU are common, offering opportunities for the provision of quality palliative and end-of-life care. Efforts to support more home-based deaths have grown (Craig & Mancini, 2013), but over 90% of infants that die do so in the hospital setting, usually after planned withdrawal of life-sustaining support (Currie et al., 2023; Fontana et al., 2013). Despite the well-documented benefits of palliation, advance directives are often initiated in the last day of life if at all, and less than one-third of infants who die receive a palliative care consult (Currie et al., 2023; Fortney et al., 2022).

End-of-Life Care of Children

For older children, research has primarily focused on characteristics of the end of life among children with cancer. The physiological symptoms associated with the end of life can vary, but children typically experience an average of 11 symptoms in the last week of life (Drake et al., 2003; Jalmsell et al., 2006; Wolfe et al., 2000). The most frequent and bothersome symptoms reported are fatigue and pain, which are nearly universal in children at the end of life (Drake et al., 2003; Pritchard et al., 2008; Theunissen et al., 2007). Other common symptoms include respiratory problems, nausea/vomiting, drowsiness, and poor appetite (Hongo et al., 2003; Jalmsell et al., 2006; Wolfe et al., 2000). Among children with complex chronic conditions, the most common symptoms near the end of life include respiratory distress, seizures, and feeding difficulties (Bao et al., 2021). These symptoms are often associated with multiorgan and neurological dysfunction, common to children with complex chronic conditions. In addition to the physiological symptoms associated with end-organ failure, children nearing death also experience psychological distress, which can manifest as sadness, anxiety, or irritability (Hongo et al., 2003). While it may be unrealistic to achieve complete symptom control for children near the end of life, there is clear evidence of poor quality of life across many domains and an urgent need for improvement, helping to inform future research and clinical interventions with this population (Huang et al., 2010; Tomlinson et al., 2011).

About half of children with life-limiting illnesses die in the hospital, with about half of those deaths occurring in the intensive care unit (ICU; Bao et al., 2021; Bradshaw et al., 2005; Wolfe et al., 2000). Most children with life-limiting conditions (or up to two-thirds of these children) have do-not-resuscitate (DNR) or allow natural death (AND) orders, usually written in the last month of life, with nearly half written in the last week prior to death (Bradshaw et al., 2005; Wolfe et al., 2000). Notably, the use of advance directives and palliative care may be higher for certain populations, such as children with complex chronic conditions (DeCourcey et al., 2018). Most children with life-limiting conditions who die in the ICU have an active DNR/AND order (Carter et al., 2004; DeCourcey et al., 2018; Drake et al., 2003).

END-OF-LIFE MODELS OF CARE: QUALITY OF DEATH, HOSPICE CARE, AND PALLIATIVE CARE MODELS

Quality of Death

Quality of death is a concept that has received increasing attention and is related to, but distinct from, symptom burden and quality of life. Quality of death is multidimensional and based on subjective, cultural, and dynamic factors during the final stages of the illness and dying process (Bhadelia et al., 2022; Hales et al., 2008). It is often defined as a death that is free from avoidable suffering, preserves one's dignity, and allows families to prepare, honor wishes, and say goodbye. A "good death" often occurs at home, with early palliative involvement, and advance directives in place, but this is primarily based on studies of adult deaths, with less research focused on children (Bluebond-Langner et al., 2013; Fortney & Steward, 2014; Moynihan et al., 2022). Most importantly, a "good death" is characterized by a death which is "goal-concordant" or consistent with the wishes of the deceased. However, goals for end-of-life care may differ among health care providers, parents, and the child (Bhadelia et al., 2022; Hales et al., 2008; Hendrickson & McCorkle, 2008). For example, many adults hope for a quick and painless death for themselves, but parents may tolerate their child having significant symptoms if it allows the possibility of having more time with them (Hales et al., 2008; Hendrickson & McCorkle, 2008). In a study of parents whose child died of a cardiac condition, a "good death" was associated with greater preparedness, having an advance care plan, non-cure-oriented goals of care, pain control, and avoidance of resuscitation efforts (Moynihan et al., 2022).

While a "good death" should be the standard of care, it remains unrealized for many individuals, and more research is needed in pediatric populations (Bhadelia et al., 2022; Hales et al., 2008). One way to help families achieve a "good death" is to consider implementing "end-of-life care models." Despite the benefits of certain specialty services, such as palliative and end-of-life care (Chong et al., 2018; Kaye et al., 2021; Marcus et al., 2020), many children with life-limiting conditions may not receive these services or receive them too late (Afonso et al., 2021; Cheng et al., 2019). Misperceptions regarding the meaning of end-of-life, hospice, and palliative care persist, with the terms often used interchangeably (Grant et al., 2021). Each is a distinct type of service to ease symptoms and suffering and to optimize quality of life.

End-of-Life-Care and Hospice Care

End-of-life care involves holistic management of a terminal condition and preparation of the family in the final months of life (Field & Behrman, 2003). Such services are often interdisciplinary (including physicians, nurses, social workers, chaplains, and psychologists) and can be provided by palliative care or hospice teams. *Hospice* is a type of end-of-life care and refers to a specialized program, often based in the home or a separate facility, for families of individuals who are typically within the last 6 months of life (von Gunten et al., 2001). There are some differences regarding which families pursue hospice or end-of-life care, with children who are White, who have cancer, and who have higher socioeconomic status being more likely to die at home (Wolff et al., 2020).

Palliative Care

Palliative care has been declared a fundamental right for children (Benini et al., 2022), and is described by the World Health Organization (2015) as comprehensive care that improves the quality of life and reduces suffering for individuals with a life-threatening condition and their families. Palliative care can coincide with curative goals and involves early identification, prevention, and treatment of physical, psychosocial, and spiritual distress. The American Academy of Pediatrics has endorsed national guidelines recommending the integration of palliative care at diagnosis, or as early as possible, to manage symptoms and to complement curative therapies for children (National Consensus Project for Quality Palliative Care, 2013). If curative therapies become less effective or fail, palliation can increase as the child's health declines and ease the transition to end-of-life care. Recognizing that families should not have to choose between palliative care and cure-directed medical care, the Affordable Care Act of 2010 made a specific provision for children to receive both at the same time, called concurrent care (Gans et al., 2016).

Benefits of palliative care. A growing body of research indicates that timely and appropriate referrals to palliative and end-of-life care can result in better outcomes for children and families. For example, one study found improvements in parents' perceptions of the child's symptoms and quality of life, communication, and access to care after referral (Vollenbroich et al., 2012). Health care providers also noted better family support, communication, and cooperation. Children who receive palliative care may spend fewer days in the hospital, receive fewer invasive interventions, and are less likely to die in the ICU (Keele et al., 2013). A recent review of palliative care for children with cancer found better symptom control and quality of life, fewer intensive procedures, higher rates of advance care planning, less time in the ICU, and a higher likelihood of dying at home (Kaye et al., 2021). Families also reported higher satisfaction with their child's care and improved communication. Other work has shown similar positive outcomes and reduced medical costs (Chong et al., 2018), but it also emphasizes the need for more research in this area (Marcus et al., 2020).

Challenges to implementation. Although historically more common, the death of a child tends to disrupt the natural order of events and is often preceded by heroic or prolonged efforts to save the child. With medical advancements, children with acute injuries or life-limiting conditions that were previously considered imminently fatal now live much longer. During this time, they may experience protracted rounds of treatment and medical interventions, as well as periods of relapses or flares, remissions, and/or refractory or quiescent disease. The unpredictability of these trajectories makes it difficult for providers to prognosticate when a condition will be life-limiting and when is the optimal time to broach the topic of palliative, end-of-life, or hospice care.

Family members and pediatric providers may avoid discussions about death due to their own discomfort, time constraints, language barriers, and a desire to protect the child from distress (Davies et al., 2008). Other challenges to providing quality palliative or end-of-life care include ethical issues, legal concerns, and financial barriers. This is amplified by a lack of U.S. Food and Drug Administration–approved medications and dosing for children, making off-label medication use common (García-López et al., 2020; Neville et al., 2014). Lastly, community-based palliative care or hospice organizations largely care for adults, who have quite different conditions and end-of-life trajectories than children. All these factors can hinder the provision of quality health care for seriously ill children. Despite these challenges, there is agreement about the benefits of end-of-life care (Kaye et al., 2021) and the importance of implementation within an ecological framework (Boyden et al., 2022).

ECOLOGICAL CONTEXTS RELEVANT TO END-OF-LIFE CARE

Based on Bronfenbrenner's ecological model (Bronfenbrenner, 1977), a multilevel framework has been described to conceptualize home-based care for children with serious illness and to guide future research (Boyden et al., 2022). Boyden et al. (2022) propose five levels of influence including individual (e.g., adherence, communication), family (e.g., caregiving, parent distress), home (e.g., language, finances), community (e.g., school-based services, spiritual support), and regional systems of care (e.g., pediatric palliative care, home health care). These levels represent more proximal to distal factors in relation to the child. Care coordination and disparities are also proposed as cross-cutting or transcendent factors that impact each level. Adverse outcomes for families result from the many interacting influences across each level that contribute to unnecessarily complex, fragmented, and poor-quality pediatric home-based care. A focus on factors at any single level or two is insufficient and instead requires a more comprehensive approach involving multilevel intervention to create meaningful and sustainable improvements in child outcomes.

Developmental Considerations in Death and Dying

Considerations around end-of-life care, and conversations with children who experience life-limiting conditions, should be individualized according to the child's developmental level. Pediatric providers and parents struggle with how and when to talk to children with life-limiting conditions and how to include them in decision making. Developmentally, children's understanding of illness and death evolves over time, particularly from the ages of 5 to 9 (Stein et al., 2019). At ages 3 or 4, children acknowledge death as an absence and part of the cycle of life. They have more concrete and temporary conceptualizations of illness and death that involve fantasy and magical thinking (e.g., death as a boogeyman or the ability to wish harm on others). At age 5, children begin to understand the permanence of death and that all living things die. Between ages 7 and 9, they gradually acquire more complex and abstract views that recognize their own mortality, appropriate causality, as well as the separation of the body and soul depending on the family's cultural or religious beliefs. However, understanding of death may occur at different ages among children and adults with neurodevelopmental disabilities.

It is now widely accepted that school-age children with life-limiting conditions should be informed about their health and treatment plan. "Truth-telling" can reduce children's uncertainty and fears, while enhancing their understanding, psychological adjustment, and adherence (Stein et al., 2019). Indeed, children want to be included in communication and decision making (Coyne & Gallagher, 2011; Lin et al., 2022; Sansom-Daly et al., 2020). Young children may have more difficulty understanding and making treatment decisions, but one-quarter of children (ages 8–12) and two-thirds of adolescents (ages 13–17) in one study wished to be involved (Ellis & Leventhal, 1993). Children have an awareness of their bodies and often observe cues from others, even if they are not explicitly or fully informed of their prognosis. They fear being alone at the end of life, and some children may feel isolated if they are aware of their impending death and are unable to talk about it (Hilden et al., 2000; Theunissen et al., 2007). Nearly all school-aged children with cancer want to be told if they are dying (Ellis & Leventhal, 1993), but they also report difficulty talking to parents about death and worry about upsetting them (Theunissen et al., 2007).

Not surprisingly, parents share more information with older children, but it is often focused on treatment and procedural details rather than disease severity (Eiser & Havermans, 1992). In a retrospective study of 139 bereaved parents in the U.S., nearly two-thirds spoke with their child about their cancer prognosis and death, and over 75% wanted support to talk to their children (Kenney et al., 2021). Half of the children had asked about death, particularly if they were older. However, in a Swedish cohort, only one-third of bereaved parents talked about death with their children who had cancer (Kreicbergs et al., 2004). Of parents who chose not to talk to their child, 27% regretted it, particularly when they sensed their child was aware of the impending death. Furthermore, regretful parents had more anxiety and depression 4 to 9 years later compared to parents who were content with their decision. Higher quality parent–child communication near diagnosis was related to better adjustment in children with advanced cancer over one year later (Keim et al., 2017). Thus, while it may not be appropriate or feasible to discuss death with all children, communicating openly can facilitate both parent and child adjustment and align goals of care.

Death, Dying, and the Family System

A family systems approach recognizes that a change in one family member (such as the experience of a child's life-limiting condition) affects all members of the family unit, and that adjustment to this process requires reorganization and adaptation (Hayslip & Page, 2013; Mehta et al., 2009). We consider this context as we examine how death and dying impact the family system through effects on parents and siblings.

Impact on parents. Limited research has focused on the well-being of parents near the end of a child's life. Parents of children in acute crisis in the emergency room or ICU may understandably experience significant anxiety and traumatic stress (Abela et al., 2020; October et al., 2018). In other cases where children may have a more protracted course before death, the family impact may vary. A qualitative study noted parents of children receiving home-based palliative care had concerns or worries in four areas: (a) ensuring that their child's remaining days were spent living well physically, emotionally, and socially; (b) uncertainty regarding their child's diagnosis, prognosis, and treatments; (c) what to expect in the dying process and when their child's death would occur; and (d) the impact on siblings and wanting to cherish as much family time as possible (Tutelman et al., 2021). Fear of the child's death and physical symptoms are frequent concerns for parents (Theunissen et al., 2007), and about half of parents of children with advanced cancer report high rates of distress (Rosenberg et al., 2013).

Caring for a seriously ill child can also negatively affect a parent's quality of life, mood, sleep, and fatigue (Klassen et al., 2008; Theunissen et al., 2007). These outcomes may be worse for parents of children with poorer health status, more intense treatment, less time since diagnosis, and more financial hardship (Klassen et al., 2008; Rosenberg et al., 2013). In one study, parents of children who had a "difficult death" (e.g., unrelieved pain, anxiety, respiratory distress, sleep disruption) reported more internalizing symptoms, more severe grief, and worse quality of life up to 9 years later (Jalmsell et al., 2010; Kreicbergs et al., 2005; van der Geest et al., 2014). Similarly, among bereaved parents whose infants died in the NICU, those who perceived greater suffering in the infant at the end of life reported higher levels of distress and feeling less satisfied with the care provided (Clark et al., 2021).

Impact on siblings. Siblings share a unique and often lifelong bond. When a child in the family has a life-limiting condition, siblings may have reduced contact with the ill child and parents, as well as additional demands for caregiving and other adult roles in the home (Gaab et al., 2014; von Essen & Enskär, 2003). Maintaining a normal routine can be a challenge, and siblings may view the illness or condition as a loss of their family's way of life (Labay & Walco, 2004; Williams et al., 2014). Exposure to a parent's distress and family disruption can significantly increase the risk for psychosocial difficulties in siblings (Long et al., 2018). Thus, it is important to consider sibling adjustment in the context of the family, as well as the developmental tasks or demands of typical children their age.

Siblings of children with life-limiting conditions may be at risk for multiple difficulties, such as internalizing problems before the death and afterward (Bolton et al., 2016; D'Alton et al., 2022; Hoffmann et al., 2018; Long et al., 2018; Vermaes et al., 2012). However, one systematic review also concluded bereaved siblings exhibited a high level of positive adjustment (D'Alton et al., 2022). While positive outcomes following the death of a sibling have been reported, such as having a better outlook on life and being kinder, more compassionate, and mature (Foster et al., 2012), a large body of literature has identified adjustment difficulties in siblings of deceased children. Specifically, bereaved siblings may have lower social competence and more internalizing and externalizing problems relative to instrument norms or controls (Bolton et al., 2016; McCown & Davies, 1995; Rosenberg et al., 2015). Self-concept can decline after the death (Eilegård et al., 2013), and bereaved siblings who are younger or male can also exhibit difficulties in peer relationships relative to classmates (Gerhardt et al., 2012). Adjustment usually improves with time, but grief symptoms can resurface as siblings reflect on the loss as they mature, highlighting the importance of longitudinal monitoring in children who have experienced the death of a sibling (Sveen et al., 2014).

SUPPORTING FAMILIES THROUGH DEATH, DYING, AND BEREAVEMENT

Grief is a universal response to loss and can be manifested through affective cognitive, behavioral, and physiological aspects, such as despair, anger, crying, agitation, and recurrent thoughts of the deceased. Parents can also experience anticipatory grief during their journey. The loss of the child's functioning, inability to attend school, and even the death of another child with a similar condition, are part of a series of cumulative losses that may precede their child's death. With critically ill neonates, anticipatory grief may result from an inability to interact with the infant outside of the hospital, experiencing fewer milestones, and missing opportunities for family or friends to meet the newborn or observe them in a parenting role (Clark, Fortney, Dunnells, Winning, et al., 2021; Currie et al., 2016). Attempts to differentiate typical and more pathological responses to grief have evolved (Gravesen & Birkelund, 2021), from traumatic or complicated grief (Horowitz et al., 2003; Shear et al., 2011) to complex bereavement disorder (American Psychiatric Association, 2022) to most recently, prolonged grief disorder (Prigerson et al., 2021, 2009). While controversial given the limitations they impose on the length and nature of grief (Gravesen & Birkelund, 2021), these diagnoses generally vary in the number, type (e.g., yearning, intense loneliness, preoccupation with the deceased), and duration of symptoms (e.g., 6–12 months), but all require clinically significant distress or functional impairment that is outside of sociocultural norms.

Compared to other types of loss, parental grief is more severe, and parents are at greater risk for complicated or prolonged grief reactions, particularly among mothers (Flach et al., 2022; Lannen et al., 2008; Lichtenthal et al., 2015; October et al., 2018). A systematic review of outcomes among fathers found that they, too, have a significant risk for persistent distress and may "navigate loss through stoicism, self-isolation, and hard work" (S. Morris et al., 2019). Other systematic reviews of bereaved parents confirm an increased risk for prolonged grief, depression, anxiety, and poor quality of life across multiple studies and types of death (Flach et al., 2022; McNeil et al., 2021; S. Morris et al., 2019; Rosenberg et al., 2012). Furthermore, bereaved parents report learning to live with fluctuations in pain as opposed to "getting over" their child's death, and grief can intensify at significant times (e.g., holidays, the anniversary of the child's death), a concept known as re-grief.

Bereaved parents can also face a crisis of meaning and identity after their child dies (Polita et al., 2020). They may struggle to make sense of the loss and to find meaning in their own and their child's life (Foster et al., 2009; Schaefer et al., 2021). After the death, their role as a caregiver to the ill child is suddenly gone, and they must reevaluate their identity and purpose, particularly as a parent. Bereaved parents often seek ways to continue their bond and connection to their child (Foster et al., 2011). This may include keeping linking objects (e.g., toys, clothes), building legacies (e.g., foundations, memorials), and other rituals (e.g., visiting gravesite) to keep their child's memory alive. Families bereaved by a violent death (e.g., firearm-related) may respond through activism or attempts to raise awareness of injustices (Cook, 2020). While continuing bonds may be adaptive, they can also interfere with other relationships if the parent is overly involved in these activities.

As individual family members grieve, they must learn new ways of being with each other (Hayslip & Page, 2013). The home may be joyless as parents and siblings withdraw into their own grief. Families may undergo significant change, with less family cohesion and greater parental and marital strain (Martinson et al., 1994; West et al., 1991). Grief among parents can be interdependent, influencing one another over time (Buyukcan-Tetik et al., 2022). While some relationships may strengthen, bereaved parents have reported lower marital satisfaction and sexual intimacy, more frequent thoughts of separation, and higher divorce rates than nonbereaved parents (Albuquerque et al., 2016; Gottlieb et al., 1996; Lang & Gottlieb, 1993; Lyngstad, 2013). However, adaptive outcomes following the death of a child have also been noted, with some parents reporting personal growth and positive outcomes, such as having greater compassion and closer relationships after their child's death (Clark, Fortney, Dunnells, Winning, et al., 2021; Flach et al., 2022; Jaaniste et al., 2017).

Factors Contributing to Risk and Resilience

Although risk and protective factors may contribute to variability in the adjustment of bereaved parents and siblings, findings have been inconsistent, likely due to methodological challenges in bereavement research. A systematic review noted that previous losses, financial hardship, greater duration and intensity of the child's treatment, less time to prepare for the child's death, perceptions of care, the child's quality of life, location and time since death, as well as other psychological comorbidities, are associated with greater difficulties among bereaved parents (Rosenberg et al., 2012). Similarly, parents' perception of symptom burden and suffering were related to greater distress after their infant's death in the NICU (Clark, Fortney, Dunnells, Gerhardt, et al., 2021). Longer stays in the ICU and financial hardship were associated with distress among bereaved family members, while greater social support and having a DNR order were associated with less distress (Tang et al., 2021). In another review, loss-oriented (e.g., multiple deaths, inability to say goodbye), interpersonal (e.g., marital disruption, less social support), and intrapersonal (e.g., female sex, less adaptive coping) factors were related to negative parent outcomes following the death of a child from other life-limiting conditions (Tang et al., 2021).

Having an opportunity to say goodbye has been associated with greater grief-related growth among siblings bereaved by cancer, while being present at the death and wishing they had done something differently were associated with both greater grief and growth in one study (Kenney et al., 2022). In another study, siblings who were dissatisfied with communication, ill-prepared for the death, unable to say goodbye, and/or felt cancer negatively affected their relationships also experienced greater long-term distress (Rosenberg et al., 2015). Adolescent females may experience greater internalizing symptoms, while adolescent males may exhibit more externalizing symptoms (D'Alton et al., 2022). Parent distress, poor family communication, negative parenting, and less social support can also contribute to worse sibling outcomes (D'Alton et al., 2022; Hoffmann et al., 2018; Howard Sharp et al., 2020; A. T. Morris et al., 2016). However, bereaved siblings may experience less grief and more growth with support from teachers and friends regardless of age, with adolescents particularly benefiting from support from close friends and peers (Howard Sharp et al., 2018).

The Importance of Communication and Goal-Directed Partnerships

Helping families navigate the experience of death, dying, and bereavement requires open communication between the health care team and families to facilitate decision making and advance care planning, and to assist families with coping and adjustment. For pediatric providers, communication with the family and other team members is an ongoing process, requiring staff support and mutually agreed upon treatment goals.

Effective communication between families and pediatric providers is central to quality care. However, parents have reported dissatisfaction with their child's medical care and communication at the end of life (Contro et al., 2002; Meyer et al., 2002). They may not feel fully informed of the situation and often have overly optimistic views of their child's prognosis (Kaye & Mack, 2013; Mack, Cronin, et al., 2020; Meyer et al., 2002; Miller et al., 2012; Rosenberg et al., 2014), particularly parents from minoritized backgrounds (Mack, Uno, et al., 2020). In one study, over half of parents felt they had little or no control over their child's final days, and nearly 25% would have made different decisions in retrospect (Meyer et al., 2002). At the same time, physicians report anxiety and reluctance to prognosticate, deliver bad news, and diminish hope in families (Meyer et al., 2002). Yet, evidence shows that physicians' discussions of prognosis do not necessarily diminish hope in parents, even when the chance of cure is low (Mack et al., 2007). Furthermore, parents' hope for a cure is unrelated to long-term grief or symptoms of depression (van der Geest et al., 2015), suggesting that provider conversations that offer honest prognoses while involving parents in decision making can create goal-directed partnerships that offer realistic hope.

There are circumstances when communication can be more difficult, such as when death occurs unexpectedly. Guidelines have been provided for managing communication and care in the context of a child's unanticipated death in the emergency room, which can be quite challenging when there is little time to establish a relationship with the family (O'Malley et al., 2014). In other circumstances, for example, in the case of a child's life-limiting condition, providers may have more time and should be prepared to have multiple conversations, usually first with parents when breaking bad news and then to assess their preference for sharing information with the child and others. Providers should meet family members at their level of understanding and comfort to help them process the information and make decisions over time. It is important to confirm family values and beliefs about death, assist parents in talking about the diagnosis and death with the child and siblings, give children time to ask questions and express themselves in developmentally appropriate ways (e.g., journaling, artwork), support shared decision making, allow the family to express feelings for one another, and prepare them to say goodbye as the end of life approaches. Consensus building and assessing family preferences for care, such as life-sustaining treatments, mechanical support, code status, and place of death, are important and foundational to building goal-directed partnerships with families. It is also important to include children with life-limiting conditions in this partnership, to allow them to have a voice in end-of-life decisions. For example, some children may wish to leave gifts or belongings to loved ones, participate in funeral planning, or make other requests as the time of death approaches (Foster et al., 2009; Sansom-Daly et al., 2020).

When providers assist with advance care planning, they should also consider the cultural, spiritual, and religious beliefs of the child and family (Kirkwood, 2005), as well as ethical and legal guidelines. Several advance directive tools (e.g., Five Wishes™, Voicing my Choices™) and family-centered interventions have been developed and can facilitate these challenging discussions (Lin et al., 2022; Lyon et al., 2013; Wiener et al., 2012; Zadeh et al., 2015). It is also important to discuss a living will and durable power of attorney with patients over 18, who have decisional capacity. Advance care plans should be documented in writing, readily accessible, and periodically revised based on changes in the child's status and re-evaluation of family needs and preferences.

Discussions about organ donation and autopsy may also occur before or soon after the death. While difficult, these discussions have the potential to promote family healing and closure, provide altruistic benefits, and minimize uncertainty or long-term regrets (Sullivan & Monagle, 2011). Given the high need and lack of "right-sized" organs in pediatric transplant, research on family decision making regarding organ donation is surprisingly limited. Notably, one study of over 2000 healthy Dutch adolescents (ages 12–15) found that two-thirds would be open to organ donation, and 75% wanted to make the decision themselves (Siebelink et al., 2012). Although physicians may be reluctant to initiate conversations about organ donation and autopsy with families, adolescents and young adults with life-limiting conditions report appreciating the opportunity to donate their body or specimens for research, while parents value helping other children and contributing to medical knowledge (Sullivan & Monagle, 2011; Wiener et al., 2012). In one study, nearly 90% of bereaved parents indicated they would have considered an autopsy had it been discussed (Wiener et al., 2014). While acknowledging the potential need for multiple discussions, most bereaved parents (87%) felt these conversations would have been valuable before the child died, with 77% preferring the discussion when death was near to aid clearer decision making, meaning making, and preparation for the death (Wiener et al., 2014).

RITUALS AFTER DEATH: FUNERALS, MEMORIALS, AND CELEBRATIONS OF LIFE

The preferences and needs of families can vary as their child nears the end of life. If possible, it is important to determine if family members have any special requests (e.g., baptism, last rites) before the child dies and if they wish to be together before or during the death. Not all family members can or want to be present at the time of death, but this should be addressed with the preferences of both the child and family in mind. Providers should prepare parents for the physical responses to death (e.g., changes in respiration, rigor mortis) if they choose to be present. Some may want to remain with the child afterward to hold them, take pictures, or prepare the body (e.g., bathing, dressing). Parents may wish to have a lock of hair, imprints of their child's hands or feet, or other mementos as well. Families should be allowed as much time as needed to say goodbye during these last moments.

While some families may have made decisions regarding memorial services, others may need the support of the health care team to make arrangements. If a family does not have spiritual or religious support in their community, hospital social workers and chaplains can assist with the choice of funeral home, types of services, and resources for financial support. Acceptance of cremation, embalming, or viewing of the body, as well as the timing of rituals and burial, can vary based on cultural or religious beliefs (Weaver et al., 2023). Parents should be encouraged to discuss arrangements with siblings and offer an opportunity for them to attend, be involved, and grieve with the family (Anderson, 2020). They should not be forced to attend or denied (Søfting et al., 2016). Siblings may wish to write a letter, draw a picture, or leave a memento with their brother or sister. Depending on their age, some siblings may want to say a few words, share a reading or poem, or participate in another aspect of the service. It is also important to discern the family's desire for future contact or openness to the attendance of health care providers at the visitation or services (Macdonald et al., 2005). Again, these decisions should be made with the family's wishes in mind, as well as the preferences of the provider and/or guidelines from the organization. Importantly, it is common practice to provide families with information on bereavement resources and support after the death.

Grief Interventions for Families and Providers

Research indicates that bereaved individuals underutilize services, and support groups may be perceived as stigmatizing or unhelpful (Cherlin et al., 2007; Hill et al., 2023; Lichtenthal et al., 2015). Currently, there is a relative lack of empirically based interventions for families of children near the end of life or for their providers.

Interventions for families. Several meta-analyses of grief interventions for bereaved parents or siblings have reached different conclusions regarding efficacy (Currier et al., 2007; Hill et al., 2023; Jordan & Neimeyer, 2003; Larson & Hoyt, 2007; Rosner et al., 2010). The largest and most persistent effects are found for cognitive behavioral approaches and when studies screen parents and siblings to include only those with elevated levels of distress. Challenges remain regarding whom to target, as well as the content, structure, and timing of interventions (Hill et al., 2023). Only 30% to 40% of bereaved parents receive formal services; most often these are bereaved mothers, who have greater distress and tend to seek medications or psychotherapy (Hill et al., 2023; Lichtenthal et al., 2015).

Several factors influence whether families seek intervention or services to address grief and bereavement. Families may not seek treatment because they are often reluctant to return to the hospital for help due to painful memories or trauma, and bereavement services may be limited in the community. Furthermore, many bereaved individuals may desire support that is specific to their child's diagnosis or situation (e.g., accidental death or illness), which may make it difficult to find individualized resources and services. Some families find support groups, books, web-based resources, or formal therapy helpful, while others prefer to process their grief alone (Hill et al., 2023). To facilitate family adjustment, there have been recent calls for greater accessibility to bereavement care in the United States, including updating the Family and Medical Leave Act to recognize child death as an eligible event for parental leave (Mulheron & Inouye, 2020). Given that Black parents experience disproportionate rates of bereavement, such policies may also support broader efforts to minimize racial health disparities (Umberson et al., 2017).

Interventions for providers. For providers caring for children with life-limiting conditions, there is recognition of the unique and compounding effects of trauma and loss in a pediatric environment. Most literature has focused on provider burnout or compassion fatigue, with less on grief-specific support (Carton & Hupcey, 2014). However, stress management, maintenance of professional boundaries, peer support, and debriefings may be helpful for pediatric providers (Melin-Johansson et al., 2014). Hospital-based interventions have been found to facilitate positive outcomes, such as closure, stress relief, team cohesion, and improved end-of-life care, but evidence has been inconsistent in reducing provider grief (Yazdan et al., 2023). For families and providers, there is recognition that grief is an intensely personal experience, and what benefits one person may not benefit another. Thus, recommendations based on the current evidence suggest services should focus on those bereaved individuals with the greatest symptoms and need.

METHODOLOGICAL CONSIDERATIONS IN RESEARCH

Despite the recent increase in palliative care research, the design and methodological rigor of bereavement studies have lagged. Most studies are retrospective and qualitative, especially those with bereaved siblings. As a result, there have been calls for prospective, longitudinal research that incorporates standardized measures of both negative effects (e.g., grief, risk for psychopathology), as well as the assessment of personal growth (Niemeyer & Hogan, 2001). Recent work has highlighted available measures for use in pediatric palliative care (Coombes et al., 2016; Friedel et al., 2019) and grief research (Coombes et al., 2016; Ennis et al., 2023; Tomita & Kitamura, 2002; Zhang et al., 2023). This more balanced approach to assessment acknowledges that both positive and negative outcomes are possible in response to stress and that they are not mutually exclusive.

Additional methodological issues include small samples, a lack of controls, and poor recruitment and retention rates. Given the rarity of some pediatric conditions, often researchers can only detect large effects, which may explain inconsistencies in the literature. Larger samples are necessary to adequately test models regarding processes that contribute to different outcomes for families. Potential ascertainment bias may be introduced by recruitment from home care or support groups. Furthermore, inclusion of only intact couples may underestimate the negative influence on partnered relationships, while disproportionately excluding families with nontraditional structures, families from minoritized racial, ethnic, and social groups, and families with lower socioeconomic status. Lastly, few studies have included multiple informants, especially fathers or patient-reported outcomes from children and siblings.

The Role of Pediatric Psychology and Developmental Pediatrics

Pediatric psychologists and developmental-behavioral pediatricians can play important and collaborative roles in the care of children with life-limiting conditions and their families, as well as in research and advocacy. For example, integrative models of care propose interdisciplinary care coordination for children with neurodevelopmental disabilities and complex medical conditions (Gall et al., 2022; Graham & Robinson, 2005). Care coordination extends beyond typical medical case management by including social and educational services in a tailored, patient-centered care plan (Gall et al., 2022). This holistic approach to improving outcomes considers other lifestyle, environmental, emotional, and spiritual factors, in which pediatric psychologists and developmental-behavioral pediatricians are well suited to partner. As guidelines for palliative, end-of-life, and bereavement care evolve, we must promote early introduction to and continuity of palliative care services for children with life-limiting and complex chronic conditions. Developmental pediatricians are highly skilled at the assessment and management of comorbidities, including psychosocial challenges, among medically complex children, and psychologists have been increasingly included in interdisciplinary teams and the provision of palliative care (Hildenbrand et al., 2021). Notably, recent work has outlined core competencies for pediatric psychologists in palliative care to recognize their unique expertise and value in this subspecialty (Thompson et al., 2023).

SUMMARY AND FUTURE DIRECTIONS

Pediatric providers frequently encounter children with life-limiting conditions and bereaved family members, who can benefit from compassionate, evidence-based care that is culturally responsive and developmentally tailored to the family's needs. Despite growing consensus concerning best clinical practices, these infants and children may not have timely access to quality palliative and end-of-life care. As a result, they may experience significant, and unique, profiles of symptom burden depending on age, presenting problems, and other factors at the end of life. Family members also report unmet needs and may underutilize psychosocial services due to limitations in access, perceived fit, and stigma. As such parents and siblings remain at elevated risk for difficulties, particularly near the end of life and over the first 2 years after a child's death. While the availability of pediatric palliative programs, hospice, and bereavement care has grown over the last 2 decades, improvements in provider education, training, and services are still needed. Rigorous controlled, prospective research, including diverse families and standardized measures, is crucial to identify risk and protective factors that can inform interventions across the continuum of care. Although children are not always able to provide self-reports, their perspectives can and should be solicited when possible. Finally, advocacy efforts are needed to address ongoing challenges related to funding of clinical care and research in this area. With focused efforts, pediatric providers, researchers, and advocates can play a pivotal role in improving care and promoting resilience among families affected by a child's life-limiting condition and death.

RESOURCES

Center to Advance Palliative Care

A national organization dedicated to increasing the availability of quality, equitable health care for people living with serious illness. In addition to family resources, they provide health care professionals and organizations with the training, tools, and technical assistance necessary to deliver effective pediatric palliative care.

https://www.capc.org/toolkits/designing-a-pediatric-palliative-care-program/

Center for Loss and Life Transition

An organization led by Dr. Alan Wolfelt, dedicated to helping people who are grieving different types of loss and those who care for them. They provide resources, educational training, and an online bookstore.

https://www.centerforloss.com/

Centering Corporation

A nonprofit organization dedicated to providing education and resources for the bereaved. They have an extensive listing of print resources and books for purchase covering different types of grief-related needs.

https://centering.org/

Coalition to Support Grieving Students

The Coalition to Support Grieving Students is a unique collaboration of the leading professional organizations representing the school community. The Coalition's purpose is to create and share a set of industry-endorsed resources that will empower school communities across America in the ongoing support of their grieving students.

https://grievingstudents.org/

The Compassionate Friends

A nonprofit organization, existing for 50+ years, offering support to every family experiencing the death of a son or daughter, brother or sister, or grandchild. There are local chapters and online resources including books on all types of grief and loss.

https://www.compassionatefriends.org/

Courageous Parents Network

Created by parents for parents of seriously ill children and the providers who care for them, Courageous Parents Network is a nonprofit organization that offers a free web-based platform accessible anytime from anywhere. It has videos, blogs, and guides produced jointly with family and professional input to help families from the point of diagnosis through bereavement.

https://courageousparentsnetwork.org/

The Dougy Center for Grieving Families and Children

An organization that is a model for providing peer support groups in a safe space where children, teens, young adults, and their families can share their experiences with grief. They also provide educational materials about children and grief to be used by schools and the greater community.

https://www.dougy.org/

Five Wishes

The nation's only advance care planning program, covering personal, spiritual, medical, and legal wishes all in one document. They provide digital or paper versions written for the lay person and available in 30 languages.

https://www.fivewishes.org/

The Grief Sensitive Health Care Project

This is a collaborative effort among the Yale Child Study Center, Child Bereavement UK, and the New York Life Foundation. The purpose is to provide educational trainings and resources to health care professionals about the many ways in which grief can be experienced and expressed in families, and how this may inform how care is provided in a sensitive manner.

https://griefsensitivehealthcare.org/

National Alliance for Children's Grief

A nonprofit professional member organization that specifically addresses childhood bereavement and offers continuing education, peer networking, an annual symposium on children's grief, and a national database of children's bereavement support programs.

https://nacg.org/

The National Coalition for Hospice and Palliative Care

This coalition is comprised of 13 national organizations dedicated to improving the care of people living with serious illness. They provide resources, including clinical practice guidelines on palliative care.

https://www.nationalcoalitionhpc.org/

National Hospice and Palliative Care Organization

The nation's largest membership organization for providers and professionals who care for people affected by serious and life-limiting illness. They provide tools and resources to support pediatric palliative and hospice care.

https://www.nhpco.org/pediatrics/

NICU Helping Hands

NICU Helping Hands provides hospital- and community-based programs to educate and support families with babies in the neonatal intensive care unit (NICU), during their transition from hospital to home, and in the event of an infant loss. They offer a family resource list, including bereavement support.

https://nicuhelpinghands.org/

Postpartum Support International

The purpose of the organization is to increase awareness among public and professional communities about the emotional changes that women experience during pregnancy and postpartum. The website includes information and resources for professionals and families related to grief and loss.

https://www.postpartum.net/get-help/loss-grief-in-pregnancy-postpartum/

> **SuperSibs**
>
> Sponsored by Alex's Lemonade Stand Foundation, SuperSibs provides support to siblings (ages 4–18) of children with cancer but applies to a broad range of families coping with pediatric conditions.
>
> https://www.alexslemonade.org/childhood-cancer/for-families/supersibs
>
> **Voicing My Choices**
>
> Based on the Five Wishes advance directive, this document empowers young people living with a serious illness to communicate to family, friends, and caregivers how they want to be comforted, supported, treated, and remembered.
>
> https://store.fivewishes.org/ShopLocal/en/p/VC-MASTER-000/voicing-my-choices

References

Abela, K. M., Wardell, D., Rozmus, C., & LoBiondo-Wood, G. (2020). Impact of pediatric critical illness and injury on families: An updated systematic review. *Journal of Pediatric Nursing, 51*, 21–31. https://doi.org/10.1016/j.pedn.2019.10.013

Afonso, N. S., Ninemire, M. R., Gowda, S. H., Jump, J. L., Lantin-Hermoso, R. L., Johnson, K. E., Puri, K., Hope, K. D., Kritz, E., Achuff, B. J., Gurganious, L., & Bhat, P. N. (2021). Redefining the relationship: Palliative care in critical perinatal and neonatal cardiac patients. *Children, 8*(7), 548. https://doi.org/10.3390/children8070548

Albuquerque, S., Pereira, M., & Narciso, I. (2016). Couple's relationship after the death of a child: A systematic review. *Journal of Child and Family Studies, 25*(1), 30–53. https://doi.org/10.1007/s10826-015-0219-2

American Psychiatric Association. (2022). *Diagnostic and statistical manual of mental disorders* (5th ed., text rev.). https://doi.org/10.1176/appi.books.9780890425787

Anderson, B. (2020). Do children belong at funerals? In D. Adams & E. Deveau (Eds.), *Beyond the innocence of childhood: Vol. 1. Factors influencing children and adolescents' perceptions and attitudes toward death*. Routledge.

Bao, D., Feichtinger, L., Andrews, G., Pawliuk, C., Steele, R., & Siden, H. H. (2021). Charting the territory: End-of-life trajectories for children with complex neurological, metabolic, and chromosomal conditions. *Journal of Pain and Symptom Management, 61*(3), 449–455, e441.

Benini, F., Papadatou, D., Bernadá, M., Craig, F., De Zen, L., Downing, J., Drake, R., Friedrichsdorf, S., Garros, D., Giacomelli, L., Lacerda, A., Lazzarin, P., Marceglia, S., Marston, J., Muckaden, M. A., Papa, S., Parravicini, E., Pellegatta, F., & Wolfe, J. (2022). International standards for pediatric palliative care: From IMPaCCT to GO-PPaCS. *Journal of Pain and Symptom Management, 63*(5), e529–e543. https://doi.org/10.1016/j.jpainsymman.2021.12.031

Bertaud, S., Montgomery, A. M., & Craig, F. (2023). Paediatric palliative care in the NICU: A new era of integration. *Seminars in Fetal and Neonatal Medicine, 28*(3), 101436. https://doi.org/10.1016/j.siny.2023.101436

Bhadelia, A., Oldfield, L. E., Cruz, J. L., Singh, R., & Finkelstein, E. A. (2022). Identifying core domains to assess the "Quality of Death": A scoping review. *Journal of Pain and Symptom Management, 63*(4), e365–e386. https://doi.org/10.1016/j.jpainsymman.2021.11.015

Bluebond-Langner, M., Beecham, E., Candy, B., Langner, R., & Jones, L. (2013). Preferred place of death for children and young people with life-limiting and life-threatening conditions: A systematic review of the literature and recommendations for future inquiry and policy. *Palliative Medicine, 27*(8), 705–713. https://doi.org/10.1177/0269216313483186

Bolton, J. M., Au, W., Chateau, D., Walld, R., Leslie, W. D., Enns, J., Martens, P. J., Katz, L. Y., Logsetty, S., & Sareen, J. (2016). Bereavement after sibling death: A population-based longitudinal case-control study. *World Psychiatry, 15*(1), 59–66. https://doi.org/10.1002/wps.20293

Boyden, J. Y., Hill, D. L., LaRagione, G., Wolfe, J., & Feudtner, C. (2022). Home-based care for children with serious illness: Ecological framework and research implications. *Children, 9*(8), 1115. https://doi.org/10.3390/children9081115

Bradshaw, G., Hinds, P. S., Lensing, S., Gattuso, J. S., & Razzouk, B. I. (2005). Cancer-related deaths in children and adolescents. *Journal of Palliative Medicine, 8*(1), 86–95. https://doi.org/10.1089/jpm.2005.8.86

Bronfenbrenner, U. (1977). Toward an experimental ecology of human development. *American Psychologist, 32*(7), 513–531. https://doi.org/10.1037/0003-066X.32.7.513

Buyukcan-Tetik, A., Albuquerque, S., Stroebe, M. S., Schut, H. A., & Eisma, M. C. (2022). Grieving together: Dyadic trajectories and reciprocal relations in parental grief after child loss. In C. L. Scott,

H. M. Williams, & S. Wilder (Eds.), *Facing death: Familial responses to illness and death* (pp. 149–168). Emerald Publishing Limited. https://doi.org/10.1108/S1530-353520220000019005

Carter, B. S., Howenstein, M., Gilmer, M. J., Throop, P., France, D., & Whitlock, J. A. (2004). Circumstances surrounding the deaths of hospitalized children: Opportunities for pediatric palliative care. *Pediatrics, 114*(3), e361–e366. https://doi.org/10.1542/peds.2003-0654-f

Carton, E. R., & Hupcey, J. E. (2014). The forgotten mourners: Addressing health care provider grief—A systematic review. *Journal of Hospice and Palliative Nursing, 16*(5), 291–303. https://doi.org/10.1097/NJH.0000000000000067

Cheng, B. T., Rost, M., De Clercq, E., Arnold, L., Elger, B. S., & Wangmo, T. (2019). Palliative care initiation in pediatric oncology patients: A systematic review. *Cancer Medicine, 8*(1), 3–12. https://doi.org/10.1002/cam4.1907

Cherlin, E. J., Barry, C. L., Prigerson, H. G., Green, D. S., Johnson-Hurzeler, R., Kasl, S. V., & Bradley, E. H. (2007). Bereavement services for family caregivers: How often used, why, and why not. *Journal of Palliative Medicine, 10*(1), 148–158. https://doi.org/10.1089/jpm.2006.0108

Chong, P. H., De Castro Molina, J. A., Teo, K., & Tan, W. S. (2018). Paediatric palliative care improves patient outcomes and reduces healthcare costs: Evaluation of a home-based program. *BMC Palliative Care, 17*(1), 11. https://doi.org/10.1186/s12904-017-0267-z

Clark, O. E., Fortney, C. A., Dunnells, Z., Winning, A. M., Gerhardt, C. A., & Baughcum, A. E. (2021). Parents' own words: Adjustment and coping following infant death in the NICU. *Clinical Practice in Pediatric Psychology, 9*(3), 261–271. https://doi.org/10.1037/cpp0000418

Clark, O. E., Fortney, C. A., Dunnells, Z. D. O., Gerhardt, C. A., & Baughcum, A. E. (2021). Parent perceptions of infant symptoms and suffering and associations with distress among bereaved parents in the NICU. *Journal of Pain and Symptom Management, 62*(3), e20–e27. https://doi.org/10.1016/j.jpainsymman.2021.02.015

Cohen, E., Berry, J. G., Camacho, X., Anderson, G., Wodchis, W., & Guttmann, A. (2012). Patterns and costs of health care use of children with medical complexity. *Pediatrics, 130*(6), e1463–e1470. https://doi.org/10.1542/peds.2012-0175

Connor, S. R., Downing, J., & Marston, J. (2017). Estimating the global need for palliative care for children: A cross-sectional analysis. *Journal of Pain and Symptom Management, 53*(2), 171–177. https://doi.org/10.1016/j.jpainsymman.2016.08.020

Contro, N., Larson, J., Scofield, S., Sourkes, B., & Cohen, H. (2002). Family perspectives on the quality of pediatric palliative care. *Archives of Pediatrics & Adolescent Medicine, 156*(1), 14–19. https://doi.org/10.1001/archpedi.156.1.14

Cook, E. A. (2020). Bereaved family activism. In J. Tapley & P. Davies (Eds.), *Victimology: Research, policy and activism* (pp. 115–134). Palgrave Macmillan, Cham. https://doi.org/10.1007/978-3-030-42288-2_5

Coombes, L. H., Wiseman, T., Lucas, G., Sangha, A., & Murtagh, F. E. (2016). Health-related quality-of-life outcome measures in paediatric palliative care: A systematic review of psychometric properties and feasibility of use. *Palliative Medicine, 30*(10), 935–949. https://doi.org/10.1177/0269216316649155

Cortezzo, D. E., Sanders, M. R., Brownell, E. A., & Moss, K. (2015). End-of-life care in the neonatal intensive care unit: Experiences of staff and parents. *American Journal of Perinatology, 32*(8), 713–724.

Coyne, I., & Gallagher, P. (2011). Participation in communication and decision-making: Children and young people's experiences in a hospital setting. *Journal of Clinical Nursing, 20*(15–16), 2334–2343.

Craig, F., & Mancini, A. (2013). Can we truly offer a choice of place of death in neonatal palliative care? *Seminars in Fetal & Neonatal Medicine, 18*(2), 93–98. https://doi.org/10.1016/j.siny.2012.10.008

Currie, E. R., Christian, B. J., Hinds, P. S., Perna, S. J., Robinson, C., Day, S., & Meneses, K. (2016). Parent perspectives of neonatal intensive care at the end-of-life. *Journal of Pediatric Nursing, 31*(5), 478–489. https://doi.org/10.1016/j.pedn.2016.03.023

Currie, E. R., Wolfe, J., Boss, R., Johnston, E. E., Paine, C., Perna, S. J., Buckingham, S., McKillip, K. M., Li, P., Dionne-Odom, J. N., Ejem, D., Morvant, A., Nichols, C., & Bakitas, M. A. (2023). Patterns of pediatric palliative and end-of-life care in neonatal intensive care patients in the southern US. *Journal of Pain and Symptom Management, 65*(6), 532–540. https://doi.org/10.1016/j.jpainsymman.2023.01.025

Currier, J. M., Holland, J. M., & Neimeyer, R. A. (2007). The effectiveness of bereavement interventions with children: A meta-analytic review of controlled outcome research. *Journal of Clinical Child and Adolescent Psychology, 36*(2), 253–259. https://doi.org/10.1080/15374410701279669

D'Alton, S. V., Ridings, L., Williams, C., & Phillips, S. (2022). The bereavement experiences of children following sibling death: An integrative review. *Journal of Pediatric Nursing, 66,* e82–e99. https://doi.org/10.1016/j.pedn.2022.05.006

Davies, B., Sehring, S. A., Partridge, J. C., Cooper, B. A., Hughes, A., Philp, J. C., Amidi-Nouri, A., & Kramer, R. F. (2008). Barriers to palliative care for children: Perceptions of pediatric health care providers. *Pediatrics, 121*(2), 282–288. https://doi.org/10.1542/peds.2006-3153

DeCourcey, D. D., Silverman, M., Oladunjoye, A., Balkin, E. M., & Wolfe, J. (2018). Patterns of care at the end of life for children and young adults with life-threatening complex chronic conditions. *The Journal of Pediatrics, 193,* 196–203. https://doi.org/10.1016/j.jpeds.2017.09.078

Drake, R., Frost, J., & Collins, J. J. (2003). The symptoms of dying children. *Journal of Pain and Symptom Management, 26*(1), 594–603. https://doi.org/10.1016/S0885-3924(03)00202-1

Eilegård, A., Steineck, G., Nyberg, T., & Kreicbergs, U. (2013). Psychological health in siblings who lost a brother or sister to cancer 2 to 9 years earlier. *Psycho-Oncology, 22*(3), 683–691. https://doi.org/10.1002/pon.3053

Eiser, C., & Havermans, T. (1992). Children's understanding of cancer. *Psycho-Oncology, 1*(3), 169–181. https://doi.org/10.1002/pon.2960010306

Ellis, R., & Leventhal, B. (1993). Information needs and decision-making preferences of children with cancer. *Psycho-Oncology, 2*(4), 277–284. https://doi.org/10.1002/pon.2960020407

Ennis, N., Bottomley, J., Sawyer, J., Moreland, A. D., & Rheingold, A. A. (2023). Measuring grief in the context of traumatic loss: A systematic review of assessment instruments. *Trauma, Violence, & Abuse, 24*(4), 2346–2362. https://doi.org/10.1177/15248380221093694

Field, M. J., & Behrman, R. E. (Eds.). (2003). *When children die: Improving palliative and end-of-life care for children and their families.* National Academies Press.

Flach, K., Gressler, N. G., Marcolino, M. A. Z., & Levandowski, D. C. (2022). Complicated grief after the loss of a baby: A systematic review about risk and protective factors for bereaved women. *Trends in Psychology, 31*(4), 777–811. https://doi.org/10.1007/s43076-021-00112-z

Fontana, M. S., Farrell, C., Gauvin, F., Lacroix, J., & Janvier, A. (2013). Modes of death in pediatrics: Differences in the ethical approach in neonatal and pediatric patients. *The Journal of Pediatrics, 162*(6), 1107–1111. https://doi.org/10.1016/j.jpeds.2012.12.008

Fortney, C. A., Baughcum, A. E., Garcia, D., Winning, A. M., Humphrey, L., Cistone, N., Moscato, E. L., Keim, M. C., Nelin, L. D., & Gerhardt, C. A. (2022). Characteristics of critically ill infants at the end of life in the neonatal intensive care unit. *Journal of Palliative Medicine, 26*(5), 674–683. https://doi.org/10.1089/jpm.2022.0408

Fortney, C. A., & Steward, D. K. (2014). A new framework to evaluate the quality of a neonatal death. *Death Studies, 38*(5), 294–301. https://doi.org/10.1080/07481187.2012.742475

Foster, T. L., Gilmer, M. J., Davies, B., Barrera, M., Fairclough, D., Vannatta, K., & Gerhardt, C. A. (2009). Bereaved parents' and siblings' reports of legacies created by children with cancer. *Journal of Pediatric Oncology Nursing, 26*(6), 369–376. https://doi.org/10.1177/1043454209340322

Foster, T. L., Gilmer, M. J., Davies, B., Dietrich, M. S., Barrera, M., Fairclough, D. L., Vannatta, K., & Gerhardt, C. A. (2011). Comparison of continuing bonds reported by parents and siblings after a child's death from cancer. *Death Studies, 35*(5), 420–440. https://doi.org/10.1080/07481187.2011.553308

Foster, T. L., Gilmer, M. J., Vannatta, K., Barrera, M., Davies, B., Dietrich, M. S., Fairclough, D. L., & Gerhardt, C. A. (2012). Changes in siblings after the death of a child from cancer. *Cancer Nursing, 35*(5), 347–354. https://doi.org/10.1097/NCC.0b013e3182365646

Friedel, M., Aujoulat, I., Dubois, A.-C., & Degryse, J.-M. (2019). Instruments to measure outcomes in pediatric palliative care: A systematic review. *Pediatrics, 143*(1), e20182379. https://doi.org/10.1542/peds.2018-2379

Gaab, E. M., Owens, G. R., & MacLeod, R. D. (2014). Siblings caring for and about pediatric palliative care patients. *Journal of Palliative Medicine, 17*(1), 62–67. https://doi.org/10.1089/jpm.2013.0117

Gall, V. N., Buchhalter, J., Antonelli, R. C., Richard, C., Yohemas, M., Lachuk, G., & Gibbard, W. B. (2022). Improving care for families and children with neurodevelopmental disorders and co-occurring chronic health conditions using a care coordination intervention. *Journal of Developmental and Behavioral Pediatrics, 43*(8), 444–453. https://doi.org/10.1097/DBP.0000000000001102

Gans, D., Hadler, M. W., Chen, X., Wu, S.-H., Dimand, R., Abramson, J. M., Ferrell, B., Diamant, A. L., & Kominski, G. F. (2016). Cost analysis and policy implications of a pediatric palliative care program. *Journal of Pain and Symptom Management, 52*(3), 329–335. https://doi.org/10.1016/j.jpainsymman.2016.02.020

García-López, I., Cuervas-Mons Vendrell, M., Martín Romero, I., de Noriega, I., Benedí González, J., & Martino-Alba, R. (2020). Off-label and unlicensed drugs in pediatric palliative care: A prospective observational study. *Journal of Pain and Symptom Management*, 60(5), 923–932. https://doi.org/10.1016/j.jpainsymman.2020.06.014

Gerhardt, C. A., Fairclough, D. L., Grossenbacher, J. C., Barrera, M., Gilmer, M. J., Foster, T. L., Compas, B. E., Davies, B., Hogan, N. S., & Vannatta, K. (2012). Peer relationships of bereaved siblings and comparison classmates after a child's death from cancer. *Journal of Pediatric Psychology*, 37(2), 209–219. https://doi.org/10.1093/jpepsy/jsr082

Goldstick, J. E., Cunningham, R. M., & Carter, P. M. (2022). Current causes of death in children and adolescents in the United States. *The New England Journal of Medicine*, 386(20), 1955–1956. https://doi.org/10.1056/NEJMc2201761

Gottlieb, L., Lang, A., & Amsel, R. (1996). The long-term effects of grief on marital intimacy following infant death. *Omega: Journal of Death and Dying*, 33(1), 1–19. https://doi.org/10.2190/T2C9-FKLK-0R4F-2VMB

Graham, R. J., & Robinson, W. M. (2005). Integrating palliative care into chronic care for children with severe neurodevelopmental disabilities. *Journal of Developmental and Behavioral Pediatrics*, 26(5), 361–365. https://doi.org/10.1097/00004703-200510000-00004

Grant, M. S., Back, A. L., & Dettmar, N. S. (2021). Public perceptions of advance care planning, palliative care, and hospice: A scoping review. *Journal of Palliative Medicine*, 24(1), 46–52. https://doi.org/10.1089/jpm.2020.0111

Gravesen, J. D., & Birkelund, R. (2021). The discursive transformation of grief throughout history. *Nursing Philosophy*, 22(3), e12351. https://doi.org/10.1111/nup.12351

Hales, S., Zimmermann, C., & Rodin, G. (2008). The quality of dying and death. *Archives of Internal Medicine*, 168(9), 912–918. https://doi.org/10.1001/archinte.168.9.912

Hayslip, B., & Page, K. S. (2013). Family characteristics and dynamics: A systems approach to grief. *Family Science*, 4(1), 50–58. https://doi.org/10.1080/19424620.2013.819679

Hendrickson, K., & McCorkle, R. (2008). A dimensional analysis of the concept: Good death of a child with cancer. *Journal of Pediatric Oncology Nursing*, 25(3), 127–138. https://doi.org/10.1177/1043454208317237

Heron, M. P. (2018). Deaths: Leading causes for 2016. *National Vital Statistics Reports*, 67(6), 1–77.

Hilden, J. M., Watterson, J., Chrastek, J., & Anderson, P. M. (2000). Tell the children. *Journal of Clinical Oncology*, 18(17), 3193–3195. https://doi.org/10.1200/jco.2000.18.17.3193

Hildenbrand, A. K., Amaro, C. M., Gramszlo, C., Alderfer, M. A., Levy, C., Ragsdale, L., Wohlheiter, K., & Marsac, M. L. (2021). Psychologists in pediatric palliative care: Clinical care models within the United States. *Clinical Practice in Pediatric Psychology*, 9(3), 229–241. https://doi.org/10.1037/cpp0000402

Hill, K. N., Olsavsky, A., Barrera, M., Gilmer, M. J., Fairclough, D. L., Akard, T. F., Compas, B. E., Vannatta, K., & Gerhardt, C. A. (2023). Factors associated with mental health service use among families bereaved by pediatric cancer. *Palliative & Supportive Care*, 21(5), 829–835. https://doi.org/10.1017/S1478951522001018

Hoffmann, R., Kaiser, J., & Kersting, A. (2018). Psychosocial outcomes in cancer-bereaved children and adolescents: A systematic review. *Psycho-Oncology*, 27(10), 2327–2338. https://doi.org/10.1002/pon.4863

Hongo, T., Watanabe, C., Okada, S., Inoue, N., Yajima, S., Fujii, Y., & Ohzeki, T. (2003). Analysis of the circumstances at the end of life in children with cancer: Symptoms, suffering and acceptance. *Pediatrics International*, 45(1), 60–64. https://doi.org/10.1046/j.1442-200X.2003.01668.x

Horowitz, M. J., Siegel, B., Holen, A., Bonanno, G. A., Milbrath, C., & Stinson, C. H. (2003). Diagnostic criteria for complicated grief disorder. *Focus—American Psychiatric Publishing*, 1(3), 290–298. https://doi.org/10.1176/foc.1.3.290

Howard Sharp, K. M., Meadows, E. A., Keim, M. C., Winning, A. M., Barrera, M., Gilmer, M. J., Akard, T. F., Compas, B. E., Fairclough, D. L., Davies, B., Hogan, N., Vannatta, K., & Gerhardt, C. A. (2020). The influence of parent distress and parenting on bereaved siblings' externalizing problems. *Journal of Child and Family Studies*, 29(4), 1081–1093. https://doi.org/10.1007/s10826-019-01640-0

Howard Sharp, K. M., Russell, C., Keim, M., Barrera, M., Gilmer, M. J., Foster Akard, T., Compas, B. E., Fairclough, D. L., Davies, B., Hogan, N., Young-Saleme, T., Vannatta, K., & Gerhardt, C. A. (2018). Grief and growth in bereaved siblings: Interactions between different sources of social support. *School Psychology Quarterly*, 33(3), 363–371. https://doi.org/10.1037/spq0000253

Huang, I. C., Shenkman, E. A., Madden, V. L., Vadaparampil, S., Quinn, G., & Knapp, C. A. (2010). Measuring quality of life in pediatric palliative care: Challenges and potential solutions. *Palliative Medicine*, 24(2), 175–182. https://doi.org/10.1177/0269216309352418

Jaaniste, T., Coombs, S., Donnelly, T. J., Kelk, N., & Beston, D. (2017). Risk and resilience factors related to parental bereavement following the death of a child with a life-limiting condition. *Children*, *4*(11), 96. https://doi.org/10.3390/children4110096

Jalmsell, L., Kreicbergs, U., Onelöv, E., Steineck, G., & Henter, J. I. (2006). Symptoms affecting children with malignancies during the last month of life: A nationwide follow-up. *Pediatrics*, *117*(4), 1314–1320. https://doi.org/10.1542/peds.2005-1479

Jalmsell, L., Kreicbergs, U., Onelöv, E., Steineck, G., & Henter, J. I. (2010). Anxiety is contagious—Symptoms of anxiety in the terminally ill child affect long-term psychological well-being in bereaved parents. *Pediatric Blood & Cancer*, *54*(5), 751–757. https://doi.org/10.1002/pbc.22418

Jordan, J. R., & Neimeyer, R. A. (2003). Does grief counseling work? *Death Studies*, *27*, 765–786.

Kaye, E., & Mack, J. W. (2013). Parent perceptions of the quality of information received about a child's cancer. *Pediatric Blood & Cancer*, *60*(11), 1896–1901. https://doi.org/10.1002/pbc.24652

Kaye, E. C., Weaver, M. S., DeWitt, L. H., Byers, E., Stevens, S. E., Lukowski, J., Shih, B., Zalud, K., Applegarth, J., Wong, H.-N., Baker, J. N., Ullrich, C. K., & AAHPM Research Committee. (2021). The impact of specialty palliative care in pediatric oncology: A systematic review. *Journal of Pain and Symptom Management*, *61*(5), 1060–1079, e1062.

Keele, L., Keenan, H. T., Sheetz, J., & Bratton, S. L. (2013). Differences in characteristics of dying children who receive and do not receive palliative care. *Pediatrics*, *132*(1), 72–78. https://doi.org/10.1542/peds.2013-0470

Keim, M. C., Lehmann, V., Shultz, E. L., Winning, A. M., Rausch, J. R., Barrera, M., Gilmer, M. J., Murphy, L. K., Vannatta, K. A., Compas, B. E., & Gerhardt, C. A. (2017). Parent–child communication and adjustment among children with advanced and non-advanced cancer in the first year following diagnosis or relapse. *Journal of Pediatric Psychology*, *42*(8), 871–881. https://doi.org/10.1093/jpepsy/jsx058

Kenney, A. E., Bedoya, S. Z., Gerhardt, C. A., Young-Saleme, T., & Wiener, L. (2021). End of life communication among caregivers of children with cancer: A qualitative approach to understanding support desired by families. *Palliative & Supportive Care*, *19*(6), 715–722. https://doi.org/10.1017/S1478951521000067

Kenney, A. E., Tutelman, P. R., Fisher, R. S., Lipak, K. G., Barrera, M., Gilmer, M. J., Fairclough, D., Akard, T. F., Compas, B. E., Davies, B., Hogan, N. S., Vannatta, K., & Gerhardt, C. A. (2022). Impact of end-of-life circumstances on the adjustment of bereaved siblings of children who died from cancer. *Journal of Clinical Psychology in Medical Settings*, *29*(1), 230–238. https://doi.org/10.1007/s10880-021-09797-x

Kirkwood, N. A. (2005). *A hospital handbook on multiculturalism and religion*. Morehouse Publishing.

Klassen, A. F., Klaassen, R., Dix, D., Pritchard, S., Yanofsky, R., O'Donnell, M., Scott, A., & Sung, L. (2008). Impact of caring for a child with cancer on parents' health-related quality of life. *Journal of Clinical Oncology*, *26*(36), 5884–5889. https://doi.org/10.1200/JCO.2007.15.2835

Kreicbergs, U., Valdimarsdóttir, U., Onelöv, E., Björk, O., Steineck, G., & Henter, J. I. (2005). Care-related distress: A nationwide study of parents who lost their child to cancer. *Journal of Clinical Oncology*, *23*(36), 9162–9171. https://doi.org/10.1200/JCO.2005.08.557

Kreicbergs, U., Valdimarsdóttir, U., Onelöv, E., Henter, J. I., & Steineck, G. (2004). Talking about death with children who have severe malignant disease. *The New England Journal of Medicine*, *351*(12), 1175–1186. https://doi.org/10.1056/NEJMoa040366

Kuo, D. Z., Houtrow, A. J., & the Council on Children with Disabilities. (2016). Recognition and management of medical complexity. *Pediatrics*, *138*(6), e20163021. https://doi.org/10.1542/peds.2016-3021

Labay, L. E., & Walco, G. A. (2004). Brief report: Empathy and psychological adjustment in siblings of children with cancer. *Journal of Pediatric Psychology*, *29*(4), 309–314. https://doi.org/10.1093/jpepsy/jsh032

Lang, A., & Gottlieb, L. (1993). Parental grief reactions and marital intimacy following infant death. *Death Studies*, *17*(3), 233–255. https://doi.org/10.1080/07481189308252620

Lannen, P. K., Wolfe, J., Prigerson, H. G., Onelov, E., & Kreicbergs, U. C. (2008). Unresolved grief in a national sample of bereaved parents: Impaired mental and physical health 4 to 9 years later. *Journal of Clinical Oncology*, *26*(36), 5870–5876. https://doi.org/10.1200/JCO.2007.14.6738

Larson, D. G., & Hoyt, W. T. (2007). What has become of grief counseling? An evaluation of the empirical foundations of the new pessimism. *Professional Psychology: Research and Practice*, *38*(4), 347–355. https://doi.org/10.1037/0735-7028.38.4.347

Lichtenthal, W. G., Corner, G. W., Sweeney, C. R., Wiener, L., Roberts, K. E., Baser, R. E., Li, Y., Breitbart, W., Kissane, D. W., & Prigerson, H. G. (2015). Mental health services for parents who lost a child to cancer: If we build them, will they come? *Journal of Clinical Oncology*, *33*(20), 2246–2253. https://doi.org/10.1200/JCO.2014.59.0406

Lin, B., Gutman, T., Hanson, C. S., Ju, A., Manera, K., Butow, P., Cohn, R. J., Dallas-Pozza, L., Greenzang, K. A., Mack, J., Wakefield, C. E., Craig, J. C., &

Tong, A. (2020). Communication during childhood cancer: Systematic review of patient perspectives. *Cancer, 126*(4), 701–716. https://doi.org/10.1002/cncr.32637

Lin, M., Sayeed, S., DeCourcey, D. D., Wolfe, J., & Cummings, C. (2022). The case for advance care planning in the NICU. *Pediatrics, 150*(6), e2022057824. https://doi.org/10.1542/peds.2022-057824

Long, K. A., Lehmann, V., Gerhardt, C. A., Carpenter, A. L., Marsland, A. L., & Alderfer, M. A. (2018). Psychosocial functioning and risk factors among siblings of children with cancer: An updated systematic review. *Psycho-Oncology, 27*(6), 1467–1479. https://doi.org/10.1002/pon.4669

Lyngstad, T. H. (2013). Bereavement and divorce: Does the death of a child affect parents' marital stability? *Family Science, 4*(1), 79–86. https://doi.org/10.1080/19424620.2013.821762

Lyon, M. E., Jacobs, S., Briggs, L., Cheng, Y. I., & Wang, J. (2013). Family-centered advance care planning for teens with cancer. *JAMA Pediatrics, 167*(5), 460–467. https://doi.org/10.1001/jamapediatrics.2013.943

Macdonald, M. E., Liben, S., Carnevale, F. A., Rennick, J. E., Wolf, S. L., Meloche, D., & Cohen, S. R. (2005). Parental perspectives on hospital staff members' acts of kindness and commemoration after a child's death. *Pediatrics, 116*(4), 884–890. https://doi.org/10.1542/peds.2004-1980

Mack, J. W., Cronin, A. M., Uno, H., Shusterman, S., Twist, C. J., Bagatell, R., Rosenberg, A., Marachelian, A., Granger, M. M., Glade Bender, J., Baker, J. N., Park, J., Cohn, S. L., Levine, A., Taddei, S., & Diller, L. R. (2020). Unrealistic parental expectations for cure in poor-prognosis childhood cancer. *Cancer, 126*(2), 416–424. https://doi.org/10.1002/cncr.32553

Mack, J. W., Uno, H., Twist, C. J., Bagatell, R., Rosenberg, A. R., Marachelian, A., Granger, M. M., Glade Bender, J., Baker, J. N., Park, J. R., Cohn, S. L., Fernandez, J. H., Diller, L. R., & Shusterman, S. (2020). Racial and ethnic differences in communication and care for children with advanced cancer. *Journal of Pain and Symptom Management, 60*(4), 782–789. https://doi.org/10.1016/j.jpainsymman.2020.04.020

Mack, J. W., Wolfe, J., Cook, E. F., Grier, H. E., Cleary, P. D., & Weeks, J. C. (2007). Hope and prognostic disclosure. *Journal of Clinical Oncology, 25*(35), 5636–5642. https://doi.org/10.1200/JCO.2007.12.6110

Marcus, K. L., Santos, G., Ciapponi, A., Comandé, D., Bilodeau, M., Wolfe, J., & Dussel, V. (2020). Impact of specialized pediatric palliative care: A systematic review. *Journal of Pain and Symptom Management, 59*(2), 339–364, e310.

Martinson, I. M., McClowry, S. G., Davies, B., & Kuhlenkamp, E. J. (1994). Changes over time: A study of family bereavement following childhood cancer. *Journal of Palliative Care, 10*(1), 19–25. https://doi.org/10.1177/082585979401000106

McCown, D. E., & Davies, B. (1995). Patterns of grief in young children following the death of a sibling. *Death Studies, 19*(1), 41–53. https://doi.org/10.1080/07481189508252712

McNeil, M. J., Baker, J. N., Snyder, I., Rosenberg, A. R., & Kaye, E. C. (2021). Grief and bereavement in fathers after the death of a child: A systematic review. *Pediatrics, 147*(4), e2020040386. https://doi.org/10.1542/peds.2020-040386

Mehta, A., Cohen, S. R., & Chan, L. S. (2009). Palliative care: A need for a family systems approach. *Palliative & Supportive Care, 7*(2), 235–243. https://doi.org/10.1017/S1478951509000303

Melin-Johansson, C., Day, A., Axelsson, I., & Forslund, I. (2014). Supportive interventions and their impact on pediatric health care professionals' emotional well-being: A systematic literature review. *Clinical Nursing Studies, 2*(4), 60–73. https://doi.org/10.5430/cns.v2n4p60

Meyer, E. C., Burns, J. P., Griffith, J. L., & Truog, R. D. (2002). Parental perspectives on end-of-life care in the pediatric intensive care unit. *Critical Care Medicine, 30*(1), 226–231. https://doi.org/10.1097/00003246-200201000-00032

Miller, K. S., Vannatta, K., Vasey, M., Yeager, N., Compas, B. E., & Gerhardt, C. A. (2012). Health literacy variables related to parents' understanding of their child's cancer prognosis. *Pediatric Blood & Cancer, 59*(5), 914–918. https://doi.org/10.1002/pbc.24146

Morris, A. T., Gabert-Quillen, C., Friebert, S., Carst, N., & Delahanty, D. L. (2016). The indirect effect of positive parenting on the relationship between parent and sibling bereavement outcomes after the death of a child. *Journal of Pain and Symptom Management, 51*(1), 60–70. https://doi.org/10.1016/j.jpainsymman.2015.08.011

Morris, S., Fletcher, K., & Goldstein, R. (2019). The grief of parents after the death of a young child. *Journal of Clinical Psychology in Medical Settings, 26*(3), 321–338. https://doi.org/10.1007/s10880-018-9590-7

Moynihan, K. M., Ziniel, S. I., Johnston, E., Morell, E., Pituch, K., & Blume, E. D. (2022). A "good death" for children with cardiac disease. *Pediatric Cardiology, 43*(4), 744–755. https://doi.org/10.1007/s00246-021-02781-0

Mulheron, J., & Inouye, S. K. (2020). Bereavement care in America is broken: A call to action [Commentary]. *NAM Perspectives*. National Academy of Medicine. https://doi.org/10.31478/202001e

National Consensus Project for Quality Palliative Care. (2013). *Clinical practice guidelines for quality palliative care* (3rd ed.).

Neville, K. A., Frattarelli, D. A., Galinkin, J. L., Green, T. P., Johnson, T. D., Paul, I. M., Van Den Anker, J. N., & the American Academy of Pediatrics Committee on Drugs. (2014). Off-label use of drugs in children. *Pediatrics*, 133(3), 563–567. https://doi.org/10.1542/peds.2013-4060

Niemeyer, R. A., & Hogan, N. S. (2001). Quantitative or quantitative? Measurement issues in the study of grief. In M. S. Stroebe, R. Hansson, W. Stroebe, & H. Schut (Eds.), *Handbook of bereavement research: Consequences, coping, and care* (pp. 89–118). American Psychological Association. https://doi.org/10.1037/10436-004

October, T., Dryden-Palmer, K., Copnell, B., & Meert, K. L. (2018). Caring for parents after the death of a child. *Pediatric Critical Care Medicine*, 19(8), S61–S68.

O'Malley, P., Barata, I., Snow, S., American Academy of Pediatrics Committee on Pediatric Emergency Medicine, American College of Emergency Physicians Pediatric Emergency Medicine Committee, & Emergency Nurses Association Pediatric Committee, Shook, J. E., Ackerman, A. D., Chun, T. H., Conners, G. P., Dudley, N. C., Fuchs, S. M., Gorelick, M. H., Lane, N. E., Moore, B. R., Wright, J. L., Benjamin, L. S., Barata, I. A., . . . Brecher, D. (2014). Death of a child in the emergency department. *Pediatrics*, 134(1), e313–e330. https://doi.org/10.1542/peds.2014-1246

Polita, N. B., de Montigny, F., Neris, R. R., Alvarenga, W. A., Silva-Rodrigues, F. M., Leite, A. C. A. B., & Nascimento, L. C. (2020). The experiences of bereaved parents after the loss of a child to cancer: A qualitative metasynthesis. *Journal of Pediatric Oncology Nursing*, 37(6), 444–457. https://doi.org/10.1177/1043454220944059

Prigerson, H. G., Boelen, P. A., Xu, J., Smith, K. V., & Maciejewski, P. K. (2021). Validation of the new *DSM-5-TR* criteria for prolonged grief disorder and the PG-13-Revised (PG-13-R) scale. *World Psychiatry*, 20(1), 96–106. https://doi.org/10.1002/wps.20823

Prigerson, H. G., Horowitz, M. J., Jacobs, S. C., Parkes, C. M., Aslan, M., Goodkin, K., Raphael, B., Marwit, S. J., Wortman, C., Neimeyer, R. A., Bonanno, G. A., Block, S. D., Kissane, D., Boelen, P., Maercker, A., Litz, B. T., Johnson, J. G., First, M. B., & Maciejewski, P. K. (2009). Prolonged grief disorder: Psychometric validation of criteria proposed for *DSM-V* and *ICD-11*. *PLOS Medicine*, 6(8), e1000121. https://doi.org/10.1371/journal.pmed.1000121

Pritchard, M., Burghen, E., Srivastava, D. K., Okuma, J., Anderson, L., Powell, B., Furman, W. L., & Hinds, P. S. (2008). Cancer-related symptoms most concerning to parents during the last week and last day of their child's life. *Pediatrics*, 121(5), e1301–e1309. https://doi.org/10.1542/peds.2007-2681

Rosenberg, A. R., Baker, K. S., Syrjala, K., & Wolfe, J. (2012). Systematic review of psychosocial morbidities among bereaved parents of children with cancer. *Pediatric Blood & Cancer*, 58(4), 503–512. https://doi.org/10.1002/pbc.23386

Rosenberg, A. R., Dussel, V., Kang, T., Geyer, J. R., Gerhardt, C. A., Feudtner, C., & Wolfe, J. (2013). Psychological distress in parents of children with advanced cancer. *JAMA Pediatrics*, 167(6), 537–543. https://doi.org/10.1001/jamapediatrics.2013.628

Rosenberg, A. R., Orellana, L., Kang, T. I., Geyer, J. R., Feudtner, C., Dussel, V., & Wolfe, J. (2014). Differences in parent-provider concordance regarding prognosis and goals of care among children with advanced cancer. *Journal of Clinical Oncology*, 32(27), 3005–3011. https://doi.org/10.1200/JCO.2014.55.4659

Rosenberg, A. R., Postier, A., Osenga, K., Kreicbergs, U., Neville, B., Dussel, V., & Wolfe, J. (2015). Long-term psychosocial outcomes among bereaved siblings of children with cancer. *Journal of Pain and Symptom Management*, 49(1), 55–65. https://doi.org/10.1016/j.jpainsymman.2014.05.006

Rosner, R., Kruse, J., & Hagl, M. (2010). A meta-analysis of interventions for bereaved children and adolescents. *Death Studies*, 34(2), 99–136. https://doi.org/10.1080/07481180903492422

Sansom-Daly, U. M., Wakefield, C. E., Patterson, P., Cohn, R. J., Rosenberg, A. R., Wiener, L., & Fardell, J. E. (2020). End-of-life communication needs for adolescents and young adults with cancer: Recommendations for research and practice. *Journal of Adolescent and Young Adult Oncology*, 9(2), 157–165. https://doi.org/10.1089/jayao.2019.0084

Schaefer, M. R., Kenney, A. E., Himelhoch, A. C., Howard Sharp, K. M., Humphrey, L., Olshefski, R., Young-Saleme, T., & Gerhardt, C. A. (2021). A quest for meaning: A qualitative exploration among children with advanced cancer and their parents. *Psycho-Oncology*, 30(4), 546–553. https://doi.org/10.1002/pon.5601

Shear, M. K., Simon, N., Wall, M., Zisook, S., Neimeyer, R., Duan, N., Reynolds, C., Lebowitz, B.,

Sung, S., Ghesquiere, A., Gorscak, B., Clayton, P., Ito, M., Nakajima, S., Konishi, T., Melhem, N., Meert, K., Schiff, M., O'Connor, M. F., . . . Keshaviah, A. (2011). Complicated grief and related bereavement issues for DSM-5. *Depression and Anxiety, 28*(2), 103–117. https://doi.org/10.1002/da.20780

Shultz, E. L., Switala, M., Winning, A. M., Keim, M. C., Baughcum, A. E., Gerhardt, C. A., & Fortney, C. A. (2017). Multiple perspectives of symptoms and suffering at end of life in the NICU. *Advances in Neonatal Care, 17*(3), 175–183. https://doi.org/10.1097/ANC.0000000000000385

Siebelink, M. J., Geerts, E. A. H. M., Albers, M. J. I. J., Roodbol, P. F., & van de Wiel, H. B. M. (2012). Children's opinions about organ donation: A first step to assent? *European Journal of Public Health, 22*(4), 529–533. https://doi.org/10.1093/eurpub/ckr088

Søfting, G. H., Dyregrov, A., & Dyregrov, K. (2016). Because I'm also part of the family. Children's participation in rituals after the loss of a parent or sibling: A qualitative study from the children's perspective. *Omega: Journal of Death and Dying, 73*(2), 141–158. https://doi.org/10.1177/0030222815575898

Stein, A., Dalton, L., Rapa, E., Bluebond-Langner, M., Hanington, L., Stein, K. F., Ziebland, S., Rochat, T., Harrop, E., Kelly, B., Bland, R., Betancourt, T., D'Souza, C., Fazel, M., Hochhauser, D., Kolucki, B., Lowney, A. C., Netsi, E., Richter, L., Yousafzai, A., & the Communication Expert Group. (2019). Communication with children and adolescents about the diagnosis of their own life-threatening condition. *The Lancet, 393*(10176), 1150–1163. https://doi.org/10.1016/S0140-6736(18)33201-X

Sullivan, J., & Monagle, P. (2011). Bereaved parents' perceptions of the autopsy examination of their child. *Pediatrics, 127*(4), e1013–e1020. https://doi.org/10.1542/peds.2009-2027

Sveen, J., Eilegård, A., Steineck, G., & Kreicbergs, U. (2014). They still grieve—A nationwide follow-up of young adults 2–9 years after losing a sibling to cancer. *Psycho-Oncology, 23*(6), 658–664. https://doi.org/10.1002/pon.3463

Tang, S. T., Huang, C.-C., Hu, T.-H., Chou, W.-C., Chuang, L.-P., & Chiang, M. C. (2021). Course and predictors of posttraumatic stress-related symptoms among family members of deceased ICU patients during the first year of bereavement. *Critical Care, 25*(1), 282. https://doi.org/10.1186/s13054-021-03719-x

Theunissen, J. M., Hoogerbrugge, P. M., van Achterberg, T., Prins, J. B., Vernooij-Dassen, M. J., & van den Ende, C. H. (2007). Symptoms in the palliative phase of children with cancer. *Pediatric Blood & Cancer, 49*(2), 160–165. https://doi.org/10.1002/pbc.21042

Thompson, A. L., Schaefer, M. R., McCarthy, S. R., Hildenbrand, A. K., Cousino, M. K., Marsac, M. L., Majeski, J., Wohlheiter, K., & Kentor, R. A. (2023). Competencies for psychology practice in pediatric palliative care. *Journal of Pediatric Psychology, 48*(7), 614–622. https://doi.org/10.1093/jpepsy/jsad007

Tomita, T., & Kitamura, T. (2002). Clinical and research measures of grief: A reconsideration. *Comprehensive Psychiatry, 43*(2), 95–102. https://doi.org/10.1053/comp.2002.30801

Tomlinson, D., Hinds, P. S., Bartels, U., Hendershot, E., & Sung, L. (2011). Parent reports of quality of life for pediatric patients with cancer with no realistic chance of cure. *Journal of Clinical Oncology, 29*(6), 639–645. https://doi.org/10.1200/JCO.2010.31.4047

Tutelman, P. R., Lipak, K. G., Adewumi, A., Fults, M. Z., Humphrey, L. M., & Gerhardt, C. A. (2021). Concerns of parents with children receiving home-based pediatric palliative care. *Journal of Pain and Symptom Management, 61*(4), 705–712. https://doi.org/10.1016/j.jpainsymman.2020.09.007

Umberson, D., Olson, J. S., Crosnoe, R., Liu, H., Pudrovska, T., & Donnelly, R. (2017). Death of family members as an overlooked source of racial disadvantage in the United States. *Proceedings of the National Academy of Sciences of the United States of America, 114*(5), 915–920. https://doi.org/10.1073/pnas.1605599114

van der Geest, I. M. M., Darlington, A. S. E., Streng, I. C., Michiels, E. M. C., Pieters, R., & van den Heuvel-Eibrink, M. M. (2014). Parents' experiences of pediatric palliative care and the impact on long-term parental grief. *Journal of Pain and Symptom Management, 47*(6), 1043–1053. https://doi.org/10.1016/j.jpainsymman.2013.07.007

van der Geest, I. M. M., van den Heuvel-Eibrink, M. M., Falkenburg, N., Michiels, E. M. C., van Vliet, L., Pieters, R., & Darlington, A. S. E. (2015). Parents' faith and hope during the pediatric palliative phase and the association with long-term parental adjustment. *Journal of Palliative Medicine, 18*(5), 402–407. https://doi.org/10.1089/jpm.2014.0287

Vermaes, I. P. R., van Susante, A. M. J., & van Bakel, H. J. A. (2012). Psychological functioning of siblings in families of children with chronic health conditions: A meta-analysis. *Journal of Pediatric Psychology, 37*(2), 166–184. https://doi.org/10.1093/jpepsy/jsr081

Vollenbroich, R., Duroux, A., Grasser, M., Brandstätter, M., Borasio, G. D., & Führer, M. (2012). Effectiveness of a pediatric palliative home care team as experienced by parents and health care professionals. *Journal of Palliative Medicine, 15*(3), 294–300. https://doi.org/10.1089/jpm.2011.0196

von Essen, L., & Enskär, K. (2003). Important aspects of care and assistance for siblings of children treated for cancer: A parent and nurse perspective. *Cancer Nursing, 26*(3), 203–210. https://doi.org/10.1097/00002820-200306000-00005

von Gunten, C. F., Ferris, F. D., Portenoy, R. K., & Glajchen, M. (Eds.). (2001). *CAPC manual: How to establish a palliative care program.* Center to Advance Palliative Care.

Weaver, M. S., Nasir, A., Lord, B. T., Starin, A., & Linebarger, J. S. (2023). Supporting the family after the death of a child or adolescent. *Pediatrics, 152*(6), e2023064426. https://doi.org/10.1542/peds.2023-064426

West, S. G., Sandler, I., Pillow, D. R., Baca, L., & Gersten, J. C. (1991). The use of structural equation modeling in generative research: Toward the design of a preventive intervention for bereaved children. *American Journal of Community Psychology, 19*(4), 459–480. https://doi.org/10.1007/BF00937987

Wiener, L., Sweeney, C., Baird, K., Merchant, M. S., Warren, K. E., Corner, G. W., Roberts, K. E., & Lichtenthal, W. G. (2014). What do parents want to know when considering autopsy for their child with cancer? *Journal of Pediatric Hematology/Oncology, 36*(6), 464–470. https://doi.org/10.1097/MPH.0000000000000078

Wiener, L., Zadeh, S., Battles, H., Baird, K., Ballard, E., Osherow, J., & Pao, M. (2012). Allowing adolescents and young adults to plan their end-of-life care. *Pediatrics, 130*(5), 897–905. https://doi.org/10.1542/peds.2012-0663

Williams, P. D., Williams, K. A., & Williams, A. R. (2014). Parental caregiving of children with cancer and family impact, economic burden: Nursing perspectives. *Issues in Comprehensive Pediatric Nursing, 37*(1), 39–60. https://doi.org/10.3109/01460862.2013.855843

Wolfe, J., Grier, H. E., Klar, N., Levin, S. B., Ellenbogen, J. M., Salem-Schatz, S., Emanuel, E. J., & Weeks, J. C. (2000). Symptoms and suffering at the end of life in children with cancer. *The New England Journal of Medicine, 342*(5), 326–333. https://doi.org/10.1056/NEJM200002033420506

Wolff, S. L., Christiansen, C. F., Nielsen, M. K., Johnsen, S. P., Schroeder, H., & Neergaard, M. A. (2020). Predictors for place of death among children: A systematic review and meta-analyses of recent literature. *European Journal of Pediatrics, 179*(8), 1227–1238. https://doi.org/10.1007/s00431-020-03689-2

World Health Organization. (2015). *Palliative care.* Retrieved May 18, 2024, from https://www.who.int/cancer/palliative/definition/en

Xu, J., Murphy, S. L., Kochanek, K. D., & Arias, E. (2022). Mortality in the United States, 2021. *NCHS Data Brief*, No. 456, 1–8.

Yazdan, R., Corey, K., Messer, S. J., Kim, E. H., Roberts, K. E., Selwyn, P. A., & Weinberger, A. H. (2023). Hospital-based interventions to address provider grief: A narrative review. *Journal of Pain and Symptom Management, 66*(1), e85–e107. https://doi.org/10.1016/j.jpainsymman.2023.03.001

Zadeh, S., Pao, M., & Wiener, L. (2015). Opening end-of-life discussions: How to introduce Voicing My CHOiCES™, an advance care planning guide for adolescents and young adults. *Palliative & Supportive Care, 13*(3), 591–599. https://doi.org/10.1017/S1478951514000054

Zhang, T., Krysinska, K., Alisic, E., & Andriessen, K. (2023). Grief instruments in children and adolescents: A systematic review. *Omega: Journal of Death and Dying, 0*(0). https://doi.org/10.1177/00302228231171188

PART II

SELECT CHILD DEVELOPMENTAL CONTEXTS, CHILD HEALTH CONDITIONS, AND THE ROLE OF PEDIATRIC PSYCHOLOGY

> # CHAPTER 6

GENDER IDENTITY, GENDER DYSPHORIA, AND GENDER-AFFIRMING MODELS IN CHILDHOOD AND ADOLESCENCE: CLINICAL AND DEVELOPMENTAL SCIENCE PERSPECTIVES

Diane Ehrensaft

The 21st century has witnessed an explosion in the numbers of children and adolescents who are exploring their gender, declaring that their gender does not match the sex designated on their birth records, and expressing their gender in ways that do not conform to the social expectations and norms for gender in their culture. To accommodate the needs of these children, groups of experts from different disciplines have convened to formulate a system of understanding and providing care, the Gender Affirmative Model (GAM; Ehrensaft, 2011, 2012, 2016). This model emphasizes gender diversity and gender health, recognizing that a child's gender can unfold in infinite combinations and permutations and is not necessarily binary. This model contrasts with previous models in which genders that did not conform to binary male–female or match the sex designated at birth were disregarded or pathologized. The concept of the "gender web" is a personcentric approach driven by children's ability to weave their own unique gender based on the three major threads of nature, nurture, and culture. The GAM was introduced to understand the trajectory of children's consolidation of their gender self over time incorporating both *gender identity* ("who I know myself to be as male, female, or other") and *gender expressions* ("how I do my gender—its outward manifestations, including appearance, choice of roles and activities, etc."). In the GAM, gender is viewed as a dynamic construct—one that is not fixed at a particular time but can shift over an individual's lifetime. This new paradigm replaces the traditional model of binary gender development based on chromosomal sex designated at birth, presenting challenges for researchers and providers. At the same time, it offers the possibility to promote the gender health of all children. *Gender health* is defined as the opportunity to live in one's authentic gender, free of social aspersion or rejection, and supported by gender acceptance.

Portions of this chapter were reprinted or adapted from "Exploring Gender Expansive Expressions Versus Asserting a Gender Identity," by D. Ehrensaft, in C. Keo-Meier and D. Ehrensaft (Eds.), *The Gender Affirmative Model: An Interdisciplinary Approach to Supporting Transgender and Gender Expansive Children* (pp. 37–53), 2018, American Psychological Association (https://doi.org/10.1037/0000095-003). Copyright 2018 by the American Psychological Association.
https://doi.org/10.1037/0000414-006
APA Handbook of Pediatric Psychology, Developmental-Behavioral Pediatrics, and Developmental Science: Vol. 2. Pediatric Psychology and Developmental-Behavioral Pediatrics: Clinical Applications of Developmental Science, P. E. Shah and M. H. Bornstein (Editors-in-Chief)
Copyright © 2025 by the American Psychological Association. All rights reserved.

This chapter considers the multifactorial contexts associated with gender health, utilizing a gender-diverse framework. It first presents theoretical models of gender identity and describes the evolution of the GAM and trajectories of the development of gender identity. It highlights the importance of cultural sensitivity in understanding children's gender in their social context and examines multilevel ecological contexts associated with adaptive versus suboptimal outcomes in children with gender diversity. The chapter revisits previous views of "gender pathology" and presents an alternate view of co-occurring mental health issues that typically result from external impingements rather than internal disorders.

The chapter proposes a paradigmatic shift—that gender pathology most likely resides in a social milieu around the child that is driven by gender rejection or aspersion and does not reside in the child (Hidalgo et al., 2013). The chapter further considers issues that emerge when the binary model of gender is replaced by a paradigm of gender infinity, including, "How does one ascertain a child's authentic gender self?", "What measures should be taken to support a child's gender health?", and "How do we define gender health?" This chapter presents the framework of gender as a spectrum, manifest as a multiple rather than binary construct, with a third genre of gender-diverse youth: nonbinary/gender-fluid children and adolescents who live between, among, or beyond the binary gender paradigm in their gender selves, creatively assembling a diverse sense of gender identity and expression. To optimize outcomes of children with gender diversity across the lifespan, we highlight the importance of a comprehensive interdisciplinary approach that encompasses the fields of developmental psychology, mental health, pediatrics, pediatric psychology, developmental-behavioral pediatrics, adolescent medicine, endocrinology, education, and social work. The roles of these disciplines in the care and management of gender-diverse individuals are briefly discussed. The chapter concludes with opportunities for research and future directions.

TRADITIONAL THEORETICAL MODELS OF GENDER AND EVOLUTION OF THE GENDER AFFIRMATIVE MODEL

Traditional theories of gender development often conflated gender identity with gender expressions. To review, *gender identity* is one's internal sense of themselves as male, female, nonbinary, or some other individualized configuration of gender. *Gender expressions* refers to the various gender-related ways one presents and acts—including physical presentation, name and pronoun choice, preferred activities, societal roles, and so forth. This conflation was embedded in the construct that the biological sex designated at birth, typically determined by observation of external genitalia, was coincident with the individual's gender. In traditional models of the evolution of gender identity, the developmental task was to first learn one's gender identity defined by binary constructs (i.e., "I am a boy" or "I am a girl"), followed by a period of sex role socialization, culminating at around 6 years of age, at which time the child's gender identity was conceived as a stable construct, with the understanding that this identity was permanent or irreversible. A child who failed to reach the developmental milestone of "gender identity" was considered "disordered" and in need of treatment, often along with parents.

The GAM provides a contrasting view by recognizing that biological sex (as defined by chromosomal genotype) does not equate with gender, and that gender expressions differ from gender identity. The GAM further adds to the complexity of this differentiation by asserting that children explore gender expressions following different pathways as, for example, (a) children who accept the gender associated with the sex assigned to them at birth but do not conform to the social expectations for gender roles and behavior, (b) children who affirm a gender identity that is other than that associated with the sex designated to them at birth, and (c) children who present a mélange of interwoven gender identity and gender expressions that do not conform to societal norms or expectations. Because the GAM diverges from traditional models of gender, several questions, informed by developmental science, have emerged:

- Can a young child genuinely know their gender identity if it differs from the one associated with the sex designated to them at birth?
- Can professionals accurately detect a child's authentic gender identity?
- Would it be in or against a child's best interests to allow a transgender and gender diverse (TGD) young child to socially transition from one gender to another gender?
- What are the predictors of persistent gender dysphoria, considering that previous clinical research has indicated that most children assessed with gender dysphoria early in life do not evidence dysphoria by the advent of puberty?

Answers to each of these questions are being addressed within the GAM by differentiating three groups of children: those who question and explore their gender identities, those who question and explore their gender expressions, and those who question and explore both gender identity and gender expression. The three groups are not fixed categories, and a child can move from one to another over a period of time or stay firmly embedded in any one of them. Further, in the spirit of gender inclusivity, developmental scientists continually identify intersections between and among individuals with divergent gender identities, individuals with gender-diverse expressions, and individuals exploring both gender identity and gender expressions.

EPIDEMIOLOGY OF GENDER DYSPHORIA IN CHILDHOOD

Researchers at the gender clinic at the Vrije Universiteit University Medical Center in Amsterdam documented trajectories of gender identity of children who came to their program for services. Using measures informed by *Diagnostic and Statistical Manual of Mental Disorders* (*DSM*) criteria, children were assessed to determine whether they met diagnostic criteria for either Gender Identity Disorder (GID) as outlined in the fourth edition of the *DSM* (*DSM-IV*; American Psychiatric Association, 1994), or, as more recently identified in the fifth edition of the *DSM* (*DSM-5*; American Psychiatric Association, 2013), for Gender Dysphoria. Based on a study of 127 adolescents receiving services at the clinic in 2011, 70% to 80% of children who met diagnostic criteria for GID (the diagnosis used at the time of the study) prior to the age of 12 no longer met *DSM* diagnostic criteria for GID. These youth were referred to as the "desisters" (Steensma et al., 2011, 2013). Moreover, the persistence of the GID diagnosis into adolescence occurred in a relatively small percentage of children, with the reported incidence being somewhere between 20% and 30%. Those who maintained the same diagnosis in prepubertal years into adolescence became known as the "persisters" (Steensma et al., 2011, 2013).

In 2013, the Dutch researchers reevaluated the prevalence data of children who persisted in the diagnosis of gender dysphoria (Steensma et al., 2013) and reported the following: (a) the percentage of children with early gender dysphoria who did not manifest gender dysphoria in adolescence was adjusted to 63% (down from previous estimates of 70%–80%), and (b) children who persisted with symptoms of gender dysphoria in adolescence had a complete childhood diagnosis of gender dysphoria at significantly higher rates ($p < .001$) than children whose gender dysphoria resolved. In addition, children with persistent gender dysphoria showed more gender nonconforming behavior, such as mode of dress, chosen activities and play preferences (i.e., gender expansive expressions) and had a greater degree of gender dysphoria throughout childhood, manifest by the articulation that they were the other gender and expressed through a greater discomfort with their sexed bodies. Specifically, the youth who persisted into adolescence exhibited a consistent feeling of incongruence between their body and gender identity. Finally, (c), in contrast to children with persistent gender dysphoria, children whose gender dysphoria abated by adolescence manifested more fluidity in their gender expressions as reflected in statements that *they wished* they were the other gender, rather than *they were* the other gender. Later, in adolescence, these children were also more likely to express attraction for people of the same gender as themselves (Steensma et al., 2013). Taken together, these data suggest that patterns of gender identity show signs of differentiation in early childhood. The trajectories of persistent gender dysphoria represent the children who coalesce a transgender identity—some, if given the opportunity—early in life.

These updated findings are consistent with rapidly accumulating clinical observations among gender-affirmative practitioners engaged with prepubertal children in recent years, as more pediatric gender clinics have come into being and more families sought supports for their gender-exploring or gender-diverse children. In the GAM, which emphasizes stages rather than ages of gender consolidation, a cluster of behaviors and feelings separated children who might benefit from a social transition to their articulated gender identity from children who need support in expressing themselves in ways that are at odds with the gender norms of their cultural context.

PROFILES AND TRAJECTORIES OF GENDER DIVERSITY IN CHILDREN

Extrapolating from the updated findings about youth who were labeled as "persisters," there are children who are indicating early in life that they are developing an understanding that the gender they know themselves to be is incongruent with the sex designated to them at birth, an understanding that remains consistent over time. Typically, they may demonstrate cross-gender identifications early in life and continue with them into and beyond puberty. The term *cross-gender* is used judiciously, in line with the common lexicon in the professional literature. From the child's point of view, they have never "crossed over" at all. Instead, the people around this set of children must change their thinking and come to the realization that the child who is consistent in articulating a gender that does not match the sex designated at birth is not the gender that the adults assumed that child to be.

These children are often referred to as "*consistent, persistent,* and *insistent*" in their affirmed gender identities, identities that do not match their sex designated at birth. Many of these children, but not all, are binary in their gender identity, which may extend to rigidly binary gender expressions as they try to communicate to others their affirmed gender identity. Over time, those gender expressions may evolve to be more fluid, affording children the opportunity for freedom in their gender expressions once they feel they have been heard about their authentic gender identity. These children's primary concern is not gender expression but gender identity—an identity, particularly in early life, that may first be communicated through gender-expansive expressions.

One indicator of a child being in the category of children who recognize a stable and consistent transgender identity early in life is that the child may typically say, "I *am* a [boy, girl, other]" rather than "I *wish I were* a [boy, girl, other]." The presence of this indicator, "to be" rather than "want to be," should be qualified by the reality that some children as young as 3 years old, or even as young as the beginning stages of expressive language development, will have already read the signals that those around them might not understand or would be upset if they were to defy social gender expectations. When that occurs, they learn to hedge their bets, so to speak, and dilute or soften their gender assertions with statements such as, "Well, maybe sometimes I would like to be a [girl, boy, other]" to avoid negative or aversive responses or to assuage their parents' anxieties. As children become increasingly cognizant of the attitudes and mores of the world around them, such dilutions can be expected to be even more in evidence for children who experience continuing stress or dysphoria related to the incongruence between their internal sense of their gender and the gender others perceive or expect them to be. This circumstance can challenge providers and caregivers who want to help the child transcend psychological defenses and access and feel more confident in expressing their authentic gender self.

Many children in the category of transgender people who discover or begin to become cognizant of their gender identity early in life express body dysphoria at a very young age. They may be displeased or distraught about the genitalia they have, experiencing their anatomy as a betrayal of the gender they know themselves to be and a signifier that perhaps they can never be a "real" person of that gender. This dysphoria increases if the child receives messages that only people with vaginas can be girls and only people with penises can be boys. Yet even without those messages, young children may express frustration or anger that "God got it wrong and made me the wrong way" or "Why can't I go back in Mommy's tummy and come out the right way next time?" In their frustration or distress, some children may attempt to mutilate their genitals, and others, particularly those still in the magic years of early childhood (Fraiberg, 1959), may insist that their vagina is actually a penis or believe that they can go to the doctor's office and trade the genitalia of their choice in exchange for the genitalia they were born with and do not want.

These children's gender expressions, although not the root of the matter, serve as an important communication tool. They may function as serious business with an important social message embedded. So, for example, a biologically male child who knows they are a girl may sneak into their sister's room and take off with her favorite school dress, not her fairy princess costume. In donning the school dress, the child is trying to tell the world that they are a girl just like their sister; such acts are not fantasy play.

In the context of nature, nurture, and culture, the three interwoven components of each child's individual gender self, nature threads appear to be quite strong for children who fall in the category defined by early and persistent recognition of their affirmed gender identity. Whether it is genetics, prenatal environmental influences (e.g., the distribution of hormones through hormone receptors in the critical fetal months of sex formation), or some other biological factors, the narrative from parents of these children is often the same: "I swear, we did not do anything to make this happen. Our child just came to us this way."

When allowed to socially transition to their affirmed gender, symptoms of anxiety, agitation, stress, and distress previously observed in these children typically dissipate (but do not necessarily disappear), replaced by increased confidence and psychological well-being. Clinicians have reported that this boost in psychological functioning following a full social transition to their authentic gender identity stands out as one of the most dramatic psychosocial changes observed among children seeking psychological services for any kind of issue (Ehrensaft & Jurkiewicz, 2024). Put another way, this youngest cohort of transgender people do well when given the opportunity to live in their authentic gender identity.

Other research findings (Olson et al., 2015) have also shown that young children expressing a transgender identity who have had the opportunity to socially transition do equally well as a comparison group of same-age nontransgender peers in several areas of psychological functioning. A reevaluation of their persister/desister data conducted by Thomas Steensma and colleagues in the Netherlands supported clinical observations of other gender specialists that the children in their study who, at a young age, indicated that they *were* the other gender rather than they *wanted to be* the other gender, showed early body dysphoria and demonstrated an early history of cross-gender interests and activities (Steensma & Cohen-Kettenis, 2018).

Because children identified as "persisters" presented their gender expansiveness early in childhood—a presentation that is "insistent, consistent, and persistent"—parents and professionals alike mistakenly believe that if a child's first assertion of a transgender identity shows up only much later, particularly in adolescence or beyond, it is not authentic (Littman, 2018; Shrier, 2020). Often this will be presented in a clinical session with a parent expressing, "I swear to you, my child never showed even the slightest sign of cross-gender interests until now.

I think he's putting us on. This couldn't be real. He's not one of the kids like Jazz" [Jennings, the transgender girl featured in her early childhood in the first Barbara Walters special on transgender children, who went on to become a young adult author and media spokesperson for transgender youth] (Goldberg, 2007). Doing a gender-affirmative assessment with this parent's child will hopefully reveal whether the youth's declarations of a gender identity are authentic. The main point is that a child can assert a transgender identity at any point in childhood, young adulthood, or beyond—one that may well remain "insistent, persistent, and consistent" as each individual consolidates an authentic gender self. In that context, the onset of puberty is often a nodal point when a youth first recognizes within themselves a transgender identity. At that moment in development that sensibility may surface, even erupt, often from the depths of unconscious repression or the layers of conscious suppression. The catalyst for this sudden motion is the youth's confrontation with the beginning signs of secondary sex characteristics (breast development, widening hips, facial hair, deepening voice) and hormone-based bodily functions (menstruation, ejaculations). The youth begins to experience an incongruence between their emerging adult body and the emergent self-realization of the gender they are, rather than the one they have been living in. In that sense, youth who articulate a transgender identity later in childhood may be no less authentic in their gender articulations than the cohort of children who know from early childhood.

Children Originally Designated as Desisters

Among the children designated as "desisters" (i.e., receiving a GID/gender dysphoria diagnosis in childhood that no longer was in evidence in adolescence) are the children who do not abide by socially inscribed gender norms in their gender presentations but do not repudiate the sex designated to them at birth, finding that the label fits as long as they are not policed in their gender expressions. In contrast to the cohort of young transgender children who will assert "I *am* a [boy, girl, other]," children who in previous research got designated as "desisters" more likely express, "I *wish I were* a [boy, girl, other]." Many of these children will later discover their gay or queer identities, and others will grow to be cisgender (having a gender that matches the sex designated at birth) gender-expansive heterosexuals; some youth who explored gender-expansive expressions earlier in life may shed their gender-nonconforming behaviors by adolescence; some will first discover their gender expansiveness as they enter adolescence. Because the developmental track of gender formation can cross with the developmental track of sexual orientation/sexual identity formation, many "protogay" children (i.e., children in the process of discovery but not yet conscious of their gay selves) explore gender on the way to affirming their sexuality. In a culture that is predominately heterosexist in its norms, young children have few opportunities to experience relationships between a male and a male or a female and a female. Even with the early 21st-century publication of books like *King and King* (De Haan & Nijland, 2002), the dominant theme in children's socialization has remained kings and queens, princes and princesses. A young boy with an awakening realization that he longs for the prince might fashion himself as the princess as the only way to fetch a prince. Thus, this young boy might don a princess costume, imagining himself as the belle of the ball and attracting the admiration of the prince, and telling his parents, "I *wish I were* a girl." As he grows older and discovers that men can love men and women can love women, he may change his earlier feminine-leaning expressions as he realizes he can be a prince loving a prince.

This group of "effeminate" boys includes those who historically have been captured in clinical and research programs (e.g., Green, 1987) that attempt to purge their cross-gender interests to avoid "homosexual" outcomes. They are also the children tagged as gender dysphoric early in childhood, mistakenly included in the same category as the so called persisters but later identified as the so-called "desisters," aka cisgender lesbian, gay, bisexual, or queer youth.

Again, not all of the children in this second category of children exploring gender expressions rather than gender identities will be protogay; some simply revel in rebelling against societal gender norms and creatively put together their own gender mosaic expressions, rather than the modes prescribed within their culture. These children tend not to repudiate their bodies or show distress about their genitals. Instead, they may engage in fantasy play or ruminations about life in another body. For example, a little girl might pack her pajama bottoms with socks to have a bulge like her brother's, giggling all the while. A little boy may borrow his sister's ballet costume, stuff the bodice with socks, and prance through the house as the buxom ballerina, giggling all the while. Their play is filled with a jouissance in celebrating the delightful and transgressive expression of gender outside binary gender boxes. In contrast with the first group, for these children play is not serious business and urgent communication about a gender identity that others may have failed to recognize.

The declaration "I wish I were a girl" is often the differentiating feature between the children establishing a gender identity and the children establishing their chosen gender expressions. The challenge for clinicians is to differentiate between "I wish" as an authentic articulation and "I wish" as a defensive strategy. In either case, time will tell: With enough open and safe space for in-depth exploration in the child–clinician relationship, genuine articulations typically surface: the child who is consolidating their gender expressions stays firm with "I wish" and eventually expresses "I am." In sum, one group is occupied most centrally with gender expressions, whereas the other is centrally occupied with gender identity, using gender expressions as a means of communication of the true gender identity as well as an authentic expression of how that child wants to express their gender.

Exploring Both Identity and Expressions Outside Binary Gender Boxes

Although research reports sought to differentiate their constructed categories of "persisters" and "desisters," it subsequently became apparent that another group of children presented themselves in a gender-creative fashion and needed to be included. These children are weaving together a gender self that includes both gender-expansive identities beyond the binary and expansive/creative gender expressions. These youth give evidence that gender exists beyond binary boxes. Until recently, they have appeared among older youth, from middle school-age and above. By the third decade of the 21st century, more children younger than that have also begun articulating a gender self that is expansive in both identities and expressions. Those in the older cohort may identify themselves as *agender* (i.e., having either no gender or any gender), *genderqueer* (identifying with all people who are expansive in identities and expressions), *gender fluid* (flowing from one gender iteration to another either over time or within themselves), *nonbinary* (living beyond binary gender boxes), *demi-girl* (part male, leaning toward female), *demi-boy* (part female, leaning toward male), or any other assignation signifying that they do not consolidate a gender self based on "either/or" but rather "all or any" (Goldner, 2011). In short, they are the gender weavers who make a tapestry of self that is neither male nor female but their own creative understanding of gender, both in identities and expressions. Professionals and parents alike may feel compelled to place these children in one of two boxes: male or female. Typically, if fortified with enough gender resilience, these children will resist. As one 9-year-old explained, "Look, I'm a boy–girl. And that's all I can tell you about me right now."

Regarding their physical selves, for the youth in this third category, bodies can be a cause for stress. In the context of a culture that equates penis with boy and vagina with girl, they may struggle to be the boy with a penis who is also a girl, and so forth. Clinical observation suggests that body dysphoria is seldom as intense in contrast to the body dysphoria of children and adolescents who strongly articulate that they are the "opposite" gender. Instead, many of the youth in this third category embrace the gender middle ground of "all and any." When this is accompanied by an expressed desire to have a body that can transcend the boundaries of male/female bodies, providers are presented with a challenge, particularly those working in medical or interdisciplinary clinics where medical interventions (puberty blockers, gender-affirming hormones, and gender-affirming surgeries) are potential provisions of care, either in adolescence (or even younger for puberty blockers) or early adulthood. If one is to abide by the gender-affirmative rubric that gender is not binary but an infinite variety of possibilities, youth who identify as nonbinary, agender, or gender fluid may push for professional practices to abide by this rubric. They may ask for just a touch of testosterone, or a small dose of estrogen, or chest surgery but no other medical intervention as they strive to embody a gender self that is uniquely theirs. Meeting the needs of this third group of young people is an area of gender care that, more than any other, requires practitioners to examine their own values, biases, discomforts, or reactions in their youth through their own self-discovery to expand beyond their training and sensibilities that informed them that gender is binary.

DEVELOPMENTAL EMERGENCE OF AUTHENTIC GENDER SELVES

Longitudinal studies have suggested that children who did not persist in what was identified as gender dysphoria at adolescence differed fundamentally from children who persisted with the diagnosis of gender dysphoria assigned to them in childhood. Using the diagnostic formulation of gender dysphoria or, earlier, gender identity disorder, has not proved to be the most accurate measurement of children's gender trajectories. Identifying their differing pathways might be clearer if proper measuring tools could be used and if the appropriate clinical/developmental question could be asked, namely, "What can you tell me and what can I learn about your gender identity and your gender expressions?"

An important question, rooted in developmental science, is whether young children know their gender and at what age gender identity emerges. Starting with these questions may be the most robust way to move on to the task of differentiating children in different gender categories and matching them with the supports and interventions most beneficial to their gender health. Typically, the question "Can young children really know their gender?" is not in reference to cisgender children (children whose gender congruent with the sex designated at birth) but rather to children who declare at an early age that their gender is neither the one everyone thinks it is nor the gender that matches the sex designated at birth.

A World Health Organization (WHO) field study surveyed transgender participants ($N = 250$) regarding their first awareness of their transgender identity and reported that symptoms of gender dysphoria emerged at a mean age of 5.6 years (Robles et al., 2016). These data suggest that young children know their gender and can self-identify experienced gender incongruence. These data also corroborate findings from an earlier study of 3,474 transgender adults (Beemyn & Rankin, 2011). In their online survey, 82.6% of the transgender respondents reported that they were aware before age 12 that they felt different. In follow-up interviews with 419 of the sample, 67% of the transgender men and 62% of the transgender women reported feeling that from a young age they were different from the gender matching the sex designated to them at birth. In this study, most respondents expressed that they hid this self-knowledge from those around them, acknowledging their transgender identity only to themselves. The reported effect was chronic psychological pain and suffering. Acknowledging the limitations of retrospective data, wherein people may have the tendency to recall their history through the tint of the historical lens, these narratives still align with collective clinical observations across pediatric gender clinics and programs internationally: Parents of transgender children report that their children indicated in word and action from a very early age (some as young as toddlerhood) that "someone had gotten it wrong" and that "they were not the gender people thought they were."

Mirroring the findings from the studies of adults, children who experience gender dysphoria also describe feelings of stress, distress, frustration, or anger, particularly if their gender-diverse feelings are dismissed or their gender articulations are denied. Children may reveal their experiences of gender diversity through play or in words. For example, a 6-year-old who had been designated male at birth but had refused anything "boy" since age 2 shared that she always knew she was a girl, even while still in diapers. When she learned boys had penises, she assumed hers would go away as soon as she changed her name from George to Ginny. That change occurred when she was 5, after which she reported that her parents "finally stopped being so silly and calling me a boy" (Ehrensaft, 2014; Malpas, 2011).

Similarly, transgender adults report having early knowledge of their gender diversity, although many note that in childhood they did not have the words or opportunity to express it given the social expectations of the era in which they grew up. This older cohort has expressed envy in face of the realization that their childhoods did not afford them the opportunity to expose their transgender self, but forced them to hide it, sometimes even from themselves. In retrospective studies, transgender adults report feeling clear about their transgender identity from an early age (Beemyn & Rankin, 2011), which raises the question regarding how to best identify children who may manifest persistent gender dysphoria with an eye to individualizing their care and optimizing adaptation and future outcomes.

Building on this framework, it may be a revolutionary rite of passage to question, explore, and create a mosaic of gender. In the 20th century, Erikson (1963) identified the developmental stage of adolescence as one in which youth strive to consolidate their identities. Whereas adult sexual selves were included in his categories of exploration, gender was not, as in that historical period of Western psychology gender was considered bedrock rather than something to be explored, questioned, or reckoned with. In the 21st century, gender is now understood to be one more identity category that youth consider ripe for Erikson's identity explorations, and not to be taken for granted. Thus, for many of the youth who present as gender fluid, particularly those in adolescence, it is helpful to think of them taking full advantage of the stage of identity versus role confusion to fully and creatively plumb the depths of their gender selves. The gender explorations of these youth within the Eriksonian expanded developmental task of Identity vs. Role Confusion can challenge providers who experience these youth as moving targets rather than as poetry in motion. For gender-fluid individuals, the cultural component of their gender selves influences their questioning and explorations of "What's my gender?" The task for clinicians working with nonbinary/gender fluid youth is to facilitate their living a gender-expansive life without prematurely pushing them into one gender category or another on the basis of being unable to answer the question—boy or girl?

FINDINGS FROM MULTICENTER STUDIES AND RELEVANCE OF THE GENDER AFFIRMATIVE MODEL

Emerging evidence suggests that, if asked the appropriate questions (e.g., questions that differentiate between gender identity and gender expressions), young children may reveal through their narratives whether or not they know themselves to be transgender at a young age and whether they demonstrate a profile of characteristics predictive of later gender trajectories. Gathering information from these questions will help better understand the different developmental pathways and identifying features of young children who present as gender diverse. Among them, the children focused on their gender identity rather than expressions may likely, but not necessarily, continue on a track of consolidating a transgender identity, possibly with accompanying gender stress along the way, depending on environmental provisions and supports. The young children who exhibit gender nonconformity not in their identities but in their expressions may also exhibit potential gender stress, typically generated by other people's reactions to them. This stress might qualify them for an early childhood diagnosis of gender dysphoria, a diagnosis that will have disappeared by adolescence, because it most likely was an inaccurate diagnosis in the beginning. For these youth, the developmental trajectory is toward being a person who is creative in how they express their gender but satisfied with the sex designated to them at birth.

Early research of children attending pediatric gender clinics was limited by a focus on measuring gender stress and distress, rather than employing measures that would measure gender identity and gender expressions. More recent research, incorporating the GAM, is measuring whether the child is primarily exploring or grappling with gender identity (who I am as boy, girl, or other), gender expressions (how I want to express my gender), or both. In this approach, measures of gender identity and gender expressions are neutral categories rather than assessments of pathology or psychological malfunctioning, as were previously described by the terms Gender Dysphoria (or Gender Identity Disorder). Research has assessed mental health correlates associated with profiles of gender identity (Olson et al., 2015, 2016). These investigations have examined children's affirmed gender identity at ages 9 and younger and evaluated associations with mental health measures of these children in comparison with two control groups (siblings and cisgender peers).

Building on this work, an ongoing four-site NIH research study of gender development in prepubertal gender-diverse children (Chen et al., 2019) is examining a combination of both categories of measures: gender identity/gender expressions and evidence of stress/distress related to gender. The aims of this research are to elucidate the child's perception of their gender and to gain a better understanding of how they experience themselves as boy, girl, or other; how they express their gender (e.g., through modes of dress, play, friendship patterns, activities, etc.); and experiences of stress or distress related to either. Employing this "wide-angle lens" is thought to be essential for research and clinical practice, leading to more "gender expansive" care.

The Evolution of Clinical Management of Gender Diversity: From Watchful Waiting to Gender Literacy and the Timing of Social Transitioning

Watchful waiting. Early research in gender identity was predicated on the notion that neither researchers, clinicians, nor parents could determine a child's authentic gender in early childhood (Cohen-Kettenis & Pfafflin, 2003). This way of thinking led to the belief that a child may be "damaged" by facilitating a social transition prior to the child's readiness that comes with the advent of puberty, and as a result, in the past, clinical recommendations took a "watchful waiting" approach: holding off on any gender transitions until a youth reached adolescence and the advent of puberty, when the understanding of the child's gender status would be in clearer focus. That orientation was guided by data that suggested gender dysphoria remitted after puberty in the vast majority of children (Steensma et al., 2011). If by adolescence children persisted in cross-gender identifications, actions could be taken to help them socially transition and receive medical interventions to better align their bodies with their transgender psyche. Before the onset of adolescence, it would be too early to determine a child's stable gender status. Because by measurements used only a small number of gender dysphoric young children continued to be gender dysphoric in adolescence, it was thought that gender dysphoria in early childhood was not a reliable predictor of later transgender outcomes.

Gender literacy. With greater acceptance of the GAM framework, clinical care of gender-diverse individuals has evolved to include a focus on "gender literacy" in childhood. This change was guided by the premise that gender does not just come in "two boxes" and is not determined by the appearance of external genitalia or the notation of F or M registered on birth records. This shift in practice was informed by three tenets of the GAM: (a) a small number of children emerge early on who are cross-gender or "another gender" in their expressions, and transgender in their identities (i.e., individuals who persist in gender diversity); (b) predictive variables exist which can identify these children and differentiate them from the children who are exploring gender expressions but not gender identity; and (c) the risks of allowing a child to socially transition at an early age are outweighed by the benefits of allowing a child to live in the gender that is most authentic to them, at the same time leaving all pathways open for evolving or new iterations of gender as they move forward in life.

Management of young children with gender divergence has focused on providing opportunities for children to explore their gender, without promoting an early and potentially premature or inappropriate gender transition. Informed by research that suggests that most children will grow out of their gender dysphoria and will not grow up to be transgender, the GAM emphasizes stages rather than ages of gender consolidation and highlights clusters of behaviors and feelings that may separate children who might benefit from a social transition to their articulated gender identity from the children who just need support in expressing themselves in ways that are at odds with the gender norms in their cultural context. This development has led to a shift in practice to encourage earlier social transitioning for children with gender diversity. The GAM recognizes that having a better understanding of which children persist with symptoms of gender dysphoria into adolescence could help inform clinical care prior to adolescence and help to identify which children would become good candidates for puberty blockers and/or gender-affirming hormones, culminating in an affirmed transgender identity.

Building on this premise, unpublished data from the parent NIH four-site study of medical and psychological effects of puberty blockers and gender-affirming hormones (Olson-Kennedy et al., 2019) indicated that close to 90% of the children eligible for puberty blockers had already socially transitioned earlier in childhood. The newly constructed chapter on childhood in the revised *Standards of Care, Version 8* released by the World Professional Association for Transgender Health (WPATH) in 2022 (Coleman et al., 2022) offers more proactive rather than cautionary guidelines for prepubertal social transitions, endorsing that some children will benefit from a social transition prior to puberty rather than following the watchful waiting approach and postponing social transition until the onset of puberty or beyond. As stated in the chapter,

> . . . social transition, when it takes place, is likely to best serve a child's well-being when it takes place thoughtfully and individually for each child. A child's social transition (and gender as well) may evolve over time and is not necessarily static, but best reflects the cross-section of the child's established self-knowledge of their present gender identity and desired actions to express that identity. (Coleman et al., 2022, p. S76)

Clinical Evaluation of Gender Diverse Children and Adolescents

Assessing and establishing a gender health plan for children can take many forms and may vary based on providers' theoretical orientation and training, resources, local statutes, or insurance requirements.

Clinical setting. Overall, the goal is the same: to get a child's gender in focus; make practice recommendations for supporting a child in their gender explorations, treating dysphoria or stress related to gender along with any co-occurring psychological issue; outline recommended interventions, including gender-affirming medical treatments for older youth (puberty blockers, gender-affirming hormones, gender-affirming surgeries); and establish a treatment plan. Accomplishing these goals requires training as a gender specialist, and optimally will include input from an interdisciplinary team, which can include a pediatric endocrinologist, nurse practitioner, adolescent medicine provider, psychologist, psychiatrist, developmental-behavioral pediatrician, social worker, and educational expert. Interdisciplinary pediatric gender clinics have expanded exponentially since the beginning of the 2000s to provide this care. This is not the only portal to care, however. Primary care providers, developmental-behavioral pediatricians, and mental health professionals may work independently or within informal networks to provide both assessment and follow-up care and support. While there is no standardized evaluation template, the recommendations provided in the WPATH *Standards of Care* along with the Endocrine Society Clinical Practice Guideline (Hembree et al., 2017) are typically used as the framework in which gender care for youth is conducted.

Clinical history. The following is an example of a child who may present to a developmental-behavioral pediatrician, pediatric psychologist, child psychiatrist, or other type of mental health provider for evaluation of gender diversity:

> Imagine two parents coming to a psychologist's office for a consultation. They are puzzled by what their 6-year-old child is attempting to tell them about the child's gender. The parents are committed to doing the right thing for their child, but they do not know what that is. Designated female at birth, their child will only wear clothes chosen from the boys' section of their local department store, has attempted to urinate standing up in imitation of their older brother, and is distraught because, according to the rules, they will not be allowed to try out for the boys' junior softball team.

Rather than immediately assessing for gender dysphoria, here is an example of questions a clinician might ask the parents about their child instead (Ehrensaft, 2016):

- How long has your child been communicating gender-expansive identifications or behaviors?
- Has this been consistent over an extended period of time?
- If your child is able to express a sense of their own gender, how does your child articulate it, and with what feeling?
- Does your child say, "I *want to be* a girl [boy] [other]," or does your child say, "I *am* a girl [boy] [other]"?
- How insistent is your child in declarations and demonstrations of gender? How persistent?
- Does your child show distress or stress about the body your child has, particularly their genitalia?
- Is your child making serious statements rather than playful gestures when gravitating toward the toys, activities, dress codes, and so on typically designated for the "other" gender within your culture?
- Does your child express distress when someone "misgenders" them?
- Does your child show delight when someone perceives your child as a gender other than the one that matches the sex designated to them at birth?
- Has your child asked for a change in name or gender pronouns?
- How do you as parents and other people in your child's life respond to your child's gender messages?

These 11 questions are just a sample of the type of queries that would begin to generate a narrative about the child's gender status, in terms of how the child knows themselves to be a boy, girl, or other, and how they "do" their gender. The same genre of queries would inform a clinician's direct interactions with the child if the child is to be seen at all.

Clinical support/management. The clinical management of gender-diverse children and adolescents has evolved over time. Regarding the timing and process of gender (social) transitions, WPATH initially adopted a cautionary stance when it released the seventh version of the *Standards of Care* (Coleman et al., 2012):

> Mental health professionals can help families to make decisions regarding the timing and process of any gender role changes [social transitions] for their young children. They should provide information and help parents to weigh the potential benefits and challenges of particular choices. Relevant in this respect are the previously described relatively low persistence rates of childhood gender dysphoria. A change back to the original gender role [assigned sex] can be highly distressing and even result in postponement of this second social transition on the child's part. For reasons such as these, parents may want to present this role change [social transition] as an exploration of living in another gender role, rather than an irreversible situation. Mental health professionals can assist parents in identifying potential in-between solutions or compromises (e.g., only when on vacation). It is also important that parents explicitly let the child know that there is a way back. (p. 17)

The WPATH concern was that children given a green light to change their gender early in life may have a hard time turning back, given that most young children do not continue on a path that results in a transgender identity. Therefore, it was suggested that professionals caring for these children (including developmental-behavioral pediatricians, pediatric psychologists, and child and adolescent psychiatrists) take a conservative stance, forestalling any social transitions until certain that the child's transgender identity is authentic.

Since that time, considerations regarding social transition for gender-diverse individuals has evolved, including within the program in the Netherlands that initially developed the watchful waiting approach. For example, in comparison to the children who are consistent from childhood into adolescence in articulating a gender-diverse identity, children who in the past were identified as "desisters" do not need to transition to another gender identity as they do not repudiate the gender identity matching the sex designated at birth. For them, in promoting gender health, it is ever necessary to open a path to nonconforming gender expressions most concordant to them rather than society and to challenge any social policing of those expressions. Parents typically report that their gender-diverse children simply come to them that way rather than being molded by them. They may say something like: "I swear, I have four children, and I've raised them all the same. And this is the only one who threw out all his trucks and demanded a Barbie doll and screamed 'Make me a girl'." Nature may certainly play its hand here in children's gender development, yet nurture and culture are also strong contributors—nurture, because the acquisition of their specific gender is established within the relational matrix of parent and child relationships, teacher and child relationships, and so forth; culture, because the norms of gender and therefore the challenges to those norms vary significantly from culture to culture and from one historical period to another. For example, in U.S. American culture, wearing a skirt may serve as a strong statement for a little boy who is gender expansive and be considered transgressive; in another culture such as Myanmar, no one would even take notice because skirts or long wraps are typically worn by males as normative gender garb.

The indicators listed are not requisites for a child to qualify as a transgender child or a child who would benefit from a social transition but rather a set of guidelines to better understand the child's "gender trajectory" as it unfolds over time. Often an *ex post facto* test enables a clinician to fully recognize who the child is and to measure whether the clinician was correct in an assessment. When allowed to socially transition to their affirmed gender, a child's symptoms of anxiety, agitation, stress, and distress typically dissipate (but not necessarily disappear), replaced by increased confidence and psychological well-being. Clinicians have reported that this boost in psychological functioning following a full social transition to their authentic gender identity stands out as one of the most dramatic psychosocial changes observed among children seeking psychological services for any kind of issue. Put another way, this youngest cohort of transgender people does well when given the opportunity to live in their authentic gender identity.

Other research findings have also shown that young gender-diverse children who have had the opportunity to socially transition do equally well as a comparison group of same-age non-transgender peers in several areas of psychological functioning, showing no higher rates of depression and no areas of mental health assessment in the clinical range except for a minimally elevated rate of anxiety (Olson et al., 2015). Furthermore, the profile of the young child asserting a transgender identity matches the findings of Steensma et al. (2013) who discovered that the children who had been identified as persisters at a young age more likely indicated that they were the other gender rather than they wanted to be the other gender, showed early body dysphoria, and demonstrated an early history of cross-gender interests and activities. Whereas some doubt the ability of young children to know their own gender, worrying about prematurely constraining children in a new gender box before they have had the rest of their childhood to explore, both clinical observations and emerging research data indicate that allowing children to socially transition once their affirmed gender is in focus, a phenomenon that can occur as early as the preschool years, appears to be in the child's best interests. Assuming that parents are accepting and supportive of the transition, giving the child the opportunity to socially transition may be the best insurance policy against psychological risk factors for a child chronically confronted with the dysphoria of being forced to live in a gender that is not their authentic one. Steensma et al.'s (2013) reevaluation of persister and desister data indicated that persisters showed more intense and consistent gender dysphoria—

which makes sense, especially if they were barred from socially transitioning to their authentic gender. As reflected in the most recent edition of the WPATH *Standards of Care*, the approach to the clinical care and support of gender-diverse individuals has evolved to include greater consideration for the benefits of early social transition.

Guidelines for Clinical Interventions for Gender-Diverse Children and Adolescents

The clinical management of children with gender diversity varies based on the age of presentation and whether the child is experiencing issues related to gender identity, to gender expressions, or both.

Children with early awareness of their gender identity. Can clinicians know with 100% accuracy that young children who articulate a transgender identity and desire a social transition, which might include name, pronoun, and gender marker change, will be stable and consistent in their transgender identity? The answer to that question is simple: No. The past WPATH *Standards of Care, Version 7* (Coleman et al., 2012), in guiding people to be cautious about prepubertal social transitions, cited a study by Steensma and Cohen-Kettenis (2011) in which a very small sample of middle-school-age girls experienced stress when shifting from a masculine presentation to a more feminine presentation. These youth reportedly exhibited gender expressions that trended toward masculine in their earlier childhood, and they experienced stress as they transitioned to a more feminine presentation. What was not documented was whether these girls had been exploring gender expressions versus gender identity and whether the stress they experienced in middle school was the result of socially induced stress as a consequence of others' negative responses to their shift to a more feminine presentation. Absent a rejecting social environment, no documented evidence to date suggests that children's psychological well-being will suffer if they either traverse back to an earlier gender identity that had been discarded or move forward to yet another one as they carve out their gender pathways, as long as they receive social supports in doing so. In the GAM, in which gender development is seen as a lifelong unfolding rather than fixed at an early age and in which pathology is perceived to lie more in the culture's repudiation of gender expansiveness than in an internal anomaly of the child, the major risk of social transitions for young gender diverse children is more likely in society's discomfort than in the child's internal gender confusion or distress.

Before the onset of puberty, the central intervention for young transgender children is social transition: the opportunity for the child to leave an ill-fitting gender behind and embrace an alternative gender identity that feels more authentic. This transition can include a change in name, gender pronouns, dress and appearance, activity and bathroom choices, particularly those that are sex-segregated, and any other aspects of daily living that a child finds useful in consolidating a true gender self. A child will be a good candidate for a social transition if:

1. Other possibilities besides gender are ruled out as being at the core of the child's presentation to others; specifically, if gender is discovered to be a symptom or signal of some other underlying problem or issue, such as a childhood psychosis or effort to escape from chronic sexual abuse.
2. The central issue for the child is determined to be gender identity, not gender expressions.
3. The child expresses a need or desire to socially transition to another gender.
4. The child possesses the emotional and cognitive capacities to comprehend the processes involved in a social transition.
5. Parents can offer positive support for their child transitioning.

If all those criteria are met, a full social transition can be considered, either everywhere, or, at least to begin, in more limited settings that are considered safe (this is particularly important for children who live in communities openly hostile or abusive to anyone who defies gender norms and in which the child would be subject to chronic maltreatment). In the latter situations, the ongoing community-based work, which should include the clinician's input, is to widen the circles of safety and acceptance for that child, so the child can move toward full expression of themselves in all situations. In the meantime, the child can be offered full opportunity to be their authentic gender self in protected spaces with the understanding that they themselves are "gender fabulous" and some other people do not yet understand that, with the objective of externalizing rather than internalizing transphobic sensibilities.

As a continuity of self, children stable in a transgender identity who arrive at the threshold of puberty should be afforded the option of puberty blockers and then later gender-affirming hormone treatment (estrogen or testosterone). Considerations of gender-affirming surgeries are also possible for these youth well into adolescence. Because fertility options will be compromised for children who receive puberty blockers before going through puberty and then followed by hormone therapy, interventions will also involve counseling about alternative family-building options for the gender-diverse youth or presently experimental procedures for freezing ovarian or testicular tissue. For those youth who have already gone through puberty before being assessed as eligible for gender-affirming hormonal treatment (testosterone, estrogen), counseling should include possibilities of gamete preservation through sperm banking or egg extraction.

Children exploring gender expressions. In some ways, this is the easiest group of children to support. If the child's gender presentation is not about core gender identity but about gender expressions, the role of the environment, including parents and providers, is to carve out space and support for the child to perform their gender in a way that suits the child, rather than society. For this group of children, no social gender transition, as defined previously, is called for. Within the context of a social system unaccepting of expansive gender expressions, a child whose central issue is gender expressions may need a safe therapeutic space to work out the stresses of defying social gender expectations in how they "do" their gender and in building gender resilience so that they can assert their gender selves with pride and confidence rather than fear and anxiety. It should be noted in this respect that much homophobic and transphobic bullying and harassment toward youth are based primarily on the individual's nonconforming gender presentations, rather than either their sexual or gender identity. In that regard, the boy in a dress may be at higher risk for maltreatment than the young transgender girl who has gone through a full social transition and appears like any other girl in her class (as long as she remains dressed). When the gender is male, as for little boys who previously in life had been identified as "desisters," the disjuncture between gender and social norms for dress may draw more fire and that child will need some added social supports, again with a promise of working toward a more gender-accepting society. The specific vulnerability for children who are diverse in their gender expressions rather than gender identity, particularly for those who are boys (in our society, due to sexism, girls are given far more leeway to be nonconforming in their appearance than boys) is a factor often overlooked when compared to the more dramatic trajectory of the children who are diverse in their gender identities, particularly when they have had the opportunity to go through a social transition.

Children exploring both gender expressions and gender identities. These youth are a mélange. Some may request or benefit from a gender transition but not necessarily a binary one. Others accept the sex designated at birth but redefine what that means. Like the children solely exploring gender expressions, they may benefit from supportive psychological services or community support groups to support their unique and diverse gender consolidations and to offer them protection against a society that may be more ill-equipped to accept them than to accept the youth who have established a binary transgender identity (boy to girl or girl to boy). When it comes to gender-affirming medical interventions (hormones and surgery), mental health professionals and medical professionals need to work together in interdisciplinary partnerships to consider the possible medical interventions that will support a youth who is neither male nor female in gender identity, gender expressions, or both, and asking for specific treatments to embody their nonbinary gender in a way that feels most authentic to them.

ANTICIPATORY GUIDANCE AND CONSIDERATIONS: GENDER STRESS, GENDER DYSPHORIA, GENDER RESILIENCE, GENDER HEALTH

Separating children who are consolidating a gender identity from those coalescing their gender expressions or those engaged in redefining both their gender identities and expressions in nonbinary ways is not a stand-alone operation. Accompanying that endeavor is a search for any signs of gender angst, gender minority stress, or gender dysphoria as each child traverses their gender journey. Gender dysphoria as used here is not to be equated with formulations constructed in diagnostic manuals such as the *DSM-5* (although they can be helpful adjunct tools). Gender dysphoria, as used here, is not a psychiatric diagnosis but refers in nonpsychiatric terms to the discomfort, stress, or cacophony between body and psyche or psyche and society a child may experience in the context of trying to consolidate an authentic gender self. This use of the term "gender dysphoria" may include to any of the following features: discomfort with one's body, the internalization of external negative or pejorative messages about one's gender, the confusion between internal feelings and cognitive messages about the definition of healthy or "real" gender (as in "girls can't have penises," penis = boy), the disappointment that parents failed to get it right, the lack of opportunity to live in their authentic gender.

Many gender-diverse children and adolescents do not suffer from gender dysphoria because they have had the opportunity to live fully in their true gender selves with abundant support around them. It is only when puberty is on the horizon and feared unwanted bodily changes are in the offing that some of those youth begin to feel dysphoric about their bodies and/or anxious about being able to continue to be gendered correctly if their bodies exhibit endogenous secondary sex characteristics. Prior to puberty, except for genitalia, children can easily construct their gender with little differentiation between the bodies of children designated female and those designated male at birth. Unfortunately, that ease is taken away when bodies start to respond to adult sex hormones—for a gender-diverse child, the appearance of breast buds in a transgender boy or the sound of a cracking voice in a transgender girl can be experienced as anywhere from an annoyance to significant trauma.

Whether the disquiet is generated from external gender minority stress, defined as social stressors such as discrimination and stigma to which gender minorities are subject (Testa et al., 2015), or internal conflicts, the role of the health care provider, such as the developmental-behavioral pediatrician, pediatric psychologist, or child and adolescent psychiatrist, is to keep a watch over any developing stress, distress, or dysphoria. The objective is to develop a gender health plan that will facilitate growth, build resilience, and reduce reactive psychological disturbances, such as anxiety or depression. Helping a child build or strengthen gender resilience, the psychological adaptive skills that protect youth from harm while simultaneously allowing them to remain confident in their affirmed gender selves, is a key, but often overlooked task for health professionals. Possessing gender resilience can contribute significantly to ensuring the physical and mental health of gender-diverse children and adolescents.

The role of the developmental scientist is to provide the professional and lay community with evidence-based knowledge about gender development, gender supports, and gender outcomes. Gender becomes disordered only when the environment fails to provide the knowledge as well as the psychosocial and later the medical supports that allow a youth to experience gender euphoria rather than dysphoria. The contribution of developmental scientists in strengthening gender resilience among gender diverse cannot be stressed enough. By sharing evidence-based knowledge with the professional community, families, the gender public, and legislative bodies, the resultant best practices and potential enhancement of societal supports will in turn allow a child of any gender to achieve gender health through living in their authentic gender with acceptance and absent aspersion.

RESEARCH AND FUTURE DIRECTIONS

The knowledge base concerning the health and welfare of gender-diverse children and adolescents has expanded exponentially in the past quarter century. Moving forward, there is a need to gather more information about the developmental progression and the long-term physical and psychological effects for children who are receiving pediatric gender care. As these children move into adulthood, more longitudinal information is needed about the outcomes for children who socially transition at an early age; youth who received puberty blockers at the onset of puberty; adolescents who choose a course of gender-affirming hormones or later, gender-affirming surgeries; and individuals who began a course of gender-affirming medical care and then discontinued that care. Best practices and standards of care are living, organic documents to be reassessed as new knowledge is accrued. Although guidelines regarding pediatric gender care are presently available, there is nonetheless controversy and debate within the pediatric field regarding the benefits and risks of the accrued best practices. The future of the field needs to leave ample room for scientific and respectful dialogue and discussion about the definition of and methods for ensuring gender health for all children. Increasingly, it will be imperative that professionals share and compare knowledge across disciplines: general practice pediatricians, pediatric endocrinologists, behavioral pediatricians, reproductive medicine specialists, child and adolescent psychologists and psychiatrists, and scientific researchers. Simultaneously, it will be important to continue learning from the life experiences of the children themselves, along with their parents.

CONCLUSION

Children at a young age, both cisgender and transgender, can definitively know their gender. The challenge for any professional working in the field of pediatric gender care, whether it be a health care provider, an academic researcher, or one who shares both roles, remains the same: to develop knowledge that translates into the tools that will allow the interdisciplinary cadre of scientists and practitioners to decipher what children are trying to communicate about their gender and to establish a health care plan to support them. By differentiating gender identity from gender expressions and using the template of the three categories of children who concentrate on one or the other or both of these components of a gender self, this complex task will hopefully become simpler as we come to a greater consensus about both the science and practice of pediatric gender care. The simpler task can happen only if there are no set timelines, and children can discover and make their gender selves known at any point in their development. Thinking about the three groups of gender-diverse children and adolescents identified, one must always remember that no child is permanently relegated to one of the three categories and not every gender-expansive child will fit neatly into one of the three categories. Like gender itself, these categories flow and meld among one another.

RESOURCES

- **American Academy of Family Physicians' Health Equity Curricular Toolkit.** Structured training modules designed to facilitate knowledge around social determinants of health, vulnerable populations, and economics and policy.

  https://www.aafp.org/family-physician/patient-care/the-everyone-project/health-equity-tools.html

- **American Academy of Pediatrics.** Ensuring comprehensive care and support for transgender and gender-diverse children and adolescents.

  Rafferty, J., Committee on Psychosocial Aspects of Child and Family Health, Committee on Adolescence, Section on Lesbian, Gay, Bisexual, and Transgender Health and Wellness, Yogman, M., Baum, R., Gambon, T. B., Lavin, A., Mattson, G., Sagin Wissow, L., Breuner, C., Alderman, E. M., Grubb, L. K., Powers, M. E., Upadhya, K., Wallace, S. B., Hunt, L., Gearhart, A. T., Harris, C., Melland Lowe, K., Taylor Rodgers, C., & Sherer, I. M. (2018). Ensuring comprehensive care and support for transgender and gender-diverse children and adolescents. *Pediatrics*, 142(4), e20182162. https://doi.org/10.1542/peds.2018-2162

- **American Medical Association's Center for Health Equity.**

  https://www.ama-assn.org/delivering-care/health-equity

- **American Psychiatric Association.** A guide for working with transgender and gender nonconforming patients.

  https://www.psychiatry.org/psychiatrists/diversity/education/transgender-and-gender-nonconforming-patients

- **American Psychological Association's Office of Equity, Diversity, and Inclusion.**

  https://www.apa.org/about/apa/equity-diversity-inclusion

- **American Psychological Association.** Guidelines for psychological practice with transgender and gender nonconforming people.

  https://www.apa.org/practice/guidelines/transgender.pdf

- **National Institutes of Health's Office of Equity, Diversity, and Inclusion.**

  https://www.edi.nih.gov

- **SAMHSA LGBTQ+ Behavioral Health Equity Center of Excellence.**

  https://www.samhsa.gov/resource/tta/lgbtq-behavioral-health-equity-center-excellence

- UCSF Center of Excellence for Transgender Health.

    https://transcare.ucsf.edu/welcome-0

- World Professional Association for Transgender Health.

    https://www.wpath.org/

- WPATH *Standards of Care, Version 8.*

    https://www.wpath.org/publications/soc

References

American Psychiatric Association. (1994). *Diagnostic and statistical manual of mental disorders* (4th ed.).

American Psychiatric Association. (2013). *Diagnostic and statistical manual of mental disorders* (5th ed.). https://doi.org/10.1176/appi.books.9780890425596

Beemyn, G., & Rankin, S. (2011). *The lives of transgender people.* Columbia University Press.

Chen, D., Ehrensaft, D., Hidalgo, M., & Tishelman, A. C. (2019). A longitudinal study of gender nonconformity in prepubescent children. National Institutes of Health.

Cohen-Kettenis, P., & Pfafflin, F. (2003). *Transgenderism and intersexuality in childhood and adolescence.* SAGE Publications.

Coleman, E., Bockting, W., Botzer, M., Cohen-Kettenis, P., DeCuypere, G., Feldman, J., Fraser, L., Green, J., Knudson, G., Meyer, W. J., Monstrey, S., Adler, R. K., Brown, G. R., Devor, A. H., Ehrbar, R., Ettner, R., Eyler, F., Garofalo, R., Karasic, D. H., . . . Zucker, K. (2012). Standards of care for the health of transsexual, transgender, and gender-nonconforming people, version 7. *International Journal of Transgenderism, 13*(4), 165–232. https://doi.org/10.1080/15532739.2011.700873

Coleman, E., Radix, A. E., Bouman, W. P., Brown, G. R., de Vries, A. L. C., Deutsch, M. B., Ettner, R., Fraser, L., Goodman, M., Green, J., Hancock, A. B., Johnson, T. W., Karasic, D. H., Knudson, G. A., Leibowitz, S. F., Meyer-Bahlburg, H. F. L., Monstrey, S. J., Motmans, J., Nahata, L., Nieder, T. O., . . . Arcelus, J. (2022). Standards of care for the health of transgender and gender diverse people, version 8. *International Journal of Transgender Health, 23*(Suppl. 1), S1–S259. https://doi.org/10.1080/26895269.2022.2100644

De Haan, L., & Nijland, S. (2002). *King and king.* Tricycle Press.

Ehrensaft, D. (2011). *Gender born, gender made: Raising healthy, gender nonconforming children.* The Experiment.

Ehrensaft, D. (2012). From gender identity disorder to gender identity creativity: True gender self child therapy. *Journal of Homosexuality, 59,* 337–356. https://doi.org/10.1080/00918369.2012.653303

Ehrensaft, D. (2014). Found in transition: Our youngest transgender people. *Contemporary Psychoanalysis, 50,* 571–592. https://doi.org/10.1080/00107530.2014.942591

Ehrensaft, D. (2016). *The gender creative child.* The Experiment.

Ehrensaft, D., & Jurkiewicz, M. (2024). Gender explained: A new Understanding of identity in a gender creative world. *The Experiment.*

Erikson, E. H. (1963). *Childhood and society.* Norton.

Fraiberg, S. H. (1959). *The magic years: Understanding and healing the problems of early childhood.* Simon & Schuster.

Goldberg, A. B. (Producer). (2007, April 27). *My secret self: A story of transgender children* [Television program]. ABC News.

Goldner, V. (2011). Trans: Gender in free fall. *Psychoanalytic Dialogues, 21,* 159–171. https://doi.org/10.1080/10481885.2011.562836

Green, R. (1987). *The "sissy boy" syndrome and the development of homosexuality.* Yale University Press. https://doi.org/10.2307/j.ctt1ww3v4c

Hembree, W. C., Cohen-Kettenis, P. T., Gooren, L., Hannema, S. E., Meyer, W. J., Murad, M. H., Rosenthal, S. M., Safer, J. D., Tangpricha, V., & T'Sjoen, G. G. (2017). Endocrine treatment of gender-dysphoric/gender-incongruent persons: An Endocrine Society Clinical Practice Guideline. *The Journal of Clinical Endocrinology and Metabolism, 102*(11), 3869–3903. https://doi.org/10.1210/jc.2017-01658

Hidalgo, M. A., Ehrensaft, D., Tishelman, A. C., Clark, L. F., Garofalo, R., Rosenthal, S. M., Spack, N. P., & Olson, J. (2013). The gender affirmative model: What we know and what we aim to learn [Editorial]. *Human Development, 56*(5), 285–290. https://doi.org/10.1159/000355235

Littman, L. (2018). Parent reports of adolescents and young adults perceived to show signs of a rapid onset of gender dysphoria. *PLOS ONE, 13*(8), e0202330. https://doi.org/10.1371/journal.pone.0202330

Malpas, J. (2011). Between pink and blue: A multi-dimensional family approach to gender nonconforming children and their families. *Family Process, 50*(4), 453–470. https://doi.org/10.1111/j.1545-5300.2011.01371.x

Olson, K. R., Durwood, L., DeMeules, M., & McLaughlin, K. A. (2016). Mental health of transgender children who are supported in their identities. *Pediatrics, 137*(3), 277–282. https://doi.org/10.1542/peds.2015-3223

Olson, K. R., Key, A. C., & Eaton, N. R. (2015). Gender cognition in transgender children. *Psychological Science, 26*(4), 467–474. https://doi.org/10.1177/0956797614568156

Olson-Kennedy, J., Chan, Y. M., Garofalo, R., Spack, N., Chen, D., Clark, L., Ehrensaft, D., Hidalgo, M., Tishelman, A., & Rosenthal, S. (2019). Impact of early medical treatment for transgender youth: Protocol for the longitudinal, observational trans youth care study. *JMIR Research Protocols, 8*(7), e14434. https://doi.org/10.2196/14434

Robles, R., Fresán, A., Vega-Ramírez, H., Cruz-Islas, J., Rodríguez-Pérez, V., Domínguez-Martínez, T., & Reed, G. M. (2016). Removing transgender identity from the classification of mental disorders: A Mexican field study for *ICD–11*. *The Lancet, 3*(9), 850–859. https://doi.org/10.1016/S2215-0366(16)30165-1

Shrier, A. (2020). *Irreversible damage: The transgender craze seducing our daughters*. Regnery Publications.

Steensma, T. D., Biemond, R., de Boer, F., & Cohen-Kettenis, P. T. (2011). Desisting and persisting gender dysphoria after childhood: A qualitative follow-up study. *Clinical Child Psychology and Psychiatry, 16*(4) 499–516. https://doi.org/10.1177/1359104510378303

Steensma, T. D., & Cohen-Kettenis, P. T. (2011). Gender transitioning before puberty? *Archives of Sexual Behavior, 40*, 649–650. https://doi.org/10.1007/s10508-011-9752-2

Steensma, T. D., & Cohen-Kettenis, P. T. (2018). A critical commentary on "A critical commentary on follow-up studies and 'desistence' theories about transgender and gender non-conforming children." *International Journal of Transgenderism, 19*(2), 225–230. https://doi.org/10.1080/15532739.2018.1468292

Steensma, T. D., McGuire, J. K., Kreukels, B. P., Beekman, A. J., & Cohen-Kettenis, P. T. (2013). Factors associated with desistence and persistence of childhood gender dysphoria: A quantitative follow-up study. *Journal of the American Academy of Child & Adolescent Psychiatry, 52*(6), 582–590. https://doi.org/10.1016/j.jaac.2013.03.016

Testa, R. J., Habarth, J., Peta, J., Balsam, K., & Bockting, W. (2015). Development of the Gender Minority Stress and Resilience Measure. *Psychology of Sexual Orientation and Gender Diversity, 2*(1), 65–77. https://doi.org/10.1037/sgd0000081

CHAPTER 7

GENETIC DISORDERS IN CHILDHOOD: CHROMOSOME 22q11.2 DELETION SYNDROME, DOWN SYNDROME, AND FRAGILE X SYNDROME

Kathleen Angkustsiri, Angela Thurman, and Randi Hagerman

In this chapter, we describe the most common genetic syndromes associated with intellectual disability (ID), Down syndrome (1 in 700), and fragile X syndrome (1 in 4,000 to 7,000). We also include chromosome 22q11.2 deletion syndrome (22q; 1 in 4,000), the most common microdeletion syndrome (i.e., a syndrome caused by the loss of genetic material too small to be detected using a conventional microscope, generally < 3 megabases [Mb]). Each section describes the prevalence, genetics, physical and behavioral phenotypes, and treatment issues associated with each syndrome. The multimodality approach to treatment is emphasized for all the disorders. We are in an age of genetic techniques for both diagnosis and, eventually as gene therapy advances, treatment, so the genetic aspects of these disorders are emphasized.

Genetic workup should be pursued for any child with an ID, developmental delay, or autism spectrum disorder (ASD; Miclea et al., 2015). First-line testing includes chromosomal microarray (CMA) and fragile X DNA testing. Identification of genetic etiology can guide management and treatment, aid with family planning, help families advocate for their children, and prevent unnecessary medical workups and procedures (Moeschler et al., 2014). A genetic cause can be found in up to 40% of individuals with developmental delay and autism (Miclea et al., 2015), although identification may improve as advances in whole-genome sequencing develop. All these genetic disorders have multiple medical, behavioral, and cognitive manifestations.

By way of organization, this chapter presents the aforementioned genetic disorders (22q, Down syndrome, and fragile X syndrome) by first discussing the prevalence and genetics of each syndrome and highlighting the syndromes' medical, developmental, and behavioral phenotypes. We then present the physical phenotype and medical, developmental, and psychological comorbidities for each condition and discuss the evaluation and clinical management, with consideration for emerging therapeutic interventions (e.g., genetics, immunotherapy, pharmacological management). Finally, recognizing the complex needs of children with 22q, Down syndrome, and fragile X syndrome, we discuss the role of multidisciplinary care of children with these conditions, highlighting the roles of pediatric

---

Support for this chapter was obtained through the Azrieli Foundation and through the MIND Institute Intellectual and Developmental Disabilities Research Center from National Institute of Child Health and Human Development P50 HD103526.

https://doi.org/10.1037/0000414-007

APA Handbook of Pediatric Psychology, Developmental-Behavioral Pediatrics, and Developmental Science: Vol. 2. Pediatric Psychology and Developmental-Behavioral Pediatrics: Clinical Applications of Developmental Science, P. E. Shah and M. H. Bornstein (Editors-in-Chief)
Copyright © 2025 by the American Psychological Association. All rights reserved.

psychologists, developmental-behavioral pediatricians, and the importance of a developmental science perspective in providing comprehensive care for these children.

CHROMOSOME 22Q11.2 DELETION SYNDROME (22Q)

Overview, Prevalence, and Genetics

Chromosome 22q11.2 deletion syndrome (22q) is caused by the deletion of genes on the long arm of chromosome 22. It is the most common microdeletion syndrome (Botto et al., 2003) and the second leading cause of developmental delay and congenital heart disease after Down syndrome (Bassett et al., 2011). It is highly variable, with over 180 possible symptoms, and was described separately before the identification of the common genetic mechanism. Overlapping presentations include DiGeorge syndrome, Velocardiofacial syndrome, Shprintzen syndrome, Opitz G/BBB, Cayler cardiofacial syndrome, and others (Exhibit 7.1). The preferred label is chromosome 22q11.2 deletion syndrome or simply "22q" to prevent confusion over the different presentations. Less is known about duplication of genes at chromosome 22q11.2 (not covered in this chapter), although initial findings suggest that the 22q11.2 duplication may be more variable and possibly more common (Grati et al., 2015).

Prevalence. 22q deletion occurs in 1 of every 2,000 to 6,000 live births (Botto et al., 2003), affects males and females equally (Kobrynski & Sullivan, 2007), and is similar across ethnic groups (Botto et al., 2003). Its actual prevalence may be higher (Grati et al., 2015), given the lack of population-based estimates and lower ascertainment of individuals without cardiac or palate anomalies.

Genetics. Individuals with 22q have one (instead of two) copies of genes located on the long arm of the 22nd chromosome. Approximately 90% of 22q deletions are *de novo* (or spontaneous) mutations, with variability in the expression of characteristic symptoms. Most individuals have a "common" 3 (2.54) Mb deletion encompassing 30 to 40 genes (McDonald-McGinn et al., 1999), and another 5% carry a smaller 1.5 Mb deletion. There is no association between deletion size and symptom presentation (McDonald-McGinn et al., 1999). Affected individuals have a 50% chance of passing along the deletion (autosomal dominant inheritance).

Diagnosis can be confirmed by CMA to quantify copy number variations (extra or missing copies of genes) in the 22q11.2 region, as well as other regions. Targeted analysis using fluorescence in-situ hybridization (FISH) and other methods can be used to identify copy number variations specifically in the 22q11.2 region. FISH is often used if 22q is highly suspected or to test relatives of an individual presenting with 22q.

Several genes in the 22q11.2 region have been identified as possible contributors to the physical and psychiatric manifestations. For example, catechol-O-methyl-transferase (COMT) is responsible for metabolizing dopamine in the prefrontal cortex and may play a role in cognition as well as the development of psychosis symptoms described in greater detail in a later section (Karayiorgou et al., 2010). Due to having only one copy of genes in the 22q11.2 region, individuals with 22q have lower COMT activity, with a presumed increase in cortical dopamine. Another gene of interest is proline dehydrogenase (PRODH), which

---

EXHIBIT 7.1

Names Associated With Chromosome 22q11.2 Deletion Syndrome

DiGeorge Syndrome
Velocardiofacial/Shprintzen Syndrome
Conotruncal Anomaly Face Syndrome
Opitz G/BBB Syndrome (autosomal dominant)
Cayler Cardiofacial Syndrome

Note. Data from McDonald-McGinn et al. (1999).

may affect glutamate and γ-aminobutyric acid (GABA; Karayiorgou et al., 2010). PRODH is also implicated in idiopathic schizophrenia and may play a role in learning difficulties, epilepsy, and schizoaffective disorder in 22q (Karayiorgou et al., 2010). T-box transcription factor-1 (TBX-1) is a regulator of growth and transcription factors in the T-box family of genes that play an important role in physical development. TBX-1 has been associated with development of physical features such as the aortic arch, thymus, parathyroid, and palate (Jyonouchi et al., 2009).

Medical, Developmental, and Behavioral Phenotype

Individuals with 22q are often identified early in life (median age 6 months) due to cardiac abnormalities (Óskarsdóttir et al., 2005), and prenatal diagnosis is also increasing due to improvements in prenatal imaging and noninvasive genetic testing. Infants often present with medical issues or motor delays, whereas school-aged children are identified due to learning difficulties, ADHD, or anxiety. Teens (and adults) are often diagnosed due to psychiatric concerns. Because of these developmental and behavioral symptoms (described in further detail later on), children with 22q can benefit from evaluation by developmental and behavioral specialists (e.g., pediatric psychologists, developmental-behavioral pediatricians, and child and adolescent psychiatrists) when concerns arise.

Physical phenotype and medical comorbidities. For a detailed review of the physical phenotype, see the practical management guidelines published by the International 22q11.2 Deletion Syndrome Consortium (Boot et al., 2023; Óskarsdóttir et al., 2023) and *Gene Reviews* (McDonald-McGinn et al., 1999). Briefly, facial features include mild dysmorphia, including hooded eyelids, narrow palpebral fissures, hypertelorism, bulbous nasal tip, and bifid uvula (see https://positiveexposure.org/album/22q11-2/; Óskarsdóttir et al., 2023). More than half have cardiac involvement, including ventricular septal defects (holes in the heart wall) and other heart anomalies such as tetralogy of Fallot (64%; McDonald-McGinn et al., 1999). Conductive and sensorineural hearing loss are reported. Ears tend to be unusually shaped (overfolded, cupped, or microtic). Palatal abnormalities (67%; McDonald-McGinn et al., 1999) include overt and submucous cleft palate, split uvula, functional problems with the palate (velopharyngeal incompetence [VPI]), and air escaping from the nose when speaking (hypernasality). Feeding difficulties are also prevalent. Immune deficiency is present in 75% of individuals and involves thymic hypoplasia, T-cell impairment, and frequent sinopulmonary infections. T-cell production is decreased, but T-cell function is usually less impaired and often improves over time (Sullivan et al., 1999). Increased risk for autoimmune conditions include juvenile rheumatoid arthritis, low platelets caused by immune problems, and decreased pigment in the skin (Sullivan, 2019). Low thyroid hormone and low calcium levels are also common and can fluctuate over time, with recurrence during periods of stress or illness (Bassett et al., 2011). Thyroid hormone can be low, but hyperthyroidism is also reported (McDonald-McGinn et al., 1999). Growth can be slow during infancy and childhood, although adults often have normal stature. Growth hormone deficiency has also been reported (Weinzimer et al., 1998). Neurologic manifestations include epilepsy in 5% to 7% of individuals (Fung et al., 2015) and structural brain differences, such as cavum septum pellucidum, polymicrogyria, cortical dysplasia, and microcephaly (Karayiorgou et al., 2010).

Developmental aspects. Developmental delays are common, including hypotonia with gross motor delay and speech/language delay (McDonald-McGinn et al., 1999). Thirty percent have mild-to-moderate ID (De Smedt et al., 2007), although mean intelligence quotient (IQ) is in the borderline range but quite variable. Full-scale IQ is often misleading due to higher verbal IQ compared to nonverbal IQ (De Smedt et al., 2007). Neurocognitive profiles include strengths in rote verbal learning, reading decoding, and spelling, along with weaknesses in visuo-spatial processing, attention, and math (Simon, 2008).

Behavioral manifestations and psychiatric comorbidities. Psychiatric conditions develop in childhood, continue into adulthood, and should be screened for and treated appropriately, as interventions are available (Jhawar et al., 2021). Anxiety is present in 35% of children and adolescents (Schneider et al., 2014). Specific phobia (fear of particular objects or situations) is most common, followed by social phobia and generalized anxiety (Jolin et al., 2012). Anxiety is often underidentified, undertreated (Tang et al., 2014), and may be misattributed to inattention, shyness, or avoidance (Angkustsiri et al., 2012). Attention deficit/hyperactivity disorder (ADHD) is also common in childhood (~35%; Schneider et al., 2014). The most common presentation is inattentive ADHD (Niarchou et al., 2015), with executive function, inhibition (Simon et al., 2005), cognitive flexibility, and organization difficulties. The prevalence of ASD varies across studies (10%–40%; Antshel et al., 2007; Fine et al., 2005) due to methodological differences, ascertainment bias, and comorbidities. A meta-analysis estimated that 11% of children with 22q have ASD (Richards et al., 2015). Many children with 22q exhibit social impairments, including social communication difficulties and restricted and repetitive behaviors, without meeting formal diagnostic criteria for ASD (Ousley et al., 2017). Mood disorders are low in childhood (3%; Schneider et al., 2014). The prevalence of bipolar disorders is not increased, affecting <1% of children and adolescents (Schneider et al., 2014).

22q is the third-highest risk factor for schizophrenia and is considered a genetic model for psychosis spectrum disorders (including schizophrenia, schizoaffective disorder, etc.), which is present in 20% to 30% of adults with 22q deletion syndrome (Bassett et al., 2011). Onset is similar to idiopathic psychosis with 21% to 42% reporting symptoms in late adolescence and early adulthood (Schneider et al., 2014). Predictors include a decline in verbal IQ, lower baseline IQ, and preexisting anxiety (Antshel et al., 2010). Negative life events and stress (Beaton & Simon, 2011) may also contribute to psychosis risk.

Management and Intervention

Pediatric and Adult Guidelines (Boot et al., 2023; Óskarsdóttir et al., 2023) are helpful in the management of medical problems and should be utilized by providers caring for an individual with 22q. Briefly, this includes assessment for medical, developmental, and psychiatric conditions at various time points during the lifespan, and highlights the importance of psychologists and developmental-behavioral pediatricians in the evaluation, management, and longitudinal monitoring of children with 22q. Regarding medical surveillance, kidney ultrasound, immune function, and palate evaluation should be performed at diagnosis, whereas a complete blood count, thyroid function, and calcium should be checked routinely. The adult guidelines (Boot et al., 2023) provide additional guidance for the identification and management of psychiatric conditions, genetic counseling, and supporting independent living skills.

Future Treatments

Studies are investigating immune tissue and blood cell transplantation for severe immune deficiency in 22q. Few randomized controlled trials have been conducted for the psychiatric manifestations, although an increasing number of trials are currently registered (see clinicaltrials.gov), including cognitive remediation to improve cognitive flexibility/executive function and possibly prevent psychosis risk (Kern et al., 2009). This method has been effective in the treatment of schizophrenia (Kern et al., 2009). Trials of novel therapeutics, such as NRC-1 (an mGluR modulator) and cannabidiol (CBD; NCT05149898), are still awaiting study results. Other ongoing trials include risperidone for neuroprotection (NCT04639960) and Concerta (a long-acting methylphenidate) for ADHD in 22q (NCT04647500). Terminated/completed trials include metyrosine for psychosis (NCT01127503) and SAMe for depression and ADHD, although no data support the use of either (Green et al., 2012).

DOWN SYNDROME

Genetics, Prevalence, and Overview of Down Syndrome

Down syndrome (DS) is the leading genetic cause of intellectual disability, with an estimated prevalence rate of 1 in 700 live births (Mégarbané et al., 2009). In 1959, karyotyping techniques confirmed that DS results from an extra copy of chromosome 21 (Mégarbané et al., 2009). Later advancements in cytogenetic techniques clarified that DS is caused by three distinct chromosomal alterations: (a) trisomy 21 (~95%), in which an extra chromosome 21 is replicated in all cells; (b) unbalanced translocation (~3%–4%), in which part of a third copy of chromosome 21 attaches to another chromosome; or (c) mosaicism (~1%–2%), in which there is a mixture of cells with either two or three copies (Mégarbané et al., 2009). Further advancements have provided additional insight into the etiology of trisomy 21 by classifying the parent of origin for the extra chromosome and more specific information regarding the type of error that occurred (Sherman et al., 2007).

The most common risk factor for DS is advanced maternal age, with the likelihood of having a child with DS rising from less than 1 in 1,000 for mothers under 30 years of age to 1 in 12 for mothers 40 years of age (Roizen, 1997). However, due to the association between birth rates and maternal age, most children with DS are born to mothers under 35 years (Olsen et al., 1996). The only other risk factor known to be associated with DS is altered recombination patterns, which predispose chromosome pairs to erroneously separate (Sherman et al., 2007).

Phenotype.

Medical. The clinical presentation of DS is complex and considerable heterogeneity is observed at all levels of description (Karmiloff-Smith et al., 2016). Nearly all individuals with DS demonstrate a characteristic set of craniofacial features, including brachycephaly (i.e., skull's length-to-width ratio is reduced), depressed nasal root, upward-slanting palpebral fissures, and epicanthal folds (i.e., upper eyelid skin that covers the inner corner of the eye). In addition, individuals with DS are at increased risk of presenting with a variety of co-occurring medical conditions (Bull & Committee on Genetics, 2011). Congenital heart disease (e.g., ventricular or atrioventricular septal defects), hearing loss, frequent ear infections, vision difficulties, hypotonia, and ligament laxity are the most common conditions (Bull & Committee on Genetics, 2011; Sherman et al., 2007). In addition, several other medical conditions are less frequent in their occurrence but also observed at higher rates relative to the general population, such as thyroid issues, seizures, hematological problems (such as anemia, iron deficiency, and leukemia), and celiac disease (Bull & Committee on Genetics, 2011; Capone et al., 2018). The American Academy of Pediatrics (AAP) has provided health supervision guidelines to facilitate early screening and progression of a variety of medical issues from the prenatal period to 21 years of age (Bull & Committee on Genetics, 2011). In general, within these guidelines, the AAP highlights consideration of age-specific co-occurring medical and developmental conditions, the child's strengths and positive family experiences, and discussing resources available (e.g., financial, medical, and educational support programs, parent support groups, etc.). Co-occurring medical conditions, such as sleep difficulties and thyroid dysfunction, can negatively impact the level of functioning and quality of life demonstrated by individuals with DS (Breslin et al., 2014; Fernandez & Reeves, 2015).

Behavioral. Children with DS are commonly described as demonstrating increased sociability. Even though the social abilities and interests demonstrated by individuals with DS are thought to reflect areas of strength, these strengths do not preclude the presence of social difficulties (Thurman & del Hoyo Soriano, 2021). For example, individuals with DS are commonly described as being at lower risk for behavioral challenges and psychiatric symptomatology relative to their peers with nonspecific ID or other genetic neurodevelopmental disorders; however, these descriptions often overshadow the fact that individuals with DS are at increased risk, relative to the general population, for presenting with a variety of behavioral conditions (Dykens, 2007; Tassé et al., 2016). In early childhood, externalizing behaviors, such as oppositionality, attentional difficulties, and impulsivity, have been noted, and Ekstein et al. (2011) found that ~44% of their sample met criteria for ADHD. Considering oppositionality, it is estimated that 10% to 15% of children with DS are diagnosed with conduct/oppositionality disorders, primarily manifested by behaviors such as noncompliance, disobedience, and low-level aggression (Dykens, 2007). Finally, individuals with DS appear to be at greater risk of presenting with symptoms of ASD, with estimates of the co-occurring presence of ASD ranging from 5% to 39% (Dimachkie Nunnally et al., 2021; Thurman & del Hoyo Soriano, 2021).

Cognitive. The DS phenotype is characterized by significant cognitive delays, although considerable heterogeneity is observed (Karmiloff-Smith et al., 2016). Early in development, differences between infants with DS and infants with typical development (TD) are relatively subtle. As children with DS transition into toddlerhood nearly all demonstrate developmental delay and across the school-age years children with DS increasingly lag behind their peers with TD, with most children with DS demonstrating cognitive levels consistent with ID (Couzens et al., 2012). Investigations that consider metrics that focus on growth in skills (versus metrics that consider performance relative to the general population) clarify that, albeit slowly, cognitive skills are indeed progressing across childhood and into early adulthood (Couzens et al., 2012).

Individuals with DS demonstrate relative strengths in the areas of nonverbal communication, gross motor skills, visual-motor integration, and visual imitation; by contrast, areas that are particularly challenging for individuals with DS include auditory short-term memory, episodic memory, aspects of executive function, and expressive language (Abbeduto et al., 2016; Daunhauer & Fidler, 2011). Advances in elucidating the DS cognitive phenotype have focused on providing potential links between the cognitive phenotypes and their neural underpinnings; for example, atypical development of the hippocampus has been associated with aspects of spatial processing and episodic memory (Edgin et al., 2015). Even though individuals with DS often have better receptive than expressive language skills, even when considering only receptive language skills, areas of strength and challenge may occur (Abbeduto et al., 2016; Thurman & del Hoyo Soriano, 2021). For example, receptive vocabulary is generally stronger than receptive grammar, and within the vocabulary, the reception of some types of words may be more challenging (e.g., relational terms) than others (Abbeduto et al., 2016).

Importantly, understanding of the DS cognitive profile has been based on group-level findings. The proportion of individuals with DS who demonstrate this specific profile remains unclear because the DS phenotype is also associated with considerable heterogeneity at every level and system of development (Karmiloff-Smith et al., 2016). Furthermore, variations in genetics, neurobiology, severity of affectedness, medical as well as psychiatric comorbidities, and developmental period have all been shown to contribute to the variable presentation of the DS phenotype (Fernandez & Reeves, 2015; Karmiloff-Smith et al., 2016; Thurman & del Hoyo Soriano, 2021).

Diagnosis and Management

Currently, it is recommended that all pregnant women, regardless of age, be offered the option to participate in minimally invasive diagnostic screening procedures, such as nuchal translucency ultrasonography and measurement of maternal serum human chorionic gonadotropin (β-hCG) and pregnancy-associated plasma protein-A. Integrated screening, or the combination of first- and second-trimester screening, will yield a detection rate of 95% (Bull & Committee on Genetics, 2011). In general, it is recommended that health providers evaluate for conditions frequently associated with the DS phenotype and routinely monitor for less frequently observed conditions to ensure early diagnosis and treatment; as described earlier, the American Psychological Association has provided thorough health supervision guidelines to facilitate early screening and progression of a variety of medical issues until 21 years of age (Bull & Committee on Genetics, 2011).

In addition to ongoing medical screening and health management, intervention services, educational supports, and vocational training are all frequently recommended to support the success of individuals across all stages of development. Advances in elucidating the behavioral phenotype associated with DS have yielded much insight into intervention targets to support development (e.g., motor skills, language, executive function, self-help skills). Because early skills set the foundation for the skills that follow, early intervention is recommended. Physical therapy, speech-language therapy, and occupational therapy can help support the development of babies and young children with DS (Daunhauer & Fidler, 2011; Fidler & Nadel, 2007). Across school-age years, the level of developmental delay is associated with academic achievement and support needs; however, children with DS benefit from mainstream schooling, with evidence that children with mainstream schooling demonstrate greater progress than peers with DS with similar cognitive levels in specialized schools (Turner et al., 2008). Taken together, because of the heterogeneity of the developmental and behavioral vulnerabilities seen in children with DS, evaluation and longitudinal monitoring by developmental-behavioral pediatricians and pediatric psychologists with expertise in school assessment can help guide interventions and educational planning across the childhood lifespan.

Brain Sciences Discoveries Guiding Targeted Treatments

Basic science discoveries using mouse models of DS (e.g., Ts65Dn) and advancements in new pharmacological interventions are yielding promising results. Indeed, a variety of pharmacological interventions has been shown to rescue, or partially rescue, learning and memory challenges associated with DS as well as ameliorate cellular and electrophysiological features uncovered in the mouse models (Stagni et al., 2015). The phenotypes associated with DS are posited to result from various factors such as dose-sensitive genes, environment (e.g., social, educational, nutritional), and/or other factors that may result from the presence of an extra chromosome (Herault et al., 2017). Mouse models have provided significant insight into genotype–phenotype associations in DS. A region of 33 genes is implicated in the cognitive impairment associated with DS, with a particular interest in *Dyrk1* (Herault et al., 2017; Olson et al., 2007). Indeed, normalization of *Dyrk1* is associated with learning improvements and improvements in hippocampal long-term potentiation (García-Cerro et al., 2014). In addition, numerous studies have considered the efficacy of potential pharmacological interventions in the mouse models of DS with positive results (Herault et al., 2017; Stagni et al., 2015). In addition, the effectiveness of neural stem cell therapies has also been considered, but limitations to the translation of this approach to humans remain (Herault et al., 2017).

Future Treatments

Advances in basic science discoveries have shed light on a wide variety of potential advances in supporting the development of individuals with DS across the lifespan (Stagni et al., 2015). Therapies targeting changes in overall cognitive ability are argued to likely be most successful when done early, with prenatal interventions believed to make the biggest impact (D'Souza & Karmiloff-Smith, 2017). There is also considerable interest in identifying treatment approaches to delay declines associated with Alzheimer's disease in individuals with DS, with interest in the impact of targeting oxidative stress and neuroinflammation on supporting adult outcomes (Bartesaghi et al., 2015). Moreover, nonpharmacological interventions, such as behavioral interventions and cognitive training, can be combined with pharmacological therapeutics to maximize treatment effects (Bartesaghi et al., 2015).

FRAGILE X SYNDROME AND PREMUTATION DISORDERS

Molecular Overview and Fragile X Spectrum Disorders

Fragile X syndrome (FXS) is caused by the full mutation (greater than 200 CGG repeats) in the fragile X messenger ribonucleoprotein 1 gene (*FMR1*), which is on the bottom end of the X chromosome. The full mutation is usually methylated such that transcription is shut down and little or no mRNA is produced, leading to little or no *FMR1* protein (FMRP). The lack of FMRP causes ID, the physical phenotype including a large head circumference, large and prominent ears (see https://positiveexposure.org/album/fragile-x-syndrome/), and hyperextensible finger joints, and the behavioral features of FXS described in the following paragraphs. The full mutation occurs in approximately 4,000 to 6,000 individuals in the general population, although the prevalence varies in different countries. For instance, the prevalence of FXS is very common in Ricaurte, Colombia, South America, where a founder effect occurs, and approximately 2 in 100 individuals in the population have FXS; other countries also have pockets of high prevalence, including Indonesia, Mexico, and Majorca (Saldarriaga et al., 2018).

Those with the premutation (55 to 200 CGG repeats) typically do not have methylation, and their level of *FMR1* mRNA is elevated compared to the normal population with a normal allele (5 to 40 CGG repeats). The higher the number of CGG repeats within the premutation range, the higher the level of mRNA; the highest level is approximately eight times normal. Individuals with the premutation usually do not suffer from ID unless there is an additional genetic mutation, although autism can occur in approximately 15% of males with the premutation, and ADHD symptoms can be seen in the majority of males. The premutation is common in the general population and approximately 1 in 150–200 females and 1 in 250–400 males have the premutation. The elevated level of mRNA in carriers of the premutation is associated with RNA toxicity because the elevated mRNA can sequester proteins that are important for neuronal and glial cell functioning.

The clinical problems occurring in premutation carriers can include early ovarian failure or insufficiency before age 40, called the fragile X-associated primary ovarian insufficiency (FXPOI), seen in approximately 20% of female carriers (Hunter et al., 2020), and fragile X-associated neuropsychiatric disorders (FXAND), which includes psychiatric disorders such as anxiety, depression, obsessive-compulsive disorder, ADHD, chronic fatigue, chronic pain, social deficits, and insomnia commonly found in carriers of the premutation (Hagerman et al., 2018). One or more of these problems occur in about 50% of premutation carriers and are often clustered with additional medical problems such as migraine headaches, fibromyalgia, autoimmune thyroid disease, and, rarely, other autoimmune problems (Allen et al., 2020).

The most severe clinical problem associated with the premutation is fragile X-associated tremor/ataxia syndrome (FXTAS), which occurs in approximately 40% of males and 16% of females with the premutation (Hagerman & Hagerman, 2016). The onset of FXTAS is usually in the early 60s and typically begins with an action tremor in the hands followed by a cerebellar ataxia, leading to frequent falling. FXTAS is a neurodegenerative syndrome characterized by white matter disease on MRI in the middle cerebellar peduncles (MCP sign), insula, periventricular areas, and the splenium of the corpus callosum. In the family history of children with FXS, typically one of the grandparents on the mother's side has FXTAS symptoms, but it is easily misdiagnosed as atypical Parkinson's disease (Hagerman & Hagerman, 2016).

Molecular and clinical association with autism. Individuals with the full mutation or the premutation can have a diagnosis of ASD. However, this diagnosis is more common in those with FXS; ASD occurs in ~60% of males and 20% of females with FXS (Thurman et al., 2014). Those with ASD typically have a lower IQ, more frequent seizures (which typically occur in 16% of males), and more behavioral problems than those with FXS without ASD (Kaufmann et al., 2017). The cause of ASD is likely related to the deficit of FMRP, which has multiple functions in the central nervous system, such as the control of translation for hundreds of mRNAs, including many that are causal for ASD when the genes are mutated (Iossifov et al., 2012); control of synaptic plasticity; and also control of multiple ion channels related to behavior (Deng & Klyachko, 2021).

ASD in those with a premutation is less common but does occur in 8% to 19% of males and approximately 1% to 4% of females (Bailey et al., 2008; Loesch et al., 2007). The etiology of ASD in premutation carriers is more complex and likely has multiple factors. FMRP may be mildly deficient in carriers with a CGG repeat over 120 because translation is stalled with a long-repeat sequence. However, the mRNA is high in premutation carriers, leading to RNA toxicity, and carriers are vulnerable to environmental toxicity because of reactive oxygen species and mitochondrial dysfunction, leading to earlier neuronal cell death. In addition, there may be a second or multiple genes that predispose to ASD in the background genetics.

Behavioral and cognitive phenotype linking to molecular pathways. The level of ID in those with FXS correlates with the level of FMRP in the blood (Kim et al., 2020; Tassone et al., 1999). However, the measure of FMRP is typically carried out in research studies and not clinically, so it is difficult to measure FMRP on a routine clinical basis (Kim et al., 2020). In females with FXS, the activation ratio (the percentage of cells with the normal X as the active X in blood) will correlate with IQ, and the higher this ratio, the higher the IQ (Tassone et al., 1999). Approximately 30% of females with the full mutation will have an IQ in the normal range, 30% will have a borderline IQ, and 30% will have an IQ in the ID range but typically only have mild ID. In males with FXS, 85% will have ID that ranges from mild to severe, and the most severe will also have ASD. The other 15% of males will have an IQ of 70 or higher, but usually their DNA lacks methylation in the full mutation range, or they will be mosaic with some cells with the premutation and some cells with the full mutation; they are therefore producing some FMRP from their premutated cells or from the cells with a lack of methylation. However, if most cells in a mosaic individual with FXS have the premutation or if the full mutation is not methylated, then the level of mRNA may be elevated, which puts the individual at risk for developing FXTAS with aging. Otherwise, those with FXS develop neither FXTAS nor FXPOI.

The behavioral phenotype of individuals with FXS includes shyness and social deficits as well as anxiety and ADHD with significant hyperactivity and impulsivity. Males with FXS and many affected females are hypersensitive to sensory stimuli, and they are unable to habituate to these stimuli, most likely related to their GABA deficits. They are easily hyperaroused, with stimuli often leading to tantrum behavior. Transitions from one environment to another are difficult for them because of the changes in stimuli.

Behavioral features of FXS include poor eye contact, hand flapping, hand biting, and sometimes self-injurious behaviors, such as head banging or self-hitting. Aggression toward others occurs in 30% to 40% of those with FXS, which can be controlled at younger ages, but for some, it can escalate with puberty, leading to aggressive acts, particularly towards their mother (Wheeler et al., 2016). Such behavior contributes significant stress and trauma to caregivers and is often the reason for out-of-home placement. For some adults, this episodic dyscontrol can occur unexpectedly without a precipitant, and it can lead to significant destruction of the household and significant injury to family members and friends. Such behavior often leads to the use of atypical antipsychotics, mood stabilizers, and even anticonvulsants and the need for behavior therapy.

Outcomes in childhood. Intellectual scores tend to decline with age in FXS; although those with FXS do not lose skills, they do not develop abstract reasoning abilities parallel to the general population. So, IQ can decline but mental age continues to improve in adolescence. As individuals with FXS age, ADHD can be a significant problem in mid-childhood, and treatment with stimulants is usually utilized until the late teen years. Then, ADHD can be less of a problem and hyperactivity improves; however, for males, attention problems linger throughout adulthood. Aggression can peak in the teenage years, related perhaps to testosterone levels, and may persist into young adulthood. Most individuals stay in school for vocational training until age 21, depending on what programs are available. Several universities and colleges have developed programs for those with ID so they can experience the social benefits of college life and further develop their self-help and vocational skills, with significant mentoring and support (Hagerman et al., 2020). As with the other genetic disorders presented, children with FXS can benefit from evaluation and longitudinal monitoring by developmental and behavioral specialists (e.g., developmental-behavioral pediatricians and pediatric psychologists), to provide baseline assessments of cognitive and behavioral functioning, and to initiate interventions when concerns arise. Such care can be provided in the context of multidisciplinary FXS clinics, described further in the next section.

Treatment of FXS. Treatment and interventions in FXS involve a team of professions working together with the family and the patient. Often the developmental and behavioral pediatrician is leading the team from a specialized clinic and there are over 25 Fragile X Treatment and Research Centers around the United States (see listings at the National Fragile X Foundation [NFXF] at https://fragileX.org). Each specialized clinic has a team of professionals that usually includes a psychologist and therapists (speech and language, OTs and PTs) in addition to educational experts. Written information on the NFXF's website has guidance information for families and professionals for each of these therapies. Behavioral interventions can be helpful with calming strategies and preparations for change and in those with FXS plus ASD. ABA therapy, particularly Early Start Denver Model, a naturalistic form of ABA can be helpful (Riley et al., 2020). Occupational therapy in addition to cognitive behavior therapy are helpful throughout school. Speech and language therapy is also essential, and improvements in communication skills help behavior (Chitwood et al., 2020).

The outcome of patients with FXS is not only dependent on the severity of involvement of the child and the quality of the interventions but also on the efforts of the family and their educational abilities also related to their socioeconomic status. Many families are stressed financially, particularly if they have to pay for the multiple interventions needed for their children. In addition, the mother may be overwhelmed by her own problems related to the premutation or perhaps to a full mutation. If the mother is intellectually impaired because of a full mutation or depressed because of the premutation and the stress of raising one or more children with FXS, this will have consequences for the child(ren). Many patients can lead semi-independent lives with the support of the treatment team and the family. The benefits of a healthy lifestyle, including daily exercise; nutritional support to avoid obesity; avoidance of harmful environmental factors such as alcohol or illicit drugs; and the use of the targeted treatments described in this chapter may be helpful to a growing group of patients as they age.

There are also targeted medical treatments that can reverse the neurobiological changes caused by the loss of FMRP. Although not targeted treatments, some medications can be very helpful for behavior, such as stimulants or guanfacine for the symptoms of ADHD, selective serotonin reuptake inhibitors (SSRIs) for anxiety, and atypical antipsychotics (aripiprazole and risperidone) for mood instability/aggression. Sleep problems are very typical in young children with FXS, and they usually respond to melatonin and sometimes clonidine as needed. A review from the Fragile X Online Registry With Accessible Research Database (FORWARD) involving 975 patients from multiple FXS clinics demonstrated that 63% were treated with a psychotropic medication. The most frequent agents were SSRIs in 43%, stimulants in 38%, and atypical antipsychotics in 33%, the latter mainly in males with ID and ASD (Dominick et al., 2021).

Many of the targeted treatments that are being studied in FXS are currently not available by prescription because they are not FDA approved for clinical use, but some medications are available by prescription. Unfortunately, no medication has been approved by the FDA specifically for treatment of FXS. So, the medications discussed can be used for FXS, but they are used off label. Minocycline, for example, can be prescribed and has limited efficacy in FXS (Leigh et al., 2013); however, the side effects of darkened teeth when it is used in patients under 8 years old can be a deterrent. Minocycline may also demonstrate occasional side effects such as a lupus-like reaction, so if a rash develops or the patient's antinuclear antibody (ANA) level is significantly increased, then it should be discontinued (Hagerman et al., 2020).

Another medication that rescued symptoms of FXS in animal models and can be helpful for behavior problems and language is metformin. Metformin is a biguanide antihyperglycemic medication used to treat Type 2 diabetes, and it down-regulates the mTOR pathway that is upregulated in FXS. Metformin is currently in a controlled trial in children and adults with FXS; early studies have shown improvement in developmental testing in young patients with FXS in an open-label trial (Biag et al., 2019). Case studies of metformin have demonstrated improvement in IQ in 2 adults with FXS (Protic, Aydin, et al., 2019) and rescue of macroorchidism when started before puberty (Protic, Kaluzhny, et al., 2019). Metformin is also helpful for overeating, facilitates weight loss, protects against many forms of cancer, reduces inflammation, protects against cerebrovascular disease, and lowers blood pressure; these benefits may be helpful in both those with FXS and premutation carriers (Romero et al., 2017). Metformin is well tolerated even in young children; however, it is important to start at a low dose that can be obtained in the generic liquid preparation of 100 mg/ml. Starting with a dose at dinner and then gradually increasing the dose each week typically helps to avoid the main side effect of diarrhea. Metformin can be given twice a day, at breakfast and at dinner, in the final dosing. If the child becomes ill and cannot eat or is scheduled for surgery, the metformin should be stopped until the patient is able to eat again to avoid lactic acidosis. It is also recommended that the patient take a multivitamin that includes vitamin B_{12} (Hagerman et al., 2020).

Another medication that is commonly used clinically in FXS is sertraline, an SSRI. Sertraline is used to treat anxiety, which typically emerges at age 2 or older. A retrospective review of young children with FXS treated with sertraline demonstrated improvement in both receptive and expressive language trajectory on the Mullen Scales of Early Learning (MSEL) compared to those not treated with sertraline (Indah Winarni et al., 2012); a controlled trial was then carried out with low-dose sertraline (2.5 to 5.0 mg/day) in children ages 2 to 6 years old for 6 months (Greiss Hess et al., 2016). This study demonstrated significant improvement on the fine motor scale and the visual perception scale, in addition to the composite T score on the MSEL. In a post hoc analysis among the patients with FXS and ASD, representing 60% of the overall 57 children who underwent the study, significant improvement was seen in the expressive language scale on sertraline compared to placebo. The Tobii eye tracker was also used in a passive receptive language paradigm in this controlled trial, and significant improvements were seen in receptive language on sertraline compared to placebo (Yoo et al., 2017). These studies have supported the clinical use of sertraline in children with FXS.

Another targeted treatment to help with anxiety is cannabidiol (CBD), the nonpsychotropic component of marijuana. Although there are anecdotal reports of CBD use in FXS where the CBD is obtained at a marijuana store or over the internet, products obtained this way are not free of the psychotropic component of marijuana, tetrahydrocannabinol (THC). The pharmaceutical company Zynerba has studied their manufactured topical CBD preparation (with no THC) in an open-label study of CBD in FXS, demonstrating benefits for many behavioral problems, including anxiety and ADHD (Heussler et al., 2019). Subsequently, an international multicenter randomized phase 3 controlled trial was carried out lasting 12 weeks in children ages 3 to 18 years old with doses of 250 to 500 mg given twice a day topically with preliminary positive results.

Diagnosis and management. The diagnosis of FXS and premutation disorders is made through fragile X DNA testing. The key behavioral features that suggest the diagnosis are a lack of language at 3 years, global developmental delay, hyperactivity, anxiety, and stereotypies such as hand flapping and hand biting. The patient may already be diagnosed with ASD because of poor eye contact and social avoidance. The physical features of FXS including a large head circumference, large, prominent ears, and hyperextensible finger joints may also suggest the diagnosis, because these features are seen in about 60% to 70% of young children with FXS (see https://positiveexposure.org/album/fragile-x-syndrome/). So, the presence of ASD, characteristic physical features, and developmental delay should key the psychologist, therapist, or physician to consider FXS and order fragile X DNA testing.

Both polymerase chain reaction and Southern blot testing are carried out routinely at most commercial and university laboratories. The laboratory will report the number of CGG repeats in *FMR1*; however, the activation ratio and the percentage of cells with or without methylation may not be provided unless tested through a research laboratory. Once a positive test is obtained, it is important for the clinician to meet with the positive individual, and preferably the whole family, to review genetic counseling or refer the family to a genetic counselor, because many more individuals in the family may be carriers or affected by the premutation or the full mutation. Further fragile X DNA testing should be carried out to find potentially positive individuals for treatment. The earlier the diagnosis is made, the sooner treatment can be started. Because *FMR1* is on the X-chromosome and can expand to a full mutation only through the mother, if a patient has the full mutation, then the mother is the carrier, or she may have the full mutation herself, whereas a male carrier will pass on the premutation to all his daughters. The siblings of the proband should also be tested. Often, the maternal grandparents are tested because one will be a carrier, which may affect their health as they age. The families should also be referred to resources listed in Resources section.

MULTIDISCIPLINARY CARE FOR CHILDREN WITH GENETIC SYNDROMES

Multiple specialists need to work together—including the pediatrician, the psychologist, and the developmental and behavioral pediatrician—along with additional specialists as needed, to give high-quality care to those with genetic syndromes.

Role of General Pediatrician

General pediatricians play an important role in diagnosing 22q, DS, and FXS, particularly for children not already identified due to existing medical conditions. For example, in 22q, children with VPI, nasal speech, or learning problems may be missed, especially in the absence of ID. General pediatricians are also responsible for routine screening (calcium, platelets, thyroid, etc.) and referrals to specialists (ENT, ophthalmology, etc.) for medical management. Developmental-behavioral pediatricians are also knowledgeable about targeted treatments and they can work with the general pediatrician to adjust the medications for those with FXS or other neurodevelopmental disorders (Hagerman et al., 2020).

Role of Pediatric Psychologists

Pediatric psychologists may care for children with genetic conditions, such as 22q, DS, and FXS, as it is important to follow neurocognitive development over time, particularly during specific developmental periods (preschool to elementary school, high school to adulthood, etc.) to consider whether educational expectations match ability level (Jhawar et al., 2021). Psychologists often diagnose learning disabilities and ID, along with behavioral health conditions (e.g., co-occurrence of ASD, ADHD, or anxiety), and some provide behavioral therapies, along with adaption to chronic illness and family support. There are no syndrome-specific treatments, and existing evidenced-based interventions for target symptoms (anxiety, ADHD, etc.) used in the general population are effective for individuals with genetic conditions. Cognitive behavior therapy has been adapted for children with other neurodevelopmental disorders, such as ASD and ID (Spence et al., 2011; Wood et al., 2009) and should be pursued for children with 22q/DS/FXS experiencing anxiety.

Role of Developmental-Behavioral Pediatrician

Developmental-behavioral pediatricians also play a critical role in evaluating and treating co-occurring conditions, such as anxiety and ADHD, and helping families advocate for school and other services. Medication management of other childhood psychiatric conditions may also be appropriate. Psychotropic medications are efficacious, but they are often underutilized in children with identified syndromes, such as 22q (Tang et al., 2014). For example, few medication studies have been published in 22q or DS, although most support the use of stimulants, selective serotonin reuptake inhibitors (SSRIs), and antipsychotics if indicated (Mosheva et al., 2020). Medication studies have been reported in FXS as summarized previously and reviewed in Hagerman et al. (2020). Stimulants for ADHD are effective, tolerated, and safe in FXS (Hagerman et al., 2020) and in 22q, although side effects, such as appetite suppression or sleep disturbance, are common (Gothelf et al., 2003). There is no evidence to support that stimulants increase psychosis risk in 22q (Mosheva et al., 2020). Over one-half of individuals with 22q treated with SSRIs show improvement (Mosheva et al., 2020). Psychosis is best managed by psychiatrists in all three disorders, but developmental-behavioral pediatricians may sometimes co-manage this. For example, up to 85% of individuals with 22q treated with antipsychotics show improvement with no serious adverse events (Mosheva et al., 2020). Mild side effects are common, including extrapyramidal symptoms and weight gain (Dori et al., 2017). Other considerations include medical susceptibility, so monitoring for heart rhythm dysfunction, low blood counts, and so on is recommended.

Role of Subspecialty Clinics

Due to the complex nature of care required to address medical, learning, and mental health concerns, multi-disciplinary teams are recommended (Dori et al., 2017). They may include specialties, such as cleft/craniofacial/ENT, cardiology, immunology, endocrinology, developmental-behavioral pediatrics, psychology, genetics, psychiatry, dental, and sometimes other specialties such as hematology or orthopedics.

Roles of School System and Community Supports

Recognizing the importance of the broader ecological contexts in which children are embedded, optimizing the school and educational environment is an important consideration for children with genetic disorders. Educational and community supports are imperative for successful function over the lifespan for all three disorders. Children with 22q as well as female children with FXS and premutation disorders may have difficulty with eligibility for special education services in the absence of ID, but many may be eligible for an Individualized Educational Plan under the heading of "other health impairment." Individuals with all three of these disorders often do better when they are comfortable socially and expectations are modified to competency level (Jhawar et al., 2021). An adult transition plan is especially important due to underestimation of needs and includes access to rehabilitative, mental health, and disability services for genetic conditions.

CONCLUSION

Children with genetic syndromes (e.g., 22q, Down syndrome and fragile X syndrome) are a heterogeneous population who often manifest developmental and behavioral vulnerabilities that can present at any point in the childhood lifespan. To optimize behavioral health outcomes for children with genetic syndromes, multidisciplinary care is recommended, which includes evaluation and management by providers with expertise in cognitive and behavioral assessment, such as pediatric psychologists, neuropsychologists, and developmental-behavioral pediatricians. Drawing from research in developmental science, support for children with genetic disorders should also consider the family system, and the broader contexts (such as the educational environment) in which children grow and develop. This multidisciplinary approach is critical to fostering optimal outcomes across the childhood lifespan for children with genetic syndromes.

RESOURCES

22q International/National Organizations

- The International 22q11.2 Foundation:
  https://22q.org/
- 22q Foundation Australia & New Zealand:
  https://www.22q.org.au/
- 22q11 Ireland:
  https://www.22q11ireland.org/
- Max Appeal (UK):
  https://www.maxappeal.org.uk/
- The 22q Family Foundation (USA):
  https://22qfamilyfoundation.org/

Down Syndrome

- National Down Syndrome Society, 8 East 41st Street, 8th Floor, New York, NY 10017, (800) 221-4602, https://www.ndss.org/
- LUMIND IDSC Foundation, 20 Mall Road, Suite 200, Burlington, MA 01803-4126, (781) 825-1300, https://www.lumindidsc.org

Fragile X

- The National Fragile X Foundation, 1861 International Drive Suite 200, McLean, VA 22102, (800) 688-8765, https://fragilex.org/
- The FRAXA Research Foundation, 10 Prince Place, Suite 203, Newburyport, MA 01950, (978) 462-1866, https://www.fraxa.org/

References

Abbeduto, L., McDuffie, A., Thurman, A. J., & Kover, S. T. (2016). Language development in individuals with intellectual and developmental disabilities: From phenotypes to treatments. *International Review of Research in Developmental Disabilities*, 50, 71–118. https://doi.org/10.1016/bs.irrdd.2016.05.006

Allen, E. G., Charen, K., Hipp, H. S., Shubeck, L., Amin, A., He, W., Hunter, J. E., & Sherman, S. L. (2020). Clustering of comorbid conditions among women who carry an FMR1 premutation. *Genetics in Medicine*, 22(4), 758–766. https://doi.org/10.1038/s41436-019-0733-5

Angkustsiri, K., Leckliter, I., Tartaglia, N., Beaton, E. A., Enriquez, J., & Simon, T. J. (2012). An examination of the relationship of anxiety and intelligence to adaptive functioning in children with chromosome 22q11.2 deletion syndrome. *Journal of Developmental and Behavioral Pediatrics*, 33(9), 713–720. https://doi.org/10.1097/DBP.0b013e318272dd24

Antshel, K. M., Aneja, A., Strunge, L., Peebles, J., Fremont, W. P., Stallone, K., Abdulsabur, N., Higgins, A. M., Shprintzen, R. J., & Kates, W. R. (2007). Autistic spectrum disorders in velo-cardio facial syndrome (22q11.2 deletion). *Journal of Autism and Developmental Disorders*, 37(9), 1776–1786. https://doi.org/10.1007/s10803-006-0308-6

Antshel, K. M., Shprintzen, R., Fremont, W., Higgins, A. M., Faraone, S. V., & Kates, W. R. (2010). Cognitive and psychiatric predictors to psychosis in velocardiofacial syndrome: A 3-year follow-up study. *Journal of the American Academy of Child & Adolescent Psychiatry*, 49(4), 333–344. https://doi.org/10.1097/00004583-201004000-00008

Bailey, D. B., Jr., Raspa, M., Olmsted, M., & Holiday, D. B. (2008). Co-occurring conditions associated with *FMR1* gene variations: Findings from a national parent survey. *American Journal of Medical Genetics. Part A, 146A*(16), 2060–2069. https://doi.org/10.1002/ajmg.a.32439

Bartesaghi, R., Haydar, T. F., Delabar, J. M., Dierssen, M., Martínez-Cué, C., & Bianchi, D. W. (2015). New perspectives for the rescue of cognitive disability in Down syndrome. *The Journal of Neuroscience, 35*(41), 13843–13852. https://doi.org/10.1523/JNEUROSCI.2775-15.2015

Bassett, A. S., McDonald-McGinn, D. M., Devriendt, K., Digilio, M. C., Goldenberg, P., Habel, A., Marino, B., Oskarsdottir, S., Philip, N., Sullivan, K., Swillen, A., Vorstman, J., & the International 22q11.2 Deletion Syndrome Consortium. (2011). Practical guidelines for managing patients with 22q11.2 deletion syndrome. *The Journal of Pediatrics, 159*(2), 332-9.E1. https://doi.org/10.1016/j.jpeds.2011.02.039

Beaton, E. A., & Simon, T. J. (2011). How might stress contribute to increased risk for schizophrenia in children with chromosome 22q11.2 deletion syndrome? *Journal of Neurodevelopmental Disorders, 3*(1), 68–75. https://doi.org/10.1007/s11689-010-9069-9

Biag, H. M. B., Potter, L. A., Wilkins, V., Afzal, S., Rosvall, A., Salcedo-Arellano, M. J., Rajaratnam, A., Manzano-Nunez, R., Schneider, A., Tassone, F., Rivera, S. M., & Hagerman, R. J. (2019). Metformin treatment in young children with fragile X syndrome. *Molecular Genetics & Genomic Medicine, 7*(11), e956. https://doi.org/10.1002/mgg3.956

Boot, E., Óskarsdóttir, S., Loo, J. C., Crowley, T. B., Orchanian-Cheff, A., Andrade, D. M., Arganbright, J. M., Castelein, R. M., Cserti-Gazdewich, C., de Reuver, S., Fiksinski, A. M., Klingberg, G., Lang, A. E., Mascarenhas, M. R., Moss, E. M., Nowakowska, B. A., Oechslin, E., Palmer, L., . . . Bassett, A. S. (2023). Updated clinical practice recommendations for managing adults with 22q11.2 deletion syndrome. *Genetics in Medicine, 25*(3), 100344. https://doi.org/10.1016/j.gim.2022.11.012

Botto, L. D., May, K., Fernhoff, P. M., Correa, A., Coleman, K., Rasmussen, S. A., Merritt, R. K., O'Leary, L. A., Wong, L. Y., Elixson, E. M., Mahle, W. T., & Campbell, R. M. (2003). A population-based study of the 22q11.2 deletion: Phenotype, incidence, and contribution to major birth defects in the population. *Pediatrics, 112*(1), 101–107. https://doi.org/10.1542/peds.112.1.101

Breslin, J., Spanò, G., Bootzin, R., Anand, P., Nadel, L., & Edgin, J. (2014). Obstructive sleep apnea syndrome and cognition in Down syndrome. *Developmental Medicine & Child Neurology, 56*(7), 657–664. https://doi.org/10.1111/dmcn.12376

Bull, M. J., & Committee on Genetics. (2011). Clinical report: Health supervision for children with Down syndrome. *Pediatrics, 128*(2), 393–406. https://doi.org/10.1542/peds.2011-1605

Capone, G. T., Chicoine, B., Bulova, P., Stephens, M., Hart, S., Crissman, B., Videlefsky, A., Myers, K., Roizen, N., Esbensen, A., Peterson, M., Santoro, S., Woodward, J., Martin, B., Smith, D., & the Down Syndrome Medical Interest Group DSMIG-USA Adult Health Care Workgroup. (2018). Co-occurring medical conditions in adults with Down syndrome: A systematic review toward the development of health care guidelines. *American Journal of Medical Genetics. Part A, 176*(1), 116–133. https://doi.org/10.1002/ajmg.a.38512

Chitwood, K., Greiss Hess, L., Diez-Juan, M., & Braden, M. (2020). Academic intervention and therapies for children with FXS. In R. Hagerman & P. Hagerman (Eds.), *Fragile X syndrome and premutation disorders: New developments and treatments* (pp. 111–136). Mac Keith Press.

Couzens, D., Haynes, M., & Cuskelly, M. (2012). Individual and environmental characteristics associated with cognitive development in Down syndrome: A longitudinal study. *Journal of Applied Research in Intellectual Disabilities, 25*(5), 396–413. https://doi.org/10.1111/j.1468-3148.2011.00673.x

D'Souza, H., & Karmiloff-Smith, A. (2017). Neurodevelopmental disorders. *WIREs Cognitive Science, 8*(1–2), e1398. https://doi.org/10.1002/wcs.1398

Daunhauer, L. A., & Fidler, D. J. (2011). The Down syndrome behavioral phenotype: Implications for practice and research in occupational therapy. *Occupational Therapy In Health Care, 25*(1), 7–25. https://doi.org/10.3109/07380577.2010.535601

De Smedt, B., Devriendt, K., Fryns, J. P., Vogels, A., Gewillig, M., & Swillen, A. (2007). Intellectual abilities in a large sample of children with Velo-Cardio-Facial Syndrome: An update. *Journal of Intellectual Disability Research, 51*(9), 666–670. https://doi.org/10.1111/j.1365-2788.2007.00955.x

Deng, P. Y., & Klyachko, V. A. (2021). Channelopathies in fragile X syndrome. *Nature Reviews Neuroscience, 22*(5), 275–289. https://doi.org/10.1038/s41583-021-00445-9

Dimachkie Nunnally, A., Nguyen, V., Anglo, C., Sterling, A., Edgin, J., Sherman, S., Berry-Kravis, E., Del Hoyo Soriano, L., Abbeduto, L., & Thurman, A. J. (2021). Symptoms of autism spectrum disorder in individuals with Down syndrome. *Brain Sciences, 11*(10), 1278. https://doi.org/10.3390/brainsci11101278

Dominick, K. C., Andrews, H. F., Kaufmann, W. E., Berry-Kravis, E., & Erickson, C. A. (2021). Psychotropic drug treatment patterns in persons with fragile X syndrome. *Journal of Child and Adolescent Psychopharmacology, 31*(10), 659–669. https://doi.org/10.1089/cap.2021.0042

Dori, N., Green, T., Weizman, A., & Gothelf, D. (2017). The effectiveness and safety of antipsychotic and antidepressant medications in individuals with 22q11.2 deletion syndrome. *Journal of Child and Adolescent Psychopharmacology, 27*(1), 83–90. https://doi.org/10.1089/cap.2014.0075

Dykens, E. M. (2007). Psychiatric and behavioral disorders in persons with Down syndrome. *Mental Retardation and Developmental Disabilities Research Reviews, 13*(3), 272–278. https://doi.org/10.1002/mrdd.20159

Edgin, J. O., Clark, C. A. C., Massand, E., & Karmiloff-Smith, A. (2015). Building an adaptive brain across development: Targets for neurorehabilitation must begin in infancy. *Frontiers in Behavioral Neuroscience, 9*(September), 232. https://doi.org/10.3389/fnbeh.2015.00232

Ekstein, S., Glick, B., Weill, M., Kay, B., & Berger, I. (2011). Down syndrome and attention-deficit/hyperactivity disorder (ADHD). *Journal of Child Neurology, 26*(10), 1290–1295. https://doi.org/10.1177/0883073811405201

Fernandez, F., & Reeves, R. H. (2015). Assessing cognitive improvement in people with Down syndrome: Important considerations for drug-efficacy trials. In K. Kantak & J. Wettstein (Eds.), *Cognitive enhancement. Handbook of experimental pharmacology* (Vol. 228, pp. 335–380). Springer. https://doi.org/10.1007/978-3-319-16522-6_12

Fidler, D. J., & Nadel, L. (2007). Education and children with Down syndrome: Neuroscience, development, and intervention. *Mental Retardation and Developmental Disabilities Research Reviews, 13*(3), 262–271. https://doi.org/10.1002/mrdd.20166

Fine, S. E., Weissman, A., Gerdes, M., Pinto-Martin, J., Zackai, E. H., McDonald-McGinn, D. M., & Emanuel, B. S. (2005). Autism spectrum disorders and symptoms in children with molecularly confirmed 22q11.2 deletion syndrome. *Journal of Autism and Developmental Disorders, 35*(4), 461–470. https://doi.org/10.1007/s10803-005-5036-9

Fung, W. L., Butcher, N. J., Costain, G., Andrade, D. M., Boot, E., Chow, E. W., Chung, B., Cytrynbaum, C., Faghfoury, H., Fishman, L., García-Miñaúr, S., George, S., Lang, A. E., Repetto, G., Shugar, A., Silversides, C., Swillen, A., van Amelsvoort, T., McDonald-McGinn, D. M., & Bassett, A. S. (2015). Practical guidelines for managing adults with 22q11.2 deletion syndrome. *Genetics in Medicine, 17*(8), 599–609. https://doi.org/10.1038/gim.2014.175

García-Cerro, S., Martínez, P., Vidal, V., Corrales, A., Flórez, J., Vidal, R., Rueda, N., Arbonés, M. L., & Martínez-Cué, C. (2014). Overexpression of Dyrk1A is implicated in several cognitive, electrophysiological and neuromorphological alterations found in a mouse model of Down syndrome. *PLOS ONE, 9*(9), e106572. https://doi.org/10.1371/journal.pone.0106572

Gothelf, D., Gruber, R., Presburger, G., Dotan, I., Brand-Gothelf, A., Burg, M., Inbar, D., Steinberg, T., Frisch, A., Apter, A., & Weizman, A. (2003). Methylphenidate treatment for attention-deficit/hyperactivity disorder in children and adolescents with velocardiofacial syndrome: An open-label study. *The Journal of Clinical Psychiatry, 64*(10), 1163–1169. https://doi.org/10.4088/JCP.v64n1004

Grati, F. R., Malvestiti, F., Grimi, B., Liuti, R., Agrati, C., Gaetani, E., Milani, S., Martinoni, L., Zanatta, V., Gallazzi, G., Maggi, F., & Simoni, G. (2015). Increased risk after noninvasive prenatal screening on cell-free DNA circulating in maternal blood: Does a new indication for invasive prenatal diagnosis require new criteria for confirmatory cytogenetic analysis? *Prenatal Diagnosis, 35*(3), 308–309. https://doi.org/10.1002/pd.4483

Green, T., Steingart, L., Frisch, A., Zarchi, O., Weizman, A., & Gothelf, D. (2012). The feasibility and safety of S-adenosyl-L-methionine (SAMe) for the treatment of neuropsychiatric symptoms in 22q11.2 deletion syndrome: A double-blind placebo-controlled trial. *Journal of Neural Transmission, 119*(11), 1417–1423. https://doi.org/10.1007/s00702-012-0831-x

Greiss Hess, L., Fitzpatrick, S. E., Nguyen, D. V., Chen, Y., Gaul, K. N., Schneider, A., Lemons Chitwood, K., Eldeeb, M. A., Polussa, J., Hessl, D., Rivera, S., & Hagerman, R. J. (2016). A randomized, double-blind, placebo-controlled trial of low-dose sertraline in young children with fragile X syndrome. *Journal of Developmental and Behavioral Pediatrics, 37*(8), 619–628. https://doi.org/10.1097/DBP.0000000000000334

Hagerman, R., Protic, D., & Berry-Kravis, E. (2020). Medical, psychopharmacological, and targeted treatment for FXS. In R. Hagerman & P. Hagerman (Eds.), *Fragile X syndrome and premutation disorders: New developments and treatments* (pp. 41–58). Mac Keith Press.

Hagerman, R. J., & Hagerman, P. (2016). Fragile X-associated tremor/ataxia syndrome—Features, mechanisms and management. *Nature Reviews: Neurology, 12*(7), 403–412. https://doi.org/10.1038/nrneurol.2016.82

Hagerman, R. J., Protic, D., Rajaratnam, A., Salcedo-Arellano, M. J., Aydin, E. Y., & Schneider, A. (2018). Fragile X-associated neuropsychiatric disorders (FXAND). *Frontiers in Psychiatry*, 9, 564. https://doi.org/10.3389/fpsyt.2018.00564

Herault, Y., Delabar, J. M., Fisher, E. M. C., Tybulewicz, V. L. J., Yu, E., & Brault, V. (2017). Rodent models in Down syndrome research: Impact and future opportunities. *Disease Models & Mechanisms*, 10(10), 1165–1186. https://doi.org/10.1242/dmm.029728

Heussler, H., Cohen, J., Silove, N., Tich, N., Bonn-Miller, M. O., Du, W., O'Neill, C., & Sebree, T. (2019). A phase 1/2, open-label assessment of the safety, tolerability, and efficacy of transdermal cannabidiol (ZYN002) for the treatment of pediatric fragile X syndrome. *Journal of Neurodevelopmental Disorders*, 11(1), 16. https://doi.org/10.1186/s11689-019-9277-x

Hunter, J., Wheeler, A., Allen, E., Wald, K., Rajkovic, A., Hagerman, R., & Sherman, S. (2020). Women's issues in Fragile X spectrum disorders. In R. Hagerman & P. Hagerman (Eds.), *Fragile X Syndrome and premutation disorders: New developments and treatments* (pp. 75–82). Mac Keith Press.

Indah Winarni, T., Chonchaiya, W., Adams, E., Au, J., Mu, Y., Rivera, S. M., Nguyen, D. V., & Hagerman, R. J. (2012). Sertraline may improve language developmental trajectory in young children with fragile X syndrome: A retrospective chart review. *Autism Research and Treatment*, 2012, 104317. https://doi.org/10.1155/2012/104317

Iossifov, I., Ronemus, M., Levy, D., Wang, Z., Hakker, I., Rosenbaum, J., Yamrom, B., Lee, Y. H., Narzisi, G., Leotta, A., Kendall, J., Grabowska, E., Ma, B., Marks, S., Rodgers, L., Stepansky, A., Troge, J., Andrews, P., Bekritsky, M., . . . Wigler, M. (2012). De novo gene disruptions in children on the autistic spectrum. *Neuron*, 74(2), 285–299. https://doi.org/10.1016/j.neuron.2012.04.009

Jhawar, N., Brown, M. J., Cutler-Landsman, D., Kates, W. R., Angkustsiri, K., & Antshel, K. M. (2021). Longitudinal psychiatric and developmental outcomes in 22q11.2 deletion syndrome: A systematic review. *Journal of Developmental and Behavioral Pediatrics*, 42(5), 415–427. https://doi.org/10.1097/DBP.0000000000000927

Jolin, E. M., Weller, R. A., & Weller, E. B. (2012). Occurrence of affective disorders compared to other psychiatric disorders in children and adolescents with 22q11.2 deletion syndrome. *Journal of Affective Disorders*, 136(3), 222–228. https://doi.org/10.1016/j.jad.2010.11.025

Jyonouchi, S., McDonald-McGinn, D. M., Bale, S., Zackai, E. H., & Sullivan, K. E. (2009). CHARGE (coloboma, heart defect, atresia choanae, retarded growth and development, genital hypoplasia, ear anomalies/deafness) syndrome and chromosome 22q11.2 deletion syndrome: A comparison of immunologic and nonimmunologic phenotypic features. *Pediatrics*, 123(5), e871–e877. https://doi.org/10.1542/peds.2008-3400

Karayiorgou, M., Simon, T. J., & Gogos, J. A. (2010). 22q11.2 microdeletions: Linking DNA structural variation to brain dysfunction and schizophrenia. *Nature Reviews Neuroscience*, 11(6), 402–416. https://doi.org/10.1038/nrn2841

Karmiloff-Smith, A., Al-Janabi, T., D'Souza, H., Groet, J., Massand, E., Mok, K., Startin, C., Fisher, E., Hardy, J., Nizetic, D., Tybulewicz, V., & Strydom, A. (2016). The importance of understanding individual differences in Down syndrome. *F1000 Research*, 5, F1000 Faculty Rev-1389. https://doi.org/10.12688/f1000research.7506.1

Kaufmann, W. E., Kidd, S. A., Andrews, H. F., Budimirovic, D. B., Esler, A., Haas-Givler, B., Stackhouse, T., Riley, C., Peacock, G., Sherman, S. L., Brown, W. T., & Berry-Kravis, E. (2017). Autism spectrum disorder in fragile X syndrome: Co-occurring conditions and current treatment. *Pediatrics*, 139(Suppl. 3), S194–S206. https://doi.org/10.1542/peds.2016-1159F

Kern, R. S., Glynn, S. M., Horan, W. P., & Marder, S. R. (2009). Psychosocial treatments to promote functional recovery in schizophrenia. *Schizophrenia Bulletin*, 35(2), 347–361. https://doi.org/10.1093/schbul/sbn177

Kim, K. M., Meng, Q., Perez de Acha, O., Mustapic, M., Cheng, A., Eren, E., Kundu, G., Piao, Y., Munk, R., Wood, W. H., III, De, S., Noh, J. H., Delannoy, M., Cheng, L., Abdelmohsen, K., Kapogiannis, D., & Gorospe, M. (2020). Mitochondrial RNA in Alzheimer's disease circulating extracellular vesicles. *Frontiers in Cell and Developmental Biology*, 8, 581882. https://doi.org/10.3389/fcell.2020.581882

Kobrynski, L. J., & Sullivan, K. E. (2007). Velocardiofacial syndrome, DiGeorge syndrome: The chromosome 22q11.2 deletion syndromes. *The Lancet*, 370(9596), 1443–1452. https://doi.org/10.1016/S0140-6736(07)61601-8

Leigh, M. J., Nguyen, D. V., Mu, Y., Winarni, T. I., Schneider, A., Chechi, T., Polussa, J., Doucet, P., Tassone, F., Rivera, S. M., Hessl, D., & Hagerman, R. J. (2013). A randomized double-blind, placebo-controlled trial of minocycline in children and adolescents with fragile X syndrome. *Journal of Developmental and Behavioral Pediatrics*, 34(3), 147–155. https://doi.org/10.1097/DBP.0b013e318287cd17

Loesch, D. Z., Bui, Q. M., Dissanayake, C., Clifford, S., Gould, E., Bulhak-Paterson, D., Tassone, F., Taylor, A. K., Hessl, D., Hagerman, R., & Huggins, R. M. (2007). Molecular and cognitive predictors of the continuum of autistic behaviours in fragile X. *Neuroscience and Biobehavioral Reviews, 31*(3), 315–326. https://doi.org/10.1016/j.neubiorev.2006.09.007

McDonald-McGinn, D. M., Hain, H. S., Emanuel, B. S., & Zackai, E. H. (1999). 22q11.2 deletion syndrome. In M. P. Adam, J. Feldman, G. M. Mirzaa, R. A. Pagon, S. E. Wallace, L. J. H. Bean, K. W. Gripp, & A. Amemiya (Eds.), *GeneReviews®* [Internet]. University of Washington. https://www.ncbi.nlm.nih.gov/books/NBK1523/

Mégarbané, A., Ravel, A., Mircher, C., Sturtz, F., Grattau, Y., Rethoré, M. O., Delabar, J. M., & Mobley, W. C. (2009). The 50th anniversary of the discovery of trisomy 21: The past, present, and future of research and treatment of Down syndrome. *Genetics in Medicine, 11*(9), 611–616. https://doi.org/10.1097/GIM.0b013e3181b2e34c

Miclea, D., Peca, L., Cuzmici, Z., & Pop, I. V. (2015). Genetic testing in patients with global developmental delay/intellectual disabilities. A review. *Clujul Medical, 88*(3), 288–292. https://doi.org/10.15386/cjmed-461

Moeschler, J. B., Shevell, M., & the Committee on Genetics. (2014). Comprehensive evaluation of the child with intellectual disability or global developmental delays. *Pediatrics, 134*(3), e903–e918. https://doi.org/10.1542/peds.2014-1839

Mosheva, M., Korotkin, L., Gur, R. E., Weizman, A., & Gothelf, D. (2020). Effectiveness and side effects of psychopharmacotherapy in individuals with 22q11.2 deletion syndrome with comorbid psychiatric disorders: A systematic review. *European Child & Adolescent Psychiatry, 29*(8), 1035–1048. https://doi.org/10.1007/s00787-019-01326-4

Niarchou, M., Martin, J., Thapar, A., Owen, M. J., & van den Bree, M. B. (2015). The clinical presentation of attention deficit-hyperactivity disorder (ADHD) in children with 22q11.2 deletion syndrome. *American Journal of Medical Genetics Part B: Neuropsychiatric Genetics, 168*(8), 730–738. https://doi.org/10.1002/ajmg.b.32378

Olsen, C. L., Cross, P. K., Gensburg, L. J., & Hughes, J. P. (1996). The effects of prenatal diagnosis, population ageing, and changing fertility rates on the live birth prevalence of Down syndrome in New York State, 1983–1992. *Prenatal Diagnosis, 16*(11), 991–1002. https://doi.org/10.1002/(SICI)1097-0223(199611)16:11<991::AID-PD977>3.0.CO;2-5

Olson, L. E., Roper, R. J., Sengstaken, C. L., Peterson, E. A., Aquino, V., Galdzicki, Z., Siarey, R., Pletnikov, M., Moran, T. H., & Reeves, R. H. (2007). Trisomy for the Down syndrome 'critical region' is necessary but not sufficient for brain phenotypes of trisomic mice. *Human Molecular Genetics, 16*(7), 774–782. https://doi.org/10.1093/hmg/ddm022

Óskarsdóttir, S., Boot, E., Crowley, T. B., Loo, J. C., Arganbright, J. M., Armando, M., Baylis, A. L., Breetvelt, E. J., Castelein, R. M., Chadehumbem, M., Cielo, C. M., de Reuver, S., Eliez, S., Fiksinski, A. M., Forbes, B. J., Gallagher, E., Hopkins, S. E., Jackson, O. A., . . . McDonald-McGinn, D. M. (2023). Updated clinical practice recommendations for managing children with 22q11.2 deletion syndrome. *Genetics in Medicine, 25*(3), 100338. https://doi.org/10.1016/j.gim.2022.11.006

Óskarsdóttir, S., Persson, C., Eriksson, B. O., & Fasth, A. (2005). Presenting phenotype in 100 children with the 22q11 deletion syndrome. *European Journal of Pediatrics, 164*(3), 146–153. https://doi.org/10.1007/s00431-004-1577-8

Ousley, O., Evans, A. N., Fernandez-Carriba, S., Smearman, E. L., Rockers, K., Morrier, M. J., Evans, D. W., Coleman, K., & Cubells, J. (2017). Examining the overlap between autism spectrum disorder and 22q11.2 deletion syndrome. *International Journal of Molecular Sciences, 18*(5), 1071. https://doi.org/10.3390/ijms18051071

Protic, D., Aydin, E. Y., Tassone, F., Tan, M. M., Hagerman, R. J., & Schneider, A. (2019). Cognitive and behavioral improvement in adults with fragile X syndrome treated with metformin-two cases. *Molecular Genetics & Genomic Medicine, 7*(7), e00745. https://doi.org/10.1002/mgg3.745

Protic, D., Kaluzhny, P., Tassone, F., & Hagerman, R. (2019). Prepubertal metformin treatment in fragile X syndrome alleviated macroorchidism: A case study. *Advances in Clinical and Translational Research, 2*, 100021. https://emrespublisher.com/open-access-pdf/prepubertal-metformin-treatment-in-fragile-x-syndrome-alleviated-macroorchidism-a-case-study-100021.pdf

Richards, C., Jones, C., Groves, L., Moss, J., & Oliver, C. (2015). Prevalence of autism spectrum disorder phenomenology in genetic disorders: A systematic review and meta-analysis. *The Lancet Psychiatry, 2*(10), 909–916. https://doi.org/10.1016/S2215-0366(15)00376-4

Riley, K., Schneider, A., Hessl, D., & Braden, M. (2020). Behavioral interventions to improve tantrums, aggression, anxiety and mood instability. In R. Hagerman & P. Hagerman (Eds.), *Fragile X syndrome and premutation disorders: New developments and treatments* (pp. 59–74). Mac Keith Press.

Roizen, N. J. (1997). Down syndrome. In M. L. Batshaw (Ed.), *Children with disabilities* (4th ed.). Paul H. Brooks.

Romero, R., Erez, O., Hüttemann, M., Maymon, E., Panaitescu, B., Conde-Agudelo, A., Pacora, P., Yoon, B. H., & Grossman, L. I. (2017). Metformin, the aspirin of the 21st century: Its role in gestational diabetes mellitus, prevention of preeclampsia and cancer, and the promotion of longevity. *American Journal of Obstetrics and Gynecology, 217*(3), 282–302. https://doi.org/10.1016/j.ajog.2017.06.003

Saldarriaga, W., Forero-Forero, J. V., González-Teshima, L. Y., Fandiño-Losada, A., Isaza, C., Tovar-Cuevas, J. R., Silva, M., Choudhary, N. S., Tang, H. T., Aguilar-Gaxiola, S., Hagerman, R. J., & Tassone, F. (2018). Genetic cluster of fragile X syndrome in a Colombian district. *Journal of Human Genetics, 63*(4), 509–516. https://doi.org/10.1038/s10038-017-0407-6

Schneider, M., Debbané, M., Bassett, A. S., Chow, E. W., Fung, W. L., van den Bree, M., Owen, M., Murphy, K. C., Niarchou, M., Kates, W. R., Antshel, K. M., Fremont, W., McDonald-McGinn, D. M., Gur, R. E., Zackai, E. H., Vorstman, J., Duijff, S. N., Klaassen, P. W., Swillen, A., . . . Eliez, S., for the International Consortium on Brain and Behavior in 22q11.2 Deletion Syndrome. (2014). Psychiatric disorders from childhood to adulthood in 22q11.2 deletion syndrome: Results from the International Consortium on Brain and Behavior in 22q11.2 Deletion Syndrome. *The American Journal of Psychiatry, 171*(6), 627–639. https://doi.org/10.1176/appi.ajp.2013.13070864

Sherman, S. L., Allen, E. G., Bean, L. H., & Freeman, S. B. (2007). Epidemiology of Down syndrome. *Mental Retardation and Developmental Disabilities Research Reviews, 13*(3), 221–227. https://doi.org/10.1002/mrdd.20157

Simon, T. J. (2008). A new account of the neurocognitive foundations of impairments in space, time and number processing in children with chromosome 22q11.2 deletion syndrome. *Developmental Disabilities Research Reviews, 14*(1), 52–58. https://doi.org/10.1002/ddrr.8

Simon, T. J., Bish, J. P., Bearden, C. E., Ding, L., Ferrante, S., Nguyen, V., Gee, J. C., McDonald-McGinn, D. M., Zackai, E. H., & Emanuel, B. S. (2005). A multilevel analysis of cognitive dysfunction and psychopathology associated with chromosome 22q11.2 deletion syndrome in children. *Development and Psychopathology, 17*(3), 753–784. https://doi.org/10.1017/S0954579405050364

Spence, S. H., Donovan, C. L., March, S., Gamble, A., Anderson, R. E., Prosser, S., & Kenardy, J. (2011). A randomized controlled trial of online versus clinic-based CBT for adolescent anxiety. *Journal of Consulting and Clinical Psychology, 79*(5), 629–642. https://doi.org/10.1037/a0024512

Stagni, F., Giacomini, A., Guidi, S., Ciani, E., & Bartesaghi, R. (2015). Timing of therapies for Down syndrome: The sooner, the better. *Frontiers in Behavioral Neuroscience, 9*, 265–265. https://doi.org/10.3389/fnbeh.2015.00265

Sullivan, K. E. (2019). Immune biomarkers of autoimmunity in chromosome 22q11.2 deletion syndrome. *The Journal of Allergy and Clinical Immunology: In Practice, 7*(7), 2377–2378. https://doi.org/10.1016/j.jaip.2019.04.051

Sullivan, K. E., McDonald-McGinn, D., Driscoll, D. A., Emanuel, B. S., Zackai, E. H., & Jawad, A. F. (1999). Longitudinal analysis of lymphocyte function and numbers in the first year of life in chromosome 22q11.2 deletion syndrome (DiGeorge syndrome/velocardiofacial syndrome). *Clinical and Diagnostic Laboratory Immunology, 6*(6), 906–911. https://doi.org/10.1128/CDLI.6.6.906-911.1999

Tang, S. X., Yi, J. J., Calkins, M. E., Whinna, D. A., Kohler, C. G., Souders, M. C., McDonald-McGinn, D. M., Zackai, E. H., Emanuel, B. S., Gur, R. C., & Gur, R. E. (2014). Psychiatric disorders in 22q11.2 deletion syndrome are prevalent but undertreated. *Psychological Medicine, 44*(6), 1267–1277. https://doi.org/10.1017/S0033291713001669

Tassé, M. J., Navas Macho, P., Havercamp, S. M., Benson, B. A., Allain, D. C., Manickam, K., & Davis, S. (2016). Psychiatric conditions prevalent among adults with Down syndrome. *Journal of Policy and Practice in Intellectual Disabilities, 13*(2), 173–180. https://doi.org/10.1111/jppi.12156

Tassone, F., Hagerman, R. J., Iklé, D. N., Dyer, P. N., Lampe, M., Willemsen, R., Oostra, B. A., & Taylor, A. K. (1999). FMRP expression as a potential prognostic indicator in fragile X syndrome. *American Journal of Medical Genetics, 84*(3), 250–261. https://www.ncbi.nlm.nih.gov/pubmed/10331602

Thurman, A. J., & del Hoyo Soriano, L. (2021). Down syndrome. In L. Cummings (Ed.), *Handbook of pragmatic language disorders*. Springer. https://doi.org/10.1007/978-3-030-74985-9_5

Thurman, A. J., McDuffie, A., Hagerman, R., & Abbeduto, L. (2014). Psychiatric symptoms in boys with fragile X syndrome: A comparison with nonsyndromic autism spectrum disorder. *Research in Developmental Disabilities, 35*(5), 1072–1086. https://doi.org/10.1016/j.ridd.2014.01.032

Turner, S., Alborz, A., & Gayle, V. (2008). Predictors of academic attainments of young people with

Down's syndrome. *Journal of Intellectual Disability Research, 52*(5), 380–392. https://doi.org/10.1111/j.1365-2788.2007.01038.x

Weinzimer, S. A., McDonald-McGinn, D. M., Driscoll, D. A., Emanuel, B. S., Zackai, E. H., & Moshang, T., Jr. (1998). Growth hormone deficiency in patients with 22q11.2 deletion: Expanding the phenotype. *Pediatrics, 101*(5), 929–932. https://doi.org/10.1542/peds.101.5.929

Wheeler, A. C., Raspa, M., Bishop, E., & Bailey, D. B., Jr. (2016). Aggression in fragile X syndrome. *Journal of Intellectual Disability Research, 60*(2), 113–125. https://doi.org/10.1111/jir.12238

Wood, J. J., Drahota, A., Sze, K., Har, K., Chiu, A., & Langer, D. A. (2009). Cognitive behavioral therapy for anxiety in children with autism spectrum disorders: A randomized, controlled trial. *Journal of Child Psychology and Psychiatry, 50*(3), 224–234. https://doi.org/10.1111/j.1469-7610.2008.01948.x

Yoo, K., Burris, J., Gaul, K., Hagerman, R., & Rivera, S. (2017). Low-dose sertraline improves receptive language in children with fragile X syndrome when eye tracking methodology is used to measure treatment outcome. *Journal of Psychology & Clinical Psychiatry, 7*(6), 00465. https://doi.org/10.15406/jpcpy.2017.07.00465

CHAPTER 8

CONGENITAL MEDICAL CONDITIONS IN CHILDHOOD AND ADOLESCENCE, STIGMA, AND PSYCHOSOCIAL ADJUSTMENT

Canice E. Crerand and Jennifer Hansen-Moore

Birth defects are estimated to affect 1 in every 33 children born in the United States each year (Centers for Disease Control and Prevention, 2008; Mai et al., 2019). These congenital differences in structural and/or physical functioning may be diagnosed at or before birth or when growth and/or development do not occur as expected. Regardless of when they are diagnosed, these conditions can have lifelong physical and psychosocial impacts for affected children and their families, including risks for stigmatization (Hansen-Moore et al., 2021). Children born with congenital differences typically require medical care and monitoring by a range of specialists often from infancy through adulthood.

This chapter will center on cleft lip and/or palate (CL/P), an example of a commonly occurring congenital condition associated with visible appearance and/or distinct speech differences, and differences of sex development (DSD), a group of less commonly occurring conditions involving genital and/or reproductive differences, to illustrate the range of effects that congenital conditions can have on affected children and their families across the lifespan. CL/P is the second most common birth defect in the United States (Mai et al., 2019) and results from the incomplete closure of the lip and/or roof of the mouth during early prenatal development. CL/P is associated with visible facial appearance and/or speech differences that may have detrimental impacts on psychosocial functioning and stigmatization. In contrast, DSD are relatively rare conditions that are associated with atypical and/or ambiguous genitalia or discordances between genetic sex (male or female sex chromosomes) and physical characteristics (e.g., masculinized genitalia in a child with female sex chromosomes). While often readily concealable from others in most settings (owing to the areas of the body that are affected), DSD are nonetheless associated with a myriad of psychosocial concerns including risks for real or feared stigmatization for both parents and affected individuals from diagnosis through adulthood. Children with DSD and CL/P may require support and monitoring from pediatric psychologists, neuropsychologists, and developmental-behavioral pediatricians to achieve optimal psychosocial outcomes. Thus, it is important for these specialists to understand factors that are associated with healthy and poor adjustment in these populations in order to provide appropriate screening and interventions.

This chapter reviews psychosocial adjustment and stigma related to CL/P and DSD, two congenital conditions with disparate impacts on appearance

https://doi.org/10.1037/0000414-008
APA Handbook of Pediatric Psychology, Developmental-Behavioral Pediatrics, and Developmental Science: Vol. 2. Pediatric Psychology and Developmental-Behavioral Pediatrics: Clinical Applications of Developmental Science, P. E. Shah and M. H. Bornstein (Editors-in-Chief)
Copyright © 2025 by the American Psychological Association. All rights reserved.

and functioning that confer risks for stigmatization across the lifespan. Drawing on contemporary theoretical frameworks of risk and resilience informed by developmental science, research on psychosocial adjustment is reviewed for both conditions, with an emphasis on how enacted and felt stigma affect children and their families across developmental stages. For example, during infancy and toddlerhood, the psychosocial effects of the child's condition are often felt most acutely by parents or caregivers, with increasing impacts observed for affected children as they develop and navigate normative transitions associated with childhood, adolescence, and adulthood. The chapter concludes with clinical implications, including interdisciplinary care needs, the role of pediatric psychologists and developmental-behavioral pediatricians in the clinical management of these disorders, and directions for future research.

OVERVIEW OF CLEFT LIP AND/OR PALATE AND DIFFERENCES OF SEX DEVELOPMENT

Cleft Lip and/or Palate

Cleft palate, with or without cleft lip, is among the most common of all congenital conditions, occurring in approximately 1 in every 800 live births in the United States (Mai et al., 2019). CL/P is associated with speech, hearing, and dental problems, and there is often some degree of residual appearance differences even after corrective surgeries. CL/P can occur either in isolation or as part of a syndrome, and both genetic and environmental factors are thought to play a role in their etiology (Losee & Kirschner, 2016). Cleft conditions can cause functional problems such as difficulties with feeding, speech, and hearing as well as dental problems (e.g., missing or misaligned teeth). Facial appearance can also be affected due to bone and soft tissue deficiencies and surgical scarring. The physical and aesthetic problems caused by CL/P can contribute to experiences of stigma and significantly affect the psychosocial functioning and quality of life for individuals with these conditions (Crerand et al., 2017; Stock & Feragen, 2016). While cleft conditions are sometimes diagnosed prenatally during routine ultrasound, diagnosis at birth remains a common experience, particularly for children with cleft palate only (Losee & Kirschner, 2016).

Differences of Sex Development

DSD is an umbrella term describing a heterogeneous group of congenital conditions that impact the course of sex determination and differentiation (Cools et al., 2018; Hughes et al., 2006). Currently, there is much controversy around terminology across health care providers and importantly, among individuals with lived experiences of DSDs (e.g., Bennecke et al., 2021; Johnson et al., 2017). While "DSD" is often favored by health care providers, individuals may prefer to use the name of their specific condition, such as congenital adrenal hyperplasia (CAH) or Turner syndrome (Lin-Su et al., 2015) or other terms like "intersex" or "variations in sex traits."

DSD are estimated to affect 1 in 4,500 births (Hughes et al., 2006) and can have a range of complex medical, psychological, and social impacts (Sandberg et al., 2012; Wisniewski et al., 2019). For example, DSD may be associated with physical differences including atypical and/or ambiguous genitalia, or sex-discordant features (e.g., sex chromosomes that do not match the gender in which the person is reared, gynecomastia, excess facial and body hair in females). In addition, individuals with DSDs experience challenges throughout their lifespan including (early in life) parents' complex proxy decision making regarding the gender of rearing and whether or when to pursue genital and/or gonadal surgery; and (later in life) infertility or impaired fertility; and sexual dysfunction (Crerand et al., 2021; Lee et al., 2016). DSD are often diagnosed at birth when genital atypicality and/or ambiguity are observed, although prenatal diagnosis is becoming more frequent (Lee et al., 2016). In other cases, DSD may not be detected until puberty does not occur as expected.

Commonalities in CL/P and DSD

Both CL/P and DSD typically involve surgical management and coordinated medical care during childhood and adolescence to improve both the function of the affected structures and to make appearance more typical (American Cleft Palate Craniofacial Association, 2018; Hughes et al., 2006). Children with CL/P are typically followed by teams of specialists including plastic surgeons, speech-language pathologists, and orthodontists, and care teams may involve other specialists including geneticists, otolaryngologists, pediatric psychologists, and potentially developmental-behavioral pediatricians beginning at birth and continuing through early adulthood (American Cleft Palate Craniofacial Association, 2018). Initial reconstructive surgery is typically performed in infancy, with secondary surgical procedures (e.g., scar revisions, rhinoplasty, orthognathic surgery) continuing through young adulthood. Families often experience significant financial and other burdens as a consequence of their child's cleft-related care (Crerand et al., 2017; Losee & Kirschner, 2016).

For children with DSD, interdisciplinary care has only recently become the standard of care. Historically, DSD management was paternalistic (Siminoff & Sandberg, 2015), meaning that decisions about care, and particularly sex and gender assignment, were often made unilaterally by physicians with little to no input from the family or patient. In accordance with the optimal gender policy, which purported that in the case of ambiguous or atypical genitalia, surgery should be performed to align and/or normalize genital appearance with sex and gender assignment (e.g., Money et al., 1955), treatment decisions were typically made by surgeons. Surgery was typically recommended and performed during infancy in order to protect the child and family from perceived stigma and psychological distress (Nordenström & Thyen, 2014; Roen & Pasterski, 2014). Although secrecy was not an explicit tenet of the optimal gender policy (Money, 1994), information about DSD diagnoses and related medical treatment was often withheld from affected individuals by physicians. Unfortunately, this secretive approach engendered shame, stigma, and distrust in health care providers and had other negative physical and psychosocial impacts for individuals treated during this era (Crerand et al., 2021).

Advances in genetics, diagnostics, and treatment approaches, combined with continued reports of dissatisfaction with care practices from advocacy groups, patients, and families, led to a meeting of patients and health care professionals and the subsequent creation of the 2006 Consensus Statement (Hughes et al., 2006). Care practices have changed significantly including recommendations for early, ongoing information sharing with affected individuals (Roen & Pasterski, 2014) to reduce the likelihood of shame and stigma associated with DSD diagnoses and detrimental effects on psychosocial adjustment (Crerand et al., 2021).

STIGMA: DEFINITIONS AND IMPLICATIONS FOR CHILDREN WITH CONGENITAL MEDICAL CONDITIONS

Stigma is "an attribute that is deeply discrediting," and that diminishes a person in the eyes of others "from a whole and usual person to a tainted, discounted one" (Goffman, 1963, p. 3). While stigma can refer to the presence of a physical appearance difference (e.g., obesity, short stature), it is also associated with any undesirable characteristics or statuses related to health (e.g., having a mental illness, HIV/AIDS); behaviors (e.g., alcohol and drug use); sexual orientation and gender identity; race or ethnicity; and many others characteristics or circumstances (e.g., history of incarceration or poverty; Pescosolido & Martin, 2015). In the broader stigma literature, there is some debate about terminology as it relates to stigma, with some expressed preference for framing stigma as discrimination due to any undesirable or socially discrediting attribute (see Pescosolido & Martin, 2015 for a review). Further, there is growing recognition of intersectionality (Carroll, 2020), that is, having multiple attributes or identities that may be stigmatizing (e.g., identifying as a nonbinary Hispanic youth with DSD).

In line with Goffman (1963), stigma can be categorized into two types: enacted stigma and felt stigma. *Enacted stigma* refers to instances of negative or unfair treatment such as discrimination (e.g., not hiring a person with a physical difference) and/or other types of unwanted attention or treatment (e.g., teasing/bullying) because of the devalued characteristic (Scambler, 2009). *Felt stigma* refers to fear of enacted stigma or anticipation of social rejection if the difference is exposed (Quinn & Earnshaw, 2013). Identification of experiences of enacted or felt stigma is important because stigma is often cited as a contributing risk factor to poor psychosocial outcomes for children born with CL/P and DSD (Crerand et al., 2021).

CL/P and DSD involve physical appearance differences and are associated with increased risk for social stigmatization, including teasing or bullying, and other forms of enacted stigma such as discriminatory behaviors. For children with CL/P or DSD, experiences of stigma can have a profound impact on their physical and psychosocial functioning, and quality of life (de Vries et al., 2019; Stock & Feragen, 2016). In children with CL/P, visible facial appearance differences due to sequelae of the cleft and/or reconstructive surgery are commonly observed along with risks for speech articulation and intelligibility problems. Collectively, these observable and/or audible differences can heighten risks for social stigmatization. DSD often impact genital appearance, with implications for gender dysphoria, sexual function, and fertility issues that are often invisible or concealable, but nonetheless carry risks for stigma and psychosocial distress. In the broader pediatric literature, stigmatization such as bullying is a known risk factor for mental health concerns, including suicidality (Arseneault, 2017; Wilson et al., 2023). To date, few studies have looked at stigma experiences and suicidality in youth with CL/P or DSD specifically, nor have studies examined whether individuals with CL/P or DSD who are bullied during childhood become bullies themselves. Future research is indicated to better understand how bullying and other stigmatizing experiences affect individuals over time.

Stigma Development and Related Factors

In the context of congenital conditions that affect physical appearance, several factors are thought to contribute to the development of stigma and related discriminatory behaviors. Physical appearance is known to have a significant impact on a person's life across a range of settings, from school to the workplace, with evidence of preferential treatment for individuals who are attractive (Hartung et al., 2019; Langlois et al., 2000). This association between attractiveness and preferential treatment has been coined the "what is beautiful is good" stereotype (Dion et al., 1972). In other words, attractive people are often viewed as being more trustworthy, smart, socially adept, and well-adjusted, along with possessing other positive personality characteristics. Many of these associations are reinforced in the mass media (e.g., advertisements, movies) where attractive individuals are portrayed positively while "evil" or "bad" characters often have physical features that are anomalous and/or "ugly" (Hartung et al., 2019).

There is growing evidence that judgments about attractiveness are made quickly and potentially outside of an individual's conscious awareness, consistent with what is known as *implicit bias*, that is, subconscious attitudes that may affect behavior (Hartung et al., 2019). Biases toward attractiveness may have their origins in evolution, including neurological responses that are preferential to facial symmetry and/or "averageness," which signify overall and reproductive health to optimize the likelihood of producing healthy offspring (Yarosh, 2019). Neuroimaging studies document that viewing attractive faces is associated with activation of brain regions associated with reward, empathy, and social cognition (Hartung et al., 2019).

While human beings appear to be hard-wired from a neurological standpoint to prefer attractive faces, there is growing evidence that there is neurological underpinning for stigmatization or a "disfigured is bad" stereotype. Specifically, Hartung and colleagues (2019) found evidence for deactivation of the anterior cingulate cortex when subjects were presented with photos of individuals with disfigurements, suggesting suppression of empathy and social cognition. They also observed greater neural responses to the occipitotemporal cortex, which correlates to attentional rather than reward properties of the face, that may relate to stigmatization behaviors including staring.

Although similar studies about the neurological underpinnings of DSD-related stigma have yet to be conducted, stigma can be associated with any difference or devalued characteristic. Even if a difference is concealable, the affected individual may fear inadvertent disclosure and related impacts on social acceptance and integration, particularly in cultures or contexts in which social norms are paramount with limited tolerance for differences in gender identity, sexual functioning, or reproduction (Ediati et al., 2016). Thus, stigma is a highly salient construct for understanding risk and resiliency in persons with DSD. In the following sections, we highlight ways in which stigma affects domains of psychosocial functioning for both individuals with CL/P or DSD and their families across the lifespan.

FRAMEWORKS FOR UNDERSTANDING RISK AND RESILIENCE IN CHILDREN WITH CONGENITAL CONDITIONS

Theoretical frameworks have been developed to understand psychosocial functioning and adjustment in children with congenital medical disorders, including CL/P and DSD. Wallander and Varni's (1992) seminal model posits that there are both risk and resistance (or resilience) factors that affect psychosocial outcomes. This model identifies the presence of a chronic medical condition as a stressor in and of itself to both the affected child and their caregivers, which requires ongoing adaptation for the child and family to function in their daily lives across the lifespan. *Risk factors* are variables that make children more vulnerable to poor outcomes across multiple areas of functioning, including the presence and severity of a chronic condition, the condition's impact on functional independence and daily activities, psychosocial stress due to medical issues (including stigmatization), or the presence of ecological or environmental stressors (e.g., family resource limitations, divorce). *Resilience factors* are conceptualized as influences that promote positive outcomes, including factors that mitigate stress (e.g., coping strategies), and multilevel socioecological factors (Bronfenbrenner, 1979), including peer and family support.

Wallander and Varni's model has been used to conceptualize psychosocial outcomes in children with CL/P (Kapp-Simon & Gaither, 2016). Specifically, application of this model to CL/P identifies *medical* (e.g., failure to thrive; hearing loss; need for multiple surgical procedures to address appearance, speech, and dental concerns; presence of a genetic syndrome), *functional* (e.g., speech and language impairment, speech intelligibility, learning disabilities), and *psychosocial* risks (e.g., stress related to surgery). Resilience factors include both family- and child-related characteristics associated with positive psychosocial outcomes in CL/P, namely child temperament and personality (e.g., having an easy-going temperament and being socially extroverted), family cohesiveness, parental emotional well-being, adequate social support, and having financial resources available to access care (Kapp-Simon & Gaither, 2016).

Biopsychosocial models such as Wallander and Varni's are also recommended for use in conceptualizing outcomes in DSD (e.g., Holmbeck & Aspinall, 2015), although less work has been done to identify condition-specific risk and resistance factors for this population in accordance with a specific theoretical model. Nonetheless, in the following sections, we review risk and resilience factors that impact adjustment to CL/P and DSD, including emotional and behavioral functioning, cognitive and school functioning, peer and family relationships, and body image and appearance concerns, with specific focus on how stigma may impact functioning in these domains for both populations.

PSYCHOSOCIAL ADJUSTMENT: CLEFT LIP AND/OR PALATE

A large body of research has developed over the past several decades regarding the impacts of CL/P on individuals and their families across the lifespan (see Collett & Speltz, 2007; Nelson et al., 2012; Stock & Feragen, 2016 for reviews). While most research has focused on psychosocial risks, in recent years, more attention has been focused on identifying factors associated with resilience and healthy adjustment in children with CL/P and their families (see Baker et al., 2009; Feragen et al., 2009).

Parent Psychosocial Adaptation to the Diagnosis of CL/P

The emotional impact of a child's CL/P diagnosis is initially felt by the child's family. Parents typically experience a range of emotions, including shock, sadness, grief, anxiety, and anger, upon learning that their child either has been or will be born with a cleft (Nelson et al., 2012). Parents typically report worries about their child's future, including whether the child will be bullied or socially excluded (Zeytinoğlu et al., 2017). They also experience stress related to their child's medical care needs (Nelson et al., 2012). Parents frequently encounter enacted stigmatization, including being asked about their child's differences in public or being stared at by strangers (Nelson et al., 2012; Nidey et al., 2016).

Contextual factors, such as a family's race, ethnicity, culture, socioeconomic status, and access to resources such as insurance may affect how parents perceive and adapt to their child's cleft and related differences (e.g., Nidey et al., 2016). Learning about the child's diagnosis during pregnancy may confer some benefits to parents' emotional adjustment, offering time to process their feelings and to develop a plan for their child's care, with greater anxiety and postpartum depressive symptoms observed in mothers who learn of the child's CL/P at birth, compared with mothers who learn of the diagnosis prenatally (Johns et al., 2018; Zeytinoğlu et al., 2017).

While most parents adjust to the child's diagnosis, parents with a history of mental health problems, who experience stressors during pregnancy, and/or who are older at the time of conception have increased risks for adjustment problems to their child's diagnosis (Stock, Costa, et al., 2020). Consistent with a transactional framework (Fiese & Sameroff, 1989), parental distress and poor adjustment during infancy are associated with child psychosocial problems in preschool- (Pope & Snyder, 2005) and school-age children (Wolodiger & Pope, 2019).

Child Psychosocial Adaptation and Emotional Functioning Related to CL/P

During childhood and adolescence, children with CL/P are at risk for internalizing problems, such as poor self-concept, social and separation anxiety, and depression as well as externalizing problems, including hyperactivity, impulsivity, oppositionality, and aggression (e.g., Collett & Speltz, 2007; Richman et al., 2012; Stock & Feragen, 2016). Psychosocial risks may be exacerbated by appearance concerns and/or social difficulties. Branson and colleagues (2024) recently conducted a systematic review and meta-analysis of studies evaluating psychosocial difficulties in children with CL/P and nonaffected children. Results of their meta-analysis, which focused on studies that used the Strengths and Difficulties Questionnaire, found that across studies, children with CL/P had increased emotional, conduct, and hyperactivity problems on this measure relative to children without CL/P (Branson et al., 2024). However, among the 41 studies included in their systematic review, most studies of overall psychological adjustment and resiliency observed that children with CL/P did not differ from nonaffected peers, although risks for teasing, appearance concerns, and anxiety and depression were noted for children with CL/P (Branson et al., 2024). Psychosocial risks appear to persist through adulthood, with some studies reporting higher rates of mental health diagnoses in individuals with CL/P (Ardouin et al., 2021) including anxiety and depression (Nicholls et al., 2018).

Given the evidence for both psychosocial risks and healthy adjustment in CL/P, research has shifted toward understanding factors associated with resilience and positive adjustment. For example, optimism, satisfaction with health care, and satisfaction with their relationship with their spouse and/or partner are associated with healthy adjustment in parents of young children with CL/P (Stock, Costa, et al., 2020). Broder et al. (2014) observed that positive self-concept and self-efficacy were associated with better oral health-related quality of life. Peer and family support and healthy coping strategies (e.g., use of approach rather than avoidance-oriented coping) are associated with better adjustment (Baker et al., 2009).

Cognitive and School Functioning Related to CL/P

Children with CL/P are at risk for developmental delays including speech and language, gross motor, and cognitive delays (Gallagher & Collett, 2019). Structural brain differences in children born with CL/P (Richman et al., 2012) have been linked to cognitive problems, including deficits in visuospatial abilities, attention and executive functioning, motor, sensorimotor function, language, and general cognitive abilities (Stock & Feragen, 2016). Children with cleft typically have average intellectual abilities although rates of learning disabilities range from 30% to 40%, most commonly with reading or verbal skills (Richman et al., 2012). Higher rates of academic problems, lower educational attainment, and use of special education services have also been documented in children with CL/P (e.g., Wehby et al., 2014). A recent systematic review (Gallagher & Collett, 2019) noted that across 31 studies, children with cleft had poorer neurodevelopmental and academic functioning relative to peers from infancy through adulthood. Palatal involvement (either cleft palate or cleft lip and palate) is implicated as a risk for lower achievement (Constantin & Wehby, 2022). Because of the risk for academic problems, children with CL/P who present with school difficulties may benefit from a developmental evaluation by a developmental-behavioral pediatrician or a psychologist with training in psychoeducational or neuropsychological assessment.

There is limited research about children with CL/P in the school setting. Early research suggested that teachers may underestimate intellectual abilities or have lower expectations for academic achievement due to facial appearance or speech differences (Constantin & Wehby, 2022), owing to implicit biases or stereotypes associated with these differences (Hartung et al., 2019). A more recent qualitative study found that while teachers were aware of CL/P-related social, emotional, and treatment-related challenges, they did not view CL/P as being a risk for children's educational achievement (Stock et al., 2019). Stock and Ridley (2018) highlighted negative social experiences, including being teased, and traditional benchmarks for school success (e.g., written and oral examinations) as factors that may contribute to feelings of "not fitting in" or being "different" from peers or having low self-confidence at school. These findings underscore the need for access to psychological supports (e.g., pediatric psychologists, school counselors) to foster self-esteem and self-image and to address risks for stigmatization in the school setting.

In adulthood, most individuals with CL/P achieve equivalent education, employment, and income levels relative to individuals without CL/P (e.g., Nicholls et al., 2018). Nonetheless, stigmatization in the workplace has been reported, including concerns about not being hired because of facial appearance and/or speech differences (Ardouin et al., 2021).

Family and Peer Relationships and Child Adjustment to CL/P

Family relationships. CL/P affects the child's relationships with their caregivers and siblings. Studies indicate bidirectional (transactional) influences with mothers of infants with CL/P, with some studies suggesting that mothers are observed to be less sensitive to their children (Murray et al., 2008), while other studies have suggested that children with CL/P are less active and disengaged in interactions with their caregivers (Frederickson et al., 2006). Despite these observations of "disconnected" dyadic interactions, similar rates of secure and insecure infant–parent attachment have been reported for CL/P infants, relative to infants without CL/P (Murray et al., 2008), although other maternal factors, including advanced maternal age and multiple parity, have been implicated as potential risk factors for parent–child interactional difficulties (Tsuchiya et al., 2019).

During childhood, positive family relationships are thought to serve as a protective factor in children with CL/P, with individuals with CL/P who report close, cohesive relationships with their families reporting protection from stigma in other social relationships (Stock & Feragen, 2016). A study that directly observed parent–child interactions during a lab-based task (completing a puzzle) found that parents of school-age children with CL/P provide more encouragement, including compliments and expressions of positive emotion, relative to parents of healthy children or children with other health conditions (Gassling et al., 2014). Relatedly, while family interactions influence outcomes of children with CL/P, children with CL/P similarly influence outcomes of the family system. Studies of sibling relationships of children with CL/P report both positive (e.g., enhanced empathy toward others with differences) and negative associations (e.g., feeling overly protective of their sibling with CL/P in social situations) related to being the sibling of a child with CL/P (Stock et al., 2016).

Peer relationships. There is some evidence that peer relationships are a potential source of vulnerability and stigma for children with CL/P. Children and adolescents with CL/P are at risk for overt stigmatization, including teasing, bullying, and unwanted attention from others (Rumsey & Harcourt, 2007) due to facial appearance and/or speech differences. Up to 67% of youth with CL/P report being teased about their speech or appearance at least once during childhood (Stock & Feragen, 2016). Social experience is a strong predictor of psychosocial adjustment in youth with CL/P (Berger & Dalton, 2011). Less satisfaction with appearance, greater perception of speech problems, and use of avoidant coping strategies are predictive of poorer social experiences in adolescents with CL/P (Berger & Dalton, 2011).

Adolescents with CL/P may experience some risks related to forming romantic relationships due to appearance and body image concerns (Feragen et al., 2016). Studies of adults with CL/P observe that while they tend to have positive, close relationships with their families and friends and marry at an age similar to nonaffected adults, there is some evidence for delays in independent living and having fewer romantic relationships (Nicholls et al., 2018). Nonetheless, studies also highlight risks for bullying and discrimination, which may persist during adulthood, including in the workplace (Ardouin et al., 2021). Taken together, there is a growing body of research suggesting that individuals with CL/P have vulnerabilities in peer and social relationships that can persist throughout the lifespan. As such, this is an area that merits close monitoring and surveillance by clinical providers (e.g., by pediatric psychologists, developmental-behavioral pediatricians, and mental health professionals) who can identify potential risks and are well-poised to initiate supports and services.

BODY IMAGE, APPEARANCE CONCERNS, AND PSYCHOSOCIAL FUNCTIONING

There is a developmental emergence regarding how body image unfolds across childhood. Early experiences with sensory, movement, and social experiences inform body image development during infancy (Lawlor & Elliot, 2012; Smolak, 2012). As children enter their toddler and preschool years, cognitive development and speech and language development, including the development of social comparison, along with increasing social relationship experiences influence their body image development (Lawlor & Elliot, 2012). Children become aware of their own and others' appearances during the preschool years (e.g., Smolak, 2012) and begin to notice that they may have appearance differences. They may be aware that others stare at them or ask their parents questions about their appearance and/or speech differences. Such differential attention can influence their self-perceptions and contribute to either positive or negative perceptions of body image.

Negative perceptions of physical appearance (i.e., body image dissatisfaction), are common among children, adolescents, and adults with CL/P, with some evidence for variation by sex. Females report more appearance-related stigma and body image dissatisfaction relative to males (Crerand et al., 2017, 2020). Perceived stigmatization is a significant predictor of body image dissatisfaction and satisfaction with facial appearance and speech in adolescents with craniofacial conditions (Crerand et al., 2020). Childhood teasing is related to greater body image dissatisfaction and depressive symptoms during adolescence in females with CL/P (Feragen & Stock, 2016). Body image dissatisfaction, specifically related to facial appearance, is related to poorer psychosocial adjustment in adolescence and adulthood (Crerand et al., 2017). For clinicians who work with children with CL/P, screening for perceptions of body image dissatisfaction and affective symptoms can help identify individuals who are at risk for worse psychosocial outcomes, and who may benefit from additional supports and services.

DIFFERENCES OF SEX DEVELOPMENT

DSD conditions are a rare and heterogeneous population to study. Treatment approaches have undergone vast changes over time, so the study of DSD continues to be an emerging field for understanding many aspects of what it means to live with one of these conditions. DSD are often diagnosed at birth or early in life. Thus, studies of emotional and behavioral functioning have primarily focused on parent and family adjustment during infancy and early childhood due to the known impacts that parents' well-being and adjustment can have on the child's psychosocial functioning.

Parent Psychosocial Adaptation to the Diagnosis of DSD

For many families, pregnancy is a time of hope and expectations for the child's future. Prenatal care often includes an anatomy scan that may describe external genitalia. Noninvasive prenatal testing can provide the genetic sex. These care experiences have led to early sharing of expected sex with family and friends, "gender reveal parties," and posting the expected sex more widely and permanently to social media. Even for those who elect to wait to learn this information at birth, there can be trauma from the uncertainty that presents with ambiguous genitalia. Specific concerns can include the immediate health of the child and considerations for name, what sex or name to put on government documents, and what to share with others. Often the first professional contacts for these families and babies are with medical providers who may not know much about DSD and are unable to normalize the situation and decrease the need for a sense of urgency with decision making. When the child is diagnosed later, families may not only mourn the loss of what they had expected for their child but also worry about their child's gender identity and future adjustment in life. Not surprisingly, current estimates suggest that about one-third of caregivers of children with DSD are at risk for psychosocial problems (Ernst et al., 2018), a rate that matches risk levels in other pediatric populations (e.g., Crerand et al., 2018). Another study reported that 21% of mothers experience posttraumatic stress symptoms related to their child's DSD diagnosis (Delozier et al., 2019). Further, a recent study identified that greater stigma perceptions among parents of children with DSD, and greater perceptions of child-focused stigma, were correlated with poorer parental adjustment, including symptoms of anxiety and depression (Traino et al., 2022). Future studies are needed to address child perceptions of stigma and relationships to child psychosocial outcomes.

Open and developmentally appropriate communication with the child about their condition is recommended to promote autonomy and agency with their bodies and to decrease shame and stigma (Weidler et al., 2023; Wisniewski et al., 2019). Nonetheless, there can often be some discomfort in having these conversations as they can involve sexual and reproductive functioning.

Caregivers may also naturally avoid discussing the condition that is associated with past distress or even traumatic stress for themselves (e.g., Delozier et al., 2019). For clinicians working with families with DSDs, including pediatricians, psychologists, and other mental health providers, it is critically important to explicitly relay the recommendation of open communication with families. Families in general express appreciation for this support. There is a strong desire among families and medical team members for the presence of psychological support and peer support during the course of treatment (Crerand et al., 2019) as evidenced by its consistent inclusion in professional and patient advocacy groups' clinical standards of care (Lee et al., 2016).

Child Psychosocial Adaptation and Emotional Functioning Related to DSD

In youth with DSD, available research suggests variation in coping and adjustment across and within diagnoses. This uncertainty is challenging as clinicians strive to be able to provide parents with good anticipatory guidance about what to expect for their children. Fortunately, consortiums have been formed (e.g., dsd-LIFE in Europe and DSD-TRN in the United States) that can capture larger participant pools to help answer some of these important questions.

Sex-chromosome aneuploidies (e.g., Turner and Klinefelter syndromes) are associated with neurodevelopmental and psychiatric issues. For instance, in Turner syndrome, approximately 25% of patients have a diagnosis of attention deficit/hyperactivity disorder (ADHD; Gravholt et al., 2017), with increased risks of anxiety (Hutaff-Lee et al., 2019) and depression in adolescents and young adults (Morris et al., 2020). Similarly, in Klinefelter syndrome, there is an increased rate of ADHD (Ross et al., 2012), and depressive symptoms in adolescents and adults (Turriff et al., 2011).

In other DSD, the research regarding child adaptation and emotional and behavioral functioning is mixed. Some research suggests individuals with DSD in general have good psychosocial functioning (Kleinemeier et al., 2010), with the presence of caring relationships with parents, and a best friend serving as protective factors to mitigate potential negative outcomes (Schweizer et al., 2017). Other studies report more significant concerns, including increased rates of suicidal ideation from 12% to 45% depending on proxy or self-report, diagnostic subgroups, and age (de Vries et al., 2019; Hansen-Moore et al., 2021; Schweizer et al., 2017). It can be challenging to discern clear patterns and predictors of adjustment as many studies examine heterogenous groups of DSD, treated in different ways and across various countries, cultures, and institutions (Traino et al., 2022).

Early surgery is a polemical topic and is hypothesized to impact overall adjustment in DSD. There is still no consensus on having surgery and the timing of surgery for specific diagnoses (Lee et al., 2016). Research in adults who received surgery in infancy or early childhood suggests individuals may not view surgical outcomes as favorably as their surgeons. Certain surgical procedures do have a higher rate of impact on quality of life, including gonadectomy, hypospadias repair, and clitoridectomy. However, by and large, individuals do not report a significantly negative impact of early surgery on their quality of life (Rapp et al., 2021).

Cognitive and school functioning. Cognitive and school functioning have received relatively limited attention in DSD populations, in part because most DSD do not appear to be associated with cognitive deficits. In some instances, as with girls with CAH, improved abilities in specific domains (e.g., spatial abilities) have been observed relative to nonaffected siblings (Berenbaum et al., 2012), owing in part to structural brain differences and potentially, effects of androgen exposure (see Beltz et al., 2023 for a review). However, as noted previously, sex chromosome aneuploidy conditions such as Turner syndrome and Klinefelter syndrome are associated with neurocognitive deficits including risks for ADHD, autism, and challenges with learning, social cognition, and executive functioning (Kremen et al., 2023; Skakkebæk et al., 2020). These deficits can affect both academic and social functioning in school settings. Youth with Turner or Klinefelter syndrome may benefit from close monitoring with pediatricians, pediatric psychologists, and neuropsychologists given these known risks.

DSD can potentially impact school performance and participation in related activities due to medical care needs (e.g., frequent medical appointments; Sandberg et al., 2001). Further, concerns about being "outed" as having atypical physical features related to DSD can occur. For example, youth and their caregivers may fear inadvertent disclosure of the child's differences when using the restroom, changing clothes for gym class, or during extracurricular activities that may require revealing attire such as leotards or swimsuits. As described previously, social stressors such as being teased or bullied by peers or even anticipatory anxiety about being rejected by peers can affect how youth with DSD perceive of and participate in school-related activities (Gravholt et al., 2017; Yau et al., 2015). Sandberg and colleagues (2017) observed that some school-age children with DSD rate their school and athletic competencies negatively. Among children with hypospadias, negative parental appraisal of the child's genitalia was associated with more school-related problems, potentially because of poorer emotional and/or behavioral adjustment in children with suboptimal cosmetic and/or functional surgical outcomes (Sandberg et al., 2001). Studies of health-related quality of life in children with DSD note deficits in school-related domain scores (e.g., Şentürk Pilan et al., 2021; Yau et al., 2015). Taken together, these findings illustrate risks for youth with DSD in school settings, with implications for screening and monitoring by pediatric psychologists, neuropsychologists, and developmental pediatricians to ensure optimal outcomes, academically and socially.

Family and Peer Relationships, and Child Adjustment to DSD

Family relationships. Consistent with a transactional framework, the parent's adjustment to their child's DSD diagnosis has implications for their children's psychological adaptation. Parental positive adjustment and normalization of their child's DSD are key to the child's own internalization of acceptance and self-image (Pasterski et al., 2014). Body image, psychological distress, and suicidal ideation can be related to perception of parental care and approach to dealing with their child's condition (Schweizer et al., 2017). Information sharing regarding the condition with extended family is often a personalized family choice depending on family culture and acceptance. While open communication works well for many, if the child will be judged or stigmatized by other family members, it is likely not in their best interest to have their information shared with those family members or to wait until the child is old enough to decide for themselves with whom they want to share their private health information.

It is natural for families to worry about how the information may be received in the child's social circle. During childhood, there is often relationship upheaval such that relationships that are seemingly close can become more distant as children approach adolescence. Given the advent of social media, it is possible that if information about a child's DSD is shared on the internet, there will be widespread knowledge about their condition that will not be able to be effectively retracted. Therefore, the risks of peer victimization with information sharing need to be balanced with the desire for children to be able to share important information about themselves safely and without shame (Tishelman et al., 2019). These issues can be discussed by family and medical team providers directly with the child in deciding how and when to talk to peers.

Peer relationships. Social concerns including real or feared rejection from peers and teasing or bullying can also affect perceptions about school (Gravholt et al., 2017). Children may not have yet directly experienced some of the differences associated with their medical conditions, which may become more salient as they mature. As is typical for adolescents in general, individuals with DSD worry about being different from their peers and fear rejection. At a time when being different can be ostracizing, girls with CAH have increased rates of aggression and "tomboyish" behavior. In other DSD populations, the patient may be the only girl in her peer group to not get a period (Bukowski et al., 2015). Girls with Turner syndrome have difficulties with social processing and initiating or maintaining friendships (Gravholt et al., 2017).

While feeling different from peers is a common theme with many pediatric populations, the issues related to diagnoses of DSDs are unique, as the differences children with DSDs experience often intersect with their basic core identity of biological sex and gender (one's self-perception of being male, female, nonbinary, transgender, or other identity). There can be a persistent fear of discovery that may lead to adolescents isolating themselves or avoiding certain activities (e.g., locker room changing) where they may feel more exposed. Social disruptions may also arise from frequent doctor visits and/or hospitalizations for surgery, which may interfere with school attendance or participation (Sandberg et al., 2001).

In terms of romantic relationships, adolescent and young adult females with a DSD tend to delay romantic relationships and initial forms of intimacy (Kleinemeier et al., 2010). This could be due in part to anxiety about sharing information regarding diagnosis and fertility with romantic partners for fear of rejection. In males with DSD, while some sexual functioning difficulties may exist, overall, they have romantic partners and report satisfaction with their relationships at the same rate as males without DSD (Tishelman et al., 2019; van der Zwan et al., 2013).

Body Image, Appearance Concerns, and Psychosocial Functioning in DSD

DSD can be associated with a range of physical differences including atypical genitalia, sex-discordant features such as gynecomastia in males with Klinefelter syndrome or excess facial hair in females with CAH, and other condition-specific differences (e.g., webbed neck in females with Turner syndrome). Very few studies have evaluated body image in children with DSD conditions. There are risks for body image dissatisfaction across DSD conditions (Kanhere et al., 2015), although not all children report concerns in this domain. Those who report concerns with genital appearance are more sexually inhibited than their peers (Schönbucher et al., 2012). Psychological discomfort with genitals, including shame and body image distress, can also impact sexual functioning and quality of life. Adolescents and adults may harbor concerns about sexual function that are embarrassing to express but may have repercussions for their willingness to engage in intimate relationships. It is important for providers to openly discuss sexual issues with youth starting in adolescence, and to create a climate that enables an adolescent to ask questions freely and express concerns.

Body image concerns can also arise when there is gender dysphoria. In general, children with DSD conditions experience higher gender identity discordance from their assigned birth sex than the general population, with this phenomenon more highly represented in some DSD diagnoses than others (Tishelman et al., 2019). Those with CAH, complete androgen insensitivity syndrome, and complete gonadal dysgenesis, who are raised as female have relatively low levels of gender dysphoria. However, patients who have 5-alpha reductase deficiency, 17 hydroxysteroid dehydrogenase deficiency, partial androgen insensitivity syndrome, and mixed gonadal dysgenesis report higher levels of gender dysphoria (Babu & Shah, 2021). Those who do report gender dysphoria are at greater risk of internalizing concerns (Kreukels et al., 2018).

CLINICAL IMPLICATIONS IN THE MANAGEMENT OF CONGENITAL MEDICAL CONDITIONS

Given the psychosocial risks associated with CL/P, the American Cleft Palate Craniofacial Association's (ACPA) *Parameters for Evaluation and Treatment of Patients with Cleft Lip/Palate or Other Craniofacial Anomalies* (2018) recommend interdisciplinary care approaches that include routine psychosocial assessments. While care parameters do not yet exist for DSD, consensus statements recognize the profound psychosocial impacts associated with these conditions and recommend interdisciplinary care including access to providers who can screen for psychosocial risks, and offer supports and interventions (e.g., psychologists, mental health providers, developmental-behavioral pediatricians; Cools et al., 2018; Hughes et al., 2006). In the following sections, we highlight clinical care practices to support children and their families and areas for future research.

Education and Support

All families need accurate information about their child's specific medical condition, treatments, and psychosocial risks. Ideally, education is provided at the time of diagnosis (including prenatally) with continued information sharing occurring as the child (and family) traverse developmental stages. Pediatricians and mental health specialists can work together to address gaps in families' understandings of their child's condition and assist with risk monitoring.

While education can be shared by providers in the context of a medical visit, caregivers and older youth may also seek information and support online. Thus, it is important that providers be aware of reputable websites and support resources (see the Resources box at the end of the chapter). Finally, some medical teams facilitate opportunities for families with similar diagnoses to connect and offer support to each other (e.g., support groups and/or social events such as family picnics).

One strategy that providers can routinely use to support resilience and decrease stigma is to utilize neutral and descriptive language when discussing diagnoses and treatment, since medical terminology can have potentially stigmatizing interpretations. For children with CL/P, it is recommended that clinicians refrain from using terms such as "defect," "malformation," or "fix" when describing procedures, as these terms may have negative connotations and imply that the child is "broken" or "defective." Providers can model the use of neutral descriptors about the child's condition for children with CL/P and their families, which in turn can promote healthy identity development (Stock, Marik, et al., 2020). Simple descriptive language can help families explain diagnoses and respond to questions. Parents can be advised to model confident nonverbal communication skills when teaching the child about their cleft-related differences, using neutral terms in much the same way as they teach them about their other body parts (Stock, Marik, et al., 2020). Siblings may need guidance about answering questions about their siblings' differences.

Similarly, in the context of DSD care, terminology can be potentially stigmatizing. Providers can normalize the child's differences by providing information about the range of differences that occur across human genotypes and phenotypes and by utilizing nonstigmatizing language (e.g., refraining from using terms such as "anomaly," "abnormality," "disorder"). The clinician can talk with youth and their families about their preferred terminology and use sensitive language in handouts, websites, and clinic names.

For families of children with DSD, information sharing can be more challenging, and they may grapple with questions such as who to tell, who not to tell, and when to share information with others and their child. Clinicians can offer guidance about sharing information using developmentally appropriate language over time. Further, they can offer information about how to describe the child's differences to other people (e.g., day care providers; Cools et al., 2018). As children age into adolescence and adulthood, clinicians can offer support and guidance around how and when to talk about their differences with other people, including romantic partners.

Psychosocial Screening, Assessment, and Intervention

Screening. Due to the risks associated with CL/P and DSD, routine psychosocial screening is recommended. Ideally, interdisciplinary care teams will include pediatric psychologists or other mental health professionals who can screen for psychosocial risks. However, professionals from a variety of disciplines, including social work, nursing, and pediatrics, can also conduct risk screenings.

There are no current standards for risk screening in either CL/P or DSD populations. For CL/P, commonly used screening instruments include the Pediatric Quality of Life Inventory (Varni et al., 2001) and Child Behavior Checklist (Achenbach & Rescorla, 2001) along with condition-specific instruments including the Psychosocial Assessment Tool-Craniofacial Version (Crerand et al., 2018) and the CLEFT-Q (Wong Riff et al., 2018), which also assess for stigmatization. Similar measures have been utilized for screening and outcomes assessments in DSD populations (Ernst et al., 2018). The Parent Stigma Scale and the Child Stigma Scale, originally developed to assess epilepsy-related stigma, have recently been adapted for DSD (Traino et al., 2021).

Screening can also provide opportunities to offer anticipatory guidance about how family and child strengths can be leveraged to support well-being and resiliency. Highlighting what is going well—in addition to acknowledging areas of struggle—can help youth and their families develop a balanced perspective about health-related stressors and consider ways that they have grown or experienced positive changes despite the challenges they have encountered.

Assessment and intervention. CL/P and DSD are associated with risks for emotional and behavioral problems that may be significant enough to warrant a formal diagnosis of mood, anxiety, or other behavioral disorders (e.g., ADHD). To evaluate such concerns, a consultation with a developmental-behavioral pediatrician, pediatric or clinical psychologists, or child and adolescent psychiatrists may be helpful. There are also elevated risks for neurodevelopmental and learning disabilities associated with CL/P and some DSD (e.g., Turner and Klinefelter syndromes), for which ongoing educational supports may be indicated. Developmental-behavioral pediatricians and neuropsychologists can provide monitoring and evaluation of cognitive and developmental concerns in these instances.

Referrals to clinical or pediatric psychologists are indicated when individuals experience significant emotional, social, or behavioral problems or have difficulty coping with their condition or treatments. Brief strategies to help ease social situations and manage stigma can be integrated into therapy. For example, parents and children can be taught to "Explain-Reassure-Distract" when asked questions about appearance differences (e.g., *I was born with a split in my lip and the doctor sewed it back together. It doesn't hurt, and I can smile just like everyone else. Hey, what did you think of the football game last night?*; Stock, Marik, et al., 2020).

There has been substantially less research on the development and testing of tailored or condition-specific interventions. To date, there are no DSD-specific interventions. Online interventions for adults (Norman et al., 2015) and adolescents with appearance-altering conditions (Williamson et al., 2019) have been developed to target appearance and social stigmatization with randomized controlled trials underway (e.g., Kling et al., 2022). Despite this progress, CL/P-specific interventions are infrequently utilized in clinical practice. Further, access to psychologists with expertise in CL/P remains limited. In the absence of condition-specific interventions, evidence-based therapies (e.g., cognitive behavior therapy) can be utilized.

Treatment Adherence

CL/P and DSD treatments vary widely by diagnosis and related sequelae, and typically, routine follow-up with interdisciplinary specialists is indicated. Studies of adherence to CL/P care have identified that surgical care delays, missed appointments, incomplete treatment or care attrition, increased surgical complications, and longer hospital stays are associated with sociodemographic variables (e.g., non-White race, ethnicity; Pfeifauf et al., 2022). There is a critical need to view adherence through a lens of intersectionality, with recognition of how sociodemographic factors affect adherence and contribute to health disparities.

Additionally, craniofacial team visits can have inadvertently negative impacts on children and their caregivers. Children may feel intimidated, frightened, or confused, with parents feeling pressured to both listen to and engage with clinicians while attending to and mitigating any negative emotional impacts of the visit for their child (Feragen et al., 2019). Stigmatizing experiences (e.g., scrutiny of facial appearance) could contribute to poor treatment adherence, although this relationship has yet to be investigated.

To date, the role of sociodemographic variables and treatment adherence in DSD has received little study. However, there is a documented history of inadequate, insensitive care practices for individuals with DSD that could result in mistrust and potentially trauma (Cools et al., 2018). Such experiences may contribute to dissatisfaction with health care which could be reasonably hypothesized to impact treatment adherence (Cools et al., 2018). Research is clearly needed to further investigate sociodemographic variables, patient perceptions of care practices, and treatment adherence in DSD. The DSD Pathways Study, which is evaluating health status and health care utilization patterns in persons with DSD (Goodman et al., 2022), will help evaluate adherence to care recommendations and factors related to adherence.

RESEARCH GAPS AND FUTURE DIRECTIONS IN THE CLINICAL CARE OF CONGENITAL MEDICAL CONDITIONS

Research is needed in key areas to ensure that individuals with CL/P or DSD achieve optimal health and psychosocial outcomes. First, much of the onus on stigma management has typically been placed on children and their families (e.g., learning how to cope with stigma). There is continued need to develop interventions at the societal level, including increasing awareness and acceptance of a range of facial and bodily appearances and developing policies that combat stigmatization and related discrimination and prejudice across the lifespan. Important advocacy work is being done to advance equitable treatment of persons with facial differences by organizations such as Face Equality International (see the Resources box). Similarly, interACT is spearheading advocacy for the human rights and well-being of intersex youth.

Implicit bias affects attitudes and behaviors toward other patient populations vulnerable to stigma including individuals with obesity (Lawrence et al., 2021). However, there is exceedingly limited research about implicit attitudes about CL/P or DSD. In one of the only studies of implicit attitudes toward people with visible differences, implicit attitudes were not negative, suggesting that other mechanisms may explain stigmatizing behaviors, including uncertainty about how to react to visible differences (Roberts et al., 2017). Future research is needed to evaluate implicit biases in relationship to stigma in both CL/P and DSD populations.

Finally, additional research is needed to center patients' voices in the context of interdisciplinary care for both DSD and CL/P as terminology and care practices can be inadvertently stigmatizing and potentially, traumatizing. Future research should also evaluate how the intersectionality of race, class, ethnicity, and sex relate to stigma in persons with DSD and CL/P (Stangl et al., 2019). Early surgery for DSD remains a controversial topic that requires additional longitudinal research to better understand the motivations for and outcomes of surgery. Future research should also focus on relationships between stigma and motivations for surgery and evaluations of surgical outcomes in both CL/P and DSD populations.

CONCLUSION

Children with CL/P and DSD and their families are vulnerable to psychosocial risks, including stigmatization. Psychosocial risks are often more salient for parents when children are young, but as children approach early childhood and school entry, vulnerabilities for internalizing and externalizing problems, social difficulties, learning problems, and challenges coping with treatment emerge and may persist through adolescence and adulthood. Interdisciplinary care that is attuned to the needs of children and their families can help mitigate risks and support resiliency through routine psychosocial screenings and referrals to psychologists, neuropsychologists, and developmental-behavioral pediatricians for assessment and interventions. Additional research is indicated to address condition-related stigma for individuals, families, and at societal and/or systems levels.

RESOURCES

Patient and family support organizations for cleft lip and/or palate (CL/P) and differences of sex development (DSD) that offer a range of educational, advocacy, and support programs include:

Organizations Focused on CL/P

- American Cleft Palate Craniofacial Association (ACPA):

  https://acpacares.org/

  ACPA supports individuals with cleft and other craniofacial conditions and craniofacial health care professionals through research, education, and advocacy.

- Changing Faces:

  https://www.changingfaces.org.uk

  This U.K.-based organization provides support, resources, and advocacy for individuals of all ages with any type of visible difference.

- Face Equality International:

  https://faceequalityinternational.org

  Face Equality International is an organization comprised of nongovernmental organizations, charities, and support groups who share a mission focused on advocacy to recognize disfigurement as a human rights issue; elimination of facial difference and disfigurement-related stigma and prejudice; cultivation of a community of organizations and individuals who strive to advocate for face equality; and advocacy for equity within society for all individuals with facial differences.

Organizations Focused on DSD

- Accord Alliance:

  https://www.accordalliance.org

  This organization is focused on the promotion of integrated care approaches for individuals with DSD and their families.

- DSD Families:

  https://dsdfamilies.org

  DSD Families is an information and peer support charity for families based in the United Kingdom.

- interACT:

  https://interactadvocates.org

  interACT is an intersex-led organization that strives to advocate for the human rights of intersex youth. They also raise awareness of and promote the inclusion of intersex individuals. They support and advocate for laws and policies to protect intersex bodily autonomy. interACT's ultimate purpose is to support intersex well-being and to end nonconsensual and medically unnecessary surgery for children with intersex traits.

References

Achenbach, T. M., & Rescorla, L. A. (2001). *Manual for the ASEBA school-age forms & profiles*. University of Vermont, Research Center for Children, Youth, and Families.

American Cleft Palate Craniofacial Association. (2018). Parameters for evaluation and treatment of patients with cleft lip/palate or other craniofacial anomalies. *The Cleft Palate Craniofacial Journal*, 55(1), 137–156. https://doi.org/10.1177/1055665617739564

Ardouin, K., Hotton, M., & Stock, N. M. (2021). Interpersonal relationship experiences in adults born with cleft lip and/or palate: A whole of life survey in the United Kingdom. *The Cleft Palate Craniofacial Journal*, 58(11), 1412–1421. https://doi.org/10.1177/1055665620987109

Arseneault, L. (2017). The long-term impact of bullying victimization on mental health. *World Psychiatry, 16*(1), 27–28. https://doi.org/10.1002/wps.20399

Babu, R., & Shah, U. (2021). Gender identity disorder (GID) in adolescents and adults with differences of sex development (DSD): A systematic review and meta-analysis. *Journal of Pediatric Urology, 17*(1), 39–47. https://doi.org/10.1016/j.jpurol.2020.11.017

Baker, S. R., Owens, J., Stern, M., & Willmot, D. (2009). Coping strategies and social support in the family impact of cleft lip and palate and parents' adjustment and psychological distress. *The Cleft Palate Craniofacial Journal, 46*(3), 229–236. https://doi.org/10.1597/08-075.1

Beltz, A. M., Demidenko, M. I., Wilson, S. J., & Berenbaum, S. A. (2023). Prenatal androgen influences on the brain: A review, critique, and illustration of research on congenital adrenal hyperplasia. *Journal of Neuroscience Research, 101*(5), 563–574. https://doi.org/10.1002/jnr.24900

Bennecke, E., Köhler, B., Röhle, R., Thyen, U., Gehrmann, K., Lee, P., Nordenström, A., Cohen-Kettenis, P., Bouvattier, C., & Wiesemann, C. (2021). Disorders or differences of sex development? Views of affected individuals on DSD terminology. *Journal of Sex Research, 58*(4), 522–531. https://doi.org/10.1080/00224499.2019.1703130

Berenbaum, S. A., Bryk, K. L., & Beltz, A. M. (2012). Early androgen effects on spatial and mechanical abilities: Evidence from congenital adrenal hyperplasia. *Behavioral Neuroscience, 126*(1), 86–96. https://doi.org/10.1037/a0026652

Berger, Z. E., & Dalton, L. J. (2011). Coping with a cleft II: Factors associated with psychosocial adjustment of adolescents with a cleft lip and palate and their parents. *The Cleft Palate Craniofacial Journal, 48*(1), 82–90. https://doi.org/10.1597/08-094

Branson, E. K., Branson, V. M., McGrath, R., Rausa, V. C., Kilpatrick, N., & Crowe, L. M. (2024). Psychological and peer difficulties of children with cleft lip and/or palate: A systematic review and meta-analysis. *The Cleft Palate Craniofacial Journal, 61*(2), 258–270. https://doi.org/10.1177/10556656221125377

Broder, H. L., Wilson-Genderson, M., Sischo, L., & Norman, R. G. (2014). Examining factors associated with oral health-related quality of life for youth with cleft. *Plastic and Reconstructive Surgery, 133*(6), 828e–834e. https://doi.org/10.1097/PRS.0000000000000221

Bronfenbrenner, U. (1979). *The ecology of human development: Experiments by nature and design.* Harvard University Press.

Bukowski, W. M., McCauley, E., & Mazur, T. (2015). Disorders of sex development (DSD): Peer relations and psychosocial well-being. *Hormone and Metabolic Research, 47*(5), 357–360. https://doi.org/10.1055/s-0035-1549884

Carroll, L. (2020). An intersectional approach to understanding potential health disparities in adolescents with a disorder of sex development/intersex. *Journal of Pediatric Nursing, 52*, 111–112. https://doi.org/10.1016/j.pedn.2020.02.026

Centers for Disease Control and Prevention (CDC). (2008). Update on overall prevalence of major birth defects—Atlanta, Georgia, 1978–2005. *MMWR: Morbidity and Mortality Weekly Report, 57*(1), 1–5.

Collett, B. R., & Speltz, M. L. (2007). A developmental approach to mental health for children and adolescents with orofacial clefts. *Orthodontics & Craniofacial Research, 10*(3), 138–148. https://doi.org/10.1111/j.1601-6343.2007.00394.x

Constantin, J., & Wehby, G. L. (2022). Academic outcomes of children with orofacial clefts: A review of the literature and recommendations for future research. *Oral Diseases, 28*(5), 1387–1399. https://doi.org/10.1111/odi.14137

Cools, M., Nordenström, A., Robeva, R., Hall, J., Westerveld, P., Flück, C., Köhler, B., Berra, M., Springer, A., Schweizer, K., Pasterski, V., & the COST Action BM1303 working group 1. (2018). Caring for individuals with a difference of sex development (DSD): A consensus statement. *Nature Reviews: Endocrinology, 14*(7), 415–429. https://doi.org/10.1038/s41574-018-0010-8

Crerand, C. E., Kapa, H. M., & Litteral, J. (2017). A review of psychosocial risks and management for children with cleft lip and/or palate. *Perspectives of the ASHA Special Interest Groups, 2*(5), 23–34. https://doi.org/10.1044/persp2.SIG5.23

Crerand, C. E., Kapa, H. M., Litteral, J., Pearson, G. D., Eastman, K., & Kirschner, R. E. (2018). Identifying psychosocial risk factors among families of children with craniofacial conditions: Validation of the Psychosocial Assessment Tool-Craniofacial Version. *The Cleft Palate Craniofacial Journal, 55*(4), 536–545. https://doi.org/10.1177/1055665617748010

Crerand, C. E., Kapa, H. M., Litteral, J. L., Nahata, L., Combs, B., Indyk, J. A., Jayanthi, V. R., Chan, Y. M., Tishelman, A. C., & Hansen-Moore, J. (2019). Parent perceptions of psychosocial care for children with differences of sex development.

Journal of Pediatric Urology, 15(5), 522.e1–522.e8. https://doi.org/10.1016/j.jpurol.2019.06.024

Crerand, C. E., Rumsey, N., Kazak, A., Clarke, A., Rausch, J., & Sarwer, D. B. (2020). Sex differences in perceived stigmatization, body image disturbance, and satisfaction with facial appearance and speech among adolescents with craniofacial conditions. *Body Image, 32*, 190–198. https://doi.org/10.1016/j.bodyim.2020.01.005

Crerand, C. E., Sarwer, D. B., Kazak, A. E., Clarke, A., & Rumsey, N. (2017). Body image and quality of life in adolescents with craniofacial conditions. *The Cleft Palate Craniofacial Journal, 54*(1), 2–12. https://doi.org/10.1597/15-167

Crerand, C. E., Suorsa-Johnson, K. I., Hansen-Moore, J. A., Ernst, M., Pennesi, C., Delozier, A., Fei, F., Johnson, J., Jewell, T., Lanphier, E., Jaffal, N., Umbaugh, H., James, L. N., Saylor, K. M., & Sandberg, D. E. (2021). Stigma and differences of sex development: A scoping review protocol. *Deep Blue.* https://doi.org/10.7302/1232

de Vries, A. L. C., Roehle, R., Marshall, L., Frisén, L., van de Grift, T. C., Kreukels, B. P. C., Bouvattier, C., Köhler, B., Thyen, U., Nordenström, A., Rapp, M., Cohen-Kettenis, P. T., & the dsd-LIFE Group. (2019). Mental health of a large group of adults with disorders of sex development in six European countries. *Psychosomatic Medicine, 81*(7), 629–640. https://doi.org/10.1097/PSY.0000000000000718

Delozier, A. M., Gamwell, K. L., Sharkey, C., Bakula, D. M., Perez, M. N., Wolfe-Christensen, C., Austin, P., Baskin, L., Bernabé, K. J., Chan, Y. M., Cheng, E. Y., Diamond, D. A., Ellens, R. E. H., Fried, A., Galan, D., Greenfield, S., Kolon, T., Kropp, B., Lakshmanan, Y., . . . Mullins, L. L. (2019). Uncertainty and posttraumatic stress: differences between mothers and fathers of infants with disorders of sex development. *Archives of Sexual Behavior, 48*(5), 1617–1624. https://doi.org/10.1007/s10508-018-1357-6

Dion, K., Berscheid, E., & Walster, E. (1972). What is beautiful is good. *Journal of Personality and Social Psychology, 24*(3), 285–290. https://doi.org/10.1037/h0033731

Ediati, A., Maharani, N., & Utari, A. (2016). Sociocultural aspects of disorders of sex development. *Birth Defects Research Part C, 108*(4), 380–383. https://doi.org/10.1002/bdrc.21144

Ernst, M. M., Gardner, M., Mara, C. A., Délot, E. C., Fechner, P. Y., Fox, M., Rutter, M. M., Speiser, P. W., Vilain, E., Weidler, E. M., Sandberg, D. E., & the DSD-Translational Research Network Leadership Group and Psychosocial Workgroup. (2018). Psychosocial screening in disorders/differences of sex development: Psychometric evaluation of the Psychosocial Assessment Tool. *Hormone Research in Paediatrics, 90*(6), 368–380. https://doi.org/10.1159/000496114

Feragen, K. B., Borge, A. I., & Rumsey, N. (2009). Social experience in 10-year-old children born with a cleft: Exploring psychosocial resilience. *The Cleft Palate Craniofacial Journal, 46*(1), 65–74. https://doi.org/10.1597/07-124.1

Feragen, K. B., Myhre, A., & Stock, N. M. (2019). "Exposed and vulnerable": Parent reports of their child's experience of multidisciplinary craniofacial consultations. *The Cleft Palate Craniofacial Journal, 56*(9), 1230–1238. https://doi.org/10.1177/1055665619851650

Feragen, K. B., & Stock, N. M. (2016). A longitudinal study of 340 young people with or without a visible difference: The impact of teasing on self-perceptions of appearance and depressive symptoms. *Body Image, 16*, 133–142. https://doi.org/10.1016/j.bodyim.2016.01.003

Feragen, K. B., Stock, N. M., Sharratt, N. D., & Kvalem, I. L. (2016). Self-perceptions of romantic appeal in adolescents with a cleft lip and/or palate. *Body Image, 18*, 143–152. https://doi.org/10.1016/j.bodyim.2016.06.009

Fiese, B. H., & Sameroff, A. J. (1989). Family context in pediatric psychology: A transactional perspective. *Journal of Pediatric Psychology, 14*(2), 293–314. https://doi.org/10.1093/jpepsy/14.2.293

Frederickson, M. S., Chapman, K. L., & Hardin-Jones, M. (2006). Conversational skills of children with cleft lip and palate: A replication and extension. *The Cleft Palate Craniofacial Journal, 43*(2), 179–188. https://doi.org/10.1597/04-086.1

Gallagher, E. R., & Collett, B. R. (2019). Neurodevelopmental and academic outcomes in children with orofacial clefts: A systematic review. *Pediatrics, 144*(1), e20184027. https://doi.org/10.1542/peds.2018-4027

Gassling, V., Christoph, C., Wahle, K., Koos, B., Wiltfang, J., Gerber, W. D., & Siniatchkin, M. (2014). Children with a cleft lip and palate: An exploratory study of the role of the parent–child interaction. *Journal of Cranio-Maxillofacial Surgery, 42*(6), 953–958. https://doi.org/10.1016/j.jcms.2014.01.016

Goffman, E. (1963). *Stigma: Notes on the management of spoiled identity.* Prentice-Hall.

Goodman, M., Yacoub, R., Getahun, D., McCracken, C. E., Vupputuri, S., Lash, T. L., Roblin, D., Contreras, R., Cromwell, L., Gardner, M. D., Hoffman, T., Hu, H., Im, T. M., Prakash Asrani, R., Robinson, B., Xie, F., Nash, R., Zhang, Q., Bhai,

S. A., Venkatakrishnan, K., . . . Sandberg, D. E. (2022). Cohort profile: Pathways to care among people with disorders of sex development (DSD). *BMJ Open, 12*(9), e063409. https://doi.org/10.1136/bmjopen-2022-063409

Gravholt, C. H., Andersen, N. H., Conway, G. S., Dekkers, O. M., Geffner, M. E., Klein, K. O., Lin, A. E., Mauras, N., Quigley, C. A., Rubin, K., Sandberg, D. E., Sas, T. C. J., Silberbach, M., Söderström-Anttila, V., Stochholm, K., van Alfen-van derVelden, J. A., Woelfle, J., Backeljauw, P. F., & the International Turner Syndrome Consensus Group. (2017). Clinical practice guidelines for the care of girls and women with Turner syndrome: Proceedings from the 2016 Cincinnati International Turner Syndrome Meeting. *European Journal of Endocrinology, 177*(3), G1–G70. https://doi.org/10.1530/EJE-17-0430

Hansen-Moore, J. A., Kapa, H. M., Litteral, J. L., Nahata, L., Indyk, J. A., Jayanthi, V. R., Chan, Y. M., Tishelman, A. C., & Crerand, C. E. (2021). Psychosocial functioning among children with and without differences of sex development. *Journal of Pediatric Psychology, 46*(1), 69–79. https://doi.org/10.1093/jpepsy/jsaa089

Hartung, F., Jamrozik, A., Rosen, M. E., Aguirre, G., Sarwer, D. B., & Chatterjee, A. (2019). Behavioural and neural responses to facial disfigurement. *Scientific Reports, 9*(1), 8021. https://doi.org/10.1038/s41598-019-44408-8

Holmbeck, G. N., & Aspinall, C. L. (2015). Disorders of sex development: Lessons to be learned from studies of spina bifida and craniofacial conditions. *Hormone and Metabolic Research, 47*(5), 380–386. https://doi.org/10.1055/s-0035-1545273

Hughes, I. A., Houk, C., Ahmed, S. F., Lee, P. A., & the Lawson Wilkins Pediatric Endocrine Society/European Society for Pediatric Endocrinology Consensus Group. (2006). Consensus statement on management of intersex disorders. *Journal of Pediatric Urology, 2*(3), 148–162. https://doi.org/10.1016/j.jpurol.2006.03.004

Hutaff-Lee, C., Bennett, E., Howell, S., & Tartaglia, N. (2019). Clinical developmental, neuropsychological, and social-emotional features of Turner syndrome. *American Journal of Medical Genetics. Part C, Seminars in Medical Genetics, 181*(1), 42–50. https://doi.org/10.1002/ajmg.c.31687

Johns, A. L., Hershfield, J. A., Seifu, N. M., & Haynes, K. A. (2018). Postpartum depression in mothers of infants with cleft lip and/or palate. *The Journal of Craniofacial Surgery, 29*(4), e354–e358. https://doi.org/10.1097/SCS.0000000000004319

Johnson, E. K., Rosoklija, I., Finlayson, C., Chen, D., Yerkes, E. B., Madonna, M. B., Holl, J. L., Baratz, A. B., Davis, G., & Cheng, E. Y. (2017). Attitudes towards "disorders of sex development" nomenclature among affected individuals. *Journal of Pediatric Urology, 13*(6), 610–611. https://doi.org/10.1016/j.jpurol.2017.04.007

Kanhere, M., Fuqua, J., Rink, R., Houk, C., Mauger, D., & Lee, P. A. (2015). Psychosexual development and quality of life outcomes in females with congenital adrenal hyperplasia. *International Journal of Pediatric Endocrinology, 2015*(1), 21. https://doi.org/10.1186/s13633-015-0017-z

Kapp-Simon, K. A., & Gaither, R. (2016). Psychological and behavioral aspects of orofacial clefting. In J. E. Losee & R. E. Kirschner (Eds.), *Comprehensive cleft care* (pp. 383–392). Thieme.

Kleinemeier, E., Jürgensen, M., Lux, A., Widenka, P. M., Thyen, U., & the Disorders of Sex Development Network Working Group. (2010). Psychological adjustment and sexual development of adolescents with disorders of sex development. *Journal of Adolescent Health, 47*(5), 463–471. https://doi.org/10.1016/j.jadohealth.2010.03.007

Kling, J., Zelihić, D., Williamson, H., & Feragen, K. B. (2022). Is it safe? Exploring positive and negative outcome changes following a web-based intervention for adolescents distressed by a visible difference (YP Face IT). *Body Image, 43*, 8–16. https://doi.org/10.1016/j.bodyim.2022.07.012

Kremen, J., Davis, S. M., Nahata, L., Kapa, H. M., Dattilo, T. M., Liu, E., Hutaff-Lee, C., Tishelman, A. C., & Crerand, C. E. (2023). Neuropsychological and mental health concerns in a multicenter clinical sample of youth with Turner syndrome. *American Journal of Medical Genetics. Part A, 191*(4), 962–976. https://doi.org/10.1002/ajmg.a.63103

Kreukels, B. P. C., Köhler, B., Nordenström, A., Roehle, R., Thyen, U., Bouvattier, C., de Vries, A. L. C., Cohen-Kettenis, P. T., & the dsd-LIFE Group. (2018). Gender dysphoria and gender change in disorders of sex development/intersex conditions: Results from the dsd-LIFE study. *Journal of Sexual Medicine, 15*(5), 777–785. https://doi.org/10.1016/j.jsxm.2018.02.021

Langlois, J. H., Kalakanis, L., Rubenstein, A. J., Larson, A., Hallam, M., & Smoot, M. (2000). Maxims or myths of beauty? A meta-analytic and theoretical review. *Psychological Bulletin, 126*(3), 390–423. https://doi.org/10.1037/0033-2909.126.3.390

Lawlor, M. C., & Elliot, M. L. (2012). Physical disability and body image in children. In T. F. Cash (Ed.), *Encyclopedia of body image and human appearance* (pp. 650–656). Academic Press.

https://doi.org/10.1016/B978-0-12-384925-0.00102-4

Lawrence, B. J., Kerr, D., Pollard, C. M., Theophilus, M., Alexander, E., Haywood, D., & O'Connor, M. (2021). Weight bias among health care professionals: A systematic review and meta-analysis. *Obesity*, 29(11), 1802–1812. https://doi.org/10.1002/oby.23266

Lee, P. A., Nordenström, A., Houk, C. P., Ahmed, S. F., Auchus, R., Baratz, A., Baratz Dalke, K., Liao, L. M., Lin-Su, K., Looijenga, L. H., III, Mazur, T., Meyer-Bahlburg, H. F., Mouriquand, P., Quigley, C. A., Sandberg, D. E., Vilain, E., Witchel, S., & the Global DSD Update Consortium. (2016). Global disorders of sex development update since 2006: Perceptions, approach, and care. *Hormone Research in Paediatrics*, 85(3), 158–180. https://doi.org/10.1159/000442975

Lin-Su, K., Lekarev, O., Poppas, D. P., & Vogiatzi, M. G. (2015). Congenital adrenal hyperplasia patient perception of 'disorders of sex development' nomenclature. *International Journal of Pediatric Endocrinology*, 2015(1), 9. https://doi.org/10.1186/s13633-015-0004-4

Losee, J. E., & Kirschner, R. E. (Eds.). (2016). *Comprehensive cleft care* (2nd ed., Vols. 1 & 2). Thieme.

Mai, C. T., Isenburg, J. L., Canfield, M. A., Meyer, R. E., Correa, A., Alverson, C. J., Lupo, P. J., Riehle-Colarusso, T., Cho, S. J., Aggarwal, D., Kirby, R. S., & the National Birth Defects Prevention Network. (2019). National population-based estimates for major birth defects, 2010–2014. *Birth Defects Research*, 111(18), 1420–1435. https://doi.org/10.1002/bdr2.1589

Money, J. (1994). *Sex errors of the body and related syndromes: A guide to counseling children, adolescents, and their families*. Paul H. Brookes Publishing.

Money, J., Hampson, J. G., & Hampson, J. L. (1955). An examination of some basic sexual concepts: The evidence of human hermaphroditism. *Johns Hopkins Hospital Bulletin*, 97(4), 301–319.

Morris, L. A., Tishelman, A. C., Kremen, J., & Ross, R. A. (2020). Depression in Turner syndrome: A systematic review. *Archives of Sexual Behavior*, 49(2), 769–786. https://doi.org/10.1007/s10508-019-01549-1

Murray, L., Hentges, F., Hill, J., Karpf, J., Mistry, B., Kreutz, M., Woodall, P., Moss, T., Goodacre, T., & the Cleft Lip and Palate Study Team. (2008). The effect of cleft lip and palate, and the timing of lip repair on mother–infant interactions and infant development. *Journal of Child Psychology and Psychiatry*, 49(2), 115–123. https://doi.org/10.1111/j.1469-7610.2007.01833.x

Nelson, P., Glenny, A. M., Kirk, S., & Caress, A. L. (2012). Parents' experiences of caring for a child with a cleft lip and/or palate: A review of the literature. *Child: Care, Health and Development*, 38(1), 6–20. https://doi.org/10.1111/j.1365-2214.2011.01244.x

Nicholls, W., Harper, C., Robinson, S., Persson, M., & Selvey, L. (2018). Adult-specific life outcomes of cleft lip and palate in a Western Australian cohort. *The Cleft Palate Craniofacial Journal*, 55(10), 1419–1429. https://doi.org/10.1177/1055665618768540

Nidey, N., Moreno Uribe, L. M., Marazita, M. M., & Wehby, G. L. (2016). Psychosocial well-being of parents of children with oral clefts. *Child: Care, Health and Development*, 42(1), 42–50. https://doi.org/10.1111/cch.12276

Nordenström, A., & Thyen, U. (2014). Improving the communication of healthcare professionals with affected children and adolescents. *Endocrine Development*, 27, 113–127. https://doi.org/10.1159/000363636

Norman, A., Persson, M., Stock, N., Rumsey, N., Sandy, J., Waylen, A., Edwards, Z., Hammond, V., Partridge, L., & Ness, A. (2015). The effectiveness of psychosocial intervention for individuals with cleft lip and/or palate. *The Cleft Palate Craniofacial Journal*, 52(3), 301–310. https://doi.org/10.1597/13-276

Pasterski, V., Mastroyannopoulou, K., Wright, D., Zucker, K. J., & Hughes, I. A. (2014). Predictors of posttraumatic stress in parents of children diagnosed with a disorder of sex development. *Archives of Sexual Behavior*, 43(2), 369–375. https://doi.org/10.1007/s10508-013-0196-8

Pescosolido, B. A., & Martin, J. K. (2015). The stigma complex. *Annual Review of Sociology*, 41(1), 87–116. https://doi.org/10.1146/annurev-soc-071312-145702

Pfeifauf, K. D., Cooper, D. C., Gibson, E., Skolnick, G. B., Naidoo, S. D., Snyder-Warwick, A. K., & Patel, K. B. (2022). Factors contributing to delay or absence of alveolar bone grafting. *American Journal of Orthodontics and Dentofacial Orthopedics*, 161(6), 820–828.e1. https://doi.org/10.1016/j.ajodo.2021.01.033

Pope, A. W., & Snyder, H. T. (2005). Psychosocial adjustment in children and adolescents with a craniofacial anomaly: Age and sex patterns. *The Cleft Palate Craniofacial Journal*, 42(4), 349–354. https://doi.org/10.1597/04-043r.1

Quinn, D. M., & Earnshaw, V. A. (2013). Concealable stigmatized identities and psychological well-being. *Social and Personality Psychology Compass*, 7(1), 40–51. https://doi.org/10.1111/spc3.12005

Rapp, M., Duranteau, L., van de Grift, T. C., Schober, J., Hirschberg, A. L., Krege, S., Nordenstrom, A., Roehle, R., Thyen, U., Bouvattier, C., Kreukels, B. P. C., Nordenskjold, A., Kohler, B., Neumann, U., Cohen-Kettenis, P., Kreukels, B., de Vries, A., Arlt, W., Wiesemann, C., . . . Szarras-Czapnik, M. (2021). Self- and proxy-reported outcomes after surgery in people with disorders/differences of sex development (DSD) in Europe (dsd-LIFE). *Journal of Pediatric Urology, 17*(3), 353–365. https://doi.org/10.1016/j.jpurol.2020.12.007

Richman, L. C., McCoy, T. E., Conrad, A. L., & Nopoulos, P. C. (2012). Neuropsychological, behavioral, and academic sequelae of cleft: Early developmental, school age, and adolescent/young adult outcomes. *The Cleft Palate Craniofacial Journal, 49*(4), 387–396. https://doi.org/10.1597/10-237

Roberts, R. M., Neate, G. M., & Gierasch, A. (2017). Implicit attitudes towards people with visible difference: Findings from an implicit association test. *Psychology, Health & Medicine, 22*(3), 352–358. https://doi.org/10.1080/13548506.2016.1163399

Roen, K., & Pasterski, V. (2014). Psychological research and intersex/DSD: Recent developments and future directions. *Psychology & Sexuality, 5*(1), 102–116. https://doi.org/10.1080/19419899.2013.831218

Ross, J. L., Roeltgen, D. P., Kushner, H., Zinn, A. R., Reiss, A., Bardsley, M. Z., McCauley, E., & Tartaglia, N. (2012). Behavioral and social phenotypes in boys with 47,XYY syndrome or 47,XXY Klinefelter syndrome. *Pediatrics, 129*(4), 769–778. https://doi.org/10.1542/peds.2011-0719

Rumsey, N., & Harcourt, D. (2007). Visible difference amongst children and adolescents: Issues and interventions. *Developmental Neurorehabilitation, 10*(2), 113–123. https://doi.org/10.1080/13638490701217396

Sandberg, D. E., Gardner, M., Callens, N., Mazur, T., & the DSD-TRN Psychosocial Workgroup, the DSD-TRN Advocacy Advisory Network, and Accord Alliance. (2017). Interdisciplinary care in disorders/differences of sex development (DSD): The psychosocial component of the DSD-Translational research network. *American Journal of Medical Genetics. Part C, Seminars in Medical Genetics, 175*(2), 279–292. https://doi.org/10.1002/ajmg.c.31561

Sandberg, D. E., Gardner, M., & Cohen-Kettenis, P. T. (2012). Psychological aspects of the treatment of patients with disorders of sex development. *Seminars in Reproductive Medicine, 30*(5), 443–452. https://doi.org/10.1055/s-0032-1324729

Sandberg, D. E., Meyer-Bahlburg, H. F., Hensle, T. W., Levitt, S. B., Kogan, S. J., & Reda, E. F. (2001). Psychosocial adaptation of middle childhood boys with hypospadias after genital surgery. *Journal of Pediatric Psychology, 26*(8), 465–475. https://doi.org/10.1093/jpepsy/26.8.465

Scambler, G. (2009). Health-related stigma. *Sociology of Health & Illness, 31*(3), 441–455. https://doi.org/10.1111/j.1467-9566.2009.01161.x

Schönbucher, V., Schweizer, K., Rustige, L., Schützmann, K., Brunner, F., & Richter-Appelt, H. (2012). Sexual quality of life of individuals with 46,XY disorders of sex development. *Journal of Sexual Medicine, 9*(12), 3154–3170. https://doi.org/10.1111/j.1743-6109.2009.01639.x

Schweizer, K., Brunner, F., Gedrose, B., Handford, C., & Richter-Appelt, H. (2017). Coping with diverse sex development: Treatment experiences and psychosocial support during childhood and adolescence and adult well-being. *Journal of Pediatric Psychology, 42*(5), 504–519. https://doi.org/10.1093/jpepsy/jsw058

Şentürk Pilan, B., Özbaran, B., Çelik, D., Özcan, I., Özen, S., Gökşen, D., Ulman, İ., Avanoğlu, A., Tiryaki, S., Onay, H., Çoğulu, Ö., Özkınay, F., & Darcan, Ş. (2021). Quality of life and psychological well-being in children and adolescents with disorders of sex development. *Journal of Clinical Research in Pediatric Endocrinology, 13*(1), 23–33. https://doi.org/10.4274/jcrpe.galenos.2020.2020.0141

Siminoff, L. A., & Sandberg, D. E. (2015). Promoting shared decision making in disorders of sex development (DSD): Decision aids and support tools. *Hormone and Metabolic Research, 47*(5), 335–339. https://doi.org/10.1055/s-0035-1545302

Skakkebæk, A., Gravholt, C. H., Chang, S., Moore, P. J., & Wallentin, M. (2020). Psychological functioning, brain morphology, and functional neuroimaging in Klinefelter syndrome. *American Journal of Medical Genetics Part C, Seminars in Medical Genetics, 184*(2), 506–517. https://doi.org/10.1002/ajmg.c.31806

Smolak, L. (2012). Body image development—Girl children. In T. F. Cash (Ed.), *Encyclopedia of body image and human appearance* (pp. 212–218). Academic Press. https://doi.org/10.1016/B978-0-12-384925-0.00033-X

Stangl, A. L., Earnshaw, V. A., Logie, C. H., van Brakel, W., Simbayi, L. C., Barré, I., & Dovidio, J. F. (2019). The Health Stigma and Discrimination Framework: A global, cross-cutting framework to inform research, intervention development, and policy on health-related stigmas. *BMC Medicine, 17*(1), 31. https://doi.org/10.1186/s12916-019-1271-3

Stock, N. M., Costa, B., White, P., & Rumsey, N. (2020). Risk and protective factors for psychological distress in families following a diagnosis of cleft lip and/or palate. *The Cleft Palate Craniofacial Journal*, 57(1), 88–98. https://doi.org/10.1177/1055665619862457

Stock, N. M., & Feragen, K. B. (2016). Psychological adjustment to cleft lip and/or palate: A narrative review of the literature. *Psychology & Health*, 31(7), 777–813. https://doi.org/10.1080/08870446.2016.1143944

Stock, N. M., Marik, P., Magee, L., Aspinall, C. L., Garcia, L., Crerand, C., & Johns, A. (2020). Facilitating positive psychosocial outcomes in craniofacial team care: Strategies for medical providers. *The Cleft Palate Craniofacial Journal*, 57(3), 333–343. https://doi.org/10.1177/1055665619868052

Stock, N. M., & Ridley, M. (2018). Young person and parent perspectives on the impact of cleft lip and/or palate within an educational setting. *The Cleft Palate Craniofacial Journal*, 55(4), 607–614. https://doi.org/10.1177/1055665617734991

Stock, N. M., Ridley, M., & Guest, E. (2019). Teachers' perspectives on the impact of cleft lip and/or palate during the school years. *The Cleft Palate Craniofacial Journal*, 56(2), 204–209. https://doi.org/10.1177/1055665618770191

Stock, N. M., Stoneman, K., Cunniffe, C., & Rumsey, N. (2016). The psychosocial impact of cleft lip and/or palate on unaffected siblings. *The Cleft Palate Craniofacial Journal*, 53(6), 670–682. https://doi.org/10.1597/15-148

Tishelman, A. C., Hansen-Moore, J., & Crerand, C. E. (2019). Disorders of sex development. In S. Hupp & J. D. Jewell (Eds.), *The encyclopedia of child and adolescent development*. John Wiley & Sons. https://doi.org/10.1002/9781119171492

Traino, K. A., Baudino, M. N., Kraft, J. D., Basile, N. L., Dattilo, T. M., Davis, M. P., Buchanan, C., Cheng, E. Y., Poppas, D. P., Wisniewski, A. B., & Mullins, L. L. (2021). Factor analysis of the Stigma Scale—Parent version in pediatric disorders/differences of sex development. *Stigma and Health*, 6(4), 390–396. https://doi.org/10.1037/sah0000346

Traino, K. A., Roberts, C. M., Fisher, R. S., Delozier, A. M., Austin, P. F., Baskin, L. S., Chan, Y. M., Cheng, E. Y., Diamond, D. A., Fried, A. J., Kropp, B., Lakshmanan, Y., Meyer, S. Z., Meyer, T., Buchanan, C., Palmer, B. W., Paradis, A., Reyes, K. J., Tishelman, A., . . . Wisniewski, A. B. (2022). Stigma, intrusiveness, and distress in parents of children with a disorder/difference of sex development. *Journal of Developmental and Behavioral Pediatrics*, 43(7), e473–e482. https://doi.org/10.1097/DBP.0000000000001077

Tsuchiya, S., Tsuchiya, M., Momma, H., Koseki, T., Igarashi, K., Nagatomi, R., Arima, T., Yaegashi, N., & the Japan Environment & Children's Study Group. (2019). Association of cleft lip and palate on mother-to-infant bonding: A cross-sectional study in the Japan Environment and Children's Study (JECS). *BMC Pediatrics*, 19(1), 505. https://doi.org/10.1186/s12887-019-1877-9

Turriff, A., Levy, H. P., & Biesecker, B. (2011). Prevalence and psychosocial correlates of depressive symptoms among adolescents and adults with Klinefelter syndrome. *Genetics in Medicine*, 13(11), 966–972. https://doi.org/10.1097/GIM.0b013e3182227576

van der Zwan, Y. G., Callens, N., van Kuppenveld, J., Kwak, K., Drop, S. L., Kortmann, B., Dessens, A. B., Wolffenbuttel, K. P., & the Dutch Study Group on DSD. (2013). Long-term outcomes in males with disorders of sex development. *The Journal of Urology*, 190(3), 1038–1042. https://doi.org/10.1016/j.juro.2013.03.029

Varni, J. W., Seid, M., & Kurtin, P. S. (2001). PedsQL 4.0: Reliability and validity of the Pediatric Quality of Life Inventory version 4.0 generic core scales in healthy and patient populations. *Medical Care*, 39(8), 800–812. https://doi.org/10.1097/00005650-200108000-00006

Wallander, J., & Varni, J. (1992). Adjustment in children with chronic physical disorders: Programmatic research on a disability-stress-coping model. In A. M. La Greca, L. J. Siegel, J. L. Wallander, & C. E. Walker (Eds.), *Stress and coping in child health* (pp. 279–298). Guilford Press.

Wehby, G. L., Collet, B., Barron, S., Romitti, P. A., Ansley, T. N., & Speltz, M. (2014). Academic achievement of children and adolescents with oral clefts. *Pediatrics*, 133(5), 785–792. https://doi.org/10.1542/peds.2013-3072

Weidler, E. M., Suorsa-Johnson, K. I., Baskin, A. S., Fagerlin, A., Gardner, M. D., Rutter, M. M., Schafer-Kalkhoff, T., van Leeuwen, K., & Sandberg, D. E. (2023). "It became easier once I knew": Stakeholder perspectives for educating children and teenagers about their difference of sex development. *Patient Education and Counseling*, 113, 107763. https://doi.org/10.1016/j.pec.2023.107763

Williamson, H., Hamlet, C., White, P., Marques, E. M. R., Paling, T., Cadogan, J., Perera, R., Rumsey, N., Hayward, L., & Harcourt, D. (2019). A web-based self-help psychosocial intervention for adolescents distressed by appearance-affecting conditions and injuries (Young Persons' Face IT): Feasibility study for a parallel randomized controlled trial. *JMIR Mental Health*, 6(11), e14776. https://doi.org/10.2196/14776

Wilson, E., Crudgington, H., Morgan, C., Hirsch, C., Prina, M., & Gayer-Anderson, C. (2023). The longitudinal course of childhood bullying victimization and associations with self-injurious thoughts and behaviors in children and young people: A systematic review of the literature. *Journal of Adolescence*, 95(1), 5–33. https://doi.org/10.1002/jad.12097

Wisniewski, A. B., Batista, R. L., Costa, E. M. F., Finlayson, C., Sircili, M. H. P., Dénes, F. T., Domenice, S., & Mendonca, B. B. (2019). Management of 46,XY differences/disorders of sex development (DSD) throughout life. *Endocrine Reviews*, 40(6), 1547–1572. https://doi.org/10.1210/er.2019-00049

Wolodiger, E. D., & Pope, A. W. (2019). Associations between parenting stress at school entry and later psychosocial adjustment: A longitudinal study of children with congenital craniofacial anomalies. *The Cleft Palate Craniofacial Journal*, 56(4), 487–494. https://doi.org/10.1177/1055665618781371

Wong Riff, K. W. Y., Tsangaris, E., Goodacre, T. E. E., Forrest, C. R., Lawson, J., Pusic, A. L., & Klassen, A. F. (2018). What matters to patients with cleft lip and/or palate: An international qualitative study informing the development of the CLEFT-Q. *The Cleft Palate Craniofacial Journal*, 55(3), 442–450. https://doi.org/10.1177/1055665617732854

Yarosh, D. B. (2019). Perception and deception: Human beauty and the brain. *Behavioral Sciences*, 9(4), 34. https://doi.org/10.3390/bs9040034

Yau, M., Vogiatzi, M., Lewkowitz-Shpuntoff, A., Nimkarn, S., & Lin-Su, K. (2015). Health-related quality of life in children with congenital adrenal hyperplasia. *Hormone Research in Paediatrics*, 84(3), 165–171. https://doi.org/10.1159/000435855

Zeytinoğlu, S., Davey, M. P., Crerand, C., Fisher, K., & Akyil, Y. (2017). Experiences of couples caring for a child born with cleft lip and/or palate: Impact of the timing of diagnosis. *Journal of Marital and Family Therapy*, 43(1), 82–99. https://doi.org/10.1111/jmft.12182

CHAPTER 9

PEDIATRIC CENTRAL NERVOUS SYSTEM DISORDERS: SPINA BIFIDA, EPILEPSY, AND TRAUMATIC BRAIN INJURY

Grayson N. Holmbeck, Dhanashree Bahulekar, Olivia E. Clark, Julie Doran, Aimee W. Smith, Amery Treble-Barna, and Adrien M. Winning

This chapter reviews three relatively common disorders of the central nervous system (CNS), namely spina bifida (SB), epilepsy, and traumatic brain injury (TBI), from the perspectives of pediatric psychology, developmental-behavioral pediatrics, and developmental science. Although there is variability both within and across these three conditions, considerable overlap has been found across these three conditions with respect to their impact on the family and child outcomes. A developmental science perspective is adopted throughout the chapter, drawing on ecological systems theory whereby multiple contexts (e.g., individual, family, community, cultural, and the health care system) are expected to impact on important child outcomes across each of these three conditions (Bronfenbrenner, 1977; Modi et al., 2012). Coverage for each condition is subdivided into the following sections: epidemiology; etiology/prognosis; clinical presentation and developmental course; diversity and equity; individual and family outcomes: a developmental perspective; risk and resilience; transition to adult health care; and clinical management. The sections on spina bifida and epilepsy also cover self-management and adherence. We also provide recommendations for clinical interventions and future research.

Throughout this chapter, linkages between pediatric psychology, developmental-behavioral pediatrics, and developmental science will be highlighted, furthering our understanding of these three CNS conditions. Pediatric psychologists often work alongside developmental-behavioral pediatricians (e.g., in integrated primary care settings; Stancin & Perrin, 2014); both of these disciplines adopt an evidence-based perspective in their work that draws extensively on research from the field of developmental science. Whereas developmental-behavioral pediatricians typically monitor overall development and health outcomes, pediatric psychologists can conduct more fine-grained assessments of neuropsychological functioning as well as screenings for mood and behavioral concerns. Moreover, pediatric psychologists can implement brief interventions focused on, for example, parenting or child behavioral concerns. Developmental-behavioral pediatricians and pediatric psychologists together serve as advocates for recommended educational and community services, based on family needs.

Completion of this chapter was supported in part by research grants from the National Institute of Child Health and Human Development (R01 HD048629) and the March of Dimes Birth Defects Foundation (12-FY13-271).

https://doi.org/10.1037/0000414-009

APA Handbook of Pediatric Psychology, Developmental-Behavioral Pediatrics, and Developmental Science: Vol. 2. Pediatric Psychology and Developmental-Behavioral Pediatrics: Clinical Applications of Developmental Science, P. E. Shah and M. H. Bornstein (Editors-in-Chief)
Copyright © 2025 by the American Psychological Association. All rights reserved.

Finally, contributions of research from the field of developmental science provide a much needed understanding of brain development over time across these three CNS conditions, as well as information on growth in cognitive and functional outcomes across differing social contexts. At the most basic level, a developmental perspective is critical to understanding the impact over time of these three conditions (Holmbeck et al., 2008). Indeed, concepts from developmental science such as developmental trajectories, resilience, and multifinality (i.e., two children with the same condition at the same level of severity often develop along differing pathways with very different medical and psychological outcomes) are critical to understanding how particular conditions unfold over time (Holmbeck, 2002).

SPINA BIFIDA

Epidemiology

SB is the most common congenital birth defect affecting the CNS, occurring in roughly 1 out of every 2758 live births in the United States (Centers for Disease Control and Prevention [CDC], 2020). Of note, there are differences in incidence across ethnic groups. Latin American women have the highest rate of SB incidence: roughly 3.80 of every 10,000 live births have SB, as compared to 2.73 of every 10,000 live births in African American populations and 3.09 of every 10,000 live births in European American populations (CDC, 2020).

Etiology/Prognosis

SB develops during early pregnancy when the neural tube fails to fully close (Copp et al., 2015). Specifically, during the formation of the nervous system, the neural tube zips up and closes from the middle (i.e., the caudal end of the hindbrain) in both directions (Sadler, 2005). In children who have SB, the posterior region of the neural tube fails to close and, as a result, the spinal cord is exposed to the amniotic fluid environment in utero. This toxic exposure leads to the death of neurons and ultimately impacts physical functioning below the level of the lesion (Copp et al., 2015). Although advancements in medical care have improved long-term survival rates, the mortality rate for individuals with SB remains significantly higher than the general population (i.e., about 1% per year from 5 to 30 years of age; Oakeshott et al., 2010).

Notably, there are four types of SB that vary in severity. *Occulta* is the mildest form in which there is a small gap in the spine, no open lesion or fluid filled sack, and generally no symptoms or associated disabilities. *Lipomeningocele* is another type of SB that is characterized by intact skin and a fatty tumor that covers the spine. It is associated with mild forms of disability, such as motor challenges and/or bladder and bowel dysfunction. A third type of SB is *meningocele*, which develops when the spinal fluid and meninges protrude through a vertebral opening into a skin-covered sack. The spinal cord remains intact; individuals with meningoceles rarely experience physical dysfunction. Finally, *myelomeningocele* is the most severe and common form of SB, in which the spinal cord and associated nerves protrude through a vertebral opening and are either exposed or covered by a fluid-filled sack, resulting in a moderate-to-severe physical disability (see a more detailed overview in the next section). Additional abnormalities in the brain and spine that commonly accompany myelomeningocele, in particular, are the Chiari II malformation (i.e., part of the cerebellum and brain stem extend into the spinal canal via foramen magnum), hydrocephalus (i.e., excessive buildup of cerebrospinal fluid on the brain, often treated with a shunt placement), and tethered cord (i.e., spinal cord becomes tethered or fixed to tissue in the spinal canal; Copp et al., 2015; Sandler, 2010).

The underlying cause of SB remains unknown. However, multiple genetic, nutritional, and environmental factors increase the risk of having a child with SB. Indeed, risk for SB is higher for children who have a sibling with the condition and among certain ethnic groups, suggesting a major genetic component in causation (Copp et al., 2015). Apart from genetics, inadequate maternal folic acid consumption and obesity have been identified as significant risk factors (Copp et al., 2015). Exposure to environmental toxins, such as pollutants, may also contribute to the development of SB (Copp et al., 2015).

Clinical Presentation and Developmental Course

There is significant variability in the clinical presentation of SB. Individuals with myelomeningocele, the most common form of SB accounting for approximately 78% of cases, generally experience motor and sensory difficulties below the level of the spinal cord lesion as well as significant neurological features (CDC, 2020; Copp et al., 2015; Driscoll, Ohanian, et al., 2018). Specifically, lower limb limitations may limit or prevent ambulation, potentially requiring use of a wheelchair, braces, and/or crutches, and increasing risk for pressure injuries. Furthermore, neurogenic bladder and bowel function require use of catheterization and bowel program adherence (Copp et al., 2015). Additional comorbidities associated with SB include latex allergy, neurobehavioral challenges (e.g., socioemotional difficulties, learning disabilities), and obesity (Copp et al., 2015; Spina Bifida Association, 2018). Corrective surgeries are beneficial (e.g., tethered cord release), and surgical techniques may offer some potential for prevention (e.g., in utero lesion repair), but SB is a lifelong condition, and complications persist throughout the lifespan. Sequelae associated with SB, and risk and protective factors associated with outcomes, are described in greater detail in later sections.

Diversity and Equity

Most past research examining the impact of SB on individuals and their families has utilized samples comprised of European American, middle-class families from Western cultures. Clearly, more attention is needed to learn how the presence of SB may impact individuals and families differently depending on the presence of various diversity characteristics (e.g., cultural, ethnicity, language, age, gender, sexual orientation, religion, geographic location, socioeconomic status (SES), education, family structure, disability status). The few studies that have examined ethnic differences among individuals with SB have found differences in health-related and psychosocial outcomes (e.g., urinary and bowel incontinence, school achievement, IQ, parenting satisfaction, perceived competence as a parent, parental perceptions of child vulnerability; Chowanadisai et al., 2013; Devine, Holbein, et al., 2012; Swartwout et al., 2010). Limited existing research also suggests that family health-related belief systems are often culturally rooted (Ohanian et al., 2018). As such, families from collectivist cultures (where the needs of the group are valued more than the needs of individuals), as opposed to more individualistic Western cultures (where individual independence is highly valued), may have different expectations regarding autonomy and independence.

Certain sociodemographic factors may also put youth at risk for poorer outcomes (Papadakis & Holmbeck, 2021). Notably, the estimated lifetime cost of a child with SB is approximately $600,000, a value composed of medical costs, special education costs, caregiver needs, and other expenses, which place individuals with limited financial means at a disadvantage when accessing treatment and resources (Copp et al., 2015). Families living in areas with minimal health care infrastructure may also experience challenges accessing necessary, coordinated care (Spina Bifida Association, 2018); such challenges could be mitigated by use of telehealth and eHealth strategies (Cushing, 2017).

Individual and Family Outcomes: A Developmental Perspective

Social-emotional outcomes and quality of life. Youth with SB are at increased risk for internalizing symptoms (e.g., anxiety, depression) and reduced health-related quality of life (HRQoL) compared to typically developing children and/or children with other medical conditions (Copp et al., 2015; Holmbeck & Devine, 2010). Internalizing symptoms tend to emerge during later childhood and adolescence, whereas reductions in HRQoL are present across development (Copp et al., 2015).

Academic achievement and educational attainment. Broadly, youth with SB demonstrate poorer school performance and grades than comparison peers (Holmbeck et al., 2003). Youth are also at risk of learning problems (Holmbeck et al., 2003), with one study finding that 60% of children with SB had a specific learning disability in reading, writing, and/or math (Mayes & Calhoun, 2006); such disabilities can be identified during developmental-behavioral pediatricians' screenings or pediatric psychologists' more detailed neuropsychological assessments. Evidence suggests that these academic problems endure from childhood into adolescence (Holmbeck et al., 2010). During adulthood, individuals with SB are less likely to attend college, and they have lower rates of employment (Copp et al., 2015).

Family relationships. Parents of youth with SB often experience higher levels of psychological distress (e.g., anxiety, depression) and stress than comparison parents who do not have a child with a chronic health condition (Holmbeck & Devine, 2010). Parents often report feeling socially isolated, less competent and satisfied as parents, and less optimistic about the future (Holmbeck & Devine, 2010). Certain groups of parents, such as those who are single, from lower SES backgrounds, and from an ethnic minority group, are at greater risk of experiencing such difficulties (Holmbeck & Devine, 2010). Overall, past work supports a resilience-disruption view of family functioning, such that families demonstrate disruptions in some domains (e.g., youth may be more dependent on parents and less likely to state their own views and opinions in family conversations) and resilience in others (e.g., youth exhibit less conflict with parents during the transition to adolescence; Lennon, Murray, et al., 2015).

Peer relationships. Children with SB master some fundamental social skills (e.g., asking a friend to get together; Devine, Holmbeck, et al., 2012; see also Volume 1, Chapter 12, this handbook). Despite this, children with SB, and especially those with more neuropsychological deficits, are also at risk for experiencing social isolation and social difficulties (e.g., fewer friendships and interactions outside of school, social skills deficits) and tend to demonstrate passivity in their interactions with others (Holbein et al., 2017; Holmbeck & Devine, 2010; Holmbeck et al., 2003). Such social difficulties can persist as youth transition into later adolescence and early adulthood. Indeed, emerging adults with SB are also less likely to be in romantic relationships than are their typically developing peers; they report needing additional support from health care providers in navigating such relationships (Heller et al., 2016; Verhoef et al., 2005).

Risk and Resilience

Risk factors. Multiple risk factors have been linked to poorer outcomes in individuals with SB. With regard to individual factors, lesion level is associated with functional outcomes, such that individuals with higher lesion levels typically experience higher levels of impairment (Schechter et al., 2015). Those shunted for hydrocephalus are also at risk for lower HRQoL (Copp et al., 2015). In early childhood, these indicators of SB severity (e.g., presence of a shunt, higher lesion level) have also been linked to fewer motor skills and slower cognitive growth over time (Lomax-Bream et al., 2007). Of note, males with SB are less likely to be continent and ambulatory than females with SB, perhaps linked to biological differences, and/or differences in societal expectations.

In terms of environmental factors, greater sociodemographic risk is broadly associated with more pain, lower HRQoL, and less family cohesion (Papadakis & Holmbeck, 2021). Individuals with SB who have private insurance tend to surpass those without private insurance regarding physical functioning (continence, ambulation), perhaps associated with differences in income that may impact access to health care services, health literacy, and community resources. Further, African American individuals with SB tend to be less continent than individuals with SB belonging to other racial/ethnic groups, although evidence is lacking and requires further investigation to understand social forces impacting this pattern of outcomes (Schechter et al., 2015).

Resilience factors. Several factors have also been identified that may support resilience in the context of SB. Specifically, older age, urological surgery, household educational status, and improved physical functioning are all positively associated with resilience in adults with SB (Showen et al., 2021). Additionally, factors such as having a college education and being employed or a full-time student have been linked to more benefit finding (i.e., deriving benefit from adversity) as individuals with SB transition into young adulthood (Kritikos et al., 2022).

Self-Management and Adherence

Youth with SB often must adhere to a complex medical regimen, which includes catheterization, bowel program management, and monitoring for pressure injuries and shunt malfunctions. Transition of responsibility for self-management tasks from caregivers to individuals with SB is essential for developing autonomy, independence, and a sense of mastery (Spina Bifida Association, 2018). Most youth with SB (roughly ⅔) gain medical responsibility over the course of late childhood and early adolescence, but those who do not are more likely to be male, have lower IQs and executive dysfunction, and come from families with higher levels of stress (Greenley, 2010; Kayle et al., 2020). Also, youth responsibility is lower in families with parents who are more intrusive or overprotective and/or perceive their children as medically more vulnerable, which itself appears to arise from higher levels of parental maladjustment (Driscoll et al., 2020).

Medical adherence is the degree to which an individual's management of their condition is consistent with treatment recommendations. Importantly, individuals with SB must adhere to a complex multicomponent treatment regimen while *at the same time* managing a unique array of cognitive and psychosocial challenges and comorbidities that hinder self-management and medical adherence (Holmbeck et al., 2021). Such adherence is improved when the individual exhibits lower levels of condition severity, fewer neuropsychological deficits, and a clear understanding of the importance of the medical regimen. Individuals also benefit from parents who have effective problem-solving skills and the ability to transfer medical responsibilities gradually (Stern et al., 2020). Both developmental-behavioral pediatricians and pediatric psychologists can assess the degree to which the self-management and adherence processes are being managed in a developmentally appropriate manner; such processes could be targets for brief interventions.

Transition to Adult Health Care

Transition to adult health care is an essential part of maintaining health and quality of life (QoL) for individuals with SB and supports independent management and direction of care throughout the lifespan (see Volume 1, Chapter 16, this handbook). Importantly, such youth endure multiple transitions to adult health care (e.g., in the areas of urology, orthopedics, neurosurgery, and primary care) that may unfold across different timeframes. Developmentally appropriate transitions can begin around age 12–14 in youth with SB, with increased child involvement with age in medical care, medical appointment-making, and navigating insurance coverage (Driscoll, Ohanian, et al., 2018). The roles of the medical team members who are instrumental in fostering this transition are described in greater detail in the following sections. Finally, three transition-related constructs need to be assessed as part of the larger transition construct, namely:

1. Transition readiness (which encompasses knowledge and behaviors related to self-care, self-advocacy, and decision-making skills that are required for a successful transition).
2. Transition completion (for the transition from pediatric to adult health care).
3. Transition success (which would occur when the transition to adult health care is accompanied by few secondary health complications).

Clinical Management

Individuals with SB require lifelong, extensive, and active treatment from an interdisciplinary team that focuses on bladder and bowel management, mobility, skin care, self-care activities and health care maintenance, psychological well-being, education and vocational counseling, social services, recreation and leisure time activities, and prevention and management of complications. Up to one-half of youth hospitalizations are due to potentially preventable conditions, such as urinary tract infections and pressure injuries (Mahmood et al., 2011). The ultimate goal in treating youth with SB is for them to experience satisfying and productive lives as independently functioning and healthy adults in society (Zebracki et al., 2010). Providing anticipatory guidance to parents and caregivers, such as long-term implications of living with a disability, is crucial as youth transition through various developmental stages.

Medical assessment. Medical assessment is the most prevalent method of SB diagnosis; prenatal anatomy scans are the primary approach to diagnosis. The fetal spine and cranial features indicative of SB can be examined at the end of the first trimester via ultrasound (Copp et al., 2015). Once SB has been diagnosed, early intervention (i.e., surgery to close the spinal cord, shunt placement if necessary) should be a priority. Ongoing medical assessment and monitoring are required to manage potential secondary complications in youth with SB.

Psychological assessment. Given the array of cognitive, psychosocial, and learning impairments that are commonly present in SB, regular comprehensive neuropsychological, psychosocial, psychoeducational, and speech and language evaluations are strongly recommended to monitor functioning and to provide recommendations for intervention and treatment (Deaton & Castaldi, 2011). Youth with SB myelomeningocele typically demonstrate strengths in rule-based processing and weaknesses in more fluid reasoning domains. Neuropsychological assessments should also evaluate social language, visual-motor integration, spatial reasoning, attention, and executive functions. In addition, youth with SB are at risk for depressive symptoms, medical adherence difficulties, social challenges, and difficulty with gaining independence, which should be monitored throughout development (Spina Bifida Association, 2018).

Based on current pediatric care models, children with SB are usually seen at least annually in a SB multidisciplinary clinic (Thibadeau et al., 2020). Brief screeners can be incorporated into multidisciplinary clinic visits to identify those with mood, behavioral, and/or cognitive concerns, and then appropriately refer these individuals for more comprehensive assessments as needed. Assessments targeting transition readiness and self-management skills are also particularly important from ages 12–17 to appropriately tailor the transition to adult health care (Fremion & Dosa, 2019). Finally, current neuropsychological guidelines recommend administering infant development scales that assess cognitive, language, motor, and social development in children with SB ages 0–3 years, particularly those with myelomeningocele or other clinical risk factors (e.g., severe Chiari II malformation). Children with such risk factors should be closely monitored as they age and undergo a full neuropsychological evaluation if concerns emerge (Spina Bifida Association, 2018).

Is diagnosis the role/responsibility of the general pediatrician? As SB is typically diagnosed during gestation, the responsibility of diagnosis typically falls to the obstetrician during anatomical scans and prenatal testing. That said, some minor cases of SB are diagnosed postnatally by the family doctor or the developmental-behavioral pediatrician (Copp et al., 2015).

What is the role of developmental-behavioral pediatricians? Developmental-behavioral pediatricians, especially those with expertise in neurodevelopmental disabilities, are uniquely situated to provide families with current evidence-based information regarding the medical needs and functional goals of those with SB across the lifespan (Spina Bifida Association, 2018). Such providers play an important role in monitoring and assessing the development of young children with SB, providing appropriate referrals and recommendations (e.g., for school services and therapies), helping families access necessary medical care, and monitoring academic, social, and functional adaptation across the lifespan.

What is the role of pediatric psychologists?
In addition to the medical team, pediatric psychologists can provide important psychoeducation about SB, common secondary health complications, and potential developmental and psychosocial challenges (Spina Bifida Association, 2018). Pediatric psychologists also play a vital role in monitoring youth for psychosocial and neuropsychological concerns as well as problems adhering to medical regimen. Their role is essential in preventing major psychosocial and medical regimen difficulties. Indeed, if difficulties within these domains are detected, pediatric psychologists can implement appropriate psychological interventions (e.g., behavioral strategies to improve medical adherence, coping skills) and make referrals for neuropsychological testing and outpatient psychotherapy. By partnering with patients and their families, psychologists can also help families openly communicate with health care providers about expectations regarding developmental milestones (e.g., responsibilities of parents vs. youth for self-care and medical self-management) and successfully transfer increasingly more medical responsibility to youth as they transition to adult health care. Pediatric psychologists often provide services within outpatient (including integrated primary care settings), multidisciplinary clinics, as well as inpatient settings.

What is the role of subspecialty/multidisciplinary clinics?
Considering the complex medical presentation of SB, an interdisciplinary team is important to promote the best possible outcomes. Multidisciplinary clinics that include providers from a variety of specialties (e.g., neurosurgery, orthopedic surgery, rehabilitation, urology, psychology) allow for immediate, open communication between providers to facilitate comprehensive clinical care. Many medical providers do not routinely care for individuals with SB, so specialized clinics ensure that the needs of those with SB are appropriately managed (Spina Bifida Association, 2018).

Recommendations for Clinical Interventions and Research

Clinical recommendations. In contrast to the extensive literature on evidence-based interventions for other chronic physical conditions (e.g., Type 1 diabetes), there is a lack of such interventions for families of young people with SB (Holmbeck et al., 2006). More generally, with only two exceptions (Betz et al., 2010; Stubberud et al., 2015), no randomized clinical trials (RCTs) have been reported for this population across all psychosocial domains. Other preliminary work points to the need for RCTs. For example, a manualized summer camp-based intervention was developed that targets independence and social skills among children, adolescents, and young adults with SB (Holbein et al., 2013; O'Mahar et al., 2010), but an RCT focused on this intervention has not yet been conducted. More generally, we need more developmentally informed psychosocial interventions across nearly every affected area of functioning for youth with SB and their families.

Recommendations for future research. The literature on family and psychosocial functioning in individuals with SB will benefit from theory-driven advances that include the following features:

- a developmental emphasis,
- a focus on both illness-specific and general family processes,
- models that examine mediational processes (e.g., social skills may mediate associations between neuropsychological deficits and depressive symptoms; Lennon, Klages, et al., 2015), and
- models that consider family-related variables (e.g., autonomy-promoting parenting) that serve as potential buffers or moderators of associations between risk factors (e.g., neurological status) and negative outcomes (e.g., academic failure).

It is also recommended that research be programmatic and longitudinal, where predictor and outcome variables are all assessed over time, particularly during key developmental periods or transition points (e.g., early childhood, transition to elementary school, early adolescent transition, transition to early adulthood; Holmbeck & Devine, 2010).

PEDIATRIC EPILEPSY

Epidemiology

Approximately 470,000 children in the United States have epilepsy (Zack & Kobau, 2017). Globally, rates are higher, around 0.9% (Olusanya et al., 2020). Epilepsy is most prevalent in Latin America and the Caribbean (1.2%) and least prevalent in Asia and Oceania (0.7%; Olusanya et al., 2020). In general, ethnicity (African American more than European American) and education (those who do not complete high school more than those who attend graduate school) impact lifetime and active epilepsy rates (Kroner et al., 2013).

Etiology/Prognosis

The etiology of a child's epilepsy diagnosis influences therapy, prognosis, and clinical outcome. Current diagnostic processes for epilepsy require consideration of etiology from first diagnosis. Etiology for epilepsy may be structural, genetic, infectious, metabolic, immune, or unknown (Scheffer et al., 2017).

The prevalence of epilepsy is somewhat higher in boys, but occurrence is evenly distributed between boys and girls. Epilepsy occurs relatively frequently in infancy, with the highest prevalence among children under the age of 12 months (Sokka et al., 2017). The prognosis for children with epilepsy is good for about 65% of children (e.g., no cognitive impairment, some experience seizure remission) whereas 35% of children with epilepsy fare less well (e.g., cognitive impairment, continued seizures; Mohanraj & Brodie, 2006; Sokka et al., 2017). Developmentally, onset at an age later than 10 or 12 years has been linked to a worse prognosis (Mohanraj & Brodie, 2013). Seizure types including infantile spasms, atonic spells, atypical absences, and simple partial seizures were related to worse outcomes compared to generalized tonic-clonic seizures (GTCS; Arts et al., 1999). Predictors associated with worse outcomes in children include the presence of psychological comorbidities (i.e., developmental delay), response to antiepileptic drugs, and number of seizures before beginning treatment (Mohanraj & Brodie, 2013).

Clinical Presentation and Developmental Course

Pediatric epilepsy is a neurological condition diagnosed by two or more unprovoked seizures. Epilepsy is diagnosed by seizure type (epileptic or nonepileptic), epilepsy type, and epilepsy syndrome. The four major types of epilepsies are *generalized, focal, combined,* and *unknown* (Scheffer et al., 2017). *Generalized onset seizures* simultaneously affect either both sides of the brain or clusters of cells on both sides of the brain. *Focal onset seizures* begin in a single region or group of cells on one side of the brain (Sokka et al., 2017). Roughly one-third of children with epilepsy fall into a distinct epilepsy syndrome category (Camfield & Camfield, 2015).

Epileptic seizures affect about 3% of people at some point in their lives, with most cases occurring during infancy (Neubauer et al., 2008). An epilepsy diagnosis can be present at birth or be diagnosed at any point in development, and in some cases may go undiagnosed for an extended period of time. The risk of sudden unexpected death in epilepsy (SUDEP) is one of the most severe potential outcomes. Risk factors for SUDEP include increased seizure frequency and seizures type, with those who exhibit nocturnal GTCS and antiseizure drug resistance being most at risk (Harden et al., 2017). SUDEP is more common in children with severe epilepsies. However, there have been a few instances of SUDEP in children with less severe seizure profiles (Doumlele et al., 2017). The inclusion of a caregiver's nighttime monitoring may minimize SUDEP risk (Harden et al., 2017).

Diversity and Equity

Incidence, disease course, and outcomes in epilepsy are affected by multilevel factors that highlight difficulties as well as intervention targets across ecological variables. Incidence rates of epilepsy are higher among rural populations and slowly developing nations than developed countries (Camfield & Camfield, 2015). Low socioeconomic level and minority status are linked to higher rates of epilepsy as well as more hospitalizations and emergency department (ED) visits (Szaflarski, 2014). Family factors such as parents' level of education and SES influence outcomes related to medication adherence and QoL in epilepsy (Huber & Weber, 2022). Health literacy is a vital modifiable factor to address, as low health literacy is linked to poor patient outcomes, higher mortality, and poor management of health care (Bautista et al., 2009). Epilepsy surgery rates are lower for those with lower SES and lower for African American patients (Sánchez Fernández et al., 2017). For review of the social determinants of epilepsy using an ecological approach consistent with developmental science, see Szaflarski (2014).

Individual and Family Outcomes: A Developmental Perspective

Social-emotional outcomes and quality of life. Children with epilepsy have worse social-emotional and academic outcomes and poorer QoL compared to the general population. For example, rates of psychiatric diagnoses in children with epilepsy are as high as 61%, but only one-third receive mental health treatment (Ott et al., 2003). Beyond childhood, people with epilepsy are significantly less likely to live independently (Kroner et al., 2013) and more likely to be unemployed (de Souza et al., 2018) compared to those without epilepsy.

Academic achievement and educational attainment. Epilepsy is prevalent in schools, with current estimates indicating approximately 6 in 1,000 school-aged children have epilepsy (CDC, 2021a). Despite the high prevalence, people with epilepsy are less likely to be educated compared to the general population (Burneo et al., 2009). Children with epilepsy are more likely to exhibit low academic achievement (Reilly et al., 2014a) and repeat a grade compared to their peers without epilepsy (Russ et al., 2012).

Family relationships. Children with epilepsy may experience challenging family dynamics. Parents of children with epilepsy have higher levels of stress compared to parents of children without disabilities (Russ et al., 2012); family stress and limited access to resources may contribute to poorer emotional well-being in children with epilepsy (Goodwin et al., 2017). As children age, adolescents may experience frustration with parental restrictions and supervision due to seizures, which may contribute to limited parent–child communication about epilepsy (O'Toole et al., 2016). Despite potential strain on family relationships, a review of qualitative studies revealed parents of children with epilepsy often desire their children to have typical childhoods and acknowledge their children's ability to manage symptoms and social relationships (Harden et al., 2016).

Peer relationships. Peer relationships may also be challenging for children and youth with epilepsy. Younger children with epilepsy have lower social competence compared to children without epilepsy (Lew et al., 2015), and adolescents may have difficulty disclosing their epilepsy status to their peers (McEwan et al., 2004). Additionally, children and adolescents often exhibit high internalized stigma regarding epilepsy, which may be exacerbated in those who are younger, worry about their condition frequently, have a higher perceived need for emotional support, and have high seizure severity (Austin et al., 2014).

Risk and Resilience

Several risk factors are associated with poor outcomes among people with epilepsy. For example, those from lower SES backgrounds often experience worse outcomes compared to those from higher SES backgrounds (Ferro, 2014). Specifically, low-SES individuals are more likely to visit the ED for seizure care, take more than one medication, have more side effects from their antiepileptic drugs, have higher rates of depression and anxiety, and report overall lower QoL (Groover et al., 2020). Beyond low SES, clinical factors such as ongoing illness, high frequency and severity of seizures, taking several antiepileptic drugs and the presence of medication side effects are associated with worse QoL (Ferro, 2014). Family factors such as high parental anxiety are also associated with poorer QoL (Ferro, 2014). Among adolescents, qualitative research has indicated that epilepsy symptomology's impact on peer relationships and level of independence can influence QoL (McEwan et al., 2004).

Many protective factors have also been identified in children with epilepsy. Clinical factors (i.e., seizure frequency) have less of an impact on QoL compared to psychosocial factors. For example, more social support from peers and families, fewer symptoms of depression among both children and their parents, as well as better verbal abilities in children were more highly associated with QoL than were clinical factors (Ferro et al., 2017).

Self-Management and Adherence

Adherence in pediatric epilepsy requires consistency with a medication regimen (typically taking a pill one to three times daily) and avoiding triggers for seizures, such as increased stress or lack of sleep. Rates of nonadherence in pediatric epilepsy range from 42% to 60%. Adherence is measured through self-report, electronic monitors, blood serum levels, and providers' estimates of adherence. Interventions to improve adherence generally consist of multicomponent interventions (e.g., education and problem solving) and have shown long-term impacts on adherence behaviors (e.g., Modi et al., 2021). A more complete review of adherence in pediatric epilepsy can be found in Smith et al. (2020).

Transition to Adult Health Care

Transitioning from pediatric to adult health care for adolescents and young adults with epilepsy is challenging and can lead to disengagement from health care (Lewis & Noyes, 2013). However, certain factors are associated with transition readiness such as more epilepsy-related knowledge and better executive functioning and communication skills, factors that are susceptible to intervention to improve outcomes (Smith et al., 2021). To assess transition readiness, clinicians can administer EpiTRAQ, a validated assessment tool specifically developed for people with epilepsy (Clark et al., 2020).

Clinical Management

The clinical management of epilepsy requires timely assessment and effective treatment of the seizures as well as associated comorbidities. There are comprehensive overviews of the assessment and treatment of epilepsy and common psychological comorbidities (e.g., Follansbee-Junger et al., 2018). Briefly, a neurologist diagnoses epilepsy, and assessment generally includes a detailed history and occasionally use of electroencephalogram to confirm seizure activity. General pediatricians may be involved through recognizing potential seizure activity (e.g., staring spells may be absence seizures) and providing appropriate referrals. In less complex epilepsy cases, primary care pediatricians may be the main epilepsy provider for some patients (for an example, see the Joshi et al., 2020, ECHO model). Finally, developmental and behavioral pediatricians are likely to encounter many youth with epilepsy, given the high rates of comorbidity between developmental concerns and epilepsy in youth. In one population-based study, up to 80% of youth with epilepsy had a comorbid cognitive or behavioral problem, with 40% meeting criteria for intellectual disability and 21% meeting criteria for autism spectrum disorder (Reilly et al., 2014b).

In addition to medical care, mental health and behavioral care is key for children with epilepsy. Pediatric psychologists are natural fits for addressing epilepsy's multiple potential mental health comorbidities through screening, diagnosis, and treatment, often in integrated medical settings and multidisciplinary clinics (e.g., Guilfoyle et al., 2019). Neuropsychologists may clarify how seizures affect specific cognitive functions or complex diagnostic combinations and neuropsychological assessments can be used to assess change across development (e.g., yearly assessments). Psychologists or neuropsychologists may provide specific recommendations for accommodations that would benefit a child with epilepsy in the school system (e.g., through a 504 plan or an individualized education program).

Recommendations for Clinical Interventions and Research

Despite great strides in the past decades regarding care for youth with epilepsy, it remains an underresearched area, particularly in addressing comorbid psychological and learning conditions in this population. One way to close this gap is to increase the number of psychological and mental health trainees who learn to work with youth with epilepsy to increase the number of behavioral health experts available to care for these patients, ideally in integrated settings to improve access to care and patient QoL. Additionally, given the disparities noted among those with lower SES, improving accessibility to mental health care for youth with epilepsy and increasing health literacy in this population will be essential in improving a range of outcomes. Future research is needed in a few key areas, but especially in the integration of technology (for at-home monitoring of seizures/adherence and delivery of psychosocial interventions) and increased diversity in samples.

TRAUMATIC BRAIN INJURY

Epidemiology

TBI, a leading cause of morbidity and mortality in childhood, is caused by a penetrating head injury or a bump, blow, or jolt to the head that disrupts the normal function of the brain. The global incidence of pediatric TBI ranges broadly by country between 47–280 per 100,000 children (Dewan et al., 2016). A bimodal age distribution is often reported, with more common injury among children under 2 years and adolescents 15–18 years (Dewan et al., 2016). In the United States, there were approximately 17,610 TBI-related hospitalizations and 2,810 TBI-related deaths among children 0–17 years of age in 2017 (CDC, 2021b). Because children with TBI can present to various clinical locations (e.g., EDs, urgent care clinics, primary care) or not seek or receive medical care at all, incidence estimates, especially for mild TBI, are likely significant underestimates.

Etiology/Prognosis

The leading causes of TBI-related hospitalizations and deaths in the United States shift across development from unintentional falls in children 0–4 years, to unintentional falls and motor vehicle traffic crashes in middle childhood, to motor vehicle traffic crashes and suicide in individuals 15–24 years of age. Sports and recreational activities are the leading cause of TBI-related ED visits among children and adolescents. Abusive head trauma, also known as nonaccidental TBI, is a mechanism of injury most often affecting children younger than 12 months (Peterson et al., 2015). TBI severity can be classified into mild, moderate, and severe categories based on initial clinical presentation and is most often measured using the Glasgow Coma Scale (GCS). The GCS assesses patients according to three aspects of responsiveness: eye-opening (1–4), motor (1–6), and verbal responses (1–5). GCS scores of 13–15 are mild, 8–12 are moderate, and less than 8 are severe. The term *concussion* is used interchangeably with mild TBI, which can also be further described as complicated mild TBI in the presence of positive neuroimaging findings (e.g., skull fracture, intracranial bleeding). Children with complicated mild TBI are often grouped together with moderate TBI in research studies due to higher morbidity in children with complicated vs. uncomplicated mild TBI. The vast majority of TBIs are categorized as mild, accounting for 70–90% of TBI-related ED visits. However, the outcome and recovery trajectories are very different for mild vs. moderate-to-severe TBI. Thus, the information in subsequent sections of this chapter is often presented separately by severity group.

In terms of estimating prognosis for the individual patient with TBI, injury severity is often considered alongside additional factors including age at injury, premorbid child function, and psychosocial and environmental factors (e.g., SES and family functioning). Despite these known predictive factors, outcomes following moderate-to-severe TBI are heterogeneous and predictive models only account for approximately 35% of this variation. Numerous studies are underway attempting to account for unexplained heterogeneity in TBI outcomes, through the examination of biomarkers, therapeutic interventions, and improved research methods and outcome measurement.

Clinical Presentation and Developmental Course

Mild TBI. By definition, children with mild TBI present with confusion or disorientation, loss of consciousness (LOC) for 30 minutes or less, posttraumatic amnesia (PTA; e.g., inability to form new continuous memories and/or a state of disorientation to time, place, and person) for less than 24 hours, and/or other transient neurological abnormalities, such as focal signs, symptoms, or seizure (also a GCS score of 13–15 after 30 minutes post injury or later upon presentation for health care). Additional symptoms of mild TBI can include headaches and dizziness as well as difficulty with thinking, memory, physical activities, mood and behavior, and sleep. These additional symptoms usually develop immediately but can also present over a few days post injury. Longitudinal studies show that the majority of children who sustain a mild TBI have symptom resolution within 6 weeks (Barlow et al., 2010; Sroufe et al., 2010). A subset of children with mild TBI, however, experience postconcussive symptoms and behavioral or psychological difficulties that persist beyond the typical recovery period, often termed *postconcussive syndrome*.

Moderate to severe TBI. Children with moderate TBI have LOC or PTA lasting 1–24 hours and GCS scores of 9 to 12; with severe TBI they have LOC or PTA greater than 24 hours and GCS scores of 3 to 8. With moderate to severe TBI, children often require immediate and intensive medical treatment. Complex and systemwide medical comorbidities are common and can include autonomic dysfunction, disorders of consciousness, headache, swelling or hydrocephalus, endocrine problems, motor dysfunction, respiratory problems, sensory issues, and seizures, among others. Moderate-to-severe TBI is often associated with a range of cognitive, motor, emotional, and behavioral difficulties that can present early or late after injury and can change over time and with development. The most rapid and significant cognitive and behavioral recovery occurs within the first 6 to 12 months post injury, typically followed by a plateau during which additional recovery is minimal. TBI-related impairments persisting around 12 months post injury tend to be chronic. Some difficulties may not emerge until years after the injury when higher-level cognitive and behavioral functioning are expected.

Diversity and Equity

There are several noted health disparities related to pediatric TBI severity and mortality, receiving medical care, and outcomes. African American, Latin American, and Native American children are more likely than European American children to sustain more severe injuries and have higher mortality rates (Linton & Kim, 2014). Children from lower SES homes and children with public insurance or who are uninsured also have higher mortality and are less likely to receive appropriate hospital care and interventional procedures, inpatient and outpatient rehabilitation, follow-up specialty care, and mental health services (Greene et al., 2014; Porter et al., 2020). Similarly, children living in rural areas are more likely to sustain a TBI and die as a result of their injury relative to children living in urban areas; children in rural areas are less likely to receive timely medical care and are more often unnecessarily transferred to another hospital (Yue et al., 2020). Minority children, children living in rural areas, and children with lower SES are less likely to receive outpatient rehabilitation and mental health services following TBI (Graves et al., 2019; Jimenez et al., 2017). Disparities also exist in short- and long-term outcomes. Latin and African American children have demonstrated greater functional impairments at discharge from inpatient rehabilitation relative to European American children (Jimenez et al., 2015). Studies of disparities in long-term outcomes following pediatric TBI have focused on psychosocial factors such as income, parental education level, and social integration into the community. Children from families of lower SES have poorer long-term outcomes in several domains, including social, emotional/behavioral, academic, and adaptive functioning (Gerring & Wade, 2012). Disparities in outcomes may be partly addressable through improving access to services, such as through telehealth interventions (Zhang et al., 2019), but injury prevention efforts for minority and rural children may offer the greatest impact on reducing disparities.

Individual and Family Outcomes: A Developmental Perspective

Mild TBI. Difficulties with social-emotional functioning, QoL, and educational functioning are common during the acute and subacute (e.g., days to weeks) period following mild TBI. However, these difficulties typically resolve within 6 weeks post injury, except for ~10% of children and adolescents who have persistent postconcussive symptoms beyond 3 months post injury (Barlow et al., 2010).

Social-emotional outcomes and quality of life. Children and adolescents can experience depressive and anxiety symptoms, fluctuations in mood, and increased disruptive behaviors (Emery et al., 2016). Sustaining a mild TBI can increase the risk of having a new affective or behavioral disorder up to 4 years after the initial injury (Delmonico et al., 2024). QoL findings in children and adolescents following mild TBI have focused on 1–12 months post injury with some studies suggesting reduced QoL, while others found no differences in QoL between children with mild TBI and orthopedically injured controls (Di Battista et al., 2012).

Educational/academic achievement/school failure/ educational attainment. Because of the acute/ subacute cognitive difficulties, especially inattention and increased hyperactivity (Emery et al., 2016), as well as the physical and emotional symptoms of mild TBI, school difficulties are common. These include interference due to postconcussion symptoms while in school, decline in academic performance and concerns about school performance, and missing school days. Fourteen percent of children with mild TBI were receiving new educational supports at 12 months post injury in a large cohort study (Rivara et al., 2012).

Family and peer relationships. Very little research has investigated family and peer relationships following mild TBI. A prospective longitudinal study found that mild TBI with LOC was associated with greater family burden relative to an orthopedic injury (OI) comparison group at 3 months post injury (Ganesalingam et al., 2008). However, other studies have found that the quality of parent–child interactions, peer relationships, and prosocial behaviors are not affected by mild TBI (Keenan et al., 2018; Lalonde et al., 2018).

Moderate to severe TBI. Although some children with moderate-to-severe TBI experience full recovery, many others suffer from chronic neurobehavioral impairments, especially in executive functioning, behavior, and social skills, which hamper their long-term academic, occupational, and social function.

Social-emotional outcomes and quality of life. It is estimated that up to 70% of children sustaining severe TBI are at risk for emotional and behavioral problems, including internalizing and externalizing difficulties (Bloom et al., 2001; Luis & Mittenberg, 2002). Attention problems, often diagnosed as secondary attention-deficit/hyperactivity disorder, are also common, with estimates around 20% of children with severe TBI (Asarnow et al., 2021). Disruptive behaviors, such as aggression, tantrums, and destructiveness, are observed in approximately 20–40% of children (Ganesalingam et al., 2007). A systematic review and meta-analysis reported mixed findings relating to QoL following severe TBI, but that reports of poor QoL slightly outnumber reports of good QoL (Di Battista et al., 2012).

Educational/academic achievement/school failure/educational attainment. Short- and long-term impairments in attention, learning and memory, and executive function, are common and impact children's ability to perform in school (Taylor et al., 2008). Children with moderate-to-severe TBI achieve lower grades, have higher rates of grade retention, and receive more special education services than their uninjured peers.

Family relationships. Caregivers of children with moderate-to-severe TBI show greater psychological distress and family injury-related burden in the short- and long-term as compared to caregivers of children with OI (Stancin et al., 2010). Video-recorded interactions of caregivers and young children with TBI in the laboratory have also shown lower caregiver warm responsiveness and more directive statements toward the child compared to caregivers of children with OI (Wade et al., 2008).

Peer relationships. Children with moderate-to-severe TBI show deficits in theory of mind skills and associated poorer communication and social skills (Ryan et al., 2020). Compared to children with OI, children with severe TBI also experience greater rejection and victimization (Hung et al., 2017) and are rated by their peers as lower in sociability, popularity, and prosocial behaviors. In addition, they are less likely to have mutual friendships (Yeates et al., 2013).

Risk and Resilience
Mild TBI.

Risk factors. Several injury and individual child factors are associated with an increased risk of persistent postconcussive symptoms and psychiatric difficulties following mild TBI. These factors include mild TBI resulting in hospitalization, history of multiple mild TBIs, higher acute postconcussive symptoms (especially cognitive symptoms), and preinjury psychiatric and neurodevelopmental disorders, especially anxiety, learning disorders, and ADHD (Emery et al., 2016).

Protective factors. Little research has examined unique protective factors following mild TBI. Psychological resilience may be protective against postconcussive syndrome (Laliberté Durish et al., 2018).

Moderate to severe TBI.

Risk factors. Several risk factors account for about one-third of the variation in outcomes following moderate-to-severe pediatric TBI. Although these broad categories overlap and have bidirectional associations, they can be broadly characterized as injury-related factors, child-related factors, and environmental factors.

Injury severity shows a dose-response relation with outcomes, with greater structural and functional abnormalities associated with greater morbidity. Additionally, children sustaining non-accidental TBI show significantly less favorable outcomes as compared to children with accidental mechanisms of injury, which is attributable to a combination of risk factors (e.g., likelihood of multiple episodes of nonaccidental TBI, more severe and more diffuse TBI, subsequent placement in foster care). In terms of child-related risk factors, children who sustain TBI during infancy or early childhood show more significant and persistent impairments relative to children injured during later childhood or adolescence (Anderson et al., 2005; Ewing-Cobbs et al., 2006). Children with lower preinjury functioning are also at greater risk for poorer recovery from moderate-to-severe TBI (Donders & Kim, 2019; Yeates et al., 2005). Finally, with regard to environmental influences, children from less optimal family environments tend to be vulnerable to worse recovery as compared to children from higher functioning or greater resourced family environments, although these effects vary by age at injury and injury severity, and may wane with time since injury (Taylor et al., 2002; Wade et al., 2016).

Protective factors. The inverse of the risk factors in each domain described above (e.g., less severe injuries, higher preinjury functioning, greater psychosocial resources) compose the knowledge base regarding protective factors for recovery from moderate-to-severe TBI.

Transition to Adult Health Care
Individuals who sustain moderate-to-severe TBI during childhood and adolescence are at an increased risk for lower achievement of adult milestones relative to individuals with other disabilities (Cameto et al., 2004), including lower rates of employment, postsecondary education, and independent living. In addition, adults with a history of TBI have higher rates of mental health difficulties (Ryan et al., 2013) and may be at an increased risk for criminal offending behavior

(McKinlay et al., 2014). The transition to adult health care may be particularly challenging for individuals with TBI because adolescents and young adults with TBI may not be consistently followed by a specialty health care provider and the individual's primary adult health care provider may not be informed about the TBI history (CDC, 2018). Evidence-based models of care for children with a history of TBI need to be developed and supported within the health care system to better facilitate the transition from pediatric to adult health care (CDC, 2018).

Clinical Management

Mild TBI. Providers are referred to the *Centers for Disease Control and Prevention Guideline on the Diagnosis and Management of Mild Traumatic Brain Injury Among Children* (Lumba-Brown et al., 2018) for the most up-to-date, comprehensive, and evidence-based guidelines for the clinical management of children with mild TBI. Key recommendations include:

- Do not routinely image patients to diagnose mild TBI.
- Use validated, age-appropriate symptom scales to diagnose mild TBI.
- Assess evidence-based risk factors for prolonged recovery.
- Provide patients with instructions on return to activity, customized to their symptoms.
- Counsel patients to return gradually to non-sports activities after no more than 2–3 days of rest.

Children with mild TBI often present to the general pediatrician who may refer to developmental-behavioral pediatricians, pediatric psychologists, and/or subspecialty/multidisciplinary clinics for clinical management, especially if postconcussive symptoms persist. Children with persisting cognitive difficulties may be referred for neuropsychological evaluation to assist in determining etiology and recommending targeted treatment. Relatedly, because children with mild TBI are at increased risk for affective disorders, ongoing screening for affective and behavioral disorders following a TBI can help identify sequelae that may interfere with recovery (Delmonico et al., 2024). Coordinated, multidisciplinary management, as well as cognitive behavioral interventions (e.g., psychoeducation, activity scheduling, relaxation, cognitive restructuring), have also shown promising results (McCarty et al., 2021; McNally et al., 2018).

The CDC guideline includes recommendations for return to school following mild TBI. Medical and school-based teams should counsel students and families regarding customized, gradual increase of duration and intensity of academic activities as tolerated. Postconcussive symptoms and academic progress should be monitored collaboratively by the student, family, health care provider, and school teams to jointly determine what modifications or accommodations are needed, and these should be adjusted on an ongoing basis until the student's academic performance has returned to preinjury levels. For students with prolonged postconcussive symptoms that interfere with academic performance, school-based teams should assess educational needs and determine the need for additional educational supports as described under pertinent federal statutes (e.g., Individuals With Disabilities Education Act, Section 504).

Moderate to severe TBI. Children with moderate-to-severe TBI often require aggressive medical management, with treatment at a certified pediatric trauma center and in adherence with acute medical management guidelines associated with better outcomes (Faul et al., 2007). Unfortunately, evidence-based treatment or management guidelines for moderate-to-severe TBI beyond the acute period are lacking. Clinical management of these children is dependent on multiple service delivery systems that are often unsystematic and poorly coordinated across the child's lifespan (CDC, 2018). Research shows substantial unmet health care needs for children with moderate-to-severe TBI in the first year post injury, especially relating to services addressing cognitive impairments (Slomine et al., 2006). Routine medical care that is family-centered and care coordination that links children and their families with appropriate services and resources, is critical for children with special health care needs.

Primary care providers and/or specialists (e.g., physiatrists, developmental-behavioral pediatricians) caring for the child across their development should regularly screen for functional impairments in areas of communication, fine and gross motor skills, cognitive and academic functioning, and social and behavioral functioning and coordinate referrals for speech/language, occupational, and physical therapies, as well as neuropsychological evaluations and behavioral health services, as needed. A multidisciplinary brain injury clinic staffed by a team composed of a pediatric rehabilitation medicine physician, a speech/language pathologist, a physical therapist, an occupational therapist, and a neuropsychologist is an optimal model of care. Continued monitoring for impairments and health care needs beyond the first year post injury is critical given that impairments can worsen or new impairments can emerge over time as developmental expectations increase.

Given the demonstrated essential role of the family in recovery following moderate-to-severe TBI in children (Taylor et al., 2002; Wade et al., 2016), interventions and supports to promote family functioning are a high priority. Interventions with the strongest evidence (Laatsch et al., 2020) include Stepping Stones Triple P combined with acceptance and commitment therapy (Brown et al., 2015) and family-centered problem-solving approaches (Wade, Kurowski, et al., 2015; Wade, Taylor, et al., 2015). Family-centered problem-solving training involves a systematic, iterative approach to addressing social challenges that includes adopting a positive orientation to problems, careful definition of the situation, brainstorming, choosing solutions that maximize positive outcomes and minimize negative ones, developing systematic action plans, and evaluating their success. This intervention has shown efficacy in improving both child and caregiver outcomes via both face-to-face and online delivery in randomized clinical trials. Health professionals can submit a request for intervention materials at https://tops4tbi.com/.

A range of supports is available for children when they are ready to return to school and to accommodate for subacute and chronic impairments affecting academic functioning. These include early intervention services, special education under the Individuals With Disabilities Education Act, and supports and accommodations through a Section 504 plan. Schools should closely monitor the student's academic performance and provide tailored accommodations and modifications appropriate to the child, which may include a functional academic curriculum that emphasizes life skills and the application of academic knowledge in real world settings to promote the child's capacity to navigate within the community and function independently. A repeat neuropsychological evaluation around 1–2 years post injury and at important transition times (e.g., before the start of kindergarten, middle school, high school, graduation) is informative for understanding chronic impairments, for detecting the emergence of new difficulties over the developmental period, and for updating recommendations for academic supports.

Recommendations for Clinical Interventions and Research

Providers are referred to the Centers for Disease Control and Prevention *Report to Congress: The Management of Traumatic Brain Injury in Children* (CDC, 2018) for a comprehensive summary of clinical and research knowledge gaps and opportunities for action to improve the care of children with moderate-to-severe TBI. Calls for action in this report focus on enhancing health care services to improve clinical management; improving children's return to school, activity, and independence; improving the transition to adulthood; improving professional training for those involved in the management of pediatric TBI; and future directions for research.

CONCLUSION

This chapter reviewed linkages between the three disciplines that are the focus of this volume (i.e., pediatric psychology, developmental-behavioral pediatrics, and developmental science) in relation to SB, epilepsy, and TBI. For all three conditions, multiple contexts in the life of the child (i.e., individual, family, community, cultural, health care related) have a significant impact on relevant family, parent, and child outcomes. Just like all children, youth with these conditions progress through a host of developmental stages, although milestone achievement is complicated and often disrupted by condition-related complications that emerge throughout the developmental process (Holmbeck et al., 2008). Such youth must manage the typical developmental milestones of childhood, adolescence, and emerging adulthood while at the same time managing their condition (e.g., the transfer of medical responsibility from parent to child, the transition from pediatric to adult health care). Clearly, pediatric psychologists, developmental-behavioral pediatricians, and developmental scientists all play unique and important roles in ongoing screening for adaptational difficulties, intervening when necessary to prevent the emergence of major developmental, psychosocial, and medical challenges, and in increasing the knowledge base for these three conditions.

RESOURCES

The following list of resources contains helpful links for relevant foundation and government fact sheets and guidelines that will be potentially useful for health professionals as well as families of children with these chronic health conditions.

Spina Bifida

- National Institutes of Health Fact Sheet:

  https://www.ninds.nih.gov/Disorders/Patient-Caregiver-Education/Fact-Sheets/Spina-Bifida-Fact-Sheet

- Got Transition:

  https://www.gottransition.org/

- Spina Bifida Association Care Guidelines:

  https://www.spinabifidaassociation.org/guidelines/

- CDC:

  https://www.cdc.gov/ncbddd/spinabifida/index.html

Epilepsy

- Centers for Disease Control and Prevention for general information:

  https://www.cdc.gov/epilepsy/index.html

- Epilepsy Foundation:

  https://www.epilepsy.com/

- Child Neurology Foundation:

  https://www.childneurologyfoundation.org/disorder/epilepsy/

- International League Against Epilepsy diagnosis tool:

  https://www.epilepsydiagnosis.org

Traumatic Brain Injury

- Centers for Disease Control's HEADS UP initiative:

  https://www.cdc.gov/headsup/youthsports

- https://www.brainline.org

- The Brain Injury Association of America (BIA) state affiliates:

  https://www.biausa.org

- Family-based intervention materials can be requested:

  https://tops4tbi.com/

References

Anderson, V., Catroppa, C., Morse, S., Haritou, F., & Rosenfeld, J. (2005). Functional plasticity or vulnerability after early brain injury? *Pediatrics*, *116*(6), 1374–1382. https://doi.org/10.1542/peds.2004-1728

Arts, W. F. M., Geerts, A. T., Brouwer, O. F., Boudewyn Peters, A. C., Stroink, H., & van Donselaar, C. A. (1999). The early prognosis of epilepsy in childhood: The prediction of a poor outcome.

The Dutch study of epilepsy in childhood. *Epilepsia*, *40*(6), 726–734. https://doi.org/10.1111/j.1528-1157.1999.tb00770.x

Asarnow, R. F., Newman, N., Weiss, R. E., & Su, E. (2021). Association of attention-deficit/hyperactivity disorder diagnoses with pediatric traumatic brain injury: A meta-analysis. *JAMA Pediatrics*, *175*(10), 1009–1016. https://doi.org/10.1001/jamapediatrics.2021.2033

Austin, J. K., Perkins, S. M., & Dunn, D. W. (2014). A model for internalized stigma in children and adolescents with epilepsy. *Epilepsy & Behavior*, *36*, 74–79. https://doi.org/10.1016/j.yebeh.2014.04.020

Barlow, K. M., Crawford, S., Stevenson, A., Sandhu, S. S., Belanger, F., & Dewey, D. (2010). Epidemiology of postconcussion syndrome in pediatric mild traumatic brain injury. *Pediatrics*, *126*(2), e374–e381. https://doi.org/10.1542/peds.2009-0925

Bautista, R. E. D., Glen, E. T., Shetty, N. K., & Wludyka, P. (2009). The association between health literacy and outcomes of care among epilepsy patients. *Seizure*, *18*(6), 400–404. https://doi.org/10.1016/j.seizure.2009.02.004

Betz, C. L., Smith, K., & Macias, K. (2010). Testing the transition preparation training program: A randomized controlled trial. *International Journal of Child and Adolescent Health*, *3*(4), 595–607.

Bloom, D. R., Levin, H. S., Ewing-Cobbs, L., Saunders, A. E., Song, J., Fletcher, J. M., & Kowatch, R. A. (2001). Lifetime and novel psychiatric disorders after pediatric traumatic brain injury. *Journal of the American Academy of Child & Adolescent Psychiatry*, *40*(5), 572–579. https://doi.org/10.1097/00004583-200105000-00017

Bronfenbrenner, U. (1977). Toward an experimental ecology of human development. *American Psychologist*, *32*(7), 513–531. https://doi.org/10.1037/0003-066X.32.7.513

Brown, F. L., Whittingham, K., Boyd, R. N., McKinlay, L., & Sofronoff, K. (2015). Does Stepping Stones Triple P plus Acceptance and Commitment Therapy improve parent, couple, and family adjustment following paediatric acquired brain injury? A randomised controlled trial. *Behaviour Research and Therapy*, *73*, 58–66. https://doi.org/10.1016/j.brat.2015.07.001

Burneo, J. G., Jette, N., Theodore, W., Begley, C., Parko, K., Thurman, D. J., Wiebe, S., the Task Force on Disparities in Epilepsy Care, & the North American Commission of the International League Against Epilepsy. (2009). Disparities in epilepsy: Report of a systematic review by the North American Commission of the International League Against Epilepsy. *Epilepsia*, *50*(10), 2285–2295. https://doi.org/10.1111/j.1528-1167.2009.02282.x

Cameto, R., Levine, P., & Wagner, M. (2004). *Transition planning for students with disabilities. A special topic of report of findings from the National Longitudinal Transition Study-2 (NLTS2)*. https://nlts2.sri.com/reports/2004_11/nlts2_report_2004_11_execsum.pdf

Camfield, P., & Camfield, C. (2015). Incidence, prevalence and aetiology of seizures and epilepsy in children. *Epileptic Disorders*, *17*(2), 117–123. https://doi.org/10.1684/epd.2015.0736

Centers for Disease Control and Prevention. (2020, September 3). *Data & statistics on spina bifida*. https://www.cdc.gov/ncbddd/spinabifida/data.html

Centers for Disease Control and Prevention. (2021a). *CDC healthy schools: Epilepsy*. Retrieved October 28, 2021, from https://www.cdc.gov/healthyschools/npao/epilepsy.htm

Centers for Disease Control and Prevention. (2021b). *Surveillance report of traumatic brain injury-related hospitalizations and deaths by age group, sex, and mechanism of injury—United States, 2016 and 2017*. https://www.cdc.gov/traumaticbraininjury/pdf/TBI-surveillance-report-2016-2017-508.pdf

Centers for Disease Control and Prevention, National Center for Injury Prevention and Control, & Division of Unintentional Injury Prevention. (2018). *Report to Congress: The management of traumatic brain injury in children—Opportunities for action*. https://www.cdc.gov/traumaticbraininjury/pdf/reportstocongress/managementoftbiinchildren/TBI-ReporttoCongress-508.pdf

Chowanadisai, M., de la Rosa Perez, D. L., Weitzenkamp, D. A., Wilcox, D. T., Clayton, G. H., & Wilson, P. E. (2013). The role of ethnicity and culture on functional status in children with spina bifida. *Journal of Pediatric Rehabilitation Medicine*, *6*(4), 203–213. https://doi.org/10.3233/PRM-140259

Clark, S. J., Beimer, N. J., Gebremariam, A., Fletcher, L. L., Patel, A. D., Carbone, L., Guyot, J. A., & Joshi, S. M. (2020). Validation of EpiTRAQ, a transition readiness assessment tool for adolescents and young adults with epilepsy. *Epilepsia Open*, *5*(3), 487–495. https://doi.org/10.1002/epi4.12427

Copp, A. J., Adzick, N. S., Chitty, L. S., Fletcher, J. M., Holmbeck, G. N., & Shaw, G. M. (2015). Spina bifida. *Nature Reviews: Disease Primers*, *1*(1), 15007. https://doi.org/10.1038/nrdp.2015.7

Cushing, C. C. (2017). eHealth applications in pediatric psychology. In M. C. Roberts & R. G. Steele (Eds.), *Handbook of pediatric psychology* (5th ed., pp. 201–211). Guilford Press.

Deaton, A. V., & Castaldi, J. (2011). The role of the child clinical psychologist in life care planning. In S. Riddick-Grisham & L. Deming (Eds.), *Pediatric life care planning and case management* (2nd ed., pp. 133–145). Taylor & Francis Group.

Delmonico, R. L., Tucker, L. Y., Theodore, B. R., Camicia, M., Filanosky, C., & Haarbauer-Krupa, J. (2024). Mild traumatic brain injuries and risk for affective and behavioral disorders. *Pediatrics, 153*(2), e2023062340. https://doi.org/10.1542/peds.2023-062340

de Souza, J. L., Faiola, A. S., Miziara, C. S. M. G., & de Manreza, M. L. G. (2018). The perceived social stigma of people with epilepsy with regard to the question of employability. *Neurology Research International, 2018*, 4140508. https://doi.org/10.1155/2018/4140508

Devine, K. A., Holbein, C. E., Psihogios, A. M., Amaro, C. M., & Holmbeck, G. N. (2012). Individual adjustment, parental functioning, and perceived social support in Hispanic and non-Hispanic White mothers and fathers of children with spina bifida. *Journal of Pediatric Psychology, 37*(7), 769–778. https://doi.org/10.1093/jpepsy/jsr083

Devine, K. A., Holmbeck, G. N., Gayes, L., & Purnell, J. Q. (2012). Friendships of children and adolescents with spina bifida: Social adjustment, social performance, and social skills. *Journal of Pediatric Psychology, 37*(2), 220–231. https://doi.org/10.1093/jpepsy/jsr075

Dewan, M. C., Mummareddy, N., Wellons, J. C., & Bonfield, C. M. (2016). Epidemiology of global pediatric traumatic brain injury: Qualitative review. *World Neurosurgery, 91*(6), 497–509.e1. https://doi.org/10.1016/j.wneu.2016.03.045

Di Battista, A., Soo, C., Catroppa, C., & Anderson, V. (2012). Quality of life in children and adolescents post-TBI: A systematic review and meta-analysis. *Journal of Neurotrauma, 29*(9), 1717–1721. https://doi.org/10.1089/neu.2011.2157

Donders, J., & Kim, E. (2019). Effect of cognitive reserve on children with traumatic brain injury. *Journal of the International Neuropsychological Society, 25*(4), 355–361. https://doi.org/10.1017/S1355617719000109

Doumlele, K., Friedman, D., Buchhalter, J., Donner, E. J., Louik, J., & Devinsky, O. (2017). Sudden unexpected death in epilepsy among patients with benign childhood epilepsy with centrotemporal spikes. *JAMA Neurology, 74*(6), 645–649. https://doi.org/10.1001/jamaneurol.2016.6126

Driscoll, C. F. B., Ohanian, D., Papadakis, J. P., Stern, A., Zabel, T. A., Zebracki, K., & Holmbeck, G. N. (2018). Spina bifida myelomeningocele. In J. Donders & S. J. Hunter (Eds.), *Neuropsychological conditions across the lifespan* (pp. 24–44). Cambridge.

Driscoll, C. F. B., Ohanian, D. M., Ridosh, M. M., Stern, A., Wartman, E. C., Starnes, M., & Holmbeck, G. N. (2020). Pathways by which maternal factors are associated with youth spina bifida-related responsibility. *Journal of Pediatric Psychology, 45*(6), 610–621. https://doi.org/10.1093/jpepsy/jsaa020

Emery, C. A., Barlow, K. M., Brooks, B. L., Max, J. E., Villavicencio-Requis, A., Gnanakumar, V., Robertson, H. L., Schneider, K., & Yeates, K. O. (2016). A systematic review of psychiatric, psychological, and behavioural outcomes following mild traumatic brain injury in children and adolescents. *Canadian Journal of Psychiatry, 61*(5), 259–269. https://doi.org/10.1177/0706743716643741

Ewing-Cobbs, L., Prasad, M. R., Kramer, L., Cox, C. S., Jr., Baumgartner, J., Fletcher, S., Mendez, D., Barnes, M., Zhang, X., & Swank, P. (2006). Late intellectual and academic outcomes following traumatic brain injury sustained during early childhood. *Journal of Neurosurgery, 105*(4), 287–296. https://doi.org/10.3171/ped.2006.105.4.287

Faul, M., Wald, M. M., Rutland-Brown, W., Sullivent, E. E., & Sattin, R. W. (2007). Using a cost-benefit analysis to estimate outcomes of a clinical treatment guideline: Testing the Brain Trauma Foundation guidelines for the treatment of severe traumatic brain injury. *The Journal of Trauma, 63*(6), 1271–1278. https://doi.org/10.1097/TA.0b013e3181493080

Ferro, M. A. (2014). Risk factors for health-related quality of life in children with epilepsy: A meta-analysis. *Epilepsia, 55*(11), 1722–1731. https://doi.org/10.1111/epi.12772

Ferro, M. A., Avery, L., Fayed, N., Streiner, D. L., Cunningham, C. E., Boyle, M. H., Lach, L., Glidden, G., Rosenbaum, P. L., Ronen, G. M., Connolly, M., Bello-Espinosa, L., Rafay, M. F., Appendino, J. P., Shevell, M., & Carmant, L. (2017). Child- and parent-reported quality of life trajectories in children with epilepsy: A prospective cohort study. *Epilepsia, 58*(7), 1277–1286. https://doi.org/10.1111/epi.13774

Follansbee-Junger, K., Smith, A. W., Guilfoyle, S. M., & Modi, A. C. (2018). Epilepsy. In S. G. Forman & J. D. Shahidullah (Eds.), *Handbook of pediatric behavioral healthcare: An interdisciplinary collaborative approach*. Springer. https://doi.org/10.1007/978-3-030-00791-1_7

Fremion, E. J., & Dosa, N. P. (2019). Spina bifida transition to adult healthcare guidelines. *Journal of Pediatric Rehabilitation Medicine, 12*(4), 423–429. https://doi.org/10.3233/PRM-190633

Ganesalingam, K., Sanson, A., Anderson, V., & Yeates, K. O. (2007). Self-regulation as a mediator of the effects of childhood traumatic brain injury on social and behavioral functioning. *Journal of the International Neuropsychological Society*, *13*(2), 298–311. https://doi.org/10.1017/S1355617707070324

Ganesalingam, K., Yeates, K. O., Ginn, M. S., Taylor, H. G., Dietrich, A., Nuss, K., & Wright, M. (2008). Family burden and parental distress following mild traumatic brain injury in children and its relationship to post-concussive symptoms. *Journal of Pediatric Psychology*, *33*(6), 621–629. https://doi.org/10.1093/jpepsy/jsm133

Gerring, J. P., & Wade, S. (2012). The essential role of psychosocial risk and protective factors in pediatric traumatic brain injury research. *Journal of Neurotrauma*, *29*(4), 621–628. https://doi.org/10.1089/neu.2011.2234

Goodwin, S. W., Wilk, P., Campbell, M. K., & Speechley, K. N. (2017). Emotional well-being in children with epilepsy: Family factors as mediators and moderators. *Epilepsia*, *58*(11), 1912–1919. https://doi.org/10.1111/epi.13900

Graves, J., Mackelprang, J., Moore, M., Abshire, D., Rivara, F., Jimenez, N., Fuentes, M., & Vavilala, M. S. (2019). Rural-urban disparities in health care costs and health service utilization following pediatric mild traumatic brain injury. *Health Services Research*, *54*(2), 337–345. https://doi.org/10.1111/1475-6773.13096

Greene, N. H., Kernic, M. A., Vavilala, M. S., & Rivara, F. P. (2014). Variation in pediatric traumatic brain injury outcomes in the United States. *Archives of Physical Medicine and Rehabilitation*, *95*(6), 1148–1155. https://doi.org/10.1016/j.apmr.2014.02.020

Greenley, R. N. (2010). Health professional expectations for self-care skill development in youth with spina bifida. *Pediatric Nursing*, *36*(2), 98–102.

Groover, O., Morton, M. L., Janocko, N. J., Teagarden, D. L., Villarreal, H. K., Drane, D. L., & Karakis, I. (2020). Mind the gap: Health disparities in families living with epilepsy are significant and linked to socioeconomic status. *Epileptic Disorders*, *22*(6), 782–789. https://doi.org/10.1684/epd.2020.1229

Guilfoyle, S. M., Mara, C. A., Follansbee-Junger, K., Smith, A. W., Hater, B., & Modi, A. C. (2019). Quality of life improves with integrated behavioral health services in pediatric new-onset epilepsy. *Epilepsy & Behavior*, *96*, 57–60. https://doi.org/10.1016/j.yebeh.2019.04.017

Harden, C., Tomson, T., Gloss, D., Buchhalter, J., Cross, J. H., Donner, E., French, J. A., Gil-Nagel, A., Hesdorffer, D. C., Smithson, W. H., Spitz, M. C., Walczak, T. S., Sander, J. W., & Ryvlin, P. (2017). Practice guideline summary: Sudden unexpected death in epilepsy incidence rates and risk factors: Report of the guideline development, dissemination, and implementation subcommittee of the American Academy of Neurology and the American Epilepsy Society. *Neurology*, *88*(17), 1674–1680. https://doi.org/10.1212/WNL.0000000000003685

Harden, J., Black, R., & Chin, R. F. M. (2016). Families' experiences of living with pediatric epilepsy: A qualitative systematic review. *Epilepsy & Behavior*, *60*, 225–237. https://doi.org/10.1016/j.yebeh.2016.04.034

Heller, M. K., Gambino, S., Church, P., Lindsay, S., Kaufman, M., & McPherson, A. C. (2016). Sexuality and relationships in young people with spina bifida and their partners. *Journal of Adolescent Health*, *59*(2), 182–188. https://doi.org/10.1016/j.jadohealth.2016.03.037

Holbein, C. E., Murray, C. B., Psihogios, A. M., Wasserman, R. M., Essner, B. S., O'Hara, L. K., & Holmbeck, G. N. (2013). A camp-based psychosocial intervention to promote independence and social function in individuals with spina bifida: Moderators of treatment effectiveness. *Journal of Pediatric Psychology*, *38*(4), 412–424. https://doi.org/10.1093/jpepsy/jst003

Holbein, C. E., Peugh, J. L., & Holmbeck, G. N. (2017). Social skills in youth with spina bifida: A longitudinal multimethod investigation comparing biopsychosocial predictors. *Journal of Pediatric Psychology*, *42*(10), 1133–1143. https://doi.org/10.1093/jpepsy/jsx069

Holmbeck, G. N. (2002). A developmental perspective on adolescent health and illness: An introduction to the special issues. *Journal of Pediatric Psychology*, *27*(5), 409–416. https://doi.org/10.1093/jpepsy/27.5.409

Holmbeck, G. N., DeLucia, C., Essner, B., Kelly, L., Zebracki, K., Friedman, D., & Jandasek, B. (2010). Trajectories of psychosocial adjustment in adolescents with spina bifida: A 6-year, four-wave longitudinal follow-up. *Journal of Consulting and Clinical Psychology*, *78*(4), 511–525. https://doi.org/10.1037/a0019599

Holmbeck, G. N., & Devine, K. A. (2010). Psychosocial and family functioning in spina bifida. *Developmental Disabilities Research Reviews*, *16*(1), 40–46. https://doi.org/10.1002/ddrr.90

Holmbeck, G. N., Greenley, R. N., Coakley, R. M., Greco, J., & Hagstrom, J. (2006). Family functioning in children and adolescents with spina bifida: An evidence-based review of research and interventions. *Journal of Developmental and Behavioral Pediatrics*, *27*(3), 249–277. https://doi.org/10.1097/00004703-200606000-00012

Holmbeck, G. N., Jandasek, B., Sparks, C., Zukerman, J., & Zurenda, L. (2008). Theoretical foundations of developmental-behavioral pediatrics. In M. L. Wolraich, P. H. Dworkin, D. Drotar, & E. Perrin (Eds.), *Developmental and behavioral pediatrics* (pp. 13–45). Elsevier.

Holmbeck, G. N., Kritikos, T. K., Stern, A., Ridosh, M., & Friedman, C. V. (2021). The transition to adult health care in youth with spina bifida: Theory, measurement, and interventions. *Journal of Nursing Scholarship*, 53(2), 198–207. https://doi.org/10.1111/jnu.12626

Holmbeck, G. N., Westhoven, V. C., Phillips, W. S., Bowers, R., Gruse, C., Nikolopoulos, T., Totura, C. M., & Davison, K. (2003). A multimethod, multi-informant, and multidimensional perspective on psychosocial adjustment in preadolescents with spina bifida. *Journal of Consulting and Clinical Psychology*, 71(4), 782–796. https://doi.org/10.1037/0022-006X.71.4.782

Huber, R., & Weber, P. (2022). Is there a relationship between socioeconomic factors and prevalence, adherence and outcome in childhood epilepsy? A systematic scoping review. *European Journal of Paediatric Neurology*, 38, 1–6. https://doi.org/10.1016/j.ejpn.2022.01.021

Hung, A. H., Cassedy, A., Schultz, H. M., Yeates, K. O., Taylor, H. G., Stancin, T., Walz, N. C., & Wade, S. L. (2017). Predictors of long-term victimization after early pediatric traumatic brain injury. *Journal of Developmental and Behavioral Pediatrics*, 38(1), 49–57. https://doi.org/10.1097/DBP.0000000000000366

Jimenez, N., Osorio, M., Ramos, J. L., Apkon, S., Ebel, B. E., & Rivara, F. P. (2015). Functional independence after inpatient rehabilitation for traumatic brain injury among minority children and adolescents. *Archives of Physical Medicine and Rehabilitation*, 96(7), 1255–1261. https://doi.org/10.1016/j.apmr.2015.02.019

Jimenez, N., Quistberg, A., Vavilala, M. S., Jaffe, K. M., & Rivara, F. P. (2017). Utilization of mental health services after mild pediatric traumatic brain injury. *Pediatrics*, 139(3), e20162462. https://doi.org/10.1542/peds.2016-2462

Joshi, S., Gali, K., Radecki, L., Shah, A., Hueneke, S., Calabrese, T., Katzenbach, A., Sachdeva, R., Brown, L., Kimball, E., White, P., McManus, P., Wood, D., Nelson, E. L., & Archuleta, P. (2020). Integrating quality improvement into the ECHO model to improve care for children and youth with epilepsy. *Epilepsia*, 61(9), 1999–2009. https://doi.org/10.1111/epi.16625

Kayle, M., Chu, D. I., Stern, A., Pan, W., & Holmbeck, G. N. (2020). Predictors of distinct trajectories of medical responsibility in youth with spina bifida. *Journal of Pediatric Psychology*, 45(10), 1153–1165. https://doi.org/10.1093/jpepsy/jsaa065

Keenan, H. T., Clark, A. E., Holubkov, R., Cox, C. S., & Ewing-Cobbs, L. (2018). Psychosocial and executive function recovery trajectories one year after pediatric traumatic brain injury: The influence of age and injury severity. *Journal of Neurotrauma*, 35(2), 286–296. https://doi.org/10.1089/neu.2017.5265

Kritikos, T. K., Stiles-Shields, C., Shapiro, J. B., & Holmbeck, G. N. (2022). Benefit-finding among young adults with spina bifida. *Journal of Health Psychology*, 27(5), 1176–1186. https://doi.org/10.1177/1359105321990804

Kroner, B. L., Fahimi, M., Kenyon, A., Thurman, D. J., & Gaillard, W. D. (2013). Racial and socioeconomic disparities in epilepsy in the District of Columbia. *Epilepsy Research*, 103(2–3), 279–287. https://doi.org/10.1016/j.eplepsyres.2012.07.005

Laatsch, L., Dodd, J., Brown, T., Ciccia, A., Connor, F., Davis, K., Doherty, M., Linden, M., Locascio, G., Lundine, J., Murphy, S., Nagele, D., Niemeier, J., Politis, A., Rode, C., Slomine, B., Smetana, R., & Yaeger, L. (2020). Evidence-based systematic review of cognitive rehabilitation, emotional, and family treatment studies for children with acquired brain injury literature: From 2006 to 2017. *Neuropsychological Rehabilitation*, 30(1), 130–161. https://doi.org/10.1080/09602011.2019.1678490

Laliberté Durish, C., Yeates, K. O., & Brooks, B. L. (2018). Psychological resilience as a predictor of persistent post-concussive symptoms in children with single and multiple concussion. *Journal of the International Neuropsychological Society*, 24(8), 759–768. https://doi.org/10.1017/S1355617718000437

Lalonde, G., Bernier, A., Beaudoin, C., Gravel, J., & Beauchamp, M. H. (2018). Investigating social functioning after early mild TBI: The quality of parent-child interactions. *Journal of Neuropsychology*, 12(1), 1–22. https://doi.org/10.1111/jnp.12104

Lennon, J. M., Klages, K. L., Amaro, C. M., Murray, C. B., & Holmbeck, G. N. (2015). Longitudinal study of neuropsychological functioning and internalizing symptoms in youth with spina bifida: Social competence as a mediator. *Journal of Pediatric Psychology*, 40(3), 336–348. https://doi.org/10.1093/jpepsy/jsu075

Lennon, J. M., Murray, C. B., Bechtel, C. F., & Holmbeck, G. N. (2015). Resilience and disruption in observed family interactions in youth with and without spina bifida: An eight-year, five-wave longitudinal study. *Journal of Pediatric Psychology*, 40(9), 943–955. https://doi.org/10.1093/jpepsy/jsv033

Lew, A. R., Lewis, C., Lunn, J., Tomlin, P., Basu, H., Roach, J., Rakshi, K., & Martland, T. (2015). Social cognition in children with epilepsy in mainstream education. *Developmental Medicine & Child Neurology*, 57(1), 53–59. https://doi.org/10.1111/dmcn.12613

Lewis, S. A., & Noyes, J. (2013). Effective process or dangerous precipice: Qualitative comparative embedded case study with young people with epilepsy and their parents during transition from children's to adult services. *BMC Pediatrics*, 13(1), 169. https://doi.org/10.1186/1471-2431-13-169

Linton, K. F., & Kim, B. J. (2014). Traumatic brain injury as a result of violence in Native American and Black communities spanning from childhood to older adulthood. *Brain Injury*, 28(8), 1076–1081. https://doi.org/10.3109/02699052.2014.901558

Lomax-Bream, L. E., Barnes, M., Copeland, K., Taylor, H. B., & Landry, S. H. (2007). The impact of spina bifida on development across the first 3 years. *Developmental Neuropsychology*, 31(1), 1–20. https://doi.org/10.1207/s15326942dn3101_1

Luis, C. A., & Mittenberg, W. (2002). Mood and anxiety disorders following pediatric traumatic brain injury: A prospective study. *Journal of Clinical and Experimental Neuropsychology*, 24(3), 270–279. https://doi.org/10.1076/jcen.24.3.270.982

Lumba-Brown, A., Yeates, K. O., Sarmiento, K., Breiding, M. J., Haegerich, T. M., Gioia, G. A., Turner, M., Benzel, E. C., Suskauer, S. J., Giza, C. C., Joseph, M., Broomand, C., Weissman, B., Gordon, W., Wright, D. W., Moser, R. S., McAvoy, K., Ewing-Cobbs, L., Duhaime, A. C., . . . Timmons, S. D. (2018). Centers for Disease Control and Prevention guideline on the diagnosis and management of mild traumatic brain injury among children. *JAMA Pediatrics*, 172(11), e182853. https://doi.org/10.1001/jamapediatrics.2018.2853

Mahmood, D., Dicianno, B., & Bellin, M. (2011). Self-management, preventable conditions and assessment of care among young adults with myelomeningocele. *Child: Care, Health and Development*, 37(6), 861–865. https://doi.org/10.1111/j.1365-2214.2011.01299.x

Mayes, S. D., & Calhoun, S. L. (2006). Frequency of reading, math, and writing disabilities in children with clinical disorders. *Learning and Individual Differences*, 16(2), 145–157. https://doi.org/10.1016/j.lindif.2005.07.004

McCarty, C. A., Zatzick, D. F., Marcynyszyn, L. A., Wang, J., Hilt, R., Jinguji, T., Quitiquit, C., Chrisman, S. P. D., & Rivara, F. P. (2021). Effect of collaborative care on persistent postconcussive symptoms in adolescents: A randomized clinical trial. *JAMA Network Open*, 4(2), e210207. https://doi.org/10.1001/jamanetworkopen.2021.0207

McEwan, M. J., Espie, C. A., Metcalfe, J., Brodie, M. J., & Wilson, M. T. (2004). Quality of life and psychosocial development in adolescents with epilepsy: A qualitative investigation using focus group methods. *Seizure*, 13(1), 15–31. https://doi.org/10.1016/S1059-1311(03)00080-3

McKinlay, A., Grace, R. C., McLellan, T., Roger, D., Clarbour, J., & MacFarlane, M. R. (2014). Predicting adult offending behavior for individuals who experienced a traumatic brain injury during childhood. *The Journal of Head Trauma Rehabilitation*, 29(6), 507–513. https://doi.org/10.1097/HTR.0000000000000000

McNally, K. A., Patrick, K. E., LaFleur, J. E., Dykstra, J. B., Monahan, K., & Hoskinson, K. R. (2018). Brief cognitive behavioral intervention for children and adolescents with persistent post-concussive symptoms: A pilot study. *Child Neuropsychology*, 24(3), 396–412. https://doi.org/10.1080/09297049.2017.1280143

Modi, A. C., Guilfoyle, S. M., Glauser, T. A., & Mara, C. A. (2021). Supporting treatment adherence regimens in children with epilepsy: A randomized clinical trial. *Epilepsia*, 62(7), 1643–1655. https://doi.org/10.1111/epi.16921

Modi, A. C., Pai, A. L., Hommel, K. A., Hood, K. K., Cortina, S., Hilliard, M. E., Guilfoyle, S. M., Gray, W. N., & Drotar, D. (2012). Pediatric self-management: A framework for research, practice, and policy. *Pediatrics*, 129(2), e473–e485. https://doi.org/10.1542/peds.2011-1635

Mohanraj, R., & Brodie, M. J. (2006). Diagnosing refractory epilepsy: Response to sequential treatment schedules. *European Journal of Neurology*, 13(3), 277–282. https://doi.org/10.1111/j.1468-1331.2006.01215.x

Mohanraj, R., & Brodie, M. J. (2013). Early predictors of outcome in newly diagnosed epilepsy. *Seizure*, 22(5), 333–344. https://doi.org/10.1016/j.seizure.2013.02.002

Neubauer, B. A., Gross, S., & Hahn, A. (2008). Epilepsy in childhood and adolescence. *Deutsches Ärzteblatt International*, 105(17), 319–327. https://doi.org/10.3238/arztebl.2008.0319

O'Mahar, K., Holmbeck, G. N., Jandasek, B., & Zukerman, J. (2010). A camp-based intervention targeting independence among individuals with spina bifida. *Journal of Pediatric Psychology*, 35(8), 848–856. https://doi.org/10.1093/jpepsy/jsp125

O'Toole, S., Lambert, V., Gallagher, P., Shahwan, A., & Austin, J. K. (2016). "I don't like talking about it because that's not who I am": Challenges children face during epilepsy-related family communication.

Chronic Illness, 12(3), 216–226. https://doi.org/10.1177/1742395316644307

Oakeshott, P., Hunt, G. M., Poulton, A., & Reid, F. (2010). Expectation of life and unexpected death in open spina bifida: A 40-year complete, non-selective, longitudinal cohort study. *Developmental Medicine & Child Neurology, 52*(8), 749–753. https://doi.org/10.1111/j.1469-8749.2009.03543.x

Ohanian, D. M., Stiles-Shields, C., Afzal, K. I., Driscoll, C. F. B., Papadakis, J. L., Stern, A., Starnes, M., & Holmbeck, G. N. (2018). Cultural considerations for autonomy and medical adherence in a young Palestinian American Muslim female with spina bifida: A longitudinal case study in a research context. *Clinical Practice in Pediatric Psychology, 6*(4), 386–397. https://doi.org/10.1037/cpp0000250

Olusanya, B. O., Wright, S. M., Nair, M. K. C., Boo, N. Y., Halpern, R., Kuper, H., Abubakar, A. A., Almasri, N. A., Arabloo, J., Arora, N. K., Backhaus, S., Berman, B. D., Breinbauer, C., Carr, G., de Vries, P. J., Del Castillo-Hegyi, C., Eftekhari, A., Gladstone, M. J., Hoekstra, R. A., ... Kassebaum, N. J. (2020). Global burden of childhood epilepsy, intellectual disability, and sensory impairments. *Pediatrics, 146*(1), e20192623. https://doi.org/10.1542/peds.2019-2623

Ott, D., Siddarth, P., Gurbani, S., Koh, S., Tournay, A., Shields, W. D., & Caplan, R. (2003). Behavioral disorders in pediatric epilepsy: Unmet psychiatric need. *Epilepsia, 44*(4), 591–597. https://doi.org/10.1046/j.1528-1157.2003.25002.x

Papadakis, J. L., & Holmbeck, G. N. (2021). Sociodemographic factors and health-related, neuropsychological, and psychosocial functioning in youth with spina bifida. *Rehabilitation Psychology, 66*(3), 286–299. https://doi.org/10.1037/rep0000381

Peterson, C., Xu, L., Florence, C., & Parks, S. E. (2015). Annual cost of U.S. hospital visits for pediatric abusive head trauma. *Child Maltreatment, 20*(3), 162–169. https://doi.org/10.1177/1077559515583549

Porter, A., Brown, C. C., Tilford, J. M., Thomas, K., Maxson, R. T., Sexton, K., Karim, S., Zohoori, N., & Rodriguez, A. (2020). Association of insurance status with treatment and outcomes in pediatric patients with severe traumatic brain injury. *Critical Care Medicine, 48*(7), e584–e591. https://doi.org/10.1097/CCM.0000000000004398

Reilly, C., Atkinson, P., Das, K. B., Chin, R. F. C., Aylett, S. E., Burch, V., Gillberg, C., Scott, R. C., & Neville, B. G. (2014a). Academic achievement in school-aged children with active epilepsy: A population-based study. *Epilepsia, 55*(12), 1910–1917. https://doi.org/10.1111/epi.12826

Reilly, C., Atkinson, P., Das, K. B., Chin, R. F., Aylett, S. E., Burch, V., Gillberg, C., Scott, R. C., & Neville, B. G. (2014b). Neurobehavioral comorbidities in children with active epilepsy: A population-based study. *Pediatrics, 133*(6), e1586–e1593. https://doi.org/10.1542/peds.2013-3787

Rivara, F. P., Koepsell, T. D., Wang, J., Temkin, N., Dorsch, A., Vavilala, M. S., Durbin, D., & Jaffe, K. M. (2012). Incidence of disability among children 12 months after traumatic brain injury. *American Journal of Public Health, 102*(11), 2074–2079. https://doi.org/10.2105/AJPH.2012.300696

Russ, S. A., Larson, K., & Halfon, N. (2012). A national profile of childhood epilepsy and seizure disorder. *Pediatrics, 129*(2), 256–264. https://doi.org/10.1542/peds.2010-1371

Ryan, N. P., Anderson, V., Godfrey, C., Eren, S., Rosema, S., Taylor, K., & Catroppa, C. (2013). Social communication mediates the relationship between emotion perception and externalizing behaviors in young adult survivors of pediatric traumatic brain injury (TBI). *International Journal of Developmental Neuroscience, 31*(8), 811–819. https://doi.org/10.1016/j.ijdevneu.2013.10.002

Ryan, N. P., Anderson, V. A., Bigler, E. D., Dennis, M., Taylor, H. G., Rubin, K. H., Vannatta, K., Gerhardt, C. A., Stancin, T., Beauchamp, M. H., Hearps, S., Catroppa, C., & Yeates, K. O. (2020). Delineating the nature and correlates of social dysfunction after childhood traumatic brain injury using common data elements: Evidence from an international multi-cohort study. *Journal of Neurotrauma, 38*(2), 252–260. https://doi.org/10.1089/neu.2020.7057

Sadler, T. W. (2005, May). Embryology of neural tube development. *American Journal of Medical Genetics Part C, Seminars in Medical Genetics, 135C*(1), 2–8. https://doi.org/10.1002/ajmg.c.30049

Sánchez Fernández, I., Stephen, C., & Loddenkemper, T. (2017). Disparities in epilepsy surgery in the United States of America. *Journal of Neurology, 264*(8), 1735–1745. https://doi.org/10.1007/s00415-017-8560-6

Sandler, A. D. (2010). Children with spina bifida: Key clinical issues. *Pediatric Clinics of North America, 57*(4), 879–892. https://doi.org/10.1016/j.pcl.2010.07.009

Schechter, M. S., Liu, T., Soe, M., Swanson, M., Ward, E., & Thibadeau, J. (2015). Sociodemographic attributes and spina bifida outcomes. *Pediatrics, 135*(4), e957–e964. https://doi.org/10.1542/peds.2014-2576

Scheffer, I. E., Berkovic, S., Capovilla, G., Connolly, M. B., French, J., Guilhoto, L., Hirsch, E., Jain, S., Mathern, G. W., Moshé, S. L., Nordli, D. R., Perucca, E., Tomson, T., Wiebe, S., Zhang, Y. H.,

& Zuberi, S. M. (2017). ILAE classification of the epilepsies: Position paper of the ILAE Commission for Classification and Terminology. *Epilepsia, 58*(4), 512–521. https://doi.org/10.1111/epi.13709

Showen, A. E., Copp, H. L., Allen, I. E., & Hampson, L. A. (2021). Resilience and associated characteristics in adults with spina bifida. *Developmental Medicine & Child Neurology, 63*(10), 1229–1235. https://doi.org/10.1111/dmcn.14919

Slomine, B. S., McCarthy, M. L., Ding, R., MacKenzie, E. J., Jaffe, K. M., Aitken, M. E., Durbin, D. R., Christensen, J. R., Dorsch, A. M., Paidas, C. N., & the CHAT Study Group. (2006). Health care utilization and needs after pediatric traumatic brain injury. *Pediatrics, 117*(4), e663–e674. https://doi.org/10.1542/peds.2005-1892

Smith, A. W., Gutierrez-Colina, A. M., Guilfoyle, S. M., & Modi, A. C. (2020). Pediatric epilepsy. In A. C. Modi & K. A. Driscoll (Eds.), *Adherence and self-management in pediatric populations* (pp. 207–233). Academic Press. https://doi.org/10.1016/B978-0-12-816000-8.00009-8

Smith, A. W., Gutierrez-Colina, A. M., Roemisch, E., Hater, B., Combs, A., Shoulberg, A. M., & Modi, A. C. (2021). Modifiable factors related to transition readiness in adolescents and young adults with epilepsy. *Epilepsy & Behavior, 115*, 107718–107718. https://doi.org/10.1016/j.yebeh.2020.107718

Sokka, A., Olsen, P., Kirjavainen, J., Harju, M., Keski-Nisula, L., Räisänen, S., Heinonen, S., & Kälviäinen, R. (2017). Etiology, syndrome diagnosis, and cognition in childhood-onset epilepsy: A population-based study. *Epilepsia Open, 2*(1), 76–83. https://doi.org/10.1002/epi4.12036

Spina Bifida Association. (2018). *Guidelines for the care of people with spina bifida*. https://www.spinabifidaassociation.org/guidelines/

Sroufe, N. S., Fuller, D. S., West, B. T., Singal, B. M., Warschausky, S. A., & Maio, R. F. (2010). Postconcussive symptoms and neurocognitive function after mild traumatic brain injury in children. *Pediatrics, 125*(6), e1331–e1339. https://doi.org/10.1542/peds.2008-2364

Stancin, T., & Perrin, E. C. (2014). Psychologists and pediatricians: Opportunities for collaboration in primary care. *American Psychologist, 69*(4), 332–343. https://doi.org/10.1037/a0036046

Stancin, T., Wade, S. L., Walz, N. C., Yeates, K. O., & Taylor, H. G. (2010). Family adaptation 18 months after traumatic brain injury in early childhood. *Journal of Developmental & Behavioral Pediatrics, 31*(4), 317–325. https://doi.org/10.1097/DBP.0b013e3181dbaf32

Stern, A., Amaral, S., Driscoll, C. F. B., Psihogios, A. M., Stiles-Shields, E. C., Zebracki, K., & Holmbeck, G. N. (2020). Spina bifida. In A. C. Modi & K. A. Driscoll (Eds.), *Adherence and self-management in pediatric populations* (pp. 235–261). Elsevier. https://doi.org/10.1016/B978-0-12-816000-8.00010-4

Stubberud, J., Langenbahn, D., Levine, B., Stanghelle, J., & Schanke, A. K. (2015). Emotional health and coping in spina bifida after goal management training: A randomized controlled trial. *Rehabilitation Psychology, 60*(1), 1–16. https://doi.org/10.1037/rep0000018

Swartwout, M. D., Garnaat, S. L., Myszka, K. A., Fletcher, J. M., & Dennis, M. (2010). Associations of ethnicity and SES with IQ and achievement in spina bifida meningomyelocele. *Journal of Pediatric Psychology, 35*(9), 927–936. https://doi.org/10.1093/jpepsy/jsq001

Szaflarski, M. (2014). Social determinants of health in epilepsy. *Epilepsy & Behavior, 41*, 283–289. https://doi.org/10.1016/j.yebeh.2014.06.013

Taylor, H. G., Swartwout, M. D., Yeates, K. O., Walz, N. C., Stancin, T., & Wade, S. L. (2008). Traumatic brain injury in young children: Post-acute effects on cognitive and school readiness skills. *Journal of the International Neuropsychological Society, 14*(5), 734–745. https://doi.org/10.1017/S1355617708081150

Taylor, H. G., Yeates, K. O., Wade, S. L., Drotar, D., Stancin, T., & Minich, N. (2002). A prospective study of short- and long-term outcomes after traumatic brain injury in children: Behavior and achievement. *Neuropsychology, 16*(1), 15–27. https://doi.org/10.1037/0894-4105.16.1.15

Thibadeau, J., Walker, W. O., Jr., Castillo, J., Dicianno, B. E., Routh, J. C., Smith, K. A., & Ouyang, L. (2020). Philosophy of care delivery for spina bifida. *Disability and Health Journal, 13*(2), 100883. https://doi.org/10.1016/j.dhjo.2019.100883

Verhoef, M., Barf, H. A., Vroege, J. A., Post, M. W., Van Asbeck, F. W., Gooskens, R. H., & Prevo, A. J. (2005). Sex education, relationships, and sexuality in young adults with spina bifida. *Archives of Physical Medicine and Rehabilitation, 86*(5), 979–987. https://doi.org/10.1016/j.apmr.2004.10.042

Wade, S. L., Kurowski, B. G., Kirkwood, M. W., Zhang, N., Cassedy, A., Brown, T. M., Nielsen, B., Stancin, T., & Taylor, H. G. (2015). Online problem-solving therapy after traumatic brain injury: A randomized controlled trial. *Pediatrics, 135*(2), e487–e495. https://doi.org/10.1542/peds.2014-1386

Wade, S. L., Taylor, H. G., Cassedy, A., Zhang, N., Kirkwood, M. W., Brown, T. M., & Stancin, T. (2015). Long-term behavioral outcomes after a randomized, clinical trial of counselor-assisted problem solving for adolescents with complicated mild-to-severe traumatic brain injury. *Journal of Neurotrauma, 32*(13), 967–975. https://doi.org/10.1089/neu.2014.3684

Wade, S. L., Taylor, H. G., Walz, N. C., Salisbury, S., Stancin, T., Bernard, L. A., Oberjohn, K., & Yeates, K. O. (2008). Parent-child interactions during the initial weeks following brain injury in young children. *Rehabilitation Psychology, 53*(2), 180–190. https://doi.org/10.1037/0090-5550.53.2.180

Wade, S. L., Zhang, N., Yeates, K. O., Stancin, T., & Taylor, H. G. (2016). Social environmental moderators of long-term functional outcomes of early childhood brain injury. *JAMA Pediatrics, 170*(4), 343–349. https://doi.org/10.1001/jamapediatrics.2015.4485

Yeates, K. O., Armstrong, K., Janusz, J., Taylor, H. G., Wade, S., Stancin, T., & Drotar, D. (2005). Long-term attention problems in children with traumatic brain injury. *Journal of the American Academy of Child & Adolescent Psychiatry, 44*(6), 574–584. https://doi.org/10.1097/01.chi.0000159947.50523.64

Yeates, K. O., Gerhardt, C. A., Bigler, E. D., Abildskov, T., Dennis, M., Rubin, K. H., Stancin, T., Taylor, H. G., & Vannatta, K. (2013). Peer relationships of children with traumatic brain injury. *Journal of the International Neuropsychological Society, 19*(5), 518–527. https://doi.org/10.1017/S1355617712001531

Yue, J. K., Upadhyayula, P. S., Avalos, L. N., & Cage, T. A. (2020). Pediatric traumatic brain injury in the United States: Rural-urban disparities and considerations. *Brain Sciences, 10*(3). https://doi.org/10.3390/brainsci10030135

Zack, M. M., & Kobau, R. (2017). National and state estimates of the numbers of adults and children with active epilepsy—United States, 2015. *MMWR: Morbidity and Mortality Weekly Report, 66*(31), 821–825. https://doi.org/10.15585/mmwr.mm6631a1

Zebracki, K., Zaccariello, M., Zelko, F., & Holmbeck, G. (2010). Adolescence and emerging adulthood in individuals with spina bifida: A developmental neuropsychological perspective. In J. Donders & S. Hunter (Eds.), *Principles and practice of lifespan developmental neuropsychology* (pp. 183–194). Cambridge University Press. https://doi.org/10.1017/CBO9780511674815.015

Zhang, N., Kaizar, E. E., Narad, M. E., Kurowski, B. G., Yeates, K. O., Taylor, H. G., & Wade, S. L. (2019). Examination of injury, host, and social-environmental moderators of online family problem solving treatment efficacy for pediatric traumatic brain injury using an individual participant data meta-analytic approach. *Journal of Neurotrauma, 36*(7), 1147–1155. https://doi.org/10.1089/neu.2018.5885

CHAPTER 10

PEDIATRIC SICKLE CELL DISEASE: IMPLICATIONS FOR CHILD HEALTH AND DEVELOPMENT

Kemar V. Prussien, Lamia P. Barakat, and Lisa A. Schwartz

Sickle cell disease (SCD) is a genetic disorder that primarily occurs in individuals of African descent and results in the production of abnormal, sickle-shaped hemoglobin that prevents sufficient oxygen delivery to tissue, muscles, and organs throughout the body. Sickle cell anemia (SCA), the most common and severe genotype of SCD (i.e., Hemoglobin SS [HbSS]), often results in chronic anemia, which has downstream effects on multiple aspects of health, including chronic pain, fatigue, organ damage, silent cerebral infarcts (SCIs), and stroke. SCD is primarily diagnosed at infancy, and both physiological and psychosocial impacts of the disease are prevalent throughout the lifespan. During childhood, medical morbidities can impact psychosocial functions including cognition, school performance, peer relationships, and overall health-related quality of life. SCD primarily occurs in individuals of African descent. Medical and psychosocial outcomes are heavily impacted by ecological contexts and social determinants of health across individual, family, institutional, and societal levels. Children with SCD, therefore, require interdisciplinary care across hematology, neurology, pediatric psychology, neuropsychology, and developmental-behavioral pediatrics to facilitate healthy development, prevent and treat sickle cell comorbidities, and address barriers to care that limit health-related quality of life.

As such, this chapter reviews medical, developmental, and psychosocial aspects of pediatric SCD. Drawing from the research in developmental science, multilevel risk and resiliency factors are described in each medical and psychosocial outcome. Further, as SCD is primarily prevalent in individuals across the African diaspora, and many immigrant or international families receive treatment in the United States, results from global studies are discussed. The chapter begins by describing the pathophysiology and epidemiology of SCD including prevalence and incidence, survival and mortality, and pharmacological treatments. A review follows with important socioecological models relevant to development, medical, and psychosocial outcomes in SCD. Further, medical morbidities such as acute and chronic pain, central nervous system (CNS) complications, and cognitive functioning will be reviewed. Psychosocial outcomes including school functioning and academic achievement, social functioning and peer relationships, emotional functioning, stigma, and self-management are also discussed. The chapter will then review particularly salient resilience factors related to improved health-related quality of life, important considerations for multidisciplinary care, including the role of developmental-behavioral pediatricians and pediatric psychologists, and assessment for

https://doi.org/10.1037/0000414-010
APA Handbook of Pediatric Psychology, Developmental-Behavioral Pediatrics, and Developmental Science: Vol. 2. Pediatric Psychology and Developmental-Behavioral Pediatrics: Clinical Applications of Developmental Science, P. E. Shah and M. H. Bornstein (Editors-in-Chief)
Copyright © 2025 by the American Psychological Association. All rights reserved.

the transition from pediatric to adult-oriented care. Important take-aways for the chapter are summarized in the conclusion, and resources for both clinicians and families are also provided.

PATHOPHYSIOLOGY AND EPIDEMIOLOGY OF SICKLE CELL DISEASE

It is critical to understand the pathophysiology and epidemiology of SCD to fully deduce the developmental-behavioral implications of the condition. This section describes SCD pathophysiology, prevalence and incidence, and survival and mortality.

Pathophysiology

SCD describes a group of hemoglobin disorders that occur in individuals who inherit a hemoglobin S (HbS) gene as well as another abnormal hemoglobin gene. The homozygous SCD genotype (HbSS; also known as SCA) is the most common genotype, and heterozygous genotypes (e.g., HbS beta thalassemias, HbSC, HbSD, HbSE, HbSO/Arab) occur with less frequency. Red blood cells with HbS carry fewer oxygen molecules and live an average of 10 to 20 days—significantly shorter than the 120-day lifespan of a cell with healthy hemoglobin A (Kanter & Kruse-Jarres, 2013). These factors contribute to the numerous medical complications of SCD, which can begin as early as 3 to 6 months of age when the infant body transitions from fetal hemoglobin (which is able to transport sufficient oxygen to tissues) to the production of adult hemoglobin with the abnormal gene. Due to the insufficient carrying capacity and transport of oxygen, children and adolescents with SCD experience both acute and chronic pain (Brandow et al., 2017). Acute pain events, called *vaso-occlusive pain crises* (VOCs), occur during periods of severe anemia caused by hemolysis, or the destruction of red blood cells (Brandow et al., 2017). Additional outcomes of hemolytic anemia (as opposed to anemia due to iron deficiency) include insufficient oxygenation of organs, including the brain. Chronic organ complications impacted by SCD include chronic kidney disease, end-stage renal disease, and pulmonary hypertension, splenic infarction (also known as splenic sequestration), avascular necrosis, retinopathy, and priapism (Ware et al., 2017).

SCA can have a significant impact on the brain via its impact on cerebral hemodynamics, which can be quantified by four measures:

1. the volume of blood being delivered to brain tissue (i.e., cerebral blood volume; mL blood/100 g tissue),
2. the rate of blood delivery to brain tissue (i.e., cerebral blood flow; mL blood/100 g tissue/min),
3. the metabolic rate of oxygen consumption (mL O_2/100 mL brain/min), and
4. the percentage of oxygen extracted from the blood by the tissue relative to the volume of oxygen delivered (i.e., oxygen extraction fraction).

Due to the lower levels of oxygen, there is a compensatory effect for blood flow such that the rate of blood delivery is increased to compensate for the hypoxic conditions. Low oxygen, compensatory increases in cerebral blood flow, and the presence of a prior infarct all increase the risk of cerebral infarcts in children with SCD (DeBaun & Kirkham, 2016).

Prevalence and Incidence

The global prevalence of SCD is estimated to be greater than 20 million (National Institutes of Health [NIH], 2021), and, due to the protective and adaptive nature of sickle cell trait (Hemoglobin AS) against malaria infection, the birth rate will likely increase by one-third from 2010 to 2050 with nations in sub-Saharan Africa carrying the greatest burden of the disease (Piel et al., 2013). There are approximately 100,000 people living with SCD in the United States, and national newborn screenings have identified that SCD occurs in 1 in 365 African American births (Brousseau, Panepinto, et al., 2010). Although nearly 90% of individuals with SCD in the United States are African American (Brousseau, Panepinto, et al., 2010), SCD is also prevalent among individuals of Hispanic, Mediterranean, Middle Eastern, and Indian descent (Piel et al., 2013).

Survival and Mortality

Survival has improved significantly for children with SCD in the United States with nearly 95% of people with SCD currently living into adulthood (Elmariah et al., 2014). Due to the deleterious impact of the disease on spleen functioning that results in the improper clearing of bacteria, infectious complications often resulted in shortened lifespan (Ware et al., 2017). Average life expectancy was less than 20 years of age in 1970, and life expectancy increased to 42 years of age for men and 48 years of age for women by the early 1990s with the initiation of newborn screening programs and improved use of penicillin prophylaxis and pneumococcal vaccination that reduces infection due to splenic sequestration (inflamed spleen due to HbS-related infarction) or resultant splenectomy (Lanzkron et al., 2013). Nevertheless, life expectancy for individuals with SCD at present in the United States remains 25 to 30 years shorter than the general population, with morbidity at its highest between age 18 and 30 years during the transition from pediatric to adult-oriented specialty care (Lanzkron et al., 2013; Volume 1, Chapter 16, this handbook). Public health programs and availability of treatments, especially during childhood, drive differential survival across the United States relative to sub-Saharan Africa where morbidity is highest during ages 0 to 5 years of age, with nearly 50% of children with SCD dying before age 5 (Nnodu et al., 2021; Piel et al., 2013).

Pharmacological Treatment

Three oral medications, hydroxyurea, L-glutamine (Endari), and voxeletor (Oxbryta), have been approved by the United States Food and Drug Administration (USFDA) as treatments for symptom management and prevention of further complications of the disease. Hydroxyurea acts to prevent the sickling of red blood cells by inducing fetal hemoglobin; L-glutamine provides antioxidants to allow red blood cells to regain flexibility; and voxeletor increases stability in HbS during an oxygenated state. Children as young as 9 months old are eligible to begin hydroxyurea, and children ages 5 years and above can begin L-glutamine separately from, or in addition to, hydroxyurea. Voxeletor is available to children ages 4 years and older, and it can be combined with hydroxyurea for children ages 12 years and older (Herity et al., 2021). Monthly crizanlizumab (Adakveo) infusions for patients aged 16 years and older was USFDA approved in 2019 to reduce frequency of VOCs by inhibiting red blood cell adhesion (Blair, 2020). Individuals with severe complications or elevated medical risk may receive chronic transfusion therapy to replace cells with HbS, or patients might become eligible for hematopoietic stem cell transplantation, which is the only available curative treatment (Khemani et al., 2019). Gene therapy is currently being studied in Phase II trials with encouraging findings, but it is not yet widely available (Khemani et al., 2019).

MULTILEVEL PREDICTORS OF HEALTH OUTCOMES AND DISPARITIES

Developmental science has underscored how child development and health outcomes unfold over time, influenced by numerous factors in the child, family, and broader ecological environment. Among the most well-known and utilized socioecological model of child development, Urie Bronfenbrenner's Ecological Systems Theory poses that children's developmental processes are impacted by a complex system of environmental levels (Bronfenbrenner, 1979), including:

- the child's individual characteristics,
- relationships within their immediate environment (e.g., parents, siblings, teachers, school peers; i.e., microsystem [Volume 1, Chapter 13, this handbook]),
- interactions among individuals within their immediate environment (e.g., parent interactions with teachers; i.e., mesosystem),
- formal and informal social structures that might indirectly impact the child through both the micro and mesosystem (e.g., parental workplace; i.e., exosystem), and
- social impacts on cultural and sociodemographic factors (e.g., socioeconomic status [SES], poverty, racial disparities; i.e., macrosystem [Volume 1, Chapters 18 and 19, this handbook]).

The final level of Bronfenbrenner's Ecological Systems Theory is the chronosystem, which describes broad environmental changes, including global and historical events, and life transitions, that influence a child's development. Therefore, this theory poses that there are individual-level, family-level, institutional-level, and broader systemic-level factors that interact with, and contribute to, children's development.

Socioecological theories have also been applied to pediatric conditions to investigate and describe risk and resilience for health and psychosocial outcomes. The Health Equity Framework emphasizes multiple interacting spheres of influence, including systems of power, relationships and networks, and physiological pathways in addition to individual factors to describe multifactorial predictors of health equity and health disparities (Peterson et al., 2021). For example, factors within systems of power can be used to promote health equity by ensuring fair access to resources and opportunities across groups, whereas systems can also increase health disparities by promoting or maintaining unfair environmental, social, and economic advantages for one group over another. Nevertheless, each of these constructs can be investigated across and within several socioecological contexts (e.g., daily interpersonal racism vs. institutional and systemic racism). In sum, health outcomes are a result of complex interactions between people and their environment.

Factors across multiple socioecological levels drive health disparities within and across disease populations (Volume 1, Chapter 18, this handbook). Among the most assessed are factors relevant to the individual (e.g., race/ethnicity, sex, gender, income, education); however, individual factors alone do not explain poor health and outcomes. As SCD primarily impacts Black individuals across the African diaspora, medical and psychosocial outcomes are impacted by intersections among social determinants of health and implicit biases within the context of systemic racism. Racial bias has been most clearly documented in the barriers to effective pain treatment, described in detail in the subsequent section "Racial Bias and Stigma" (see also Volume 1, Chapter 19, this handbook). Further, children and adolescents with SCD experience significant health disparities related to limited access to health care and elevated reliance on emergency medicine. In the United States comprehensive care for SCD is significantly limited relative to other genetic conditions with lower prevalence, such as cystic fibrosis, and poor outcomes in nonspecialized hospitals are related to lack of hematologists with expertise in SCD (McCavit et al., 2011). Relatedly, compared to other diseases, research in SCD is underfunded, which contributes to disparities in treatment and health outcomes (Farooq et al., 2020).

Insufficient federal and foundation funding has hampered efforts to develop effective treatments for SCD relative to other pediatric populations. For example, cystic fibrosis, a disease that primarily occurs in the non-Hispanic White population, obtains 3.4 times more funding as SCD from the National Institutes of Health and 75 times more funding from national foundations, despite cystic fibrosis having approximately one-third the prevalence of SCD in the United States (Farooq et al., 2020). There have been direct calls to reduce racism in the care of individuals with SCD (Power-Hays & McGann, 2020).

Suboptimal medical and psychosocial outcomes in SCD have been associated with ecological risk factors at the individual level (e.g., biological risks), family level (e.g., SES, psychosocial factors, parental factors), and systemic level (e.g., implicit bias and stigma), and these influences will be discussed in greater detail within each subsequent section of this chapter.

MEDICAL MORBIDITIES ASSOCIATED WITH SICKLE CELL DISEASE

Despite incremental medical advances, children and adolescents with SCD are at risk for lifelong disability and significant morbidity. The primary areas of medical and neurological risk in SCD are acute and chronic pain, CNS complications via silent cerebral infarcts and strokes, and deficits in cognitive function.

Acute and Chronic Pain

Children and adolescents with SCD often experience both acute and chronic pain (Brandow et al., 2017). Acute pain events, VOCs, occur abruptly causing severe and debilitating pain that can last one week or more (Brandow et al., 2017). VOCs can begin in infants as young as 6 months of age, during the period when fetal hemoglobin in replaced by abnormal HbS (Brandow et al., 2017). Pain crises in infants and toddlers often present in swollen hands and feet (i.e., dactylitis; Ware et al., 2017), which is often confused with trauma or injury; yet this presentation reduces during childhood and shifts to a more invisible disease, which can contribute to implicit bias regarding recognition and timely management of pain crises, described in a subsequent section. Nevertheless, crises increase in number, duration, and severity with age, such that adolescents report greater pain relative to children (Brandow et al., 2017; Panepinto et al., 2005). VOCs, as well as hemolysis-related anemia, are triggered by illness, dehydration, and cold temperatures, high wind speeds, and high barometric pressure; however, there is often no clear precipitant, making VOCs unpredictable and difficult to prevent (Brandow et al., 2017). As such, VOCs are the leading cause of emergency department (ED) visits and hospital admissions for the SCD population (Brandow et al., 2017).

Pain treatments range from oral and intravenous medications to cognitive behavior therapies, relaxation, and mindfulness. Intravenous opioids are the primary treatment for VOCs, and, due to the lifelong treatment of episodes, individuals with SCD often require higher opioid doses over time (Crawford et al., 2006). Given the stark rise of opioid-related deaths from 1999 to 2018, medical institutions have increased suspicion of drug abuse among patients that request or require opioid medications. Regarding the impact of systemic-level and interpersonal racial bias on health outcomes within the context of the opioid crisis, Black and African Americans are significantly less likely than non-Hispanic White individuals to receive adequate pain management within the health care system (Lee et al., 2019). Despite findings that patients with SCD do not show increased risk for drug abuse or opioid-related death (Ballas, 2021; Ehrentraut et al., 2014), the impact and outcomes of racial bias heightens negative experiences with suspicion from the medical system. Adolescents and young adults with SCD are often viewed as drug-seeking when stating accurate knowledge of effective medications and their pain plan was developed with the hematology team (Stollon et al., 2015). Of note, a multicenter retrospective study revealed that children and adolescents with SCD who presented to the ED with acute pain often waited 70 to 75 minutes longer than guideline recommendations to receive analgesics (Tanabe et al., 2007), further highlighting inadequate pain treatment that this population receives.

Moreover, children and adolescents with SCD are at a greater risk for developing chronic pain that can be due to, or independent from, acute crises. Up to 40% of children and adolescents with SCD have chronic pain, with 35% reporting daily pain (Sil, Cohen, et al., 2016). Greater VOCs and *pain catastrophizing*, defined as persistent rumination on painful experiences and describing it in exaggerated or limitless terms (e.g., "It's terrible, and I think it's never going to get any better"), among children with SCD and their parents are related to chronic pain frequency and intensity (Brandow et al., 2017; Sil, Dampier, et al., 2016). For example, when assessing individual and family-level risk and resilience factors, Sil, Dampier, and Cohen (2016) found that having a parent with low pain catastrophizing acts as a protective factor for disability only when the child also has low catastrophizing. In contrast, children with low levels of catastrophizing show moderate pain disability when their parents report high catastrophizing. In fact, children of high catastrophizing parents show moderate pain disability regardless of whether the child's catastrophizing is high or low. Yet, low parent catastrophizing paired with high child catastrophizing results in the greatest level of disability. These findings suggest that high levels of parent catastrophizing and incongruence between parent and child catastrophizing are related to poor functional outcomes. High parental catastrophizing might trigger additional anxiety and worry about pain, which can then amplify the child's pain experience and behavior, which then contribute to feedback loop of negative emotions and outcomes between the parent and child. Incongruence, however, is likely related to feelings of invalidation, frustration, poor communication, and conflicting opinions in pain management strategies.

Cognitive behavior therapy, with core components of relaxation, guided imagery, and cognitive restructuring related to catastrophizing and other maladaptive thinking patterns, has been identified as a potentially effective treatment for chronic pain in SCD and improved daily functioning (Chen et al., 2004; Gil et al., 2001). Although other psychosocial interventions effective for other chronic and acute pain conditions (e.g., hypnosis, biofeedback) have been tested in pediatric SCD with promising outcomes, findings are limited by nonrandomized research methods and lack of replication (Chen et al., 2004).

Central Nervous System Complications

Cerebral infarction is the most common cause of neurological damage in children with SCD, with broad impacts on functional outcomes in motor, cognitive, and psychological functioning (DeBaun & Kirkham, 2016; Ware et al., 2017). Stroke occurs in 11% of children with SCD by 18 years of age (Ohene-Frempong et al., 1998), and silent cerebral infarcts (i.e., infarcts that do not have immediate and visible clinical symptoms) occur in up to 30% of children with SCD prior to 6 years of age and 39% of children by 18 years (Bernaudin et al., 2015; Kwiatkowski et al., 2009). Hemorrhagic strokes are significantly less common, occurring in approximately 3% of children with SCD (Kossorotoff et al., 2015).

Several hemodynamic risk factors have been investigated in relation to silent cerebral infarcts and stroke. Central nervous system vasculopathy, elevated cerebral blood flow, lower cerebrovascular reserve, and lower oxygen saturation coupled with greater oxygen demand are additional risk factors for stroke (DeBaun & Kirkham, 2016). Children with low baseline hemoglobin, hypertension, acute anemia, and evidence of cerebrovascular disease on intracranial and extracranial magnetic resonance angiography are at greater risk for silent cerebral infarct (Bernaudin et al., 2015). Despite these well-studied risk factors, accurate prediction of cerebral infarction remains difficult (DeBaun & Kirkham, 2016). Randomized controlled trials have shown that monthly blood transfusion therapy is an effective treatment for primary stroke prevention for children with abnormally elevated cerebral flood flow velocity (i.e., ≥ 200 cm/sec), measured by transcranial Doppler ultrasound, and secondary stroke prevention in children who have already experienced a silent cerebral infarct or stroke (DeBaun et al., 2014; Ware et al., 2012).

Cognitive Function

A comprehensive meta-analysis of cognitive function in SCD across the lifespan showed that children and adolescents with SCD are at risk for deficits in several domains of cognitive function (Prussien et al., 2019). Deficits in Full Scale IQ (FSIQ), verbal reasoning, and executive function relative to the normative mean emerged during preschool years. On average, young children with SCD obtain scores 6 to 10 points below the mean on tests of cognitive function ($M = 100$, $SD = 15$). Although this is a statistically significant, these scores are still in the average range. School-aged samples of children with SCD showed large deficits in FSIQ, verbal reasoning, perceptual reasoning, executive function, and processing speed of verbal and visual information relative to the normative mean, with scores falling in the low average range (13 to 18 points below the mean). School-aged children show medium to large effects compared with siblings or healthy controls. The magnitude of these SCD-associated cognitive deficits appear to increase with age, with school-aged children showing greater deficits in FSIQ, verbal reasoning, and perceptual reasoning relative to preschool samples (King et al., 2014). These cognitive deficits which are amplified with age highlight the importance of longitudinal monitoring of academic and school functioning by pediatric professionals with expertise in assessing these domains (e.g., neuropsychologists and developmental-behavioral pediatricians).

There are several disease-related physiological risks for cognitive deficits including neurological injury such as silent cerebral infarct and overt stroke (King et al., 2014; Prussien et al., 2019). Cerebral infarcts increase the risk and severity of cognitive impairment, but deficits still occur in those without a history of silent cerebral infarct or stroke. Individuals with SCD HbSS with normal magnetic resonance imaging, silent cerebral infarct, and strokes had mean FSIQ scores of 91, 85, and 73, respectively. Samples without neurological injury show large deficits relative to the normative mean across FSIQ, verbal reasoning, perceptual reasoning, executive functions, and processing speed (Prussien et al., 2019). Chronic disease-related hemodynamic risks for infarction, such as anemia and elevated transcranial Doppler velocity (Bakker et al., 2014), cerebral blood flow (Prussien, Compas, et al., 2021), and oxygen extraction fraction (Prussien, Compas, et al., 2021) may contribute to cognitive impairment in individuals with SCD with and without an acute insult to the brain.

Consistent with research in developmental science, sociodemographic factors also predict cognitive function above and beyond silent cerebral infarcts. King et al. (2014) found that parental education was a significant predictor of FSIQ within this population. In a sample of 150 children with SCD, children living with a parent who had some college education scored 6.2 IQ points higher than children living with a parent who had no college education. Children with a silent infarct whose head of household had some college education performed better compared to children without a silent cerebral infarct whose primary caregiver had a high school degree or less. Another study found that the association of chronic anemia and cognitive performance in children with SCD depended on their family's SES, suggesting interdependence of disease-related and environmental risks, and the potential moderating role of sociodemographic factors on outcomes associated with SCD (Schatz et al., 2004).

Familial psychosocial factors have also been associated with differences in cognitive outcomes of children with SCD. Parental stress related to financial hardship and stress related to caring for a child with a chronic illness have been identified as correlates of lower cognitive function in pediatric SCD. Over 50% of children with SCD live at or below the poverty line, and King et al. (2014) showed that each additional $1000 per capita is associated with a 0.33-point increase in FSIQ. Maternal financial stress is related to lower self-reported positive parenting and compromised multiple domains of cognitive function in children with SCD (Yarboi et al., 2017). Furthermore, Yarboi et al. (2019) found that caregivers who reported greater socioeconomic and pediatric disease-related stress engaged in less responsive parenting behaviors, and school-aged children of less responsive parents had lower scores on cognitive assessments. These findings further highlight the complex, interactive effects of socioecological factors, including social determinants of health, on outcomes such as cognitive functioning. Parents and caregivers of children with SCD, who are also at risk for socioeconomic disadvantage, can experience a double hit to their ability to provide responsive parenting to encourage cognitive development in children.

ACADEMIC, EMOTIONAL, AND PSYCHOSOCIAL MORBIDITIES ASSOCIATED WITH SICKLE CELL DISEASE

Due to their experiences with pain, CNS complications, and neurocognitive sequelae, children and adolescents with SCD are also at risk for academic, emotional, and psychosocial morbidities. This includes difficulty with school functioning and academic achievement, social functioning and peer relationships, emotional functioning, racial bias and stigma, and self-management.

School Functioning and Academic Achievement

SCD-related morbidity such as VOCs, chronic pain, and related outpatient visits, ED visits, and hospitalizations are associated with increased risk for school absenteeism and lower school performance in children and adolescents with SCD (Schatz, 2004). Students with SCD miss approximately 12% to 21% of school days due to pain, fatigue, and frequent outpatient visits (Schwartz et al., 2009; Shapiro et al., 1995), and nearly 30% do not graduate from high school (Farber et al., 1985). Furthermore, students with SCD are 10 times more likely to repeat a grade relative to U.S. data for African American students (Heitzer et al., 2021). A meta-analysis showed that students with SCD scored lower on standardized tests of reading, math, and spelling relative to the normative mean, and they had medium deficits in these academic domains relative to sibling or healthy controls (Heitzer et al., 2021). The meta-analysis also found that student FSIQ explained large proportions of the variance in reading and math, and students with silent cerebral infarct or stroke performed worse on academic tests compared to students without neurological injury.

Given the well-documented challenges with academic achievement and attainment that occur early in their development, children with SCD would benefit from early intervention to improve outcomes, and longitudinal surveillance and assessment to monitor for deficits as they emerge over time. Preliminary findings from a school-based intervention targeting SCD education for teachers and students demonstrated improvement in both teacher and peer knowledge of SCD, and students with SCD in the intervention group had fewer school absences than students who obtained only routine services (Koontz et al., 2004). Although this intervention is promising, targeted interventions are still needed to address the range of academic needs of students with SCD. All students with SCD are eligible to receive accommodations to eliminate logistical barriers to learning under Section 504 of the U.S. Rehabilitation Act of 1973, but only 20% of students with SCD have a 504 plan (Karkoska et al., 2021). Students with documented cognitive deficits or learning disabilities might also be eligible for special education services through an individualized education plan (IEP) under the Individuals With Disabilities Education Act. Despite the high prevalence of cognitive and academic impairment in children with SCD, only 31% of students with SCD have an IEP (Karkoska et al., 2021).

Social Functioning and Peer Relationships

Social functioning is often measured using subscales from validated measures such as the Behavior Assessment System for Children, Third Edition (BASC-3; Reynolds & Kamphaus, 2015), or the Achenbach System of Empirically Based Assessment (ASEBA; Achenbach & Rescorla, 2001). The BASC assesses social skills by asking youth, parents, and teachers to rate how often the child or adolescent engages in common prosocial behaviors (e.g., making positive comments about others, showing interest in others' ideas, and accepting people who are different from themself). Multireporter ratings on ASEBA scales assess social problems by asking how true a behavioral statement is for the child (e.g., complains of loneliness, doesn't get along with other kids, is easily jealous). Findings of social functioning in youth with SCD differ based on the reporter. In self-assessments, children and adolescents with SCD report poor interpersonal skills (Rodrigue et al., 1996) that are amplified when they also report depressive and anxious symptoms (Valrie et al., 2020). Parent reports also suggest that children with SCD have social skills deficits due in part to executive dysfunction, even after accounting for the effect of intelligence (Hensler et al., 2014; Trzepacz et al., 2004). Further, in peer nomination studies, during which children are asked to identify or rank individuals in their peer group based on various characteristics, children with SCD are perceived as more isolated than their peers (Noll et al., 2007); however, both peers and teachers also rate children with SCD as more prosocial and less aggressive than their classmates, suggesting that perceptions of social functioning in children with SCD can vary across settings.

Several SCD-related factors impact peer relationships for children and adolescents with SCD. For example, acute and chronic pain events and school absenteeism can limit peer interactions and foster a sense of isolation (Poku et al., 2018). Furthermore, children and adolescents with SCD have reported that differences in physical appearance, such as the presence of jaundiced eyes (a result of buildup of bilirubin after breakdown of fragile sickled cells), distended abdomen (related red cell buildup in the spleen), or small developmental stature can impact the quality of social relationships and contribute to bullying from peers (Buser et al., 2021; Volume 1, Chapter 14, this handbook). Many adolescents express reluctance to disclose SCD diagnosis to their peers due to fear of rejection and being stereotyped (Buser et al., 2021; Derlega et al., 2018), yet some youth are motivated to disclose for social support-seeking and educating others (Derlega et al., 2018). Unfortunately, predictors of disclosure are unclear and it is also unknown if disclosure actually leads to greater social support, resilience, or posttraumatic growth.

Emotional Functioning

Chronic illness poses disease-related stress for children and adolescents in addition to normative developmental stressors, much of it outside of their personal control (Compas et al., 2012). Although many previous studies investigating stress in pediatric SCD focused primarily on pain crises (Gil et al., 1991; Mitchell et al., 2007), children with SCD are also affected by other stressors that include, but are not limited to, pain. Multi-informant semistructured interviews with children and their caregivers reveal that families experience stress related to medical complications (i.e., pain, bedwetting), treatment and side effects (i.e., taking medications, hospital visits/stays), disruption in daily routines and activities (i.e., missing school, inability to participate in activities), emotional reactions and communication issues (i.e., speaking with doctors, telling friends about SCD), social challenges (i.e., feeling or looking different from others), and concerns about the future (i.e., transition to adulthood, adult health; Hildenbrand et al., 2015).

Children who experience high rates of disease-related stress are at greater risk for experiencing symptoms of depression and anxiety (Compas et al., 2012); however, findings on rates of internalizing symptoms for children and adolescents with SCD are inconsistent. In a comprehensive review (Moody et al., 2019), prevalence of depression in youth with SCD was estimated between 4% and 46% across 13 studies using a range of clinical instruments. Studies that assessed depression that used only a self-reported rating scale estimated a prevalence rate between 4% and 27%, whereas studies that used both a self-report screening tool and a structured clinical interview found that 10% to 13% of the sample met criteria for depression.

In addition, although some studies show that children and adolescents with SCD are at higher risk for experiencing symptoms of distress and internalizing problems relative to healthy peers or siblings (Trzepacz et al., 2004), other studies have concluded that youth with SCD are at lower risk (Benton et al., 2007). As such, health care clinicians of youth with SCD are urged to interpret self-reported screening tools for depression with caution (Moody et al., 2019). For example, similar to the discrepancy in prevalence rates of depression across studies, Yang et al. (1994) found that 29% of adolescents with SCD were in the clinical range for depression on the Children's Depression Rating Scale–Revised (Poznanski et al., 1985), where 12% of the healthy controls obtained clinical scores; yet only 13% of the sample met clinical criteria in a follow-up semistructured clinical interview. Scores of adolescents with SCD were inflated by SCD-related symptoms (e.g., fatigue); thus, the reported difference from controls was not clinically meaningful.

RACIAL BIAS AND STIGMA

Implicit bias and stigma associated with SCD have contributed to suboptimal outcomes in SCD. Inequities in the health care system as well as other experiences with structural systems of power are related to occurrence of racial bias and health-related stigma for youth with SCD, particularly during adolescence and young adulthood (Mulchan et al., 2016; Porter et al., 2017; Stollon et al., 2015). Most adolescents with SCD report high occurrences of racial bias and health-related stigma (Wakefield et al., 2017). Greater experience with racial bias is related to greater pain burden (Wakefield et al., 2017), and high health-related stigma is related to less pain reduction in the hospital and greater pain interference (Martin et al., 2018). Adolescents and young adults who report more experiences with health-related stigma also report lower health-related quality of life (Martin et al., 2018; Wakefield et al., 2017), with symptoms of depression serving as a significant mediator. Therefore, greater perceived racism predicts greater symptoms of depression, which in turn relates to poor health-related quality of life. Experiencing health-related stigma is not unique to adolescents and young adults with SCD in the United States. Stigma might be greater in sub-Saharan Africa where the prevalence of SCD is higher. Studies conducted Uganda and Ghana reported negative biases and stereotypes contributing to SCD stigma, including that SCD is caused by an ancestral curse and that individuals with SCD should not be integrated in social life or given equal rights. These factors contribute to increased bullying, fear of diagnosis disclosure, and neglect for children with SCD (Buser et al., 2021; Tusuubira et al., 2019).

Self-Management

For adolescents with SCD, medical challenges often worsen during this developmental period when they take on more responsibilities for their disease management and their parents step back. *Self-management* describes health behaviors that a patient and their support system engage in to care for an illness. Important self-management behaviors for youth with SCD include monitoring for fevers, attending appointments, managing medications, tracking health, managing daily activities, and communicating with a medical team. Despite the growing importance of self-management skills during adolescence, adolescents with SCD often struggle to maintain behaviors that require significant use of problem-solving and executive functions. Crosby et al. (2020) reported preliminary findings for a technology-based self-management intervention to improve behavioral activation. Significant effects were found for tracking health such that adolescents with SCD in the mobile intervention group had significant improved tracking behaviors at postintervention relative to the health education group, suggesting that skills can improve over time with appropriate intervention.

Other constructs relevant to self-management include coping and adherence. *Coping* includes many volitional cognitive and behavioral actions in response to a stressor, such as problem-solving, cognitive reappraisal, distraction, and avoidance, which can impact the uptake or utilization of important self-management behaviors. *Adherence* to medication management is a specific subset of self-management behaviors that has critical impact on disease course and morbidities, and there is an important emphasis in SCD and across all pediatric populations to identify and remove barriers to adherence.

Coping. Research on coping in children and adolescents with SCD is divided in two areas: one specifically focused on coping with pain and another focused on coping with disease-related stressors including, but not limited to, pain. Gil et al.'s (1991) model of SCD pain coping, widely used in the SCD literature, is composed of three components: (a) coping attempts (diverting attention, reinterpreting pain sensations, ignoring pain sensations, calming self-statements, and increased behavior activity), (b) negative thinking (catastrophizing and fearful self-statements, angry self-statements, and isolation), and (c) passive adherence coping (resting, taking fluids, praying and hoping, and applying heat, cold, or massage). These components of pain coping are assessed on the Coping Strategies Questionnaire for SCD (Gil et al., 1991), with studies providing an updated factor structure and expanded delineation of the coping model (Barakat, Patterson, et al., 2007; Gil et al., 1993). Gil et al. (1993) did a longitudinal descriptive study that showed coping attempts were more stable over time for younger children and more variable for adolescents, and research from the broader field of child and adolescent psychology suggests that this change in variability might be due to the increased range of stressors and improved cognitive resources, emotional development, and social development experienced by adolescents relative to younger children.

SCD pain coping has been associated with health care utilization, daily functioning, and psychosocial outcomes. *Active coping attempts* are significantly associated with more involvement in school, the home, and social activities during pain crises, and *passive adherence coping* is related to positive family functioning and fewer ED visits (Mitchell et al., 2007). In contrast, negative thinking has been associated with more interactions with the health care system (Gil et al., 2001), greater psychological distress and internalizing problems, and mediating the relation between pain intensity and depressive symptoms (Barakat, Schwartz, et al., 2007). Therefore, negative thinking patterns have been identified as a potential target of intervention to reduce internalization problems and pain in youth with SCD.

Although pain is the hallmark of SCD, it remains important to assess how children cope with other stressors related to SCD. The control-based model of coping emphasizes the adaptive nature of coping skills relative to the controllability of the stressor (Compas et al., 2012). Prussien et al. (2018) found that children and adolescents with SCD who use secondary control coping mechanisms (i.e., cognitive reappraisal, positive thinking, acceptance, and distraction) to cope with a broad range of SCD-related stressors report fewer symptoms of depression; however, Prussien et al. did not directly assess controllability of stressors. When assessing how adolescents and young adults with SCD cope with peer-related stress, studies show that secondary control coping was related to fewer symptoms of depression only when individuals perceived peer stressors as uncontrollable (Prussien, Siciliano, et al., 2021). Therefore, how a child copes with stress is related to mood and adjustment. Yet, in another example of the interconnected complexities of SCD-related outcomes, a child's ability to use adaptive coping mechanisms for disease-related stress is also impacted by disease-related cognitive sequelae. Lower verbal reasoning skills are related to lower use of secondary control coping mechanisms, and lower scores on working memory tasks are related to greater depressive/anxious symptoms (Prussien et al., 2018). Cognitive deficits associated with the disease can make it harder to adaptively cope with disease-related stress.

Adherence. Adherence to medication and health behaviors are challenging for youth with SCD, with tasks that include medication management as well as behaviors to reduce pain triggers (e.g., avoiding exposure to cold temperatures, staying hydrated) and clinic attendance. In a systematic review and meta-analysis of adherence in SCD, Loiselle et al. (2016) reported that rates of medication adherence ranged from 12% to 100% across medications, and nonadherence to individual treatment plans was found to increase disease complications and ED visits. Furthermore, adherence was lowest for prophylactic antibiotics (e.g., penicillin) and iron chelators relative to hydroxyurea and other medications. When examining hydroxyurea, only 35% to 50% of pediatric patients adhere at the rates attained in clinical trials, and nonadherence limits clinical effectiveness (Candrilli et al., 2011; Thornburg et al., 2011). Adolescents report that they shared the responsibility of tasks related to hydroxyurea adherence; however, few parent–child dyads agreed on how to complete treatment tasks (Creary et al., 2019). Barriers to medication adherence include perceived memory challenges, negative beliefs about medication effectiveness, fear of side effects and stigma, difficulty accessing medication, and lack of confidence in the ability to manage SCD (Alberts et al., 2020; Badawy et al., 2017).

Given suboptimal rates of adherence and identified barriers, development and testing of interventions to improve adherence are necessary. Creary et al. (2019) tested a 6-month mobile health (mHealth) intervention that included daily text messages with small monetary incentives to improve hydroxyurea adherence in children with SCD. After completing the mHealth intervention, medication possession increased from 61.7% to 84.4% and hydroxyurea adherence (on 80% of days) improved from 30% to 67%, suggesting promising efficacy. Other mobile interventions targeting improved self-management and adherence have also demonstrated increased medication possession ratio; however, the small sample size across studies and lack of control groups limit interpretation of intervention effects.

RESILIENCE AND HEALTH-RELATED QUALITY OF LIFE

Resilience is defined as an individual's ability to persevere in the face of a challenge, including a physical illness (Stewart & Yuen, 2011), and health-related quality of life is often used as an indicator for resilience across pediatric populations (Volume 1, Chapter 15, this handbook). Health-related quality of life is not only an absence of a deficit, but the model emphasizes positive functioning across physical, social, emotional, and academic domains. Children with SCD experience lower health-related quality of life relative to their peers on self- and parent reports. Risks for lower health-related quality of life include experiencing stigma or racism, greater pain frequency and intensity (Brito da Cunha et al., 2020), lower parental education (Ragab et al., 2021), and negative family functioning (Psihogios et al., 2018); however, a number of protective factors against reduced quality of life have been identified.

Better health-related quality of life among children and adolescents with SCD is associated with having heightened school support and greater adaptive behaviors (Koontz et al., 2004; Ziadni et al., 2011). Parent and family functioning, parent support, and parent problem-solving skills are consistently described as resilience factors for children and adolescents with SCD (Barakat et al., 2014; Raphael et al., 2013). A meta-analysis of family functioning and medical adherence across pediatric populations revealed several family-level resilience factors, including lower family conflict, greater family cohesion, greater family flexibility, more positive communication, and better overall family problem-solving skills (Psihogios et al., 2018). Parents who report higher satisfaction with social support also report less stress and are more likely to attend routine outpatient health care visits with their child, whereas children of parents with less social support incur greater health care costs through higher emergency care utilization (Barakat et al., 2014; Raphael et al., 2013). Parents who feel less stressed and have more perceived support are likely to utilize effective problem-solving (Barakat et al., 2014).

MULTIDISCIPLINARY CARE AND ASSESSMENT

As described previously, children and adolescents with SCD experience significant health and psychosocial challenges that require support from multiple clinicians with care coordinated through the pediatric hematologist. A quality improvement report in pediatric SCD asserted that comprehensive multidisciplinary care and intervention with representation from pediatric hematology, child psychology, child psychiatry, adolescent medicine, pain medicine, pediatric emergency medicine, nursing, social work, and child life can reduce health care utilization and hospital costs (Balsamo et al., 2019). Multidisciplinary screening, assessment, and intervention are critical in helping children and adolescents with SCD reduce medical and psychosocial risks and access necessary resources. American Society of Hematology (ASH) guidelines for the management of acute and chronic pain in SCD (Brandow et al., 2020) also emphasize the importance for multidisciplinary care to create and implement appropriate care plans. For example, ASH states that a multidisciplinary approach to pain treatment for individuals with SCD should include the hematologist and primary care team, nursing, integrative health, pain medicine, social work, psychology, and physical therapy/rehabilitation (Brandow et al., 2020). Although all-in-one clinics have not been explicitly outlined in guidelines or standard of care for this population, frequent communication and collaboration across specialties are critical.

Although there are known multifactorial risks to cognitive function and school achievement in this population, it is unclear how many patients meet the criteria for specific learning disorders or intellectual disability. Current ASH guidelines for the prevention, diagnosis, and treatment of cerebrovascular disease in children and adults with SCD (DeBaun et al., 2020) recommend surveillance for developmental delays in preschool children (recommendation 8.1) and formal referral to a psychologist or pediatrician/developmental-behavioral pediatrician for additional screening or evaluation for children with elevated risks for CNS complications (recommendation 8.2). Specific ages for evaluation or frequency of neurocognitive surveillance were not included in the guidelines. Nevertheless, early assessment is generally recommended in the fields of clinical and neuropsychology to implement early intervention. Pediatric psychologists and neuropsychologists are necessary members of the broader care team, as their ability to provide cognitive and educational assessments is vital. Developmental-behavioral pediatricians can also help children with learning needs navigate the educational system. Assessments are necessary for those who qualify to receive an IEP to assist students in educational achievements. Despite recommendations, children in this population face many barriers in accessing these services. Support from additional members of the psychosocial team, including social workers, is integral in assisting families in overcoming barriers in access to evaluation and acquiring a 504 plan, for which all students with SCD in public school are eligible. In addition to providing comprehensive mental health screenings and assessments, pediatric psychologists are adept in providing mental health interventions for disease-related stress and coping or behavioral challenges with medical adjustment or adherence. Furthermore, collaboration with child and adolescent psychiatrists is often useful when addressing the impact of broader significant psychopathology or psychiatric disturbance.

Developmental-behavioral pediatricians are central members of any pediatric multidisciplinary team. In addition to their ability to advocate for neurocognitive evaluations and educational accommodations alongside psychologists, the relevance of developmental-behavioral pediatricians' expertise is heightened for children and adolescents with SCD due to the intersection among SCD outcomes and behavioral challenges. For example, children and adolescents with SCD are at greater risk for attention deficits and executive dysfunction, and these challenges overlap with attention deficit/hyperactivity disorder (ADHD). Prevalence of ADHD diagnoses is estimated up to 24% children with SCD (Acquazzino et al., 2017), which is greater than both the diagnostic rate for African American children and the general child population in the United States (Cénat et al., 2021). However, given that ADHD is often over-diagnosed in Black and African American children due to racial and socioeconomic bias (Cénat et al., 2021), culturally and medically informed differential diagnosis is necessary to ensure that children are accurately diagnosed and receive appropriate services. Additional key diagnoses under the purview of developmental-behavioral pediatricians, such as autism spectrum disorder, cerebral palsy, and other developmental disabilities that do not occur in SCD at greater rates relative to the general population might still have physical and behavioral sequelae that impact SCD-related outcomes such as medical adherence or treatment adjustment.

Finally, the primary care provider and/or pediatrician plays an integral role in creating a patient-centered medical home for youth with SCD. Pediatricians have the unique position of interacting with families of children with SCD frequently throughout their years of development and can monitor and identify developmental trajectories that are either in line with or deviate from normative development. The patient-centered medical home is also a useful environment to enhance pain management through multidisciplinary care. Raphael and Oyeku (2013) outlined multiple applications of the patient-centered medical home model to pain management in SCD. For example, increased access to care and information through same-day appointments, after-hours coverage, and electronic visits can assist with monitoring and treatment for early pain symptoms and prevent delays in care or unnecessary emergency care. Other patient-centered medical home elements relevant to SCD pain management include practice-based services (e.g., the multidisciplinary approach to pain management and routine screening of precipitators), care management (creation of SCD registry to practice site), care coordination (e.g., community connections, collaborative relationships with ED, specialists, case management, care transitions), and practice-based care teams (e.g., health care clinician-led multidisciplinary team).

Lifelong Management in Sickle Cell Disease and Transition to Adult Care

Although diagnosed in infancy and early childhood, SCD is a lifelong condition requiring ongoing care beyond adolescence. Many adolescents and young adults with SCD do not successfully transfer to an adult hematology provider after leaving the pediatric setting (Saulsberry et al., 2019), resulting in increased disease severity and SCD-related health conditions during later adolescence and young adulthood (Blinder et al., 2013; Brousseau, Owens, et al., 2010). Likely related to lack of transfer, adolescents and young adults often receive inadequate treatment for SCD. Transfusion rates among patients peak at 16 years of age and engagement in transfusions reduces significantly until age 26 despite eligibility for continued treatment (Blinder et al., 2013). As preventative care decreases post transfer, health costs and patient reliance on acute care increase (Blinder et al., 2013; Brousseau, Owens, et al., 2010). Unsurprisingly, the transition period from pediatric to adult health care settings is associated with the highest rate of morbidity and mortality for this population (Lanzkron et al., 2013). This care transition in SCD, and resulting challenges with obtaining appropriate treatment, are increasingly worrisome as over 95% of children with SCD in the United States now live into adulthood (Elmariah et al., 2014).

There are common barriers to transition across pediatric conditions, including suboptimal knowledge about the transition process, low self-management ability, fear of leaving familiar providers, and concerns about costs of treatment (Gray et al., 2018), and many challenges are magnified for adolescents and young adults with SCD. Qualitative findings from adolescents and young adults with SCD and their providers suggest that adolescents and young adults experience many barriers identified in the Socio-ecological Model of Adolescent and Young Adult Readiness for Transition (Schwartz et al., 2011, 2013). However, additional concepts must be taken into consideration for this population including the impact of race or culture, pain management, societal stigma, and limited number of adult providers who have expert knowledge in SCD (Mulchan et al., 2016). Furthermore, very little rigorous research has investigated the effectiveness of transition programs despite the critical need to address this gap in care. Nevertheless, experts have stated that transition programming for SCD should include an emphasis on

- creating a transition policy that informs adolescents of timing and process;
- tracking and monitoring progress;
- assessing transition readiness via readiness assessments, disease education, and self-management skills training;
- planning for adult care via neurocognitive screening, academic support, and community involvement;
- transferring to adult care; and
- integrating adolescents and young adults into adult care (Saulsberry et al., 2019).

Preliminary evidence suggests that programs that implement these elements have improved transfer success and higher early adult care engagement (Saulsberry et al., 2019).

Multidisciplinary collaboration among hematologists, social workers, psychologists, and developmental-behavioral pediatricians is critical in assisting adolescents with developmental differences to prepare for the transition to adulthood as a broad concept, in addition to the specific transition of medical services. Given the high morbidity and mortality rates during the transition from pediatric- to adult-oriented care in this population, support during this transition from multiple clinicians is beneficial to ensure a successful transition.

CONCLUSION

SCD is a genetic disorder that has widespread impact on health and psychosocial outcomes. Children and adolescents should be monitored for several medical outcomes including acute and chronic pain, silent cerebral infarcts and strokes, neurocognitive impairment, and difficulties during the transition to adult-oriented care. Improvements in medical screenings and treatments have significantly reduced the risk of these morbidities over the last several decades, and curative therapies are on the horizon. Nevertheless, psychosocial outcomes are still important to monitor, as children and adolescents with SCD are at risk for challenges with academic achievement, social functioning, stigma, and successful self-management. More research is required about resilience factors, yet research shows promising findings on the positive impact of family functioning and low parental stress.

Each of the outcomes reviewed in this chapter must be considered in the context of socioecological factors relevant to health equity and disparities. Youth with SCD are faced with significant stress related to stigma and bias, and institutional- and systemic-level systems of power can drive individual differences in morbidity and mortality. Individual and family level factors may be protective against the disease-related and systems-level risks for poor outcomes, and increasing multidisciplinary care is an important step in increasing health equity.

RESOURCES

Web-based resources for families provide information about the health condition and available treatments, education about psychosocial considerations including support, and tangible resources to mitigate the costs of accessing treatments. Here, we highlight trustworthy websites to recommend to families.

- Sickle Cell Disease Association of America is the primary advocacy and support organization with local chapters that offer services and support groups:

  https://www.sicklecelldisease.org

- Sickle Cell Disease Coalition offers a range of resources that can be filtered for patients, providers, and researchers:

  https://www.scdcoalition.org

- Centers for Disease Control and Prevention has compiled vetted resources on sickle cell disease:

  https://www.cdc.gov/sickle-cell/scdc/index.html

- Association of Pediatric Hematology/Oncology Nurses offers handbooks for families on hematologic and oncologic conditions:

  https://aphon.org/education/patient-family-resources

References

Achenbach, T. M., & Rescorla, L. A. (2001). *Manual for the ASEBA school-age forms and profiles*. University of Vermont, Research Center for Children, Youth, and Families.

Acquazzino, M. A., Miller, M., Myrvik, M., Newby, R., & Scott, J. P. (2017). Attention deficit hyperactivity disorder in children with sickle cell disease referred for an evaluation. *Journal of Pediatric Hematology/Oncology, 39*(5), 350–354. https://doi.org/10.1097/MPH.0000000000000847

Alberts, N. M., Badawy, S. M., Hodges, J., Estepp, J. H., Nwosu, C., Khan, H., Smeltzer, M. P., Homayouni, R., Norell, S., Klesges, L., Porter, J. S., & Hankins, J. S. (2020). Development of the InCharge health mobile app to improve adherence to hydroxyurea in patients with sickle cell disease: User-centered design approach. *JMIR mHealth and uHealth, 8*(5), e14884. https://doi.org/10.2196/14884

Badawy, S. M., Thompson, A. A., Penedo, F. J., Lai, J. S., Rychlik, K., & Liem, R. I. (2017). Barriers to hydroxyurea adherence and health-related quality of life in adolescents and young adults with sickle cell disease. *European Journal of Haematology, 98*(6), 608–614. https://doi.org/10.1111/ejh.12878

Bakker, M. J., Hofmann, J., Churches, O. F., Badcock, N. A., Kohler, M., & Keage, H. A. (2014). Cerebrovascular function and cognition in childhood: A systematic review of transcranial Doppler studies. *BMC Neurology, 14*(1), 43. https://doi.org/10.1186/1471-2377-14-43

Ballas, S. K. (2021). Opioids are not a major cause of death of patients with sickle cell disease. *Annals of Hematology, 100*(5), 1133–1138. https://doi.org/10.1007/s00277-021-04502-2

Balsamo, L., Shabanova, V., Carbonella, J., Szondy, M. V., Kalbfeld, K., Thomas, D. A., Santucci, K., Grossman, M., & Pashankar, F. (2019). Improving care for sickle cell pain crisis using a multidisciplinary approach. *Pediatrics, 143*(5), e20182218. https://doi.org/10.1542/peds.2018-2218

Barakat, L. P., Daniel, L. C., Smith, K., Renée Robinson, M., & Patterson, C. A. (2014). Parental problem-solving abilities and the association of sickle cell disease complications with health-related quality of life for school-age children. *Journal of Clinical Psychology in Medical Settings, 21*(1), 56–65. https://doi.org/10.1007/s10880-013-9379-7

Barakat, L. P., Patterson, C. A., Weinberger, B. S., Simon, K., Gonzalez, E. R., & Dampier, C. (2007). A prospective study of the role of coping and family functioning in health outcomes for adolescents with sickle cell disease. *Journal of Pediatric Hematology/Oncology, 29*(11), 752–760. https://doi.org/10.1097/MPH.0b013e318157fdac

Barakat, L. P., Schwartz, L. A., Simon, K., & Radcliffe, J. (2007). Negative thinking as a coping strategy mediator of pain and internalizing symptoms in adolescents with sickle cell disease. *Journal of Behavioral Medicine, 30*(3), 199–208. https://doi.org/10.1007/s10865-007-9103-x

Benton, T. D., Ifeagwu, J. A., & Smith-Whitley, K. (2007). Anxiety and depression in children and adolescents with sickle cell disease. *Current Psychiatry Reports, 9*(2), 114–121. https://doi.org/10.1007/s11920-007-0080-0

Bernaudin, F., Verlhac, S., Arnaud, C., Kamdem, A., Vasile, M., Kasbi, F., Hau, I., Madhi, F., Fourmaux, C., Biscardi, S., Epaud, R., & Pondarré, C. (2015). Chronic and acute anemia and extracranial internal carotid stenosis are risk factors for silent cerebral infarcts in sickle cell anemia. *Blood, 125*(10), 1653–1661. https://doi.org/10.1182/blood-2014-09-599852

Blair, H. A. (2020). Crizanlizumab: First approval. *Drugs, 80*(1), 79–84. https://doi.org/10.1007/s40265-019-01254-2

Blinder, M. A., Vekeman, F., Sasane, M., Trahey, A., Paley, C., & Duh, M. S. (2013). Age-related treatment patterns in sickle cell disease patients and the associated sickle cell complications and healthcare costs. *Pediatric Blood & Cancer, 60*(5), 828–835. https://doi.org/10.1002/pbc.24459

Brandow, A. M., Carroll, C. P., Creary, S., Edwards-Elliott, R., Glassberg, J., Hurley, R. W., Kutlar, A., Seisa, M., Stinson, J., Strouse, J. J., Yusuf, F., Zempsky, W., & Lang, E. (2020). American Society of Hematology 2020 guidelines for sickle cell disease: Management of acute and chronic pain. *Blood Advances, 4*(12), 2656–2701. https://doi.org/10.1182/bloodadvances.2020001851

Brandow, A. M., Zappia, K. J., & Stucky, C. L. (2017). Sickle cell disease: A natural model of acute and chronic pain. *Pain, 158*(1), S79–S84. https://doi.org/10.1097/j.pain.0000000000000824

Brito da Cunha, V., Freitas de Andrade Rodrigues, C., Alves Rodrigues, T., Silva Gomes de Oliveira, E. J., & Santos Garcia, J. B. (2020). Self-report for assessment of pain and quality of life in children with sickle cell anemia in a developing country. *Journal of Pain Research, 13*, 3171–3180. https://doi.org/10.2147/JPR.S261605

Bronfenbrenner, U. (1979). *The ecology of human development: Experiments by nature and design*. Harvard University Press.

Brousseau, D. C., Owens, P. L., Mosso, A. L., Panepinto, J. A., & Steiner, C. A. (2010). Acute care utilization and rehospitalizations for sickle cell disease. *JAMA: Journal of the American Medical Association, 303*(13), 1288–1294. https://doi.org/10.1001/jama.2010.378

Brousseau, D. C., Panepinto, J. A., Nimmer, M., & Hoffmann, R. G. (2010). The number of people with sickle-cell disease in the United States: National and state estimates. *American Journal of Hematology, 85*(1), 77–78. https://doi.org/10.1002/ajh.21570

Buser, J. M., Bakari, A., Seidu, A. A., Paintsil, V., Osei-Akoto, A., Amoah, R., Otoo, B., & Moyer, C. A. (2021). Stigma associated with sickle cell disease in Kumasi, Ghana. *Journal of Transcultural Nursing, 32*(6), 757–764. https://doi.org/10.1177/10436596211008216

Candrilli, S. D., O'Brien, S. H., Ware, R. E., Nahata, M. C. S., Seiber, E. E., & Balkrishnan, R. (2011). Hydroxyurea adherence and associated outcomes among Medicaid enrollees with sickle cell disease. *American Journal of Hematology, 86*(3), 273–277. https://doi.org/10.1002/ajh.21968

Cénat, J. M., Blais-Rochette, C., Morse, C., Vandette, M. P., Noorishad, P. G., Kogan, C., Ndengeyingoma, A., & Labelle, P. R. (2021).

Prevalence and risk factors associated with attention-deficit/hyperactivity disorder among US Black individuals: A systematic review and meta-analysis. *JAMA Psychiatry, 78*(1), 21–28. https://doi.org/10.1001/jamapsychiatry.2020.2788

Chen, E., Cole, S. W., & Kato, P. M. (2004). A review of empirically supported psychosocial interventions for pain and adherence outcomes in sickle cell disease. *Journal of Pediatric Psychology, 29*(3), 197–209. https://doi.org/10.1093/jpepsy/jsh021

Compas, B. E., Jaser, S. S., Dunn, M. J., & Rodriguez, E. M. (2012). Coping with chronic illness in childhood and adolescence. *Annual Review of Clinical Psychology, 8*(1), 455–480. https://doi.org/10.1146/annurev-clinpsy-032511-143108

Crawford, M. W., Galton, S., & Naser, B. (2006). Postoperative morphine consumption in children with sickle-cell disease. *Paediatric Anaesthesia, 16*(2), 152–157. https://doi.org/10.1111/j.1460-9592.2005.01705.x

Creary, S., Chisolm, D., Stanek, J., Hankins, J., & O'Brien, S. H. (2019). A multidimensional electronic hydroxyurea adherence intervention for children with sickle cell disease: Single-arm before-after study. *JMIR mHealth and uHealth, 7*(8), e13452. https://doi.org/10.2196/13452

Crosby, L. E., Hood, A., Kidwell, K., Nwankwo, C., Peugh, J., Strong, H., Quinn, C., & Britto, M. T. (2020). Improving self-management in adolescents with sickle cell disease. *Pediatric Blood & Cancer, 67*(10), e28492. https://doi.org/10.1002/pbc.28492

DeBaun, M. R., Gordon, M., McKinstry, R. C., Noetzel, M. J., White, D. A., Sarnaik, S. A., Meier, E. R., Howard, T. H., Majumdar, S., Inusa, B. P., Telfer, P. T., Kirby-Allen, M., McCavit, T. L., Kamdem, A., Airewele, G., Woods, G. M., Berman, B., Panepinto, J. A., Fuh, B. R., . . . Casella, J. F. (2014). Controlled trial of transfusions for silent cerebral infarcts in sickle cell anemia. *The New England Journal of Medicine, 371*(8), 699–710. https://doi.org/10.1056/NEJMoa1401731

DeBaun, M. R., Jordan, L. C., King, A. A., Schatz, J., Vichinsky, E., Fox, C. K., McKinstry, R. C., Telfer, P., Kraut, M. A., Daraz, L., Kirkham, F. J., & Murad, M. H. (2020). American Society of Hematology 2020 guidelines for sickle cell disease: Prevention, diagnosis, and treatment of cerebrovascular disease in children and adults. *Blood Advances, 4*(8), 1554–1588. https://doi.org/10.1182/bloodadvances.2019001142

DeBaun, M. R., & Kirkham, F. J. (2016). Central nervous system complications and management in sickle cell disease. *Blood, 127*(7), 829–838. https://doi.org/10.1182/blood-2015-09-618579

Derlega, V. J., Maduro, R. S., Janda, L. H., Chen, I. A., & Goodman, B. M., III. (2018). What motivates individuals with sickle cell disease to talk with others about their illness? Reasons for and against sickle cell disease disclosure. *Journal of Health Psychology, 23*(1), 103–113. https://doi.org/10.1177/1359105316649786

Ehrentraut, J. H., Kern, K. D., Long, S. A., An, A. Q., Faughnan, L. G., & Anghelescu, D. L. (2014). Opioid misuse behaviors in adolescents and young adults in a hematology/oncology setting. *Journal of Pediatric Psychology, 39*(10), 1149–1160. https://doi.org/10.1093/jpepsy/jsu072

Elmariah, H., Garrett, M. E., De Castro, L. M., Jonassaint, J. C., Ataga, K. I., Eckman, J. R., Ashley-Koch, A. E., & Telen, M. J. (2014). Factors associated with survival in a contemporary adult sickle cell disease cohort. *American Journal of Hematology, 89*(5), 530–535. https://doi.org/10.1002/ajh.23683

Farber, M. D., Koshy, M., Kinney, T. R., & The Cooperative Study of Sickle Cell Disease. (1985). Cooperative study of sickle cell disease: Demographic and socioeconomic characteristics of patients and families with sickle cell disease. *Journal of Chronic Diseases, 38*(6), 495–505. https://doi.org/10.1016/0021-9681(85)90033-5

Farooq, F., Mogayzel, P. J., Lanzkron, S., Haywood, C., & Strouse, J. J. (2020). Comparison of US federal and foundation funding of research for sickle cell disease and cystic fibrosis and factors associated with research productivity. *JAMA Network Open, 3*(3), e201737. https://doi.org/10.1001/jamanetworkopen.2020.1737

Gil, K. M., Anthony, K. K., Carson, J. W., Redding-Lallinger, R., Daeschner, C. W., & Ware, R. E. (2001). Daily coping practice predicts treatment effects in children with sickle cell disease. *Journal of Pediatric Psychology, 26*(3), 163–173. https://doi.org/10.1093/jpepsy/26.3.163

Gil, K. M., Thompson, R. J., Jr., Keith, B. R., Tota-Faucette, M., Noll, S., & Kinney, T. R. (1993). Sickle cell disease pain in children and adolescents: Change in pain frequency and coping strategies over time. *Journal of Pediatric Psychology, 18*(5), 621–637. https://doi.org/10.1093/jpepsy/18.5.621

Gil, K. M., Williams, D. A., Thompson, R. J., Jr., & Kinney, T. R. (1991). Sickle cell disease in children and adolescents: The relation of child and parent pain coping strategies to adjustment. *Journal of Pediatric Psychology, 16*(5), 643–663. https://doi.org/10.1093/jpepsy/16.5.643

Gray, W. N., Schaefer, M. R., Resmini-Rawlinson, A., & Wagoner, S. T. (2018). Barriers to transition from pediatric to adult care: A systematic review.

Journal of Pediatric Psychology, 43(5), 488–502. https://doi.org/10.1093/jpepsy/jsx142

Heitzer, A. M., Hamilton, L., Stafford, C., Gossett, J., Ouellette, L., Trpchevska, A., King, A. A., Kang, G., & Hankins, J. S. (2021). Academic performance of children with sickle cell disease in the United States: A meta-analysis. *Frontiers in Neurology*, 12, 786065. https://doi.org/10.3389/fneur.2021.786065

Hensler, M., Wolfe, K., Lebensburger, J., Nieman, J., Barnes, M., Nolan, W., King, A., & Madan-Swain, A. (2014). Social skills and executive function among youth with sickle cell disease: A preliminary investigation. *Journal of Pediatric Psychology*, 39(5), 493–500. https://doi.org/10.1093%2Fjpepsy%2Fjst138

Herity, L. B., Vaughan, D. M., Rodriguez, L. R., & Lowe, D. K. (2021). Voxelotor: A novel treatment for sickle cell disease. *The Annals of Pharmacotherapy*, 55(2), 240–245. https://doi.org/10.1177/1060028020943059

Hildenbrand, A. K., Barakat, L. P., Alderfer, M. A., & Marsac, M. L. (2015). Coping and coping assistance among children with sickle cell disease and their parents. *Journal of Pediatric Hematology/Oncology*, 37(1), 25–34. https://doi.org/10.1097/MPH.0000000000000092

Kanter, J., & Kruse-Jarres, R. (2013). Management of sickle cell disease from childhood through adulthood. *Blood Reviews*, 27(6), 279–287. https://doi.org/10.1016/j.blre.2013.09.001

Karkoska, K. A., Haber, K., Elam, M., Strong, S., & McGann, P. T. (2021). Academic challenges and school service utilization in children with sickle cell disease. *The Journal of Pediatrics*, 230, 182–190. https://doi.org/10.1016/j.jpeds.2020.11.062

Khemani, K., Katoch, D., & Krishnamurti, L. (2019). Curative therapies for sickle cell disease. *The Ochsner Journal*, 19(2), 131–137. https://doi.org/10.31486/toj.18.0044

King, A. A., Strouse, J. J., Rodeghier, M. J., Compas, B. E., Casella, J. F., McKinstry, R. C., Noetzel, M. J., Quinn, C. T., Ichord, R., Dowling, M. M., Miller, J. P., & Debaun, M. R. (2014). Parent education and biologic factors influence on cognition in sickle cell anemia. *American Journal of Hematology*, 89(2), 162–167. https://doi.org/10.1002/ajh.23604

Koontz, K., Short, A. D., Kalinyak, K., & Noll, R. B. (2004). A randomized, controlled pilot trial of a school intervention for children with sickle cell anemia. *Journal of Pediatric Psychology*, 29(1), 7–17. https://doi.org/10.1093/jpepsy/jsh002

Kossorotoff, M., Brousse, V., Grevent, D., Naggara, O., Brunelle, F., Blauwblomme, T., Gaussem, P., Desguerre, I., & De Montalembert, M. (2015). Cerebral haemorrhagic risk in children with sickle-cell disease. *Developmental Medicine & Child Neurology*, 57(2), 187–193. https://doi.org/10.1111/dmcn.12571

Kwiatkowski, J. L., Zimmerman, R. A., Pollock, A. N., Seto, W., Smith-Whitley, K., Shults, J., Blackwood-Chirchir, A., & Ohene-Frempong, K. (2009). Silent infarcts in young children with sickle cell disease. *British Journal of Haematology*, 146(3), 300–305. https://doi.org/10.1111/j.1365-2141.2009.07753.x

Lanzkron, S., Carroll, C. P., & Haywood, C., Jr. (2013). Mortality rates and age at death from sickle cell disease: U.S., 1979–2005. *Public Health Reports*, 128(2), 110–116.

Lee, P., Le Saux, M., Siegel, R., Goyal, M., Chen, C., Ma, Y., & Meltzer, A. C. (2019). Racial and ethnic disparities in the management of acute pain in US emergency departments: Meta-analysis and systematic review. *The American Journal of Emergency Medicine*, 37(9), 1770–1777. https://doi.org/10.1016/j.ajem.2019.06.014

Loiselle, K., Lee, J. L., Szulczewski, L., Drake, S., Crosby, L. E., & Pai, A. L. (2016). Systematic and meta-analytic review: Medication adherence among pediatric patients with sickle cell disease. *Journal of Pediatric Psychology*, 41(4), 406–418. https://doi.org/10.1093/jpepsy/jsv084

Martin, S. R., Cohen, L. L., Mougianis, I., Griffin, A., Sil, S., & Dampier, C. (2018). Stigma and pain in adolescents hospitalized for sickle cell vaso-occlusive pain episodes. *The Clinical Journal of Pain*, 34(5), 438–444. https://doi.org/10.1097/AJP.0000000000000553

McCavit, T. L., Lin, H., Zhang, S., Ahn, C., Quinn, C. T., & Flores, G. (2011). Hospital volume, hospital teaching status, patient socioeconomic status, and outcomes in patients hospitalized with sickle cell disease. *American Journal of Hematology*, 86(4), 377–380. https://doi.org/10.1002/ajh.21977

Mitchell, M. J., Lemanek, K., Palermo, T. M., Crosby, L. E., Nichols, A., & Powers, S. W. (2007). Parent perspectives on pain management, coping, and family functioning in pediatric sickle cell disease. *Clinical Pediatrics*, 46(4), 311–319. https://doi.org/10.1177/0009922806293985

Moody, K. L., Mercer, K., & Glass, M. (2019). An integrative review of the prevalence of depression among pediatric patients with sickle cell disease. *Social Work in Public Health*, 34(4), 343–352. https://doi.org/10.1080/19371918.2019.1606754

Mulchan, S. S., Valenzuela, J. M., Crosby, L. E., & Diaz Pow Sang, C. (2016). Applicability of the SMART model of transition readiness for sickle-cell disease. *Journal of Pediatric Psychology, 41*(5), 543–554. https://doi.org/10.1093/jpepsy/jsv120

NIH. (2021). *Cure sickle cell initiative.* https://www.nhlbi.nih.gov/science/cure-sickle-cell-initiative

Nnodu, O. E., Oron, A. P., Sopekan, A., Akaba, G. O., Piel, F. B., & Chao, D. L. (2021). Child mortality from sickle cell disease in Nigeria: A model-estimated, population-level analysis of data from the 2018 demographic and health survey. *The Lancet Haematology, 8*(10), e723–e731. https://doi.org/10.1016/S2352-3026(21)00216-7

Noll, R. B., Reiter-Purtill, J., Vannatta, K., Gerhardt, C. A., & Short, A. (2007). Peer relationships and emotional well-being of children with sickle cell disease: A controlled replication. *Child Neuropsychology, 13*(2), 173–187. https://doi.org/10.1080/09297040500473706

Ohene-Frempong, K., Weiner, S. J., Sleeper, L. A., Miller, S. T., Embury, S., Moohr, J. W., Wethers, D. L., Pegelow, C. H., & Gill, F. M. (1998). Cerebrovascular accidents in sickle cell disease: Rates and risk factors. *Blood, 91*(1), 288–294. https://doi.org/10.1182/blood.V91.1.288

Panepinto, J. A., Brousseau, D. C., Hillery, C. A., & Scott, J. P. (2005). Variation in hospitalizations and hospital length of stay in children with vaso-occlusive crises in sickle cell disease. *Pediatric Blood & Cancer, 44*(2), 182–186. https://doi.org/10.1002/pbc.20180

Peterson, A., Charles, V., Yeung, D., & Coyle, K. (2021). The health equity framework: A science- and justice-based model for public health researchers and practitioners. *Health Promotion Practice, 22*(6), 741–746. https://doi.org/10.1177/1524839920950730

Piel, F. B., Hay, S. I., Gupta, S., Weatherall, D. J., & Williams, T. N. (2013). Global burden of sickle cell anaemia in children under five, 2010–2050: Modelling based on demographics, excess mortality, and interventions. *PLOS Medicine, 10*(7), e1001484. https://doi.org/10.1371/journal.pmed.1001484

Poku, B. A., Caress, A. L., & Kirk, S. (2018). Adolescents' experiences of living with sickle cell disease: An integrative narrative review of the literature. *International Journal of Nursing Studies, 80*, 20–28. https://doi.org/10.1016/j.ijnurstu.2017.12.008

Porter, J. S., Wesley, K. M., Zhao, M. S., Rupff, R. J., & Hankins, J. S. (2017). Pediatric to adult care transition: perspectives of young adults with sickle cell disease. *Journal of Pediatric Psychology, 42*(9), 1016–1027. https://doi.org/10.1093/jpepsy/jsx088

Power-Hays, A., & McGann, P. T. (2020). When actions speak louder than words—Racism and sickle cell disease. *The New England Journal of Medicine, 383*(20), 1902–1903. https://doi.org/10.1056/NEJMp2022125

Poznanski, E. O., Freeman, L. N., & Mokros, H. B. (1985). Children's depression rating scale–Revised. *Psychopharmacology Bulletin, 21*, 979–989.

Prussien, K. V., Compas, B. E., Siciliano, R. E., Ciriegio, A. E., Lee, C. A., Kassim, A. A., DeBaun, M. R., Donahue, M. J., & Jordan, L. C. (2021). Cerebral hemodynamics and executive function in sickle cell anemia. *Stroke, 52*(5), 1830–1834. https://doi.org/10.1161/STROKEAHA.120.032741

Prussien, K. V., DeBaun, M. R., Yarboi, J., Bemis, H., McNally, C., Williams, E., & Compas, B. E. (2018). Cognitive function, coping, and depressive symptoms in children and adolescents with sickle cell disease. *Journal of Pediatric Psychology, 43*(5), 543–551. https://doi.org/10.1093/jpepsy/jsx141

Prussien, K. V., Jordan, L. C., DeBaun, M. R., & Compas, B. E. (2019). Cognitive function in sickle cell disease across domains, cerebral infarct status, and the lifespan: A meta-analysis. *Journal of Pediatric Psychology, 44*(8), 948–958. https://doi.org/10.1093/jpepsy/jsz031

Prussien, K. V., Siciliano, R. E., Ciriegio, A. E., Lee, C. A., DeBaun, M. R., Jordan, L. C., & Compas, B. E. (2021). Preliminary study of coping, perceived control, and depressive symptoms in youth with sickle cell anemia. *Journal of Developmental and Behavioral Pediatrics, 42*(6), 485–489. https://doi.org/10.1097/DBP.0000000000000922

Psihogios, A. M., Daniel, L. C., Tarazi, R., Smith-Whitley, K., Patterson, C. A., & Barakat, L. P. (2018). Family functioning, medical self-management, and health outcomes among school-aged children with sickle cell disease: A mediation model. *Journal of Pediatric Psychology, 43*(4), 423–433. https://doi.org/10.1093/jpepsy/jsx120

Ragab, I. A., Ellabody, M. A., Ramy, H. A., Mahmoud, N. F., & Sayed, S. M. (2021). Evaluation of sickle cell module for quality of life in Egyptian children and adolescents patients: Impact of psychiatric and disease specific variables. *Indian Journal of Hematology & Blood Transfusion, 37*(4), 616–622. https://doi.org/10.1007/s12288-021-01396-y

Raphael, J. L., Butler, A. M., Rattler, T. L., Kowalkowski, M. A., Mueller, B. U., & Giordano, T. P. (2013). Parental information, motivation, and adherence behaviors among children with sickle cell disease. *Pediatric Blood & Cancer, 60*(7), 1204–1210. https://doi.org/10.1002/pbc.24466

Raphael, J. L., & Oyeku, S. O. (2013). Sickle cell disease pain management and the medical home.

Hematology, 2013(1), 433–438. https://doi.org/10.1182/asheducation.V2013.1.433.3850724

Reynolds, C. R., & Kamphaus, R. W. (2015). *Behavior assessment system for children* (3rd ed.). Pearson.

Rodrigue, J. R., Streisand, R., Banko, C., Kedar, A., & Pitel, P. A. (1996). Social functioning, peer relations, and internalizing and externalizing problems among youth with sickle cell disease. *Children's Health Care, 25*(1), 37–52. https://doi.org/10.1207/s15326888chc2501_4

Saulsberry, A. C., Porter, J. S., & Hankins, J. S. (2019). A program of transition to adult care for sickle cell disease. *Hematology, 2019*(1), 496–504. https://doi.org/10.1182/hematology.2019000054

Schatz, J. (2004). Brief report: Academic attainment in children with sickle cell disease. *Journal of Pediatric Psychology, 29*(8), 627–633. https://doi.org/10.1093/jpepsy/jsh065

Schatz, J., Finke, R., & Roberts, C. W. (2004). Interactions of biomedical and environmental risk factors for cognitive development: A preliminary study of sickle cell disease. *Journal of Developmental & Behavioral Pediatrics, 25*(5), 303–310. https://doi.org/10.1097/00004703-200410000-00001

Schwartz, L. A., Brumley, L. D., Tuchman, L. K., Barakat, L. P., Hobbie, W. L., Ginsberg, J. P., Daniel, L. C., Kazak, A. E., Bevans, K., & Deatrick, J. A. (2013). Stakeholder validation of a model of readiness for transition to adult care. *JAMA Pediatrics, 167*(10), 939–946. https://doi.org/10.1001/jamapediatrics.2013.2223

Schwartz, L. A., Radcliffe, J., & Barakat, L. P. (2009). Associates of school absenteeism in adolescents with sickle cell disease. *Pediatric Blood & Cancer, 52*(1), 92–96. https://doi.org/10.1002/pbc.21819

Schwartz, L. A., Tuchman, L. K., Hobbie, W. L., & Ginsberg, J. P. (2011). A social-ecological model of readiness for transition to adult-oriented care for adolescents and young adults with chronic health conditions. *Child: Care, Health and Development, 37*(6), 883–895. https://doi.org/10.1111/j.1365-2214.2011.01282.x

Shapiro, B. S., Dinges, D. F., Orne, E. C., Bauer, N., Reilly, L. B., Whitehouse, W. G., Ohene-Frempong, K., & Orne, M. T. (1995). Home management of sickle cell-related pain in children and adolescents: Natural history and impact on school attendance. *Pain, 61*(1), 139–144. https://doi.org/10.1016/0304-3959(94)00164-A

Sil, S., Cohen, L. L., & Dampier, C. (2016). Psychosocial and functional outcomes in youth with chronic sickle cell pain. *The Clinical Journal of Pain, 32*(6), 527–533. https://doi.org/10.1097/AJP.0000000000000289

Sil, S., Dampier, C., & Cohen, L. L. (2016). Pediatric sickle cell disease and parent and child catastrophizing. *The Journal of Pain, 17*(9), 963–971. https://doi.org/10.1016/j.jpain.2016.05.008

Stewart, D. E., & Yuen, T. (2011). A systematic review of resilience in the physically ill. *Psychosomatics, 52*(3), 199–209. https://doi.org/10.1016/j.psym.2011.01.036

Stollon, N. B., Paine, C. W., Rabelais, E., Brumley, L. D., Poole, E. S., Peyton, T., Grant, A. W., Jan, S., Trachtenberg, S., Zander, M., Bonafide, C. P., & Schwartz, L. A. (2015). Transitioning adolescents and young adults with sickle cell disease from pediatric to adult health care: Provider perspectives. *Journal of Pediatric Hematology/Oncology, 37*(8), 577–583. https://doi.org/10.1097/MPH.0000000000000427

Tanabe, P., Myers, R., Zosel, A., Brice, J., Ansari, A. H., Evans, J., Martinovich, Z., Todd, K. H., & Paice, J. A. (2007). Emergency department management of acute pain episodes in sickle cell disease. *Academic Emergency Medicine, 14*(5), 419–425. https://doi.org/10.1111/j.1553-2712.2007.tb01801.x

Thornburg, C. D., Calatroni, A., & Panepinto, J. A. (2011). Differences in health-related quality of life in children with sickle cell disease receiving hydroxyurea. *Journal of Pediatric Hematology/Oncology, 33*(4), 251–254. https://doi.org/10.1097/MPH.0b013e3182114c54

Trzepacz, A. M., Vannatta, K., Gerhardt, C. A., Ramey, C., & Noll, R. B. (2004). Emotional, social, and behavioral functioning of children with sickle cell disease and comparison peers. *Journal of Pediatric Hematology/Oncology, 26*(10), 642–648. https://doi.org/10.1097/01.mph.0000139456.12036.8d

Tusuubira, S. K., Naggawa, T., & Nakamoga, V. (2019). To join or not to join? A case of sickle cell clubs, stigma and discrimination in secondary schools in Butambala district, Uganda. *Adolescent Health, Medicine and Therapeutics, 10*, 145–152. https://doi.org/10.2147/AHMT.S223956

Valrie, C., Floyd, A., Sisler, I., Redding-Lallinger, R., & Fuh, B. (2020). Depression and anxiety as moderators of the pain-social functioning relationship in youth with sickle cell disease. *Journal of Pain Research, 13*, 729–736. https://doi.org/10.2147/JPR.S238115

Wakefield, E. O., Popp, J. M., Dale, L. P., Santanelli, J. P., Pantaleao, A., & Zempsky, W. T. (2017). Perceived racial bias and health-related stigma among youth with sickle cell disease. *Journal of Developmental and Behavioral Pediatrics, 38*(2), 129–134. https://doi.org/10.1097/DBP.0000000000000381

Ware, R. E., de Montalembert, M., Tshilolo, L., & Abboud, M. R. (2017). Sickle cell disease. *The Lancet, 390*(10091), 311–323. https://doi.org/10.1016/S0140-6736(17)30193-9

Ware, R. E., Helms, R. W., & the SWiTCH Investigators. (2012). Stroke with transfusions changing to hydroxyurea (SWiTCH). *Blood, 119*(17), 3925–3932. https://doi.org/10.1182/blood-2011-11-392340

Yang, Y. M., Cepeda, M., Price, C., Shah, A., & Mankad, V. (1994). Depression in children and adolescents with sickle-cell disease. *Archives of Pediatrics & Adolescent Medicine, 148*(5), 457–460. https://doi.org/10.1001/archpedi.1994.02170050015003

Yarboi, J., Compas, B. E., Brody, G. H., White, D., Rees Patterson, J., Ziara, K., & King, A. (2017). Association of social-environmental factors with cognitive function in children with sickle cell disease. *Child Neuropsychology, 23*(3), 343–360. https://doi.org/10.1080/09297049.2015.1111318

Yarboi, J., Prussien, K. V., Bemis, H., Williams, E., Watson, K. H., McNally, C., Henry, L., King, A. A., DeBaun, M. R., & Compas, B. E. (2019). Responsive parenting behaviors and cognitive function in children with sickle cell disease. *Journal of Pediatric Psychology, 44*(10), 1234–1243. https://doi.org/10.1093/jpepsy/jsz065

Ziadni, M. S., Patterson, C. A., Pulgarón, E. R., Robinson, M. R., & Barakat, L. P. (2011). Health-related quality of life and adaptive behaviors of adolescents with sickle cell disease: Stress processing moderators. *Journal of Clinical Psychology in Medical Settings, 18*(4), 335–344. https://doi.org/10.1007/s10880-011-9254-3

CHAPTER 11

CHILDHOOD CANCER: PROMOTING HEALTH AND WELL-BEING THROUGH PEDIATRIC MULTIDISCIPLINARY CARE

Lisa A. Schwartz, Katie Darabos, Megan N. Perez, Branlyn DeRosa, Kemar V. Prussien, Meredith E. MacGregor, and Lamia P. Barakat

Cancer is a disease characterized by an uncontrolled division of abnormal cells in any part of the body that can occur at any age. It is a heterogenous diagnosis that includes cancers of the blood or solid tumors, with the potential to originate from and impact any organ system. Pediatric cancer, inclusive of adolescent cancer, is relatively rare. Yet, beyond infancy, cancer is the leading cause of disease-related death among children in the United States (American Cancer Society, 2021). Pediatric cancer may differ from adult cancers in terms of disease characteristics, treatment, and outcomes. Cancer in childhood is mostly caused by a randomly acquired (not inherited) DNA mutation. Compared to cancer in adults, childhood cancer is less likely to be caused by exposures from the environment (e.g., chemical exposure) or health harming behaviors (e.g., tobacco). Survival in pediatric cancer is also higher than in adults, with about 80% surviving into adulthood, representing significant gains in survival in recent decades (Curtin et al., 2016).

Despite the prospect of cure for most cases, childhood cancer has a major impact on the patient and family that endures beyond treatment and cure. The onset of cancer often leads to abrupt changes in physical and psychosocial functioning, requiring an adjustment to a "new normal." Treatment for cancer is intense from the standpoint of time and length, often lasting years, and sometimes with long inpatient stays or daily treatments (e.g., daily radiation or chemotherapy). Further, the treatment is often intense physically, given the toxic nature of many cancer curing treatments that result in significant side effects such as nausea, fatigue, pain, and mucositis. Such intensity impacts the patient and the whole family in terms of disruptions in work, school, and social functioning; financial burden; and physical and psychological well-being. Survivors post treatment may continue to experience or be at risk for long-term physical, psychosocial, and cognitive morbidities known as late effects. While many patients and families demonstrate significant resilience, the many cumulative stressors such as illness uncertainty, treatment intensity, and delayed developmental milestones are burdensome for the duration of cancer and beyond.

The significant impact of cancer on development, well-being, and family functioning requires multidisciplinary teams to treat and support resiliency. Beyond oncologists and related providers taking care of children with cancer (e.g., nurse practitioners, physician assistants, hospitalists),

https://doi.org/10.1037/0000414-011
APA Handbook of Pediatric Psychology, Developmental-Behavioral Pediatrics, and Developmental Science: Vol. 2. Pediatric Psychology and Developmental-Behavioral Pediatrics: Clinical Applications of Developmental Science, P. E. Shah and M. H. Bornstein (Editors-in-Chief)
Copyright © 2025 by the American Psychological Association. All rights reserved.

other experts attending to the behavioral, psychosocial, and developmental outcomes of the patient and family are needed to optimize well-being and long-term outcomes. In this chapter, we highlight the challenges of children and their families managing cancer, as well as outcomes, beyond cancer survival. We review the epidemiology of childhood cancer, including prevalence and incidence, survival and mortality, health outcomes and psychosocial outcomes. Drawing from research in developmental science, we consider the relevant multilevel influences associated with risk and resilience, and we present related models of care. We also highlight the role of providers with expertise in development and behavior, including pediatric psychologists and psychiatrists, and developmental-behavioral pediatricians who can partner with medical teams in the management of children with cancer.

EPIDEMIOLOGY OF CANCER

Cancer is not a homogeneous disease. It represents many diagnoses with many treatment options and outcomes.

Etiology, Prevalence, and Incidence

Cancer in children is most often a sporadic event with an unknown cause. However, there is increasing understanding and discovery of genetic links to childhood cancer, and it is now believed that more than 10% of pediatric cancer patients harbor a germline mutation in a cancer predisposition gene (Brodeur et al., 2017). There are known genetic disorders that relate to an increased risk of cancer in addition to being linked to developmental and intellectual differences such as Down syndrome and PTEN hamartoma tumor syndrome. For these families, the need to manage multiple comorbidities and risks is burdensome, especially for those with linked family history of genetic risk.

Pediatric cancer rates have slightly increased over the past several decades, such that over 15,000 new cases of cancer among children and adolescents were estimated to be diagnosed in the United States in 2021 (American Cancer Society, 2021). The most common cancers in childhood are leukemias (28%) and brain and other nervous system tumors (27%; which includes benign and borderline malignant tumors), whereas brain and other nervous system tumors (21%) and lymphomas (19%) are the most frequently diagnosed cancers in adolescence (American Cancer Society, 2021). Other cancers that tend to emerge in infancy and early childhood include neuroblastoma (6%), Wilms tumor (5%), and retinoblastoma (2%; American Cancer Society, 2019). Bone cancers, including osteosarcoma and Ewing sarcoma, are more common among teens and make up about 3% of childhood cancer (American Cancer Society, 2019). Certain cancers more commonly found among adults, such as thyroid and melanoma, are also common in adolescents, accounting for 11% and 3% of cases, respectively, compared to 2% and 1% in children. (American Cancer Society, 2021).

Diagnosis, Treatment, and Survival

Delays in diagnosis of childhood cancer are common, as many symptoms (e.g., swollen lymph nodes, limb pain or headaches, fevers, fatigue) of cancer are mistaken for other more common problems, including behavioral. In one study, 52% of 364 cases received an initial incorrect nononcological diagnosis (Chen & Mullen, 2017). The role of symptoms on diagnosis delay may be mediated by age with older patients more at risk. They are less reliant on parent report and have cancers with more diffuse symptom presentation than young children (e.g., abdominal mass of Wilms tumor in young child is more obvious compared to fatigue and pain in an older child; Dang-Tan & Franco, 2007). Thus, providers should be careful not to dismiss symptoms that may signal cancer, especially among teens. This is especially true for pediatricians and behavioral health providers that may be assessing psychosomatic complaints without obvious associations.

Through advances in cancer treatments, optimization of current treatment regimens, and access to clinical trials, survival rates have improved to an average of 84% for children and 85% for adolescents across all types of cancers (American

Cancer Society, 2021). Multimodal treatment can include intensive chemotherapy, surgical resection, radiation, hematopoietic transplant, and immunotherapies that last months to years in inpatient and outpatient settings, resulting in multiple side effects and adverse events during treatment. Treatment often includes enrollment in clinical trials, a contributing factor to the improvement in survival rates throughout the years. Trials may range from Phase 3 (therapeutic trials to compare to standard of care) to very experimental Phase 1 trials that involve assessment of safety and dosage of new possible treatments. Adolescents are less likely to enroll in clinical trials than children, necessitating greater understanding of and interventions for adolescent decision making. Adolescents may have unique values and perspectives about treatment-related decisions yet may defer to adults when making decisions. This highlights the important role of developmentally attuned providers in understanding adolescent cognitive capacity to participate in decision making and optimizing adolescent engagement to the extent that it is congruent with their values and goals.

HEALTH DISPARITIES

Cancer disparities are differences that occur in health measures of cancer, such as rates of screening, incidence, stage at diagnosis, morbidity, mortality, survival, and quality of life in survivorship. Both incidence and survival rates differ by sex, yet these differences change across the developmental trajectory. In childhood cancer (birth to 14 years), boys have approximately 10% greater risk of a cancer diagnosis than girls; however, by adolescence (15–19), diagnostic rates even out with comparable incidence between boys and girls (American Cancer Society, 2014; Miller et al., 2020). Mortality rates are higher for males than females across childhood and adolescence (American Cancer Society, 2014; Miller et al., 2020) and these mortality differences may be explained in part by the type of cancers that are more common in males (American Cancer Society, 2014). Furthermore, survival within diagnoses varies based on age such that acute lymphocytic leukemia survival is greater for children at 91% but 75% for adolescents and rhabdomyosarcoma survival for children at 70% but adolescents 46% (Miller et al., 2020). Further, the risk for morbidities is greater for survivors diagnosed during childhood compared to diagnosis in adolescence, but the risk of death from progression or relapse is greater for adolescent survivors than child survivors (Miller et al., 2020; Ward et al., 2014).

Cancer disparities have also been identified across races and ethnicities. Overall, cancer prevalence is greater for non-Hispanic White and Hispanic children and adolescents and lowest among American Indian/Alaskan Natives (American Cancer Society, 2014; Miller et al., 2020; Ward et al., 2014). However, non-Hispanic White patients experience better 5-year survival rates as compared with communities of color (American Cancer Society, 2014; Aristizabal et al., 2021; Miller et al., 2020), and non-Hispanic Black and Hispanic children with cancer experience greater rates of relapse, earlier death, and higher rates of death from infections than non-Hispanic White children (Aristizabal et al., 2021).

Multilevel Risk Factors

Research in developmental science has helped inform our understanding of the multilevel factors associated with risks and disparities in cancer outcomes. Discernment of the mechanisms through which cancer disparities occur is complicated by the intersection of social determinants of health with the social constructs of race and ethnicity, such that structural racism influences socioeconomic status (SES) and access to care. Consequently, distinguishing the distinct influence of an individual social determinant of health on cancer outcomes from other racial, ethnic, or genetic differences is complex (Aristizabal et al., 2021). Factors specific to pediatric cancer survival disparities include family SES, health insurance status, parent education, access to quality treatment, cancer knowledge, supportive care (American Cancer Society, 2014; Ward et al., 2014), and quality of communication between caregivers and medical staff (Bhatia, 2011). These factors affect timeliness of diagnosis, rates of clinical trials enrollment, and adherence to medical treatments, which can impact cancer outcomes (Aristizabal et al., 2021; Bhatia, 2011).

Notably, health insurance status affects access to care, children living in high-poverty areas have greater risk of relapse compared to those who live in low-poverty areas (Aristizabal et al., 2021; Bona et al., 2016), and SES explains a significant portion of the disparities in racial and ethnic survival rates (Kehm et al., 2018; Volume 1, Chapter 18, this handbook). For example, children and adolescents with Medicaid coverage are more likely to have delays in diagnosis, be diagnosed with a late-stage cancer, and, thus, have worse survival outcomes than children with private health insurance (Aristizabal et al., 2021). Also, adolescence and early adulthood add cumulative risk of deleterious outcomes for multiple reasons including unique biology, delayed diagnosis, less availability of clinical trials, and behavioral risk factors (e.g., poor adherence, less adult supervision). Health disparities also exist for off-treatment survivors for many reasons. A confluence of sociodemographic determinants as well as limited knowledge of health care providers related to the significance of long-term follow-up care for monitoring and managing late effects, influences less than optimal uptake of follow-up care (Mobley et al., 2021).

MEDICAL CONSIDERATIONS

Despite cure, childhood cancer has a lasting impact on health, necessitating follow-up care and self-management.

Acute and Late Effects

The treatment of cancer is often more debilitating and toxic than the cancer alone. Side effects of treatment are numerous such as nausea, pain, mouth sores, neuropathy, gastrointestinal symptoms, headache, anemia, infections, and skin changes. These symptoms can impact adherence and distress (described in later sections). Such adverse symptoms are often more pronounced in adolescents for numerous reasons including more intensive treatments, different biology, and better reporting. Although pharmacological treatments are often the first line of defense for supportive care, pediatric psychologists can play a significant role in helping to mitigate such acute symptoms and, in fact, parents prefer to incorporate behavioral interventions (Tutelman et al., 2018). Parents also play a key role in helping to manage their child's symptoms and modeling positive coping behaviors.

The toxicity of treatment also may cause physical late effects and increase risk for second cancers. Such late effects may evolve over time and may emerge years after treatment ends, with the potential to impact any organ system, including pulmonary, cardiac, endocrine, reproductive, and nervous system. Among over 10,000 survivors of childhood cancer from the National Cancer Institute–funded largescale Childhood Cancer Survivor Study, 62.3% had at least one chronic condition; 27.5% had a severe or life-threatening condition (Oeffinger et al., 2006). Late effects can also be more diffuse symptoms such as fatigue and pain. Late effects may limit functional abilities (e.g., stamina, ambulation, senses), impacting normative developmental tasks (e.g., work and school). Emerging evidence indicates that newer targeted and less toxic therapies (e.g., proton radiation, immunotherapy) may reduce risk of long-term late effects and risk for second cancers.

Although it is well established that survivor late effects are related to the cancer and treatment, including a dose-response effect, this risk is modified by many factors that are not directly linked to cancer history. Research evaluating the influence of patient-specific demographic and genetic factors, premorbid and comorbid conditions, health behaviors, and aging has identified additional risk factors that influence cancer treatment-related toxicity and possible targets for intervention in this population (Dixon et al., 2018). For example, because childhood is a period of critical growth and development, the age of cancer diagnosis and treatment can impact the risk of subsequent treatment-related late effects. As an example, the impact of cranial irradiation on cognitive function is particularly apparent among younger children in earlier stages of brain development. Another example is the interaction of demographic risk factors, health behaviors, and late effects whereby low educational attainment (i.e., less than a high school education) and lower household income among survivors have been associated with risky health behaviors, including physical inactivity, smoking, and drinking (Dixon et al., 2018).

Follow-Up and Transition Care for Survivors

At the end of treatment, survivors are expected to return to the clinic for surveillance of recurrence and management of any morbidities related to treatment. Such follow-up care is tapered from, on average, about once per month to once every six months. This represents a transition off active treatment that, while momentous, can also be anxiety-provoking to families. Patients and parents often feel like broader supports from behavioral health and supportive care are also tapered off while simultaneously experiencing stress and anxiety related to the uncertainty of surveillance for cancer recurrence (sometimes referred to as scanxiety) and getting back to normal. During this time, patients and families are also learning to manage any disabilities and morbidities (temporary or permanent) as a result of treatment (e.g., avascular necrosis causing mobility difficulty, lasting fatigue) that may make reentry into normal life difficult. Thus, while supportive care may seem to be tapering off along with oncology care, there remains a need for broad multidisciplinary support around adjustment, management of late effects, and reentry to school and other contexts, including accommodations.

Eventually, it is expected that the follow-up care will shift from surveillance of cancer recurrence to surveillance and management of late effects and second cancers, which can emerge long after cancer treatment ends. Long-term survivorship care, known as *risk-based care* (considering the individual treatment profile and other risk factors), is recommended annually (see guidelines from Children's Oncology Group). Survivors who remain engaged in follow-up care are more knowledgeable about their diagnosis/treatment, more accurate in their perception of late-effects risk, receive more regular surveillance/screening, have more late effects detected, and have fewer emergency department visits (Signorelli et al., 2017). Lifelong follow-up care eventually requires and transfers to an adult provider. Unfortunately, childhood cancer survivors are often lost in transition, resulting in less than half receiving appropriate follow-up care in adulthood (Nathan et al., 2008; Szalda et al., 2016).

Reasons for poor uptake of long-term follow-up care are multifactorial and can be informed by the social-ecological model of young adult readiness for transition (SMART), which was developed for childhood cancer survivors (although it is generalizable; Schwartz et al., 2013). SMART emphasizes the importance of understanding the social-ecology of the transition process. This includes sociodemographic and disease-related factors less amenable to change (sociodemographic/culture, access/insurance, medical status/risk, and neurocognitive functioning/IQ) and more modifiable factors (knowledge, beliefs/expectations, goals/motivations, skills/self-efficacy, relationships/communication, and psychosocial functioning/emotions) of multiple stakeholders (patient, parent, and provider), as well as the developmental maturity of the patient. This model is intended to inform targets of intervention in adolescence to prepare survivors to assume greater responsibility for their health and health care, facilitating a smooth transition to adult follow-up care that begins with preparation earlier in adolescence. It reflects the importance of not only targeting a teen patient, but also their parents and providers who play a vital role in helping them manage their health and adjust to new medical challenges and environments.

Self-Management and Adherence

Self-management involves using a range of strategies, such as decision-making, problem-solving, or resource management to maintain a sense of wellness, rather than illness (Lorig & Holman, 2003). An aspect of self-management involves adherence to recommended cancer treatment protocols. Children with cancer and their families are often required to self-manage a complex treatment regimen that includes the administration of multiple medications at varied dosing schedules, regular clinic attendance, symptom monitoring, and engaging in certain lifestyle recommendations (e.g., physical activity, dietary modifications; Psihogios et al., 2019). Nonadherence is often high (50–75%) and can result in several negative outcomes including poor disease control, increased risk of relapse, reduced health-related quality of life (HRQoL), increased health care utilization and health care spending, and cancer-related complications (McGrady & Hommel, 2016). An emerging body of evidence supports routinely assessing adherence as a standard of clinical care in pediatric oncology to optimize treatment adherence and reduce negative health outcomes (Pai & McGrady, 2015). Adherence to medical guidelines and surveillance is also important for the management of late effects from cancer treatment. Factors associated with self-management and adherence are multifactorial as described in the Pediatric Self-Management Model and highlighted in the chapter on pediatric treatment adherence (Chapter 2, this volume). Multidisciplinary providers may assist caregivers in scaffolding their children's abilities and recognizing limitations due to a priori or cancer-related cognitive issues.

PSYCHOSOCIAL OUTCOMES ASSOCIATED WITH CANCER

Childhood cancer is a life-altering event that impacts the trajectory and well-being of the child and their family.

Cognitive Impact, School Functioning, and Academic Achievement

Cancer may impact cognitive functioning and educational and vocational outcomes most often due to treatments impacting the central nervous system (CNS) and the cumulative impact of missed school. It is estimated that one-third of all survivors and most brain tumor survivors experience cognitive impairment (Phillips et al., 2021).

Cognitive late effects may include diminished IQ, attention and concentration, processing speed, visual perceptual skills, executive functioning, memory, cognitive fatigue, and overall acquisition of new information and skills, which in turn can contribute to poor academic performance, low education attainment, and low levels of employment (Krull et al., 2018; Phillips et al., 2021). Cognitive impact can be seen during treatment in children as young as 3 and younger, even in non-CNS cancers, as evidenced by findings of deficits compared to healthy controls in motor, mental, and language development (Bornstein et al., 2012). Notably, better health status and mother-rated behavior was related to better motor and mental performance.

Most research has demonstrated that the effects of cancer and cancer treatment on neurocognitive functioning are often delayed, becoming evident one or more years post treatment. The specific pattern of neurocognitive deficits depends in part on age at diagnosis (younger), type of cancer (CNS malignancies), type of cancer treatment (cranial radiation therapy, intrathecal therapy, hematopoietic transplant), and tumor size/site or surgical complications (impacting relevant surrounding structures). Other factors that may moderate neuropsychological outcomes include child-specific factors (e.g., higher baseline cognitive functioning, female gender) and family factors (e.g., lower SES, higher parent stress, lower parental education; Paltin, Burgers, et al., 2018). Neurocognitive assessment is essential for monitoring changing neurocognitive abilities over the course of development and treatment, and for planning for home, school, and community supports (Paltin, Burgers, et al., 2018). This ideally would include evaluation around diagnosis, as well as repeated evaluations during treatment and into survivorship. Interpretation of results of testing must also consider the potential confounding effects of fatigue and sleep disturbance, mood and anxiety, medication effects, and symptoms such as anemia.

The cognitive impact, as well as treatment of pediatric cancer, can impact school experiences and academic achievement across the continuum of treatment. At diagnosis, absenteeism and reduced academic performance as a result of cancer treatment (e.g., chemotherapy, radiation) and treatment-related side effects (e.g., fatigue, nausea, lower immune system functioning; Eiser & Vance, 2002; Gerhardt et al., 2007) may contribute to declines in academic achievement, delayed academic milestones, and disrupted peer relationships (Robinson et al., 2010). Further, neurocognitive late effects secondary to cancer and cancer treatments have been linked to adverse effects on school engagement and academic achievement. For example, compared to controls, survivors of brain tumors and acute lymphoblastic leukemia have been shown to perform significantly worse on reading, spelling, and math tasks (Paltin, Burgers, et al., 2018). Moreover, children with cancer who are less integrated into school often perceive cancer-related stressors as more stressful, have fewer friends, display more negative thinking, and have reduced self-image compared to those who are more integrated into school (Hockenberry-Eaton et al., 1997). Research has found some links between maternal adjustment and children's cognitive skills and school functioning (Sultan et al., 2016). Yet, this may also reflect the effect of children's limitations on parental distress and common factors such as intensity of treatment.

Developmental-behavioral care for children with cancer. Multidisciplinary approaches to address cognitive and academic impact are critical. Developmental-behavioral pediatricians can contribute to evaluations of neurocognitive late effects such as attention and executive functioning skills and with consideration of prescription of pharmacological interventions. For example, medication to address attention deficits (e.g., methylphenidate) can improve cognitive and psychosocial functioning (Paltin, Schofield, et al., 2018). Computerized cognitive training such as Cogmed has also shown promise for improving working memory, attention, and processing speed with some modest gains in academic achievement (Butler et al., 2008; Paltin, Schofield, et al., 2018). Computerized programs help reduce burden on families by limiting the need for in-person cognitive rehabilitation and caregiver coaching. As for school absenteeism and accommodations, a team approach is necessary that involves the family, multidisciplinary providers, and school staff (Hocking et al., 2018). Children and adolescents may require formalized accommodations and interventions via 504 accommodation plans and individualized education plans. Further, the patient's providers can help educate the school about cancer treatment, cognitive late effects, and other enduring impacts of treatment.

Physical Appearance and Stigma

Children with cancer often experience appearance changes that can include hair loss due to chemotherapy, weight gain or weight loss, disfigurement, amputation, and/or scars from surgery or radiation treatment (Eiser, 1998; Vani et al., 2021; Wallace et al., 2007). These appearance changes can bring a host of psychosocial challenges, including withdrawal from social interactions and peer relationships; feeling different and unattractive compared with their peers; reduced self-esteem; increased self-consciousness; body image concerns; and increases in social isolation that negatively affect HRQoL particularly for adolescents (Pahl et al., 2021; van Erp et al., 2021). Yet, children have reported adopting adaptive coping strategies for appearance changes, such as wearing jewelry and using humor (Vani et al., 2021; Williamson et al., 2010).

Social Functioning

In addition to experiencing cancer-related appearance changes that can impact interactions with peers, missed opportunities for socialization due to extended school absences (Robinson et al., 2010) and the cognitive impact of treatments on social competence (Moyer et al., 2012) may negatively impact social functioning. Among children with cancer, younger age is associated with greater impairments in social functioning due to fewer opportunities to learn foundational social skills from preschool and other activities (Brinkman et al., 2012; Willard et al., 2021). Adolescents with cancer may also experience difficulties in social functioning, such as less satisfaction with friends at school than their peers (Winterling et al., 2015) which is particularly problematic given the importance of peer relationships during this developmental stage. In addition, youth with central nervous system-directed treatments/brain tumors are at greater risk for problems in social functioning than youth with non-CNS directed treatments, at different points in the cancer care continuum (Hocking et al., 2020) and during adolescence (Pahl et al., 2021). Unfortunately, youth with cancer appear to experience higher rates of bullying than peers, with verbal bullying being cited as the most common form (Collins et al., 2019), perhaps due to changes in appearance, school absences, and school accommodations that make them targets (Collins et al., 2019; Volume 1, Chapter 18, this handbook). Peer relationships and social functioning are also impacted for adolescent and young adult (AYA) survivors. Challenges include identify development (e.g., identifying as a survivor or dismissing prior cancer history), how and when to disclose information related to their health, having a history of relationship disruptions or less opportunity to develop relationships, and potential changes in appearance that become more salient to a survivor with age (Schwartz et al., 2020). Social skills groups have shown some success at improving social competence, especially with brain tumor survivors (Barrera et al., 2018).

Emotional Functioning

Although children and adolescents with cancer are generally resilient, symptoms of anxiety, including posttraumatic stress symptoms (PTSS), and depression may be evident throughout treatment and into survivorship. Aside from the initial shock of the diagnosis, other traumatic triggers may include hair loss or other appearance changes already noted, painful procedures, adverse events from treatment, and missed time with peers and in school. Survivors may also experience traumatic triggers such as scans for surveillance, threat of future cancers or late effects, late effects, and losses such as diminished cognitive, social, and reproductive capacity. As such, a posttraumatic stress framework is useful for understanding the short- and long-term psychosocial impact of childhood cancer. Cancer, after all, is a trauma that entails initial shock, adjustment, and ongoing life-threat.

For children and adolescents in treatment, it can be difficult to tease apart psychological from physical changes. Specifically, cancer treatment can cause symptoms such as changes in appetite and weight, fatigue, stomachaches and nausea, headaches, externalizing behaviors (often from corticosteroids), and irritability, making differential diagnosis challenging (Vannatta & Salley, 2017). Furthermore, it is not uncommon for children and adolescents with cancer to have frequent thoughts of death given the intensity of treatment they may experience and potential life threat. Anxiety may also increase during treatment, especially with anticipatory anxiety around clinic appointments or procedures.

For the most part, children with cancer and their parents (noted in the following sections) experience significant distress soon after the diagnosis, which then subsides to levels similar to that of the general population (Sultan et al., 2016). Younger children especially seem to be resilient. Most do not exhibit elevated psychological symptoms although behavioral dysregulation and PTSS may be present in some, with increased risk related to negative affectivity (temperament) and parental PTSS (Sultan et al., 2016).

Depression and anxiety, as well as PTSS, have been identified more often in older survivors. Rates of survivors' anxiety are 13–14% at 5 years' survival (Phillips et al., 2015) and may be exacerbated by fear of cancer recurrence. One study found 13% reported suicidality (Recklitis et al., 2006). PTSS are also relatively common, with about 12% of survivors experiencing severe symptom burden (Allen et al., 2018; Langeveld et al., 2004) although researchers have cautioned to not assume cancer is the most traumatic event on which people report (Allen et al., 2018). PTSS may include intrusive thoughts, increased arousal when thinking or talking about cancer, avoidance of thinking or talking about cancer, avoidance of health care settings or doing things to take care of health, and hypervigilance of body and symptoms (Schwartz et al., 2020). Across studies, various demographic, psychosocial, and disease-related characteristics confer greater risk for distress outcomes. For example, being diagnosed with cancer in adolescence is associated with more prevalent moderate PTSS, increased withdrawn/depressed scores, and worse psychosocial outcomes at long-term follow-up than those diagnosed at younger ages (Kazak et al., 2010; Kwak et al., 2013).

Caregiver Distress, Impact on Child, and Related Multilevel Associates

Caregivers of children with cancer navigate many challenges including managing their child's life-threatening disease, learning how to balance medical treatment demands, caring for all family members, and addressing financial and other family concerns. Caregivers endorse distress, anxiety, and intrusive thoughts about cancer (Norberg & Boman, 2008; Pai et al., 2007).

Caregivers are more likely to be distressed than the child, and a small subset continue to suffer throughout treatment and beyond (Kazak et al., 2004). However, as noted, most caregivers also experience reduced distress over time since diagnosis. A meta-analysis demonstrated the incredible variability of caregiver distress, ranging from 5% to 65% for anxiety, 7% to 91% for depression, and 4% to 75% for posttraumatic stress disorder (van Warmerdam et al., 2019). Furthermore, these caregiver prevalence rates exceed those of adult cancer survivors (Bruce, 2006). Parents may retain traumatic memories of caring for their sick children and may have lasting fear and illness uncertainty.

Child and parent adaptation to a pediatric cancer diagnosis are closely linked (Bakula et al., 2019; Fedele et al., 2013; Sultan et al., 2016). This has mostly been researched among mothers, but is also true for fathers (Robinson et al., 2007; Sultan et al., 2016). Further, acute distress of the parent has been linked to long-term child adjustment (Robinson et al., 2007; Sultan et al., 2016). One review paper reported that parental distress, anxiety, depression, and traumatic stress within the first year post diagnosis predicted multiple indices of higher child distress and social competence problems up to 7 years post diagnosis (Sultan et al., 2016).

Findings related to disease-related variables are mixed, with some evidence that treatment intensity, proximity to diagnosis, and relapse relate to parent distress (Sultan et al., 2016). However, inconsistent with the general trauma literature is the finding that objective disease variables such as intensity and severity fail to consistently predict PTSS (Bruce, 2006). The finding of female gender as a risk factor for survivor and caregiver PTSS is more consistent with trauma literature. Poorer family functioning, negative affectivity, and low self-esteem have also been found to relate to distress over time for caregivers (Sultan et al., 2016). On the other hand, family cohesion may buffer parental and child distress, especially in the case of father distress (Robinson et al., 2007). Other stressors, especially ones that predated the cancer (e.g., divorce, job change) and general stressors that are cumulative with cancer stressors confer risk for distress (Bemis et al., 2015) for caregivers and children. However, there has been mixed evidence for the independent role of education and income in caregiver and child distress outcomes, which may be confounded by more direct influence of situational variables such as stressors and single parenthood.

ADAPTIVE OUTCOMES

Youth and their families experience a range of adaptive outcomes that impact well-being.

Health-Related Quality of Life

HRQoL refers to the youth's and/or caregiver's perception of functioning/adaptation across multiple domains (e.g., physical, social, emotional, and school) and is an indicator of resilience (Salamon et al., 2016). HRQoL tends to decrease during active treatment, but typically improves throughout treatment (Vannatta & Salley, 2017), with survivors experiencing relatively positive long-term outcomes (Barakat et al., 2009). Children with CNS involvement, including brain tumors, appear to experience worse HRQoL than other diagnoses (Maunsell et al., 2006). This may be attributed to experiencing more intense treatments with subsequent functional disability as well as more restrictions due to immunosuppression (Salamon et al., 2016). Adolescents with cancer typically have worse HRQoL than same age peers as well as younger patients. This also may be related to experiencing greater toxicity from more intense treatment typical of adolescent cancer, which in turn limits the ability to engage in typical adolescent developmental tasks such as building autonomy and relationships. Alternatively, that many report positive HRQoL is, to some degree, thought to be related to response shift. As such, their perspective of well-being may be made relative to others who had cancer and peers who were not ever ill (O'Leary et al., 2007). They can identify positive impacts of their cancer (e.g., greater appreciation of life), find meaning in the traumatic event, and develop enhanced coping abilities to bounce back after adversity (Barakat et al., 2006; Salamon et al., 2016; Zebrack & Butler, 2012).

Resilience and Growth

As evidenced by the variability in distress and HRQoL outcomes over time, many children and caregivers traverse childhood cancer with resilience (Hullmann et al., 2014; Kazak et al., 2015; Kearney et al., 2015; Van Schoors et al., 2015). Resilience is the result of complex interactions of disease as well as patient, family, social, and environmental characteristics (Salamon et al., 2016) necessitating ongoing assessment to identify the psychosocial factors (e.g., coping, psychological adjustment, self-esteem, mastery, emotional, and financial resources) that influence adaptation to cancer both at diagnosis and throughout the cancer continuum (see Volume 1, Chapter 15, this handbook). Among caregivers, *resilience* has been defined in multiple ways to include low levels of distress, presence of positive affect, high levels of HRQoL, and benefit-finding (Gardner et al., 2017; Willard et al., 2016). Adversity may lead to growth, often referred to as benefit-finding or posttraumatic growth.

Research has also shown that survivors continue adaptive coping strategies, including posttraumatic growth (Barakat et al., 2006) and perceived positive impact (Zebrack et al., 2012).

It has been argued that searching for psychopathology among caregivers in childhood cancer has led to bias in research design and lack of appropriate controls (Phipps et al., 2015). As such, a study of caregivers responding to a structured psychiatric interview of PTSS compared to control group found no differences in rates, yet evidenced higher posttraumatic growth (Phipps et al., 2015). It is possible that cohort effects exist, whereby newer treatments in recent decades that have reduced mortality and treatment intensity along with greater supportive care, have reduced the traumatic nature of childhood cancer. Positive spiritual coping, optimism, and illness impact, uniquely, have predicted overall benefit finding for caregivers of childhood cancer survivors (Gardner et al., 2017).

Coping

Coping strategies often target aspects of the cancer that can be controlled, such as practicing acceptance (of the cancer, of social difficulties), using cognitive control strategies (e.g., avoiding finding out too much, distraction), adopting a healthier lifestyle (e.g., avoiding negative health behaviors, drinking more water), and goal and action setting (e.g., planning daily activities, setting future goals; Brown et al., 2021). By engaging in strategies that target aspects of the cancer and cancer treatment that are controllable, children with cancer and caregivers may cope better with the challenges that arise throughout their cancer experience.

Secondary control coping (e.g., acceptance, cognitive reappraisal) for children in early phases of cancer treatment may be adaptive and buffer symptoms of anxiety and depression (Compas et al., 2014). For both mothers and fathers, primary control coping (e.g., problem solving, emotional modulation) and secondary control coping were associated with lower depressive symptoms (Compas et al., 2015). Mothers' and fathers' coping as well as depressive symptoms were significantly correlated. These results are consistent with that of others as many studies indicate that adopting an active (problem-focused) coping style as opposed to a passive/emotional style may be beneficial (Sultan et al., 2016).

MODELS OF CARE: THE ROLE OF PEDIATRIC PSYCHOLOGY AND BEHAVIORAL HEALTH SUPPORTS

There are standards of care and frameworks that guide relevant multidisciplinary care to address the psychosocial needs of children with cancer.

Psychosocial Standards of Care for Children With Cancer and Their Families

Despite patient and family psychosocial stressors across the pediatric cancer trajectory, and a need for psychosocial support, psychosocial screening and intervention services have not been consistently implemented, and there are disparities in access to psychosocial resources and care (Wiener et al., 2015). Thus, a well-supported set of standards of care is vital to secure government support for universal psychosocial care for pediatric cancer families (Wiener et al., 2015). The Psychosocial Standards of Care Project for Childhood Cancer was formed to establish these standards (Wiener et al., 2015) based on 15 evidence- and consensus-based standards. They present guidance for care that is deemed essential and a minimum of care that should be provided to all children and families in pediatric cancer across cancer treatment settings to ensure optimal medical and psychosocial outcomes (Wiener et al., 2015; see Exhibit 11.1). These standards create a foundation for psychosocial care in pediatric cancer that pediatric psychologists and other behavioral health providers, as well as developmental-behavioral pediatricians, can support. Furthermore, guidelines to facilitate the implementation of these standards have been published to include a matrix for a thorough institutional assessment of one's current practice of the psychosocial standards of care, as well as guidelines for implementation of these

---

EXHIBIT 11.1

Brief Description of the Psychosocial Standards of Care for Childhood Cancer

1. Routine and systematic screening of patient and family psychosocial needs
2. Monitoring of neuropsychological deficits for patients with brain tumor or other cancers with high risk for neuropsychological deficits
3. Yearly psychosocial screening for long-term survivors of child and adolescent cancers
4. Access to psychosocial support interventions for patients and their families, throughout their cancer trajectory
5. Assessment of risk for financial hardship
6. Ongoing assessment of mental health needs for parents and caregivers
7. Psychoeducation, information, and anticipatory guidance of disease, treatment, acute and long-term effects, hospitalization, procedures, and psychosocial adaptation
8. Preparatory information and psychological interventions for invasive medical procedures
9. Opportunities for social interaction
10. Supportive services for siblings of a child with cancer
11. School reentry support
12. Assessment of medical adherence
13. Introduction to palliative care concepts regardless of disease status
14. Contact with the family after a child's death to assess family needs
15. Open communication among medical providers and specialized training of providers

Note. Data from Wiener et al. (2015).

---

standards, in which specific actions, strategies, and resources for each standard are defined (Wiener et al., 2020).

Pediatric Psychosocial Preventative Health Model

Another important consideration in pediatric oncology is the allocation of resources that match the needs of the patient and family. As such, the Pediatric Psychosocial Preventative Health Model (PPPHM) provides a framework, guided by a socioecological perspective on child health, that includes a 3-tiered model based on a public health orientation (Kazak et al., 2015). The largest group of families, Universal, consists of competent and adaptive families. A smaller group of families, Targeted, shows some elevated risk for ongoing psychosocial difficulties. The smallest group of families, Clinical/Treatment, exhibits more troublesome symptomatology that requires more tailored and intensive intervention, often by a psychologist and/or psychiatrists. Developmental-behavioral pediatricians can also provide targeted and clinical intervention, often in the form of medication management (e.g., for attention difficulties) or patient/family assessment and education on developmental and cognitive impact. The Psychosocial Assessment Tool (PAT) is a brief parent report screener of psychosocial risk based on the PPPHM that can be used for families of infants through adolescents. The scores indicate the level of support needed, with indications that one-half to two-thirds of families score at the Universal level of risk based on the PAT (Kazak et al., 2015). Standardizing assessment across all patients/families with a template for allocation of resources can reduce health disparities and ensure consistent care for all.

Multidisciplinary Care: Partnerships With Pediatric Psychology, Developmental-Behavioral Pediatrics, and General Pediatrics

As we have indicated throughout, the significant stress and demands of managing cancer require care from multiple providers, not just the pediatric oncologist. Pediatric psychologists and additional psychosocial providers (those trained in social work and child life) can help to mitigate short- and long-term stressors, barriers to care and adherence, and distress. As previously noted, a minority of patients may experience more severe psychiatric distress. Child and adolescent psychiatrists have experience with providing psychiatric care to medically ill children and adolescents as a required part of their training. Psychiatrists can be helpful in these populations to diagnose and treat psychiatric comorbidities both related and unrelated to the cancer. Developmental-behavioral pediatricians diagnose and care for children with a variety of conditions. Some diagnoses, such as autism spectrum disorder (ASD) or attention deficit/hyperactivity disorder (ADHD), may be unrelated to the cancer, but may complicate treatment due to associated behavioral symptoms or difficulty tolerating the medical setting. A developmental-behavioral pediatrician can make recommendations for interventions, potentially including medications, that can decrease distress and allow for improved adherence during treatment. Psychologists and developmental-behavioral pediatricians can also help to identify learning needs, advocate for accommodations such as individualized education plans, support families in adapting to their new demands, and help to educate broader teams about developmental and behavioral needs and challenges. The general pediatrician plays a critical role in the care of these patients as well. For children and adolescents with cancer, they may be the first to suspect diagnosis and to resume ongoing preventative care after planned cancer treatment has been completed. This may include monitoring for late effects of treatment and referring to additional subspecialists, particularly for cancer survivors who do not have access to dedicated long-term follow-up clinics. In many parts of the world, access to behavioral health and developmental-behavioral specialists may be limited and/or involve extensive wait times, so it is not unusual for general pediatricians to do basic diagnosis and treatment of mood, anxiety, and developmental disorders such as ADHD and ASD.

CONCLUSION

Pediatric cancer is a heterogeneous disease, representing many types, treatments, and possible genetic etiologies. Additionally, the late effects of cancer have significant long-term physical effects for the patient and psychosocial impact on the patient and family. In other words, it is a complex diagnosis that impacts the developing child and their family across the lifespan, and well beyond cure. Furthermore, evidence is emerging that multilevel determinants of health contribute to health disparities related to diagnosis, access to care, and outcomes (see Volume 1, Chapter 18, this handbook). For example, poverty impacts child outcomes of treatment, and financial toxicity of cancer impacts long-term adjustment of families and survivors (see Volume 1, Chapter 24, this handbook). Further, emerging treatment advances and emphasis on precision medicine to improve cure rates and reduce long-term late effects is only effective if they are delivered equitably to patients with adequate support. For example, there is emerging evidence that some cancers such as acute myeloid leukemia (AML) can be treated at home rather than the traditional mode for AML of inpatient care. However, this is only possible with instrumental and psychosocial support that is equitably delivered to ensure optimal outcomes for all patients. More research is needed to understand the omics of pediatric cancer and the complex interaction of genetics, social determinants of health, diagnosis and biology, and treatment in terms of outcomes of treatment and long-term late effects.

Given the complexity of pediatric cancer and long-term late effects, research and care must be multidisciplinary, incorporating perspectives of pediatric psychologists, developmental and behavioral pediatricians, and other behavioral health and pediatric specialists. These perspectives and areas of expertise are critical for improving family-centered and psychosocially minded care. They are also critical for understanding outcomes of treatment in terms of how aspects of the child, family, environment, and policies impact treatment access, disease management, and outcomes. Developmental science is key for considering how children and the systems in which they are embedded influence and change overtime in the context of cancer. There are likely transactional effects that influence the long-term trajectory of outcomes and well-being for those with cancer and long-term survivors.

RESOURCES

Web-based resources for families provide information about the health condition and available treatments and education about psychosocial considerations including support, and tangible resources to mitigate the costs of accessing treatments. Here, we highlight trustworthy websites to recommend to families.

- CureSearch for Children's Cancer:

  https://curesearch.org/

  Funds childhood cancer research projects with a focus on projects that will result in pediatric clinical trials. Provides resources for patients and families and includes information on clinical trials, videos, and statistics on pediatric cancer, Brave Barbie requests, and coping strategies.

- American Cancer Society:

  https://www.cancer.org/

  Funds and conducts cancer research and provides support to cancer patients and their families. Provides information on types of cancer, risk and prevention, coping strategies, and finances. Offers different programs, including, but not limited to, free rides, free housing, and helplines.

- Alex's Lemonade Stand Foundation:

  https://www.alexslemonade.org/

  Funds pediatric cancer research, raises awareness, and supports cancer patients and their families. Includes general information on pediatric cancer and resources on coping and helping children cope, travel support, sibling support, cancer guides, providers, and clinical trials. Has an information packet with stories from other families and resources on family services, clinical trials, and more.

- National Children's Cancer Society:

  https://theccs.org/

  Provides emotional, financial, and educational support to children with cancer, their families, and survivors. Includes resources on all aspects of pediatric cancer, including, but not limited to, camps, clinical trials, disabilities, education, emotional support, health care, and finances. Has links to foundations, tips/guides, tools, and books, webinars, articles, and news related to childhood cancer.

- Teen Cancer America:

  https://teencanceramerica.org/

  Provides health systems with specialized programs for adolescent and young adult (AYA) cancer patients. Includes stories from AYA cancer patients and survivors, information on their Play It Back music program, general information on cancer and living with cancer, and educational, financial, lifestyle, and support resources.

- Elephants and Tea:

  https://elephantsandtea.com/

  Has materials written for and by the adolescent and young adult (AYA) cancer community. Provides digital issues of the magazine and additional stories by cancer patients going through treatment. Includes information and resources on camps, education, research, advocacy, blogs. Has a weekly online happy hour for AYA cancer patients and survivors. Offers educational and resources information for providers on its program.

- Leukemia & Lymphoma Society:

  https://www.lls.org/

  Funds research, provides education and support, and participates in policy change to cure blood cancers and improve quality of life. Has information on the types of blood cancers and treatment, general information for adolescents and young adults and those recently diagnosed, ways to manage cancer, and educational resources like webcasts, videos, and support resources for peers, caregivers, groups, finances, nutrition, etc. Has free educational resources and video lectures for providers.

- Coalition Against Childhood Cancer:

  https://cac2.org/

  Raises awareness, supports research, and provides support. For families has information on their different support groups, including family and survivorship groups, information on the Hope Portal (database that provides families with resources related to childhood cancer), and a list of scholarships for childhood cancer survivors and patients.

- Momcology:

  https://momcology.org/

  Is a nonprofit that provides peer support to other caregivers of children with cancer. Has information on how to join an online support group, retreats, and in-hospital support groups; provides outside resources, including the Hope Portal and handbooks/guidelines from the Children's Oncology Group.

- American Society of Pediatric Hematology/Oncology:

  https://aspho.org/

  Includes information on their conferences and career development; provides virtual webinars, quizzes, and papers on different topics for hematology/oncology providers. For society members, provides access to the *Pediatric Blood & Cancer Journal*.

- Children's Oncology Group:

  https://childrensoncologygroup.org/

  Is an organization that focuses on pediatric cancer research. Provides information on their member institutions, range of research, and collaborations.

- International Society of Pediatric Oncology:

  https://siop-online.org/

  Aims to improve the quality of life of pediatric cancer patients through education and research. Provides information on their different committees, events, grants/awards, and has general knowledge center and educational materials (journals, webcasts, lectures).

References

Allen, J., Willard, V. W., Klosky, J. L., Li, C., Srivastava, D. K., Robison, L. L., Hudson, M. M., & Phipps, S. (2018). Posttraumatic stress-related psychological functioning in adult survivors of childhood cancer. *Journal of Cancer Survivorship*, *12*(2), 216–223. https://doi.org/10.1007/s11764-017-0660-x

American Cancer Society. (2014). *Special section: Cancer in children & adolescents.* https://www.cancer.org/content/dam/cancer-org/research/cancer-facts-and-statistics/annual-cancer-facts-and-figures/2014/special-section-cancer-in-children-and-adolescents-cancer-facts-and-figures-2014.pdf

American Cancer Society. (2019). *Types of cancer that develop in children.* https://www.cancer.org/cancer/cancer-in-children/types-of-childhood-cancers.html

American Cancer Society. (2021). *Cancer facts & figures, 2021.* https://www.cancer.org/research/cancer-facts-statistics/all-cancer-facts-figures/cancer-facts-figures-2021.html

Aristizabal, P., Winestone, L. E., Umaretiya, P., & Bona, K. (2021). Disparities in pediatric oncology: The 21st century opportunity to improve outcomes for children and adolescents with cancer. *American Society of Clinical Oncology Educational Book*, *41*(41), e315–e326. https://doi.org/10.1200/EDBK_320499

Bakula, D. M., Sharkey, C. M., Perez, M. N., Espeleta, H. C., Gamwell, K. L., Baudino, M., Delozier, A. M., Chaney, J. M., Alderson, M. R., & Mullins, L. L. (2019). The relationship between parent and child distress in pediatric cancer: A meta-analysis. *Journal of Pediatric Psychology*, *44*(10), 1121–1136. https://doi.org/10.1093/jpepsy/jsz051

Barakat, L. P., Alderfer, M. A., & Kazak, A. E. (2006). Posttraumatic growth in adolescent survivors of cancer and their mothers and fathers. *Journal of Pediatric Psychology*, *31*(4), 413–419. https://doi.org/10.1093/jpepsy/jsj058

Barakat, L. P., Pulgaron, E. R., & Daniel, L. C. (2009). Positive psychology in pediatric psychology. In M. C. Roberts & R. G. Steele (Eds.), *Handbook of pediatric psychology* (4th ed., pp. 763–773). Guilford Press.

Barrera, M., Atenafu, E. G., Sung, L., Bartels, U., Schulte, F., Chung, J., Cataudella, D., Hancock, K., Janzen, L., Saleh, A., Strother, D., Downie, A., Zelcer, S., Hukin, J., & McConnell, D. (2018). A randomized control intervention trial to improve social skills and quality of life in pediatric brain tumor survivors. *Psycho-Oncology*, *27*(1), 91–98. https://doi.org/10.1002/pon.4385

Bemis, H., Yarboi, J., Gerhardt, C. A., Vannatta, K., Desjardins, L., Murphy, L. K., Rodriguez, E. M., & Compas, B. E. (2015). Childhood cancer in context: Sociodemographic factors, stress, and psychological distress among mothers and children. *Journal of Pediatric Psychology*, *40*(8), 733–743. https://doi.org/10.1093/jpepsy/jsv024

Bhatia, S. (2011). Disparities in cancer outcomes: Lessons learned from children with cancer. *Pediatric Blood & Cancer*, *56*(6), 994–1002. https://doi.org/10.1002/pbc.23078

Bona, K., Blonquist, T. M., Neuberg, D. S., Silverman, L. B., & Wolfe, J. (2016). Impact of socioeconomic status on timing of relapse and overall survival for children treated on Dana-Farber Cancer Institute ALL consortium protocols (2000–2010). *Pediatric Blood & Cancer*, *63*(6), 1012–1018. https://doi.org/10.1002/pbc.25928

Bornstein, M. H., Scrimin, S., Putnick, D. L., Capello, F., Haynes, O. M., de Falco, S., Carli, M., & Pillon, M. (2012). Neurodevelopmental functioning in very young children undergoing treatment for non-CNS cancers. *Journal of Pediatric Psychology*, *37*(6), 660–673. https://doi.org/10.1093/jpepsy/jss003

Brinkman, T. M., Palmer, S. L., Chen, S., Zhang, H., Evankovich, K., Swain, M. A., Bonner, M. J., Janzen, L., Knight, S., Armstrong, C. L., Boyle, R., & Gajjar, A. (2012). Parent-reported social outcomes after treatment for pediatric embryonal tumors: A prospective longitudinal study. *Journal of Clinical Oncology*, *30*(33), 4134–4140. https://doi.org/10.1200/JCO.2011.40.6702

Brodeur, G. M., Nichols, K. E., Plon, S. E., Schiffman, J. D., & Malkin, D. (2017). Pediatric cancer predisposition and surveillance: An overview, and a tribute to Alfred G. Knudson Jr. *Clinical Cancer Research*, *23*(11), e1–e5. https://doi.org/10.1158/1078-0432.CCR-17-0702

Brown, M. C., Haste, A., Araújo-Soares, V., Skinner, R., & Sharp, L. (2021). Identifying and exploring the self-management strategies used by childhood cancer survivors. *Journal of Cancer Survivorship*, *15*(2), 344–357. https://doi.org/10.1007/s11764-020-00935-2

Bruce, M. (2006). A systematic and conceptual review of posttraumatic stress in childhood cancer survivors and their parents. *Clinical Psychology Review*, *26*(3), 233–256. https://doi.org/10.1016/j.cpr.2005.10.002

Butler, R. W., Copeland, D. R., Fairclough, D. L., Mulhern, R. K., Katz, E. R., Kazak, A. E., Noll, R. B., Patel, S. K., & Sahler, O. J. Z. (2008). A multicenter, randomized clinical trial of a cognitive remediation program for childhood survivors of a pediatric malignancy. *Journal of Consulting and Clinical Psychology*, *76*(3), 367–378. https://doi.org/10.1037/0022-006X.76.3.367

Chen, J., & Mullen, C. A. (2017). Patterns of diagnosis and misdiagnosis in pediatric cancer and relationship to survival. *Journal of Pediatric Hematology/Oncology, 39*(3), e110–e115. https://doi.org/10.1097/MPH.0000000000000688

Collins, D. E., Ellis, S. J., Janin, M. M., Wakefield, C. E., Bussey, K., Cohn, R. J., Lah, S., & Fardell, J. E. (2019). A systematic review summarizing the state of evidence on bullying in childhood cancer patients/survivors. *Journal of Pediatric Oncology Nursing, 36*(1), 55–68. https://doi.org/10.1177/1043454218810136

Compas, B. E., Bemis, H., Gerhardt, C. A., Dunn, M. J., Rodriguez, E. M., Desjardins, L., Preacher, K. J., Manring, S., & Vannatta, K. (2015). Mothers and fathers coping with their children's cancer: Individual and interpersonal processes. *Health Psychology, 34*(8), 783–793. https://doi.org/10.1037/hea0000202

Compas, B. E., Desjardins, L., Vannatta, K., Young-Saleme, T., Rodriguez, E. M., Dunn, M., Bemis, H., Snyder, S., & Gerhardt, C. A. (2014). Children and adolescents coping with cancer: Self- and parent reports of coping and anxiety/depression. *Health Psychology, 33*(8), 853–861. https://doi.org/10.1037/hea0000083

Curtin, S. C., Minino, A. M., & Anderson, R. N. (2016). Declines in cancer death rates among children and adolescents in the United States, 1999–2014. *NCHS Data Brief*, (257), 1–8.

Dang-Tan, T., & Franco, E. L. (2007). Diagnosis delays in childhood cancer. *Cancer, 110*(4), 703–713. https://doi.org/10.1002/cncr.22849

Dixon, S. B., Bjornard, K. L., Alberts, N. M., Armstrong, G. T., Brinkman, T. M., Chemaitilly, W., Ehrhardt, M. J., Fernandez-Pineda, I., Force, L. M., Gibson, T. M., Green, D. M., Howell, C. R., Kaste, S. C., Kirchhoff, A. C., Klosky, J. L., Krull, K. R., Lucas, J. T., Jr., Mulrooney, D. A., Ness, K. K., . . . Hudson, M. M. (2018). Factors influencing risk-based care of the childhood cancer survivor in the 21st century. *CA: A Cancer Journal for Clinicians, 68*(2), 133–152. https://doi.org/10.3322/caac.21445

Eiser, C. (1998). Practitioner review: Long-term consequences of childhood cancer. *Journal of Child Psychology and Psychiatry, 39*(5), 621–633. https://doi.org/10.1111/1469-7610.00362

Eiser, C., & Vance, Y. H. (2002). Implications of cancer for school attendance and behavior. *Medical and Pediatric Oncology, 38*(5), 317–319. https://doi.org/10.1002/mpo.1341

Fedele, D. A., Hullmann, S. E., Chaffin, M., Kenner, C., Fisher, M. J., Kirk, K., Eddington, A. R., Phipps, S., McNall-Knapp, R. Y., & Mullins, L. L. (2013). Impact of a parent-based interdisciplinary intervention for mothers on adjustment in children newly diagnosed with cancer. *Journal of Pediatric Psychology, 38*(5), 531–540. https://doi.org/10.1093/jpepsy/jst010

Gardner, M. H., Mrug, S., Schwebel, D. C., Phipps, S., Whelan, K., & Madan-Swain, A. (2017). Demographic, medical, and psychosocial predictors of benefit finding among caregivers of childhood cancer survivors. *Psycho-Oncology, 26*(1), 125–132. https://doi.org/10.1002/pon.4014

Gerhardt, C. A., Dixon, M., Miller, K., Vannatta, K., Valerius, K. S., Correll, J., & Noll, R. B. (2007). Educational and occupational outcomes among survivors of childhood cancer during the transition to emerging adulthood. *Journal of Developmental and Behavioral Pediatrics, 28*(6), 448–455. https://doi.org/10.1097/DBP.0b013e31811ff8e1

Hockenberry-Eaton, M., Manteuffel, B., & Bottomley, S. (1997). Development of two instruments examining stress and adjustment in children with cancer. *Journal of Pediatric Oncology Nursing, 14*(3), 178–185. https://doi.org/10.1016/S1043-4542(97)90054-0

Hocking, M. C., Noll, R. B., Kazak, A. E., Brodsky, C., Phillips, P., & Barakat, L. P. (2020). Friendships in pediatric brain tumor survivors and non-central nervous system tumor survivors. *Journal of Pediatric Psychology, 45*(2), 194–202. https://doi.org/10.1093/jpepsy/jsz101

Hocking, M. C., Paltin, I., Belasco, C., & Barakat, L. P. (2018). Parent perspectives on the educational barriers and unmet needs of children with cancer. *Children's Health Care, 47*(3), 261–274. https://doi.org/10.1080/02739615.2017.1337516

Hullmann, S. E., Fedele, D. A., Molzon, E. S., Mayes, S., & Mullins, L. L. (2014). Posttraumatic growth and hope in parents of children with cancer. *Journal of Psychosocial Oncology, 32*(6), 696–707. https://doi.org/10.1080/07347332.2014.955241

Kazak, A. E., Alderfer, M., Rourke, M. T., Simms, S., Streisand, R., & Grossman, J. R. (2004). Posttraumatic stress disorder (PTSD) and posttraumatic stress symptoms (PTSS) in families of adolescent childhood cancer survivors. *Journal of Pediatric Psychology, 29*(3), 211–219. https://doi.org/10.1093/jpepsy/jsh022

Kazak, A. E., Derosa, B. W., Schwartz, L. A., Hobbie, W., Carlson, C., Ittenbach, R. F., Mao, J. J., & Ginsberg, J. P. (2010). Psychological outcomes and health beliefs in adolescent and young adult survivors of childhood cancer and controls. *Journal of Clinical Oncology, 28*(12), 2002–2007. https://doi.org/10.1200/JCO.2009.25.9564

Kazak, A. E., Schneider, S., Didonato, S., & Pai, A. L. (2015). Family psychosocial risk screening guided by the pediatric psychosocial preventative health model (PPPHM) using the Psychosocial Assessment Tool (PAT). *Acta Oncologica, 54*(5), 574–580. https://doi.org/10.3109/0284186X.2014.995774

Kearney, J. A., Salley, C. G., & Muriel, A. C. (2015). Standards of psychosocial care for parents of children with cancer. *Pediatric Blood & Cancer, 62*(S5), S632–683. https://doi.org/10.1002/pbc.25761

Kehm, R. D., Spector, L. G., Poynter, J. N., Vock, D. M., Altekruse, S. F., & Osypuk, T. L. (2018). Does socioeconomic status account for racial and ethnic disparities in childhood cancer survival? *Cancer, 124*(20), 4090–4097. https://doi.org/10.1002/cncr.31560

Krull, K. R., Hardy, K. K., Kahalley, L. S., Schuitema, I., & Kesler, S. R. (2018). Neurocognitive outcomes and interventions in long-term survivors of childhood cancer. *Journal of Clinical Oncology, 36*(21), 2181–2189. https://doi.org/10.1200/JCO.2017.76.4696

Kwak, M., Zebrack, B. J., Meeske, K. A., Embry, L., Aguilar, C., Block, R., Hayes-Lattin, B., Li, Y., Butler, M., & Cole, S. (2013). Trajectories of psychological distress in adolescent and young adult patients with cancer: A 1-year longitudinal study. *Journal of Clinical Oncology, 31*(17), 2160–2166. https://doi.org/10.1200/JCO.2012.45.9222

Langeveld, N. E., Grootenhuis, M. A., Voûte, P. A., & de Haan, R. J. (2004). Posttraumatic stress symptoms in adult survivors of childhood cancer. *Pediatric Blood & Cancer, 42*(7), 604–610. https://doi.org/10.1002/pbc.20024

Lorig, K. R., & Holman, H. (2003). Self-management education: History, definition, outcomes, and mechanisms. *Annals of Behavioral Medicine, 26*(1), 1–7. https://doi.org/10.1207/S15324796ABM2601_01

Maunsell, E., Pogany, L., Barrera, M., Shaw, A. K., & Speechley, K. N. (2006). Quality of life among long-term adolescent and adult survivors of childhood cancer. *Journal of Clinical Oncology, 24*(16), 2527–2535. https://doi.org/10.1200/JCO.2005.03.9297

McGrady, M. E., & Hommel, K. A. (2016). Targeting health behaviors to reduce health care costs in pediatric psychology: Descriptive review and recommendations. *Journal of Pediatric Psychology, 41*(8), 835–848. https://doi.org/10.1093/jpepsy/jsv083

Miller, K. D., Fidler-Benaoudia, M., Keegan, T. H., Hipp, H. S., Jemal, A., & Siegel, R. L. (2020). Cancer statistics for adolescents and young adults, 2020. *CA: A Cancer Journal for Clinicians, 70*(6), 443–459. https://doi.org/10.3322/caac.21637

Mobley, E. M., Moke, D. J., Milam, J., Ochoa, C. Y., Stal, J., Osazuwa, N., Bolshakova, M., Kemp, J., Dinalo, J. E., Motala, A., Baluyot, D., & Hempel, S. (2021). *Disparities and barriers to pediatric cancer survivorship care* [Technical Brief No. 39]. Agency for Health Care Research and Quality. https://doi.org/10.23970/AHRQEPCTB39

Moyer, K. H., Willard, V. W., Gross, A. M., Netson, K. L., Ashford, J. M., Kahalley, L. S., Wu, S., Xiong, X., & Conklin, H. M. (2012). The impact of attention on social functioning in survivors of pediatric acute lymphoblastic leukemia and brain tumors. *Pediatric Blood & Cancer, 59*(7), 1290–1295. https://doi.org/10.1002/pbc.24256

Nathan, P. C., Greenberg, M. L., Ness, K. K., Hudson, M. M., Mertens, A. C., Mahoney, M. C., Gurney, J. G., Donaldson, S. S., Leisenring, W. M., Robison, L. L., & Oeffinger, K. C. (2008). Medical care in long-term survivors of childhood cancer: A report from the childhood cancer survivor study. *Journal of Clinical Oncology, 26*(27), 4401–4409. https://doi.org/10.1200/JCO.2008.16.9607

Norberg, A. L., & Boman, K. K. (2008). Parent distress in childhood cancer: A comparative evaluation of posttraumatic stress symptoms, depression and anxiety. *Acta Oncologica, 47*(2), 267–274. https://doi.org/10.1080/02841860701558773

O'Leary, T. E., Diller, L., & Recklitis, C. J. (2007). The effects of response bias on self-reported quality of life among childhood cancer survivors. *Quality of Life Research, 16*(7), 1211–1220. https://doi.org/10.1007/s11136-007-9231-3

Oeffinger, K. C., Mertens, A. C., Sklar, C. A., Kawashima, T., Hudson, M. M., Meadows, A. T., Friedman, D. L., Marina, N., Hobbie, W., Kadan-Lottick, N. S., Schwartz, C. L., Leisenring, W., Robison, L. L., & the Childhood Cancer Survivor Study. (2006). Chronic health conditions in adult survivors of childhood cancer. *The New England Journal of Medicine, 355*(15), 1572–1582. https://doi.org/10.1056/NEJMsa060185

Pahl, D. A., Wieder, M. S., & Steinberg, D. M. (2021). Social isolation and connection in adolescents with cancer and survivors of childhood cancer: A systematic review. *Journal of Adolescence, 87*(1), 15–27. https://doi.org/10.1016/j.adolescence.2020.12.010

Pai, A. L., Greenley, R. N., Lewandowski, A., Drotar, D., Youngstrom, E., & Peterson, C. C. (2007). A meta-analytic review of the influence of pediatric cancer on parent and family functioning. *Journal of Family Psychology, 21*(3), 407–415. https://doi.org/10.1037/0893-3200.21.3.407

Pai, A. L., & McGrady, M. E. (2015). Assessing medication adherence as a standard of care in pediatric oncology. *Pediatric Blood & Cancer, 62*(S5), S818–S828. https://doi.org/10.1002/pbc.25795

Paltin, I., Burgers, D. E., Gragert, M., & Noggle, C. (2018). Cancer. In J. Donders & S. J. Hunter (Eds.), *Neuropsychological conditions across the lifespan* (pp. 162–185). Cambridge University Press. https://doi.org/10.1017/9781316996751.010

Paltin, I., Schofield, H.-L., & Baran, J. (2018). Rehabilitation and pediatric oncology: Supporting patients and families during and after treatment. *Current Physical Medicine and Rehabilitation Reports*, 6(2), 107–114. https://doi.org/10.1007/s40141-018-0181-1

Phillips, N. S., Duke, E. S., Schofield, H. T., & Ullrich, N. J. (2021). Neurotoxic effects of childhood cancer therapy and its potential neurocognitive impact. *Journal of Clinical Oncology*, 39(16), 1752–1765. https://doi.org/10.1200/JCO.20.02533

Phillips, S. M., Padgett, L. S., Leisenring, W. M., Stratton, K. K., Bishop, K., Krull, K. R., Alfano, C. M., Gibson, T. M., de Moor, J. S., Hartigan, D. B., Armstrong, G. T., Robison, L. L., Rowland, J. H., Oeffinger, K. C., & Mariotto, A. B. (2015). Survivors of childhood cancer in the United States: Prevalence and burden of morbidity. *Cancer Epidemiology, Biomarkers & Prevention*, 24(4), 653–663. https://doi.org/10.1158/1055-9965.EPI-14-1418

Phipps, S., Long, A., Willard, V. W., Okado, Y., Hudson, M., Huang, Q., Zhang, H., & Noll, R. (2015). Parents of children with cancer: At-risk or resilient? *Journal of Pediatric Psychology*, 40(9), 914–925. https://doi.org/10.1093/jpepsy/jsv047

Psihogios, A. M., Fellmeth, H., Schwartz, L. A., & Barakat, L. P. (2019). Family functioning and medical adherence across children and adolescents with chronic health conditions: A meta-analysis. *Journal of Pediatric Psychology*, 44(1), 84–97. https://doi.org/10.1093/jpepsy/jsy044

Recklitis, C. J., Lockwood, R. A., Rothwell, M. A., & Diller, L. R. (2006). Suicidal ideation and attempts in adult survivors of childhood cancer. *Journal of Clinical Oncology*, 24(24), 3852–3857. https://doi.org/10.1200/JCO.2006.06.5409

Robinson, K. E., Gerhardt, C. A., Vannatta, K., & Noll, R. B. (2007). Parent and family factors associated with child adjustment to pediatric cancer. *Journal of Pediatric Psychology*, 32(4), 400–410. https://doi.org/10.1093/jpepsy/jsl038

Robinson, K. E., Kuttesch, J. F., Champion, J. E., Andreotti, C. F., Hipp, D. W., Bettis, A., Barnwell, A., & Compas, B. E. (2010). A quantitative meta-analysis of neurocognitive sequelae in survivors of pediatric brain tumors. *Pediatric Blood & Cancer*, 55(3), 525–531. https://doi.org/10.1002/pbc.22568

Salamon, K. S., Schwartz, L. A., & Barakat, L. P. (2016). Resilience in pediatric sickle cell disease and cancer: Social ecology indicators of health-related quality of life. In C. DeMichelis & M. Ferrari (Eds.), *Child and adolescent resilience within medical contexts: Integrating research and practice M.* (pp. 77–101). Springer. https://doi.org/10.1007/978-3-319-32223-0_5

Schwartz, L. A., Brumley, L. D., Tuchman, L. K., Barakat, L. P., Hobbie, W. L., Ginsberg, J. P., Daniel, L. C., Kazak, A. E., Bevans, K., & Deatrick, J. A. (2013). Stakeholder validation of a model of readiness for transition to adult care. *JAMA Pediatrics*, 167(10), 939–946. https://doi.org/10.1001/jamapediatrics.2013.2223

Schwartz, L. A., Wakefield, C., McCloone, J., DeRosa, B., & Kazak, A. E. (2020). Adult survivors of childhood cancer. In W. Breitbart, P. Butow, P. Jacobsen, W. Lam, M. Lazenby, & M. Loscalzo (Eds.), *Psycho-oncology* (4th ed., pp. 767–772). Oxford University Press. https://doi.org/10.1093/med/9780190097653.003.0096

Signorelli, C., Wakefield, C. E., Fardell, J. E., Wallace, W. H. B., Robertson, E. G., McLoone, J. K., & Cohn, R. J. (2017). The impact of long-term follow-up care for childhood cancer survivors: A systematic review. *Critical Reviews in Oncology/Hematology*, 114, 131–138. https://doi.org/10.1016/j.critrevonc.2017.04.007

Sultan, S., Leclair, T., Rondeau, É., Burns, W., & Abate, C. (2016). A systematic review on factors and consequences of parental distress as related to childhood cancer. *European Journal of Cancer Care*, 25(4), 616–637. https://doi.org/10.1111/ecc.12361

Szalda, D., Pierce, L., Hobbie, W., Ginsberg, J. P., Brumley, L., Wasik, M., Li, Y., & Schwartz, L. A. (2016). Engagement and experience with cancer-related follow-up care among young adult survivors of childhood cancer after transfer to adult care. *Journal of Cancer Survivorship*, 10(2), 342–350. https://doi.org/10.1007/s11764-015-0480-9

Tutelman, P. R., Chambers, C. T., Stinson, J. N., Parker, J. A., Fernandez, C. V., Witteman, H. O., Nathan, P. C., Barwick, M., Campbell, F., Jibb, L. A., & Irwin, K. (2018). Pain in children with cancer: Prevalence, characteristics, and parent management. *The Clinical Journal of Pain*, 34(3), 198–206. https://doi.org/10.1097/AJP.0000000000000531

van Erp, L. M. E., Maurice-Stam, H., Kremer, L. C. M., Tissing, W. J. E., van der Pal, H. J. H., de Vries, A. C. H., van den Heuvel-Eibrink, M. M., Versluys, B. A. B., van der Heiden-van der Loo, M., Huizinga, G. A., & Grootenhuis, M. A. (2021). A vulnerable age group: The impact of cancer on the psychosocial well-being of young adult childhood cancer survivors. *Supportive Care in Cancer*, 29(8), 4751–4761. https://doi.org/10.1007/s00520-021-06009-y

Van Schoors, M., Caes, L., Verhofstadt, L. L., Goubert, L., & Alderfer, M. A. (2015). Systematic review: Family resilience after pediatric cancer diagnosis. *Journal of Pediatric Psychology, 40*(9), 856–868. https://doi.org/10.1093/jpepsy/jsv055

van Warmerdam, J., Zabih, V., Kurdyak, P., Sutradhar, R., Nathan, P. C., & Gupta, S. (2019). Prevalence of anxiety, depression, and posttraumatic stress disorder in parents of children with cancer: A meta-analysis. *Pediatric Blood & Cancer, 66*(6), 1–8. https://doi.org/10.1002/pbc.27677

Vani, M. F., Lucibello, K. M., Trinh, L., Santa Mina, D., & Sabiston, C. M. (2021). Body image among adolescents and young adults diagnosed with cancer: A scoping review. *Psycho-Oncology, 30*(8), 1278–1293. https://doi.org/10.1002/pon.5698

Vannatta, K., & Salley, C. G. (2017). Pediatric cancer. In M. C. Roberts & R. G. Steele (Eds.), *Handbook of pediatric psychology* (5th ed., pp. 284–297). Guilford Press.

Wallace, M. L., Harcourt, D., Rumsey, N., & Foot, A. (2007). Managing appearance changes resulting from cancer treatment: Resilience in adolescent females. *Psycho-Oncology, 16*(11), 1019–1027. https://doi.org/10.1002/pon.1176

Ward, E., DeSantis, C., Robbins, A., Kohler, B., & Jemal, A. (2014). Childhood and adolescent cancer statistics, 2014. *CA: A Cancer Journal for Clinicians, 64*(2), 83–103. https://doi.org/10.3322/caac.21219

Wiener, L., Devine, K. A., & Thompson, A. L. (2020). Advances in pediatric psychooncology. *Current Opinion in Pediatrics, 32*(1), 41–47. https://doi.org/10.1097/MOP.0000000000000851

Wiener, L., Kazak, A. E., Noll, R. B., Patenaude, A. F., & Kupst, M. J. (2015). Standards for the psychosocial care of children with cancer and their families: An introduction to the special issue. *Pediatric Blood & Cancer, 62*(Suppl. 5), S419–S424. https://doi.org/10.1002/pbc.25675

Willard, V. W., Gordon, M. L., Means, B., Brennan, R. C., Conklin, H. M., Merchant, T. E., Vinitsky, A., & Harman, J. L. (2021). Social-emotional functioning in preschool-aged children with cancer: Comparisons between children with brain and non-CNS solid tumors. *Journal of Pediatric Psychology, 46*(7), 790–800. https://doi.org/10.1093/jpepsy/jsab018

Willard, V. W., Hostetter, S. A., Hutchinson, K. C., Bonner, M. J., & Hardy, K. K. (2016). Benefit finding in maternal caregivers of pediatric cancer survivors: A mixed methods approach. *Journal of Pediatric Oncology Nursing, 33*(5), 353–360. https://doi.org/10.1177/1043454215620119

Williamson, H., Harcourt, D., Halliwell, E., Frith, H., & Wallace, M. (2010). Adolescents' and parents' experiences of managing the psychosocial impact of appearance change during cancer treatment. *Journal of Pediatric Oncology Nursing, 27*(3), 168–175. https://doi.org/10.1177/1043454209357923

Winterling, J., Jervaeus, A., Af Sandeberg, M., Johansson, E., & Wettergren, L. (2015). Perceptions of school among childhood cancer survivors: A comparison with peers. *Journal of Pediatric Oncology Nursing, 32*(4), 201–208. https://doi.org/10.1177/1043454214563405

Zebrack, B., & Butler, M. (2012). Context for understanding psychosocial outcomes and behavior among adolescents and young adults with cancer. *JNCCN: Journal of the National Comprehensive Cancer Network, 10*(9), 1151–1156. https://doi.org/10.6004/jnccn.2012.0118

Zebrack, B. J., Stuber, M. L., Meeske, K. A., Phipps, S., Krull, K. R., Liu, Q., Yasui, Y., Parry, C., Hamilton, R., Robison, L. L., & Zeltzer, L. K. (2012). Perceived positive impact of cancer among long-term survivors of childhood cancer: A report from the childhood cancer survivor study. *Psycho-Oncology, 21*(6), 630–639. https://doi.org/10.1002/pon.1959

CHAPTER 12

PULMONARY DISORDERS: ASTHMA AND CYSTIC FIBROSIS, CONSIDERATIONS FOR CHILD HEALTH AND WELL-BEING

Emily F. Muther, Courtney Lynn, Emily Skeen, and Monica Federico

Pediatric pulmonary illness impacts children across all areas of functioning and across each stage of development. Two of the most common pulmonary conditions affecting children include asthma (i.e., reactive airway disease) and cystic fibrosis (CF). Although the pathophysiology of the two conditions are notably different, children with these conditions are at greater risk of ongoing medical and psychosocial sequelae that can occur throughout the developmental spectrum. Medical, psychosocial, and neurodevelopmental outcomes for children living with chronic pulmonary conditions such as asthma and CF are directly related to multilevel ecological contexts and are influenced by biological, cultural, psychological, social, and behavioral factors. For example, while the risk for asthma or CF may be related to individual biological factors (including genetic and autoimmune factors), the expression and severity of disease and associated disease-related adverse outcomes can vary due to multiple factors, including conditions in the proximal living environment, access to subspecialty medical care, race/ethnicity, social-societal determinants of health, and socioeconomic-related health inequities. Conversely, more positive outcomes, including adaptation to living with a chronic pulmonary condition, and factors associated with resilience include well-described multilevel protective factors

such as health-related quality of life (HRQoL), the presence of family and peer social support, level of family functioning, and mental and behavioral health (see Volume 1, Chapters 13 and 15, this handbook). To foster adaptive outcomes—including better adherence to treatment recommendations, more optimal management of disease symptoms, and academic and psychological resilience in children with chronic pulmonary conditions—an integrated, multidisciplinary approach is required. Critically, optimizing child health and well-being for children with asthma and/or CF requires an eco-biopsychosocial approach, informed by developmental science, and implemented by pediatric psychologists and developmental-behavioral pediatricians who are tasked with helping children with pulmonary conditions thrive across settings.

This chapter will focus on the current state of medical care and management of pediatric asthma and CF using an integrated, multidisciplinary approach bridging the fields of developmental science, pediatric psychology, and developmental-behavioral pediatrics. An overview discusses the significance of these conditions, including epidemiology and pathophysiology; the role of social determinants of health on outcomes; the clinical diagnosis of asthma and outcomes associated with asthma and CF across the childhood

https://doi.org/10.1037/0000414-012
APA Handbook of Pediatric Psychology, Developmental-Behavioral Pediatrics, and Developmental Science: Vol. 2. Pediatric Psychology and Developmental-Behavioral Pediatrics: Clinical Applications of Developmental Science, P. E. Shah and M. H. Bornstein (Editors-in-Chief)
Copyright © 2025 by the American Psychological Association. All rights reserved.

lifespan including adherence, academic outcomes, and mental well-being; and the multilevel factors associated with resilience and optimal adaptation. The chapter concludes with future directions to promote resilience, the implications of social, cultural, and psychosocial factors on coping and daily symptom management, and the role of developmental-behavioral pediatrics and pediatric psychology in the care and management of children with asthma and CF to optimize outcomes across the childhood lifespan.

BACKGROUND AND SIGNIFICANCE

While there are similarities in the management of illness, complexities of treatment, and biopsychosocial impact of both asthma and CF, important differences exist. The significance of both of these diagnoses are discussed in detail.

Asthma

The global prevalence, morbidity, and mortality related to childhood asthma has increased significantly over the last 40 years (Serebrisky & Wiznia, 2019). Asthma is the most common chronic condition in children under the age of 18 in the United States and is the leading cause of childhood hospitalizations globally, especially in low-and middle-income countries (Asher & Pearce, 2014; Bellin et al., 2017; Ferrante & La Grutta, 2018). Despite this recognition, there remain issues of underdiagnosis and undertreatment worldwide. The World Health Organization has estimated that approximately 300 million people across the globe currently have asthma; current trends are rising, and it is estimated to reach 400 million by 2025 (Masoli et al., 2004; Serebrisky & Wiznia, 2019).

Asthma is a chronic airway disease characterized by intermittent and recurrent reversible obstruction of air flow, bronchial hyperreactivity (defined as the tendency of the bronchi to narrow in response to specific triggers), and airway inflammation (National Heart, Lung, & Blood Institute, 2007). For individuals with asthma, chronic inflammation of the airways leads to recurrent episodes of wheezing, chest tightness, and coughing. In children with asthma, there is a wide spectrum of clinical symptoms ranging from intermittent to persistent daily symptoms and life-threatening disease (Kuruvilla et al., 2019). The key components of the asthma diagnosis are that these symptoms are chronic (recurrent), at least partially respond to a bronchodilator, and often have specific triggers. There is no reference standard for the diagnosis of asthma (Papi et al., 2018). As such, the diagnosis is made clinically by considering symptoms, response to therapy, and, if available, an objective assessment of expiratory airflow limitation that is at least partially reversible. Airflow obstruction is measured using pulmonary function testing (PFTs), which can be performed in the outpatient setting in children over 7 years old. Although PFTs can be used to confirm the diagnosis, a negative test does not rule out the diagnosis (Gershon et al., 2012; National Institutes of Health, 1991). Thus, although common, living with asthma can place children at greater risk of ongoing medical and psychosocial conditions. This increased risk on the physical health, family, social, cultural, emotional, and ecological contexts is an overarching theme and specifics for both asthma and CF will be highlighted throughout this chapter.

Cystic Fibrosis

CF is the most common rare genetic disorder, with a prevalence of 1 in 3,000 in North America and 1 in 25 individuals carrying the CF gene worldwide (O'Sullivan & Freedman, 2009). It is estimated to affect 70,000–90,000 people worldwide (Montemayor & Jain, 2022). CF is an autosomal recessive disease caused by mutations in the CF transmembrane conductance regulator (CFTR) gene, which regulates movement of chloride, sodium, and bicarbonate across epithelial cell membranes (Montemayor & Jain, 2022). This genetic mutation creates a negative impact on many systems in the body, including chronic lung infections, gastrointestinal abnormalities that create malabsorption and difficulty growing and maintaining weight, impairment of sexual health and reproduction that require lifelong treatments and result in a shortened life expectancy

(Cogen & Ramsey, 2020). Numerous additional developmental and psychosocial comorbidities exist such as behavioral issues with feeding and increased rates of anxiety and depression for children and their caregivers. Based on data from the Cystic Fibrosis Foundation's 2020 *Patient Registry Annual Data Report*, the predicted median age of survival for a child born in the United States with CF is now 59 years of age (Cystic Fibrosis Foundation, 2021). Data from the registries of the United Kingdom, Canada, Belgium, Europe, Australia, France, and Ireland show a range of median survival age from 44 to 53 years (Scotet et al., 2020). This increase in life expectancy over the past several decades has been one of the greatest triumphs in modern medicine and is a result of the development of new pharmaceuticals and therapies (McBennett et al., 2022).

Prevalence and Public Health Impacts

While the prevalence of asthma and CF varies widely, the social, financial, and cultural impacts of both diseases greatly affect children and families of diverse backgrounds.

Asthma. Asthma is a significant health concern worldwide. Approximately 8% of the U.S. population has a current diagnosis of asthma (Pate et al., 2021), and 10% of children in Europe carry the diagnosis (Cope et al., 2008). Although mortality from asthma is low, morbidity is high—particularly in children (Pate et al., 2021). Asthma accounts for nearly half of pediatric emergency department (ED) visits and a third of admissions (Johnson et al., 2018; Lee et al., 2020). Asthma is also one of the top causes of missed school days for children ages 5–17, and poorly controlled asthma may impair a child's academic performance (Centers for Disease Control and Prevention, 2015). This results in a significant impact on families, with missed work for caregivers and the high medical costs of ED visits and hospitalizations. Additionally, medical providers, in particular developmental-behavioral pediatricians, must consider whether family functioning and a child's academic functioning, is associated with a chronic illness such as asthma.

When children with a chronic illness are seen by primary or specialty health care providers with impairment in academic, social, or emotional functioning, how well controlled the child's symptoms are should be monitored and considered as a primary factor in any functional impairment that might exist. Yaghoubi et al. (2019) reported that the direct and indirect costs of poorly controlled asthma will be more than 48 billion dollars per year over the next 20 years. Additionally, the symptoms of asthma can lead to exercise or play avoidance and can therefore contribute to obesity (Lu et al., 2016). Fortunately, for most patients with asthma, evidence shows that symptoms and exacerbations can be effectively controlled with treatment, but this can itself be challenging and adherence with therapy is often poor (Gray et al., 2018).

Cystic fibrosis. Although CF has long been considered most prevalent in individuals of White, European descent, evidence over the last decade has shown the disease is present in all parts of the world, including the Middle East, Asia, Latin America, and Africa (Guo et al., 2022). A public health impact of this historical preconception that CF is a disease most prevalent among people of Northern European descent is that the establishment of national and/or international CF patient registries, which allow for the epidemiological study of CF across populations, has only occurred in fully developed and higher income countries (Jackson & Goss, 2018). This exclusion of individuals with CF from non-Western countries should be a focus of great importance to ensure representation in research and clinical outcomes. As a result, little is known about the epidemiology of CF in low- and middle-income countries, and while estimates are around 90,000 individuals worldwide with the disease, this is likely an underestimate given the number of patients living in regions without established registries (Bell et al., 2020; Scotet et al., 2020).

In the United States, the Hispanic/Latino population makes up 9.6% of people living with CF, whereas African Americans account for 4.7%, and other ethnic minority populations continue to grow in identification (Cystic Fibrosis Foundation, 2021). A notable disparity is in the racial inequity of the diagnosis of CF. Unfortunately, individuals from these communities are often diagnosed late and tend to have worse overall outcomes than non-Hispanic White people (Hamosh et al., 1998; Pique et al., 2017; Rho et al., 2018; Watts et al., 2012) due to the lack of identification of the disease across all racial and ethnic populations. One of the greatest worldwide public health efforts in recent years has been the commitment to making sure a high proportion of the population in underrepresented countries is captured within a registry, which minimizes the likelihood of ascertainment bias and allows accurate and equitable conclusions to be drawn (Bell et al., 2020). More accurate patient registries also directly contribute to better access to diagnostic procedures and more accurate diagnosis, clinical care, and therapeutic options to treat and manage symptoms.

Pathophysiology of Asthma and Cystic Fibrosis

Treatments and management of asthma and CF are geared towards the changes in the body that occur as a result of the disease processes. The consequences of both extend beyond the lungs and can affect many systems in the body.

Asthma. *Asthma* is a chronic inflammatory disorder of the airways. This inflammation leads to airway hyperresponsiveness and airflow limitation. It is a disease exclusive to the respiratory system; however, comorbid conditions such as obesity, allergic rhinosinusitis, and obstructive sleep apnea can exacerbate asthma symptoms (Papi et al., 2018). The etiology of asthma is multifactorial, and consists of genetic, environmental, and sociodemographic factors. There is no single genetic cause of asthma as in cystic fibrosis; however, there is heritability among families and differences in genes controlling immune function have been identified (Papi et al., 2018). *Atopy*, which is often thought of as a term that refers to clusters of allergic conditions such as hay fever, asthma, and eczema, is the strongest identifiable predisposing factor for developing asthma, and at least 80% of children with asthma have an allergic predisposition (National Heart, Lung, & Blood Institute, 2007; Pearce et al., 1999).

Cystic fibrosis. As described previously, CF is caused by genetic mutations in the CFTR protein. These CFTR dysfunctions lead to dehydration on the surface of the epithelial cells in tissues and organs throughout the body. In the airways, CFTR dysfunction leads to increased secretions, impaired mucociliary clearance, chronic respiratory infections, and progressive airflow obstruction that commonly results in early mortality (Montemayor & Jain, 2022). Other common manifestations include pancreatic insufficiency from blocked pancreatic ducts, intestinal obstruction from dehydrated stool, and infertility in males due to ciliary dyskinesia and negative impact on the vas deferens in utero.

SOCIAL DETERMINANTS OF HEALTH, CULTURAL IMPLICATIONS, AND HEALTH EQUITY

Inequities and cultural implications exist in the diagnosis and treatment of both asthma and CF. As treatments and outcomes improve, sociocultural differences must be addressed.

Ecological Factors Associated With Disease Severity—Considerations From Developmental Science

Asthma. As a multifactorial disease, asthma is influenced by biological, social, and environmental exposures throughout the life course. There is strong evidence to link both the development and severity of asthma to structural and social determinants of health (described later in further detail; Almqvist et al., 2005; Sullivan & Thakur, 2020; Thakur et al., 2013). These factors include intermediary determinants of health, such as housing, that exist between the patient and the upstream structural determinants of health, like housing policies in the United States or reduced access to housing in developing countries (Sullivan & Thakur, 2020). These structural determinants lead to social stratification and inequities in the development and progression of asthma. Across the world, asthma rates reflect global health disparities. It disproportionately impacts marginalized communities including those with low socioeconomic status (SES) and communities of color (Sloand et al., 2021), who also experience higher asthma-related morbidity and mortality (Akinbami et al., 2012; Vangeepuram et al., 2012; see also Volume 1, Chapter 18, this handbook). Race/ethnicity and access to housing have consistently proven to be a profound driver of asthma disparities, with cumulative risk from many overlapping social determinants. For example, not only is access to housing associated with disease severity, but the housing conditions are of extreme importance. This connection offers a critical opportunity for interdisciplinary collaboration between pediatric psychologists, developmental-behavioral pediatricians, and medical-legal partnerships (MLPs) to address these factors. For example, collaborations between developmental-behavioral pediatrics and MLP can lead to housing remediation or relocation (Beck et al., 2012; Mainardi et al., 2023; Sullivan & Thakur, 2020), which can help address the environmental conditions contributing to the pathogenesis of asthma.

Socioeconomic risk factors associated with asthma are also well documented. Asthma prevalence is disproportionately high among children from low-income backgrounds, including children who live in inner-city neighborhoods, experience poor air quality, indoor allergens, and a lack of education (Halfon & Newacheck, 1993). Furthermore, the impact of socioeconomic factors on the health of children with asthma extends beyond just the effects of income. It also includes factors related to social structure, family characteristics, and the access to and use of health resources (Cope et al., 2008). As with any chronic disease, emotional health, psychological functioning, and development can serve as a risk factor for outcomes associated with asthma. A variety of psychological factors can play a role in asthma management and coping. Children with asthma have been shown to be at increased risk of behavioral and emotional problems, particularly experiencing higher risk for internalizing problems such as anxiety and depression, which can impact adherence, quality of life, and disease severity and progression (McQuaid et al., 2001). While both psychological and socioeconomic risk factors are clearly present, there are also protective factors, such as social support and embedded wraparound services within the communities where those most at risk live, that can reduce the extent of impact.

Cystic fibrosis. Although CF is a heritable genetic disease, SES is an important predictor of health outcomes and has been shown to result in a three times higher likelihood of mortality for those from a lower SES background (Schechter et al., 2001). Children with CF tend to have difficulty with growth and maintaining nutritional status resulting from the impact of the disease on the digestive system and the pancreas. As such, one of the longstanding predictors of positive health outcomes in CF is weight gain, with a well-monitored goal of a BMI around the 50th percentile throughout childhood and into adulthood. Children with CF on Medicaid have been reported to have lower lung function, lower body mass index (BMI), and more frequent hospitalizations and pulmonary exacerbations compared to those who are not on Medicaid (Schechter et al., 2001). As is the case with asthma, income is not thought to be the primary driver in the discrepancies in health status, but rather the relationship to reduced access to early interventions and treatments, poorer environmental factors, and the impact of stress on physical health—a clear social determinant of health outcome for those with CF.

Social Determinants of Health and Health Equity

According to the World Health Organization, *social determinants of health* are the nonmedical factors such as conditions in which people are born, grow up, live, work, and age, that influence health outcomes. As such, social determinants of health have an important influence on health inequities (World Health Organization, n.d.) in both asthma and CF. Structural racism is the "totality of ways in which society fosters discrimination by creating and reinforcing inequitable systems through intentional policies and practices sanctioned by various levels of government and institutions" (Martinez et al., 2021, p. 2). The ways in which youth with asthma and CF, and their families, experience the world around them and the health care system can directly impact the course of their illness and their collective quality of life.

The impact of social determinants of health and structural racism on children with asthma and CF is clear and children experience the negative impacts of such factors on their caregivers as well. The impact of environmental stressors, chronic or acute trauma, and societal and systemic racism have a profound impact on the outcomes of children living with asthma and CF. Additionally, ongoing exposure to environmental irritants such as tobacco smoke and allergic triggers both at home and in school lead to increased exacerbations and poor symptom control in both asthma and CF (see Figure 12.1; Martinez et al., 2021).

Asthma. Environmental tobacco smoke exposure is a major determinant of asthma severity in children and cigarette smoking has been clearly associated with persistent asthma in adulthood (O'Connor et al., 2018; Strachan et al., 1996). Similarly, ambient air pollutants have been associated with worse asthma severity and children living proximally to roadways have worse lung function and asthma symptoms (Urman et al., 2018). Exposure to these exacerbating factors is not distributed uniformly across the population and children living in poverty and from historically disadvantaged backgrounds are disproportionately impacted contributing to higher disease severity in these children (Volume 1, Chapter 24, this handbook).

Several studies have demonstrated that both systemic stressors (e.g., poverty, violence, racism) and psychological stress (acute and/or chronic) contribute to greater airway inflammation and worse asthma control (Akinbami et al., 2014; Beck et al., 2016; O'Connor et al., 2018). Asthma control, quality of life, health beliefs, and medications beliefs are impacted not only by race/ethnic background but also by the stress of socioeconomic, environmental, and psychosocial factors, which are amplified in families experiencing socioeconomic disadvantage or health inequity.

The impact of mental health alone on asthma outcomes is not exactly clear because asthma exacerbations often have multifactorial triggers (Kulikova et al., 2021). Although strong emotions can trigger exacerbations directly, there is also a high comorbidity between asthma and psychiatric disease including anxiety and depression, and there may be a bidirectional relationship between the two (Averill et al., 2023). Recent studies of stress may elucidate the underlying physiology. Stress was shown to lead to diminished expression of genes encoding glucocorticoid receptor and beta-2 adrenergic receptor in children with asthma (Miller & Chen, 2006). Fewer glucocorticoid receptors and beta-2 receptors may lead to poor response to therapies frequently used for asthma. In Black/African American adolescents who report the stress of discrimination and racism, there are accounts of worse asthma control (Thakur et al., 2017). Follow-up studies show that adolescents who report discrimination have increased bronchial hyperreactivity on pulmonary function testing in a specific phenotype of asthma that is less responsive to bronchodilator therapy (beta-2 agonists; Carlson et al., 2017).

African American children are also affected by asthma more than any other racial and ethnic groups in the United States, with higher rates of diagnosis, hospitalizations, morbidity, and mortality (Hughes et al., 2017). Although Hispanic and White children in the United States have similar asthma prevalence, Hispanic children have higher rates of asthma-related ED visits and hospitalizations (Zahran et al., 2018). Furthermore, experiencing inadequate health care access and/or low-quality health care can play a significant role in a delayed asthma diagnosis for African American and Hispanic children (Akinbami et al., 2014). There is strong evidence to link both the development and severity of asthma to social determinants of health and structural racism across urban and nonurban settings (Almqvist et al., 2005; Martinez et al., 2021; Stempel et al., 2019; Sullivan & Thakur, 2020; Thakur et al., 2013).

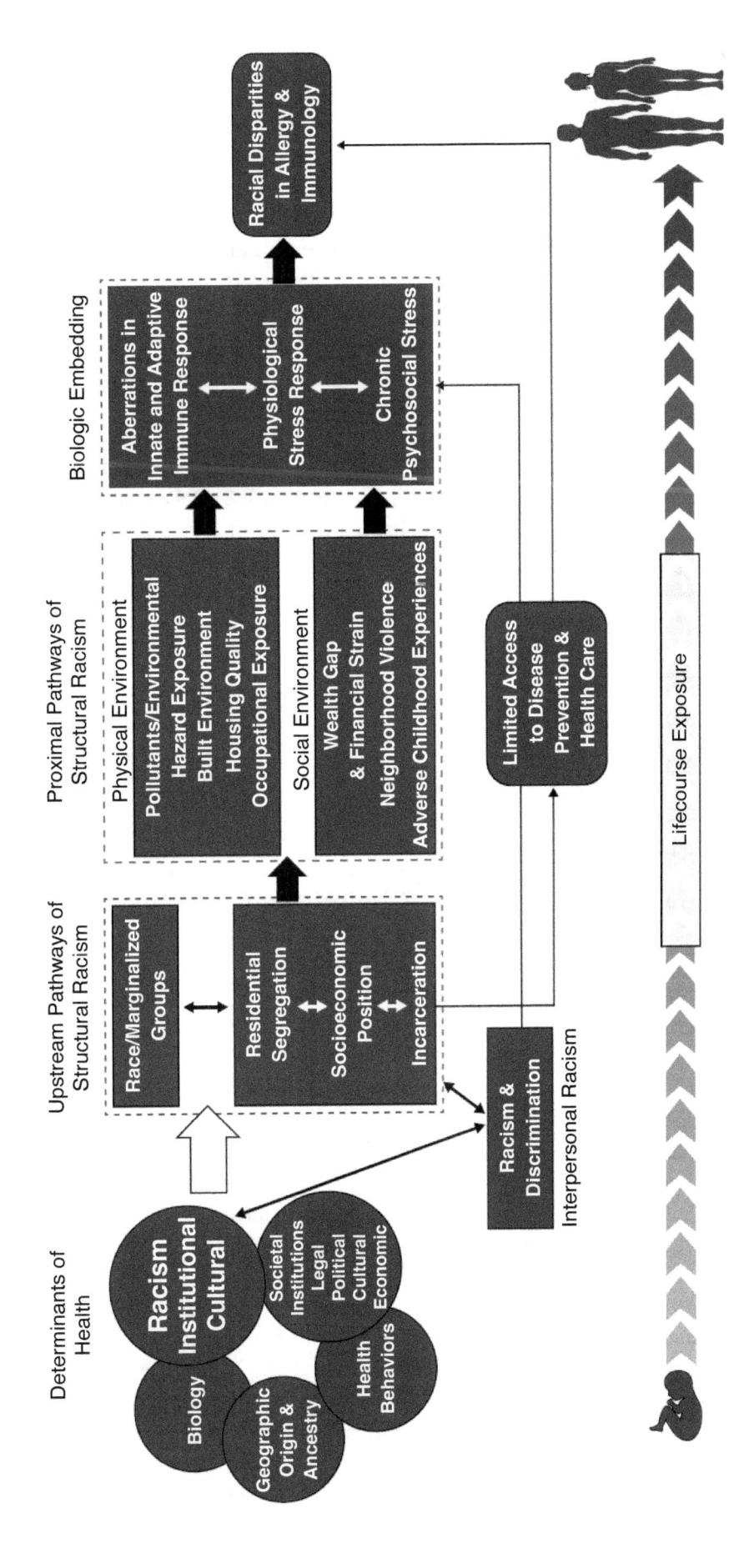

FIGURE 12.1. Structural racism as a root cause of allergy and immunology disparities. From "Structural Racism and Its Pathways to Asthma and Atopic Dermatitis," by A. Martinez, R. de la Rosa, M. Mujahid, and N. Thakur, 2021, *The Journal of Allergy and Clinical Immunology*, 148(5), p. 1114 (https://doi.org/10.1016/j.jaci.2021.09.020). Copyright 2021 by Elsevier. Reprinted with permission. Original figure converted from color.

Matsui et al. (2019) suggest that to understand causal pathways in asthma, investigators should consider using the biopsychosocial model and other conceptual frameworks from developmental science to integrate the influence of societal, environmental, psychosocial factors on the biology and phenotypes of asthma. As seen in Figure 12.1, the biopsychosocial model needs to include systems and policies that perpetuate poverty and marginalize populations.

Cystic fibrosis. As mentioned previously, while newborn screening has improved the outcome of infants diagnosed with CF by allowing early intervention, the most common newborn screening algorithms and genetic mutations tested introduce racial inequality in diagnosis (McBennett et al., 2022). The process most often used in the United States involves testing for the 23–40 most common genetic mutations of the CFTR protein that causes CF, which are not the most prevalent mutations in other ethnic and racial groups across the globe (Pique et al., 2017). While there have been perceptions and reports in the past of CF being more common among those identified as White, it is being recognized more frequently among diverse ethnic groups, with the frequency of CFTR mutations varying by ethnic group and geographic location (De Boeck, 2020; Schrijver et al., 2016).

The recognition of population-specific and individually rare CFTR variants in different racial and ethnic groups accentuates disparity in health outcomes as those variants are often absent from prenatal and newborn screening (NBS), causing a delayed diagnosis (Januska et al., 2020). Expanded NBS mutation panels can improve CF carrier detection rates within specific populations. A 69-mutation NBS is available, and although not universally used across the United States and internationally, it has been shown to increase detection of CF diagnoses and carrier status in members of African American and Hispanic American individuals, compared to the more commonly used 32-mutation NBS panel (Zvereff et al., 2014).

People with CF who have similar CF genotypes have been shown to have significantly different outcomes due to SES (Oates & Schechter, 2016; Schechter et al., 2001). Lower SES contributes to significantly poorer outcomes in weight, lung function, and pulmonary exacerbations for children with CF (Schechter et al., 2001). Low SES is also associated with disease severity, increased requirement of antibiotics to treat infections, greater health care utilization, and decreased survival in CF (O'Connor et al., 2003; Schechter & Margolis, 1998; Schechter et al., 2009) Previous studies on food insecurity in the CF community show that anywhere from 26–33% of families experience food insecurity and over 40% of adults with CF worry about being able to afford food (Brown et al., 2018; McDonald et al., 2009), which has a great impact on worse adherence to airway clearance treatments and oral medications and more weight loss than food-secure people with CF (Lim et al., 2022).

CURRENT STATE OF MEDICAL TREATMENT

As advances in detection and treatment of asthma and CF have evolved, so too have the clinical care guidelines associated with the management of each of these diseases.

Clinical Guidelines and Standards of Care

Asthma. Standard pediatric asthma care has been shown to improve outcomes, but asthma care quality can be variable, and standardization can be difficult to achieve (Johnson et al., 2018). Expert consensus has produced numerous national asthma guidelines to guide medical care. Current guidelines focus on an emphasis of the use of multiple measures to assess and monitor both *current impairment,* frequency and intensity of symptoms, low lung function and limitations of daily activities, and *future risk,* the likelihood of exacerbations, progressive loss of lung function, or adverse side effects from medications (Cloutier et al., 2020). New recommendations and approaches to managing and treating asthma emphasize strategies to promote adherence that include teaching and empowering patients to learn skills to monitor and manage their asthma, such as the use of written asthma action plans with instructions for daily management and response to worsening symptoms. Newer recommendations also encourage the expansion of educational opportunities to reach patients across a variety of settings, including pharmacies, schools, community centers, and patients' homes. Although current guidelines include acknowledgment of social determinants of health in the discussion of difficult-to-control asthma, structural racism and other cultural and ethnic factors are not mentioned and are areas for future consideration.

Cystic fibrosis. Clinical guidelines for CF exist for both the diagnosis and treatment of the multiple organ systems impacted by the disease. NBS for CF is the most common way CF is currently diagnosed, yet NBS around the world has been implemented somewhat inconsistently (Lang et al., 2011). NBS allows for the identification of the disease before the onset of symptoms, which has significantly contributed to improvements in the management of the illness and in life expectancy (Grimaldi et al., 2015). Children identified as having a positive NBS are almost always referred for a diagnostic sweat test, which is important to support the diagnosis of CF.

In 2006 the Cystic Fibrosis Foundation established guidelines for the use of sweat testing in the diagnosis of CF (LeGrys et al., 2007). The sweat test is considered the most reliable for diagnosing CF and produces a quantitative measurement of electrolytes in the sweat and an analysis of the sweat chloride, which can be indicative of a dysfunction of the CFTR protein. The guidelines suggest that a diagnosis of CF is based on at least two positive results, together with an appropriate clinical presentation and/or NBS (LeGrys, 1996).

Numerous clinical guidelines for the management and treatment of CF exist, each recommending screening and intervention for various aspects of the body system impacted. National and international guidelines address topics such as the treatment of pulmonary exacerbations, the screening and treatment of cystic fibrosis-related diabetes, maintaining growth and nutritional status, the management of gastrointestinal disorders and symptoms in CF, the screening of mental health symptoms in people with CF and their caregivers, managing chronic sinus disease, and reproductive health and fertility.

Symptom Management

Asthma. Asthma is a chronic disease that has no cure; however, for all but the most severe cases, the goal of treatment is to be symptom-free with full participation in all activities including school and athletics, and to optimize the HRQoL (Papi et al., 2018). Treatment does not modify the long-term disease state, nor does it alter pulmonary function over time, but it does improve symptoms and risk of hospitalization and severe exacerbation (Covar et al., 2012). As such, the two objectives of asthma therapy are symptom control and risk mitigation (prevention of severe exacerbation).

Pharmacologic treatment of asthma involves both the use of *controller* medications designed to prevent symptoms/exacerbations and the use of *reliever* medications that can rapidly treat symptoms when they occur. *Reliever medications* are rapid onset bronchodilators that are typically administered via inhalation. Short-acting beta-2 adrenergic agonists are the preferred agent and onset of action is typically felt within minutes and have a duration of effect from 4 to 6 hours. *Controller medications* are typically anti-inflammatory agents, most often inhaled corticosteroids (ICSs). At typical doses, most ICSs have high local potency (e.g., significant decrease in airway inflammation), but minimal systemic effects due to low absorption and/or rapid metabolism. To be effective, these medicines require once to twice daily use even when the individual is well (Papi et al., 2018). As asthma is a disease with intermittent exacerbations, successful asthma management relies heavily on patient education including self-monitoring for symptoms and knowledge of when and how to escalate treatment as needed.

Cystic fibrosis. The daily clinical management of CF involves time-intensive interventions that are complex and tedious (Sanders et al., 1991; Smith & Wood, 2007). The treatments for CF fall into multiple categories and differ in terms of their impact on the symptoms of this disease as well as the time and effort required to adhere to the therapy. These include nutritional treatments such as pancreatic enzyme replacement, fat-soluble vitamin replacement, high-caloric density and high-fat diets; inhaled treatments such as mucolytics, bronchodilators, antibiotics, and corticosteroids; chest physiotherapy and airway clearance; exercise; oral antibiotics; insulin for CF-related diabetes; and most recently, CFTR modulators (Kettler et al., 2002; Savage et al., 2011; Sawicki et al., 2009; Shakkottai et al., 2015). Most youth with CF (YwCF) are asked to incorporate a combination of many of the aforementioned treatments into their daily routines and can take up to several hours per day, frequently disrupting typical routines and activities (Sawicki et al., 2015). The major goals of treatment are to promote good nutrition and optimize growth, to delay or decelerate the development of lung disease by treating infections and clearing mucus from the lungs, and to recognize and treat the complications of CF (Colin & Wohl, 1994).

Over the past two decades, new treatments and therapies have emerged in CF, as advances in drug development and technology have occurred (Muther et al., 2020). These advances have caused enormous improvements in the lives of YwCF. The most significant development has been that of the small molecule therapies (i.e., CFTR modulators) directed at the abnormal CFTR protein that causes CF and all its associated symptoms (Guimbellot et al., 2021; Konstan et al., 2017). Even though more time is needed to continue evaluating the long-term benefit of these modulator therapies on disease progression and survival in CF, the evidence is clear that it is dramatically improving the health and quality of life of children living with CF and helping them reach adulthood with an increased promise of a better future. The advancements of the past few decades have improved symptom management and the quality of life for many YwCF; however, CF continues to be one of the most challenging and burdensome diseases to manage. Given the higher prevalence of anxiety and depression in YwCF, the relationship between psychological functioning and physical health should be incorporated in all aspects of medical management. It is clear that genetics and symptom management are not the only factors impacting disease outcomes; psychological, behavioral, and social factors play a role in long-term outcomes and adherence to daily care, necessitating multidisciplinary care for youth with CF.

Ecological Contexts Associated With Pulmonary Outcomes: The Role of Race/Ethnicity, Socioeconomic Status, and Access to Care

Asthma and CF outcomes vary along racial/ethnic and socioeconomic lines. There are notable disparities in asthma mortality and Black and Puerto Rican patients of all ages are more likely to die from their asthma (Akinbami et al., 2014). Black/African American children ages 8–21 with asthma have worse asthma control across the socioeconomic spectrum, although children with low SES report worse control (Thakur et al., 2013). Children insured by Medicaid who live in urban or poor neighborhoods and those who are Black/African American are more likely to have increased numbers of ED visits and hospitalizations due to asthma (Keet et al., 2017). Studies and clinical experience indicate social determinants of health and other psychosocial factors are responsible for more than 50% of difficult-to-treat and poorly controlled asthma (Bush et al., 2017). Studies in both asthma and CF show increased exacerbations leading to ED visits and hospitalizations of children with adverse exposure to environmental irritants (Ong et al., 2017). For example, poor housing quality and living in homes with housing code violations are associated with increased morbidity (Beck et al., 2014; Hughes et al., 2017; Volume 1, Chapter 24, this handbook). Particulate matter air pollution and increased level of irritants including nitrogen dioxide and secondhand smoke are also associated with poor asthma outcomes (Nardone et al., 2018).

Asthma. One of the factors associated with more optimal health outcomes for children with asthma is access to high-quality medical and subspecialty care. Studies indicate that patients who have strong relationships with their primary care providers are more likely to adhere to medication therapy and have better asthma control (Tackett et al., 2021). Specialty care for asthma also leads to improved asthma control due to improved adherence to asthma care guidelines and decreased asthma exacerbations (Harish et al., 2001). Children who live in the inner city are less likely to be referred to a specialist for asthma (Warman & Silver, 2018). Studies indicate that Black/African American children who live in urban areas are less likely than other populations to be referred to an asthma specialist (Flores et al., 2009). Better population health measures, such as school-based programs, in-home nursing, and/or asthma educators are needed to reduce these disparities in diagnoses and access to treatments.

Cystic fibrosis. Access to quality care is also associated with outcomes in cystic fibrosis. The presence of population-specific and individually rare CFTR variants for individuals of non-White backgrounds further accentuates disparities in early detection and diagnosis, which causes barriers to early access to care (Januska et al., 2020). As advances in medical treatments and therapies exist for the majority of YwCF, the less common CFTR variants that exist for individuals of non-White backgrounds further limit access to the highly effective modulator medications (Januska et al., 2020). Furthermore, starting in 2020 access to care was disproportionately impacted by the COVID-19 pandemic for racial and ethnic minority YwCF. During the global pandemic, much of health care saw an uptick in telehealth services and transition of traditional medical testing and visits to virtual formats. Individuals of racial and ethnic minority backgrounds were less likely to receive telemedicine services, and individuals of lower SES found the transition to increases in telehealth more difficult to navigate and were less likely to think that their concerns or questions were addressed in virtual medical visits (Albon et al., 2021).

When national care guidelines are followed, children living with asthma or CF experience better symptom control; however, not all children receive guidelines-based therapy due to lack of access to high-quality care. McQuaid (2018) found that social determinants of health including socioeconomic, environmental, and psychosocial factors impact not only access to health care, but also adherence to care plans and medications. Using Maslow's hierarchy, patients who have significant concerns about fundamental needs such as shelter or safety may have a difficult time structuring their time to prioritize adherence to daily medications (De Keyser et al., 2020).

CLINICAL IMPLICATIONS ACROSS DEVELOPMENTAL STAGES

As chronic illnesses, asthma and CF both require a focus on risk factors, comorbidities, and stressors that can grow and change across the lifespan. Clinical care of these pulmonary diseases necessitates behavioral and psychological treatments to ensure positive outcomes.

Adherence

Medication adherence has been shown to be a significant problem in many childhood chronic illnesses, and both asthma and CF are especially difficult to manage. Good adherence to medical regimen is most commonly defined as taking between 70–80% of prescribed medication and daily treatments (Jochmann et al., 2017; Santos et al., 2008). Although any cut point for adherence is quite arbitrary, there is some evidence of clinical effect when adherence falls below certain thresholds. Adolescence is a period of vulnerability for youth living with asthma and CF alike.

Asthma. Adolescents with asthma begin to take increasing control over their daily self-management, but often underestimate the severity of their symptoms and overestimate their ability to control them (Wildhaber et al., 2012). They also have different priorities compared to their caregivers, which can lead to difficulty creating and adhering to asthma management plans. Ungar et al. (2015) found that youth with asthma cared most about physical activity limitations while their parents cared most about the nighttime symptoms and avoiding multiple ED visits. Difficulty remembering to take the medications and trouble using an inhaler correctly are associated with youth-reported adherence to their medications (Sleath et al., 2018).

Pediatric asthma creates a heavy burden on children and their families. A recent study found that youth with asthma and their caregivers both reported that the child took their asthma medication exactly as prescribed less than 70% of the time (Sleath et al., 2018). Treatment burden is a significant predictor of adherence and self-management (Sloand et al., 2021). To be well-controlled, asthma requires proper education, reduced exposure to triggers, and medical management. Many barriers such as transportation difficulties, interference on parental work and family activities, limited health care office hours, individual health knowledge and/or beliefs, and negative care experiences can all impact adherence.

Cystic fibrosis. Although significant advancements in the treatment of CF have led to drastically improved medical outcomes and increased life expectancy for YwCF, managing the daily care remains burdensome and complex. A time-intensive daily CF treatment regimen is difficult to maintain and can interfere with many aspects of one's life. With the development of new therapies, high treatment adherence is often necessary for patients to experience the clinical benefit (Johnson et al., 2001; Sawicki et al., 2009). Many factors impact how well an individual adheres to recommendations of their health care team. Understanding the barriers and facilitators of treatment adherence in CF is critical as well as the interventions available to help those with this disease live better lives while managing their health.

Adolescence is a time that is typically characterized by a decline in lung function for YwCF, with epidemiologic data suggesting that the steepest decline in pulmonary function, measured by forced expiratory volume in 1 second (known in the literature as FEV_1), occurs during the adolescent and young adult ages of 13–21 years (Cystic Fibrosis Foundation, 2015). While the foundations for successful daily management of CF begin at an early age, learning how to manage one's health is important throughout development. The responsibility of management of daily CF-related care begins to shift in adolescence, correlating with a time when difficulties with adherence to the medical regimen are common. Many challenges to adherence with CF treatments exist, including the developmental task of increasing autonomy and decreased parental involvement, competing demands and lack of effective time management skills, treatment complexity and the disruption of daily routines, and the adolescent perceptions of illness and importance of required treatments (Muther et al., 2020). Despite the drastic advances and benefits of CF treatments, medication adherence among youth with CF remains low, ranging from 33% to 76% depending on type of measurement (i.e., subjective reports, pharmacy refill data, medication tracking devices; Burrows et al., 2002; Modi et al., 2006; Muther et al., 2020; Zindani et al., 2006).

Interventions to improve adherence. There have been very few evaluations on the efficacy of adherence promotion interventions in asthma and CF across childhood and adolescence. It appears that there is no one-size-fits-all approach, and that across numerous studies, interventions that are flexible and tailored to an individual's unique needs are the most acceptable and effective. Additionally, given the significant number of barriers to daily self-care in both asthma and CF, adherence interventions should include education *and* behavior management techniques (Muther et al., 2020). Meta-analyses have concluded that there have been minimal studies of sufficient quality to determine if any adherence or self-management intervention stands out above and beyond others as notably effective (Goldbeck et al., 2014; Savage et al., 2014).

Nonetheless, many different types of interventions aimed at improving daily management of asthma and CF exist. Electronic reminders are some of the most common types of interventions that clinicians use. Youth and their families are often encouraged to set reminders and alarms on their cell phones and other electronic devices to avoid one of the most common challenges: forgetting to take medications and/or do treatments. A meta-analysis involving several pediatric chronic illnesses reported that reminders are associated with a small, but helpful, improvement in medication adherence (Tao et al., 2015). Other supports such as enhanced pharmacist support, problem solving during medical appointments, positive reinforcement and incentive use, and psychological interventions have also had modest and intermittent success (Muther et al., 2020; Zobell et al., 2017).

Mental Health and Emotional Well-Being

Emotional health and psychological functioning are critical aspects of the overall care and treatment of chronic illnesses such as asthma and CF. Physical health and positive medical outcomes can never fully be achieved without considering mental health as part of an individual's health care.

Relationship between emotional functioning and chronic illness. Children with chronic medical conditions, especially asthma and CF, are at an increased risk for depression, anxiety, and other mental health comorbidities (Buchanan et al., 2015), and one of the most significant risk factors is the relationship between chronic illness and youth emotional health and well-being. Increased prevalence of mental health-related symptoms interfere with a child's ability to cope with their illness, medical stressors, and can lead to decreased motivation to engage in self-care behaviors (Dantzer et al., 2003; Korbel et al., 2007). For example, youth with CF who are experiencing mental health symptoms tend to have more difficulties sustaining daily medical care, are more likely to have lower lung function and BMI, miss clinic appointments, have high health care utilization, and report worse HRQoL (DiMatteo et al., 2000; Dowson et al., 2004; VandenBranden et al., 2012). Additionally, the impact of isolation and reduced opportunities to receive social support from others with a similar experience can negatively impact quality of life. Youth living with CF often experience social isolation as a result of infection control guidelines that prohibit close in-person contact with anyone else living with the disease. Therefore, social support, social connectedness, and validation of experience that are all known to be beneficial are severely reduced in CF (Kirk & Milnes, 2016). Social support is a critical predictor of quality of life and a known buffer against symptoms of depression, adherence-related problems, and declining health status (Frisina et al., 2004; Kaaya et al., 2013).

Children with asthma and CF will typically benefit physically from improvements in their psychological health (Bregnballe et al., 2011). Given the heavy burden of living with asthma and CF, psychosocial functioning is an integral component of a child's overall health and well-being and has led to a need for increased understanding of the risk factors associated with living with these conditions. A clear understanding of these risk factors leads to a more sustainable approach to implementing multidisciplinary interventions and strategies to overcome the identified risks.

Guidelines and recommendations for the integration of psychosocial support as well as psychological assessment and intervention into the routine care for children with pulmonary disorders exist. The International Committee on Mental Health in CF has developed recommendations for the identification and treatment of mental health risk factors in CF centers internationally (Quittner et al., 2016), which have been modeled in other conditions such as asthma. These recommendations include annual screening of depression and anxiety in YwCF and at least one parent caregiver of children under 18 years, along with preventative psychoeducational support, formal developmental-behavioral assessment and evidence-based psychological and pharmacological intervention when indicated (Muther et al., 2018).

Impact of Disease on Academic and Social Functioning

Academic functioning. Studies of children living with chronic illnesses have shown disruptions to schooling due to hospitalizations, treatments, and illness (Crump et al., 2013). While it is widely recognized that chronic illness can have an impact on a child's academic functioning, the health and educational systems are often siloed from one another, so children's health and educational needs are always well integrated. Children with asthma are more prone to school absences than their healthy peers, and those children with poorly controlled asthma are at greater risk for declines in their academic performance (Diette et al., 2000; Horner et al., 2011; Koinis-Mitchell et al., 2019; Moonie et al., 2006). Urban minority children with asthma are at an even greater risk of negative impacts on academic functioning. Another way in which asthma can affect academic performance is through its impact on sleep in children (Koinis-Mitchell et al., 2019). Asthma can affect children's sleep quality and the amount of sleep, which can interfere with attention in school and impact the quality of schoolwork (Koinis-Mitchell et al., 2017). As such, children with asthma who are demonstrating school failure may benefit from an evaluation by a developmental-behavioral pediatrician or psychologist to assess for asthma-related contributors to poor school performance.

Children with CF often miss school due to pulmonary exacerbations or hospitalizations, which is correlated with lower GPA (Grieve et al., 2011). In a study comparing YwCF to healthy controls on measures of attention and memory, YwCF had more errors on a test of attention, had higher rates of fluctuation in concentration, and made more mistakes and had fewer correct answers on a test of memory (Piasecki et al., 2017). One factor significantly associated with attention and memory performance is sleep (Paruthi et al., 2016). Children with CF also have impaired sleep quality, decreased sleep efficiency, daytime sleepiness, and sleep disordered breathing likely due to multiple causes including nocturnal cough, gastrointestinal symptoms, and time-consuming treatments among others (Reiter et al., 2022). Given the potential impact of asthma and CF on academic and emotional functioning, behavioral health providers, in particular developmental-behavioral pediatricians and psychologists, should consider a formal assessment for sleep, learning, and school performance, if children present with impairments in academic, social, or emotional functioning.

Social functioning. Given that children with asthma do not have the same infection precautions as YwCF, fewer studies have examined the social functioning of children with asthma. Several studies have suggested that the social functioning of children with asthma can be predicted by how well controlled their asthma symptoms are (Dean et al., 2010). Social support is an important construct for children with asthma and lower perceived social support has been associated with lower medication adherence (Sloand et al., 2021). Children with moderate-to-severe asthma experience more symptoms that can limit their activity, which can cause feelings of social isolation and loneliness (Dean et al., 2010).

Infection control guidelines for YwCF recommend they remain at least 6 feet apart from each other (Saiman et al., 2014). Given the limitations on interactions with other peers with CF, YwCF often engage in online platforms that allow for communication (Kirk & Milnes, 2016). These online groups allow for sharing different management strategies for treatments, emotions, and relationships, and ways to fit CF into their lives (Kirk & Milnes, 2016). Despite limited interactions with peers with CF, individuals with CF often receive support from non-CF friends around exercise and managing social networks when they are sick (Barker et al., 2012).

Caregiver and Family Functioning—Factors Associated With Risk and Resilience

There are longstanding associations between family functioning, treatment adherence, and quality of life in many pediatric chronic conditions, including asthma and CF (Drotar & Bonner, 2009; Lewin et al., 2006; Muther et al.,

2018). Being a parent of a child with any chronic illness is extremely demanding. Parents learn to implement time-intensive daily CF and asthma treatments, and typical childhood behaviors can significantly impact the stress of the parent. From the time of diagnosis, families and caregivers experience psychosocial challenges that often continue throughout development and into adulthood. During early childhood, caregivers are tasked with promoting normal child development in the setting of a very burdensome chronic disease, which can result in unique psychosocial stressors for the family such as social isolation and avoidance of common socialization opportunities (i.e., early play dates) due to risk of infection exposure (Muther et al., 2018). Even typical developmental behavioral challenges (i.e., tantrums, toilet training, picky eating) can impact daily treatments and a family's ability to sustain a complicated daily medical regimen. The increased likelihood of psychological risk factors related to coping with CF or asthma highlight the important roles of subspecialty partners (e.g., pediatric psychology, developmental-behavioral pediatrics, and child and adolescent psychology and psychiatry) to help address the comorbidities that can affect adaptation and health-related outcomes. Caregivers who have children with chronic pulmonary conditions must navigate the complexities of the health care system, including communicating with medical providers, insurance companies, pharmacies, and ongoing interactions with school staff to ensure understanding of medical requirements (Filigno et al., 2019). Interactions and relationships between family members also can be impacted given the significant burden of daily treatment and unpredictability of the illness (Filigno et al., 2019).

Incorporating family-centered care into the diagnosis and treatment of children with asthma helps reduce the long-term impact of poorer family functioning across the childhood developmental lifespan. Early family-based interventions in the care of pediatric asthma and CF, including the identification of parental mental health needs, during the toddler and preschool years may enhance family interactions over time and mitigate risk as children grow into adolescence and young adulthood.

FUTURE DIRECTIONS: A MULTIDISCIPLINARY APPROACH TO PROMOTING RESILIENCE

Efforts aimed at identifying biological, cultural, psychosocial, and developmental risk factors for youth coping with CF and asthma are essential in promoting resilience and an ideal role for developmental-behavioral pediatricians and pediatric psychologists alike. The underlying relationship that is formed with these specific health care providers is one of the most important tools in reducing risk and promoting resilience in youth with CF and asthma, and their families. *Resilience* is defined by the American Psychological Association (APA) as the process of adapting well under adverse circumstances or significant stress (2022). Because of the continuous need to confront uncertainty that comes with living with asthma and CF, many youth experience emotion regulation strategies that contribute to resilience and an acceptance of one's health (Mitmansgruber et al., 2016). The APA has highlighted numerous strategies for building resilience, including self-care, outlook/perspective modification, realistic goal setting, and decisive action, all of which are relevant to children with asthma and CF as well as their caregivers (see Table 12.1; APA, 2022; and Volume 1, Chapter 15, this handbook).

Coping

Two of the most salient issues facing children with asthma and CF and their families, are coping and adjustment. Children with these conditions are required to manage the burden of a new medical diagnosis, deal with ongoing invasive and time-consuming treatments and procedures, and adjust to changes in functioning that impact both the child and the entire family. During childhood, caregivers of children with asthma and/or CF are tasked with promoting normal development in the setting of a chronic disease that interrupts typical routines. This challenge can result in difficulties

TABLE 12.1
Strategies to Promote Resilience

Strategy	Definition
Make connections	■ Keep good relationships with close family members and friends ■ Accept help and support from others ■ Join and be active in groups (faith-based, civic, etc.) ■ Help others in their time of need
Avoid seeing crises as insurmountable problems	■ Focus on what you can control ■ Make changes to how you interpret and respond to stress ■ Look to how things may improve in the future ■ Acknowledge subtle ways you might already be dealing with stress
Accept that change is a part of living	■ Accept circumstances that cannot be changed, allowing you to focus on things you can control
Move toward your goals	■ Develop realistic and measurable goals ■ Do something regularly, even if it seems small ■ Ask yourself, "What is one thing I know I can accomplish today that helps me move in the direction I want to go?"
Take decisive actions	■ Act on problems and stressors rather than detaching or wishing they would just go away
Look for opportunities for self-discovery	■ Realize that people learn from and find evidence of growth as a result of stress or loss (e.g., better relationships, new sense of strength, increased self-worth, heightened appreciation for life, spirituality)
Nurture a positive view of yourself	■ Develop confidence in your ability to solve problems ■ Trust your instincts
Keep things in perspective	■ Try to keep a long-term perspective even in the face of pain and significant stress
Maintain a hopeful outlook	■ Be optimistic because it allows you to expect that good things will happen in your life ■ Visualize what you want rather than worrying about what you fear
Take care of yourself	■ Pay attention to your needs and feelings ■ Engage in activities that you enjoy ■ Exercise regularly

Note. Data from American Psychological Association (2022).

coping. Research has supported interventions aimed to address the increased stress associated with living with a chronic condition, such as psychoeducation and/or evidence-based psychological interventions (i.e., cognitive behavior therapy) to improve coping and adjustment to both asthma and CF as well as reduce medical hospitalizations and exacerbations in symptoms (Varni et al., 2007; Wallander & Varni, 1992).

Coping mechanisms and styles employed by YwCF and asthma can serve either as a buffer or a risk factor for psychological problems and poor HRQoL (Elliot et al., 2011; McHugh et al., 2016; Mitmansgruber et al., 2016). Passive or avoidant coping strategies (e.g., disengagement, self-distraction, substance use) have been shown to be associated with increased risk of mental health symptoms and lower quality of life for individuals with CF and asthma (Hesselink et al., 2004; McHugh et al., 2016) as they tend to divert attention away from the illness and promote poorer self-efficacy (Abbott et al., 2011). In contrast, more active coping styles such as acceptance, seeking and maintaining social support, and planning have all predicted better quality of life and improved self-management in YwCF and asthma (Hesselink et al., 2004; Maslow et al., 2011; McHugh et al., 2016).

Personal practices to improve health coping and resilience may also include techniques such as spiritual coping, meditation, and/or physical movement (Muther et al., 2018). Of these spiritual coping has the most empirical evidence in children and families with both asthma and CF. Spiritual beliefs can help provide a framework to find meaning in experiences, increase social support, and provide a sense of belonging, as well as play an important role in managing aspects of chronic illness (Park, 2007; Reynolds et al., 2014). Additional coping strategies such as mindfulness meditation, have been well demonstrated to subjectively reduce stress and improve physical health by decreasing inflammation (Creswell et al., 2016; Muther et al., 2018).

Social Support

Social support is a critical aspect of positive coping with the chronic pulmonary conditions of asthma and CF. Social isolation has been linked to an increase in many risk factors, including mental health problems and poorer adherence to medical care (Kirk & Milnes, 2016; Sloand et al., 2021). New technologies such as internet-based forums and social media have been helpful in reducing infection control barriers to social contact and have drastically increased the social support youth with CF can now experience. Additionally, as a result of the COVID-19 pandemic, many shifts from traditional in-person mechanisms for support to virtual gatherings have increased accessibility and comfort in seeking support through new means.

Studies of youth with asthma and CF have shown that both family support and peer support are strong predictors of good disease control and higher quality of life (Rhee et al., 2010; Scheckner et al., 2015; Weber et al., 2010), which also extend to youth of diverse racial and socioeconomic status (Rhee et al., 2010). Social support is believed to be very powerful because it can improve negative perceptions adolescents may have and promote more positive beliefs about coping and self-care, ultimately enhancing treatment adherence (Sloand et al., 2021). The experience of perceived support includes not only the relationship with peers, but also extends to the amount and type of support youth perceive with their parents, extended family members, coaches, teachers, and health care providers (Knight, 2005). These findings provide hope to counter the burden that can be associated with a lifelong disease. Utilizing interventions and strategies to identify and increase supportive relationships in youths' lives can be a critical factor to improve the outcome for children living with asthma.

CONCLUSION

Living with the pediatric pulmonary conditions of asthma and CF can be burdensome for the child, their caregivers, extended family members, and the health care system as a whole. Each disease has a unique set of complicated risk factors that can make the diagnosis and management of symptoms more difficult. Each of these diseases are best treated through a multidisciplinary approach, involving care from the medical team, pediatric psychologists, developmental-behavioral pediatricians, and child and adolescent psychiatrists and psychologists who can address cultural and systemic barriers and deal with the psychological and social comorbidities across the stages of development. Although many challenges related to managing daily symptoms and maintaining all aspects of functioning exist, there is hope that as better patient and family partnerships exist with medical teams, rates of survival and quality of life will continue to improve. Drawing from research in developmental science, early intervention at the time of diagnosis, and supports for the family and environmental systems can have a profound impact for the course of illness throughout life. Finally, children, their families, and the health care system will benefit from recommendations, interventions, and policies aimed to better promote the resilience of those impacted by asthma and CF.

RESOURCES

Asthma

- American Academy of Allergy, Asthma, and Immunology is an academic and clinical organization for allergies, asthma, and immune deficiency disorders.

    https://www.aaaai.org/tools-for-the-public/school-tools

    https://www.aaaai.org/tools-for-the-public/video-library/asthma-videos

- American Lung Association is a nonprofit organization with the mission to save lives by improving lung health and preventing lung disease through research, education, and advocacy.

https://www.lung.org/lung-health-diseases/lung-disease-lookup/asthma/managing-asthma/children-and-asthma

https://www.lung.org/lung-health-diseases/lung-disease-lookup/asthma

- American Thoracic Society is a nonprofit organization focused on improving care for pulmonary diseases.

  https://www.thoracic.org/

- Centers for Disease Control and Prevention (CDC) is the national public health agency of the United States. It is a U.S. federal agency under the Department of Health and Human Services that works to protect the public's health.

  https://www.cdc.gov

Resources for Parents

- CDC—Asthma—Parents provides information and resources on the treatment and management of asthma.

  https://www.cdc.gov/asthma/

Resources for Providers

- Global Initiative for Asthma (GINA)—GINA aims to improve the diagnosis, management, and prevention of asthma by providing evidence-based strategies, tools and resources for clinicians worldwide.

  https://ginasthma.org

- Podcasts in English and Spanish

  https://www.childrenscolorado.org/health-professionals/professional-resources/charting-pediatrics-podcast

  - Sample podcast episodes include "Applying Updated Guidelines for Pediatric Asthma Primary Care" and "Asthma and Other Common Respiratory Diseases During COVID-19"

Cystic Fibrosis

- Cystic Fibrosis Foundation, USA supports a broad range of research and clinical initiatives with the primary mission to cure cystic fibrosis.

  https://www.cff.org

- European Cystic Fibrosis Society is an international community of scientific and clinical professionals committed to improving survival and quality of life for people living with cystic fibrosis.

  https://www.ecfs.eu/

- Cystic Fibrosis Research Institute is a nonprofit organization that funds research and offers education, advocacy and psychosocial support to the cystic fibrosis community.

  https://www.cfri.org

Resources for Providers

- Indiana University School of Medicine, Division of Continuing Medical Education Continuing Education in Healthcare Professions

  Online course in Cystic Fibrosis (free): Cystic Fibrosis Clinical Care Education

  https://medicine.iu.edu/cme/clinical-care-education/cystic-fibrosis

References

Abbott, J., Hart, A., Havermans, T., Matossian, A., Goldbeck, L., Barreto, C., Bergsten-Brucefors, A., Besier, T., Catastini, P., Lupi, F., & Staab, D. (2011). Measuring health-related quality of life in clinical trials in cystic fibrosis. *Journal of Cystic Fibrosis*, *10*(Suppl. 2), S82–S85. https://doi.org/10.1016/S1569-1993(11)60013-1

Akinbami, L. J., Moorman, J. E., Bailey, C., Zahran, H. S., King, M., Johnson, C. A., & Liu, X. (2012). Trends in asthma prevalence, health care use, and mortality in the United States, 2001–2010. *NCHS Data Brief*, (94), 1–8. https://www.ncbi.nlm.nih.gov/pubmed/22617340

Akinbami, L. J., Moorman, J. E., Simon, A. E., & Schoendorf, K. C. (2014). Trends in racial disparities for asthma outcomes among children 0 to 17 years, 2001–2010. *Journal of Allergy and Clinical Immunology, 134*(3), 547–553. e545. https://doi.org/10.1016/j.jaci.2014.05.037

Albon, D., Van Citters, A. D., Ong, T., Dieni, O., Dowd, C., Willis, A., Sabadosa, K. A., Scalia, P., Reno, K., Oates, G. R., & Schechter, M. S. (2021). Telehealth use in cystic fibrosis during COVID-19: Association with race, ethnicity, and socioeconomic factors. *Journal of Cystic Fibrosis, 20*(S 3), 49–54. https://doi.org/10.1016/j.jcf.2021.09.006

Almqvist, C., Pershagen, G., & Wickman, M. (2005). Low socioeconomic status as a risk factor for asthma, rhinitis and sensitization at 4 years in a birth cohort. *Clinical and Experimental Allergy, 35*(5), 612–618. https://doi.org/10.1111/j.1365-2222.2005.02243.x

American Psychological Association. (2022). *Resilience*. Retrieved April 29, 2023, from https://www.apa.org/topics/resilience

Asher, I., & Pearce, N. (2014). Global burden of asthma among children. *The International Journal of Tuberculosis and Lung Disease, 18*(11), 1269–1278. https://doi.org/10.5588/ijtld.14.0170

Averill, S., McQuillan, M., Slaven, J., Weist, A., Kloepfer, K., & Krupp, N. (2023). Assessment of anxiety and depression in a pediatric high-risk asthma clinic. *The Journal of Allergy and Clinical Immunology, 151*(2, Suppl.), AB159. https://doi.org/10.1016/j.jaci.2022.12.497

Barker, D. H., Driscoll, K. A., Modi, A. C., Light, M. J., & Quittner, A. L. (2012). Supporting cystic fibrosis disease management during adolescence: The role of family and friends. *Child: Care, Health and Development, 38*(4), 497–504. https://doi.org/10.1111/j.1365-2214.2011.01286.x

Beck, A. F., Huang, B., Auger, K. A., Ryan, P. H., Chen, C., & Kahn, R. S. (2016). Explaining racial disparities in child asthma readmission using a causal inference approach. *JAMA Pediatrics, 170*(7), 695–703. https://doi.org/10.1001/jamapediatrics.2016.0269

Beck, A. F., Huang, B., Chundur, R., & Kahn, R. S. (2014). Housing code violation density associated with emergency department and hospital use by children with asthma. *Health Affairs, 33*(11), 1993–2002. https://doi.org/10.1377/hlthaff.2014.0496

Beck, A. F., Klein, M. D., Schaffzin, J. K., Tallent, V., Gillam, M., & Kahn, R. S. (2012). Identifying and treating a substandard housing cluster using a medical-legal partnership. *Pediatrics, 130*(5), 831–838. https://doi.org/10.1542/peds.2012-0769

Bell, S. C., Mall, M. A., Gutierrez, H., Macek, M., Madge, S., Davies, J. C., Burgel, P.-R., Tullis, E., Castaños, C., Castellani, C., Byrnes, C. A., Cathcart, F., Chotirmall, S. H., Cosgriff, R., Eichler, I., Fajac, I., Goss, C. H., Drevinek, P., Farrell, P. M., . . . Ratjen, F. (2020). The future of cystic fibrosis care: A global perspective. *The Lancet Respiratory Medicine, 8*(1), 65–124. https://doi.org/10.1016/S2213-2600(19)30337-6

Bellin, M. H., Collins, K. S., Osteen, P., Kub, J., Bollinger, M. E., Newsome, A., Lewis-Land, C., & Butz, A. M. (2017). Characterization of stress in low-income, inner-city mothers of children with poorly controlled asthma. *Journal of Urban Health, 94*(6), 814–823. https://doi.org/10.1007/s11524-017-0162-1

Bregnballe, V., Schiøtz, P. O., Boisen, K. A., Pressler, T., & Thastum, M. (2011). Barriers to adherence in adolescents and young adults with cystic fibrosis: A questionnaire study in young patients and their parents. *Patient Preference and Adherence, 5*, 507–515. https://doi.org/10.2147/PPA.S25308

Brown, P. S., Durham, D., Tivis, R. D., Stamper, S., Waldren, C., Toevs, S. E., Gordon, B., & Robb, T. A. (2018). Evaluation of food insecurity in adults and children with cystic fibrosis: Community case study. *Frontiers in Public Health, 6*, 348. https://doi.org/10.3389/fpubh.2018.00348

Buchanan, C. L., Lindwall, J., Edlynn, E., & Muther, E. (2015). Behavioral health and children with chronic medical conditions or physical illnesses. *Colorado Journal of Psychiatry & Psychology, 1*(1), 99–134. https://www.ucdenver.edu/docs/librariesprovider45/default-document-library/cjppv1n1.pdf

Burrows, J. A., Bunting, J. P., Masel, P. J., & Bell, S. C. (2002). Nebulised dornase alpha: Adherence in adults with cystic fibrosis. *Journal of Cystic Fibrosis, 1*(4), 255–259. https://doi.org/10.1016/S1569-1993(02)00095-4

Bush, A., Fleming, L., & Saglani, S. (2017). Severe asthma in children. *Respirology, 22*(5), 886–897. https://doi.org/10.1111/resp.13085

Carlson, S. M., Kim, J., Khan, D. A., King, K., Lucarelli, R. T., McColl, R., Peshock, R., & Brown, E. S. (2017). Hippocampal volume in patients with asthma: Results from the Dallas Heart Study. *Journal of Asthma, 54*(1), 9–16. https://doi.org/10.1080/02770903.2016.1186174

Centers for Disease Control and Prevention. (2015). *Asthma-related missed school days among children aged 5–17 years*. https://www.cdc.gov/asthma/asthma_stats/missing_days.htm#print

Cloutier, M. M., Baptist, A. P., Blake, K. V., Brooks, E. G., Bryant-Stephens, T., DiMango, E., Dixon,

A. E., Elward, K. S., Hartert, T., Krishnan, J. A., Lemanske, R. F., Jr., Ouellette, D. R., Pace, W. D., Schatz, M., Skolnik, N. S., Stout, J. W., Teach, S. J., Umscheid, C. A., Walsh, C. G., & the Expert Panel Working Group of the National Heart, Lung, and Blood Institute. (2020). 2020 focused updates to the asthma management guidelines: A report from the national asthma education and prevention program coordinating committee expert panel working group. *The Journal of Allergy and Clinical Immunology, 146*(6), 1217–1270. https://doi.org/10.1016/j.jaci.2020.10.003

Cogen, J. D., & Ramsey, B. W. (2020). The changing face of cystic fibrosis. In S. D. Davis, M. Rosenfeld, & J. Chmiel (Eds.), *Cystic fibrosis: A multi-organ system approach* (pp. 3–16). Springer International. https://doi.org/10.1007/978-3-030-42382-7_1

Colin, A. A., & Wohl, M. E. (1994). Cystic fibrosis. *Pediatrics in Review, 15*(5), 192–200. https://doi.org/10.1542/pir.15.5.192

Cope, S. F., Ungar, W. J., & Glazier, R. H. (2008). Socioeconomic factors and asthma control in children. *Pediatric Pulmonology, 43*(8), 745–752. https://doi.org/10.1002/ppul.20847

Covar, R. A., Fuhlbrigge, A. L., Williams, P., Kelly, H. W., & Childhood Asthma Management Program Research Group. (2012). The childhood asthma management program (CAMP): Contributions to the understanding of therapy and the natural history of childhood asthma. *Current Respiratory Care Reports, 1*(4), 243–250. https://doi.org/10.1007/s13665-012-0026-9

Creswell, J. D., Taren, A. A., Lindsay, E. K., Greco, C. M., Gianaros, P. J., Fairgrieve, A., Marsland, A. L., Brown, K. W., Way, B. M., Rosen, R. K., & Ferris, J. L. (2016). Alterations in resting-state functional connectivity link mindfulness meditation with reduced Interleukin-6: A randomized controlled trial. *Biological Psychiatry, 80*(1), 53–61. https://doi.org/10.1016/j.biopsych.2016.01.008

Crump, C., Rivera, D., London, R., Landau, M., Erlendson, B., & Rodriguez, E. (2013). Chronic health conditions and school performance among children and youth. *Annals of Epidemiology, 23*(4), 179–184. https://doi.org/10.1016/j.annepidem.2013.01.001

Cystic Fibrosis Foundation. (2015). Highlights of the 2014 patient registry data. https://www.cffamilyconnection.org/wp-content/uploads/2016/03/Highlights-of-the-2014-Patient-Registry-Data.pdf

Cystic Fibrosis Foundation. (2021). *Patient registry 2020 annual data report* [Report]. https://www.cff.org/sites/default/files/2021-10/2019-Patient-Registry-Annual-Data-Report.pdf

Dantzer, C., Swendsen, J., Maurice-Tison, S., & Salamon, R. (2003). Anxiety and depression in juvenile diabetes: A critical review. *Clinical Psychology Review, 23*(6), 787–800. https://doi.org/10.1016/S0272-7358(03)00069-2

De Boeck, K. (2020). Cystic fibrosis in the year 2020: A disease with a new face. *Acta Paediatrica, 109*(5), 893–899. https://doi.org/10.1111/apa.15155

De Keyser, H. H., Ramsey, R., & Federico, M. J. (2020). They just don't take their medicines: Reframing medication adherence in asthma from frustration to opportunity. *Pediatric Pulmonology, 55*(3), 818–825. https://doi.org/10.1002/ppul.24643

Dean, B. B., Calimlim, B. C., Sacco, P., Aguilar, D., Maykut, R., & Tinkelman, D. (2010). Uncontrolled asthma among children: Impairment in social functioning and sleep. *Journal of Asthma, 47*(5), 539–544. https://doi.org/10.3109/02770900903580868

Diette, G. B., Markson, L., Skinner, E. A., Nguyen, T. T., Algatt-Bergstrom, P., & Wu, A. W. (2000). Nocturnal asthma in children affects school attendance, school performance, and parents' work attendance. *Archives of Pediatrics & Adolescent Medicine, 154*(9), 923–928. https://doi.org/10.1001/archpedi.154.9.923

DiMatteo, M. R., Lepper, H. S., & Croghan, T. W. (2000). Depression is a risk factor for noncompliance with medical treatment: Meta-analysis of the effects of anxiety and depression on patient adherence. *Archives of Internal Medicine, 160*(14), 2101–2107. https://doi.org/10.1001/archinte.160.14.2101

Dowson, C. A., Kuijer, R. G., & Mulder, R. T. (2004). Anxiety and self-management behaviour in chronic obstructive pulmonary disease: What has been learned? *Chronic Respiratory Disease, 1*(4), 213–220. https://doi.org/10.1191/1479972304cd032rs

Drotar, D., & Bonner, M. S. (2009). Influences on adherence to pediatric asthma treatment: A review of correlates and predictors. *Journal of Developmental and Behavioral Pediatrics, 30*(6), 574–582. https://doi.org/10.1097/DBP.0b013e3181c3c3bb

Elliot, A. J., Thrash, T. M., & Murayama, K. (2011). A longitudinal analysis of self-regulation and well-being: Avoidance personal goals, avoidance coping, stress generation, and subjective well-being. *Journal of Personality, 79*(3), 643–674. https://doi.org/10.1111/j.1467-6494.2011.00694.x

Ferrante, G., & La Grutta, S. (2018). The burden of pediatric asthma. *Frontiers in Pediatrics, 6*, 186. https://doi.org/10.3389/fped.2018.00186

Filigno, S. S., Miller, J., Moore, S., Peugh, J., Weiland, J., Backstrom, J., & Borschuk, A. (2019). Assessing psychosocial risk in pediatric cystic fibrosis.

Flores, G., Bridon, C., Torres, S., Perez, R., Walter, T., Brotanek, J., Lin, H., & Tomany-Korman, S. (2009). Improving asthma outcomes in minority children: A randomized, controlled trial of parent mentors. *Pediatrics, 124*(6), 1522–1532. https://doi.org/10.1542/peds.2009-0230

Frisina, P. G., Borod, J. C., & Lepore, S. J. (2004). A meta-analysis of the effects of written emotional disclosure on the health outcomes of clinical populations. *Journal of Nervous and Mental Disease, 192*(9), 629–634. https://doi.org/10.1097/01.nmd.0000138317.30764.63

Gershon, A. S., Victor, J. C., Guan, J., Aaron, S. D., & To, T. (2012). Pulmonary function testing in the diagnosis of asthma: A population study. *Chest, 141*(5), 1190–1196. https://doi.org/10.1378/chest.11-0831

Goldbeck, L., Fidika, A., Herle, M., & Quittner, A. L. (2014). Psychological interventions for individuals with cystic fibrosis and their families. *Cochrane Database of Systematic Reviews, 2014*(6), CD003148. https://doi.org/10.1002/14651858.CD003148.pub3

Gray, W. N., Netz, M., McConville, A., Fedele, D., Wagoner, S. T., & Schaefer, M. R. (2018). Medication adherence in pediatric asthma: A systematic review of the literature. *Pediatric Pulmonology, 53*(5), 668–684. https://doi.org/10.1002/ppul.23966

Grieve, A. J., Tluczek, A., Racine-Gilles, C. N., Laxova, A., Albers, C. A., & Farrell, P. M. (2011). Associations between academic achievement and psychosocial variables in adolescents with cystic fibrosis. *Journal of School Health, 81*(11), 713–720. https://doi.org/10.1111/j.1746-1561.2011.00648.x

Grimaldi, C., Brémont, F., Berlioz-Baudoin, M., Brouard, J., Corvol, H., Couderc, L., Lezmi, G., Pin, I., Petit, I., Reix, P., Remus, N., Schweitzer, C., Thumerelle, C., & Dubus, J. C. (2015). Sweat test practice in pediatric pulmonology after introduction of cystic fibrosis newborn screening. *European Journal of Pediatrics, 174*(12), 1613–1620. https://doi.org/10.1007/s00431-015-2579-4

Guimbellot, J. S., Baines, A., Paynter, A., Heltshe, S. L., VanDalfsen, J., Jain, M., Rowe, S. M., Sagel, S. D., & the GOAL-e2 Investigators. (2021). Long term clinical effectiveness of ivacaftor in people with the $G_{551}D$ CFTR mutation. *Journal of Cystic Fibrosis, 20*(2), 213–219. https://doi.org/10.1016/j.jcf.2020.11.008

Guo, J., Garratt, A., & Hill, A. (2022). Worldwide rates of diagnosis and effective treatment for cystic fibrosis. *Journal of Cystic Fibrosis, 21*(3), 456–462. https://doi.org/10.1016/j.jcf.2022.01.009

Halfon, N., & Newacheck, P. W. (1993). Childhood asthma and poverty: Differential impacts and utilization of health services. *Pediatrics, 91*(1), 56–61. https://doi.org/10.1542/peds.91.1.56

Hamosh, A., FitzSimmons, S. C., Macek, M., Jr., Knowles, M. R., Rosenstein, B. J., & Cutting, G. R. (1998). Comparison of the clinical manifestations of cystic fibrosis in Black and White patients. *The Journal of Pediatrics, 132*(2), 255–259. https://doi.org/10.1016/S0022-3476(98)70441-X

Harish, Z., Bregante, A. C., Morgan, C., Fann, C. S. J., Callaghan, C. M., Witt, M. A., Levinson, K. A., & Caspe, W. B. (2001). A comprehensive inner-city asthma program reduces hospital and emergency room utilization. *Annals of Allergy, Asthma & Immunology, 86*(2), 185–189. https://doi.org/10.1016/S1081-1206(10)62689-0

Hesselink, A. E., Penninx, B. W. J. H., Schlösser, M. A. G., Wijnhoven, H. A. H., van der Windt, D. A. W. M., Kriegsman, D. M. W., & van Eijk, J. T. M. (2004). The role of coping resources and coping style in quality of life of patients with asthma or COPD. *Quality of Life Research, 13*(2), 509–518. https://doi.org/10.1023/B:QURE.0000018474.14094.2f

Horner, C. C., Mauger, D., Strunk, R. C., Graber, N. J., Lemanske, R. F., Jr., Sorkness, C. A., Szefler, S. J., Zeiger, R. S., Taussig, L. M., & Bacharier, L. B. (2011). Most nocturnal asthma symptoms occur outside of exacerbations and associate with morbidity. *Journal of Allergy and Clinical Immunology, 128*(5), 977–982.e971–972. https://doi.org/10.1016/j.jaci.2011.07.018

Hughes, H. K., Matsui, E. C., Tschudy, M. M., Pollack, C. E., & Keet, C. A. (2017). Pediatric asthma health disparities: Race, hardship, housing, and asthma in a national survey. *Academic Pediatrics, 17*(2), 127–134. https://doi.org/10.1016/j.acap.2016.11.011

Jackson, A. D., & Goss, C. H. (2018). Epidemiology of CF: How registries can be used to advance our understanding of the CF population. *Journal of Cystic Fibrosis, 17*(3), 297–305. https://doi.org/10.1016/j.jcf.2017.11.013

Januska, M. N., Marx, L., Walker, P. A., Berdella, M. N., & Langfelder-Schwind, E. (2020). The *CFTR* variant profile of Hispanic patients with cystic fibrosis: Impact on access to effective screening, diagnosis, and personalized medicine. *Journal of Genetic Counseling, 29*(4), 607–615. https://doi.org/10.1002/jgc4.1271

Jochmann, A., Artusio, L., Jamalzadeh, A., Nagakumar, P., Delgado-Eckert, E., Saglani, S., Bush, A., Frey, U., & Fleming, L. J. (2017).

Electronic monitoring of adherence to inhaled corticosteroids: An essential tool in identifying severe asthma in children. *The European Respiratory Journal*, *50*(6), 1700910. https://doi.org/10.1183/13993003.00910-2017

Johnson, D. P., Arnold, D. H., Gay, J. C., Grisso, A., O'Connor, M. G., O'Kelley, E., & Moore, P. E. (2018). Implementation and improvement of pediatric asthma guideline improves hospital-based care. *Pediatrics*, *141*(2), e20171630. https://doi.org/10.1542/peds.2017-1630

Johnson, K. B., Ravert, R. D., & Everton, A. (2001). Hopkins teen central: Assessment of an internet-based support system for children with cystic fibrosis. *Pediatrics*, *107*(2), e24. https://doi.org/10.1542/peds.107.2.e24

Kaaya, S. F., Blander, J., Antelman, G., Cyprian, F., Emmons, K. M., Matsumoto, K., Chopyak, E., Levine, M., & Smith Fawzi, M. C. (2013). Randomized controlled trial evaluating the effect of an interactive group counseling intervention for HIV-positive women on prenatal depression and disclosure of HIV status. *AIDS Care*, *25*(7), 854–862. https://doi.org/10.1080/09540121.2013.763891

Keet, C. A., Matsui, E. C., McCormack, M. C., & Peng, R. D. (2017). Urban residence, neighborhood poverty, race/ethnicity, and asthma morbidity among children on Medicaid. *The Journal of Allergy and Clinical Immunology*, *140*(3), 822–827. https://doi.org/10.1016/j.jaci.2017.01.036

Kettler, L. J., Sawyer, S. M., Winefield, H. R., & Greville, H. W. (2002). Determinants of adherence in adults with cystic fibrosis. *Thorax*, *57*(5), 459–464. https://doi.org/10.1136/thorax.57.5.459

Kirk, S., & Milnes, L. (2016). An exploration of how young people and parents use online support in the context of living with cystic fibrosis. *Health Expectations*, *19*(2), 309–321. https://doi.org/10.1111/hex.12352

Knight, D. (2005). Beliefs and self-care practices of adolescents with asthma. *Issues in Comprehensive Pediatric Nursing*, *28*(2), 71–81. https://doi.org/10.1080/01460860590950845

Koinis-Mitchell, D., Kopel, S. J., Farrow, M. L., McQuaid, E. L., & Nassau, J. H. (2019). Asthma and academic performance in urban children. *Annals of Allergy, Asthma & Immunology*, *122*(5), 471–477. https://doi.org/10.1016/j.anai.2019.02.030

Koinis-Mitchell, D., Kopel, S. J., Seifer, R., LeBourgeois, M., McQuaid, E. L., Esteban, C. A., Boergers, J., Nassau, J., Farrow, M., Fritz, G. K., & Klein, R. B. (2017). Asthma-related lung function, sleep quality, and sleep duration in urban children. *Sleep Health*, *3*(3), 148–156. https://doi.org/10.1016/j.sleh.2017.03.008

Konstan, M. W., McKone, E. F., Moss, R. B., Marigowda, G., Tian, S., Waltz, D., Huang, X., Lubarsky, B., Rubin, J., Millar, S. J., Pasta, D. J., Mayer-Hamblett, N., Goss, C. H., Morgan, W., & Sawicki, G. S. (2017). Assessment of safety and efficacy of long-term treatment with combination lumacaftor and ivacaftor therapy in patients with cystic fibrosis homozygous for the *F508del-CFTR* mutation (PROGRESS): A phase 3, extension study. *The Lancet Respiratory Medicine*, *5*(2), 107–118. https://doi.org/10.1016/S2213-2600(16)30427-1

Korbel, C. D., Wiebe, D. J., Berg, C. A., & Palmer, D. L. (2007). Gender differences in adherence to Type 1 diabetes management across adolescence: The mediating role of depression. *Children's Health Care*, *36*(1), 83–98. https://doi.org/10.1080/02739610701316936

Kulikova, A., Lopez, J., Antony, A., Khan, D. A., Persaud, D., Tiro, J., Ivleva, E. I., Nakamura, A., Patel, Z., Tipton, S., Lloyd, T., Allen, K., Kaur, S., Owitz, M. S., Pak, R. J., Adragna, M. S., Chankalal, R., Humayun, Q., Lehman, H. K., . . . Brown, E. S. (2021). Multivariate association of child depression and anxiety with asthma outcomes. *The Journal of Allergy and Clinical Immunology: In Practice*, *9*(6), 2399–2405. https://doi.org/10.1016/j.jaip.2021.02.043

Kuruvilla, M. E., Lee, F. E.-H., & Lee, G. B. (2019). Understanding asthma phenotypes, endotypes, and mechanisms of disease. *Clinical Reviews in Allergy & Immunology*, *56*(2), 219–233. https://doi.org/10.1007/s12016-018-8712-1

Lang, C. W., McColley, S. A., Lester, L. A., & Ross, L. F. (2011). Parental understanding of newborn screening for cystic fibrosis after a negative sweat-test. *Pediatrics*, *127*(2), 276–283. https://doi.org/10.1542/peds.2010-2284

Lee, M. O., Sivasankar, S., Pokrajac, N., Smith, C., & Lumba-Brown, A. (2020). Emergency department treatment of asthma in children: A review. *Journal of the American College of Emergency Physicians: Open*, *1*(6), 1552–1561. https://doi.org/10.1002/emp2.12224

LeGrys, V. A. (1996). Sweat testing for the diagnosis of cystic fibrosis: Practical considerations. *The Journal of Pediatrics*, *129*(6), 892–897. https://doi.org/10.1016/S0022-3476(96)70034-3

LeGrys, V. A., Yankaskas, J. R., Quittell, L. M., Marshall, B. C., & Mogayzel, P. J., Jr. (2007). Diagnostic sweat testing: The Cystic Fibrosis Foundation guidelines. *The Journal of Pediatrics*, *151*(1), 85–89. https://doi.org/10.1016/j.jpeds.2007.03.002

Lewin, A. B., Heidgerken, A. D., Geffken, G. R., Williams, L. B., Storch, E. A., Gelfand, K. M., &

Silverstein, J. H. (2006). The relation between family factors and metabolic control: The role of diabetes adherence. *Journal of Pediatric Psychology, 31*(2), 174–183. https://doi.org/10.1093/jpepsy/jsj004

Lim, J. T., Ly, N. P., Willen, S. M., Iwanaga, K., Gibb, E. R., Chan, M., Church, G. D., Neemuchwala, F., & McGarry, M. E. (2022). Food insecurity and mental health during the COVID-19 pandemic in cystic fibrosis households. *Pediatric Pulmonology, 57*(5), 1238–1244. https://doi.org/10.1002/ppul.25850

Lu, K. D., Manoukian, K., Radom-Aizik, S., Cooper, D. M., & Galant, S. P. (2016). Obesity, asthma, and exercise in child and adolescent health. *Pediatric Exercise Science, 28*(2), 264–274. https://doi.org/10.1123/pes.2015-0122

Mainardi, A. S., Harris, D., Rosenthal, A., Redlich, C. A., Hu, B., & Fenick, A. M. (2023). Reducing asthma exacerbations in vulnerable children through a medical-legal partnership. *The Journal of Asthma, 60*(2), 262–269. https://doi.org/10.1080/02770903.2022.2045307

Martinez, A., de la Rosa, R., Mujahid, M., & Thakur, N. (2021). Structural racism and its pathways to asthma and atopic dermatitis. *The Journal of Allergy and Clinical Immunology, 148*(5), 1112–1120. https://doi.org/10.1016/j.jaci.2021.09.020

Maslow, G. R., Haydon, A., McRee, A. L., Ford, C. A., & Halpern, C. T. (2011). Growing up with a chronic illness: Social success, educational/vocational distress. *Journal of Adolescent Health, 49*(2), 206–212. https://doi.org/10.1016/j.jadohealth.2010.12.001

Masoli, M., Fabian, D., Holt, S., Beasley, R., & the Global Initiative for Asthma (GINA) Program. (2004). The global burden of asthma: Executive summary of the GINA Dissemination Committee report. *Allergy, 59*(5), 469–478. https://doi.org/10.1111/j.1398-9995.2004.00526.x

Matsui, E. C., Adamson, A. S., & Peng, R. D. (2019). Time's up to adopt a biopsychosocial model to address racial and ethnic disparities in asthma outcomes. *The Journal of Allergy and Clinical Immunology, 143*(6), 2024–2025. https://doi.org/10.1016/j.jaci.2019.03.015

McBennett, K. A., Davis, P. B., & Konstan, M. W. (2022). Increasing life expectancy in cystic fibrosis: Advances and challenges. *Pediatric Pulmonology, 57*(Suppl. 1), S5–S12. https://doi.org/10.1002/ppul.25733

McDonald, C. M., Christensen, N. K., Lingard, C., Peet, K. A., & Walker, S. (2009). Nutrition knowledge and confidence levels of parents of children with cystic fibrosis. *ICAN: Infant, Child, && Adolescent Nutrition, 1*(6), 325–331. https://doi.org/10.1177/1941406409355192

McHugh, R., Mc Feeters, D., Boyda, D., & O'Neill, S. (2016). Coping styles in adults with cystic fibrosis: Implications for emotional and social quality of life. *Psychology, Health & Medicine, 21*(1), 102–112. https://doi.org/10.1080/13548506.2015.1020317

McQuaid, E. L. (2018). Barriers to medication adherence in asthma: The importance of culture and context. *Annals of Allergy, Asthma & Immunology, 121*(1), 37–42. https://doi.org/10.1016/j.anai.2018.03.024

McQuaid, E. L., Kopel, S. J., & Nassau, J. H. (2001). Behavioral adjustment in children with asthma: A meta-analysis. *Journal of Developmental and Behavioral Pediatrics, 22*(6), 430–439. https://doi.org/10.1097/00004703-200112000-00011

Miller, G. E., & Chen, E. (2006). Life stress and diminished expression of genes encoding glucocorticoid receptor and β_2-adrenergic receptor in children with asthma. *Proceedings of the National Academy of Sciences of the United States of America, 103*(14), 5496–5501. https://doi.org/10.1073/pnas.0506312103

Mitmansgruber, H., Smrekar, U., Rabanser, B., Beck, T., Eder, J., & Ellemunter, H. (2016). Psychological resilience and intolerance of uncertainty in coping with cystic fibrosis. *Journal of Cystic Fibrosis, 15*(5), 689–695. https://doi.org/10.1016/j.jcf.2015.11.011

Modi, A. C., Lim, C. S., Yu, N., Geller, D., Wagner, M. H., & Quittner, A. L. (2006). A multi-method assessment of treatment adherence for children with cystic fibrosis. *Journal of Cystic Fibrosis, 5*(3), 177–185. https://doi.org/10.1016/j.jcf.2006.03.002

Montemayor, K., & Jain, R. (2022). Cystic fibrosis: Highly effective targeted therapeutics and the impact on sex and racial disparities. *The Medical Clinics of North America, 106*(6), 1001–1012. https://doi.org/10.1016/j.mcna.2022.07.005

Moonie, S. A., Sterling, D. A., Figgs, L., & Castro, M. (2006). Asthma status and severity affects missed school days. *The Journal of School Health, 76*(1), 18–24. https://doi.org/10.1111/j.1746-1561.2006.00062.x

Muther, E. F., Butcher, J. L., & Riekert, K. A. (2020). Understanding treatment adherence in cystic fibrosis: Challenges and opportunities. In S. D. Davis, M. Rosenfeld, & J. Chmiel (Eds.), *Cystic fibrosis: A multi-organ system approach* (pp. 449–463). Springer. https://doi.org/10.1007/978-3-030-42382-7_22

Muther, E. F., Polineni, D., & Sawicki, G. S. (2018). Overcoming psychosocial challenges in cystic fibrosis: Promoting resilience. *Pediatric Pulmonology*, 53(S3), S86–S92. https://doi.org/10.1002/ppul.24127

Nardone, A., Neophytou, A. M., Balmes, J., & Thakur, N. (2018). Ambient air pollution and asthma-related outcomes in Children of Color of the USA: A scoping review of literature published between 2013 and 2017. *Current Allergy and Asthma Reports*, 18(5), 29. https://doi.org/10.1007/s11882-018-0782-x

National Heart, Lung, and Blood Institute. (2007). *Expert Panel report 3: Guidelines for the diagnosis and management of asthma.* https://www.nhlbi.nih.gov/sites/default/files/media/docs/EPR-3_Asthma_Full_Report_2007.pdf

National Institutes of Health. (1991, August). *National Asthma Education and Prevention Program, Expert Panel: Guidelines for the diagnosis and management of asthma* [NIH Pub. No. 91-3042]. U.S. Government Printing Office. https://www.nhlbi.nih.gov/health-topics/guidelines-for-diagnosis-management-of-asthma

O'Connor, G. T., Lynch, S. V., Bloomberg, G. R., Kattan, M., Wood, R. A., Gergen, P. J., Jaffee, K. F., Calatroni, A., Bacharier, L. B., Beigelman, A., Sandel, M. T., Johnson, C. C., Faruqi, A., Santee, C., Fujimura, K. E., Fadrosh, D., Boushey, H., Visness, C. M., & Gern, J. E. (2018). Early-life home environment and risk of asthma among inner-city children. *The Journal of Allergy and Clinical Immunology*, 141(4), 1468–1475. https://doi.org/10.1016/j.jaci.2017.06.040

O'Connor, G. T., Quinton, H. B., Kneeland, T., Kahn, R., Lever, T., Maddock, J., Robichaud, P., Detzer, M., & Swartz, D. R. (2003). Median household income and mortality rate in cystic fibrosis. *Pediatrics*, 111(4), e333–e339. https://doi.org/10.1542/peds.111.4.e333

O'Sullivan, B. P., & Freedman, S. D. (2009). Cystic fibrosis. *The Lancet*, 373(9678), 1891–1904. https://doi.org/10.1016/S0140-6736(09)60327-5

Oates, G. R., & Schechter, M. S. (2016). Socioeconomic status and health outcomes: Cystic fibrosis as a model. *Expert Review of Respiratory Medicine*, 10(9), 967–977. https://doi.org/10.1080/17476348.2016.1196140

Ong, T., Schechter, M., Yang, J., Peng, L., Emerson, J., Gibson, R. L., Morgan, W., Rosenfeld, M., & the EPIC Study Group. (2017). Socioeconomic status, smoke exposure, and health outcomes in young children with cystic fibrosis. *Pediatrics*, 139(2), e20162730. https://doi.org/10.1542/peds.2016-2730

Papi, A., Brightling, C., Pedersen, S. E., & Reddel, H. K. (2018). Asthma. *The Lancet*, 391(10122), 783–800. https://doi.org/10.1016/S0140-6736(17)33311-1

Park, C. L. (2007). Religiousness/spirituality and health: A meaning systems perspective. *Journal of Behavioral Medicine*, 30(4), 319–328. https://doi.org/10.1007/s10865-007-9111-x

Paruthi, S., Brooks, L. J., D'Ambrosio, C., Hall, W. A., Kotagal, S., Lloyd, R. M., Malow, B. A., Maski, K., Nichols, C., Quan, S. F., Rosen, C. L., Troester, M. M., & Wise, M. S. (2016). Consensus statement of the American Academy of Sleep Medicine on the recommended amount of sleep for healthy children: Methodology and discussion. *Journal of Clinical Sleep Medicine*, 12(11), 1549–1561. https://doi.org/10.5664/jcsm.6288

Pate, C. A., Zahran, H. S., Qin, X., Johnson, C., Hummelman, E., & Malilay, J. (2021). Asthma surveillance–United States, 2006–2018. *MMWR: Surveillance Summaries*, 70(5), 1–32. https://doi.org/10.15585/mmwr.ss7005a1

Pearce, N., Pekkanen, J., & Beasley, R. (1999). How much asthma is really attributable to atopy? *Thorax*, 54(3), 268–272. https://doi.org/10.1136/thx.54.3.268

Piasecki, B., Stanisławska-Kubiak, M., Strzelecki, W., & Mojs, E. (2017). Attention and memory impairments in pediatric patients with cystic fibrosis and inflammatory bowel disease in comparison to healthy controls. *Journal of Investigative Medicine*, 65(7), 1062–1067. https://doi.org/10.1136/jim-2017-000486

Pique, L., Graham, S., Pearl, M., Kharrazi, M., & Schrijver, I. (2017). Cystic fibrosis newborn screening programs: Implications of the *CFTR* variant spectrum in nonWhite patients. *Genetics in Medicine*, 19(1), 36–44. https://doi.org/10.1038/gim.2016.48

Quittner, A. L., Abbott, J., Georgiopoulos, A. M., Goldbeck, L., Smith, B., Hempstead, S. E., Marshall, B., Sabadosa, K. A., Elborn, S., & the International Committee on Mental Health, & the EPOS Trial Study Group. (2016). International Committee on Mental Health in Cystic Fibrosis: Cystic Fibrosis Foundation and European Cystic Fibrosis Society consensus statements for screening and treating depression and anxiety. *Thorax*, 71(1), 26–34. https://doi.org/10.1136/thoraxjnl-2015-207488

Reiter, J., Breuer, O., Cohen-Cymberknoh, M., Forno, E., & Gileles-Hillel, A. (2022). Sleep in children with cystic fibrosis: More under the covers. *Pediatric Pulmonology*, 57(8), 1944–1951. https://doi.org/10.1002/ppul.25462

Reynolds, N., Mrug, S., Britton, L., Guion, K., Wolfe, K., & Gutierrez, H. (2014). Spiritual coping predicts 5-year health outcomes in adolescents with cystic fibrosis. *Journal of Cystic Fibrosis*, 13(5), 593–600. https://doi.org/10.1016/j.jcf.2014.01.013

Rhee, H., Belyea, M. J., & Brasch, J. (2010). Family support and asthma outcomes in adolescents: Barriers to adherence as a mediator. *Journal of Adolescent Health*, *47*(5), 472–478. https://doi.org/10.1016/j.jadohealth.2010.03.009

Rho, J., Ahn, C., Gao, A., Sawicki, G. S., Keller, A., & Jain, R. (2018). Disparities in mortality of Hispanic patients with cystic fibrosis in the United States. A national and regional cohort study. *American Journal of Respiratory and Critical Care Medicine*, *198*(8), 1055–1063. https://doi.org/10.1164/rccm.201711-2357OC

Saiman, L., Siegel, J. D., LiPuma, J. J., Brown, R. F., Bryson, E. A., Chambers, M. J., Downer, V. S., Fliege, J., Hazle, L. A., Jain, M., Marshall, B. C., O'Malley, C., Pattee, S. R., Potter-Bynoe, G., Reid, S., Robinson, K. A., Sabadosa, K. A., Schmidt, H. J., Tullis, E., . . . Weber, D. J. (2014). Infection prevention and control guideline for cystic fibrosis: 2013 update. *Infection Control & Hospital Epidemiology*, *35*(Suppl. 1), S1–S67. https://doi.org/10.1086/676882

Sanders, M. R., Gravestock, F. M., Wanstall, K., & Dunne, M. (1991). The relationship between children's treatment-related behaviour problems, age and clinical status in cystic fibrosis. *Journal of Paediatrics and Child Health*, *27*(5), 290–294. https://doi.org/10.1111/j.1440-1754.1991.tb02540.x

Santos, P. M., D'Oliveira, A., Jr., Noblat, L. A., Machado, A. S., Noblat, A. C., & Cruz, Á. A. (2008). Predictors of adherence to treatment in patients with severe asthma treated at a referral center in Bahia, Brazil. *Jornal Brasileiro de Pneumologia*, *34*(12), 995–1002. https://doi.org/10.1590/S1806-37132008001200003

Savage, E., Beirne, P. V., Ni Chroinin, M., Duff, A., Fitzgerald, T., & Farrell, D. (2011). Self-management education for cystic fibrosis. *Cochrane Database of Systematic Reviews*, *2011*(7), CD007641. https://doi.org/10.1002/14651858.CD007641.pub2

Savage, E., Beirne, P. V., Ni Chroinin, M., Duff, A., Fitzgerald, T., & Farrell, D. (2014). Self-management education for cystic fibrosis. *Cochrane Database of Systematic Reviews*, *2014*(9), CD007641. https://doi.org/10.1002/14651858.CD007641.pub3

Sawicki, G. S., Heller, K. S., Demars, N., & Robinson, W. M. (2015). Motivating adherence among adolescents with cystic fibrosis: Youth and parent perspectives. *Pediatric Pulmonology*, *50*(2), 127–136. https://doi.org/10.1002/ppul.23017

Sawicki, G. S., Sellers, D. E., & Robinson, W. M. (2009). High treatment burden in adults with cystic fibrosis: Challenges to disease self-management. *Journal of Cystic Fibrosis*, *8*(2), 91–96. https://doi.org/10.1016/j.jcf.2008.09.007

Schechter, M. S., & Margolis, P. A. (1998). Relationship between socioeconomic status and disease severity in cystic fibrosis. *The Journal of Pediatrics*, *132*(2), 260–264. https://doi.org/10.1016/S0022-3476(98)70442-1

Schechter, M. S., McColley, S. A., Silva, S., Haselkorn, T., Konstan, M. W., Wagener, J. S., & the Investigators and Coordinators of the Epidemiologic Study of Cystic Fibrosis and the North American Scientific Advisory Group for ESCF. (2009). Association of socioeconomic status with the use of chronic therapies and healthcare utilization in children with cystic fibrosis. *The Journal of Pediatrics*, *155*(5), 634–639.e4. https://doi.org/10.1016/j.jpeds.2009.04.059

Schechter, M. S., Shelton, B. J., Margolis, P. A., & Fitzsimmons, S. C. (2001). The association of socioeconomic status with outcomes in cystic fibrosis patients in the United States. *American Journal of Respiratory and Critical Care Medicine*, *163*(6), 1331–1337. https://doi.org/10.1164/ajrccm.163.6.9912100

Scheckner, B., Arcoleo, K., & Feldman, J. M. (2015). The effect of parental social support and acculturation on childhood asthma control. *Journal of Asthma*, *52*(6), 606–613. https://doi.org/10.3109/02770903.2014.991969

Schrijver, I., Pique, L., Graham, S., Pearl, M., Cherry, A., & Kharrazi, M. (2016). The spectrum of *CFTR* variants in nonWhite cystic fibrosis patients: Implications for molecular diagnostic testing. *The Journal of Molecular Diagnostics*, *18*(1), 39–50. https://doi.org/10.1016/j.jmoldx.2015.07.005

Scotet, V., L'Hostis, C., & Férec, C. (2020). The changing epidemiology of cystic fibrosis: Incidence, survival and impact of the *CFTR* gene discovery. *Genes*, *11*(6), 589. https://doi.org/10.3390/genes11060589

Serebrisky, D., & Wiznia, A. (2019). Pediatric asthma: A global epidemic. *Annals of Global Health*, *85*(1), 6. https://doi.org/10.5334/aogh.2416

Shakkottai, A., Kidwell, K. M., Townsend, M., & Nasr, S. Z. (2015). A five-year retrospective analysis of adherence in cystic fibrosis. *Pediatric Pulmonology*, *50*(12), 1224–1229. https://doi.org/10.1002/ppul.23307

Sleath, B., Gratie, D., Carpenter, D., Davis, S. A., Lee, C., Loughlin, C. E., Garcia, N., Reuland, D. S., & Tudor, G. (2018). Reported problems and adherence in using asthma medications among adolescents and their caregivers. *The Annals of Pharmacotherapy*, *52*(9), 855–861. https://doi.org/10.1177/1060028018766603

Sloand, E., Butz, A., Rhee, H., Walters, L., Breuninger, K., Pozzo, R. A., Barnes, C. M., Wicks, M. N., &

Tumiel-Berhalter, L. (2021). Influence of social support on asthma self-management in adolescents. *Journal of Asthma*, 58(3), 386–394. https://doi.org/10.1080/02770903.2019.1698601

Smith, B. A., & Wood, B. L. (2007). Psychological factors affecting disease activity in children and adolescents with cystic fibrosis: Medical adherence as a mediator. *Current Opinion in Pediatrics*, 19(5), 553–558. https://doi.org/10.1097/MOP.0b013e3282ef480a

Stempel, H., Federico, M. J., & Szefler, S. J. (2019). Applying a biopsychosocial model to inner city asthma: Recent approaches to address pediatric asthma health disparities. *Paediatric Respiratory Reviews*, 32, 10–15. https://doi.org/10.1016/j.prrv.2019.07.001

Strachan, D. P., Butland, B. K., & Anderson, H. R. (1996). Incidence and prognosis of asthma and wheezing illness from early childhood to age 33 in a national British cohort. *BMJ: British Medical Journal*, 312(7040), 1195–1199. https://doi.org/10.1136/bmj.312.7040.1195

Sullivan, K., & Thakur, N. (2020). Structural and social determinants of health in asthma in developed economies: A scoping review of literature published between 2014 and 2019. *Current Allergy and Asthma Reports*, 20(5), 5. https://doi.org/10.1007/s11882-020-0899-6

Tackett, A. P., Farrow, M., Kopel, S. J., Coutinho, M. T., Koinis-Mitchell, D., & McQuaid, E. L. (2021). Racial/ethnic differences in pediatric asthma management: The importance of asthma knowledge, symptom assessment, and family-provider collaboration. *Journal of Asthma*, 58(10), 1395–1406. https://doi.org/10.1080/02770903.2020.1784191

Tao, D., Xie, L., Wang, T., & Wang, T. (2015). A meta-analysis of the use of electronic reminders for patient adherence to medication in chronic disease care. *Journal of Telemedicine and Telecare*, 21(1), 3–13. https://doi.org/10.1177/1357633X14541041

Thakur, N., Barcelo, N. E., Borrell, L. N., Singh, S., Eng, C., Davis, A., Meade, K., LeNoir, M. A., Avila, P. C., Farber, H. J., Serebrisky, D., Brigino-Buenaventura, E., Rodriguez-Cintron, W., Thyne, S., Rodriguez-Santana, J. R., Sen, S., Bibbins-Domingo, K., & Burchard, E. G. (2017). Perceived discrimination associated with asthma and related outcomes in minority youth: The GALA II and SAGE II studies. *Chest*, 151(4), 804–812. https://doi.org/10.1016/j.chest.2016.11.027

Thakur, N., Oh, S. S., Nguyen, E. A., Martin, M., Roth, L. A., Galanter, J., Gignoux, C. R., Eng, C., Davis, A., Meade, K., LeNoir, M. A., Avila, P. C., Farber, H. J., Serebrisky, D., Brigino-Buenaventura, E., Rodriguez-Cintron, W., Kumar, R., Williams, L. K., Bibbins-Domingo, K., . . . Burchard, E. G. (2013). Socioeconomic status and childhood asthma in urban minority youths. The GALA II and SAGE II studies. *American Journal of Respiratory and Critical Care Medicine*, 188(10), 1202–1209. https://doi.org/10.1164/rccm.201306-1016OC

Ungar, W. J., Hadioonzadeh, A., Najafzadeh, M., Tsao, N. W., Dell, S., & Lynd, L. D. (2015). Parents and adolescents preferences for asthma control: A best-worst scaling choice experiment using an orthogonal main effects design. *BMC Pulmonary Medicine*, 15(1), 146. https://doi.org/10.1186/s12890-015-0141-9

Urman, R., Eckel, S., Deng, H., Berhane, K., Avol, E., Lurmann, F., McConnell, R., & Gilliland, F. (2018). Risk effects of near-roadway pollutants and asthma status on bronchitic symptoms in children. *Environmental Epidemiology*, 2(2), e012. https://doi.org/10.1097/EE9.0000000000000012

VandenBranden, S. L., McMullen, A., Schechter, M. S., Pasta, D. J., Michaelis, R. L., Konstan, M. W., Wagener, J. S., Morgan, W. J., McColley, S. A., & the Investigators and Coordinators of the Epidemiologic Study of Cystic Fibrosis. (2012). Lung function decline from adolescence to young adulthood in cystic fibrosis. *Pediatric Pulmonology*, 47(2), 135–143. https://doi.org/10.1002/ppul.21526

Vangeepuram, N., Galvez, M. P., Teitelbaum, S. L., Brenner, B., & Wolff, M. S. (2012). The association between parental perception of neighborhood safety and asthma diagnosis in ethnic minority urban children. *Journal of Urban Health*, 89(5), 758–768. https://doi.org/10.1007/s11524-012-9679-5

Varni, J. W., Limbers, C. A., & Burwinkle, T. M. (2007). Impaired health-related quality of life in children and adolescents with chronic conditions: A comparative analysis of 10 disease clusters and 33 disease categories/severities utilizing the PedsQL™ 4.0 Generic Core Scales. *Health and Quality of Life Outcomes*, 5(1), 43. https://doi.org/10.1186/1477-7525-5-43

Wallander, J. L., & Varni, J. W. (1992). Adjustment in children with chronic physical disorders: Programmatic research on a disability-stress-coping model. In A. M. La Greca, L. J. Siegel, J. L. Wallander, & C. E. Walker (Eds.), *Stress and coping in child health* (pp. 279–298). Guilford Press.

Warman, K. L., & Silver, E. J. (2018). Are inner-city children with asthma receiving specialty care as recommended in national asthma guidelines? *The Journal of Asthma*, 55(5), 517–524. https://doi.org/10.1080/02770903.2017.1350966

Watts, K. D., Layne, B., Harris, A., & McColley, S. A. (2012). Hispanic infants with cystic fibrosis show low *CFTR* mutation detection rates in the Illinois newborn screening program. *Journal of Genetic Counseling, 21*(5), 671–675. https://doi.org/10.1007/s10897-012-9481-2

Weber, S., Puskar, K. R., & Ren, D. (2010). Relationships between depressive symptoms and perceived social support, self-esteem, & optimism in a sample of rural adolescents. *Issues in Mental Health Nursing, 31*(9), 584–588. https://doi.org/10.3109/01612841003775061

Wildhaber, J., Carroll, W. D., & Brand, P. L. (2012). Global impact of asthma on children and adolescents' daily lives: The room to breathe survey. *Pediatric Pulmonology, 47*(4), 346–357. https://doi.org/10.1002/ppul.21557

World Health Organization. (n.d.). *Social determinants of health*. Retrieved April 20, 2022, from https://www.who.int/health-topics/social-determinants-of-health#tab=tab_1

Yaghoubi, M., Adibi, A., Safari, A., FitzGerald, J. M., & Sadatsafavi, M. (2019). The projected economic and health burden of uncontrolled asthma in the United States. *American Journal of Respiratory and Critical Care Medicine, 200*(9), 1102–1112. https://doi.org/10.1164/rccm.201901-0016OC

Zahran, H. S., Bailey, C. M., Damon, S. A., Garbe, P. L., & Breysse, P. N. (2018). Vital signs: Asthma in children—United States, 2001–2016. *MMWR: Morbidity and Mortality Weekly Report, 67*(5), 149–155. https://doi.org/10.15585/mmwr.mm6705e1

Zindani, G. N., Streetman, D. D., Streetman, D. S., & Nasr, S. Z. (2006). Adherence to treatment in children and adolescent patients with cystic fibrosis. *Journal of Adolescent Health, 38*(1), 13–17. https://doi.org/10.1016/j.jadohealth.2004.09.013

Zobell, J. T., Schwab, E., Collingridge, D. S., Ball, C., Nohavec, R., & Asfour, F. (2017). Impact of pharmacy services on cystic fibrosis medication adherence. *Pediatric Pulmonology, 52*(8), 1006–1012. https://doi.org/10.1002/ppul.23743

Zvereff, V. V., Faruki, H., Edwards, M., & Friedman, K. J. (2014). Cystic fibrosis carrier screening in a North American population. *Genetics in Medicine, 16*(7), 539–546. https://doi.org/10.1038/gim.2013.188

CHAPTER 13

PEDIATRIC AND CONGENITAL HEART DISEASE

Jennifer L. Butcher, Laurel M. Bear, Cheryl L. Brosig Soto, Colette Gramszlo, Erica Sood, and Samantha Butler

Congenital heart disease (CHD) is the most common birth defect, impacting an estimated 1% of live births (10.8 per 1,000; Egbe et al., 2014). CHD involves structural defects in the heart that occur during fetal development and fall along a spectrum ranging from mild defects requiring early monitoring that resolve without intervention (e.g., simple atrial septal defect) to severe lesions requiring surgery in early infancy followed by lifelong cardiac care including medications, subsequent surgeries, close monitoring, and in some cases heart transplant (Egbe et al., 2014). The term *complex CHD* refers to structural defects within the moderate-to-severe categories and is often characterized by the need for cardiac surgery during infancy (e.g., single ventricle defects such as hypoplastic left heart syndrome, tetralogy of Fallot, transposition of the great arteries). Heart disease may also be acquired during childhood (e.g., myocarditis, cardiomyopathy, heart failure, hypertension, syncope). Prenatal detection and advancements in medical and surgical care have contributed to a reduction in mortality, with an estimated 85% of children surviving into adulthood (Marino et al., 2012).

Subsequent to reductions in mortality, there has been increased emphasis placed on reducing morbidity. Currently, neurodevelopmental and psychosocial challenges are the most common burdens of pediatric heart disease through the lifespan. Complex CHD places children at highest risk for developmental sequelae throughout childhood, such as delays in achievement of early motor milestones and executive function deficits in adolescence (Marino et al., 2012). An estimated one-quarter to one-half of children with complex CHD experience some type of neurodevelopmental impairment, ranging from mild to severe, with higher risk among those with CHD of greater complexity and children with comorbid genetic diagnoses (Marino et al., 2012). Additionally, between one-third and one-half of children with complex CHD experience emotional, behavioral, and social challenges (Latal et al., 2009), with impacts on the entire family system (see Volume 1, Chapter 12, this handbook, and Chapter 1, this volume). One-quarter to one-half of parents report symptoms of depression and anxiety and even more experience significant psychological distress (Woolf-King et al., 2017).

Given the risk from complex CHD to the child and family system, the role of developmental experts in research and care of these children is crucial. The current standard of practice from a combined scientific statement from the American Heart Association (AHA) and American Academy

The authors have no known conflicts of interest to disclose.
https://doi.org/10.1037/0000414-013
APA Handbook of Pediatric Psychology, Developmental-Behavioral Pediatrics, and Developmental Science: Vol. 2. Pediatric Psychology and Developmental-Behavioral Pediatrics: Clinical Applications of Developmental Science, P. E. Shah and M. H. Bornstein (Editors-in-Chief)
Copyright © 2025 by the American Psychological Association. All rights reserved.

of Pediatrics (AAP) (see Assessment and Care Coordination section) is for children with complex CHD to undergo routine developmental consultation and evaluation (Marino et al., 2012). Cardiac neurodevelopmental follow-up programs are typically multidisciplinary, with 83% including a pediatric psychologist/neuropsychologist and 48% including a developmental-behavioral pediatrician (Miller et al., 2020).

While much is known about developmental outcomes, more research to understand factors that promote resiliency is greatly needed (Cassidy et al., 2021) with developmental scientists at the forefront of this research. Many individuals with CHD thrive, but greater knowledge of protective factors is needed. Further, better understanding of the role of nonmodifiable factors, such as genetic conditions or in utero neurological injury, would help triage support needs as well as target interventions. Identification, prevention/risk reduction, and intervention for modifiable influences on neurodevelopmental and psychosocial functioning, such as social determinants of health, and family functioning may mitigate risk and help most individuals with CHD achieve optimal functioning. Developmental scientists play a crucial role in cardiac neurodevelopmental research and care given the complex relationships between genetic, neurologic, developmental, and family factors resulting in the need for multispecialty expertise in the care and management of these children throughout childhood.

In this chapter, we present an overview of pediatric congenital heart disease, beginning with epidemiology and pathways associated with risk. We highlight the developmental concerns associated with CHD across the childhood lifespan, and the factors associated with risk, resilience, and health outcomes, including the role of health disparities, as informed by a developmental science framework. We discuss child and family outcomes from infancy to adolescence, and present models of assessment and care coordination, with an emphasis on the role of interdisciplinary care, including the roles of pediatricians, pediatric psychologists, and developmental-behavioral pediatricians. Finally, building on research in developmental science, we conclude with a discussion of interventions to mitigate risks and foster resilience. Resources are also included to support parents and providers caring for children with CHD.

EPIDEMIOLOGY AND FACTORS ASSOCIATED WITH RISK

Neurologic risk from CHD begins in utero; up to 59% of full-term infants with CHD show decreased brain development and brain abnormality preoperatively. Further risk of brain injury occurs during surgery, especially in early life (Khalil et al., 2014). Postsurgical complications also pose risks of neurological injury (Marino et al., 2012) along with environmental risk secondary to the harsh hospital environment that limits parental engagement and touch (Butler et al., 2017). Once children are discharged home, families often lose support services provided in the hospital and may receive suboptimal early intervention services (see Assessment and Care Coordination Section), which are too often tied to the family's socioeconomic environment (Bucholz et al., 2020; Cassidy et al., 2018; see Figure 13.1). As children enter and move through the school system, the common deficits associated with CHD are often underrecognized by the school system, and children may lack proper school supports (Marino et al., 2012). Behavioral and social-emotional challenges may also similarly go underrecognized.

In this chapter, we review what is known about neurodevelopmental and psychosocial risk from CHD across childhood, discuss the role of ecological contexts (family systems, socioeconomic) in mitigating or elevating this risk, and discuss best practices for assessment, care coordination, and interventions to promote resiliency among these children.

NEURODEVELOPMENTAL RISK

Individuals with complex CHD are at significantly increased risk for deficits in the areas of cognition, academic achievement, language, attention,

Demographic Psychosocial
- Socioeconomic status
- Parent education
- Male sex
- Family stress and anxiety

Pre-Operative
- Preterm birth
- Early term birth
- Low birthweight
- Prenatal diagnosis
- Genetics

Peri-Operative
- Brain dysmaturity
- Medical instability
- Cerebral oxygenation
- Acidosis/hematocrit
- Cardiopulmonary bypass time
- Circulatory arrest time
- Anesthesia
- Extracorporeal membrane oxygenation
- Length of hospital stay
- Neurological abnormalities/insults (e.g., stroke, seizures)

Current Cardiac Function
- Oxygen saturation
- Aortic obstruction/atresia
- Oxygen intake during exercise

Developmental & Neuropsychological Outcomes

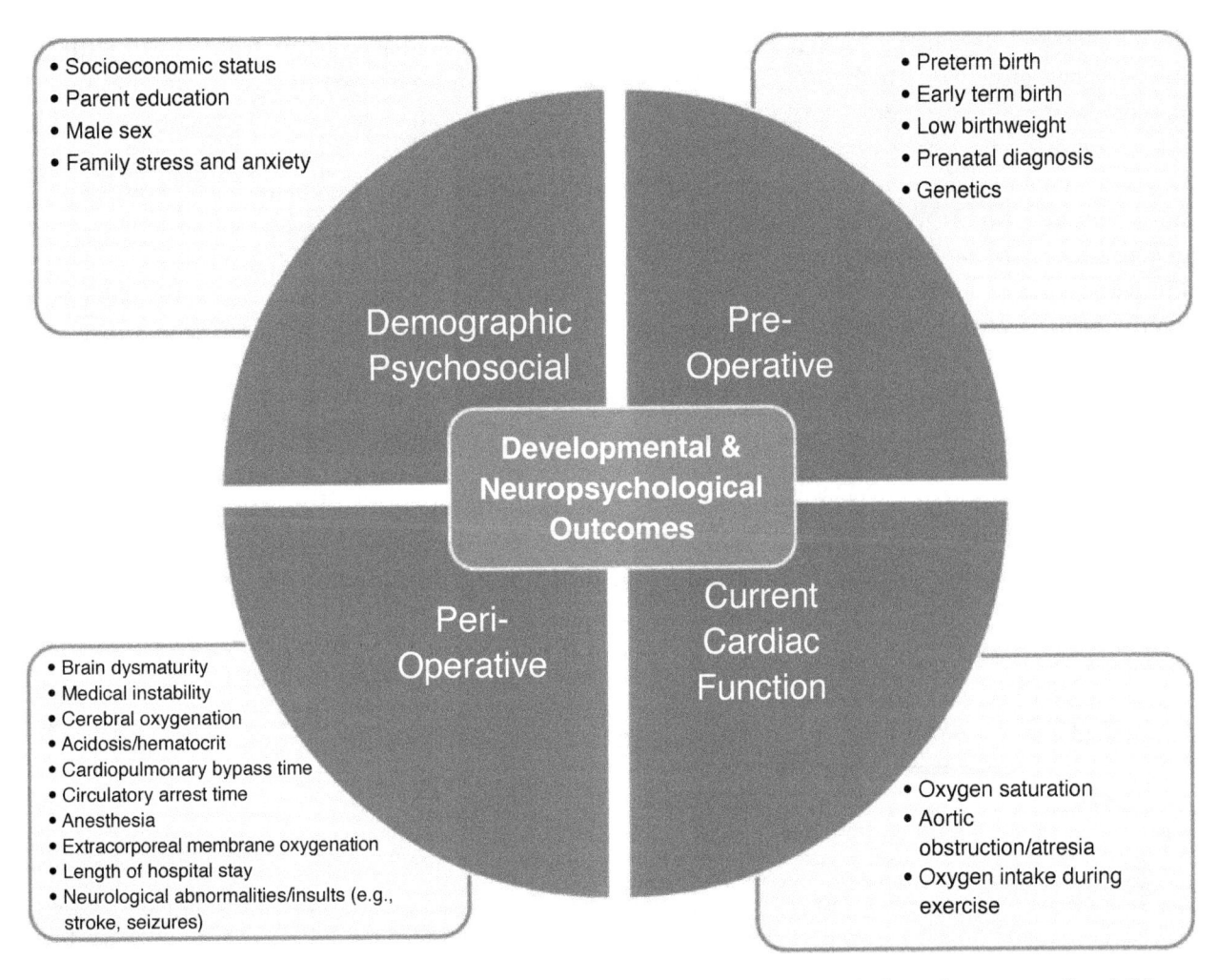

FIGURE 13.1. Factors that affect variability in developmental and neuropsychological outcomes for children and adolescents with CHD. From "Congenital Heart Disease: A Primer for the Pediatric Neuropsychologist," by A. R. Cassidy, D. Ilardi, S. R. Bowen, L. E. Hampton, K. P. Heinrich, M. M. Loman, J. H. Sanz, and K. R. Wolfe, 2018, *Child Neuropsychology*, 24(7), p. 877 (https://doi.org/10.1080/09297049.2017.1373758). Copyright 2018 by Taylor & Francis. Reprinted with permission.

executive functioning, and motor skills compared to the overall population (Marino et al., 2012). Multiple factors impact neurodevelopmental risk, including complexity of the CHD. For example, only a minority of children with single ventricle heart disease avoid neurodevelopmental sequelae (Marino et al., 2012). There is also an increased risk for developmental deficits when CHD is associated with a comorbid medical condition, such as preterm birth or a genetic syndrome. Genetic conditions, which cooccur with cardiac conditions in 30% of individuals, cause significant neurodevelopmental risk (Fahed et al., 2013; Fuller et al., 2009). The most common genetic syndromes associated with both CHD and developmental deficits are Alagille, CHARGE, Downs, 22q11.2 deletion/DiGeorge, Jacobsen deletion, Noonan, Turner, VACTERL, and Williams (Marino et al., 2012; see also Chapter 7, this volume).

Physiological abnormalities noted in the fetal and newborn period are associated with CHD and impact long-term developmental outcomes. It is becoming increasingly evident that placental structure and function is impaired in CHD. Placentas of newborns with CHD are smaller than those without CHD and manifest several vascular abnormalities (Rychik et al., 2018). Placental dysfunction in CHD contributes to decreased fetal cerebral oxygen delivery resulting in poor brain growth, brain abnormalities, and impaired neurodevelopment (Leon et al., 2022). Structural differences are seen in the fetal and newborn brain impacted by CHD, including smaller brain volumes, structural brain abnormalities, and altered brain metabolism (Licht et al., 2004; Limperopoulos et al., 2010). These differences alter ongoing brain development, thus impacting long-term outcomes.

Increased neurodevelopmental risk is also associated with earlier timing of surgery and complications related to surgery and hospitalization that result in an increased number of days in the hospital (Limperopoulos et al., 2002). In addition, neurologic sequelae (e.g., seizures, hypotonia, hypertonia, or stroke) during the preoperative, perioperative, or postoperative periods for infants with CHD are associated with higher risk for long-term developmental deficits (see Figure 13.2; Butler et al., 2022; Wernovsky & Licht, 2016).

Neurodevelopmental Concerns Across Developmental Stages of Childhood

Infancy through preschool. During infancy, individuals with complex CHD have difficulties in calming and state regulation, become easily overwhelmed by social and sensory stimulation, show difficulty establishing organization between their physiologic and behavioral systems (state organization), and require support to settle

Potential Etiologies for Central Nervous System Abnormalities

Prenatal	Preoperative	Intraoperative	Postoperative	Childhood
Genetic Abnormalities	Abnormal Cerebral Vascular Resistance	Embolism	Embolism	Repeat Surgeries
Abnormal Placenta	Decreased Oxygen Delivery	Inadequate Perfusion	Low Cardiac Output	Cardiac Arrest
Abnormal Cerebral Vascular Resistance	Decreased Substrate Delivery	Decreased Oxygen Delivery	Hypoxemia	Total Anesthesia Exposure
Decreased Oxygen Delivery	Increased CMRO$_2$	Decreased Substrate Delivery	Seizures	Total Narcotic Dose
Decreased Substrate Delivery	Birth Asphyxia	Anesthetic Exposure	Hyperventilation/Alkalosis	Total Benzodiazepine Dose
Environmental Exposures		Abnormal Oxygen Consumption	Abnormal Oxygen Consumption	Low Socioeconomic Status
Transitional Circulation		Reperfusion Injury	Dopamine, Narcotics and Benzodiazepines Exposures	Maternal Depression
		Circulatory Arrest	ICU Exposures (Infections, Thrombosis)	Parental Stress
		Regional Cerebral Perfusion		Patient Anxiety/Stress
				Patient Self/Body Image

Potential Neurological and/or Developmental Findings

Prenatal/Birth	Perioperative/ICU	Childhood
Immature Cortical Folding	Increased or New White Matter Injury	Delayed Motor Milestones
White Matter Injury	Seizures	Delay and Apraxia of Speech
Delayed Myelination	Coma	Visual-Motor Difficulties
Hemorrhage	Stroke and Thrombosis	Visual-Spatial Difficulties
Open Operculum	Hemorrhage	Clumsiness
Microcephaly	Poor Brain Growth	Autism Spectrum Disorders
Structural Brain Abnormalities	Abnormal Mental Status	Attention Deficit/Hyperactivity Disorder
	Poor Oral-Motor Coordination	Impaired Memory
		Executive Function Abnormalities
		Anxiety
		Depression
		Diminished Social Cognition

FIGURE 13.2. Potential etiologies for central nervous system abnormalities and potential neurological and/or developmental findings for children and adolescents with congenital heart disease. ICU = intensive care unit. From "Neurodevelopmental Outcomes in Children With Congenital Heart Disease—What Can We Impact?," by G. Wernovsky and D. J. Licht, 2016, *Pediatric Critical Care Medicine, 17*(8 Suppl. 1), p. S234 (https://doi.org/10.1097/PCC.0000000000000800). Copyright © 2016 by Wolters Kluwer Health. Reprinted with permission.

(Butler et al., 2019). Infants with CHD are also noted to withdraw from stimulation and interact less with their environment (Butler et al., 2019).

Challenges in motor functioning, including hypotonia, hypertonia, and asymmetry, are also observed in infancy (Butler et al., 2019). Poor oral-motor skills are common and contribute to difficulties with oral feeding and the need for feeding tube support (Jones et al., 2021). In toddlerhood, neurological concerns continue, and new concerns can be noted in atypical cognitive, language, and motor development (Cassidy et al., 2018). During preschool, children with CHD are at increased risk for deficits in motor and language functioning which contribute to poorer visual-motor skills and slower early academic achievement (Cassidy et al., 2018).

School age and adolescence. At school age, cognitive abilities typically fall in the low-average to mid-average range for intelligence quotient, but lower than expected scores are reported in academic achievement, and there is an increase in need for school-based support services (Cassidy et al., 2018). School-age children with CHD demonstrate difficulties with their attention, activity level, social cognition, and executive functioning, which negatively impact academic achievement (Cassidy et al., 2018). They also demonstrate impairments in their sensorimotor, fine motor, and visual-spatial skills (Bellinger et al., 2003). Adolescents with complex CHD demonstrate similar cognitive concerns and have elevated rates of special education and grade retention (Bellinger et al., 2011).

Practice considerations informed by developmental science. Currently, our knowledge of the risks for neurodevelopmental delay and disability for individuals with CHD outweighs our knowledge of how to mitigate those risks. Environmental factors likely impact development, and it is recommended that children with CHD receive individualized developmental care and family-centered care during hospitalization (Butler et al., 2017; Lisanti et al., 2019). Such care may include inpatient developmental assessment/screening, physical therapy, occupational therapy, feeding therapy, speech and language therapy, child life services, and music therapy to support motor skills, attention, self-regulation, feeding, and sleep. Specific aspects of developmental care, such as skin-to-skin contact, interdisciplinary developmental care rounds, cue-based care, family support, and education for providers, are thought to improve neurodevelopmental outcomes (Butler et al., 2017; Lisanti et al., 2019). The use of breast milk/breast feeding can also support infant growth and oral feeding (Combs & Marino, 1993). In addition, parents of infants born with CHD experience high stress from the time of infant diagnosis through subsequent surgical hospitalizations and beyond (Lisanti et al., 2019). Infants are often separated from parents, thus altering attachment and bonding. Parents experience increased stress, anxiety, and depression, which can negatively influence child functioning (Sood et al., 2021). Concerns for family functioning and the impact on child development highlight the necessity for ongoing family-centered care and support of the family in the inpatient setting. Psychologists, pediatricians, and developmental specialists are integral in providing child developmental support and assessment along with supporting parent behavioral health.

Following AHA and AAP recommendations, many centers have established neurodevelopmental clinics to evaluate and follow children with CHD to support their long term developmental outcomes (Ilardi et al., 2020; Ware et al., 2020). These programs help to facilitate outpatient and school interventions. Early intervention or other forms of outpatient developmental therapy are often recommended for young children with CHD after discharge home (see Assessment and Care Coordination section). Furthermore, children with CHD often require school-based services including within and outside classroom support or full-time special education classrooms (Cassidy et al., 2018).

Methodological Issues in Predicting Developmental Outcomes

Currently, no single diagnostic or treatment characteristic reliably predicts developmental outcomes. Despite intense study, individual and treatment-related factors, such as diagnosis, birth history, and perioperative events, typically account for less than 40% of the variance in developmental outcomes in children with CHD (Tabbutt et al., 2012). Clearly many other factors relate to developmental outcomes, such as environmental supports, family and social supports, and therapy, which can be challenging to control or measure.

In addition, each child with CHD displays different patterns of developmental competencies over time; many neurodevelopmental deficits are not detectable in infancy and only become apparent at school-age and beyond (Cassidy et al., 2018). This is not a failing of developmental assessment tools but reflects neural plasticity in early childhood contributing to compensatory development and neurodevelopmental functions which are not expressed until later childhood. Therefore, children with CHD require ongoing neurodevelopmental evaluations into late adolescence. Despite decades of research evaluating neurodevelopmental interventions for other medical populations, the feasibility and effectiveness of interventions to support long-term development for individuals with CHD are largely unknown. Providers recommend therapeutic services, developmental care, and school-based services with little to no evidence for their positive long-term effects in this population. Overall, more research is needed to understand resilience and optimization of developmental outcomes for individuals with CHD.

Psychosocial Outcomes

Children with CHD are at higher risk for psychosocial problems when compared to those without CHD (Abda et al., 2019). Up to 40% of children with CHD have internalizing (anxiety, depression), externalizing (attention problems, oppositional behavior), and/or social problems (Latal et al., 2009). Impaired quality of life (QoL) has also been reported by children with CHD and their parents (Ladak et al., 2019). However, results are not consistent across studies, outcomes vary by age, and risk and resilience factors impact findings.

Many risk factors are associated with worse psychosocial outcomes and poorer QoL for children and adolescents with CHD. With respect to disease-related factors, which are largely unmodifiable, those with more complex CHD have more emotional and behavioral problems than those with less complex CHD (Dahlawi et al., 2020) as well as more problematic behaviors than those without CHD (Abda et al., 2019). Greater numbers of cardiac procedures and lesion complexity are associated with worse self-reported QoL (Abassi et al., 2020) and higher likelihood of mental illness diagnosis (Khanna et al., 2019). The presence of comorbid medical or genetic conditions that result in physical impairment are also associated with poorer psychosocial outcomes (Clancy et al., 2020; Ferguson & Kovacs, 2013).

Other risk factors that are not related to the disease itself are associated with poorer psychosocial outcomes and worse QoL for children and adolescents with CHD. Mental health problems in those with CHD and their parents and lack of social support are associated with lower QoL for those with CHD (Ferguson & Kovacs, 2013). Notably, these factors are potentially modifiable and may be amenable to intervention.

Psychosocial Concerns Across Developmental Stages of Childhood

Early childhood and school age. In young children with CHD (less than 7 years), the most common finding is emotional and behavioral dysregulation (Clancy et al., 2020). Parents also report lower health-related QoL for young children with CHD compared to those without CHD (Abassi et al., 2020). During school-age, children with CHD are at higher risk for anxiety, depression, withdrawal, and social problems compared to those without CHD (Dahlawi et al., 2020; Gonzalez et al., 2021). Parents of school-age children with CHD rate their children's QoL lower than the children themselves report (Drakouli et al., 2015).

Adolescence. Adolescents with CHD shower higher rates of lifetime psychiatric diagnosis compared to those without CHD, including anxiety disorders, impulse control disorders, and mood disorders (Khanna et al., 2019). They are also more likely to have challenges with social relationships, have lower educational attainment, and have higher rates of unemployment, resulting in an increased likelihood to live with their parents into later adulthood (Kovacs & Bellinger, 2021; see Volume 1, Chapter 16, this handbook). Despite these concerns, adolescents with CHD tend to self-report QoL that is similar or even better than same-aged peers without CHD (Kovacs & Bellinger, 2021).

Practice Considerations Informed by Developmental Science

Because children with CHD are at higher risk for psychosocial problems, screening for these types of problems is recommended as part of standard cardiac care (Marino et al., 2012). Developmental-behavioral pediatricians and pediatric psychologists, with their background in developmental science and understanding of family systems theory, are well-suited to do this type of assessment and are frequently part of multidisciplinary cardiac care teams. Despite a plethora of research that describes the psychosocial problems most often seen in children with CHD and the factors that place children at greater risk, studies investigating resilience factors and effective psychosocial interventions with this population are lacking (Tesson et al., 2019). Although some risk factors are not modifiable (e.g., CHD complexity, presence of genetic conditions), others may be amenable to interventions (e.g., lack of social support, presence of parent mental health problems, stressors in the inpatient environment) and may lead to better psychosocial outcomes. Consideration of ecological contexts, including risk and protective factors within the families and communities where these children reside should be considered when designing interventions (Waller, 2001). Collaboration between the medical team and school is also needed, as school personnel are often unaware of the child's CHD diagnosis and how early medical history may be related to psychosocial concerns present in the school environment.

Methodological Issues in Predicting Psychosocial Outcomes

Research findings are limited by use of single center, cross-sectional designs that utilize different measures to assess similar constructs. Longitudinal studies, qualitative studies, and use of measures that do not rely solely on self-report are needed. Research on interventions that result in improved psychosocial outcomes for the CHD population is lacking. A research agenda and recommendations for psychosocial interventions for individuals has been proposed by the Cardiac Neurodevelopmental Outcome Collaborative (CNOC; Cassidy et al., 2021; see also Assessment and Care Coordination section). Studies are needed that not only focus on risk factors for poor psychosocial outcomes, but also identify factors that promote resilience. Finally, more attention is needed in designing interventions that are acceptable and effective for individuals with CHD of diverse cultural backgrounds who may be less likely to participate in research.

MULTILEVEL (ECOLOGICAL) CONTEXTS ASSOCIATED WITH OUTCOMES IN CONGENITAL HEART DISEASE

Parent Mental Health and Family Functioning

For the most part, children with CHD spend their developing years out of the hospital with their parents, family members, and other social networks. Relationships and interactions within a child's microsystem are known to affect child development, either positively or negatively (Bronfenbrenner, 1977). Consistent with developmental science, studies of children with CHD and their families demonstrate the central role of parental mental health, parenting behaviors, and family functioning for child neurodevelopmental and behavioral outcomes (Sood et al., 2021). Recognition of the need to proactively support parent mental health, parenting, and family functioning following a diagnosis of CHD to promote parent, family, and child well-being has increased substantially (Kasparian et al., 2019; Utens et al., 2018). However, parents and families continue to report critical unmet psychosocial needs throughout their child's medical journey (Sood et al., 2021).

Parent mental health. Parental mental health can be substantially affected by a diagnosis of CHD. Based on a systematic review of mental health symptoms in parents of children with CHD, over 80% of parents report clinically significant symptoms of posttraumatic stress, 30–80% report severe psychological distress, and 25–50% report depression and/or anxiety (Woolf-King et al., 2017). Many parents experience events related to their child's CHD as traumatic, including the initial diagnosis, invasive procedures, and life-threatening complications (McWhorter et al., 2022). Trauma associated with CHD is often chronic, given the lifelong nature of the diagnosis, the likelihood of additional procedures and hospitalizations, and the uncertainty regarding clinical course. Parenting a child with CHD can be emotionally and physically demanding due to feeding challenges, frequent medical appointments, need for medications/close monitoring at home, and financial strain, with high rates of parenting stress reported across studies (Golfenshtein et al., 2017). Most studies include primarily mothers, and therefore, less is known about fathers' stress responses. However, those studies that focus on fathers suggest that they tend to experience the stress of CHD differently from mothers (e.g., stress associated with societal expectations for fatherhood and feeling overlooked as a partner in their child's care) and access different types of support (Hoffman et al., 2020; Sood et al., 2018).

Consistent with research and theory on developmental cascades (Masten & Cicchetti, 2010), mental health symptoms and parenting stress among parents of children with CHD are associated with a range of child outcomes across the lifespan, including emotional and behavioral problems, global psychosocial functioning, neurodevelopment, and QoL. Further, parental mental health has been found to be a stronger predictor of child psychosocial outcomes than medical or surgical factors (DeMaso et al., 2014; McCusker et al., 2013).

Parenting behaviors. Relationships in a microsystem are bidirectional, and parenting behaviors can be affected by child characteristics. The CHD diagnosis and initial interventions often occur during the prenatal and early postnatal periods, a time when parenting styles and parent–child relationships are forming. Infants with CHD are often fragile and physiologically unstable, particularly following cardiac surgery. Parents often witness their infant's oxygen levels drop with distress or discomfort and may be advised to prevent their infant from crying to minimize these desaturations. These early experiences can contribute to parental perceptions of their child as vulnerable. Not surprisingly, overprotective parenting, hypervigilance, and difficulties with limit setting are common among parents of children with CHD and can be further exacerbated by parental mental health challenges (McWhorter et al., 2022). Overprotective parenting mediates the relationship between parental post-traumatic stress and child emotional and behavioral outcomes (McWhorter et al., 2022), suggesting that parenting behaviors may be an important intervention.

Family functioning. Family functioning encompasses many aspects of the family environment including relationships among family members and levels of conflict, cohesion, adaptation, and communication (Sood et al., 2021; see also Volume 1, Chapter 13, this handbook). Families of children with CHD experience significant stressors that can negatively influence family functioning, including physical separation during hospitalization, disruption to family routine and employment, and financial burden. Many families report challenges with communication and increased conflict following a diagnosis of CHD, while others report greater family cohesion, highlighting variability in how families adapt to CHD (Sood et al., 2021).

Parent and family concerns recognized across development. A diagnosis of CHD can affect parents and families in different ways across phases of medical care (e.g., initial diagnosis, hospitalization, transition from hospital to home) and stages of development. Each phase of medical care is associated with unique stressors but also supports that can serve as risks and resiliencies for parents and families. Similarly, risks and resiliencies for parent and family outcomes differ across stages of child development.

Prenatal through infancy. Many parents describe the initial prenatal or postnatal diagnosis as one of the most traumatic experiences associated with their child's CHD (McWhorter et al., 2022) often dividing their life into distinct "before diagnosis" and "after diagnosis" phases. The days and weeks following diagnosis are often characterized by high-stakes medical decisions, commonly within the context of unfamiliar medical terminology. For parents receiving a prenatal diagnosis, their experience of the pregnancy tends to be substantially altered by uncertainty about the prognosis and clinical course and feelings of distress, social isolation, and helplessness (Sood et al., 2022). In the intensive care setting, parents often describe feeling helpless and report significant stress associated with alterations to the traditional parental role (e.g., limited holding, feeding, and challenges to protecting their infant when ill), sights and sounds of the intensive care unit (e.g., tubes and lines, monitors, alarms), and their infant's appearance (Lisanti et al., 2017). Parents are exposed to life-threatening events (e.g., cardiac arrest, cardiopulmonary resuscitation) in their own infant or other infants in the hospital unit. The transition to home is also commonly described as highly stressful as parents adjust to providing independent care for their baby without nursing staff or monitors (March, 2017). Feeding challenges, early developmental challenges, and related therapies can result in substantial parenting stress (Golfenshtein et al., 2017).

Preschool through school age. As children with CHD progress to preschool and school-age, the frequency and intensity of medical care may lessen, although some children require additional surgeries during this time. When parental mental health difficulties resulting from early CHD-related experiences, including traumatic stress, are not addressed, these difficulties may become more distressing as less time and attention are focused on acute medical needs. The preschool and school-age developmental stages are also characterized by neurodevelopmental and academic challenges that introduce new stressors for parents and families who may struggle to access needed services and supports for their child (Williams et al., 2019).

Adolescence. Adolescents with CHD often exhibit difficulties with executive functioning, adaptive skills, anxiety, and depression, which complicate the transition to independent adulthood (Tyagi et al., 2014). They may also lack a comprehensive understanding of their complex medical history, particularly those events that occurred during infancy (Van Deyk et al., 2010). As a result, parents and families may struggle with the balance of promoting autonomy versus protecting their adolescent with CHD and worry about their child's ability to function and care for their health independently (Delaney et al., 2021). This can pose a strain on the family as parents and their maturing child negotiate roles within the context of a complex medical illness.

Practice considerations informed by developmental science. Given the transactional relationships between parent and family well-being and child outcomes, it is important to identify parent and family concerns to provide support and intervention (Utens et al., 2018). The feasibility of implementing formalized psychosocial screening for families affected by CHD has been demonstrated (Sood et al., 2021). However, more work is needed to identify optimal screening tools and time-points that capture risk and opportunities for promotion of child and family well-being.

Methodological issues in predicting parent and family outcomes. Most studies have examined parent mental health and parenting behaviors at a single point in time, providing only a snapshot of how CHD is associated with parenting (Sood et al., 2021). Additionally, most studies examining relations among parent mental health, parenting, and child outcomes use cross-sectional designs, limiting what we know about causal relations and underlying mechanisms. Future longitudinal research is needed to more thoroughly investigate parent mental health over time and its relations to child outcomes. At this time, there is a paucity of research on the risk and resilience factors that predict which parents and families will adapt to the stress of CHD with universal supports and which require targeted interventions and resources to prevent or reduce negative outcomes. Studies examining the impact of psychosocial intervention for paternal mental health, parenting behaviors, and family functioning in CHD are needed. Finally, little is known about the impact of CHD on siblings, who are at risk for decreased family support during hospitalizations and are likely affected by changes to the family dynamic (see Chapter 1, this volume, and Volume 1, Chapter 13, this handbook).

Health Disparities Associated With Outcomes in Congenital Heart Disease

Morbidity and mortality outcomes have improved over the last several decades, but non-Hispanic Black and Hispanic children and their families continue to experience a disproportionate burden of CHD (Lopez et al., 2020). Mortality resulting from CHD has declined almost 40% in the last 20 years; however, this rate of change is significantly greater for non-Hispanic White, as compared to non-Hispanic Black, individuals. Infants with CHD born to Black mothers are at 40% greater mortality risk prior to one year of age as compared to those born to White mothers (Collins et al., 2017). Disparities in access to and quality of care following diagnosis likely account for these trends (Davey et al., 2021; see also Volume 1, Chapter 18, this handbook). Non-Hispanic Black and Hispanic children with CHD are significantly more likely to experience preterm birth (Castellanos et al., 2020), unplanned or emergent hospital readmissions (Peyvandi et al., 2018), and adverse cardiac events (Tillman et al., 2021). Family socioeconomic status also contributes to health disparities for individuals with CHD. Poverty is consistently associated with infant mortality (Kucik et al., 2014), transplant-free survival rates (Tashiro et al., 2014), unplanned readmissions (Lushaj et al., 2020), and length of hospital admissions (Peterson et al., 2017).

For individuals with CHD, disparities in neurodevelopmental outcomes exist as well. Children with CHD, who are already at risk for neurodevelopmental differences, may be particularly impacted by risk factors within the micro (e.g., neighborhood factors) and macro (e.g., social context) systems that surround them (Bronfenbrenner, 1977). Children with CHD who live in neighborhoods with lower average household incomes tend to experience greater motor and cognitive delays; more difficulties with adaptive skills; and worse social, emotional, and behavioral functioning. Gaps in development between the highest and lowest income groups widen as children age (Bucholz et al., 2020). Although an extensive body of literature has identified perioperative factors that impact cardiac neurodevelopmental outcomes (Marino et al., 2012), individual factors, including race and socioeconomic status, have a greater impact on cardiac neurodevelopmental outcomes (Goldberg et al., 2019). Improvement in surgical and related clinical care techniques, although crucial to ensuring survival for those with CHD, may have a limited impact on complex, long-term outcomes such as problem-solving abilities or social skills. The persistence of disparities based on sociodemographic factors points toward inequitable implementation of the clinical care techniques that have contributed to overall improvement in outcomes for children with CHD. Consideration to the social context in which cardiac care is provided is essential for understanding and addressing health disparities (Volume 1, Chapter 18, this handbook).

Social determinants of health contribute to the relation between individual and family characteristics and clinical outcomes for children and adolescents with CHD and are the conditions and structures that surround people through development and daily life that impact health and QoL outcomes (Davey et al., 2021). Social determinants of health impact children with CHD and their families from the time of diagnosis. Families from lower income households are less likely to receive a CHD diagnosis prenatally (Purkey et al., 2019) leaving less time to prepare medically, emotionally, or financially for the birth of a child with complex medical needs. Families that already have access to fewer resources then bear a larger economic burden as they navigate post-surgical hospitalization after the birth of their child with CHD.

Families from lower income households are more likely to experience insurance barriers, difficulty accessing reliable transportation and care for siblings, and housing instability, all of which have been associated with greater morbidity or mortality outcomes for children with CHD (Davey et al., 2021; see also Volume 1, Chapter 24, this handbook). These barriers may prevent family members from spending time at bedside, bonding, and engaging in developmental care during hospitalizations. Separation from parents during the first year of life contributes to autonomic dysregulation in infants with CHD and stress for parents (Lisanti, 2018). Over time, these barriers may inhibit families from adhering to outpatient cardiac care on the recommended schedule. Families with public insurance are at particular risk for missed cardiology appointments (Lu et al., 2017). Without routine care, children with CHD may be vulnerable to experiencing adverse cardiac events and unplanned hospital admissions.

Practice considerations informed by developmental science. Poverty, racism, and other social determinants of health contribute to significant stress for children with CHD and their families (Lisanti, 2018). CHD research has thoroughly documented disparities in health outcomes and now must move toward developing and testing interventions that address these disparities. Although no interventions yet exist, clinical care that considers the unique culture, values, and needs of families is likely to address existing inequities.

Screening for social determinants of health should be a routine and standard part of care in cardiac centers (at prenatal appointments, during planned and unplanned hospital admissions, and regularly during outpatient care) to identify and address resource needs and to reduce barriers to accessing timely cardiac care (Wong et al., 2018). Transitions in care are particularly important opportunities for social determinants of health screening. Screening for social determinants of health during the transition from pediatric to adult care may provide an opportunity to optimize CHD outcomes into adulthood.

Even when controlling for access to care, ethnic disparities in CHD outcomes persist (Oster et al., 2011). Racism is a core social determinant of health and providers should attend to potential cultural bias when selecting assessment measures and interpreting results (Council of National Psychological Associations for the Advancement of Ethnic Minority Interests, 2016). Assessment feedback and education should always be presented in a family's preferred language (Sanz et al., 2021). Finally, providers should adhere to principles of family-centered care and shared decision making (Derrington et al., 2018). Shared decision making, a process during which providers, individuals with CHD, and their families share information and cultural preferences to collaboratively reach consensus, has the potential to build trust between families, share power among parties, and ultimately ensure that children with CHD and their families are valued and respected partners in their cardiac care (Derrington et al., 2018).

Methodological issues associated with health disparities research in congenital heart disease. As is the current state for many disciplines addressing health disparities, research in CHD has primarily focused on documenting disparities. In their framework for addressing disparities in health care settings, Kilbourne and colleagues recommended that research agendas should turn toward (a) understanding the mechanisms driving disparities, and (b) reducing disparities through intervention once disparities have been detected (Kilbourne et al., 2006). Qualitative research methods may be particularly useful for understanding the mediators and moderators that give rise to and maintain inequitable outcomes for children with CHD and their families. Future research should seek to understand individual and family preferences in cardiac care and integrate them into the development of interventions that reduce or eliminate disparities for families based on ethnicity or socioeconomic status.

Assessment and Care Coordination

The AHA's 2012 scientific statement on the evaluation and management of neurodevelopmental outcomes in children with CHD provides the framework for identifying children who are at highest risk for adverse neurodevelopmental outcomes (Marino et al., 2012). CNOC is a

> multicenter, multinational, multidisciplinary inclusive group of health care professionals committed to working together and partnering with families to optimize neurodevelopmental outcomes for individuals with pediatric and congenital heart disease through clinical, quality, and research initiatives, intending to maximize quality of life for every individual across the lifespan. (Marino et al., 2020, para. 1)

They developed recommendations for appropriate identification of evaluation tools based on the understanding that children with CHD who may or may not have been identified in infancy often have deficits that persist as the child matures (Ilardi et al., 2020; Ware et al., 2020). These impairments cross developmental domains and can affect multiple functional abilities. Areas of assessment are focused on those domains that are known to be most impacted in individuals with CHD (see Table 13.1).

There is no standardized program format for following infants with CHD. Program design is often based on the resources available at individual institutions. The programs may be free-standing, but it is not unusual to see them as part of other formalized programs for developmental care such as neonatal intensive care unit follow-up programs, developmental-behavioral clinics, and neuropsychology. There is a variety of providers that may be included in these evaluations including developmental-behavioral pediatricians, pediatric psychologists, cardiologists, neurologists, nursing, and occupational/physical/speech therapists.

Assessment and Care Coordination Across Development: Early Intervention and School-Based Supports

Infancy. Early intervention programs were established by Congress in 1986 as part of the Individuals With Disabilities Education Act (2004). The purpose was to enhance the development of infants and toddlers with disabilities, reduce

TABLE 13.1

Core Neurodevelopmental Assessment Battery by Target Age and Domain

	18–24 months	33–39 months	54–64 months	School age (8–18 years)
Cognition	X	X	X	X
Language	X	X	X	X
Motor	X	X		
Autism/social communication	X	X	X	
Adaptive skills	X	X	X	X
Social-emotional	X	X	X	X
Caregiver mental health	X	X	X	
Attention/behavior		X	X	X
Executive function		X	X	X
Academics			X	X
Memory/learning				X
Visual-motor integration			X	X

educational cost by minimizing the need for special education through intervention, minimize the likelihood of institutionalization and maximize independent living as well as enhance the capacity of families to meet their children's needs. The federal grant program assists states in operating early intervention programs from birth to three years of age. Federal regulations require that providers deliver all services in the child's "natural environment." An individualized family service plan is developed by an interdisciplinary team the includes the child's family. The plan provides a description of outcomes, strategies, supports, and services appropriate to meet the needs of the child and family and the natural environment settings where services will be provided.

Preschool, school-age, and adolescence. For children with complex developmental needs, public school involvement begins when a child turns 3 years of age. This is the transition point from early intervention to the special education services provided through the school system. Initial services are provided through the early childhood program (ages 3–5 years) and then continue as traditional special education services through the age of 21 years if necessary. The individual education program, which is developed with the input of educational specialists (teachers, psychologists) and family members, provides the framework for these services. This process is governed by federal and state laws that oversee parents' and guardians' legal rights.

Practice Considerations Informed by Developmental Science: The Role of the Medical Home and Multidisciplinary Care

The role of the primary care provider is paramount when caring for individuals with CHD. The AAP's 2006 policy statement proposed an algorithm for developmental surveillance and screening in the medical home (Council on Children With Disabilities et al., 2006). They recommend that children diagnosed with a developmental disorder should also be identified with special health care needs, thus initiating chronic condition management. To serve these needs, the primary care provider is required to establish a collaborative relationship with state and local programs, services, and resources for all children with developmental disorders.

In addition to primary care providers, myriad specialists are also involved with the care of children with CHD including psychologists, developmental-behavioral pediatricians, pediatric therapists, dietitians, social workers neurologists, and physiatrists (Miller et al., 2020). Families are first introduced to these professionals at the time of diagnosis, and they may include maternal fetal specialists, neonatologists, cardiologists, geneticists, and psychologists/neuropsychologists. Once the child with CHD requires surgery, the specialist list expands and includes cardiovascular surgeons, intensivists, hospital nursing providers, advanced practice nurses, therapists, child-life specialists, social workers, chaplaincy, and case managers. Throughout, it is important to recognize the central role that the family plays in caring for their child.

The Agency for Healthcare Research and Quality's (AHRQ) mission is to produce evidence to make health care safer, higher quality, more accessible, equitable, and affordable, and to work within the U.S. Department of Health and Human Services and with other partners to make sure that the evidence is understood and used. AHRQ defines *care coordination* as the deliberate organization of care activities between two or more participants (including the individual with chronic illness) involved in care to facilitate the appropriate delivery of health care services. This organized care involves all personnel and other resources that may be needed to engage in all required care activities and includes exchanges of information among all people responsible for the various aspects of care. The coordination of care for the pediatric population is different from that provided for adults. The focus of adult care coordination is chronic disease, whereas the care of children and youth must focus not only on the disease states but the more comprehensive needs of the family, child, and youth. Families must be at the forefront for the identification and development of any plan of care coordination (Antonelli et al., 2009).

RESILIENCE AND INTERVENTION

Knowledge of the obstacles toward optimal neurodevelopmental, psychosocial, and family functioning for individuals with CHD, as discussed previously in this chapter, far exceed our understanding of factors that contribute to resilience and which interventions can help to ameliorate challenges. Despite the challenges, many individuals with CHD thrive. They embody the concept of resilience (or other growth-through-adversity concepts such as grit, hardiness, or post-traumatic growth). *Resilience*, or "adaptation when there is exposure to adversity" is considered a process, or capacity, that develops over time and not an inherent personality trait (Ungar, 2015, p. 1; Volume 1, Chapter 15, this handbook). One theory is that resilience emerges from ordinary processes, or basic human systems, and thus creates the task of understanding how adaptive systems develop, how they operate under diverse conditions, and how they work for or against a given child and family (Masten & Cicchetti, 2010). Key concepts that promote resilience (Newman & Blackburn, 2002) are as follows:

- strong social support networks,
- the presence of at least one unconditionally supportive caregiver,
- a committed mentor or other person from outside the family,
- positive school experiences,
- a sense of mastery and a belief that one's own efforts can make a difference,
- participation in a range of extra-curricular activities that promote self-esteem,
- the capacity to reframe adversities so that the beneficial a well as the damaging effects are recognized,
- the ability/opportunity to make a difference by altruistic activities such as volunteering,
- the desire not to be excessively sheltered from challenging situations that provide opportunities to develop coping skills. (pp. 8–9)

Resilience has been associated with improved health and psychosocial outcomes among the general population (Traub & Boynton-Jarrett, 2017), better self-management for those with chronic illnesses (Sharkey et al., 2018), and lower levels of depressive symptoms for individuals with CHD (Moon et al., 2009). Thus, interventions to support the development of this capacity among those with CHD would be highly beneficial.

To date, research examining ways to directly promote resilience in CHD is limited to one feasibility study (Kovacs et al., 2015). Outcomes of CHD camp-based programs and exercise training programs have demonstrated improvements in components of resilience, but resilience was not directly measured (Cassidy et al., 2021). Promising resilience interventions with other populations, such as youth with cancer (Rosenberg et al., 2018), children with elevated negative affect (Sabin et al., 2023), and children with developmental disabilities (Park et al., 2020), have been developed and may have direct applicability for future resilience interventions in CHD.

Research examining the effects of intervention on neurodevelopmental outcomes in individuals with CHD is lacking (Cassidy et al., 2021). Following preferred reporting items for systematic review and meta-analyses guidelines, Tesson and colleagues completed a systematic review of English-language studies from six electronic databases from their start through 2017 and identified nine unique "Controlled trials evaluating a psychological intervention for people of any age with a pediatric diagnosis (i.e., 0–18 years) of congenital heart disease, an inherited arrhythmia or cardiomyopathy, or their family members" (Tesson et al., 2019, p. 152). They concluded there were significant methodological differences among studies and most trials had a significant risk of bias (89%). Four of these studies included adolescents or adults. Five studies targeted infants and school-aged children and also included parents as intervention targets in recognition of the critical role of parental mental health in successful outcomes for individuals with CHD (Sood et al., 2021). Most studies were delivered in the hospital setting with mothers as the primary participants. They used a variety of intervention approaches (e.g., parenting skills training, promoting parent–infant interaction and bonding, early palliative care involvement). Tested interventions generally demonstrated reductions in maternal anxiety, with mixed evidence for preventing or reducing other parent mental health challenges (e.g., depression) or improving child (e.g., neurodevelopment, feeding) outcomes. Psychosocial interventions delivered during pregnancy to parents who have received a prenatal diagnosis of CHD are also in the process of being tested (Sood et al., 2023).

Kasparian and colleagues completed a systematic review of parent interventions while infants are hospitalized in intensive care units and identified four intervention studies in CHD and one in gastrointestinal disease. Although the overall quality of the studies was variable, reductions were seen in maternal anxiety and improvements were seen in maternal-infant attachment, early infant mental development, and maternal coping, confidence, and satisfaction with medical care (Kasparian et al., 2019).

Phillips and Longoria synthesized the literature on neurodevelopmental interventions in CHD and concluded that, although these interventions are most likely to be provided in early childhood, impairment may not become evident until preschool age or older, and the educational needs of older children with CHD are largely underserved. Their review identified some evidence for executive functioning interventions, family-based interventions for improving child behavioral functioning, mindfulness training for reducing stress in CHD, and the use of stimulant medications for those with comorbid CHD and attention deficit/hyperactivity disorder (ADHD) (Phillips & Longoria, 2020).

Interventions Across Developmental Stages

There is preliminary evidence for infant interventions during hospitalization showing improvements in oral eating, weight gain, length of stay, and physiological regulation (Cassidy et al., 2021). From infancy through early childhood, there is some support for a family program called the Congenital Heart Disease Intervention Project (CHIP) for improving infant functioning at age 6 months (McCusker et al., 2010), and resulting in gains in family functioning and fewer days of missed school among children aged 4–6 (McCusker et al., 2012), but a similar trial found nonsignificant differences between those receiving CHIP and standard care (van der Mheen et al., 2019). In childhood through adolescence, computer-based training (Calderon et al., 2020) and aerobic exercise interventions (Dulfer et al., 2017) show promise in improving specific aspects of cognitive and psychosocial functioning. Among adolescents with CHD, single center interventions (psychotropic medication prescription, having psychologists embedded in cardiology clinic, mindfulness training, and exercise programs) have shown reductions in reports of depression, anxiety, and stress, and improved QoL (Cassidy et al., 2021). To support family functioning, group-based interventions for children with CHD along with their parents, siblings, and other caregivers may improve peer support, social skills, and be an efficient way to engage in preventative care by teaching effective coping strategies (Kovacs et al., 2015). Finally, interventions focused on improving transition between pediatric and adult care are needed (Volume 1, Chapter 16, this handbook). Transition is a high-risk time for care disruptions with 40–60% of individuals with CHD experiencing lapses in medical care during this time (Gurvitz et al., 2013). One single-center, educational-based transition intervention program demonstrated increased knowledge, self-management skills, and medical follow-up, but further study is needed to examine generalizability to other centers (Mackie et al., 2018).

Practice considerations informed by developmental science. Although not in itself a direct intervention, the use of data registries is becoming increasingly common in CHD and can be a useful tool for benchmarking between cardiac neurodevelopment centers, inspiring quality improvement projects as centers learn from each other's successes. In other complex pediatric illnesses, national registries have been the impetus for significant improvements in health and QoL outcomes (Bouchardy et al., 2014; Fink et al., 2017). The National Pediatric Cardiology Quality Improvement Collaborative (Clauss et al., 2015) and CNOC (Marino et al., 2020) are two organizations using registries to track neurodevelopmental outcomes in CHD and beginning work in benchmarking.

Because there are few CHD-specific empirically supported interventions at this time, one strategy is to adapt existing interventions that target the areas of known neurodevelopmental and psychosocial risk to research the CHD population. One population with similar early risk factors are children born very preterm. Individualized developmental care is a promising form of early intervention for improving long-term neurodevelopmental outcomes in children born preterm and has direct applicability to the CHD population (Lisanti et al., 2019). A specific neurodevelopmental care program, the Newborn Individualized Developmental Care and Assessment Program (NIDCAP) is the only evidence-based individualized developmental care program that has demonstrated efficacy in several multi-center, randomized controlled trials (Ohlsson & Jacobs, 2013). Preterm infants who participated in NIDCAP demonstrated faster transition to oral feeding, improved weight gain, shorter hospitalization, and higher infant neurobehavioral functioning compared to the control group. Families receiving NIDCAP also reported decreased parental stress (Ohlsson & Jacobs, 2013). Trauma-informed care is another promising approach for children and families experiencing adverse childhood events, such as hospitalization and surgery, that has applicability to those with CHD (Bargeman et al., 2021).

In neurodevelopmental interventions, early intervention programs have shown evidence for improving outcomes for children who have or are at risk for developmental disabilities in early childhood (Aboud et al., 2018). Empirically supported interventions addressing the mental health and psychosocial risks seen in children with CHD have been developed for the general pediatric population including treatments for ADHD and mood, anxiety, and social skills disorders (Christophersen & Mortweet VanScoyoc, 2013). These treatments could be adapted for individuals with CHD with illness-specific accommodations, such as specific cardiovascular monitoring for medications. Although there are concerns that using ADHD medications in children with CHD poses an increased risk of sudden cardiac death, these medications do not increase the risk of significant adverse cardiovascular events (Pierick et al., 2021). Finally, interventions developed to aid children with other pediatric chronic illnesses to adapt and thrive may be modified for use with individuals with CHD including those addressing coping with a medical illness, adherence to medical care, transition to adult care, and medical trauma (Roberts & Steele, 2017).

Methodological Issues Regarding Intervention Research in Congenital Heart Disease

For children with CHD experiencing adverse neurodevelopmental and psychosocial impacts, interventions have largely been limited to single-center efficacy trials with highly variable methodologies (Cassidy et al., 2021). Additional research is needed to understand the effectiveness of these interventions across the range of individuals with CHD, especially for children with comorbid conditions impacting development, such as genetic diagnoses and neurological injury, and children at higher risk for experiencing health inequities. Additionally, as family functioning is crucial for optimizing child resilience and adaptation, more research into family interventions in CHD is also needed (Sood et al., 2021) as are interventions that include fathers and siblings of children with CHD.

CONCLUSION

Neurodevelopmental risk for individuals with CHD begins in utero with alterations in brain growth and abnormalities in placental functioning, and continues into infancy and beyond with post-surgical complications, environmental concerns, and psychosocial challenges. Identification, prevention/risk reduction, and intervention for modifiable influences may mitigate risk and help individuals with CHD and their families achieve optimal functioning.

Individuals with CHD require ongoing neurodevelopmental evaluations and secondary prevention services, which begin in infancy and continue through adulthood. In addition, families of individuals with CHD require ongoing screening and support. Positively impacting long-term outcomes depends on evidence-based practices, consideration of cultural preferences, and multidimensional community action. Unfortunately, knowledge of the obstacles toward optimal neurodevelopmental, psychosocial, and family functioning for individuals with CHD is much greater than current understanding of factors that contribute to resilience and effective interventions to support long-term development.

Future directions in cardiac neurodevelopmental care include initiating developmental interventions and early access to services, expanding the focus of care to include greater outreach efforts from the fetal period through the balance of development, supporting families, and engaging individuals from all cultural backgrounds and with various medical comorbidities. The field of CHD research must move toward developing and testing interventions that address health disparities, identify opportunities to promote well-being, improve psychosocial outcomes for the CHD population and their families, longitudinally examine parent mental health and its relations to child outcomes, and identify risk and resilience factors for developmental success. A multidisciplinary team of providers including those that service the medical condition along with developmental specialists, developmental behavioral pediatricians, and pediatric psychologists are integral in providing the developmental and family-based support necessary to improve the long-term outcomes and QoL for individuals with CHD and their families.

Taken together, these strategies will move the field of study forward and provide the support needed to help individuals with complex CHD not just survive, but also thrive.

RESOURCES

Professional Resources

- Cardiac Neurodevelopmental Outcomes Collaborative:

  https://cardiacneuro.org/

- Rollins, C. K., & Newburger, J. W. (2014). Neurodevelopmental outcomes in congenital heart disease. *Circulation, 130*(14). https://doi.org/10.1161/CIRCULATIONAHA.114.008556

- Marino, B. S., Lipkin, P. H., Newburger, J. W., Peacock, G., Gerdes, M., Gaynor, J. W., Mussatto, K. A., Uzark, K., Goldberg, C. S., Johnson, W. H., Jr., Li, J., Smith, S. E., Bellinger, D. C., & Mahle, W. T., on behalf of the American Heart Association Congenital Heart Defects Committee of the Council on Cardiovascular Disease in the Young, Council on Cardiovascular Nursing, and Stroke Council. (2012). Neurodevelopmental outcomes in children with congenital heart disease: Evaluation and management: A scientific statement from the American Heart Association. *Circulation, 126*(9), 1143–1172. https://doi.org/10.1161/CIR.0b013e318265ee8a

- Kovacs, A. H., Brouillette, J., Ibeziako, P., Jackson, J. L., Kasparian, N. A., Kim, Y. Y., Livecchi, T., Sillman, C., & Kochilas, L. K., on behalf of the American Heart Association Council on Lifelong Congenital Heart Disease and Heart Health in the Young; and Stroke Council. (2022). Psychological outcomes and interventions for individuals with congenital heart disease: A scientific statement from the American Heart Association. *Circulation: Cardiovascular Quality and Outcomes, 15*(8). https://doi.org/10.1161/HCQ.0000000000000110

- Lisanti, A. J., Uzark, K. C., Harrison, T. M., Peterson, J. K., Butler, S. C., Miller, T. A., Allen, K. Y., Miller, S. P., & Jones, C. E., the American Heart Association Pediatric

Cardiovascular Nursing Committee of the Council on Cardiovascular and Stroke Nursing; Council on Lifelong Congenital Heart Disease and Heart Health in the Young; and Council on Hypertension. (2023). Developmental care for hospitalized infants with complex congenital heart disease: A science advisory from the American Heart Association. *JAHA: Journal of the American Heart Association*, *12*(3). https://doi.org/10.1161/JAHA.122.028489

- The Roadmap Project:
  https://www.roadmapforemotionalhealth.org/
- Pediatric Heart Network:
  https://www.pediatricheartnetwork.org/
- National Pediatric Cardiology Quality Improvement Network:
  https://www.npcqic.org/

Family Resources

- Psychological aspects of living with congenital heart disease: Information for patients and families:
  https://professional.heart.org/-/media/PHD-Files-2/Science-News/p/Psychological-Aspects-of-Congenital-Heart-Disease-Information-for-Patients-and-Families.pdf
- Brosig, C., Butcher, J., Ilardi, D. L., Sananes, R., Sanz, J. H., Sood, E., Struemph, K., & Ware, J. (2014). Supporting development in children with congenital heart disease. *Circulation*, *130*(20). https://doi.org/10.1161/CIRCULATIONAHA.114.010064
- Children's Heart Foundation:
  https://www.childrensheartfoundation.org/
- Conquering CHD:
  https://www.conqueringchd.org/
- Mended Hearts:
  https://mendedhearts.org/
- Sisters by Heart:
  https://www.sistersbyheart.org/

References

Abassi, H., Huguet, H., Picot, M.-C., Vincenti, M., Guillaumont, S., Auer, A., Werner, O., De La Villeon, G., Lavastre, K., Gavotto, A., Auquier, P., & Amedro, P. (2020). Health-related quality of life in children with congenital heart disease aged 5 to 7 years: A multicentre controlled cross-sectional study. *Health and Quality of Life Outcomes*, *18*(1), 366. https://doi.org/10.1186/s12955-020-01615-6

Abda, A., Bolduc, M.-E., Tsimicalis, A., Rennick, J., Vatcher, D., & Brossard-Racine, M. (2019). Psychosocial outcomes of children and adolescents with severe congenital heart defect: A systematic review and meta-analysis. *Journal of Pediatric Psychology*, *44*(4), 463–477. https://doi.org/10.1093/jpepsy/jsy085

Aboud, F. E., Yousafzai, A. K., & Nores, M. (2018). State of the science on implementation research in early child development and future directions. *Annals of the New York Academy of Sciences*, *1419*(1), 264–271. https://doi.org/10.1111/nyas.13722

Antonelli, R., Mcallister, J., & Popp, J. (2009). *Making care coordination a critical component of the pediatric health system: A multidisciplinary framework*. The Commonwealth Fund.

Bargeman, M., Smith, S., & Wekerle, C. (2021). Trauma-informed care as a rights-based "standard of care": A critical review. *Child Abuse & Neglect*, *119*(Pt. 1), 104762. https://doi.org/10.1016/j.chiabu.2020.104762

Bellinger, D. C., Wypij, D., duPlessis, A. J., Rappaport, L. A., Jonas, R. A., Wernovsky, G., & Newburger, J. W. (2003). Neurodevelopmental status at eight years in children with dextro-transposition of the great arteries: The Boston Circulatory Arrest Trial. *The Journal of Thoracic and Cardiovascular Surgery*, *126*(5), 1385–1396. https://doi.org/10.1016/S0022-5223(03)00711-6

Bellinger, D. C., Wypij, D., Rivkin, M. J., DeMaso, D. R., Robertson, R. L., Jr., Dunbar-Masterson, C., Rappaport, L. A., Wernovsky, G., Jonas, R. A., & Newburger, J. W. (2011). Adolescents with d-transposition of the great arteries corrected with the arterial switch procedure: Neuropsychological assessment and structural brain imaging. *Circulation*, *124*(12), 1361–1369. https://doi.org/10.1161/CIRCULATIONAHA.111.026963

Bouchardy, C., Rapiti, E., & Benhamou, S. (2014). Cancer registries can provide evidence-based data to improve quality of care and prevent cancer deaths. *eCancer: Medical Science*, *8*, 413. https://doi.org/10.3332%2Fecancer.2014.413

Bronfenbrenner, U. (1977). Toward an experimental ecology of human development. *American Psychologist*, *32*(7), 513–531. https://doi.org/10.1037/0003-066X.32.7.513

Bucholz, E. M., Sleeper, L. A., Goldberg, C. S., Pasquali, S. K., Anderson, B. R., Gaynor, J. W., Cnota, J. F., & Newburger, J. W. (2020). Socioeconomic status and long-term outcomes in single ventricle heart disease. *Pediatrics, 146*(4), e20201240. https://doi.org/10.1542/peds.2020-1240

Butler, S. C., Huyler, K., Kaza, A., & Rachwal, C. (2017). Filling a significant gap in the cardiac ICU: Implementation of individualised developmental care. *Cardiology in the Young, 27*(9), 1797–1806. https://doi.org/10.1017/S1047951117001469

Butler, S. C., Sadhwani, A., Rofeberg, V., Cassidy, A. R., Singer, J., Calderon, J., Wypij, D., Newburger, J. W., Rollins, C. K., & the Cardiac Neurodevelopmental Program at Boston Children's Hospital Group. (2022). Neurological features in infants with congenital heart disease. *Developmental Medicine & Child Neurology, 64*(6), 762–770. https://doi.org/10.1111/dmcn.15128

Butler, S. C., Sadhwani, A., Stopp, C., Singer, J., Wypij, D., Dunbar-Masterson, C., Ware, J., & Newburger, J. W. (2019). Neurodevelopmental assessment of infants with congenital heart disease in the early postoperative period. *Congenital Heart Disease, 14*(2), 236–245. https://doi.org/10.1111/chd.12686

Calderon, J., Wypij, D., Rofeberg, V., Stopp, C., Roseman, A., Albers, D., Newburger, J. W., & Bellinger, D. C. (2020). Randomized controlled trial of working memory intervention in congenital heart disease. *The Journal of Pediatrics, 227*, 191–198.e3. https://doi.org/10.1016/j.jpeds.2020.08.038

Cassidy, A. R., Butler, S. C., Briend, J., Calderon, J., Casey, F., Crosby, L. E., Fogel, J., Gauthier, N., Raimondi, C., Marino, B. S., Sood, E., & Butcher, J. L. (2021). Neurodevelopmental and psychosocial interventions for individuals with CHD: A research agenda and recommendations from the Cardiac Neurodevelopmental Outcome Collaborative. *Cardiology in the Young, 31*(6), 888–899. https://doi.org/10.1017/S1047951121002158

Cassidy, A. R., Ilardi, D., Bowen, S. R., Hampton, L. E., Heinrich, K. P., Loman, M. M., Sanz, J. H., & Wolfe, K. R. (2018). Congenital heart disease: A primer for the pediatric neuropsychologist. *Child Neuropsychology, 24*(7), 859–902. https://doi.org/10.1080/09297049.2017.1373758

Castellanos, D. A., Lopez, K. N., Salemi, J. L., Shamshirsaz, A. A., Wang, Y., & Morris, S. A. (2020). Trends in preterm delivery among singleton gestations with critical congenital heart disease. *The Journal of Pediatrics, 222*, 28–34.e4. https://doi.org/10.1016/j.jpeds.2020.03.003

Christophersen, E., & Mortweet VanScoyoc, S. (Eds.). (2013). *Treatments that work with children: Empirically supported strategies for managing childhood problems* (2nd ed.). American Psychological Association.

Clancy, T., Jordan, B., de Weerth, C., & Muscara, F. (2020). Early emotional, behavioural and social development of infants and young children with congenital heart disease: A systematic review. *Journal of Clinical Psychology in Medical Settings, 27*(4), 686–703. https://doi.org/10.1007/s10880-019-09651-1

Clauss, S. B., Anderson, J. B., Lannon, C., Lihn, S., Beekman, R. H., Kugler, J. D., & Martin, G. R. (2015). Quality improvement through collaboration: The National Pediatric Quality Improvement Collaborative Initiative. *Current Opinion in Pediatrics, 27*(5), 555–562. https://doi.org/10.1097/MOP.0000000000000263

Collins, J. W., Jr., Soskolne, G., Rankin, K. M., Ibrahim, A., & Matoba, N. (2017). African-American:White disparity in infant mortality due to congenital heart disease. *The Journal of Pediatrics, 181*, 131–136. https://doi.org/10.1016/j.jpeds.2016.10.023

Combs, V. L., & Marino, B. L. (1993). A comparison of growth patterns in breast and bottle-fed infants with congenital heart disease. *Pediatric Nursing, 19*(2), 175–179.

Council of National Psychological Associations for the Advancement of Ethnic Minority Interests. (2016). *Testing and assessment with persons & communities of color.* https://www.apa.org/pi/oema/resources/testing-assessment-monograph.pdf

Council on Children With Disabilities, Section on Developmental Behavioral Pediatrics, Bright Futures Steering Committee, & Medical Home Initiatives for Children With Special Needs Project Advisory Committee. (2006). Identifying infants and young children with developmental disorders in the medical home: An algorithm for developmental surveillance and screening. *Pediatrics, 118*(1), 405–420. https://doi.org/10.1542/peds.2006-1231

Dahlawi, N., Milnes, L. J., & Swallow, V. (2020). Behaviour and emotions of children and young people with congenital heart disease: A literature review. *Journal of Child Health Care, 24*(2), 317–332. https://doi.org/10.1177/1367493519878550

Davey, B., Sinha, R., Lee, J. H., Gauthier, M., & Flores, G. (2021). Social determinants of health and outcomes for children and adults with congenital heart disease: A systematic review. *Pediatric Research, 89*(2), 275–294. https://doi.org/10.1038/s41390-020-01196-6

Delaney, A. E., Qiu, J. M., Lee, C. S., Lyons, K. S., Vessey, J. A., & Fu, M. R. (2021). Parents' perceptions of emerging adults with congenital heart disease: An integrative review of qualitative studies. *Journal of Pediatric Health Care, 35*(4), 362–376. https://doi.org/10.1016/j.pedhc.2020.11.009

DeMaso, D. R., Labella, M., Taylor, G. A., Forbes, P. W., Stopp, C., Bellinger, D. C., Rivkin, M. J., Wypij, D., & Newburger, J. W. (2014). Psychiatric disorders and function in adolescents with d-transposition of the great arteries. *The Journal of Pediatrics, 165*(4), 760–766. https://doi.org/10.1016/j.jpeds.2014.06.029

Derrington, S. F., Paquette, E., & Johnson, K. A. (2018). Cross-cultural interactions and shared decision-making. *Pediatrics, 142*(Suppl. 3), S187–S192. https://doi.org/10.1542/peds.2018-0516J

Drakouli, M., Petsios, K., Giannakopoulou, M., Patiraki, E., Voutoufianaki, I., & Matziou, V. (2015). Determinants of quality of life in children and adolescents with CHD: A systematic review. *Cardiology in the Young, 25*(6), 1027–1036. https://doi.org/10.1017/S1047951115000086

Dulfer, K., Helbing, W. A., & Utens, E. M. W. J. (2017). The influence of exercise training on quality of life and psychosocial functioning in children with congenital heart disease: A review of intervention studies. *Sports, 5*(1), 13. https://doi.org/10.3390/sports5010013

Egbe, A., Uppu, S., Stroustrup, A., Lee, S., Ho, D., & Srivastava, S. (2014). Incidences and sociodemographics of specific congenital heart diseases in the United States of America: An evaluation of hospital discharge diagnoses. *Pediatric Cardiology, 35*(6), 975–982. https://doi.org/10.1007/s00246-014-0884-8

Fahed, A. C., Gelb, B. D., Seidman, J. G., & Seidman, C. E. (2013). Genetics of congenital heart disease: The glass half empty. *Circulation Research, 112*(4), 707–720. https://doi.org/10.1161/CIRCRESAHA.112.300853

Ferguson, M. K., & Kovacs, A. H. (2013). Quality of life in children and young adults with cardiac conditions. *Current Opinion in Cardiology, 28*(2), 115–121. https://doi.org/10.1097/HCO.0b013e32835d7eba

Fink, A. K., Loeffler, D. R., Marshall, B. C., Goss, C. H., & Morgan, W. J. (2017). Data that empower: The success and promise of CF patient registries. *Pediatric Pulmonology, 52*(S48), S44–S51. https://doi.org/10.1002/ppul.23790

Fuller, S., Nord, A. S., Gerdes, M., Wernovsky, G., Jarvik, G. P., Bernbaum, J., Zackai, E., & Gaynor, J. W. (2009). Predictors of impaired neurodevelopmental outcomes at one year of age after infant cardiac surgery. *European Journal of Cardio-Thoracic Surgery, 36*(1), 40–48. https://doi.org/10.1016/j.ejcts.2009.02.047

Goldberg, C. S., Hu, C., Brosig, C., Gaynor, J. W., Mahle, W. T., Miller, T., Mussatto, K. A., Sananes, R., Uzark, K., Trachtenberg, F., Pizarro, C., Pemberton, V. L., Lewis, A. B., Li, J. S., Jacobs, J. P., Cnota, J., Atz, A. M., Lai, W. W., Bellinger, D., Newburger, J. W., & PHN Investigators. (2019). Behavior and quality of life at 6 years for children with hypoplastic left heart syndrome. *Pediatrics, 144*(5), e20191010. https://doi.org/10.1542/peds.2019-1010

Golfenshtein, N., Hanlon, A. L., Deatrick, J. A., & Medoff-Cooper, B. (2017). Parenting stress in parents of infants with congenital heart disease and parents of healthy infants: The first year of life. *Comprehensive Child and Adolescent Nursing, 40*(4), 294–314. https://doi.org/10.1080/24694193.2017.1372532

Gonzalez, V. J., Kimbro, R. T., Cutitta, K. E., Shabosky, J. C., Bilal, M. F., Penny, D. J., & Lopez, K. N. (2021). Mental health disorders in children with congenital heart disease. *Pediatrics, 147*(2), e20201693. https://doi.org/10.1542/peds.2020-1693

Gurvitz, M., Valente, A. M., Broberg, C., Cook, S., Stout, K., Kay, J., Ting, J., Kuehl, K., Earing, M., Webb, G., Houser, L., Opotowsky, A., Harmon, A., Graham, D., Khairy, P., Gianola, A., Verstappen, A., Landzberg, M., & Alliance for Adult Research in Congenital Cardiology (AARCC) and Adult Congenital Heart Association. (2013). Prevalence and predictors of gaps in care among adult congenital heart disease patients: HEART-ACHD (The Health, Education, and Access Research Trial). *Journal of the American College of Cardiology, 61*(21), 2180–2184. https://doi.org/10.1016/j.jacc.2013.02.048

Hoffman, M. F., Karpyn, A., Christofferson, J., Neely, T., McWhorter, L. G., Demianczyk, A. C., James, R., Hafer, J., Kazak, A. E., & Sood, E. (2020). Fathers of children with congenital heart disease: Sources of stress and opportunities for intervention. *Pediatric Critical Care Medicine, 21*(11), e1002–e1009. https://doi.org/10.1097/PCC.0000000000002388

Ilardi, D., Sanz, J. H., Cassidy, A. R., Sananes, R., Rollins, C. K., Ullman Shade, C., Carroll, G., & Bellinger, D. C. (2020). Neurodevelopmental evaluation for school-age children with congenital heart disease: Recommendations from the cardiac neurodevelopmental outcome collaborative. *Cardiology in the Young, 30*(11), 1623–1636. https://doi.org/10.1017/S1047951120003546

Individuals With Disabilities Education Act, 20 U.S.C., § 1400, and (2004).

Jones, C. E., Desai, H., Fogel, J. L., Negrin, K. A., Torzone, A., Willette, S., Fridgen, J. L., Doody, L. R., Morris, K., Engstler, K., Slater, N. L., Medoff-Cooper, B., Smith, J., Harris, B. D., & Butler, S. C. (2021). Disruptions in the development of feeding for infants with congenital heart disease. *Cardiology in the Young, 31*(4), 589–596. https://doi.org/10.1017/S1047951120004382

Kasparian, N. A., Kan, J. M., Sood, E., Wray, J., Pincus, H. A., & Newburger, J. W. (2019). Mental health care for parents of babies with congenital heart disease during intensive care unit admission: Systematic review and statement of best practice. *Early Human Development, 139,* 104837. https://doi.org/10.1016/j.earlhumdev.2019.104837

Khalil, A., Suff, N., Thilaganathan, B., Hurrell, A., Cooper, D., & Carvalho, J. S. (2014). Brain abnormalities and neurodevelopmental delay in congenital heart disease: Systematic review and meta-analysis. *Ultrasound in Obstetrics & Gynecology, 43*(1), 14–24. https://doi.org/10.1002/uog.12526

Khanna, A. D., Duca, L. M., Kay, J. D., Shore, J., Kelly, S. L., & Crume, T. (2019). Prevalence of mental illness in adolescents and adults with congenital heart disease from the Colorado Congenital Heart Defect Surveillance System. *The American Journal of Cardiology, 124*(4), 618–626. https://doi.org/10.1016/j.amjcard.2019.05.023

Kilbourne, A. M., Switzer, G., Hyman, K., Crowley-Matoka, M., & Fine, M. J. (2006). Advancing health disparities research within the health care system: A conceptual framework. *American Journal of Public Health, 96*(12), 2113–2121. https://doi.org/10.2105/AJPH.2005.077628

Kovacs, A. H., Bandyopadhyay, M., Grace, S. L., Kentner, A. C., Nolan, R. P., Silversides, C. K., & Irvine, M. J. (2015). Adult Congenital Heart Disease-Coping And REsilience (ACHD-CARE): Rationale and methodology of a pilot randomized controlled trial. *Contemporary Clinical Trials, 45*(Pt. B), 385–393. https://doi.org/10.1016/j.cct.2015.11.002

Kovacs, A. H., & Bellinger, D. C. (2021). Neurocognitive and psychosocial outcomes in adult congenital heart disease: A lifespan approach. *Heart, 107*(2), 159–167. https://doi.org/10.1136/heartjnl-2016-310862

Kucik, J. E., Nembhard, W. N., Donohue, P., Devine, O., Wang, Y., Minkovitz, C. S., & Burke, T. (2014). Community socioeconomic disadvantage and the survival of infants with congenital heart defects. *American Journal of Public Health, 104*(11), e150–e157. https://doi.org/10.2105/AJPH.2014.302099

Ladak, L. A., Hasan, B. S., Gullick, J., & Gallagher, R. (2019). Health-related quality of life in congenital heart disease surgery in children and young adults: A systematic review and meta-analysis. *Archives of Disease in Childhood, 104*(4), 340–347. https://doi.org/10.1136/archdischild-2017-313653

Latal, B., Helfricht, S., Fischer, J. E., Bauersfeld, U., & Landolt, M. A. (2009). Psychological adjustment and quality of life in children and adolescents following open-heart surgery for congenital heart disease: A systematic review. *BMC Pediatrics, 9*(1), 6. https://doi.org/10.1186/1471-2431-9-6

Leon, R. L., Mir, I. N., Herrera, C. L., Sharma, K., Spong, C. Y., Twickler, D. M., & Chalak, L. F. (2022). Neuroplacentology in congenital heart disease: Placental connections to neurodevelopmental outcomes. *Pediatric Research, 91,* 787–794. https://doi.org/10.1038/s41390-021-01521-7

Licht, D. J., Wang, J., Silvestre, D. W., Nicolson, S. C., Montenegro, L. M., Wernovsky, G., Tabbutt, S., Durning, S. M., Shera, D. M., Gaynor, J. W., Spray, T. L., Clancy, R. R., Zimmerman, R. A., & Detre, J. A. (2004). Preoperative cerebral blood flow is diminished in neonates with severe congenital heart defects. *Journal of Thoracic and Cardiovascular Surgery, 128*(6), 841–849. https://doi.org/10.1016/j.jtcvs.2004.07.022

Limperopoulos, C., Majnemer, A., Shevell, M. I., Rohlicek, C., Rosenblatt, B., Tchervenkov, C., & Darwish, H. Z. (2002). Predictors of developmental disabilities after open heart surgery in young children with congenital heart defects. *The Journal of Pediatrics, 141*(1), 51–58. https://doi.org/10.1067/mpd.2002.125227

Limperopoulos, C., Tworetzky, W., McElhinney, D. B., Newburger, J. W., Brown, D. W., Robertson, R. L., Jr., Guizard, N., McGrath, E., Geva, J., Annese, D., Dunbar-Masterson, C., Trainor, B., Laussen, P. C., & du Plessis, A. J. (2010). Brain volume and metabolism in fetuses with congenital heart disease: Evaluation with quantitative magnetic resonance imaging and spectroscopy. *Circulation, 121*(1), 26–33. https://doi.org/10.1161/CIRCULATIONAHA.109.865568

Lisanti, A. J. (2018). Parental stress and resilience in CHD: A new frontier for health disparities research. *Cardiology in the Young, 28*(9), 1142–1150. https://doi.org/10.1017/S1047951118000963

Lisanti, A. J., Allen, L. R., Kelly, L., & Medoff-Cooper, B. (2017). Maternal stress and anxiety in the pediatric cardiac intensive care unit. *American Journal of Critical Care, 26*(2), 118–125. https://doi.org/10.4037/ajcc2017266

Lisanti, A. J., Vittner, D., Medoff-Cooper, B., Fogel, J., Wernovsky, G., & Butler, S. (2019). Individualized family-centered developmental care: An essential model to address the unique needs of infants with congenital heart disease. *Journal of Cardiovascular Nursing, 34*(1), 85–93. https://doi.org/10.1097/JCN.0000000000000546

Lopez, K. N., Morris, S. A., Sexson Tejtel, S. K., Espaillat, A., & Salemi, J. L. (2020). US mortality attributable to congenital heart disease across the lifespan from 1999 through 2017 exposes persistent racial/ethnic disparities. *Circulation*, *142*(12), 1132–1147. https://doi.org/10.1161/CIRCULATIONAHA.120.046822

Lu, J. C., Lowery, R., Yu, S., Ghadimi Mahani, M., Agarwal, P. P., & Dorfman, A. L. (2017). Predictors of missed appointments in patients referred for congenital or pediatric cardiac magnetic resonance. *Pediatric Radiology*, *47*(8), 911–916. https://doi.org/10.1007/s00247-017-3851-8

Lushaj, E. B., Hermsen, J., Leverson, G., MacLellan-Tobert, S. G., Nelson, K., Amond, K., & Anagnostopoulos, P. V. (2020). Beyond 30 Days: Analysis of unplanned readmissions during the first year following congenital heart surgery. *World Journal for Pediatric & Congenital Heart Surgery*, *11*(2), 177–182. https://doi.org/10.1177/2150135119895212

Mackie, A. S., Rempel, G. R., Kovacs, A. H., Kaufman, M., Rankin, K. N., Jelen, A., Yaskina, M., Sananes, R., Oechslin, E., Dragieva, D., Mustafa, S., Williams, E., Schuh, M., Manlhiot, C., Anthony, S. J., Magill-Evans, J., Nicholas, D., & McCrindle, B. W. (2018). Transition intervention for adolescents with congenital heart disease. *Journal of the American College of Cardiology*, *71*(16), 1768–1777. https://doi.org/10.1016/j.jacc.2018.02.043

March, S. (2017). Parents' perceptions during the transition to home for their child with a congenital heart defect: How can we support families of children with hypoplastic left heart syndrome? *Journal for Specialists in Pediatric Nursing*, *22*(3), e12185. https://doi.org/10.1111/jspn.12185

Marino, B. S., Lipkin, P. H., Newburger, J. W., Peacock, G., Gerdes, M., Gaynor, J. W., Mussatto, K. A., Uzark, K., Goldberg, C. S., Johnson, W. H., Jr., Li, J., Smith, S. E., Bellinger, D. C., Mahle, W. T., & the American Heart Association Congenital Heart Defects Committee, Council on Cardiovascular Disease in the Young, Council on Cardiovascular Nursing, and Stroke Council. (2012). Neurodevelopmental outcomes in children with congenital heart disease: Evaluation and management: A scientific statement from the American Heart Association. *Circulation*, *126*(9), 1143–1172. https://doi.org/10.1161/CIR.0b013e318265ee8a

Marino, B. S., Sood, E., Cassidy, A. R., Miller, T. A., Sanz, J. H., Bellinger, D., Newburger, J., & Goldberg, C. S. (2020). The origins and development of the cardiac neurodevelopment outcome collaborative: Creating innovative clinical, quality improvement, and research opportunities. *Cardiology in the Young*, *30*(11), 1597–1602. https://doi.org/10.1017/S1047951120003510

Masten, A. S., & Cicchetti, D. (2010). Developmental cascades. *Development and Psychopathology*, *22*(3), 491–495. https://doi.org/10.1017/S0954579410000222

McCusker, C. G., Armstrong, M. P., Mullen, M., Doherty, N. N., & Casey, F. A. (2013). A sibling-controlled, prospective study of outcomes at home and school in children with severe congenital heart disease. *Cardiology in the Young*, *23*(4), 507–516. https://doi.org/10.1017/S1047951112001667

McCusker, C. G., Doherty, N. N., Molloy, B., Rooney, N., Mulholland, C., Sands, A., Craig, B., Stewart, M., & Casey, F. (2010). A controlled trial of early interventions to promote maternal adjustment and development in infants born with severe congenital heart disease. *Child: Care, Health and Development*, *36*(1), 110–117. https://doi.org/10.1111/j.1365-2214.2009.01026.x

McCusker, C. G., Doherty, N. N., Molloy, B., Rooney, N., Mulholland, C., Sands, A., Craig, B., Stewart, M., & Casey, F. (2012). A randomized controlled trial of interventions to promote adjustment in children with congenital heart disease entering school and their families. *Journal of Pediatric Psychology*, *37*(10), 1089–1103. https://doi.org/10.1093/jpepsy/jss092

McWhorter, L. G., Christofferson, J., Neely, T., Hildenbrand, A. K., Alderfer, M. A., Randall, A., Kazak, A. E., & Sood, E. (2022). Parental post-traumatic stress, overprotective parenting, and emotional and behavioural problems for children with critical congenital heart disease. *Cardiology in the Young*, *32*(5), 738–745. https://doi.org/10.1017/S1047951121002912

Miller, T. A., Sadhwani, A., Sanz, J., Sood, E., Ilardi, D., Newburger, J. W., Goldberg, C. S., Wypij, D., Gaynor, J. W., & Marino, B. S. (2020). Variations in practice in cardiac neurodevelopmental follow-up programs. *Cardiology in the Young*, *30*(11), 1603–1608. https://doi.org/10.1017/S1047951120003522

Moon, J. R., Huh, J., Kang, I.-S., Park, S. W., Jun, T.-G., & Lee, H. J. (2009). Factors influencing depression in adolescents with congenital heart disease. *Heart & Lung*, *38*(5), 419–426. https://doi.org/10.1016/j.hrtlng.2008.11.005

Newman, T., & Blackburn, S. (2002). *Transitions in the lives of children and young people: Resilience factors.* Interchange 78. https://eric.ed.gov/?id=ED472541

Ohlsson, A., & Jacobs, S. E. (2013). NIDCAP: A systematic review and meta-analyses of randomized controlled trials. *Pediatrics*, *131*(3), e881–e893. https://doi.org/10.1542/peds.2012-2121

Oster, M. E., Strickland, M. J., & Mahle, W. T. (2011). Racial and ethnic disparities in post-operative mortality following congenital heart surgery. *The Journal of Pediatrics, 159*(2), 222–226. https://doi.org/10.1016/j.jpeds.2011.01.060

Park, E. R., Perez, G. K., Millstein, R. A., Luberto, C. M., Traeger, L., Proszynski, J., Chad-Friedman, E., & Kuhlthau, K. A. (2020). A virtual resiliency intervention promoting resiliency for parents of children with learning and attentional disabilities: A randomized pilot trial. *Maternal and Child Health Journal, 24*(1), 39–53. https://doi.org/10.1007/s10995-019-02815-3

Peterson, J. K., Chen, Y., Nguyen, D. V., & Setty, S. P. (2017). Current trends in racial, ethnic, and healthcare disparities associated with pediatric cardiac surgery outcomes. *Congenital Heart Disease, 12*(4), 520–532. https://doi.org/10.1111/chd.12475

Peyvandi, S., Baer, R. J., Moon-Grady, A. J., Oltman, S. P., Chambers, C. D., Norton, M. E., Rajagopal, S., Ryckman, K. K., Jelliffe-Pawlowski, L. L., & Steurer, M. A. (2018). Socioeconomic mediators of racial and ethnic disparities in congenital heart disease outcomes: A population-based study in California. *Journal of the American Heart Association, 7*(20), e010342. https://doi.org/10.1161/JAHA.118.010342

Phillips, J. M., & Longoria, J. N. (2020). Addressing the neurodevelopmental needs of children and adolescents with congenital heart disease: A review of the existing intervention literature. *Child Neuropsychology, 26*(4), 433–459. https://doi.org/10.1080/09297049.2019.1682131

Pierick, A. R., Lynn, M., McCracken, C. M., Oster, M. E., & Iannucci, G. J. (2021). Treatment of attention deficit/hyperactivity disorder in children with CHD. *Cardiology in the Young, 31*(6), 969–972. https://doi.org/10.1017/S1047951120004965

Purkey, N. J., Axelrod, D. M., McElhinney, D. B., Rigdon, J., Qin, F., Desai, M., Shin, A. Y., Chock, V. Y., & Lee, H. C. (2019). Birth location of infants with critical congenital heart disease in California. *Pediatric Cardiology, 40*(2), 310–318. https://doi.org/10.1007/s00246-018-2019-0

Roberts, M., & Steele, R. (2017). *Handbook of pediatric psychology* (5th ed.). Guilford Press.

Rosenberg, A. R., Bradford, M. C., McCauley, E., Curtis, J. R., Wolfe, J., Baker, K. S., & Yi-Frazier, J. P. (2018). Promoting resilience in adolescents and young adults with cancer: Results from the PRISM randomized controlled trial. *Cancer, 124*(19), 3909–3917. https://doi.org/10.1002/cncr.31666

Rychik, J., Goff, D., McKay, E., Mott, A., Tian, Z., Licht, D. J., & Gaynor, J. W. (2018). Characterization of the placenta in the newborn with congenital heart disease: Distinctions based on type of cardiac malformation. *Pediatric Cardiology, 39*(6), 1165–1171. https://doi.org/10.1007/s00246-018-1876-x

Sabin, C., Bowen, A. E., Heberlein, E., Pyle, E., Lund, L., Studts, C. R., Shomaker, L. B., Simon, S. L., & Kaar, J. L. (2023). The impact of a universal mental health intervention on youth with elevated negative affectivity: Building resilience for healthy kids. *Contemporary School Psychology, 27*, 53–60. https://doi.org/10.1007/s40688-021-00388-z

Sanz, J. H., Anixt, J., Bear, L., Basken, A., Beca, J., Marino, B. S., Mussatto, K. A., Nembhard, W. N., Sadhwani, A., Sananes, R., Shekerdemian, L. S., Sood, E., Uzark, K., Willen, E., & Ilardi, D. (2021). Characterisation of neurodevelopmental and psychological outcomes in CHD: A research agenda and recommendations from the Cardiac Neurodevelopmental Outcome Collaborative. *Cardiology in the Young, 31*(6), 876–887. https://doi.org/10.1017/S1047951121002146

Sharkey, C. M., Bakula, D. M., Baraldi, A. N., Perez, M. N., Suorsa, K. I., Chaney, J. M., & Mullins, L. L. (2018). Grit, illness-related distress, and psychosocial outcomes in college students with a chronic medical condition: A path analysis. *Journal of Pediatric Psychology, 43*(5), 552–560. https://doi.org/10.1093/jpepsy/jsx145

Sood, E., Gramszlo, C., Perez Ramirez, A., Braley, K., Butler, S. C., Davis, J. A., Divanovic, A. A., Edwards, L. A., Kasparian, N., Kelly, S. L., Neely, T., Ortinau, C. M., Riegel, E., Shillingford, A. J., & Kazak, A. E. (2022). Partnering with stakeholders to inform the co-design of a psychosocial intervention for prenatally diagnosed congenital heart disease. *Journal of Patient Experience, 9*. https://doi.org/10.1177/23743735221092488

Sood, E., Karpyn, A., Demianczyk, A. C., Ryan, J., Delaplane, E. A., Neely, T., Frazier, A. H., & Kazak, A. E. (2018). Mothers and fathers experience stress of congenital heart disease differently: Recommendations for pediatric critical care. *Pediatric Critical Care Medicine, 19*(7), 626–634. https://doi.org/10.1097/PCC.0000000000001528

Sood, E., Kenowitz, J., Goldberg, S. W., & Butler, S. C. (2023). Normalize-ask-pause-connect: A clinical approach to address the emotional health of pediatric patients with chronic conditions and their families. *The Journal of Pediatrics, 255*, 247–252. https://doi.org/10.1016/j.jpeds.2022.10.019

Sood, E., Lisanti, A. J., Woolf-King, S. E., Wray, J., Kasparian, N., Jackson, E., Gregory, M. R., Lopez, K. N., Marino, B. S., Neely, T., Randall, A., Zyblewski, S. C., & Brosig, C. L. (2021). Parent mental health and family functioning following diagnosis of CHD: A research agenda and recommendations from the Cardiac Neurodevelopmental

Outcome Collaborative. *Cardiology in the Young*, *31*(6), 900–914. https://doi.org/10.1017/S1047951121002134

Tabbutt, S., Gaynor, J. W., & Newburger, J. W. (2012). Neurodevelopmental outcomes after congenital heart surgery and strategies for improvement. *Current Opinion in Cardiology*, *27*(2), 82–91. https://doi.org/10.1097/HCO.0b013e328350197b

Tashiro, J., Wang, B., Sola, J. E., Hogan, A. R., Neville, H. L., & Perez, E. A. (2014). Patent ductus arteriosus ligation in premature infants in the United States. *The Journal of Surgical Research*, *190*(2), 613–622. https://doi.org/10.1016/j.jss.2014.02.003

Tesson, S., Butow, P. N., Sholler, G. F., Sharpe, L., Kovacs, A. H., & Kasparian, N. A. (2019). Psychological interventions for people affected by childhood-onset heart disease: A systematic review. *Health Psychology*, *8*(2), 151–161. https://doi.org/10.1037/hea0000704

Tillman, A. R., Colborn, K. L., Scott, K. A., Davidson, A. J., Khanna, A., Kao, D., McKenzie, L., Ong, T., Rausch, C. M., Duca, L. M., Daley, M. F., Coleman, S., Costa, E., III, Fernie, E., & Crume, T. L. (2021). Associations between socioeconomic context and congenital heart disease related outcomes in adolescents and adults. *The American Journal of Cardiology*, *139*, 105–115. https://doi.org/10.1016/j.amjcard.2020.10.040

Traub, F., & Boynton-Jarrett, R. (2017). Modifiable resilience factors to childhood adversity for clinical pediatric practice. *Pediatrics*, *139*(5), e20162569. https://doi.org/10.1542/peds.2016-2569

Tyagi, M., Austin, K., Stygall, J., Deanfield, J., Cullen, S., & Newman, S. P. (2014). What do we know about cognitive functioning in adult congenital heart disease? *Cardiology in the Young*, *24*(1), 13–19. https://doi.org/10.1017/S1047951113000747

Ungar, M. (2015). Practitioner review: Diagnosing childhood resilience—A systemic approach to the diagnosis of adaptation in adverse social and physical ecologies. *Journal of Child Psychology and Psychiatry*, *56*(1), 4–17. https://doi.org/10.1111/jcpp.12306

Utens, E. M. W. J., Callus, E., Levert, E. M., Groote, K., & Casey, F. (2018). Multidisciplinary family-centred psychosocial care for patients with CHD: Consensus recommendations from the AEPC Psychosocial Working Group. *Cardiology in the Young*, *28*(2), 192–198. https://doi.org/10.1017/S1047951117001378

van der Mheen, M., Meentken, M. G., van Beynum, I. M., van der Ende, J., van Galen, E., Zirar, A., Aendekerk, E. W. C., van den Adel, T. P. L., Bogers, A. J. J. C., McCusker, C. G., Hillegers, M. H. J., Helbing, W. A., & Utens, E. M. W. J. (2019). CHIP-Family intervention to improve the psychosocial well-being of young children with congenital heart disease and their families: Results of a randomised controlled trial. *Cardiology in the Young*, *29*(9), 1172–1182. https://doi.org/10.1017/S1047951119001732

Van Deyk, K., Pelgrims, E., Troost, E., Goossens, E., Budts, W., Gewillig, M., & Moons, P. (2010). Adolescents' understanding of their congenital heart disease on transfer to adult-focused care. *The American Journal of Cardiology*, *106*(12), 1803–1807. https://doi.org/10.1016/j.amjcard.2010.08.020

Waller, M. A. (2001). Resilience in ecosystemic context: Evolution of the concept. *American Journal of Orthopsychiatry*, *71*(3), 290–297. https://doi.org/10.1037/0002-9432.71.3.290

Ware, J., Butcher, J. L., Latal, B., Sadhwani, A., Rollins, C. K., Brosig Soto, C. L., Butler, S. C., Eiler-Sims, P. B., Ullman Shade, C. V., & Wernovsky, G. (2020). Neurodevelopmental evaluation strategies for children with congenital heart disease aged birth through 5 years: Recommendations from the cardiac neurodevelopmental outcome collaborative. *Cardiology in the Young*, *30*(11), 1609–1622. https://doi.org/10.1017/S1047951120003534

Wernovsky, G., & Licht, D. J. (2016). Neurodevelopmental outcomes in children with congenital heart disease—What can we impact? *Pediatric Critical Care*, *17*(8 Suppl. 1), S232–S242. https://doi.org/10.1097/PCC.0000000000000800

Williams, T. S., McDonald, K. P., Roberts, S. D., Chau, V., Seed, M., Miller, S. P., & Sananes, R. (2019). From diagnoses to ongoing journey: Parent experiences following congenital heart disease diagnoses. *Journal of Pediatric Psychology*, *44*(8), 924–936. https://doi.org/10.1093/jpepsy/jsz055

Wong, P., Denburg, A., Dave, M., Levin, L., Morinis, J. O., Suleman, S., Wong, J., Ford-Jones, E., & Moore, A. M. (2018). Early life environment and social determinants of cardiac health in children with congenital heart disease. *Paediatrics & Child Health*, *23*(2), 92–95. https://doi.org/10.1093/pch/pxx146

Woolf-King, S. E., Anger, A., Arnold, E. A., Weiss, S. J., & Teitel, D. (2017). Mental health among parents of children with critical congenital heart defects: A systematic review. *Journal of the American Heart Association*, *6*(2), e004862. https://doi.org/10.1161/JAHA.116.004862

CHAPTER 14

TYPE 1 AND TYPE 2 DIABETES: INTERDISCIPLINARY MANAGEMENT IN PEDIATRIC SETTINGS

Luiza Mali, Gabriela Guevara, and Alan M. Delamater

This chapter focuses on behavioral and psychosocial aspects of diabetes mellitus in children and adolescents, the etiological factors associated with risk, the modifiable factors that can promote resilience and more optimal outcomes across the lifespan, and the role of subspecialists (e.g., pediatric psychologists, developmental-behavioral pediatricians, and child and adolescent psychiatrists) who can help optimize adaptation and outcomes.

Type 1 diabetes (T1D) is diagnosed mostly during childhood or adolescence, while Type 2 diabetes (T2D), a condition historically affecting adults, has increased dramatically in older children and adolescents in association with the rising incidence of obesity in recent years. These two major types of diabetes differ substantially in their clinical presentations, pathophysiology, and medical management (Daneman, 2020). T1D is an autoimmune disorder resulting in an absolute insufficiency of insulin, which requires exogenous insulin administration for survival. T2D is characterized by a relative insufficiency of insulin, along with insulin resistance and glucose intolerance, which is associated with many medical conditions including obesity.

For both T1D and T2D, there are multifactorial risks underlying etiology and pathophysiology. Importantly, optimal adaptation to these chronic diseases requires multilevel supports to address the medical and psychosocial needs of the individual and family across the lifespan. Successful adaptation to these complex diseases is predicated upon an understanding of the ecological contexts contributing to risk and pathophysiology, an awareness of the effects of the diagnosis and disease upon the child and family, and a consideration of the factors to promote medical adherence, behavioral health, and school functioning across the childhood lifespan. Management of diabetes requires input and comanagement by multiple specialties. Typically, pediatric endocrinologists lead an interdisciplinary team consisting of nurses, dietitians, and behavioral health professionals such as pediatric psychologists and/or social workers. Team members often have special training in diabetes education leading to them being recognized as having certification as a diabetes educator. It is important that the team also have access to other subspecialists including developmental-behavioral pediatricians and child and adolescent psychiatrists, particularly to address specific psychiatric disorders that may require medications (such as attention-deficit/hyperactivity disorder [ADHD], depression, and eating disorders). Successful adaptation to living with diabetes should address individual and family factors associated with risk, and identify school,

https://doi.org/10.1037/0000414-014
APA Handbook of Pediatric Psychology, Developmental-Behavioral Pediatrics, and Developmental Science: Vol. 2. Pediatric Psychology and Developmental-Behavioral Pediatrics: Clinical Applications of Developmental Science, P. E. Shah and M. H. Bornstein (Editors-in-Chief)
Copyright © 2025 by the American Psychological Association. All rights reserved.

health, and community resources to promote resilience and a sense of agency for individuals living with this diagnosis.

In this chapter, we discuss research findings concerning the behavioral and psychosocial aspects of diabetes in children and adolescents, first focusing on T1D and then T2D. We will first present the epidemiology of both T1D and T2D and discuss issues associated with health equity and disparities associated with outcomes. Drawing from research in developmental science, we will then use the socioecological framework (Bronfenbrenner, 1979) to review individual psychological factors, family and social, and medical and health system-level factors associated with diabetes management and quality of life in children and adolescents (Delamater & Marrero, 2020). We will then highlight behavioral and psychological sequelae associated with T1D and T2D, and we will discuss risk and resilience factors associated with outcomes. We will address the clinical management of T1D and T2D, including psychosocial screening and assessment, and behavioral and psychosocial interventions, and discuss the roles of pediatric psychologists, developmental-behavioral pediatricians, and child and adolescent psychiatrists in the management of these diseases. We will highlight select evidence-based interventions including individual, family, peer, and group interventions, medical team interventions, and interventions delivered via the internet and other digital technologies. The chapter will conclude with recommendations for clinical practice and future research and include resources for parents and providers.

TYPE 1 DIABETES

T1D is the most common type of diabetes affecting children in the United States (Lawrence et al., 2021) and worldwide. A large observational study of youth under the age of 20 years reported that of those diagnosed with diabetes, 97% below the age of 10, 62% of those aged 10 to 14, and 42% of those aged 15 to 19 had T1D (Dabelea et al., 2014).

Epidemiology and Health Equity

Over the years, the incidence and prevalence of T1D have increased (American Diabetes Association, 2022; Lawrence et al., 2021), with an estimated worldwide prevalence of 1.1 million children and adolescents (International Diabetes Federation, 2019). Prevalence rates differ around the world (Green et al., 2021), with Europe and North America accounting for around half of all cases, and the United States, India, and Brazil being the countries with the highest number (International Diabetes Federation, 2019).

Diabetes disproportionately affects racial/ethnic minorities and groups of lower socioeconomic status (SES; CDC, 2022). Even though T1D still remains more common among the non-Hispanic White subgroup, prevalence has increased in all sex, age, and racial/ethnic subgroups, with the greatest increase in those who are non-Hispanic White and Black (Lawrence et al., 2021). The landmark Diabetes Control and Complications Trial (DCCT Study Group et al., 1993) showed that effective glycemic control in youth and adolescents, as measured by glycosylated hemoglobin A1c (HbA1c), significantly reduced the risk of health complications such as retinopathy, nephropathy, and neuropathy. Despite this knowledge, 30 years later, the translation of these findings into clinical practice remains a challenge. Ethnic minorities with T1D are more likely to develop chronic health complications. Among children with T1D, racial/ethnic minorities and those with lower SES have higher HbA1c levels than their non-Hispanic White and higher SES counterparts (Borschuk & Everhart, 2015), and Black youth are at higher risk for mortality (Saydah et al., 2017), and have higher rates of diabetic ketoacidosis (DKA) and severe hypoglycemia and lower use of technology (Majidi et al., 2021; Willi et al., 2015) compared to their non-Black counterparts.

There is also evidence of racial disparities in regimen adherence, with Black youths having lower levels of adherence than White youths (Auslander et al., 1997). While disparities in regimen adherence may be partially explained by several demographic factors (e.g., single-parent status, lower SES, and less educational attainment), issues related to health equity may also be a contributing factor. Regarding the medical regimen prescribed to children with T1D, there is some evidence suggesting that lower-income ethnic minority children are prescribed intensive insulin regimens less often (Paris et al., 2009; Valenzuela et al., 2011; Willi et al., 2015). Health care provider factors may underlie some of the observed health disparities in pediatric T1D, in which ethnic minority children may receive suboptimal, less culturally competent care (Mironovici et al., 2020).

T1D poses a significant public health problem affecting youth: compared to those diagnosed in adulthood, youth with T1D are more likely to develop earlier complications, comorbidities, and excess mortality, with significant health disparities apparent in minority groups (Lawrence et al., 2021). This also results in considerable economic costs: it was estimated in 2022 that the cost of diabetes (T2D as well as T1D) was $412.9 billion, including $306.6 billion in direct medical costs as well as $106.3 billion in reduced productivity, amounting to about 1 in 4 health care dollars in the United States going for care for people with diabetes (Parker et al., 2024). This represents a 7% increase since 2017 (American Diabetes Association, 2018, 2023). The global costs are also large, with estimates of the economic burden increasing from $1.3 trillion to $2.2 trillion by 2030 (Bommer et al., 2018). Although people with T1D represent approximately 5% of the total population of people with diabetes, the cost of managing T1D is roughly 25% higher per year than the average cost of T2D management, so T1D patients bear a disproportionate burden of direct health care costs (Joish et al., 2020).

Ecological Factors Associated With Type 1 Diabetes: Family, Social, and Medical Factors

There is an extensive literature (c.f., Datye & Jaser, 2020; de Wit et al., 2022) on the important role of multilevel ecological factors (i.e., family, social, medical, and community factors) in the adaptation to and management of T1D and its associated conditions. These factors act independently and interactively to influence individual outcomes (e.g., medication adherence, glycemic control, family function) in children with T1D.

Family factors. An extensive research literature has documented the significant role of family factors in pediatric diabetes management (Butler et al., 2020). Studies spanning the past four decades have documented that optimal regimen adherence and glycemic control are more likely in children with families in which there is cohesion, authoritative parenting, clear responsibilities, and good communication, while worse outcomes are more likely with family conflict and poor communication about diabetes (e.g., Davis et al., 2001; Miller-Johnson et al., 1994). In addition, diabetes-specific stress in the parent–youth relationship, particularly around diet, has been associated with suboptimal glycemic control (Delamater et al., 2013). Greater social support from family members has been associated with better regimen adherence (La Greca et al., 1995), underscoring the importance of parental involvement and monitoring (Ellis et al., 2007).

Collaborative parent–child relationships with shared responsibilities for diabetes management has been associated with both greater levels of regimen adherence and improved emotional functioning in youth (Trojanowski et al., 2021). Parental involvement in their youth's diabetes management throughout adolescence and the use of supportive communication which fosters autonomy has also been associated with beneficial health behaviors and T1D outcomes (Goethals et al., 2017, 2020). Conversely, earlier cessation of parental monitoring and less involvement in their youths' daily diabetes care have been associated with suboptimal diabetes outcomes (Anderson, 2012). Longitudinal research has demonstrated that throughout adolescence, regimen adherence typically declines when parents decrease their monitoring and involvement in their child's diabetes management (King et al., 2014).

Parental stress and adjustment. Psychological distress among parents of children with T1D is common and is greater than in parents whose children do not have diabetes (Van Gampelaere, Luyckx, van der Straaten, et al., 2020). Many parents report psychological distress and difficulty coping with disease management after the diagnosis of T1D in their children (Jaser et al., 2014; Noser et al., 2019), with symptoms in some parents persisting for several years after the diagnosis. While one-third of parents report distress at the time of T1D diagnosis, nearly one in five parents report continued distress up to 4 years after diagnosis (Whittemore et al., 2012). In addition, many parents continue to report significant symptoms of depression and anxiety (74% and 59% respectively) in the month following diagnosis (Streisand et al., 2008), with a notable percentage of parents (24% of mothers and 22% of fathers) reporting significant post-traumatic stress symptoms 6 weeks after diagnosis (Landolt et al., 2002).

A meta-analysis including 19 studies concluded that parental stress is common and is linked with suboptimal diabetes management (Rechenberg, Grey, et al., 2017), and it may also contribute to child behavioral adjustment difficulties (Lohan et al., 2017). Parental stress and anxiety have been associated with maladaptive parent–child interactions during mealtime in school-age children, with implications for glycemic control in their children with T1D (Van Gampelaere, Luyckx, Goethals, et al., 2020). Psychological maladjustment of fathers predicted suboptimal glycemic control in children 5 years after diagnosis (Forsander et al., 1998), and avoidant coping in fathers was related to increased parenting stress when they were more involved in diabetes management (Teasdale & Limbers, 2018). Fear of hypoglycemia is a common issue for parents (Barnard et al., 2010) and has been associated with emotional distress and suboptimal glycemic control in children (Haugstvedt et al., 2010). Taken together, converging evidence suggests that providing psychological support to parents after the diagnosis of T1D in their child is an important step to help parents more effectively manage their child's diabetes (Sullivan-Bolyai et al., 2010). Potential targets for intervention can include enhancing social support and teaching mindfulness techniques to parents. Greater social support has been associated with less stress in parents of children with recent diagnosis of T1D (Wang et al., 2021), and strategies to promote mindfulness have been shown to reduce parents' stress related to their child's diabetes (Van Gampelaere et al., 2019).

Social factors: Family and peer social support. Emotional support from family and peers is especially important for youth with T1D (Wysocki & Greco, 2006). The support of friends is important to youths' psychological well-being, and complements the support provided by parents (Raymaekers et al., 2017). Conflict in peer relationships is thought to have adverse effects on youths' diabetes management (Palladino & Helgeson, 2012), although the role of peer relationships and diabetes outcomes is still relatively understudied and is an area in need of further research (Van Vleet & Helgeson, 2020).

Medical system factors: Interdisciplinary and integrated health care. Professional organizations such as the International Society for Pediatric and Adolescent Diabetes (ISPAD) have long recommended that optimal care for T1D in children and adolescents be delivered by interdisciplinary teams of health care professionals (Delamater et al., 2018; de Wit et al., 2022). Such teams are composed of pediatric endocrinologists, nurses and certified diabetes educators, dietitians, and mental health professionals including psychologists and social workers, as well as access to child psychiatrists when clinically indicated (Delamater, 2012; Thompson et al., 2012). The ISPAD consensus guidelines for psychological care of children and adolescents with T1D specifically state that psychosocial care should be integrated with collaborative person-centered medical care and that mental and behavioral health professionals should be included in the health care team and be available to interact with youth and families at clinic visits to conduct psychosocial screenings and deliver psychosocial interventions as needed (de Wit et al., 2022).

Despite the importance of these recommendations, an international survey of physicians caring for pediatric patients with T1D found that mental health professionals participated in routine clinical care as part of interdisciplinary teams in only 43% of clinics, and 30% of treatment teams reported that they did not have access to mental health professionals (de Wit et al., 2014). Relatedly, the results of a survey of Dutch youth with T1D revealed that only 28% of patients who had significant depression reported receiving any psychological services (de Wit & Snoek, 2011), suggesting that access to integrated care models is an important context associated with T1D outcomes. Studies have also shown that problems with metabolic control are more likely in children with infrequent and irregular visits with the health care team (Jacobson et al., 1997; Kaufman et al., 1999). Therefore, regular contact with the health care team is essential for youth with T1D, as the interdisciplinary team has the potential to recognize diabetes management problems and provide appropriate interventions before complications develop.

Successful applications of collaborative care based on the chronic disease model have been reported in pediatric primary care settings (Campo et al., 2015), resulting in improved outcomes for behavioral problems and depression (Kolko et al., 2014). Pediatric psychologists have increasingly been recognized as essential members of interdisciplinary health care teams (McDaniel & deGruy, 2014) and play an important role in addressing the behavioral and psychosocial factors that are so integral to effective diabetes management. Findings from a meta-analysis of 31 randomized controlled trials demonstrated that the integration of behavioral health specialists, not only in primary care but also in the care of youth with chronic health conditions (Kolko & Perrin, 2014), has been associated with improved mental health outcomes for children and adolescents experiencing depression, anxiety, and behavioral problems compared to pediatric primary care alone (Asarnow et al., 2015).

Integrated care models involving pediatric psychologists within the interdisciplinary health care team have also been associated with better subsequent glycemic control for T1D patients, as well as reduced health care costs (Caccavale et al., 2020). Despite these benefits, there are many structural, economic and policy barriers to providing integrated care (Delamater, Guzman, et al., 2017), although medical system-based care for T1D in youth is increasingly adopting the chronic care model to improve health outcomes using quality improvement methods and should be considered in future directions for care delivery for T1D (Corathers et al., 2015).

Behavioral and Psychological Sequelae Associated With Type 1 Diabetes

Research has focused on psychological and psychiatric disorders and the impact of these conditions on diabetes management, as well as specific psychological sequelae such as diabetes-related distress, stress and coping styles, executive functioning, neurocognitive functioning, stigma, and bullying. There is evidence that children and adolescents with T1D have greater rates of depression, anxiety, and eating disorders than their peers without chronic health conditions (Butwicka et al., 2015; Datye & Jaser, 2020). The psychological and behavioral morbidities associated with T1D underscore the importance of interdisciplinary care, and the role of behavioral health providers (e.g., pediatric psychologists, developmental-behavioral pediatricians, and other mental health professionals) to optimize psychological outcomes.

Depression. Depression is associated with suboptimal glycemic control and increased diabetes-related hospitalizations (Lawrence et al., 2006), as well as less frequent blood glucose monitoring (Hood et al., 2006). The results of a meta-analysis showed that depression was associated with lower levels of regimen adherence (Kongkaew et al., 2014). Depression has also been shown in prospective studies to predict less frequent blood glucose monitoring, lower quality of life, and suboptimal glycemic control

(Hilliard et al., 2013). Anxiety, which often co-occurs with depression, has also been shown to have adverse effects on self-management behaviors, glycemic control, and quality of life (Buchberger et al., 2016; Galler et al., 2021; Nguyen et al., 2021).

Stress, coping, and adaptation. "Diabetes distress" is a term that describes the emotional response to living with and managing the demands of T1D, and is very common in adolescents with T1D, with about one-third of patients experiencing elevated levels of HbA1c (Hagger et al., 2016). High distress may have adverse effects on regimen adherence and glycemic control and can persist over time (Iturralde et al., 2019). General life stress has also been examined in and is commonly reported in youth with T1D, especially in coping with the everyday demands of self-management, dealing with emotions, diabetes-related family conflict, and relationships with peers (Chao et al., 2016; Rechenberg, Whittemore, et al., 2017). Studies have found associations between greater life stress and diabetes-specific stress with suboptimal glycemic control (Delamater et al., 2013; Helgeson et al., 2010). Research has shown that maladaptive avoidant coping can undermine effective self-management and glycemic control, while adaptive coping with self-efficacy and resilience can promote better diabetes management and glycemic control (Iturralde, Weissberg-Benchell, et al., 2017; Jaser et al., 2017; Yi-Frazier et al., 2015).

Eating disorders. Rates of disordered eating behaviors and diagnosed eating disorders are greater in youth with T1D than in peers without T1D (Young et al., 2013), with studies indicating that up to 10% of youth with T1D have an eating disorder (Butwicka et al., 2015). Disordered eating behaviors such as dietary restriction and insulin omission are more common than eating disorders, with about 40% of girls and up to 20% of boys affected. Insulin omission is often associated with intentions to control weight, especially in girls (Broadley et al., 2020). The SEARCH study found 21.2% of youth with T1D reported disordered eating behaviors, which were associated with greater depression, lower quality of life, and more frequent episodes of DKA (Nip et al., 2019). Disordered eating behaviors were also associated with negative affect, which has been associated with poorer self-management and glycemic control (Rose et al., 2020). Insulin manipulation is associated with greater rates of psychiatric disorders, including depression and eating disorders (Wagner & Karwautz, 2020). Because these behaviors may have an adverse impact on glycemic control and increase the likelihood for diabetes-related health risks, these young patients require special attention from mental health care providers to screen, assess, and treat these problems (Datye & Jaser, 2020).

Attention-deficit/hyperactivity disorder. Another psychological disorder associated with T1D that may impact T1D management is ADHD. Relatively little research has focused on the comorbidity of T1D and ADHD, but one large national registry study conducted in Germany with over 56,000 young patients revealed that 2.83% of patients with T1D also had a diagnosis of ADHD. Youth with T1D and ADHD had significantly more episodes of DKA and higher HbA1c, suggesting that youth with T1D and ADHD are at increased risk for poor health outcomes (Hilgard et al., 2017). In another study of 230 young patients with T1D, those with ADHD had higher HbA1c levels, more diabetes-related emergency department and hospital admissions, and greater health care costs compared to youth with T1D alone (Vinker-Shuster et al., 2019). Consistent with these findings are other reports in youth with T1D that focused on executive functioning—a key problem in ADHD. These findings indicated that executive functioning problems were associated with lower levels of regimen adherence and higher HbA1c (Berg et al., 2018; Vloemans et al., 2019). For individuals with T1D and ADHD, comanagement with pediatric psychologists and developmental-behavioral pediatricians or child and adolescent psychiatrists may be indicated to optimize neurobehavioral functioning and T1D management.

Neurocognitive functioning. Many studies have considered neurocognitive functioning in youth with T1D (Northam, 2020). In general, these studies have shown that T1D poses some risks for pathophysiological brain development including some deficits in learning and information processing such as attention, memory, and processing speed (Cameron et al., 2019; He et al., 2018; Mauras et al., 2021). Risk factors for neurocognitive deficits include early age of T1D diagnosis and more frequent occurrence of serious hypoglycemia, chronic hyperglycemia, and DKA (Aye et al., 2019; He et al., 2020; Mauras et al., 2021). Although early studies suggested decreased academic achievement, more recent research indicates similar school performance in youth with T1D compared with their peers (Begum et al., 2020; Mitchell et al., 2022). For individuals with T1D, concerns about executive function or academic performance should prompt a referral to a developmental-behavioral pediatrician or a pediatric psychologist to assess academic and school functioning.

Stigma and bullying. Two areas of social relationships affecting youth with T1D are stigma and bullying, with two-thirds of adolescents with T1D reporting diabetes-related stigma from their peers (Crespo-Ramos et al., 2018). Among adolescents with T1D, the prevalence of diabetes-related stigma was 65.5%, with experiences of stigma associated with suboptimal glycemic control (Brazeau et al., 2018). Among T1D adolescents (10–18 years old) in Turkey, a fear of stigmatization was common, with many youth preferring to inject insulin while alone instead of in the presence of their peers, reinforcing negative perceptions about insulin use (Arda Sürücü et al., 2020). There is limited research on bullying and youth with T1D (Andrade & Alves, 2019), but across studies, high rates of victimization among youth with T1D have been reported and have been associated with suboptimal glycemic control (Storch et al., 2004, 2006). Taken together, youth with T1D are at risk for stigmatization and bullying and may manifest vulnerabilities in socialization, social support, and acceptance of diabetes by peers, thus highlighting the need for supports by mental health specialists to foster optimal outcomes.

Risk and Resilience

Research has identified a number of factors that increase the risk of youth with T1D for suboptimal outcomes.

Risk factors: Considerations from ecological models. It is helpful to consider these risk factors from a socioecological perspective, including demographic, personal, family, medical system, and community-level factors (Delamater & Marrero, 2020). For example, studies have consistently shown that ethnic minority youths are much more likely to have suboptimal glycemic control than their majority counterparts (Delamater et al., 1999; Mironovici et al., 2020; Petitti et al., 2009). There are several potential explanations for ethnic disparities in glycemic control, including racial differences in sociodemographic risk factors, regimen adherence, and psychosocial variables including health beliefs, family structure and functioning, as well as the potential effects of structural racism and neighborhood-level poverty (Mironovici et al., 2020; Naranjo et al., 2015).

Select sociodemographic risk factors including family and neighborhood characteristics have been associated with unfavorable health outcomes in youth with T1D. Lower levels of parent education and single-parent marital status are associated with suboptimal glycemic control (Thompson et al., 2001). Relatedly, poorer family functioning characterized by diabetes-related conflict and/or lack of appropriate parental monitoring, lower involvement in diabetes management, and parental depression and stress, are also well-described psychosocial risk factors for poorer T1D outcomes (Butler et al., 2020). Individual-level risk factors for diabetes management include the child's history of depression, anxiety, and distress, eating disorders, or behavioral problems (Datye & Jaser, 2020; de Wit et al., 2022; Evans et al., 2020). At-risk neighborhood-level environments characterized by poverty, crime, and social disadvantage (defined by zip codes and census tracts) have also been implicated in suboptimal glycemic control (Mironovici et al., 2020).

Protective factors associated with resilience. There are also a number of multilevel protective factors associated with increased resilience manifest as more effective diabetes management, more optimal family functioning, and better individual coping strategies (Hilliard et al., 2012). Regarding diabetes management, health behaviors that are protective include increased frequency of blood glucose monitoring and use of continuous glucose monitoring (CGM), which have been associated with improved glycemic control (Laffel et al., 2020; Miller et al., 2013). A recent study demonstrated that six essential diabetes management habits were associated with improved glycemic control, including checking glucose at least four times per day or use of CGM, giving at least three insulin boluses per day, using an insulin pump, delivering boluses before meals, reviewing glucose data since the last clinic visit, and changing insulin doses since the last clinic visit. However, only 8.7% of patients performed all six habits (Lee et al., 2021).

One of the most significant protective factors for T1D outcomes is related to the quality of family functioning. Family functioning is characterized by cohesion, autonomy supportive parenting with warmth and empathy, clear communication about diabetes responsibilities, appropriate levels of monitoring and involvement in daily diabetes care, and regular family routines; having two involved caretakers (versus living in a single-parent household) is a protective factor associated with more optimal T1D outcomes (Butler et al., 2020). Individual factors associated with more optimal management of T1D include having effective coping strategies (e.g., better problem-solving skills, adaptive emotional regulation skills) and increased self-efficacy. Having general well-being and prosocial relationships, stronger cognitive abilities, diabetes knowledge, and good executive functioning are additional individual-level protective factors; having supportive peer relationships and school staff has also been associated with better diabetes outcomes (Hilliard et al., 2012). These protective individual factors, and lack of risk factors, are also associated with greater levels of intrinsic motivation for diabetes management, which predicts better diabetes self-management behaviors and glycemic control (Delamater, Daigre, et al., 2017).

Clinical Management of Type 1 Diabetes

The treatment regimen for T1D is complex, including multiple daily administrations of insulin via injections or through use of an insulin pump (with continuous subcutaneous insulin infusion), frequent monitoring of blood glucose (via capillary blood samples and glucose meters or by using CGM), accounting for dietary intake—particularly carbohydrates—in determining meal-time insulin doses, and monitoring of blood glucose before, during, and after bouts of physical activity (Daneman, 2020). Probably the most important health behavior risk factor is inappropriate insulin use, including omission of meal boluses (Burdick et al., 2004) and/or underdosing and overdosing (Schober et al., 2011).

Medical treatment of Type 1 diabetes: Optimizing glycemic control. Management of T1D is focused on effective glycemic control with intensive insulin regimens in patients. Adolescents and young adults typically have high rates of suboptimal glycemic control, with only 17% of adolescents and 21% of young adults achieving glycemic targets of HbA1c less than 7.5% for adolescents and 7.0% for young adults (Foster et al., 2019). Although in recent years, more patients have been using insulin pumps and CGM, which have been associated with some improvements in glycemic control, for many patients with T1D, optimal glycemic control remains elusive. While the current glycemic target for children and adolescents is HbA1c less than 7%, the SEARCH for Diabetes in Youth Study has documented worse glycemic control in a cohort of patients from 2014–2019 compared with a cohort from 2002–2007, with a mean HbA1c of 8.8% (Malik et al., 2022). Taken together, management of T1D has evolved to include psychosocial interventions to address impediments to optimal glycemic control.

Psychosocial screening and assessment. Given the high rate of diabetes management difficulties and suboptimal glycemic control, the ISPAD guidelines (Delamater et al., 2018; de Wit et al., 2022) have long recommended that psychosocial screening be conducted for patients at regular intervals during clinic visits. Despite these recommendations, psychosocial screening occurs in only approximately half of the clinics, with screening predominantly focused on global psychological functioning or quality of life (de Wit et al., 2014). Recent studies have focused on screening for depression (Marker et al., 2019; Mulvaney et al., 2021) and anxiety (Watson et al., 2020), with evidence that screening can be readily accomplished in the context of clinic flow (Iturralde, Adams, et al., 2017). When psychosocial screening has included assessments for family conflict, disordered eating, diabetes stress, and intrinsic motivation for diabetes management, results indicate that 75% of patients scored high in at least one area (Brodar et al., 2021). This supports the belief that comprehensive screening for psychosocial problems can be implemented in routine pediatric diabetes care and should include both youth and parent reports in the screening process (Barry-Menkhaus, Stoner, et al., 2020). National guidelines have supported the integration of psychosocial screening programs into diabetes clinics, as recently reported by investigators participating in the Type 1 Diabetes Exchange Quality Improvement Network (Corathers et al., 2023).

Behavioral and Psychosocial Interventions

A variety of approaches have been used for behavioral and psychosocial interventions. These include work with individual patients that utilizes cognitive behavior therapy (CBT) and motivational intervention, family-based interventions that aim to reduce diabetes-related conflict and build family teamwork and support for diabetes management behaviors, as well as peer group interventions for youth with T1D. Interventions have been delivered outside of outpatient clinic visits, integrated with clinic visits, or delivered via digital approaches, as discussed in this section. Interventions have also been developed and evaluated for parents of youth with T1D.

Timing of intervention. The time period after diagnosis provides an important opportunity to provide psychosocial interventions as this is a stressful time for both the child and the family. In an early randomized study with newly diagnosed children, increasing parental support for children and promoting problem-solving skills by utilizing results of blood glucose monitoring resulted in improved glycemic control 2 years after diagnosis (Delamater et al., 1990). In another study that examined the effects of a psychosocial intervention delivered after diagnosis, family functioning improved but without effects on glycemic control (Sundelin et al., 1996). This suggests that the time of a new diagnosis of T1D may be a "sensitive period" in which interventions, when implemented, may have greater efficacy.

Individual patient approaches. The most commonly used individual intervention approach for youth with T1D is CBT. A recent review of 14 studies of CBT with youth with T1D concluded that this approach is feasible and acceptable, with improvements noted in psychosocial functioning (Rechenberg & Koerner, 2021). Some psychological intervention studies have focused on increasing motivation for diabetes management. Intrinsic motivation for diabetes management is an important construct that can be measured reliably and validly, and research has demonstrated that higher levels of intrinsic management predict improved diabetes management, glycemic control, and psychosocial functioning (Delamater, Daigre, et al., 2017). Motivational interviewing aims to increase intrinsic motivation and pilot studies showed improved glycemic control in adolescents with T1D (Stanger et al., 2013). The findings from a multicenter randomized trial with adolescents showed that motivational interviewing had long-term improvements in glycemic control and quality of life (Channon et al., 2007), with improved glycemic control demonstrated in older adolescents (Nansel, Iannotti, et al., 2009).

Meta-analytic reviews provide support for the use of motivational interviewing with various pediatric populations (Borrelli et al., 2015;

Gayes & Steele, 2014), with these psychological interventions generally delivered by mental or behavioral health professionals with specialty training in this approach. Interventions delivered by nonpsychologist health care providers did not show improvements in glycemic control, suggesting that advanced training and specific counseling skills are needed to effect behavioral change (Robling et al., 2012). Motivational interviewing, combined with problem-solving training, has been associated with significant improvements in motivation, problem solving, diabetes management, quality of life, and reduced family conflict (Mayer-Davis et al., 2018). A recent randomized study examined the impact of a motivational intervention delivered by a nurse during home visits for adolescents and results showed significant improvements in glycemic control (Bakır et al., 2021). Increasing motivation for diabetes management has also been attempted through provision of monetary reinforcement, suggesting behavioral economics may help to improve self-management behaviors (Nally et al., 2021).

Individual psychosocial interventions have also focused on the prevention of diabetes-associated distress and depression. In a randomized controlled trial, results of an eight-session diabetes distress and depression prevention program for adolescents demonstrated significant reductions in diabetes distress for adolescents receiving the intervention (Hood et al., 2018), with continued reductions in diabetes distress and depression observed 3 years after the intervention (Weissberg-Benchell et al., 2020). More details concerning individual-level interventions for youth with T1D can be found in a recent chapter (Channon & Gregory, 2020).

Family-based approaches. Research examining effects of family-based interventions have shown reduced diabetes-related conflict as well as improved regimen adherence and sometimes improved glycemic control (Delamater et al., 2018; de Wit et al., 2022; Feldman et al., 2018). Family-based behavioral interventions include the use of a number of strategies, including self-monitoring of diabetes management behaviors, setting goals, clear communication about responsibilities for diabetes tasks, parental praise for regimen-related behaviors, use of behavioral contracts, problem-solving discussions, and appropriate parental involvement and collaborative support. In randomized controlled trials, behavioral family systems therapy with diabetes-specific tailoring and behavioral contracting reduced family conflict, improved regimen adherence, and improved glycemic control over 18 months; parent–adolescent communication and problem solving was also improved, leading to improved glycemic control (Wysocki, Harris, et al., 2007, 2008).

Youth are more likely to have difficulties with diabetes management when parents allow them to have self-management autonomy without sufficient cognitive and social maturity. Longitudinal research has shown that as parents decrease their monitoring of and involvement with their child's daily self-care, regimen adherence typically declines over time (King et al., 2014). Thus, family-based approaches should encourage parents to remain involved and supportive in their children's daily diabetes management without being intrusive and argumentative (Babler & Strickland, 2015). Positive parenting strategies have been associated with improved parent and family outcomes, and improved emotional and behavioral adjustment in children (Westrupp et al., 2015).

Psychosocial interventions during clinic visits. Delivering brief psychosocial interventions during routine outpatient clinic visits has been shown to be both feasible and effective. Having a "care ambassador" in the clinic deliver a psychoeducational intervention focused on common issues related to diabetes management has been associated with less hypoglycemia and emergency department visits (Svoren et al., 2003). In-clinic interventions to foster family teamwork have been associated with more positive parental involvement, less family conflict related to diabetes, and significant improvements in glycemic control especially for younger adolescents (Nansel et al., 2012). Clinic interventions that addressed quality of life issues with adolescent patients have been associated with improvements in later psychosocial functioning (de Wit et al., 2008), and clinic-based cognitive behavioral interventions have been associated with improved psychosocial well-being, albeit without improved glycemic control (Serlachius et al., 2016). Family-based interventions implemented in clinic with a focus on problem solving, communication skills, and appropriate sharing of responsibilities for diabetes management was associated with improved glycemic control and parental involvement, but only when families participated in at least two sessions over the course of the trial (Murphy et al., 2007).

Peer group interventions. Interventions targeting adolescent peer groups that focused on fostering peer support, coping skills training, and problem solving have been associated with improved glycemic control and quality of life (Boland et al., 1999; Grey et al., 2000). Stress management and coping skills training conducted with peer groups has also been shown to reduce diabetes-related stress (Hains et al., 2000), improve social relationships (Méndez & Beléndez, 1997), and increase blood glucose monitoring and improve glycemic control (Cook et al., 2002). Coping skills interventions have also been studied with school-age children with T1D with associated improvements to the child's quality of life and family functioning (Ambrosino et al., 2008). There is also some evidence from a study conducted in China that suggests coping skills training is more effective for school-age children compared with adolescents with T1D (Guo et al., 2020).

Digital interventions. A number of studies have been conducted to deliver behavioral and psychosocial interventions using the internet and other digital modalities. Interventions targeting diabetes problem solving have been associated with improvements in problem solving and more effective diabetes management (Mulvaney et al., 2010, 2011). In a large, multisite randomized controlled trial, results showed that both coping skills and a diabetes education program, when delivered through the internet resulted in improvements in both groups, supporting the concept that the internet can be a useful way to deliver effective interventions to larger groups of adolescent patients (Grey et al., 2013).

Other internet-based digital modalities including video messaging platforms (Harris et al., 2015), text messaging (Bergner et al., 2018; Wagner et al., 2017), and participation in chat rooms (Troncone et al., 2019) have been used with adolescents with T1D and have been associated with improved outcomes. Psychosocial interventions are now routinely being delivered by telehealth, with an associated reduction in fear of hypoglycemia and distress in both school-age children and their parents (Monzon et al., 2024). An online multicomponent motivational and cognitive intervention focused on youth with emotional dysregulation and suboptimal glycemic control resulted in increased frequency of blood glucose monitoring, as well as improved working memory and glycemic control (Stanger et al., 2018), with the greatest improvements demonstrated in the patients with the most emotional dysregulation (Lansing et al., 2019). Although the results of a recent review of internet and digital interventions suggest that these interventions are beneficial, this literature excludes other aspects of diabetes management, including diet, physical activity, or insulin use (Knox et al., 2019). Taken together, more research using theory-based approaches and stronger methodologies is needed (Garner et al., 2022).

Interventions for patients with chronically suboptimal metabolic control. A subset of youth with T1D exhibit chronically poor metabolic control and are at high risk for both short-term health complications (such as severe hypoglycemia or DKA) and long-term microvascular and macrovascular health complications. Youth at risk for suboptimal outcomes have been targeted based on their chronic suboptimal glycemic control as well as risk factors including low income and ethnic minority status. Intensive home-based, multisystemic therapy addressing the adolescent, their family, and broader community systems (such as the school and health care system) have resulted in improved blood glucose monitoring and glycemic control, and reduced health care utilization and medical costs (Ellis et al., 2008). The available research suggests that these patients require frequent, high-intensity contact with various means of communication in order to achieve improvements in diabetes management outcomes (Barry-Menkhaus, Koskela, et al., 2020; Harris et al., 2016; Wagner et al., 2015).

Interventions for parents. The stress and adjustment of parents is an important issue for clinicians to address in the management of T1D. Coping skills training for parents of young children has been shown to be helpful (Grey et al., 2011), with interventions focused on building communication and coping skills associated with reductions in distress and family conflict (Jaser et al., 2018). Video-based telehealth interventions have demonstrated efficacy in reducing fear of hypoglycemia and parenting stress (Patton et al., 2020). Websites designed for and by parents have also resulted in improved parental knowledge about managing diabetes and greater life satisfaction (Holtz et al., 2020). Taken together, multimodal interventions can help foster adaptation and adherence to T1D, with benefits to the family system.

TYPE 2 DIABETES

While T2D was seen rarely in youth before the 1990s, in recent years, there has been an increased incidence in the diagnosis of T2D (Dabelea et al., 2014). T2D disproportionately affects certain demographic groups and ethnic minorities, with increased incidence among Blacks, Hispanics, Asians/Pacific Islanders, and Native Americans compared to non-Hispanic Whites (Dabelea et al., 2014; Lawrence et al., 2021). The incidence and prevalence of T2D are also greater among individuals with lower SES (Pulgaron & Delamater, 2014) and Black and Hispanic youth are more likely to have suboptimal glycemic control when T2D is diagnosed (Bacha et al., 2021). The prevalence of T2D in youth has also increased worldwide (International Diabetes Federation, 2019), with the highest number of cases from China, India, and the United States (Wu et al., 2022).

Epidemiology and Health Equity

T2D in youth also represents a significant public health problem, with increased risk for health complications and mortality compared to individuals diagnosed with T2D in adulthood (Catherine et al., 2021). Compared to individuals with T1D, complications and comorbidities are higher in the youth with T2D (Dabelea et al., 2007). Furthermore, T2D progresses more aggressively to complications than T1D (Rao & Jensen, 2020). Health disparities in youth of minority groups are also much more apparent than in T1D (Bacha et al., 2021). As with T1D, serious health problems, disability, and economic costs are increasing with T2D in youth in the United States and worldwide (Bommer et al., 2018).

Ecological Factors Associated With Type 2 Diabetes

T2D is a complex disease with numerous contributing factors—including social, family, and medical risk factors as well as health system factors—that interact to set the stage for T2D onset and comprise the key challenges for management in pediatric patients.

Sociodemographic risk factors. Several sociodemographic factors have been found in association with T2D in youth. The prevalence of T2D has been shown to be disproportionately high among ethnic minority groups including Native Americans, African Americans, Hispanics, East and South Asians, Middle Eastern, and Pacific Islander populations (Shah et al., 2022), with the majority of new cases of T2D in the United States among Hispanic, African American, Asian and Pacific Islander, and Native American youth (Dabelea et al., 2007).

Family and peer factors. Several family factors have been associated with suboptimal T2D outcomes. A parental history of T2D was associated with higher baseline HbA1c and poorer glycemic control in youth with T2D (Weinstock et al., 2015).

Relatedly, when family members with T2D have a history of health complications, youth may perceive these complications as inevitable, and may become unmotivated to improve adherence to diabetes regimen (Jones, 1998). Parental involvement and the "dietary home environment" are also important correlates of glycemic control. Parents who are less involved in caring for their child's diabetes (Anderson et al., 2005) and parents who keep high-sugar foods in the home and consume them in the presence of their children are more likely to have T2D youth with suboptimal glycemic control (Wicklow et al., 2021). Peer support is also an important factor in T2D management, as diabetes disclosure has been associated with fears of stigmatization for children with T2D who lack peer support (Brouwer et al., 2012; St. George et al., 2017).

Medical risk factors. Several medical comorbidities are associated with increased risk for T2D. Obesity is a risk factor for T2D, with the majority of youth with T2D being classified as obese or overweight (Liu et al., 2010). Dietary factors such as consumption of high fructose corn syrup have also been implicated in the risk of T2D (Goran et al., 2013). Other lifestyle factors contributing to obesity, insulin resistance, and T2D risk include low physical activity, high sedentary behavior, and excess screen time (Pulgaron et al., 2020). Other medical comorbidities seen in youth with T2D include dyslipidemia, polycystic ovary syndrome, and obstructive sleep apnea, which, if present, can help serve as markers to identify youth with T2D (Shah et al., 2022).

Health system factors: Interdisciplinary and integrated health care. An important barrier to effective diabetes management is engagement with health care providers. A single-site study examining the association between clinic attendance and health outcomes of youth with T2D reported that nearly 80% of the patients missed clinic appointments at least once during the study period; missing regularly scheduled clinic visits was associated with suboptimal glycemic control (Pulgaron et al., 2015). Results from the Treatment Options for Type 2 Diabetes in Adolescents and Youth (TODAY) study regarding engagement with a behavioral health program in the context of a clinical trial indicated that only 54% of participants in the medication plus lifestyle intervention arm attended 75% or more of the scheduled lifestyle intervention sessions over the course of the trial, suggesting attendance to behavioral health consultations is another barrier to be overcome (Berkowitz et al., 2018).

Behavioral and Psychological Sequelae Associated With Type 2 Diabetes

Youth with T2D are at risk for numerous psychological sequelae including mood disorders, ADHD, and schizophrenia (Levitt Katz et al., 2005).

Depression. The most common psychiatric condition in youth with T2D is depression, with an estimated prevalence of at least 20% (Akbarizadeh et al., 2022). Risk factors associated with greater depressive symptoms in youth with T2D include older age, shorter diabetes duration, higher HbA1c, being non-Hispanic White, being prescribed oral medications, having a history of less psychosocial support, and family history of T2D (McVoy et al., 2023, Monaghan et al., 2021). Other risk factors for depression in youth with T2D include requiring insulin, use of public health insurance, and a history of high rates of diabetes distress (Roberts et al., 2021). Depressive symptoms are thought to impact glycemic control through their association with lower medication adherence and disordered eating behaviors, including binge eating or compensatory behaviors to change body weight (Gulley & Shomaker, 2020). Poor sleep quality has also been proposed as a mechanism underlying the association between depressive symptoms and glycemic control (Gabbs et al., 2022). Relatedly, diabetes-associated distress has also been associated with lower medication adherence and impaired psychosocial functioning (Walders-Abramson et al., 2014).

Neurocognitive functioning. Youth with T2D were found to have differences in gray matter, volume, and microstructural integrity, suggesting cerebrovascular impairment (Redel et al., 2019), as well as lower global cerebral flow in multiple brain regions compared to youth without T2D (Redel et al., 2022). Youth with T2D have been found to have lower scores in executive functions and memory (Redel et al., 2019), and lower academic achievement (Brady et al., 2017). For youth with T2D with academic or school difficulties, a referral to a developmental-behavioral pediatrician or pediatric psychologist can be helpful in evaluating for signs of diabetes-related school failure and assisting with educational planning and accommodations.

Quality of life and disordered eating. Reduced quality of life has also been documented in youth with T2D and is associated with suboptimal glycemic control (Varni et al., 2018). Lower quality of life has also been associated with being female and overweight (Naughton et al., 2014). T2D is also a risk for disordered eating behaviors: 20% of youth with T2D report subclinical, and 6% report clinically significant binge eating, which has been associated with greater obesity, more depression, and lower quality of life (TODAY Study Group, 2011).

Risk and Resilience: Considerations From Ecological Models

Socioecological considerations provide a context for understanding risk factors and protective factors or resilience, including demographic, individual, family, and health care system factors that affect T2D and its management (Delamater & Marrero, 2020).

Risk factors. Several biological risk factors have been implicated in the pathogenesis of T2D. *In utero* exposure to hyperglycemia (Shaw, 2007) as well as maternal under-nutrition, intrauterine growth retardation, and low birthweight have been found to increase the risk of obesity and T2D in later life (Shah et al., 2022). The onset of puberty is also associated with the development of T2D, as T2D is rarely observed in children under the age of 10 (Shah et al., 2022). Relatedly, the construct of "allostatic load," describing the cumulative negative effects of chronic exposure to social and environmental stressors on body weight, metabolism, blood pressure, and the sympathetic nervous system has been linked with increased T2D risk. Greater socioeconomic adversity and higher allostatic load are associated with greater prevalence of T2D among Hispanics and youth living in socially disadvantaged households (Gallo et al., 2019).

Protective factors. Protective factors such as changes in lifestyle for weight control, increasing physical activity, and eating healthy foods have been associated with better outcomes in T2D (Pulgaron et al., 2020). Certain psychological characteristics are also associated with more optimal outcomes in T2D. Higher self-efficacy has been associated with increased life satisfaction, better adaptation, reduced depression, and better glycemic control (Sacco & Bykowski, 2010). Higher resilience (via increased levels of self-awareness, problem solving, anger control, coping with stress, and positive thinking skills) has been shown to improve self-efficacy in adults with T2D (Torabizadeh et al., 2019). Promoting psychological factors associated with resilience is an important intervention target for youth with T2D, and highlights the important role that pediatric psychologists may play in optimizing outcomes for youth with T2D.

Clinical Management of Type 2 Diabetes

Clinical management of T2D includes medical monitoring and interventions as well as lifestyle changes focusing on healthful dietary intake, physical activity, and regimen adherence. Interdisciplinary collaboration is key, particularly with behavioral health providers who can aid in identifying psychological comorbidities that might impact adherence and support implementation of lifestyle modifications.

Medical treatment of Type 2 diabetes. In T2D, the medical regimen emphasizes adherence to glucose-lowering medications, regular glucose monitoring, and modification of dietary and physical activity habits for weight management. Although insulin may also be prescribed, usually a once-per-day long-acting basal insulin (Daneman, 2020), most youth with T2D can be weaned off insulin after glycemic targets are reached (Shah et al., 2022).

Adherence. Successful management of T2D requires adherence to medication and dietary guidelines. While there is some evidence that youth with T2D demonstrate fairly good medication adherence, with 80% of youth reporting in a telephone survey that they took their oral medication at least 75% of the time, and 59% reporting they monitored their blood glucose twice daily, most patients also reported poor dietary adherence, manifest by frequent overeating, drinking sweetened beverages, eating fast food, and having high rates of sedentary behavior (Rothman et al., 2008). In a large, multisite national study examining medication adherence in youth with T2D, oral medication adherence declined over time: while 72% took their medication 80% of the time 2 months after the trial began, only 56% demonstrated adherence after 48 months (Katz et al., 2016). These data suggest that promoting adherence to medication and lifestyle interventions is important in the clinical management of T2D.

Despite well-delineated treatment targets, physicians caring for patients with T2D describe high rates of nonadherence to medical treatment and diet and exercise prescriptions among adolescents with T2D, contributing to failure to lose weight, poor glycemic control, or treatment dropout. Adherence challenges may be related to the developmental period of adolescence in which the diagnosis of T2D is made and subsequent adjustment occurs (Pulgaron et al., 2015). Adolescence is a time of emerging autonomy, when youth with T2D are expected to manage their health more independently but is also a time in which they may be concerned about engaging in diabetes tasks that might make them stand out from peers. A fear of peer rejection and a lack of cognitive maturity that fails to associate unhealthy behaviors with negative health outcomes are potential barriers to adherence, contributing to suboptimal management of T2D (Auslander et al., 2010; St. George et al., 2017).

Interdisciplinary team management. Given the complex interplay of psychosocial, behavioral, and family factors that contribute to the management of T2D, interdisciplinary care coordination is necessary to help patients meet glycemic goals and achieve optimal psychosocial outcomes. An interdisciplinary team including endocrinologists, nurses, diabetes educators, dietitians, psychologists, and social workers is essential to address the multifaceted aspects of diabetes care and to integrate patient-centered strategies into clinical care. Interdisciplinary care approaches including shared decision-making, shared medical appointments, and the use of motivational interviewing to enhance behavior change are important to achieving optimal outcomes (Powell et al., 2015). In addition, within the context of an interdisciplinary team, patients with T2D can (and should) be evaluated for the psychological comorbidities of T2D, which can impact adherence, adaptation, and health-related outcomes.

Psychosocial screening, assessment and management. The ISPAD clinical practice consensus guidelines recommend that youth with T2D be screened for the most common psychosocial comorbidities, including depression, diabetes distress, and disordered eating at the time of diagnosis and at regular follow-ups (Shah et al., 2022). Those identified with mental health concerns can be referred to clinic-based or community mental health supports. To build a therapeutic alliance, providers should avoid stigmatizing language, and promote education that helps contextualize illness within a biopsychosocial framework. Providers should consider cultural, social, geographic, and economic factors when devising treatment plans and actively seek to identify and problem solve barriers to implementing behavior change, particularly those relating to food insecurity, housing instability, and financial challenges.

Screening tools can be incorporated into clinical care to assess psychological functioning of youth with T2D. The Diabetes Distress Scale, the PHQ-9, the Kessler distress score (K6), the Unger resiliency scales, and the Psychological Stress Score are among those recommended by ISPAD (Shah et al., 2022). Research has also shown that the Pediatric Quality of Life Inventory (PedsQL) 3.2 Diabetes Module Diabetes Symptoms Summary Score and Type 2–specific Diabetes Management Summary Score provide objective assessments of adherence, symptoms, and quality of life, which are useful in clinical practice (Varni et al., 2018).

Behavioral and Psychosocial Interventions

The goal of treatment for T2D is achieving normal blood glucose levels. To accomplish this treatment goal, guidelines published by the ISPAD recommend a combination of medical and lifestyle interventions (Shah et al., 2022). Youth with T2D frequently overeat, drink sweetened beverages, eat fast food, have lower rates of physical activity, and tend to be more sedentary (Kriska et al., 2013; Rothman et al., 2008). Interventions focused on lifestyle changes have primarily addressed dietary intake and exercise, as well as alternative targets (e.g., sleep, substance use) for effective T2D management (Shah et al., 2022).

Individual patient approaches. Individual interventions have focused on dietary changes to reduce or eliminate sugary soft drinks and juices to promote weight loss. Other dietary recommendations have included increasing vegetable intake, reducing portion sizes, and eliminating intake of foods made from refined, simple sugars and high fructose corn syrup. The use of other types of diets (e.g., very low calorie, low carbohydrate, ketogenic, or intermittent fasting) has a limited evidence base for youth with T2D (Shah et al., 2022). Because increasing physical activity has been associated with improved blood glucose levels, lower cardiovascular risk, weight loss, and improved well-being, exercise prescriptions are often employed and should include setting limits on sedentary behavior, such as using screens and electronic entertainment.

Family, peer, and group interventions. The family system plays an important role in helping children adopt healthy lifestyle behaviors. Parents and family members can support youth by modeling healthy eating habits, implementing meal schedules that minimize grazing, limiting distractions during meals, and discouraging overly restrictive food intake (Shah et al., 2022). A limited number of peer interventions have been studied to date. One after-school, peer-supported, community-based intervention utilized behavior modification, motivational interviewing, and peer mentoring approaches to promote behavior change (weight loss, physical activity, and impulse control). While participation in the program was not associated with changes in the anthropometric or cardiometabolic risk factors studied, reductions in HbA1c and systolic blood pressure were observed. Participants have also described being part of a group and engagement in non-competitive activities as facilitators of physical activity (Huynh et al., 2015).

Medical team interventions. The TODAY randomized controlled clinical trial examined the effectiveness of three interventions (metformin, metformin plus rosiglitazone, and metformin plus a family lifestyle program) on glycemic control in a racially, ethnically, and geographically diverse group of youth with T2D (TODAY Study Group, 2012). Results over a mean follow-up of 3.9 years indicated that nearly half of the patients had durable glycemic control with metformin alone. The addition of lifestyle intervention to metformin did not impact glycemic control but was associated with a decreased body mass index. The TODAY study also examined lifestyle interventions (characterized by changes in diet and cardiovascular fitness) on T2D outcomes and found that while only a few youth improved their fitness and/or diet over time, those who did showed a positive impact on glycemic outcomes (Kriska et al., 2018). These findings suggested that increasing physical activity, decreasing intake of sweetened beverages, increasing fiber and decreasing saturated fat may be additional intervention targets to achieve better results.

Another study from the TODAY trial examined how parenting behaviors and family conflict relate to T2D in youth and found that youth who perceive more autonomy in day-to-day and diabetes management tasks were more likely to adhere to medication regimens (Saletsky et al., 2014). Relatedly, a study examining the association of behavioral adherence to the lifestyle program (i.e., attendance at intervention sessions, rates of self-monitoring of diet and physical activity by participants and their caregivers) with changes in glycemic control and obesity, found that while behavioral adherence to lifestyle modifications was not associated with improved glycemic control, reductions in percent overweight were observed (Berkowitz et al., 2018). Taken together, at this time, empirical evidence does not fully support the efficacy of lifestyle interventions for youth with T2D, despite studies suggesting that lifestyle interventions including diet and exercise can elicit potentially meaningful changes in adiposity and cardiometabolic risk in obese children and adolescents (McGavock et al., 2015).

Medical/surgical interventions. The use of a medically supervised very-low-calorie diet and bariatric surgery are additional approaches that have been proposed for the treatment of youth with T2D. Research suggests that a very low-calorie diet for 2 months can result in a significant reduction of HbA1c and medication use in youth (Willi et al., 2004). Bariatric surgery for severely obese youth with T2D may also reverse diabetes and improve cardiovascular risk factors (Inge et al., 2009).

RECOMMENDATIONS FOR CLINICAL PRACTICE AND THE ROLE OF DEVELOPMENTAL-BEHAVIORAL PEDIATRICIANS AND PEDIATRIC PSYCHOLOGISTS

The findings from controlled research have demonstrated a number of evidence-based interventions to improve outcomes in children and adolescents with T1D and T2D (de Wit et al., 2022; Hilliard et al., 2016). Studies addressing family-based intervention approaches have shown improved regimen adherence and family relationships, while sometimes improving glycemic control as well. These interventions typically utilize positive reinforcement and behavioral contracts, communication and problem-solving skills training, and negotiation of diabetes management goals to improve collaborative parental monitoring and involvement in daily diabetes management tasks. Research findings have also shown that parents benefit from psychosocial interventions to reduce their stress.

Peer group intervention approaches to improve coping and stress management skills also may have positive effects on regimen adherence, glycemic control, and quality of life. Psychological interventions with individual adolescents have shown that CBT and motivational interviewing can improve psychosocial outcomes, quality of life, and in some studies also improve glycemic control. In a meta-analysis of intervention studies to improve regimen adherence, results from 15 studies showed stronger effects for multicomponent interventions that addressed psychosocial and emotional functioning, with small effect sizes for improvements in glycemic control (Hood et al., 2010). The representative research reviewed and discussed in this chapter strongly supports the concept that behavioral, psychological, and social factors are integral to the management of T1D and T2D in children and adolescents, as outlined in recent consensus guidelines by the ISPAD (de Wit et al., 2022), and has a number of essential clinical implications. These can be summarized as including the following: (a) having professionals with expertise in mental and behavioral health within the interdisciplinary health care team; (b) assessing adjustment to and understanding of diabetes management principles; identifying psychosocial adjustment and quality of life problems at planned intervals through periodic screening; (c) assessing general and diabetes-specific family functioning; (d) providing evidence-based psychosocial interventions for patients and families exhibiting conflict, behavioral or psychiatric difficulties, or adherence problems affecting glycemic control; and (e) implementing preventive interventions at key developmental times such as soon after diagnosis, late childhood to early adolescence, and late adolescence during the transition to more independent care in the adult health care system. Taken together, these findings highlight the importance of interdisciplinary teams and collaborations to optimize outcomes of individuals with T1D and T2D. Developmental-behavioral pediatricians, child and adolescent psychiatrists, and pediatric psychologists can help address the psychological and educational comorbidities associated with diabetes (e.g., ADHD, affective disorders, deficits in learning and academic achievement), and can initiate interventions to optimize outcomes. Pediatric psychologists can screen for psychological comorbidities, monitor for adherence, and initiate family-based interventions to foster adherence, adaptation, and coping in children and families affected by T1D and T2D.

FUTURE DIRECTIONS IN RESEARCH

There is a need for improved methodological quality in psychosocial and behavioral intervention research, and to identify factors associated with suboptimal outcomes in select patient populations. For example, in the TODAY trial, failure rates were greatest among Black and Hispanic youth, indicating that this patient population might benefit from additional treatments or culturally adapted approaches. Future research should address the socioecological factors associated with suboptimal psychosocial functioning and adherence in select patient populations. This can be achieved through purposeful sampling with an aim to include more high-risk patients in study samples, with a focus on low-income, ethnic minority, and single-parent youth (Morone, 2019), as well as the inclusion of very young children with diabetes (Rose et al., 2018). An additional priority for future research is to evaluate the cost-effectiveness of brief clinic-based behavioral interventions that can be delivered during routine outpatient care which can address barriers to effective self-management, reduction of diabetes distress, and improvements in family teamwork and potential for scalability through integrated behavioral health systems of care (Barry-Menkhaus, Wagner, & Riley, 2020).

There are a number of other significant issues to address in future research. One of the most important is the translation of the Diabetes Control and Complications Trial (DCCT), which showed the importance of controlling blood glucose to reduce the development of complications in T1D. Despite all the medical advances and technologies developed since the DCCT, most youth with T1D fail to achieve glycemic targets. We need more intervention research to help young patients meet glycemic targets using person-centered approaches that account for ecological factors and social determinants of health. To increase reach to various patient populations, more research is needed that focuses on utilization of m-Health digital technologies (including telehealth and innovative apps to improve self-management) and social marketing strategies. The external validity of findings from intervention research can be enhanced by studies conducted in real-world clinical settings; such research can benefit from using flexible, adaptive research designs.

Health disparities remain another significant public health issue. Intervention research that demonstrates how to reduce and remove the disparities gap is urgently needed so that low-income and ethnic minority patients can attain optimal diabetes management, avoid health complications, and improve their quality of life. Another crucial issue for translational research, given the increasing incidence of T2D in youth and the risk of early health complications, is to effectively disseminate the Diabetes Prevention Program specific to pediatric populations (Pulgaron et al., 2020). Additionally, because most youth with T2D do not achieve optimal glycemic control, there is a need for intervention research to help them meet glucose targets, improve lifestyle dietary and physical activity behaviors, reduce overweight and obesity, and improve their quality of life.

CONCLUSION

Both T1D and T2D are increasing in incidence worldwide. The medical regimens for effective management of diabetes are complex and adherence problems are common. While there have been many advances in medical technologies in recent years that offer the potential for optimal glycemic control, most children and adolescents with diabetes do not achieve glycemic targets and are at increased risk for eventual health complications and reduced quality of life. Much is known about psychosocial factors related to effective diabetes management, with research demonstrating that adherence and glycemic control problems are related to modifiable factors. Barriers to effective diabetes management include psychological factors such as depression, anxiety, and eating disorders, and psychosocial factors such as family conflict and lack of supportive teamwork around the daily tasks of self-care. Diabetes distress is common and stigmatization concerns may also be significant for some youth and are associated with suboptimal psychological adjustment and diabetes management.

Another major barrier is the lack of integration of medical with behavioral health care. Health disparities exist, with lower-income and ethnic minority youth at risk for suboptimal glycemic control. Research has shown that many behavioral and psychosocial interventions can improve outcomes, but most youth—including lower-income and ethnic minority youth—do not receive evidence-based interventions to improve diabetes outcomes. Patient-centered collaborative models of care that recognize patient and family autonomy and build and support intrinsic motivation and family teamwork offer skillful approaches to improve outcomes for children and adolescents, as well as their parents. Such care models should include pediatric psychologists to foster adherence and adaptation using a family-based approach and involve developmental-behavioral pediatricians and child and adolescent psychiatrists as needed to address vulnerabilities in educational and behavioral functioning and potential medications addressing psychiatric disorders that disrupt T1D management.

More research is needed to demonstrate the effectiveness and cost-offsets of integrated behavioral health care models. The translation of behavioral interventions into clinical practice settings remains a priority and challenge, but progress is being made through quality improvement programs that incorporate psychosocial screening programs into routine care. Youth with T2D present unique treatment challenges considering their obesity, high-risk lifestyle behaviors, and emotional and family issues, as well as difficulties with regimen adherence and staying engaged in medical follow-up treatment; more work is needed to understand how to effectively intervene with these youth and ultimately to prevent T2D. Until diabetes is effectively prevented and/or cured, psychosocial and behavioral issues will remain significant in the management of both T1D and T2D in children and adolescents.

RESOURCES

Resources for Parents

- **American Diabetes Association (ADA):**

  https://diabetes.org/

  The ADA website contains authoritative information about the latest technologies for effective diabetes management and provides access to the ADA bookstore which has many books for parents and children with diabetes. Through the ADA, parents can also find local support groups, summer camps for children, and a directory of mental health professionals trained in diabetes and its management.

- **Children With Diabetes:**

  https://childrenwithdiabetes.com/

  This site provides the latest information on diabetes management, nutrition, new technologies and provides opportunities for interactions with experts in diabetes care. This organization also has a library with family resources for children, adolescents, parents, and resources on food and nutrition. This organization also conducts yearly conferences that connects health care professionals to parents and children with diabetes and provides opportunities for youth to interact with other youth who have diabetes through on-line supports.

- **Breakthrough Type 1 Diabetes:**

  https://www.breakthroughT1D.org

  Breakthrough Type 1 Diabetes provides authoritative information and resources for children and parents, including community forums, virtual connections to webinars, and access to local chapters for building a network of social supports. Their website also provides information for newly diagnosed patients on the basics of diabetes management, the latest technologies, and special topics such as parenting, mental health, school plans, driving, navigating health insurance, and advocacy.

Resources for Providers

- **American Diabetes Association—Professional Resources**
  In addition to its website listed (https://diabetes.org/), the ADA has a yearly scientific meeting and publishes several journals featuring behavioral and psychosocial research such as *Diabetes Care*, *Diabetes Spectrum*, and *Clinical Diabetes*. Membership in the ADA offers continuing opportunities for health professionals to stay current with the latest research advances and has special interest groups focusing on diabetes in children and youth and behavioral medicine and psychology.

- **ADA–APA Collaboration**
  Several years ago, the ADA developed, in collaboration with the American Psychological Association (APA), an online course specifically for mental health providers in order to increase the national workforce capacity in addressing behavioral health issues in diabetes. At present, continuing education courses are provided through ADA. Psychologists and other mental health professionals can learn about how to skillfully work with their young patients who have diabetes and earn continuing education credits at no charge. Online toolkits, questionnaires, and patient handouts are also available.

  https://professional.diabetes.org/journals-resources/behavioral-health-resources

- **The International Society for Pediatric and Adolescent Diabetes (ISPAD):**

  https://www.ispad.org/

  For mental health professionals engaged in work with patients who have diabetes, ISPAD is a resource dedicated to the latest advances in diabetes research as well as network with other professionals. ISPAD also has an annual scientific conference and regularly publishes clinical consensus guidelines and research articles in their journal *Pediatric Diabetes*.

- **The Association of Diabetes Care and Education Specialists:**

  https://www.adces.org/

  The Association of Diabetes Care and Education Specialists offers many online resources, publishes clinical research articles in *The Diabetes Educator*, and has an annual conference featuring research and clinical workshops.

References

Akbarizadeh, M., Naderi Far, M., & Ghaljaei, F. (2022). Prevalence of depression and anxiety among children with Type 1 and Type 2 diabetes: A systematic review and meta-analysis. *World Journal of Pediatrics, 18*(1), 16–26. https://doi.org/10.1007/s12519-021-00485-2

Ambrosino, J. M., Fennie, K., Whittemore, R., Jaser, S., Dowd, M. F., & Grey, M. (2008). Short-term effects of coping skills training in school-age children with Type 1 diabetes. *Pediatric Diabetes, 9*(3 Pt. 2), 74–82. https://doi.org/10.1111/j.1399-5448.2007.00356.x

American Diabetes Association. (2018). Economic costs of diabetes in the U.S. in 2017. *Diabetes*

Care, 41(5), 917–928. https://doi.org/10.2337/dci18-0007

American Diabetes Association. (2022). *Statistics about diabetes.* Retrieved May 10, 2024, from https://diabetes.org/about-us/statistics/about-diabetes

American Diabetes Association. (2023). New American Diabetes Association report finds annual costs of diabetes to be $412.9 billion [Press release]. https://diabetes.org/newsroom/press-releases/new-american-diabetes-association-report-finds-annual-costs-diabetes-be

Anderson, B. J. (2012). Behavioral research in pediatric diabetes: Putting the evidence to work for advocacy and education. *Pediatric Diabetes, 13*(1), 77–80. https://doi.org/10.1111/j.1399-5448.2011.00778.x

Anderson, B. J., Cullen, K., & McKay, S. (2005). Quality of life, family behavior, and health outcomes in children with Type 2 diabetes. *Pediatric Annals, 34*(9), 722–729. https://doi.org/10.3928/0090-4481-20050901-12

Andrade, C. J. D. N., & Alves, C. A. D. (2019). Relationship between bullying and Type 1 diabetes mellitus in children and adolescents: A systematic review. *Jornal de Pediatria, 95*(5), 509–518. https://doi.org/10.1016/j.jped.2018.10.003

Arda Sürücü, H., Baran Durmaz, G., & Turan, E. (2020). Does Type 1 diabetic adolescents' fear of stigmatization predict a negative perception insulin treatment? *Clinical Nursing Research, 29*(4), 235–242. https://doi.org/10.1177/1054773818815258

Asarnow, J. R., Rozenman, M., Wiblin, J., & Zeltzer, L. (2015). Integrated medical-behavioral care compared with usual primary care for child and adolescent behavioral health: A meta-analysis. *JAMA Pediatrics, 169*(10), 929–937. https://doi.org/10.1001/jamapediatrics.2015.1141

Auslander, W. F., Sterzing, P. R., Zayas, L. E., & White, N. H. (2010). Psychosocial resources and barriers to self-management in African American adolescents with Type 2 diabetes: A qualitative analysis. *The Diabetes Educator, 36*(4), 613–622. https://doi.org/10.1177/0145721710369706

Auslander, W. F., Thompson, S., Dreitzer, D., White, N. H., & Santiago, J. V. (1997). Disparity in glycemic control and adherence between African-American and Caucasian youths with diabetes: Family and community contexts. *Diabetes Care, 20*(10), 1569–1575. https://doi.org/10.2337/diacare.20.10.1569

Aye, T., Mazaika, P. K., Mauras, N., Marzelli, M. J., Shen, H., Hershey, T., Cato, A., Weinzimer, S. A., White, N. H., Tsalikian, E., Jo, B., & Reiss, A. L. (2019). Impact of early diabetic ketoacidosis on the developing brain. *Diabetes Care, 42*(3), 443–449. https://doi.org/10.2337/dc18-1405

Babler, E., & Strickland, C. J. (2015). Moving the journey towards independence: Adolescents transitioning to successful diabetes self-management. *Journal of Pediatric Nursing, 30*(5), 648–660. https://doi.org/10.1016/j.pedn.2015.06.005

Bacha, F., Cheng, P., Gal, R. L., Beaulieu, L. C., Kollman, C., Adolph, A., Shoemaker, A. H., Wolf, R., Klingensmith, G. J., & Tamborlane, W. V. (2021). Racial and ethnic disparities in comorbidities in youth with Type 2 diabetes in the Pediatric Diabetes Consortium (PDC). *Diabetes Care, 44*(10), 2245–2251. https://doi.org/10.2337/dc21-0143

Bakır, E., Çavuşoğlu, H., & Mengen, E. (2021). Effects of the information-motivation-behavioral skills model on metabolic control of adolescents with Type 1 diabetes in Turkey: Randomized controlled study. *Journal of Pediatric Nursing, 58,* e19–e27. https://doi.org/10.1016/j.pedn.2020.11.019

Barnard, K., Thomas, S., Royle, P., Noyes, K., & Waugh, N. (2010). Fear of hypoglycaemia in parents of young children with Type 1 diabetes: A systematic review. *BMC Pediatrics, 10*(1), 50. https://doi.org/10.1186/1471-2431-10-50

Barry-Menkhaus, S. A., Koskela, N., Wagner, D. V., Burch, R., & Harris, M. A. (2020). System overload: Interventions that target the multiple systems in which youth with Type 1 diabetes live. In A. Delamater & D. Marrero (Eds.), *Behavioral diabetes* (pp. 139–152). Springer Nature. https://doi.org/10.1007/978-3-030-33286-0_11

Barry-Menkhaus, S. A., Stoner, A. M., MacGregor, K. L., & Soyka, L. A. (2020). Special considerations in the systematic psychosocial screening of youth with Type 1 diabetes. *Journal of Pediatric Psychology, 45*(3), 299–310. https://doi.org/10.1093/jpepsy/jsz089

Barry-Menkhaus, S. A., Wagner, D. V., & Riley, A. R. (2020). Small interventions for big change: Brief strategies for distress and self-management amongst youth with Type 1 diabetes. *Current Diabetes Reports, 20*(1), 3. https://doi.org/10.1007/s11892-020-1290-7

Begum, M., Chittleborough, C., Pilkington, R., Mittinty, M., Lynch, J., Penno, M., & Smithers, L. (2020). Educational outcomes among children with Type 1 diabetes: Whole-of-population linked-data study. *Pediatric Diabetes, 21*(7), 1353–1361. https://doi.org/10.1111/pedi.13107

Berg, C. A., Wiebe, D. J., Suchy, Y., Turner, S. L., Butner, J., Munion, A., Lansing, A. H., White, P. C., & Murray, M. (2018). Executive function predicting longitudinal change in Type 1 diabetes management during the transition to emerging adulthood. *Diabetes Care, 41*(11), 2281–2288. https://doi.org/10.2337/dc18-0351

Bergner, E. M., Whittemore, R., Patel, N. J., Savin, K. L., Hamburger, E. R., & Jaser, S. S. (2018). Participants' experience and engagement in Check It!: A positive psychology intervention for adolescents with Type 1 diabetes. *Translational Issues in Psychological Science, 4*(3), 215–227. https://doi.org/10.1037/tps0000161

Berkowitz, R. I., Marcus, M. D., Anderson, B. J., Delahanty, L., Grover, N., Kriska, A., Laffel, L., Syme, A., Venditti, E., Van Buren, D. J., Wilfley, D. E., Yasuda, P., Hirst, K., & the TODAY Study Group. (2018). Adherence to a lifestyle program for youth with Type 2 diabetes and its association with treatment outcome in the TODAY clinical trial. *Pediatric Diabetes, 19*(2), 191–198. https://doi.org/10.1111/pedi.12555

Boland, E. A., Grey, M., Oesterle, A., Fredrickson, L., & Tamborlane, W. V. (1999). Continuous subcutaneous insulin infusion. A new way to lower risk of severe hypoglycemia, improve metabolic control, and enhance coping in adolescents with Type 1 diabetes. *Diabetes Care, 22*(11), 1779–1784. https://doi.org/10.2337/diacare.22.11.1779

Bommer, C., Sagalova, V., Heesemann, E., Manne-Goehler, J., Atun, R., Bärnighausen, T., Davies, J., & Vollmer, S. (2018). Global economic burden of diabetes in adults: Projections from 2015 to 2030. *Diabetes Care, 41*(5), 963–970. https://doi.org/10.2337/dc17-1962

Borrelli, B., Tooley, E. M., & Scott-Sheldon, L. A. (2015). Motivational interviewing for parent-child health interventions: A systematic review and meta-analysis. *Pediatric Dentistry, 37*(3), 254–265.

Borschuk, A. P., & Everhart, R. S. (2015). Health disparities among youth with Type 1 diabetes: A systematic review of the current literature. *Families, Systems, & Health, 33*(3), 297–313. https://doi.org/10.1037/fsh0000134

Brady, C. C., Vannest, J. J., Dolan, L. M., Kadis, D. S., Lee, G. R., Holland, S. K., Khoury, J. C., & Shah, A. S. (2017). Obese adolescents with Type 2 diabetes perform worse than controls on cognitive and behavioral assessments. *Pediatric Diabetes, 18*(4), 297–303. https://doi.org/10.1111/pedi.12383

Brazeau, A. S., Nakhla, M., Wright, M., Henderson, M., Panagiotopoulos, C., Pacaud, D., Kearns, P., Rahme, E., Da Costa, D., & Dasgupta, K. (2018). Stigma and its association with glycemic control and hypoglycemia in adolescents and young adults with Type 1 diabetes: Cross-sectional study. *Journal of Medical Internet Research, 20*(4), e151. https://doi.org/10.2196/jmir.9432

Broadley, M. M., Zaremba, N., Andrew, B., Ismail, K., Treasure, J., White, M. J., & Stadler, M. (2020). 25 Years of psychological research investigating disordered eating in people with diabetes: What have we learnt? *Diabetic Medicine, 37*(3), 401–408. https://doi.org/10.1111/dme.14197

Brodar, K. E., Davis, E. M., Lynn, C., Starr-Glass, L., Lui, J. H. L., Sanchez, J., & Delamater, A. M. (2021). Comprehensive psychosocial screening in a pediatric diabetes clinic. *Pediatric Diabetes, 22*(4), 656–666. https://doi.org/10.1111/pedi.13193

Bronfenbrenner, U. (1979). *The ecology of human development*. Harvard University Press.

Brouwer, A. M., Salamon, K. S., Olson, K. A., Fox, M. M., Yelich-Koth, S. L., Fleischman, K. M., Hains, A. A., Davies, W. H., & Kichler, J. C. (2012). Adolescents and Type 2 diabetes mellitus: A qualitative analysis of the experience of social support. *Clinical Pediatrics, 51*(12), 1130–1139. https://doi.org/10.1177/0009922812460914

Buchberger, B., Huppertz, H., Krabbe, L., Lux, B., Mattivi, J. T., & Siafarikas, A. (2016). Symptoms of depression and anxiety in youth with Type 1 diabetes: A systematic review and meta-analysis. *Psychoneuroendocrinology, 70*, 70–84. https://doi.org/10.1016/j.psyneuen.2016.04.019

Burdick, J., Chase, H. P., Slover, R. H., Knievel, K., Scrimgeour, L., Maniatis, A. K., & Klingensmith, G. J. (2004). Missed insulin meal boluses and elevated hemoglobin A1c levels in children receiving insulin pump therapy. *Pediatrics, 113*(3), e221–e224. https://doi.org/10.1542/peds.113.3.e221

Butler, A. M., Georges, T., & Anderson, B. J. (2020). Family influences. In A. Delamater & D. Marrero (Eds.), *Behavioral diabetes* (pp. 105–120). Springer Nature. https://doi.org/10.1007/978-3-030-33286-0_9

Butwicka, A., Frisén, L., Almqvist, C., Zethelius, B., & Lichtenstein, P. (2015). Risks of psychiatric disorders and suicide attempts in children and adolescents with Type 1 diabetes: A population-based cohort study. *Diabetes Care, 38*(3), 453–459. https://doi.org/10.2337/dc14-0262

Caccavale, L. J., Bernstein, R., Yarbro, J. L., Rushton, H., Gelfand, K. M., & Schwimmer, B. A. (2020). Impact and cost-effectiveness of integrated psychology services in a pediatric endocrinology clinic. *Journal of Clinical Psychology in Medical Settings, 27*(3), 615–621. https://doi.org/10.1007/s10880-019-09645-z

Cameron, F. J., Northam, E. A., & Ryan, C. M. (2019). The effect of Type 1 diabetes on the developing brain. *The Lancet Child & Adolescent Health*, *3*(6), 427–436. https://doi.org/10.1016/S2352-4642(19)30055-0

Campo, J. V., Bridge, J. A., & Fontanella, C. A. (2015). Access to mental health services: Implementing an integrated solution. *JAMA Pediatrics*, *169*(4), 299–300. https://doi.org/10.1001/jamapediatrics.2014.3558

Catherine, J. P., Russell, M. V., & Peter, C. H. (2021). The impact of race and socioeconomic factors on paediatric diabetes. *EClinicalMedicine*, *42*, 101186. https://doi.org/10.1016/j.eclinm.2021.101186

Centers for Disease Control and Prevention. (2022). *Advancing health equity*. https://www.cdc.gov/diabetes/health-equity/index.html

Channon, S., & Gregory, J. W. (2020). Individual-level intervention approaches in pediatric diabetes management. In A. Delamater & D. Marrero (Eds.), *Behavioral diabetes* (pp. 91–101). Springer Nature. https://doi.org/10.1007/978-3-030-33286-0_8

Channon, S. J., Huws-Thomas, M. V., Rollnick, S., Hood, K., Cannings-John, R. L., Rogers, C., & Gregory, J. W. (2007). A multicenter randomized controlled trial of motivational interviewing in teenagers with diabetes. *Diabetes Care*, *30*(6), 1390–1395. https://doi.org/10.2337/dc06-2260

Chao, A. M., Minges, K. E., Park, C., Dumser, S., Murphy, K. M., Grey, M., & Whittemore, R. (2016). General life and diabetes-related stressors in early adolescents with Type 1 diabetes. *Journal of Pediatric Health Care*, *30*(2), 133–142. https://doi.org/10.1016/j.pedhc.2015.06.005

Cook, S., Herold, K., Edidin, D. V., & Briars, R. (2002). Increasing problem solving in adolescents with Type 1 diabetes: The choices diabetes program. *The Diabetes Educator*, *28*(1), 115–124. https://doi.org/10.1177/014572170202800113

Corathers, S., Williford, D. N., Kichler, J., Smith, L., Ospelt, E., Rompicherla, S., Roberts, A., Prahalad, P., Basina, M., Muñoz, C., & Ebekozien, O. (2023). Implementation of psychosocial screening into diabetes clinics: Experience from the Type 1 Diabetes Exchange Quality Improvement Network. *Current Diabetes Reports*, *23*(2), 19–28. https://doi.org/10.1007/s11892-022-01497-6

Corathers, S. D., Schoettker, P. J., Clements, M. A., List, B. A., Mullen, D., Ohmer, A., Shah, A., & Lee, J. (2015). Health-system-based interventions to improve care in pediatric and adolescent Type 1 diabetes. *Current Diabetes Reports*, *15*(11), 91. https://doi.org/10.1007/s11892-015-0664-8

Crespo-Ramos, G., Cumba-Avilés, E., & Quiles-Jiménez, M. (2018). "They called me a terrorist": Social and internalized stigma in Latino youth with Type 1 diabetes. *Health Psychology Report*, *6*(4), 307–320. https://doi.org/10.5114/hpr.2018.80004

Dabelea, D., Bell, R. A., D'Agostino, R. B., Jr., Imperatore, G., Johansen, J. M., Linder, B., Liu, L. L., Loots, B., Marcovina, S., Mayer-Davis, E. J., Pettitt, D. J., Waitzfelder, B., & the Writing Group for the SEARCH for Diabetes in Youth Study Group. (2007). Incidence of diabetes in youth in the United States. *JAMA: Journal of the American Medical Association*, *297*(24), 2716–2724. https://doi.org/10.1001/jama.297.24.2716

Dabelea, D., Mayer-Davis, E. J., Saydah, S., Imperatore, G., Linder, B., Divers, J., Bell, R., Badaru, A., Talton, J. W., Crume, T., Liese, A. D., Merchant, A. T., Lawrence, J. M., Reynolds, K., Dolan, L., Liu, L. L., Hamman, R. F., & the SEARCH for Diabetes in Youth Study. (2014). Prevalence of Type 1 and Type 2 diabetes among children and adolescents from 2001 to 2009. *JAMA: Journal of the American Medical Association*, *311*(17), 1778–1786. https://doi.org/10.1001/jama.2014.3201

Daneman, D. (2020). Update on medical management of diabetes in children and adolescents: Epidemiology and treatment. In A. Delamater & D. Marrero (Eds.), *Behavioral diabetes* (pp. 7–16). Springer Nature. https://doi.org/10.1007/978-3-030-33286-0_2

Datye, K. A., & Jaser, S. S. (2020). Eating disorders in youth with diabetes. In A. Delamater & D. Marrero (Eds.), *Behavioral diabetes* (pp. 67–77). Springer Nature. https://doi.org/10.1007/978-3-030-33286-0_6

Davis, C. L., Delamater, A. M., Shaw, K. H., La Greca, A. M., Eidson, M. S., Perez-Rodriguez, J. E., & Nemery, R. (2001). Parenting styles, regimen adherence, and glycemic control in 4- to 10-year-old children with diabetes. *Journal of Pediatric Psychology*, *26*(2), 123–129. https://doi.org/10.1093/jpepsy/26.2.123

Delamater, A. M. (2012). Successful team management of Type 1 diabetes in children and young people: Key psychosocial issues. *Diabetes Care for Children & Young People*, *1*, 10–16.

Delamater, A. M., Bubb, J., Davis, S. G., Smith, J. A., Schmidt, L., White, N. H., & Santiago, J. V. (1990). Randomized prospective study of self-management training with newly diagnosed diabetic children. *Diabetes Care*, *13*(5), 492–498. https://doi.org/10.2337/diacare.13.5.492

Delamater, A. M., Daigre, A. L., Marchante, A. N., Pulgarón, E. R., Patiño-Fernandez, A. M., & Sanchez, J. (2017). Intrinsic motivation in ethnic minority youth with Type 1 diabetes. *Children's Health Care*, *46*(3), 215–229. https://doi.org/10.1080/02739615.2015.1124777

Delamater, A. M., de Wit, M., McDarby, V., Malik, J. A., Hilliard, M. E., Northam, E., & Acerini, C. L. (2018). ISPAD Clinical Practice Consensus Guidelines 2018: Psychological care of children and adolescents with Type 1 diabetes. *Pediatric Diabetes, 19*(Suppl. 27), 237–249. https://doi.org/10.1111/pedi.12736

Delamater, A. M., Guzman, A., & Aparicio, K. (2017). Mental health issues in children and adolescents with chronic illness. *International Journal of Human Rights in Healthcare, 10*(3), 163–173. https://doi.org/10.1108/IJHRH-05-2017-0020

Delamater, A. M., & Marrero, D. G. (Eds.). (2020). *Behavioral diabetes: Social ecological perspectives for pediatric and adult populations.* Springer Nature. https://doi.org/10.1007/978-3-030-33286-0

Delamater, A. M., Patiño-Fernández, A. M., Smith, K. E., & Bubb, J. (2013). Measurement of diabetes stress in older children and adolescents with Type 1 diabetes mellitus. *Pediatric Diabetes, 14*(1), 50–56. https://doi.org/10.1111/j.1399-5448.2012.00894.x

Delamater, A. M., Shaw, K. H., Applegate, E. B., Pratt, I. A., Eidson, M., Lancelotta, G. X., Gonzalez-Mendoza, L., & Richton, S. (1999). Risk for metabolic control problems in minority youth with diabetes. *Diabetes Care, 22*(5), 700–705. https://doi.org/10.2337/diacare.22.5.700

de Wit, M., Delemarre-van de Waal, H. A., Bokma, J. A., Haasnoot, K., Houdijk, M. C., Gemke, R. J., & Snoek, F. J. (2008). Monitoring and discussing health-related quality of life in adolescents with Type 1 diabetes improve psychosocial well-being: A randomized controlled trial. *Diabetes Care, 31*(8), 1521–1526. https://doi.org/10.2337/dc08-0394

de Wit, M., Gajewska, K. A., Goethals, E. R., McDarby, V., Zhao, X., Hapunda, G., Delamater, A. M., & DiMeglio, L. A. (2022). ISPAD Clinical Practice Consensus Guidelines 2022: Psychological care of children, adolescents and young adults with diabetes. *Pediatric Diabetes, 23*(8), 1373–1389. https://doi.org/10.1111/pedi.13428

de Wit, M., Pulgaron, E. R., Pattino-Fernandez, A. M., & Delamater, A. M. (2014). Psychological support for children with diabetes: Are the guidelines being met? *Journal of Clinical Psychology in Medical Settings, 21*(2), 190–199. https://doi.org/10.1007/s10880-014-9395-2

de Wit, M., & Snoek, F. J. (2011). Depressive symptoms and unmet psychological needs of Dutch youth with Type 1 diabetes: Results of a web-survey. *Pediatric Diabetes, 12*(3 Pt. 1), 172–176. https://doi.org/10.1111/j.1399-5448.2010.00673.x

Diabetes Control and Complications Trial Research Group. (1993). The effect of intensive treatment of diabetes on the development and progression of long-term complications in insulin-dependent diabetes mellitus. *The New England Journal of Medicine, 329*(14), 977–986. https://doi.org/10.1056/NEJM199309303291401

Ellis, D., Naar-King, S., Templin, T., Frey, M., Cunningham, P., Sheidow, A., Cakan, N., & Idalski, A. (2008). Multisystemic therapy for adolescents with poorly controlled Type 1 diabetes: Reduced diabetic ketoacidosis admissions and related costs over 24 months. *Diabetes Care, 31*(9), 1746–1747. https://doi.org/10.2337/dc07-2094

Ellis, D. A., Podolski, C. L., Frey, M., Naar-King, S., Wang, B., & Moltz, K. (2007). The role of parental monitoring in adolescent health outcomes: Impact on regimen adherence in youth with Type 1 diabetes. *Journal of Pediatric Psychology, 32*(8), 907–917. https://doi.org/10.1093/jpepsy/jsm009

Evans, M. A., Vesco, A. T., & Weissberg-Benchell, J. (2020). Depression, diabetes-related distress, and anxiety in pediatric diabetes. In A. Delamater & D. Marrero (Eds.), *Behavioral diabetes.* Springer Nature. https://doi.org/10.1007/978-3-030-33286-0_5

Feldman, M. A., Anderson, L. M., Shapiro, J. B., Jedraszko, A. M., Evans, M., Weil, L. E. G., Garza, K. P., & Weissberg-Benchell, J. (2018). Family-based interventions targeting improvements in health and family outcomes of children and adolescents with Type 1 diabetes: A systematic review. *Current Diabetes Reports, 18*(3), 15. https://doi.org/10.1007/s11892-018-0981-9

Forsander, G., Persson, B., Sundelin, J., Berglund, E., Snellman, K., & Hellström, R. (1998). Metabolic control in children with insulin-dependent diabetes mellitus 5 y after diagnosis. Early detection of patients at risk for poor metabolic control. *Acta Paediatrica, 87*(8), 857–864. https://doi.org/10.1080/080352598750013635

Foster, N. C., Beck, R. W., Miller, K. M., Clements, M. A., Rickels, M. R., DiMeglio, L. A., Maahs, D. M., Tamborlane, W. V., Bergenstal, R., Smith, E., Olson, B. A., & Garg, S. K. (2019). State of Type 1 diabetes management and outcomes from the T1D Exchange in 2016–2018. *Diabetes Technology & Therapeutics, 21*(2), 66–72. https://doi.org/10.1089/dia.2018.0384

Gabbs, M. H. J., Dart, A. B., Woo, M. R., Pinto, T., & Wicklow, B. A. (2022). Poor sleep, increased stress and metabolic comorbidity in adolescents and youth with Type 2 diabetes. *Canadian Journal of Diabetes, 46*(2), 142–149. https://doi.org/10.1016/j.jcjd.2021.07.005

Galler, A., Tittel, S. R., Baumeister, H., Reinauer, C., Brosig, B., Becker, M., Haberland, H., Hilgard, D.,

Jivan, M., Mirza, J., Schwab, J., & Holl, R. W. (2021). Worse glycemic control, higher rates of diabetic ketoacidosis, and more hospitalizations in children, adolescents, and young adults with Type 1 diabetes and anxiety disorders. *Pediatric Diabetes, 22*(3), 519–528. https://doi.org/10.1111/pedi.13177

Gallo, L. C., Roesch, S. C., Bravin, J. I., Savin, K. L., Perreira, K. M., Carnethon, M. R., Delamater, A. M., Salazar, C. R., Lopez-Gurrola, M., & Isasi, C. R. (2019). Socioeconomic adversity, social resources, and allostatic load among Hispanic/Latino youth: The Study of Latino Youth. *Psychosomatic Medicine, 81*(3), 305–312. https://doi.org/10.1097/PSY.0000000000000668

Garner, K., Boggiss, A., Jefferies, C., & Serlachius, A. (2022). Digital health interventions for improving mental health outcomes and wellbeing for youth with Type 1 diabetes: A systematic review. *Pediatric Diabetes, 23*(2), 258–269. https://doi.org/10.1111/pedi.13304

Gayes, L. A., & Steele, R. G. (2014). A meta-analysis of motivational interviewing interventions for pediatric health behavior change. *Journal of Consulting and Clinical Psychology, 82*(3), 521–535. https://doi.org/10.1037/a0035917

Goethals, E. R., Jaser, S. S., Verhaak, C., Prikken, S., Casteels, K., Luyckx, K., & Delamater, A. M. (2020). Communication matters: The role of autonomy-supportive communication by health care providers and parents in adolescents with Type 1 diabetes. *Diabetes Research and Clinical Practice, 163*, 108153. https://doi.org/10.1016/j.diabres.2020.108153

Goethals, E. R., Oris, L., Soenens, B., Berg, C. A., Prikken, S., Van Broeck, N., Weets, I., Casteels, K., & Luyckx, K. (2017). Parenting and treatment adherence in Type 1 diabetes throughout adolescence and emerging adulthood. *Journal of Pediatric Psychology, 42*(9), 922–932. https://doi.org/10.1093/jpepsy/jsx053

Goran, M. I., Ulijaszek, S. J., & Ventura, E. E. (2013). High fructose corn syrup and diabetes prevalence: A global perspective. *Global Public Health, Policy and Practice, 8*(1), 55–64. https://doi.org/10.1080/17441692.2012.736257

Green, A., Hede, S. M., Patterson, C. C., Wild, S. H., Imperatore, G., Roglic, G., & Beran, D. (2021). Type 1 diabetes in 2017: Global estimates of incident and prevalent cases in children and adults. *Diabetologia, 64*(12), 2741–2750. https://doi.org/10.1007/s00125-021-05571-8

Grey, M., Boland, E. A., Davidson, M., Li, J., & Tamborlane, W. V. (2000). Coping skills training for youth with diabetes mellitus has long-lasting effects on metabolic control and quality of life. *The Journal of Pediatrics, 137*(1), 107–113. https://doi.org/10.1067/mpd.2000.106568

Grey, M., Jaser, S. S., Whittemore, R., Jeon, S., & Lindemann, E. (2011). Coping skills training for parents of children with Type 1 diabetes: 12-month outcomes. *Nursing Research, 60*(3), 173–181. https://doi.org/10.1097/NNR.0b013e3182159c8f

Grey, M., Whittemore, R., Jeon, S., Murphy, K., Faulkner, M. S., Delamater, A., & the TeenCope Study Group. (2013). Internet psycho-education programs improve outcomes in youth with Type 1 diabetes. *Diabetes Care, 36*(9), 2475–2482. https://doi.org/10.2337/dc12-2199

Gulley, L. D., & Shomaker, L. B. (2020). Depression in youth-onset Type 2 diabetes. *Current Diabetes Reports, 20*(10), 51. https://doi.org/10.1007/s11892-020-01334-8

Guo, J., Luo, J., Yang, J., Huang, L., Wiley, J., Liu, F., Li, X., Zhou, Z., & Whittemore, R. (2020). School-aged children with Type 1 diabetes benefit more from a coping skills training program than adolescents in China: 12-month outcomes of a randomized clinical trial. *Pediatric Diabetes, 21*(3), 524–532. https://doi.org/10.1111/pedi.12975

Hagger, V., Hendrieckx, C., Sturt, J., Skinner, T. C., & Speight, J. (2016). Diabetes distress among adolescents with Type 1 diabetes: A systematic review. *Current Diabetes Reports, 16*(1), 9. https://doi.org/10.1007/s11892-015-0694-2

Hains, A. A., Davies, W. H., Parton, E., Totka, J., & Amoroso-Camarata, J. (2000). A stress management intervention for adolescents with Type 1 diabetes. *The Diabetes Educator, 26*(3), 417–424. https://doi.org/10.1177/014572170002600309

Harris, M. A., Freeman, K. A., & Duke, D. C. (2015). Seeing is believing: Using Skype to improve diabetes outcomes in youth. *Diabetes Care, 38*(8), 1427–1434. https://doi.org/10.2337/dc14-2469

Harris, M. A., Wagner, D. V., & Dukhovny, D. (2016). Commentary: Demon$trating (our) value. *Journal of Pediatric Psychology, 41*(8), 898–901. https://doi.org/10.1093/jpepsy/jsw029

Haugstvedt, A., Wentzel-Larsen, T., Graue, M., Søvik, O., & Rokne, B. (2010). Fear of hypoglycaemia in mothers and fathers of children with Type 1 diabetes is associated with poor glycaemic control and parental emotional distress: A population-based study. *Diabetic Medicine, 27*(1), 72–78. https://doi.org/10.1111/j.1464-5491.2009.02867.x

He, J., Ryder, A. G., Li, S., Liu, W., & Zhu, X. (2018). Glycemic extremes are related to cognitive dysfunction in children with Type 1 diabetes: A meta-analysis. *Journal of Diabetes Investigation, 9*(6), 1342–1353. https://doi.org/10.1111/jdi.12840

He, J., Zhu, J., Xie, Y., Du, H., Li, S., Li, S., He, W., Li, X., Zhou, Z., & Zhu, X. (2020). Effects of diabetic ketoacidosis on executive function in children with Type 1 diabetes: Evidence from Wisconsin card sorting test performance. *Psychosomatic Medicine*, 82(4), 359–365. https://doi.org/10.1097/PSY.0000000000000797

Helgeson, V. S., Escobar, O., Siminerio, L., & Becker, D. (2010). Relation of stressful life events to metabolic control among adolescents with diabetes: 5-year longitudinal study. *Health Psychology*, 29(2), 153–159. https://doi.org/10.1037/a0018163

Hilgard, D., Konrad, K., Meusers, M., Bartus, B., Otto, K. P., Lepler, R., Schober, E., Bollow, E., Holl, R. W., & the German/Austrian DPV Study Group, the Working Group on Psychiatric, Psychotherapeutic Psychological Aspects of Paediatric Diabetology (PPAG e.V.) and the BMBF Competence Network Diabetes, Germany. (2017). Comorbidity of attention deficit hyperactivity disorder and Type 1 diabetes in children and adolescents: Analysis based on the multicentre DPV registry. *Pediatric Diabetes*, 18(8), 706–713. https://doi.org/10.1111/pedi.12431

Hilliard, M. E., Harris, M. A., & Weissberg-Benchell, J. (2012). Diabetes resilience: A model of risk and protection in Type 1 diabetes. *Current Diabetes Reports*, 12(6), 739–748. https://doi.org/10.1007/s11892-012-0314-3

Hilliard, M. E., Powell, P. W., & Anderson, B. J. (2016). Evidence-based behavioral interventions to promote diabetes management in children, adolescents, and families. *American Psychologist*, 71(7), 590–601. https://doi.org/10.1037/a0040359

Hilliard, M. E., Wu, Y. P., Rausch, J., Dolan, L. M., & Hood, K. K. (2013). Predictors of deteriorations in diabetes management and control in adolescents with Type 1 diabetes. *The Journal of Adolescent Health*, 52(1), 28–34. https://doi.org/10.1016/j.jadohealth.2012.05.009

Holtz, B. E., Mitchell, K. M., Nuttall, A. K., Cotten, S. R., Hershey, D. D., Dunneback, J. K., & Wood, M. A. (2020). Using user-feedback to develop a website: MyT1DHope, for parents of children with T1D. *Health Communication*, 35(3), 281–288. https://doi.org/10.1080/10410236.2018.1560579

Hood, K. K., Huestis, S., Maher, A., Butler, D., Volkening, L., & Laffel, L. M. (2006). Depressive symptoms in children and adolescents with Type 1 diabetes: Association with diabetes-specific characteristics. *Diabetes Care*, 29(6), 1389–1391. https://doi.org/10.2337/dc06-0087

Hood, K. K., Iturralde, E., Rausch, J., & Weissberg-Benchell, J. (2018). Preventing diabetes distress in adolescents with Type 1 diabetes: Results 1 year after participation in the STePS Program. *Diabetes Care*, 41(8), 1623–1630. https://doi.org/10.2337/dc17-2556

Hood, K. K., Rohan, J. M., Peterson, C. M., & Drotar, D. (2010). Interventions with adherence-promoting components in pediatric Type 1 diabetes: Meta-analysis of their impact on glycemic control. *Diabetes Care*, 33(7), 1658–1664. https://doi.org/10.2337/dc09-2268

Huynh, E., Rand, D., McNeill, C., Brown, S., Senechal, M., Wicklow, B., Dart, A., Sellers, E., Dean, H., Blydt-Hansen, T., & McGavock, J. (2015). Beating diabetes together: A mixed-methods analysis of a feasibility study of intensive lifestyle intervention for youth with Type 2 diabetes. *Canadian Journal of Diabetes*, 39(6), 484–490. https://doi.org/10.1016/j.jcjd.2015.09.093

Inge, T. H., Miyano, G., Bean, J., Helmrath, M., Courcoulas, A., Harmon, C. M., Chen, M. K., Wilson, K., Daniels, S. R., Garcia, V. F., Brandt, M. L., & Dolan, L. M. (2009). Reversal of Type 2 diabetes mellitus and improvements in cardiovascular risk factors after surgical weight loss in adolescents. *Pediatrics*, 123(1), 214–222. https://doi.org/10.1542/peds.2008-0522

International Diabetes Federation. (2019). *IDF diabetes atlas* (9th ed.). https://diabetesatlas.org/upload/resources/material/20200302_133351_IDFATLAS9e-final-web.pdf

Iturralde, E., Adams, R. N., Barley, R. C., Bensen, R., Christofferson, M., Hanes, S. J., Maahs, D. M., Milla, C., Naranjo, D., Shah, A. C., Tanenbaum, M. L., Veeravalli, S., Park, K. T., & Hood, K. K. (2017). Implementation of depression screening and global health assessment in pediatric sub-specialty clinics. *The Journal of Adolescent Health*, 61(5), 591–598. https://doi.org/10.1016/j.jadohealth.2017.05.030

Iturralde, E., Rausch, J. R., Weissberg-Benchell, J., & Hood, K. K. (2019). Diabetes-related emotional distress over time. *Pediatrics*, 143(6), e20183011. https://doi.org/10.1542/peds.2018-3011

Iturralde, E., Weissberg-Benchell, J., & Hood, K. K. (2017). Avoidant coping and diabetes-related distress: Pathways to adolescents' Type 1 diabetes outcomes. *Health Psychology*, 36(3), 236–244. https://doi.org/10.1037/hea0000445

Jacobson, A. M., Hauser, S. T., Willett, J., Wolfsdorf, J. I., & Herman, L. (1997). Consequences of irregular versus continuous medical follow-up in children and adolescents with insulin-dependent diabetes mellitus. *The Journal of Pediatrics*, 131(5), 727–733. https://doi.org/10.1016/S0022-3476(97)70101-X

Jaser, S. S., Linsky, R., & Grey, M. (2014). Coping and psychological distress in mothers of adolescents with Type 1 diabetes. *Maternal and Child Health Journal, 18*(1), 101–108. https://doi.org/10.1007/s10995-013-1239-4

Jaser, S. S., Lord, J. H., Savin, K., Gruhn, M., & Rumburg, T. (2018). Developing and testing an intervention to reduce distress in mothers of adolescents with Type 1 diabetes. *Clinical Practice in Pediatric Psychology, 6*(1), 19–30. https://doi.org/10.1037/cpp0000220

Jaser, S. S., Patel, N., Xu, M., Tamborlane, W. V., & Grey, M. (2017). Stress and coping predicts adjustment and glycemic control in adolescents with Type 1 diabetes. *Annals of Behavioral Medicine, 51*(1), 30–38. https://doi.org/10.1007/s12160-016-9825-5

Joish, V. N., Zhou, F. L., Preblick, R., Lin, D., Deshpande, M., Verma, S., Davies, M. J., Paranjape, S., & Pettus, J. (2020). Estimation of annual health care costs for adults with Type 1 diabetes in the United States. *Journal of Managed Care & Specialty Pharmacy, 26*(3), 311–318. https://doi.org/10.18553/jmcp.2020.26.3.311

Jones, K. L. (1998). Non-insulin dependent diabetes in children and adolescents: The therapeutic challenge. *Clinical Pediatrics, 37*(2), 103–110. https://doi.org/10.1177/000992289803700207

Katz, L. L., Anderson, B. J., McKay, S. V., Izquierdo, R., Casey, T. L., Higgins, L. A., Wauters, A., Hirst, K., Nadeau, K. J., & the TODAY Study Group. (2016). Correlates of medication adherence in the TODAY cohort of youth with Type 2 diabetes. *Diabetes Care, 39*(11), 1956–1962. https://doi.org/10.2337/dc15-2296

Kaufman, F. R., Halvorson, M., & Carpenter, S. (1999). Association between diabetes control and visits to a multidisciplinary pediatric diabetes clinic. *Pediatrics, 103*(5), 948–951. https://doi.org/10.1542/peds.103.5.948

King, P. S., Berg, C. A., Butner, J., Butler, J. M., & Wiebe, D. J. (2014). Longitudinal trajectories of parental involvement in Type 1 diabetes and adolescents' adherence. *Health Psychology, 33*(5), 424–432. https://doi.org/10.1037/a0032804

Knox, E. C. L., Quirk, H., Glazebrook, C., Randell, T., & Blake, H. (2019). Impact of technology-based interventions for children and young people with Type 1 diabetes on key diabetes self-management behaviours and prerequisites: A systematic review. *BMC Endocrine Disorders, 19*(1), 7. https://doi.org/10.1186/s12902-018-0331-6

Kolko, D. J., Campo, J., Kilbourne, A. M., Hart, J., Sakolsky, D., & Wisniewski, S. (2014). Collaborative care outcomes for pediatric behavioral health problems: A cluster randomized trial. *Pediatrics, 133*(4), e981–e992. https://doi.org/10.1542/peds.2013-2516

Kolko, D. J., & Perrin, E. (2014). The integration of behavioral health interventions in children's health care: Services, science, and suggestions. *Journal of Clinical Child and Adolescent Psychology, 43*(2), 216–228. https://doi.org/10.1080/15374416.2013.862804

Kongkaew, C., Jampachaisri, K., Chaturongkul, C. A., & Scholfield, C. N. (2014). Depression and adherence to treatment in diabetic children and adolescents: A systematic review and meta-analysis of observational studies. *European Journal of Pediatrics, 173*(2), 203–212. https://doi.org/10.1007/s00431-013-2128-y

Kriska, A., Delahanty, L., Edelstein, S., Amodei, N., Chadwick, J., Copeland, K., Galvin, B., El ghormli, L., Haymond, M., Kelsey, M., Lassiter, C., Mayer-Davis, E., Milaszewski, K., & Syme, A. (2013). Sedentary behavior and physical activity in youth with recent onset of Type 2 diabetes. *Pediatrics, 131*(3), e850–e856. https://doi.org/10.1542/peds.2012-0620

Kriska, A., El ghormli, L., Copeland, K. C., Higgins, J., Ievers-Landis, C. E., Levitt Katz, L. E., Trief, P. M., Wauters, A. D., Yasuda, P. M., Delahanty, L. M., & the TODAY Study Group. (2018). Impact of lifestyle behavior change on glycemic control in youth with Type 2 diabetes. *Pediatric Diabetes, 19*(1), 36–44. https://doi.org/10.1111/pedi.12526

Laffel, L. M., Kanapka, L. G., Beck, R. W., Bergamo, K., Clements, M. A., Criego, A., DeSalvo, D. J., Goland, R., Hood, K., Liljenquist, D., Messer, L. H., Monzavi, R., Mouse, T. J., Prahalad, P., Sherr, J., Simmons, J. H., Wadwa, R. P., Weinstock, R. S., Willi, S. M., Miller, K. M., & the CGM Intervention in Teens and Young Adults with T1D (CITY) Study Group, & the CDE10. (2020). Effect of continuous glucose monitoring on glycemic control in adolescents and young adults with Type 1 diabetes: A randomized clinical trial. *JAMA: Journal of the American Medical Association, 323*(23), 2388–2396. https://doi.org/10.1001/jama.2020.6940

La Greca, A. M., Auslander, W. F., Greco, P., Spetter, D., Fisher, E. B., Jr., & Santiago, J. V. (1995). I get by with a little help from my family and friends: Adolescents' support for diabetes care. *Journal of Pediatric Psychology, 20*(4), 449–476. https://doi.org/10.1093/jpepsy/20.4.449

Landolt, M. A., Ribi, K., Laimbacher, J., Vollrath, M., Gnehm, H. E., & Sennhauser, F. H. (2002). Posttraumatic stress disorder in parents of children with newly diagnosed Type 1 diabetes. *Journal of Pediatric Psychology, 27*(7), 647–652. https://doi.org/10.1093/jpepsy/27.7.647

Lansing, A. H., Stoianova, M., & Stanger, C. (2019). Adolescent emotional control moderates benefits of a multicomponent intervention to improve Type 1 diabetes adherence: A pilot randomized controlled trial. *Journal of Pediatric Psychology, 44*(1), 126–136. https://doi.org/10.1093/jpepsy/jsy071

Lawrence, J. M., Divers, J., Isom, S., Saydah, S., Imperatore, G., Pihoker, C., Marcovina, S. M., Mayer-Davis, E. J., Hamman, R. F., Dolan, L., Dabelea, D., Pettitt, D. J., Liese, A. D., & the SEARCH for Diabetes in Youth Study Group. (2021). Trends in prevalence of Type 1 and Type 2 diabetes in children and adolescents in the US, 2001–2017. *JAMA: Journal of the American Medical Association, 326*(8), 717–727. https://doi.org/10.1001/jama.2021.11165

Lawrence, J. M., Standiford, D. A., Loots, B., Klingensmith, G. J., Williams, D. E., Ruggiero, A., Liese, A. D., Bell, R. A., Waitzfelder, B. E., McKeown, R. E., & the SEARCH for Diabetes in Youth Study. (2006). Prevalence and correlates of depressed mood among youth with diabetes: The SEARCH for Diabetes in Youth study. *Pediatrics, 117*(4), 1348–1358. https://doi.org/10.1542/peds.2005-1398

Lee, J. M., Rusnak, A., Garrity, A., Hirschfeld, E., Thomas, I. H., Wichorek, M., Lee, J. E., Rioles, N. A., Ebekozien, O., & Corathers, S. D. (2021). Feasibility of electronic health record assessment of 6 pediatric Type 1 diabetes self-management habits and their association with glycemic outcomes. *JAMA Network Open, 4*(10), e2131278. https://doi.org/10.1001/jamanetworkopen.2021.31278

Levitt Katz, L. E., Swami, S., Abraham, M., Murphy, K. M., Jawad, A. F., McKnight-Menci, H., & Berkowitz, R. (2005). Neuropsychiatric disorders at the presentation of Type 2 diabetes mellitus in children. *Pediatric Diabetes, 6*(2), 84–89. https://doi.org/10.1111/j.1399-543X.2005.00105.x

Liu, L. L., Lawrence, J. M., Davis, C., Liese, A. D., Pettitt, D. J., Pihoker, C., Dabelea, D., Hamman, R., Waitzfelder, B., Kahn, H. S., & SEARCH for Diabetes in Youth Study Group. (2010). Prevalence of overweight and obesity in youth with diabetes in USA: The SEARCH for Diabetes in Youth study. *Pediatric Diabetes, 11*(1), 4–11. https://doi.org/10.1111/j.1399-5448.2009.00519.x

Lohan, A., Morawska, A., & Mitchell, A. (2017). Association between parental factors and child diabetes-management-related behaviors. *Journal of Developmental and Behavioral Pediatrics, 38*(5), 330–338. https://doi.org/10.1097/DBP.0000000000000447

Majidi, S., Ebekozien, O., Noor, N., Lyons, S. K., McDonough, R., Gandhi, K., Izquierdo, R., Demeterco-Berggren, C., Polsky, S., Basina, M., Desimone, M., Thomas, I., Rioles, N., Jimenez-Vega, J., Malik, F. S., Miyazaki, B., Albanese-O'Neill, A., & Jones, N. Y. (2021). Inequities in health outcomes in children and adults with Type 1 diabetes: Data from the T1D Exchange Quality Improvement Collaborative. *Clinical Diabetes, 39*(3), 278–283. https://doi.org/10.2337/cd21-0028

Malik, F. S., Sauder, K. A., Isom, S., Reboussin, B. A., Dabelea, D., Lawrence, J. M., Roberts, A., Mayer-Davis, E. J., Marcovina, S., Dolan, L., Igudesman, D., Pihoker, C., SEARCH for Diabetes in Youth Study: Malik, F. S., Sauder, K. A., Isom, S., Reboussin, B. A., Dabelea, D., Lawrence, J. M., Roberts, A., Mayer-Davis, E. J., Marcovina, S., Dolan, L., Igudesman, D., Pihoker, C., & the SEARCH for Diabetes in Youth Study. (2022). Trends in glycemic control among youth and young adults with diabetes: The SEARCH for Diabetes in Youth Study. *Diabetes Care, 45*(2), 285–294. https://doi.org/10.2337/dc21-0507

Marker, A. M., Patton, S. R., McDonough, R. J., Feingold, H., Simon, L., & Clements, M. A. (2019). Implementing clinic-wide depression screening for pediatric diabetes: An initiative to improve healthcare processes. *Pediatric Diabetes, 20*(7), 964–973. https://doi.org/10.1111/pedi.12886

Mauras, N., Buckingham, B., White, N. H., Tsalikian, E., Weinzimer, S. A., Jo, B., Cato, A., Fox, L. A., Aye, T., Arbelaez, A. M., Hershey, T., Tansey, M., Tamborlane, W., Foland-Ross, L. C., Shen, H., Englert, K., Mazaika, P., Marzelli, M., Reiss, A. L., & the Diabetes Research in Children Network (DirecNet). (2021). Impact of Type 1 diabetes in the developing brain in children: A longitudinal study. *Diabetes Care, 44*(4), 983–992. https://doi.org/10.2337/dc20-2125

Mayer-Davis, E. J., Maahs, D. M., Seid, M., Crandell, J., Bishop, F. K., Driscoll, K. A., Hunter, C. M., Kichler, J. C., Standiford, D., Thomas, J. M., Bishop, F., Bouffard, A., Clay, M., Crandell, J., Dolan, L., Driscoll, K., Grossoehme, D., Hull, M., Hunter, C., . . . Zickler, M. (2018). Efficacy of the Flexible Lifestyles Empowering Change intervention on metabolic and psychosocial outcomes in adolescents with Type 1 diabetes (FLEX): A randomised controlled trial. *The Lancet Child & Adolescent Health, 2*(9), 635–646. https://doi.org/10.1016/S2352-4642(18)30208-6

McDaniel, S. H., & deGruy, F. V., III. (2014). An introduction to primary care and psychology. *American Psychologist, 69*(4), 325–331. https://doi.org/10.1037/a0036222

McGavock, J., Dart, A., & Wicklow, B. (2015). Lifestyle therapy for the treatment of youth with Type 2 diabetes. *Current Diabetes Reports, 15*(1), 568. https://doi.org/10.1007/s11892-014-0568-z

McVoy, M., Hardin, H., Fulchiero, E., Caforio, K., Briggs, F., Neudecker, M., & Sajatovic, M. (2023). Mental health comorbidity and youth onset Type 2 diabetes: A systematic review of the literature. *International Journal of Psychiatry in Medicine, 58*(1), 37–55. https://doi.org/10.1177/00912174211067335

Méndez, F. J., & Beléndez, M. (1997). Effects of a behavioral intervention on treatment adherence and stress management in adolescents with IDDM. *Diabetes Care, 20*(9), 1370–1375. https://doi.org/10.2337/diacare.20.9.1370

Miller, K. M., Beck, R. W., Bergenstal, R. M., Goland, R. S., Haller, M. J., McGill, J. B., Rodriguez, H., Simmons, J. H., Hirsch, I. B., & the T1D Exchange Clinic Network. (2013). Evidence of a strong association between frequency of self-monitoring of blood glucose and hemoglobin A1c levels in T1D exchange clinic registry participants. *Diabetes Care, 36*(7), 2009–2014. https://doi.org/10.2337/dc12-1770

Miller-Johnson, S., Emery, R. E., Marvin, R. S., Clarke, W., Lovinger, R., & Martin, M. (1994). Parent-child relationships and the management of insulin-dependent diabetes mellitus. *Journal of Consulting and Clinical Psychology, 62*(3), 603–610. https://doi.org/10.1037/0022-006X.62.3.603

Mironovici, C., Kepper, M., Scribner, R., & Chalew, S. (2020). Demographic influences and health disparities. In A. Delamater & D. Marrero (Eds.), *Behavioral diabetes* (pp. 169–197). Springer Nature. https://doi.org/10.1007/978-3-030-33286-0_13

Mitchell, R. J., McMaugh, A., Woodhead, H., Lystad, R. P., Zurynski, Y., Badgery-Parker, T., Cameron, C. M., & Hng, T. M. (2022). The impact of Type 1 diabetes mellitus in childhood on academic performance: A matched population-based cohort study. *Pediatric Diabetes, 23*(3), 411–420. https://doi.org/10.1111/pedi.13317

Monaghan, M., Mara, C. A., Kichler, J. C., Westen, S. C., Rawlinson, A., Jacobsen, L. M., Adams, R. N., Stone, J. Y., Hood, K. K., & Mulvaney, S. A. (2021). Multisite examination of depression screening scores and correlates among adolescents and young adults with Type 2 diabetes. *Canadian Journal of Diabetes, 45*(5), 411–416. https://doi.org/10.1016/j.jcjd.2021.01.011

Monzon, A. D., Clements, M. A., & Patton, S. R. (2024). Group engagement in parent-focused telehealth interventions for families of children with Type 1 diabetes. *Journal of Telemedicine and Telecare, 30*(3), 505–513. https://doi.org/10.1177/1357633X211067

Morone, J. (2019). Systematic review of sociodemographic representation and cultural responsiveness in psychosocial and behavioral interventions with adolescents with Type 1 diabetes. *Journal of Diabetes, 11*(7), 582–592. https://doi.org/10.1111/1753-0407.12889

Mulvaney, S. A., Mara, C. A., Kichler, J. C., Majidi, S., Driscoll, K. A., Westen, S. C., Rawlinson, A., Jacobsen, L. M., Adams, R. N., Hood, K. K., & Monaghan, M. (2021). A retrospective multisite examination of depression screening practices, scores, and correlates in pediatric diabetes care. *Translational Behavioral Medicine, 11*(1), 122–131. https://doi.org/10.1093/tbm/ibz171

Mulvaney, S. A., Rothman, R. L., Osborn, C. Y., Lybarger, C., Dietrich, M. S., & Wallston, K. A. (2011). Self-management problem solving for adolescents with Type 1 diabetes: Intervention processes associated with an internet program. *Patient Education and Counseling, 85*(2), 140–142. https://doi.org/10.1016/j.pec.2010.09.018

Mulvaney, S. A., Rothman, R. L., Wallston, K. A., Lybarger, C., & Dietrich, M. S. (2010). An internet-based program to improve self-management in adolescents with Type 1 diabetes. *Diabetes Care, 33*(3), 602–604. https://doi.org/10.2337/dc09-1881

Murphy, H. R., Wadham, C., Rayman, G., & Skinner, T. C. (2007). Approaches to integrating paediatric diabetes care and structured education: Experiences from the Families, Adolescents, and Children's Teamwork Study (FACTS). *Diabetic Medicine, 24*(11), 1261–1268. https://doi.org/10.1111/j.1464-5491.2007.02229.x

Nally, L. M., Wagner, J., Sherr, J., Tichy, E., Weyman, K., Ginley, M. K., Zajac, K., Desousa, M., Shabanova, V., Petry, N. M., Tamborlane, W. V., & Van Name, M. (2021). A pilot study of youth with Type 1 diabetes initiating use of a hybrid closed-loop system while receiving a behavioral economics intervention. *Endocrine Practice, 27*(6), 545–551. https://doi.org/10.1016/j.eprac.2020.11.017

Nansel, T. R., Iannotti, R. J., & Liu, A. (2012). Clinic-integrated behavioral intervention for families of youth with Type 1 diabetes: Randomized clinical trial. *Pediatrics, 129*(4), e866–e873. https://doi.org/10.1542/peds.2011-2858

Nansel, T. R., Iannotti, R. J., Simons-Morton, B. G., Plotnick, L. P., Clark, L. M., & Zeitzoff, L. (2009). Long-term maintenance of treatment outcomes: Diabetes personal trainer intervention for youth with Type 1 diabetes. *Diabetes Care, 32*(5), 807–809. https://doi.org/10.2337/dc08-1968

Naranjo, D., Schwartz, D. D., & Delamater, A. M. (2015). Diabetes in ethnically diverse youth: Disparate burden and intervention approaches. *Current Diabetes Reviews, 11*(4), 251–260. https://doi.org/10.2174/1573399811666150421115846

Naughton, M. J., Joyce, P., Morgan, T. M., Seid, M., Lawrence, J. M., Klingensmith, G. J., Waitzfelder, B., Standiford, D. A., & Loots, B. (2014). Longitudinal associations between sex, diabetes self-care, and health-related quality of life among youth with Type 1 or Type 2 diabetes mellitus. *The Journal of Pediatrics*, 164(6), 1376–1383. https://doi.org/10.1016/j.jpeds.2014.01.027

Nguyen, L. A., Pouwer, F., Winterdijk, P., Hartman, E., Nuboer, R., Sas, T., de Kruijff, I., Bakker-Van Waarde, W., Aanstoot, H. J., & Nefs, G. (2021). Prevalence and course of mood and anxiety disorders, and correlates of symptom severity in adolescents with Type 1 diabetes: Results from diabetes LEAP. *Pediatric Diabetes*, 22(4), 638–648. https://doi.org/10.1111/pedi.13174

Nip, A. S. Y., Reboussin, B. A., Dabelea, D., Bellatorre, A., Mayer-Davis, E. J., Kahkoska, A. R., Lawrence, J. M., Peterson, C. M., Dolan, L., & Pihoker, C. (2019). Disordered eating behaviors in youth and young adults with Type 1 or Type 2 diabetes receiving insulin therapy: The SEARCH for Diabetes in Youth Study. *Diabetes Care*, 42(5), 859–866. https://doi.org/10.2337/dc18-2420

Northam, E. (2020). Effects of diabetes on neuro-cognitive function of children. In A. Delamater & D. Marrero (Eds.), *Behavioral diabetes*. Springer Nature. https://doi.org/10.1007/978-3-030-33286-0_7

Noser, A. E., Dai, H., Marker, A. M., Raymond, J. K., Majidi, S., Clements, M. A., Stanek, K. R., & Patton, S. R. (2019). Parental depression and diabetes-specific distress after the onset of Type 1 diabetes in children. *Health Psychology*, 38(2), 103–112. https://doi.org/10.1037/hea0000699

Palladino, D. K., & Helgeson, V. S. (2012). Friends or foes? A review of peer influence on self-care and glycemic control in adolescents with Type 1 diabetes. *Journal of Pediatric Psychology*, 37(5), 591–603. https://doi.org/10.1093/jpepsy/jss009

Paris, C. A., Imperatore, G., Klingensmith, G., Petitti, D., Rodriguez, B., Anderson, A. M., Schwartz, I. D., Standiford, D. A., & Pihoker, C. (2009). Predictors of insulin regimens and impact on outcomes in youth with Type 1 diabetes: The SEARCH for Diabetes in Youth study. *The Journal of Pediatrics*, 155(2), 183–189.E1. https://doi.org/10.1016/j.jpeds.2009.01.063

Parker, E. D., Lin, J., Mahoney, T., Ume, N., Yang, G., Gabbay, R. A., ElSayed, N. A., & Bannuru, R. R. (2024). Economic costs of diabetes in the U.S. in 2022. *Diabetes Care*, 47(1), 26–43. https://doi.org/10.2337/dci23-0085

Patton, S. R., Clements, M. A., Marker, A. M., & Nelson, E. L. (2020). Intervention to reduce hypoglycemia fear in parents of young kids using video-based telehealth (REDCHiP). *Pediatric Diabetes*, 21(1), 112–119. https://doi.org/10.1111/pedi.12934

Petitti, D. B., Klingensmith, G. J., Bell, R. A., Andrews, J. S., Dabelea, D., Imperatore, G., Marcovina, S., Pihoker, C., Standiford, D., Waitzfelder, B., & Mayer-Davis, E. (2009). Glycemic control in youth with diabetes: The SEARCH for Diabetes in Youth Study. *The Journal of Pediatrics*, 155(5), 668–672.e1, 3. https://doi.org/10.1016/j.jpeds.2009.05.025

Powell, P. W., Corathers, S. D., Raymond, J., & Streisand, R. (2015). New approaches to providing individualized diabetes care in the 21st century. *Current Diabetes Reviews*, 11(4), 222–230. https://doi.org/10.2174/1573399811666150421110316

Pulgaron, E. R., & Delamater, A. M. (2014). Obesity and Type 2 diabetes in children: Epidemiology and treatment. *Current Diabetes Reports*, 14(8), 508. https://doi.org/10.1007/s11892-014-0508-y

Pulgaron, E. R., Hernandez, J., Dehaan, H., Patiño-Fernandez, A. M., Carrillo, A., Sanchez, J., & Delamater, A. M. (2015). Clinic attendance and health outcomes of youth with Type 2 diabetes mellitus. *International Journal of Adolescent Medicine and Health*, 27(3), 271–274. https://doi.org/10.1515/ijamh-2014-0021

Pulgaron, E. R., Valledor, V. L., Aparicio, K. L., & Delamater, A. M. (2020). Diabetes prevention in schools and communities. In A. Delamater & D. Marrero (Eds.), *Behavioral diabetes* (pp. 213–224). Springer Nature. https://doi.org/10.1007/978-3-030-33286-0_15

Rao, G., & Jensen, E. T. (2020). Type 2 diabetes in youth. *Global pediatric health*, 7. https://doi.org/10.1177/2333794X20981343

Raymaekers, K., Oris, L., Prikken, S., Moons, P., Goossens, E., Weets, I., & Luyckx, K. (2017). The role of peers for diabetes management in adolescents and emerging adults with Type 1 diabetes: A longitudinal study. *Diabetes Care*, 40(12), 1678–1684. https://doi.org/10.2337/dc17-0643

Rechenberg, K., Grey, M., & Sadler, L. (2017). Stress and posttraumatic stress in mothers of children with Type 1 diabetes. *Journal of Family Nursing*, 23(2), 201–225. https://doi.org/10.1177/1074840716687543

Rechenberg, K., & Koerner, R. (2021). Cognitive behavioral therapy in adolescents with Type 1 diabetes: An integrative review. *Journal of Pediatric Nursing*, 60, 190–197. https://doi.org/10.1016/j.pedn.2021.06.019

Rechenberg, K., Whittemore, R., Holland, M., & Grey, M. (2017). General and diabetes-specific stress in adolescents with Type 1 diabetes. *Diabetes Research and Clinical Practice, 130*, 1–8. https://doi.org/10.1016/j.diabres.2017.05.003

Redel, J. M., DiFrancesco, M., Lee, G. R., Ziv, A., Dolan, L. M., Brady, C. C., & Shah, A. S. (2022). Cerebral blood flow is lower in youth with Type 2 diabetes compared to obese controls: A pilot study. *Pediatric Diabetes, 23*(3), 291–300. https://doi.org/10.1111/pedi.13313

Redel, J. M., Dolan, L. M., DiFrancesco, M., Vannest, J., & Shah, A. S. (2019). Youth-onset Type 2 diabetes and the developing brain. *Current Diabetes Reports, 19*(1), 3. https://doi.org/10.1007/s11892-019-1120-y

Roberts, A. J., Bao, H., Qu, P., Moss, A., Kim, G., Yi-Frazier, J. P., Pihoker, C., & Malik, F. (2021). Mental health comorbidities in adolescents and young adults with Type 2 diabetes. *Journal of Pediatric Nursing, 61*, 280–283. https://doi.org/10.1016/j.pedn.2021.07.028

Robling, M., McNamara, R., Bennert, K., Butler, C. C., Channon, S., Cohen, D., Crowne, E., Hambly, H., Hawthorne, K., Hood, K., Longo, M., Lowes, L., Pickles, T., Playle, R., Rollnick, S., Thomas-Jones, E., & Gregory, J. W. (2012). The effect of the Talking Diabetes consulting skills intervention on glycaemic control and quality of life in children with Type 1 diabetes: Cluster randomised controlled trial (DEPICTED study). *BMJ: British Medical Journal, 344*, e2359. https://doi.org/10.1136/bmj.e2359

Rose, M., Aronow, L., Breen, S., Tully, C., Hilliard, M. E., Butler, A. M., & Streisand, R. (2018). Considering culture: A review of pediatric behavioral intervention research in Type 1 diabetes. *Current Diabetes Reports, 18*(4), 16. https://doi.org/10.1007/s11892-018-0987-3

Rose, M., Streisand, R., Tully, C., Clary, L., Monaghan, M., Wang, J., & Mackey, E. (2020). Risk of disordered eating behaviors in adolescents with Type 1 diabetes. *Journal of Pediatric Psychology, 45*(5), 583–591. https://doi.org/10.1093/jpepsy/jsaa027

Rothman, R. L., Mulvaney, S., Elasy, T. A., VanderWoude, A., Gebretsadik, T., Shintani, A., Potter, A., Russell, W. E., & Schlundt, D. (2008). Self-management behaviors, racial disparities, and glycemic control among adolescents with Type 2 diabetes. *Pediatrics, 121*(4), e912–e919. https://doi.org/10.1542/peds.2007-1484

Sacco, W. P., & Bykowski, C. A. (2010). Depression and hemoglobin A1c in Type 1 and Type 2 diabetes: The role of self-efficacy. *Diabetes Research and Clinical Practice, 90*(2), 141–146. https://doi.org/10.1016/j.diabres.2010.06.026

Saletsky, R. D., Trief, P. M., Anderson, B. J., Rosenbaum, P., & Weinstock, R. S. (2014). Parenting style, parent-youth conflict, and medication adherence in youth with Type 2 diabetes participating in an intensive lifestyle change intervention. *Families, Systems, & Health, 32*(2), 176–185. https://doi.org/10.1037/fsh0000008

Saydah, S., Imperatore, G., Cheng, Y., Geiss, L. S., & Albright, A. (2017). Disparities in diabetes deaths among children and adolescents—United States, 2000-2014. *MMWR: Morbidity and Mortality Weekly Report, 66*(19), 502–505. https://doi.org/10.15585/mmwr.mm6619a4

Schober, E., Wagner, G., Berger, G., Gerber, D., Mengl, M., Sonnenstatter, S., Barrientos, I., Rami, B., Karwautz, A., Fritsch, M., & the Austrian Diabetic Incidence Study Group. (2011). Prevalence of intentional under- and overdosing of insulin in children and adolescents with Type 1 diabetes. *Pediatric Diabetes, 12*(7), 627–631. https://doi.org/10.1111/j.1399-5448.2011.00759.x

Serlachius, A. S., Scratch, S. E., Northam, E. A., Frydenberg, E., Lee, K. J., & Cameron, F. J. (2016). A randomized controlled trial of cognitive behaviour therapy to improve glycaemic control and psychosocial wellbeing in adolescents with Type 1 diabetes. *Journal of Health Psychology, 21*(6), 1157–1169. https://doi.org/10.1177/1359105314547940

Shah, A. S., Zeitler, P. S., Wong, J., Pena, A. S., Wicklow, B., Arslanian, S., Chang, N., Fu, J., Dabadghao, P., Pinhas-Hamiel, O., Urakami, T., & Craig, M. E. (2022). ISPAD Clinical Practice Consensus Guidelines 2022: Type 2 diabetes in children and adolescents. *Pediatric Diabetes, 23*(7), 872–902. https://doi.org/10.1111/pedi.13409

Shaw, J. (2007). Epidemiology of childhood Type 2 diabetes and obesity. *Pediatric Diabetes, 8*(s9, Suppl. 9), 7–15. https://doi.org/10.1111/j.1399-5448.2007.00329.x

St. George, S. M., Pulgaron, E. R., Ferranti, D., Agosto, Y., Toro, M. I., Ramseur, K. C., & Delamater, A. M. (2017). A qualitative study of cognitive, behavioral, and psychosocial challenges associated with pediatric Type 2 diabetes in ethnic minority parents and adolescents. *The Diabetes Educator, 43*(2), 180–189. https://doi.org/10.1177/0145721717691146

Stanger, C., Lansing, A. H., Scherer, E., Budney, A., Christiano, A. S., & Casella, S. J. (2018). A web-delivered multicomponent intervention for adolescents with poorly controlled Type 1 diabetes: A pilot randomized controlled trial. *Annals of Behavioral Medicine, 52*(12), 1010–1022. https://doi.org/10.1093/abm/kay005

Stanger, C., Ryan, S. R., Delhey, L. M., Thrailkill, K., Li, Z., Li, Z., & Budney, A. J. (2013). A multicomponent motivational intervention to improve adherence among adolescents with poorly controlled Type 1 diabetes: A pilot study. *Journal of Pediatric Psychology, 38*(6), 629–637. https://doi.org/10.1093/jpepsy/jst032

Storch, E. A., Heidgerken, A. D., Geffken, G. R., Lewin, A. B., Ohleyer, V., Freddo, M., & Silverstein, J. H. (2006). Bullying, regimen self-management, and metabolic control in youth with Type I diabetes. *The Journal of Pediatrics, 148*(6), 784–787. https://doi.org/10.1016/j.jpeds.2006.01.007

Storch, E. A., Lewin, A., Silverstein, J. H., Heidgerken, A. D., Strawser, M. S., Baumeister, A., & Geffken, G. R. (2004). Peer victimization and psychosocial adjustment in children with Type 1 diabetes. *Clinical Pediatrics, 43*(5), 467–471. https://doi.org/10.1177/000992280404300508

Streisand, R., Mackey, E. R., Elliot, B. M., Mednick, L., Slaughter, I. M., Turek, J., & Austin, A. (2008). Parental anxiety and depression associated with caring for a child newly diagnosed with Type 1 diabetes: Opportunities for education and counseling. *Patient Education and Counseling, 73*(2), 333–338. https://doi.org/10.1016/j.pec.2008.06.014

Sullivan-Bolyai, S., Bova, C., Leung, K., Trudeau, A., Lee, M., & Gruppuso, P. (2010). Social Support to Empower Parents (STEP). *The Diabetes Educator, 36*(1), 88–97. https://doi.org/10.1177/0145721709352384

Sundelin, J., Forsander, G., & Mattsson, S. E. (1996). Family-oriented support at the onset of diabetes mellitus: A comparison of two group conditions during 2 years following diagnosis. *Acta Paediatrica, 85*(1), 49–55. https://doi.org/10.1111/j.1651-2227.1996.tb13889.x

Svoren, B. M., Butler, D., Levine, B. S., Anderson, B. J., & Laffel, L. M. (2003). Reducing acute adverse outcomes in youths with Type 1 diabetes: A randomized, controlled trial. *Pediatrics, 112*(4), 914–922. https://doi.org/10.1542/peds.112.4.914

Teasdale, A., & Limbers, C. (2018). Avoidant coping moderates the relationship between paternal involvement in the child's Type 1 diabetes (T1D) care and parenting stress. *Journal of Child Health Care, 22*(4), 606–618. https://doi.org/10.1177/1367493518767068

Thompson, R., Delamater, A. M., Gebert, R., & Christie, D. (2012). Integrated care and multidisciplinary teamwork: The role of the different professionals. In D. Christie & C. Martin (Eds.), *Psychological aspects of diabetes*. Radcliff.

Thompson, S. J., Auslander, W. F., & White, N. H. (2001). Comparison of single-mother and two-parent families on metabolic control of children with diabetes. *Diabetes Care, 24*(2), 234–238. https://doi.org/10.2337/diacare.24.2.234

The TODAY Study Group. (2011). Binge eating, mood, and quality of life in youth with Type 2 diabetes: Baseline data from the TODAY study. *Diabetes Care, 34*(4), 858–860. https://doi.org/10.2337/dc10-1704

The TODAY Study Group. (2012). A clinical trial to maintain glycemic control in youth with Type 2 diabetes. *The New England Journal of Medicine, 366*(24), 2247–2256. https://doi.org/10.1056/NEJMoa1109333

Torabizadeh, C., Asadabadi Poor, Z., & Shaygan, M. (2019). The effects of resilience training on the self-efficacy of patients with Type 2 diabetes: A randomized controlled clinical trial. *International Journal of Community Based Nursing and Midwifery, 7*(3), 211–221. https://doi.org/10.30476/IJCBNM.2019.44996

Trojanowski, P. J., Niehaus, C. E., Fischer, S., & Mehlenbeck, R. (2021). Parenting and psychological health in youth with Type 1 diabetes: Systematic review. *Journal of Pediatric Psychology, 46*(10), 1213–1237. https://doi.org/10.1093/jpepsy/jsab064

Troncone, A., Cascella, C., Chianese, A., di Leva, A., Confetto, S., Zanfardino, A., & Iafusco, D. (2019). Psychological support for adolescents with Type 1 diabetes provided by adolescents with Type 1 diabetes: The chat line experience. *Pediatric Diabetes, 20*(6), 800–810. https://doi.org/10.1111/pedi.12873

Valenzuela, J. M., La Greca, A. M., Hsin, O., Taylor, C., & Delamater, A. M. (2011). Prescribed regimen intensity in diverse youth with Type 1 diabetes: Role of family and provider perceptions. *Pediatric Diabetes, 12*(8), 696–703. https://doi.org/10.1111/j.1399-5448.2011.00766.x

Van Gampelaere, C., Luyckx, K., Goethals, E. R., van der Straaten, S., Laridaen, J., Casteels, K., Vanbesien, J., Depoorter, S., Klink, D., Cools, M., & Goubert, L. (2020). Parental stress, anxiety and trait mindfulness: Associations with parent-child mealtime interactions in children with Type 1 diabetes. *Journal of Behavioral Medicine, 43*(3), 448–459. https://doi.org/10.1007/s10865-020-00144-3

Van Gampelaere, C., Luyckx, K., van der Straaten, S., Laridaen, J., Goethals, E. R., Casteels, K., Vanbesien, J., den Brinker, M., Depoorter, S., Klink, D., Cools, M., Goubert, L., & the Ghent University. (2020). Families with pediatric Type 1 diabetes: A comparison with the general population on child well-being, parental distress, and parenting behavior. *Pediatric Diabetes, 21*(2), 395–408. https://doi.org/10.1111/pedi.12942

Van Gampelaere, C., Luyckx, K., Van Ryckeghem, D. M. L., van der Straaten, S., Laridaen, J.,

Goethals, E. R., Casteels, K., Vanbesien, J., den Brinker, M., Cools, M., & Goubert, L. (2019). Mindfulness, worries, and parenting in parents of children with Type 1 diabetes. *Journal of Pediatric Psychology*, 44(4), 499–508. https://doi.org/10.1093/jpepsy/jsy094

Van Vleet, M., & Helgeson, V. S. (2020). Friend and Peer Relationships Among Youth with Type 1 Diabetes. In A. Delamater & D. Marrero (Eds.), *Behavioral diabetes* (pp. 121–138). Springer Nature. https://doi.org/10.1007/978-3-030-33286-0_10

Varni, J. W., Delamater, A. M., Hood, K. K., Raymond, J. K., Driscoll, K. A., Wong, J. C., Adi, S., Yi-Frazier, J. P., Grishman, E. K., Faith, M. A., Corathers, S. D., Kichler, J. C., Miller, J. L., Doskey, E. M., Aguirre, V. P., Heffer, R. W., Wilson, D. P., & the Pediatric Quality of Life Inventory™ 3.2 Diabetes Module Testing Study Consortium. (2018). Diabetes symptoms predictors of health-related quality of life in adolescents and young adults with Type 1 or Type 2 diabetes. *Quality of Life Research*, 27(9), 2295–2303. https://doi.org/10.1007/s11136-018-1884-6

Vinker-Shuster, M., Golan-Cohen, A., Merhasin, I., & Merzon, E. (2019). Attention-deficit hyperactivity disorder in pediatric patients with Type 1 diabetes mellitus: Clinical outcomes and diabetes control. *Journal of Developmental and Behavioral Pediatrics*, 40(5), 330–334. https://doi.org/10.1097/DBP.0000000000000670

Vloemans, A. F., Eilander, M. M. A., Rotteveel, J., Bakker-van Waarde, W. M., Houdijk, E. C. A. M., Nuboer, R., Winterdijk, P., Snoek, F. J., & De Wit, M. (2019). Youth with Type 1 diabetes taking responsibility for self-management: The importance of executive functioning in achieving glycemic control: Results from the longitudinal DINO Study. *Diabetes Care*, 42(2), 225–231. https://doi.org/10.2337/dc18-1143

Wagner, D. V., Barry, S. A., Stoeckel, M., Teplitsky, L., & Harris, M. A. (2017). NICH at its best for diabetes at its worst: Texting teens and their caregivers for better outcomes. *Journal of Diabetes Science and Technology*, 11(3), 468–475. https://doi.org/10.1177/1932296817695337

Wagner, D. V., Stoeckel, M., Tudor, M. E., & Harris, M. A. (2015). Treating the most vulnerable and costly in diabetes. *Current Diabetes Reports*, 15(6), 606. https://doi.org/10.1007/s11892-015-0606-5

Wagner, G., & Karwautz, A. (2020). Eating disorders in adolescents with Type 1 diabetes mellitus. *Current Opinion in Psychiatry*, 33(6), 602–610. https://doi.org/10.1097/YCO.0000000000000650

Walders-Abramson, N., Venditti, E. M., Ievers-Landis, C. E., Anderson, B., El Ghormli, L., Geffner, M., Kaplan, J., Koontz, M. B., Saletsky, R., Payan, M., Yasuda, P., & the Treatment Options for Type 2 Diabetes in Adolescents and Youth (TODAY) Study Group. (2014). Relationships among stressful life events and physiological markers, treatment adherence, and psychosocial functioning among youth with Type 2 diabetes. *The Journal of Pediatrics*, 165(3), 504–508.e1. https://doi.org/10.1016/j.jpeds.2014.05.020

Wang, C. H., Tully, C., Monaghan, M., Hilliard, M. E., & Streisand, R. (2021). Source-specific social support and psychosocial stress among mothers and fathers during initial diagnosis of Type 1 diabetes in young children. *Families, Systems, & Health*, 39(2), 358–362. https://doi.org/10.1037/fsh0000610

Watson, S. E., Spurling, S. E., Fieldhouse, A. M., Montgomery, V. L., & Wintergerst, K. A. (2020). Depression and anxiety screening in adolescents with diabetes. *Clinical Pediatrics*, 59(4–5), 445–449. https://doi.org/10.1177/0009922820905861

Weinstock, R. S., Trief, P. M., El Ghormli, L., Goland, R., McKay, S., Milaszewski, K., Preske, J., Willi, S., & Yasuda, P. M. (2015). Parental characteristics associated with outcomes in youth with Type 2 diabetes: Results from the TODAY clinical trial. *Diabetes Care*, 38(5), 784–792. https://doi.org/10.2337/dc14-2393

Weissberg-Benchell, J., Shapiro, J. B., Bryant, F. B., & Hood, K. K. (2020). Supporting Teen Problem-Solving (STEPS) 3 year outcomes: Preventing diabetes-specific emotional distress and depressive symptoms in adolescents with Type 1 diabetes. *Journal of Consulting and Clinical Psychology*, 88(11), 1019–1031. https://doi.org/10.1037/ccp0000608

Westrupp, E. M., Northam, E., Lee, K. J., Scratch, S. E., & Cameron, F. (2015). Reducing and preventing internalizing and externalizing behavior problems in children with Type 1 diabetes: A randomized controlled trial of the Triple P-Positive Parenting Program. *Pediatric Diabetes*, 16(7), 554–563. https://doi.org/10.1111/pedi.12205

Whittemore, R., Jaser, S., Chao, A., Jang, M., & Grey, M. (2012). Psychological experience of parents of children with Type 1 diabetes: A systematic mixed-studies review. *The Diabetes Educator*, 38(4), 562–579. https://doi.org/10.1177/0145721712445216

Wicklow, B., Dart, A., McKee, J., Griffiths, A., Malik, S., Quoquat, S., & Bruce, S. (2021). Experiences of First Nations adolescents living with Type 2 diabetes: A focus group study. *CMAJ: Canadian Medical Association Journal*, 193(12), E403–E409. https://doi.org/10.1503/cmaj.201685

Willi, S. M., Martin, K., Datko, F. M., & Brant, B. P. (2004). Treatment of Type 2 diabetes in childhood using a very-low-calorie diet. *Diabetes Care*, 27(2), 348–353. https://doi.org/10.2337/diacare.27.2.348

Willi, S. M., Miller, K. M., DiMeglio, L. A., Klingensmith, G. J., Simmons, J. H., Tamborlane, W. V., Nadeau, K. J., Kittelsrud, J. M., Huckfeldt, P., Beck, R. W., Lipman, T. H., & the T1D Exchange Clinic Network. (2015). Racial-ethnic disparities in management and outcomes among children with Type 1 diabetes. *Pediatrics*, 135(3), 424–434. https://doi.org/10.1542/peds.2014-1774

Wu, H., Patterson, C. C., Zhang, X., Ghani, R. B. A., Magliano, D. J., Boyko, E. J., Ogle, G. D., & Luk, A. O. Y. (2022). Worldwide estimates of incidence of Type 2 diabetes in children and adolescents in 2021. *Diabetes Research and Clinical Practice*, 185, 109785. https://doi.org/10.1016/j.diabres.2022.109785

Wysocki, T., & Greco, P. (2006). Social support and diabetes management in childhood and adolescence: Influence of parents and friends. *Current Diabetes Reports*, 6(2), 117–122. https://doi.org/10.1007/s11892-006-0022-y

Wysocki, T., Harris, M. A., Buckloh, L. M., Mertlich, D., Lochrie, A. S., Mauras, N., & White, N. H. (2007). Randomized trial of behavioral family systems therapy for diabetes: Maintenance of effects on diabetes outcomes in adolescents. *Diabetes Care*, 30(3), 555–560. https://doi.org/10.2337/dc06-1613

Wysocki, T., Harris, M. A., Buckloh, L. M., Mertlich, D., Lochrie, A. S., Taylor, A., Sadler, M., & White, N. H. (2008). Randomized, controlled trial of Behavioral Family Systems Therapy for Diabetes: Maintenance and generalization of effects on parent-adolescent communication. *Behavior Therapy*, 39(1), 33–46. https://doi.org/10.1016/j.beth.2007.04.001

Yi-Frazier, J. P., Yaptangco, M., Semana, S., Buscaino, E., Thompson, V., Cochrane, K., Tabile, M., Alving, E., & Rosenberg, A. R. (2015). The association of personal resilience with stress, coping, and diabetes outcomes in adolescents with Type 1 diabetes: Variable- and person-focused approaches. *Journal of Health Psychology*, 20(9), 1196–1206. https://doi.org/10.1177/1359105313509846

Young, V., Eiser, C., Johnson, B., Brierley, S., Epton, T., Elliott, J., & Heller, S. (2013). Eating problems in adolescents with Type 1 diabetes: A systematic review with meta-analysis. *Diabetic Medicine*, 30(2), 189–198. https://doi.org/10.1111/j.1464-5491.2012.03771.x

CHAPTER 15

PEDIATRIC OBESITY AND IMPLICATIONS FOR CHILD HEALTH AND WELL-BEING

Bethany J. Gaffka, Susan J. Woolford, Hurley O. Riley, and Alison L. Miller

Childhood obesity is a public health priority that has garnered much attention due to the rapid increase in prevalence and impact on health over the life course (Ogden et al., 2016). Children with excess weight are more likely to become adults with excess weight (Guo et al., 2002) and to suffer from illnesses such as Type 2 diabetes (Must & Strauss, 1999), coronary artery disease (Srinivasan et al., 1996), and many types of cancer (Renehan et al., 2008). Overall, excess weight during childhood is associated with poorer quality of life (QoL) and ultimately with premature death (Dietz, 1998).

Obesity does not only lead to health problems later in life, it also puts millions of children at risk for comorbidities during their youth. The role of excess weight in undermining the immune system was seen during the COVID-19 pandemic in which patients with obesity generally experienced poorer outcomes (Popkin et al., 2020). Children with excess weight have been more likely to contract the multi-inflammatory syndrome of childhood and to have long-term complications of their infection (Acevedo et al., 2021), adding to the list of well-established comorbidities seen more frequently in youth with excess weight compared to their peers, including metabolic disease, orthopedic problems, hypertension (Estrada et al., 2014), anxiety (Gariepy et al., 2010) and depression (Reeves et al., 2008).

The physical and mental health consequences of childhood obesity have significant individual and societal ramifications. At an individual level, while findings vary by race/ethnicity and sex, overall, children with obesity are at risk for poorer cognitive outcomes and lifelong earning potential (Segal et al., 2021). At a societal level, the cost of caring for children with obesity as a diagnosis is greater than for those without obesity included among their diagnoses both in outpatient (Hampl et al., 2007) and inpatient settings (Woolford et al., 2007). Indeed, the incremental lifetime health care costs for a child with excess weight compared to youth without excess weight is on average between $12,660 to $19,000 extra per individual (Finkelstein et al., 2014). Thus, the benefits of investing in efforts to address the problem of childhood obesity will be garnered at individual, family, and societal levels.

Factors contributing to the development of obesity are complex and interactional across social, cultural, and ecological contexts. There are at least three developmental periods of growth that are associated with a higher risk of obesity that extends into adulthood: gestation, postnatal (first year of life), and adiposity rebound

https://doi.org/10.1037/0000414-015
APA Handbook of Pediatric Psychology, Developmental-Behavioral Pediatrics, and Developmental Science: Vol. 2. Pediatric Psychology and Developmental-Behavioral Pediatrics: Clinical Applications of Developmental Science, P. E. Shah and M. H. Bornstein (Editors-in-Chief)
Copyright © 2025 by the American Psychological Association. All rights reserved.

(ages 5 to 7 years). Children who experience rapid weight gain during these critical periods are at higher risk of developing persistent obesity and the associated well-established comorbidities. Results from the Early Prevention of Childhood Obesity (EPOCH) trials suggest that behavioral and lifestyle interventions can be implemented during the potentially critical time periods of pregnancy and infancy to reduce toddler body mass index (BMI) scores (Askie et al., 2020). Longitudinal research will need to examine whether intervention during these sensitive time periods can change growth trajectories and reverse negative outcomes.

Integration of research from the disciplines of developmental science, developmental-behavioral pediatrics, and pediatric psychology is essential, and will ultimately inform the creation of effective interventions that will reduce health and psychosocial risks associated with pediatric obesity. All three disciplines share a deep appreciation of child development and fostering optimal child and family functioning. Developmental-behavioral pediatrics has a rich tradition of conducting developmental and biopsychosocial research associated with pediatric obesity and illuminating the influence of the family and stress on child development. Given the psychosocial complexity associated with obesity, pediatric psychologists are often well-positioned to address and consider these issues through a developmental lens, examine individual and family strengths and risk factors, and offer developmentally appropriate strategies for behavior change that are tailored to youth within the context of their family. The foundation of child development within the discipline of developmental science enriches the clinical work of pediatric psychologists and pediatricians, identifies potential modifiable targets (e.g., parenting, child management of stress, and feeding practices), and provides a theoretical compass to guide the integration of theory and practice.

In this chapter, we begin with an overview of the diagnosis and prevalence of pediatric obesity, as well as disparities and the role of ecological contexts. Theoretical models of pediatric obesity are then presented, with a discussion of risk and resilience factors at multiple levels (biological, psychological, and social) and youth health and social-emotional outcomes associated with obesity. Finally, we discuss the clinical management of pediatric obesity, including screening practices, interventions, and the role of pediatricians and pediatric psychologists.

DEFINITION AND DIAGNOSIS OF EXCESS WEIGHT IN CHILDREN

The diagnosis of pediatric obesity is often made in the context of a medical evaluation by a pediatrician, who may also initiate management in the primary care setting. However, the impact of primary care interventions is often insufficient to reverse obesity. Thus, weight management efforts frequently require a multidisciplinary approach, to address the physical and behavioral health outcomes and family system factors that contribute to its pathogenesis.

The World Health Organization (WHO; n.d.) defines obesity as abnormal or excessive fat accumulation that presents a risk to health. The most accurate methods of assessing body fat, also called adiposity, such as hydrostatic weighing, dual-energy x-ray absorptiometry, and caliper measurements of skin folds, are complex, inconvenient, and often viewed as uncomfortable for patients. Thus, the most commonly used means to screen for obesity is to calculate the BMI, which is a measure of weight (in kilograms [kg]) divided by height (in square meters [m^2]).

For children, the BMI cut points used to determine weight status vary by age and by sex and are based on percentiles. The percentiles used in the Centers for Disease Control (CDC) growth charts were normed on National Health Examination Survey (NHANES) data collected between 1963 and 1994 from a nationally representative sample of 2- to 20-year-old youth. For children 2 years of age up to age 17, a BMI equal to or more than the 95th percentile for age and for sex (or equal to or greater than 30 kg/m^2, whichever is lower) is classified as obesity. When the degree of obesity is severe, using the BMI percentile score is not an optimal measure, as there is a ceiling effect (Skinner et al., 2018). Thus, the CDC recommends using comparative metrics such as "percent of the 95th percentile" with severe obesity being a BMI equal to or greater than 120% of the 95th percentile (Freedman et al., 2017).

For children younger than 2 years of age, rather than using BMI percentiles, weight status is determined using weight-for-length percentiles. Furthermore, the terminology used for excess weight in this age group is not the same as for older youth. Children under 2 years of age with a weight-for-length at or above the 95th percentile are classified as being in the overweight category rather than the obese category, as would be the case of older age groups. This difference is due in part to an effort to avoid the stigma associated with the term obesity.

GLOBAL PREVALENCE OF PEDIATRIC OBESITY

The prevalence and patterns of obesity vary by country and region, but the problem of pediatric obesity is not limited to the United States or to well-resourced countries. It is indeed a pandemic with a global impact that has worsened since the 1970s. In 1975, an estimated 11 million children 5 to 19 years old worldwide were living with obesity. By 2016, this number was estimated to be more than 11 times larger, at 124 million (NCD Risk Factor Collaboration, 2017). This increase in prevalence has been most notable in some regions (such as Polynesia and Micronesia) and has resulted in many low-income countries facing the dilemma of twin epidemics of undernutrition and obesity concurrently (NCD Risk Factor Collaboration, 2017).

The etiology of excess weight globally points to the familiar culprits of decreased physical activity (often being replaced by increased time devoted to screens; Aubert et al., 2021) and consumption of energy-dense, low-nutrient foods. Sadly, the increase in obesity has led to the expected increase in cardiometabolic illnesses, including Type 2 diabetes and hypertension (Song et al., 2019). The rise in chronic illness is particularly dire in many low-income countries that lack the resources to absorb the resulting swell in health care needs (Akseer et al., 2020).

PREVALENCE OF OBESITY IN THE UNITED STATES

In the United States, 2015–2016 NHANES data indicate that 18.5% of youth 2 to 19 years old meet criteria for obesity (i.e., BMI equal to or greater than the 95th percentile), with a higher prevalence of excess weight for older compared to younger children (20.5% for 16- to 19-year-olds vs. 13.7% for 2- to 5-year-olds; Ogden et al., 2018). Differences are also noted by ethnicity and by gender. African American girls have the highest prevalence of obesity at 25.1%, followed by Hispanic/Latina girls at 23.5%, with European American girls at 13.6% and the lowest prevalence among Asian American girls at 10.1%. For males, Hispanic/Latino boys had the highest prevalence at 28.0%, followed by African American boys at 19.3%, European American boys at 14.7% and Asian American boys the lowest at 11.2%. For Native American youth (who are not reported as a category in NHANES data) the prevalence of obesity is even greater. Data from 2015 reveal that 18.5% of Native American youth ages 2 to 19 were overweight and 29.7% were classified as obese (Bullock et al., 2017).

The prevalence of severe obesity has also increased, and populations of color are disproportionately represented (Skinner et al., 2018). Hispanic/Latinx (9.1%) and African American youth (9.0%) have the highest prevalence of Class II (i.e., BMI equal to or greater than 120% of the 95th percentile) and III (BMI equal to or greater than 140% of the 95th percentile) obesity compared to European American (3.9%) and Asian American (1.4%) youth.

DISPARITIES AND THE ROLE OF ECOLOGICAL CONTEXTS AND SOCIAL DETERMINANTS OF HEALTH

Communities of color in the United States bear a disproportionate burden of obesity. Not only are they more likely to live with obesity, but they are also more likely to be in the severely obese category and consequently to suffer from comorbidities of obesity (Ogden et al., 2018; Skinner et al., 2018). Contributors to these disparities include limited access to healthy foods and safe spaces for exercise as well as the cumulative effect of social determinants of health (i.e., the conditions, such as poverty, in which individuals are born, grow, and live) that impact choices and increase stress for children (Kumanyika, 2008).

Socioeconomic status is significantly related to obesity with children in high-income countries whose parents have fewer years of education being more likely to develop obesity (Cohen et al., 2013). The impact of poverty appears to vary by child ethnicity and sex, but in general, income and excess weight have an inverse relation in the United States (Assari, 2018).

In addition to bearing the greatest burden of excess weight, children of color are less likely to access treatment including nutrition and exercise programs, behavior modification interventions, medication, and weight reduction surgeries (Johnson et al., 2021). Furthermore, outcomes from treatment for youth of color are poorer than for their European American peers (Zeller et al., 2004). This difference in outcome may be influenced by the need for targeted interventions as personal relevance is necessary to achieve behavior change. Yet treatment content and materials may reflect the majority culture, and the level of personal relevance of interventions may be lower for children of color (Noar et al., 2007).

THEORETICAL MODELS OF PEDIATRIC OBESITY

Multiple theoretical models have been invoked to conceptualize the causes and consequences of obesity emerging in childhood and adolescence (Bohnert et al., 2020). From developmental science, biopsychosocial and developmental ecological models can be particularly helpful in understanding pediatric obesity from a prevention perspective. Both models seek to characterize the processes that can explain associations among factors internal and external to the child and risk of developing obesity (Russell & Russell, 2019).

Biopsychosocial perspectives suggest that pediatric obesity risk is influenced by biological factors such as genetic predispositions, psychological factors such as capacity to cope with stress, and social factors such as parenting or peer pressure, in addition to broader cultural traditions, such as food preparation and preferences. The biopsychosocial model also emphasizes the transactional nature of these biological, psychological, and sociocultural contextual influences in shaping child development and risk for obesity (Russell & Russell, 2019). Beyond their biological contributions, parents' own psychology, including beliefs about feeding, eating, and capacity for stress management, is also shaped by their family history and sociocultural food traditions, which in turn can drive both feeding practices and general parenting (Malhotra et al., 2013), each of which has been linked to pediatric obesity and present risk for intergenerational transmission (Sleddens et al., 2011). Such complex processes highlight the need for multidisciplinary treatment approaches that also engage the family system.

A developmental-ecological perspective further details how pediatric obesity risk is influenced by layers of embedded ecological contexts to which a child is exposed throughout development. The "Six C's" model which details potential influences on childhood obesity risk across six contextual levels (Cell, Child, Clan, Community, Country, and Culture) is a good example, as it identifies potential points for intervention at each level, such as self-regulation at the level of "child," household routines at the level of "clan," and food policy at the level of "country" (Harrison et al., 2011). Influences that occur early in development are often the most formative as they lay the foundations for later development across many domains relevant to obesity, including biological (e.g., microbiome), behavioral (e.g., stress coping), and social functioning (e.g., interpersonal relationships). Even before birth, a fetus is shaped by genetic and intrauterine environmental factors that can increase obesity risk via prenatal programming (known as the Developmental Origins of Health and Disease, or DOHAD, hypothesis; Armitage et al., 2008). For example, maternal pre-pregnancy BMI can predispose a child to excessive weight gain during infancy (Woo Baidal et al., 2016). Child factors such as eating behavior (e.g., propensity toward food reward; Carnell & Wardle, 2007) can shape individual behavioral patterns that increase risk. Parents can shape routines and practices relevant for obesity prevention such as family mealtimes and regular bedtimes (Anzman et al., 2010; Fiese et al., 2012). As the child gets older and interacts more with actors outside the family, factors in the wider social environment such as peers and social media can exert more prominent influences (Harrison et al., 2011).

Finally, the broader sociocultural context(s) in which children and families are situated include social determinants of health such as food insecurity, housing stability, neighborhood safety, racism, stress, and exposures to environmental toxicants that may enhance risk for child obesity. As these social determinants are inequitably distributed, children living in historically marginalized communities and populations are at greatest risk (Kumanyika, 2019). Indeed, calls to address childhood obesity risk emphasize the importance of understanding impacts of social determinants across multiple levels of the developmental-ecological context, including parent–child relationships and structural influences such as the broader food environment (Campbell, 2016; Kumanyika, 2019).

RISK AND RESILIENCE FACTORS RELATED TO PEDIATRIC OBESITY

Child, family, and broader social-contextual factors may also confer or mitigate risk for obesity and these factors emerge across development. Some prominent factors at each level have been studied extensively, but much work remains correlational and observational, rather than experimental in nature. Thus, bidirectional associations may exist between obesity and the risk and protective factors mentioned herein.

Biological Factors

Genetic factors. Several processes linking biology and obesity have been proposed. Genetic factors may predispose some children to obesity. A meta-analysis of twin studies found that genetic factors strongly influenced BMI across childhood and adolescence (Silventoinen et al., 2010). Genes had less of an effect on BMI during middle childhood compared to during adolescence (Silventoinen et al., 2010). The role of genetics in obesity risk is complicated, however. Epigenetics are heritable biological markers that modify gene expression and can be affected by environmental exposures (Alvarado-Cruz et al., 2018); epigenetic changes such as methylation or histone modification can alter the expression of genes that regulate growth, so these are relevant for obesity risk (Herrera et al., 2011). No single gene is responsible for obesity; however, polygenic risk scores, which consider over 2 million genetic variants, can predict weight and obesity risk at birth (Khera et al., 2019). Researchers have uncovered protective factors that interact with the epigenome to reduce obesity risk. For example, a balanced maternal diet during the prenatal period may serve as a protective factor, as overnutrition (e.g., high fat diets) and undernutrition (e.g., low-protein diets) may cause epigenetic changes in the developing fetus which can contribute to obesity (Li, 2018). Further, reducing exposures to environmental contaminants such as tobacco smoke can reduce epigenetic changes that may contribute to obesity (Alvarado-Cruz et al., 2018).

Microbiome. Trillions of microorganisms reside in the intestinal tract, known as the gut microbiome. Specific gut microbiota are associated with later weight (Koleva et al., 2015), potentially through metabolism regulation (Martin et al., 2019). For instance, a lower presence of *Bifidobacteria* and higher presence of *S. aureus* in infant fecal samples are associated with an increased risk of overweight at age 7 years (Kalliomäki et al., 2008). Reducing antibiotic use and consuming a balanced, anti-inflammatory diet can promote a gut microbiome composition that protects against obesity (Petraroli et al., 2021).

Stress biology. Prolonged exposure to chronic stress may overactivate the hypothalamic–pituitary–adrenal (HPA) axis, the primary biological system responsible for stress responses (Miller et al., 2011). Overactivation of the HPA axis may increase cortisol levels, which can promote eating and fat deposition (Tomiyama, 2019). Early life stress exposure may also interact with other biological pathways, such as reward processing, hormones, inflammatory processes, epigenetics, microbiota, and the body's metabolite profile, which can increase risk for developing obesity over time (Miller & Lumeng, 2018; Tomiyama, 2019). Reducing stress exposure and teaching positive stress-coping strategies to children, however, can mitigate stress-induced obesity risk.

Psychological Factors

Self-regulation. Self-regulation, which involves controlling thoughts, behaviors, and emotions in pursuit of goals, is a psychological construct that develops across childhood and has implications for obesity (Miller et al., 2016). Poor self-regulation of emotion and behavior during toddlerhood predicted obesity during early childhood (Graziano et al., 2010). Difficulty regulating emotions during infancy and early childhood has also been associated with greater obesity risk (Anzman-Frasca et al., 2012; Miller et al., 2016). Several processes may explain this association, but individuals with poor emotional regulation may engage in more emotional eating and stress-eating (Dohle et al., 2018). In a meta-analysis, children with poorer behavioral self-regulation (ability to delay gratification) had increased risk for overweight or obesity (Caleza et al., 2016). A systematic review of executive functions, or cognitive aspects of self-regulation, and obesity found that children and adolescents with overweight or obesity had poorer inhibitory control, working memory, and cognitive flexibility than children and adolescents without overweight or obesity (Mamrot & Hanć, 2019). Individuals with poorer executive functioning may experience poorer self-control and decision-making, which can result in behaviors such as eating in the absence of hunger, eating more obesogenic foods, and overeating (Francis & Riggs, 2018). Supporting parents to provide a routine and structured environment can help children practice regulating their behavior, which may strengthen self-regulation skills.

Stigma. Internalized weight stigma has emerged as an area of research interest and potential psychological contributor to obesity. Weight stigmatization is often overlooked as an obesity risk factor, but it has been estimated that 25% to 50% of youth have been bullied for their body weight (Puhl & Lessard, 2020). Weight stigma can lead to psychological distress, social isolation, and maladaptive eating behaviors (Puhl & Lessard, 2020). More frequent weight-related abuse (i.e., bullying or victimization due to one's weight) predicts more frequent binge eating, emotional eating, and unhealthy weight control—disordered eating behaviors that can further exacerbate obesity (Salwen et al., 2015). To reduce weight stigma, it is important to promote positive body image from early life, for example, by avoiding stigmatizing imagery and language.

Stress and trauma. Exposure to stress and trauma is related to psychological functioning and may increase the risk for obesity through multiple pathways. Adverse childhood experiences (ACEs) are traumatic events that may lead to childhood obesity by hindering psychosocial and neuroendocrine development (Schroeder et al., 2021). Experiencing ACEs heightens attention to threatening stimuli (Dannlowski et al., 2012), HPA axis dysregulation (Iob et al., 2021), and psychological distress (Manyema et al., 2018). ACEs can result in obesogenic behaviors such as emotional eating, poor sleep quality, and impulsivity (Schroeder et al., 2021). Some of these behaviors (e.g., emotional eating) can be considered coping mechanisms that may allow short-term relief but over time can damage health. The obesity-related effects of ACEs may not become apparent for at least 2 years (Schroeder et al., 2021). To this point, it is important to note that the developmental timing and dose of risk and protective factors may differentially affect obesity risk. For instance, a Dutch study found that ACEs experienced during early adolescence have the greatest effect on body weight (Riem & Karreman, 2019). Regarding dose, individuals who have experienced more ACEs are more likely to develop obesity (Anda et al., 2006). However, supports for families who have experienced ACEs, for example, through trauma-informed practices may help protect children against the obesogenic effects of ACEs (Schroeder et al., 2021).

Social Factors

Family functioning and parenting. Family functioning characterized by high family conflict, low family cohesion, limited behavior control, and poor communication styles are associated with increased weight in childhood and adolescence (Halliday et al., 2014). In contrast, higher family functioning has been associated with more positive health behaviors (e.g., fruit and vegetable intake, family meals, physical activity), fewer unhealthy behaviors (e.g., sedentary activity, fast-food consumption), and lower BMI during adolescence (Berge et al., 2013).

Three additional dimensions of the family context have been studied in relation to obesity risk: stress, emotional climate, and parenting style (Kitzmann et al., 2008). Beyond stress affecting the HPA axis, parental work stress can result in less time spent preparing food, less frequent family meals, and a less healthful family food environment (Bauer et al., 2012). Parents of youth with obesity have reported higher family conflict than parents of youth without overweight or obesity (Zeller et al., 2007). Unpacking this association, families reporting low conflict had more self-regulated eating among children and consumed less fat, more fruits and vegetables, and fewer salty and fatty snacks (Martin-Biggers et al., 2018). An authoritative parenting style can help children become more resilient to obesity. A systematic review found that authoritative parenting is associated with children eating more healthful foods, being more physically active, and having lower BMIs than children of parents practicing authoritarian, permissive/indulgent, or uninvolved/neglectful parenting styles (Sleddens et al., 2011).

Food-specific parenting. Researchers have also examined food-specific parenting in association with obesity risk. Children whose parents engage in more food restriction and pressure-to-eat tend to consume more sugar-sweetened beverages and calorie-dense foods (Loth, 2016). Although results from randomized controlled trials (e.g., INSIGHT) suggest that parental feeding practices such as responsive feeding may have some positive effects on child eating behaviors, associations with obesity risk are not clear (Paul et al., 2018). Parent modeling is another way in which parents can reduce child obesity risk; children are more likely to have a healthier diet if their parent also eats healthy foods, for example (Ventura & Birch, 2008), whereas parents who model disinhibited eating or dietary restraint may increase risk for disordered eating and obesity in their child (Hood et al., 2000; Neumark-Sztainer et al., 2010). As children gain autonomy across development, different aspects of food parenting may wax and wane in their influence (Balantekin et al., 2020).

Household. Household-level chaos, which reflects the degree of organization, structure, and crowding in the home, is associated with child obesity across development (Bates et al., 2018). Disorganized homes may result in poorer health behaviors such as worse sleep and fewer family mealtimes, whereas families residing in more organized homes may have more consistent sleep schedules and routine mealtimes and engage in appropriate limit setting (e.g., screen time limitations), which may mitigate obesity risk. Similar to parenting style, household chaos is thought to compromise self-regulation development as children in chaotic homes experience unpredictability and a lack of routines (Martin et al., 2012). In contrast, households characterized by routines, such as regular bedtimes and mealtimes, provide opportunities for children to practice self-regulation and develop healthy habits in a structured and predictable environment.

Screen time. Children and adolescents who engage in over 2 hours of screen time per day are at greater risk for overweight and obesity (Fang et al., 2019). Screen time may displace physical activity, reduce sleep, and lead to greater consumption via food advertising and eating while viewing (Robinson et al., 2017). Young children are especially vulnerable to the effects of food advertising potentially given their limited ability to evaluate advertisements, which tend to promote energy-dense, nutrient-poor, and highly processed foods (Story & French, 2004). Adolescent brains respond differently to food versus nonfood advertisements, and food advertisements may stimulate reward-based eating behavior (Gearhardt et al., 2020). Simulation models have estimated that banning food advertisements on television may reduce the prevalence of obesity among U.S. children by approximately 3 to 7 percentage points (Veerman et al., 2009). In addition to banning food advertisements, incorporating physical activity, healthy sleep, and a balanced diet can help protect against the effects of excess screen time.

Peers/school. Beyond the family, peers and the school environment affect child obesity risk. Positive peer experiences may foster physical activity, which can reduce obesity risk, whereas negative peer experiences may discourage physical activity (Salvy & Bowker, 2014). Peers also have a social influence on child food intake. For example, preschoolers consumed 30% more food when eating snacks in a large group of nine children versus eating in a small group of three children (Lumeng & Hillman, 2007). During adolescence, friends' snack and soft drink consumption predicts adolescents' snack and soft drink consumption (Wouters et al., 2010). Positive peer experiences and positive peer modeling may reduce obesity risk across childhood and adolescence.

Neighborhood. At a broader level, children living in socially disadvantaged neighborhoods are more likely to have obesity (Greves Grow et al., 2010). Neighborhoods can shape risk in many ways. Specifically, the neighborhood's food environment, availability of safe places for physical activity, and the built environment (e.g., walkability or bike paths) have ramifications for behaviors associated with obesity (Lipek et al., 2015). Sensitivity to the obesogenic effects of neighborhoods seem to be more prominent during adolescence given the increased autonomy and interaction with the neighborhood during this time (Alvarado, 2019).

OUTCOMES FOR YOUTH WITH OBESITY

Much research has focused on identifying biological, psychological, and social risk factors for obesity, but there is also a broad base of research examining youth and adult outcomes associated with obesity during childhood.

Long-Term Health Complications

Excess weight during childhood is associated with numerous long-term consequences some of which remain regardless of whether weight loss occurs during the adult years. The impact of obesity is wide-ranging. For example, young girls with obesity are more likely to have an early onset of puberty (Lee et al., 2007) and therefore a shorter overall period of growth, resulting in them becoming shorter-stature adults. Early maturation and less linear growth occur in addition to the well-established association between childhood obesity and the development of cardiovascular disease, hypertension, Type 2 diabetes, and many cancers (Reilly et al., 2003).

Social and Emotional Functioning

In addition to health complications associated with obesity, social and emotional functioning are also negatively impacted, underscoring the need for interdisciplinary research collaborations to better understand the interplay among biological and psychological risk and resiliency factors.

Peer victimization. Children with overweight or obesity are more likely to report peer relationship challenges, such as peer victimization, being neglected or socially isolated, and experiencing difficulty developing friendships (Rupp & McCoy, 2019). A longitudinal study examining friendships and BMI in children from age 3 to 15 years found higher BMI z-scores at 3 years predicted lower ratings of peer competence at 15 years (Sutter et al., 2020), demonstrating that excess weight at a young age may impact development of social skills that are important for developing and maintaining friendships over time.

Academic functioning/academic attainment. Peer victimization (bullying) appears to influence development of social competence and impacts academic functioning. Children and adolescents with obesity who are victimized have lower rates of school attendance, and adolescents are less likely to complete homework compared to healthy-weight peers (Rupp & McCoy, 2021). Differences in the impact of obesity on school performance may differ by age. Two systematic reviews of longitudinal studies reported weak associations between obesity in school-aged children and poor academic performance, but a stronger association between obesity and less educational achievement was reported for adolescents and young adults (Martin et al., 2017; Santana et al., 2017). Adolescents with obesity are more likely to have a history of repeating a grade and are less likely to earn a college degree, compared to youth without excess weight.

Self-esteem and quality of life. A growing body of literature has found lower self-esteem and poor body image among adolescents with obesity (Rankin et al., 2016). Girls are more likely to experience negative body image and poor self-esteem compared to boys (Shriver et al., 2013). A systematic review of studies examining QoL in youth with overweight or obesity suggests impaired QoL in comparison to healthy-weight youth, as well as greater impairment in QoL as the severity of obesity increases (Buttitta et al., 2014). A 12-year longitudinal study conducted in Australia revealed a similar pattern of poorer health-related QoL as age increases and weight status worsens (Killedar et al., 2020).

Internalizing disorders. Internalizing disorders, such as depression and anxiety, have also been explored in youth with obesity. Adolescents are more likely to report symptoms of depression and have a 34% higher risk of developing depression by young adulthood compared to healthy-weight peers (Quek et al., 2017). The association between youth weight and anxiety appears weaker, although a meta-analysis demonstrated a stronger association between anxiety and weight status for children versus adolescents (Burke & Storch, 2015). Gender differences also emerged with females reporting higher rates of anxiety as weight status increased compared to males (Burke & Storch, 2015).

Taken together, youth with obesity face myriad challenges related to their physical and mental well-being as they grow older. Intervention efforts are critical to decrease risks associated with excess weight.

SCREENING AND ASSESSMENT OF PEDIATRIC OBESITY

Nationally, many disciplines collaboratively care for children with obesity, recognizing that expertise in multiple domains is often necessary to assist youth and their family with identifying what changes to make and ultimately how to make them sustainable. The composition of teams typically includes medical providers (e.g., pediatricians, pediatric endocrinologists, developmental-behavioral pediatricians), behavioral health providers (e.g., pediatric psychologists, social workers), registered dietitians, and exercise physiologists or physical therapists.

Each provider's discipline has a unique role in the management of pediatric obesity. For example, pediatricians in the primary care setting typically conduct initial medical screenings and assist families with determining when to involve other disciplines, such as pediatric psychology, social work, nutrition, and exercise physiology. It is less common for developmental-behavioral pediatricians to be involved in the primary medical management of children with obesity. While some developmental-behavioral pediatricians are integrated as providers within clinical obesity assessment and treatment clinics, many others are involved in important developmental and biobehavioral research associated with pediatric obesity. In turn, this research informs clinical interventions. Pediatric psychologists obtain the current and past history of psychosocial functioning, assess motivation/readiness to make changes, and implement/tailor behavioral interventions to the unique characteristics of the child and family. Dietitians conduct dietary assessments and make nutrition recommendations, and exercise specialists assess and assist families with creating plans for physical activity.

Screening Tools

The American Academy of Pediatrics guidelines recommend that height (measured via a wall-mounted stadiometer with patients standing in stockinged feet) and weight (in light clothing) should be obtained annually starting at age 2 years (Hagan et al., 2017) and plotted on an appropriate growth chart from the Centers for Disease Control (CDC). For children under age 2, weight for length should be plotted at each well-child visit using growth charts from the World Health Organization (WHO). Youth who are documented as having excess weight are more likely to receive appropriate counseling (O'Brien et al., 2004).

In addition to reviewing the BMI percentile, the screening process involves assessing factors such as the BMI trajectory, which can give an early warning sign of impending weight-related problems, and eliciting a family history of weight-related comorbidities/excess weight (which is a stronger predictor of future poor health outcomes for young children than is their own BMI). A psychosocial history, identification of adverse childhood events that might impact care, and an exploration of social determinants of health will also help inform treatment decisions.

Screening for nutrition, physical activity, sedentary activity, and sleep behaviors should also occur annually to

- ensure children's weight-related habits are in keeping with current recommendations (e.g., the "5, 2, 1, 0" message of five servings of fruits and vegetables each day, less than 2 hours of screen time per day, 1 hour per day of physical activity, and zero sugar-sweetened beverages),
- determine motivation to adopt healthy habits, and
- assess for any barriers to making positive changes.

Finally, a complete physical exam will help to identify potential contributors to the patient's excess weight (e.g., thyroid disease) and comorbidities (e.g., insulin resistance, elevated blood pressure). The physical exam along with the history will guide referrals and laboratory testing (Barlow & the Expert Committee, 2007).

Growth Chart Discussions

Growth charts are widely used from birth onward to assess growth parameters, make comparisons with the population at large, and aid in the prediction of health outcomes. They were introduced in the 1970s and have become an essential tool in pediatric primary care. These tools are visual aids that facilitate communication of concepts that are not just mathematically complex but also emotionally sensitive. Hence, care should be taken to discuss them in compassionate and non-stigmatizing ways (Skelton et al., 2021). Helping parents to have an awareness that their children have excess weight is a pivotal part of weight management efforts. Identifying ways to facilitate the discussion of growth charts may help providers and families.

TREATMENT AND INTERVENTIONS IN CLINICAL PRACTICE

Determination whether to initiate treatment should take into account multiple factors including the patient/family level of motivation to engage in lifestyle changes, the age of the child and their level of maturity, the severity of the excess weight, the presence of comorbidities, the degree of family support, and the availability of treatment options. Despite decades of attention to the worsening problem of pediatric obesity, treatment outcomes have in general been modest, making prevention vitally important (Daniels et al., 2015) and the results of the EPOCH trials for early prevention during pregnancy and/or infancy promising (Askie et al., 2020).

Staged Approach to Treatment

The 2007 Expert Committee recommendations outline four stages of treatment. The recommended treatment starts with Prevention Plus, in which primary care providers are encouraged to focus on the prevention messages with more frequent contact based on patient/family motivation (Barlow & the Expert Committee, 2007). If Prevention Plus efforts are not sufficiently successful after 3 to 6 months, patients may then advance to Stage 2 treatment, which adopts a more structured approach and incorporates referrals to exercise specialists, dietitians, or behavioral specialists. At this stage, providers may encourage families to set goals, ask them to engage in self-monitoring and scheduling follow-up visits to assess the outcomes of the planned changes, and offer additional help as needed. In addition, the use of counseling strategies such as motivational interviewing may help families make healthy lifestyle changes. If this is not successful after 3 to 6 months, and if patients and their parents are sufficiently motivated, referral to a Stage 3, multidisciplinary program should be considered with parental consent and patient assent (if old enough). These multidisciplinary teams typically consist of a pediatrician and a psychologist who specialize in obesity care, along with registered dietitians, exercise specialists, and social workers. The treatment offered by pediatric multidisciplinary programs includes medical monitoring, cognitive behavior therapy, individualized nutrition and exercise plans, group activities (e.g., exercise classes and cooking classes), along with care management and coaching. Ultimately, for older patients with severe obesity, if Stage 3 multidisciplinary care does not achieve the desired results, involvement in Stage 4 interventions such as the use of medications, very-low-calorie diets, or surgical interventions may be warranted.

Attrition from weight management interventions is substantial, with dropout rates as high as 73% reported in the literature (Skelton et al., 2011). Reasons for attrition are myriad: lack of resources such as transportation, child care for siblings not involved in the treatment program, the need to miss work or school to attend multiple in-person visits, and the need for extensive travel if programs are not available locally, all have been identified as barriers to care (Hampl et al., 2013; Sallinen Gaffka et al., 2013). In all stages of treatment, the primary care provider is essential to coordinate care, monitor the patient's progress, and provide support as a trusted partner who has a rapport with the patient and who has a view of the patient's overall health in mind.

Role of the Pediatrician

Pediatricians are well-positioned to partner with families to prevent and treat pediatric obesity (Daniels et al., 2015). Frequent measurements of height and weight in the era of electronic health records (EHR) and best practice alerts (BPAs) facilitate rapid identification of patients with BMI measurements that cross major percentiles, allowing pediatricians to intervene prior to children entering the obese category.

Pediatricians can assess risk by considering prenatal risk factors (e.g., gestational diabetes and maternal excess weight) and family history, along with factors that may indicate increased risk as the child grows (e.g., rapid weight gain as an infant). Prevention messages can be promoted at the earliest ages such as the promotion of exclusive breastfeeding until 6 months of age, and a diet low in added sugars but high in fiber, including at least five servings of fruits and vegetables per day (with guidance about the serving size by age group).

Pediatricians may also consider their influence as advocates and partners with community organizations that also work to improve the health of children in their region. Involvement with schools, places of worship and local governments may provide ways to impact population health beyond the walls of the primary care office to improve the health of the community. Developmental-behavioral pediatricians who are involved with interdisciplinary weight management clinics, or who work clinically with children and families who are managing excess weight in addition to other medical concerns, play a critical role in obesity management and can help manage family-level factors and stress, which are associated with increased obesity rates and risk.

Role of the Pediatric Psychologist

The staged approach to treatment calls on additional providers to become involved in intervention after Stage 1 is not sufficient to produce change. When youth are referred by their pediatrician for additional intervention, pediatric psychologists are uniquely positioned to assess for individual and family factors that may influence motivation and readiness to change and develop a treatment plan to enhance motivation to engage in healthy behaviors and manage or overcome any identified barriers.

A group of psychologists in Stage 3 pediatric obesity programs published practice recommendations for psychologists working on interprofessional obesity treatment teams (Cadieux et al., 2016). Evidence-based assessment and treatment recommendations were described. The psychologist on an interprofessional obesity team conducts comprehensive psychosocial assessments to better understand how current and past emotional and behavioral functioning may impact weight management efforts. There is a focus on the assessment of specific factors that may increase challenges with adherence to recommendations, be associated with worse prognosis, and/or necessitate additional specialized intervention. For example, psychologists are encouraged to assess for any maladaptive eating behaviors such as sneaking or hiding food, eating in the absence of hunger (boredom and emotional triggers), food selectivity, binge eating, or disordered eating practices. Pediatric psychologists are well-positioned to incorporate additional evidence-based intervention for maladaptive eating behaviors into weight management treatment for those youth who would benefit. Similarly, if mood symptoms or behavior problems may impact weight management treatment plans, psychologists need to engage in decision making with the family about when to consider treatment for underlying concerns (Cadieux et al., 2016). Timing of psychological treatment targeting mood, behavior, and/or maladaptive eating behaviors is important to discuss with the family. Based on clinic structure and feasibility, additional psychological treatment may occur in conjunction with obesity intervention, or separately from weight management treatment. Future research examining how best to integrate treatments for mood or behavior with weight management treatment is very much needed to help guide psychologists in making evidence-based recommendations to families.

Family/Parent as the Agent of Change Interventions

Pediatric psychologists play an important role in developing, implementing, and assessing the efficacy of interventions. Family-based behavioral weight management interventions have been the standard pediatric obesity treatment for many years. Family-based interventions typically involve caregivers and youth participating in treatment together to make family dietary and/or activity modifications using behavioral strategies such as self-monitoring, goal setting, parental modeling, stimulus control, and contingency management. The mode of intervention may include groups, individual sessions with an interventionist, or a combination of both.

Janicke et al. (2014) reported results of a meta-analysis of randomized control trials of comprehensive behavioral family lifestyle interventions (CBFLI), which included interventions that address dietary intake, physical activity, and behavior strategies. Results demonstrated improvements in child weight status with a small effect size. Interventions that were longer in duration, had more treatment sessions, were individual in format, and included children who were older, were associated with greater improvements in weight.

A growing literature describes parent-based weight management interventions where interventionists work exclusively with parents to teach them behavioral strategies to modify their child's dietary and activity habits (Janicke et al., 2008). Results are encouraging and suggest that parent-based treatments and family-based treatments are equally effective (Boutelle et al., 2011). Furthermore, parent-based treatments are more cost-effective than family-based treatments (Janicke et al., 2009). However, parent-based treatment may be less acceptable to families than interventions that include parents and children attending sessions together, and this warrants further investigation. Similarly, the parent-based treatments cited previously were conducted as research protocols. In clinical settings, there may be challenges associated with insurance coverage if the child is not present for the intervention.

Interest in early prevention of obesity has led to development of some promising infancy-based interventions that are focused on healthy feeding and parenting practices. A systematic review of prevention programs starting before the age of 2 years suggests that targeting diet quality and parental responsiveness to feeding cues may be particularly promising (Redsell et al., 2016). Similarly, the prospective meta-analysis of four randomized control trials of an early childhood obesity prevention program in Australia and New Zealand (EPOCH) showed lower BMI z-scores at ages 18 and 24 months, compared to standard care (Askie et al., 2020). Topics covered within these trials were related to breastfeeding, dietary intake, introduction of solids, and activity/tummy time.

School-Based Interventions and the Educational System

Many researchers have published on school-based obesity prevention and intervention efforts. Several reviews and meta-analyses suggest improvements in physical activity, dietary intake, sedentary behavior, nutrition knowledge, and self-efficacy, but BMI change is inconsistent (Kanekar & Sharma, 2009). There is some evidence that prevention programs that include more than one component, such as physical activity and nutrition education, may be more effective at reducing BMI than programs that target only one component (Shirley et al., 2015). A systematic review of school-based prevention programs that included parent involvement demonstrated small reductions in weight status and improvements in physical activity and sedentary behavior (Verjans-Janssen et al., 2018).

In the school setting, some youth may qualify for accommodations related to excess weight. Physical accommodations for safe seating to support weight may be necessary. If mobility is a concern, extra time to ambulate between classes and/or modifications to physical education may take place. For children with excessive food-seeking behaviors, it may be appropriate to have specific plans outlined for how teachers respond to food requests outside of scheduled meal and snack times. Further, for youth who are teased or bullied about their weight, it is important to teach families how to advocate and work with school staff to address the issue.

U.S. Federal Nutrition Programs

Federal programs have the potential to mitigate risk factors for obesity. In 2009, there was a mandated change in food packages received by mothers in the Special Supplemental Nutrition Program for Women, Infants, and Children (WIC) to include more fruits, vegetables, and whole grains, less formula for breastfeeding infants, and less juice and whole milk. Researchers examined the impact of the new food package on children enrolled in WIC in Los Angeles County between 2003 and 2016 and found lower obesity risk for children receiving the new food package compared to children receiving the old food package (Chaparro et al., 2019). These results are encouraging and may impart significant future health benefits for thousands of children if weight trajectories are modified early.

Potentially impacting school-aged children nationwide, in 2012 the National School Lunch Program made changes to what is served during the school day to improve nutrition and reduce hunger (Food and Nutrition Service, 2012). One study found that children increased the selection of vegetables by 16.2% and selection of fruit by 23% (Cohen et al., 2014). In 2018, the U.S. Department of Agriculture (USDA) loosened some of the requirements, allowing fewer whole grains, flavored low-fat milks, and higher sodium content of foods. More research is necessary to better understand how to have a positive impact on youth nutrition with these well-established federal programs.

CONCLUSION AND RECOMMENDATIONS

Decades of research have demonstrated the complexity of the development of pediatric obesity and its serious sequelae. Moving forward, there is a need for interdisciplinary and longitudinal studies and collaborations to more clearly elucidate factors that confer risk to youth and to develop and test interventions informed by developmental models targeting these risk factors across multiple—and interacting—contextual levels. Collaborations among developmental scientists, pediatric psychologists, pediatricians, and developmental-behavioral pediatricians are critical for developing interventions that are developmentally appropriate and incorporate components that specifically target modifiable risk and resilience factors. There is a great need for diverse samples to better understand the nuances of risk and resilience and to develop more culturally modified interventions. Collaborating with implementation scientists who engage community stakeholders would represent an important step towards creating relevant and acceptable interventions that will positively impact more youth and families.

Youth with obesity have higher rates of depression and lower social-emotional functioning compared to youth without excess weight, but many of the current interventions do not specifically target these areas of concern. Reducing BMI via participation in traditional weight management treatment may not be sufficient to significantly improve emotional functioning. Referrals to trained mental health providers for youth to engage in evidence-based treatment for depression or other mental health concerns are certainly appropriate, and it may be helpful to determine how to incorporate this treatment into obesity interventions rather than treating weight and psychopathology in separate silos.

RESOURCES

For Practitioners

- American Psychological Association: Clinical Practice Guideline for the Treatment of Obesity and Overweight in Children and Adolescents:

  https://www.apa.org/obesity-guideline/parents-and-kids

  Provides an overview of assessment and treatment recommendations, as well as links to additional resources for nutrition, physical activity, and talking about weight with children.

- American Academy of Pediatrics Institute for Healthy Childhood Weight:

  https://ihcw.aap.org/Pages/default.aspx

  Professional resources for continuing education, tools to use in clinic, and policy/advocacy opportunities.

For Parents

- Obesity Action Coalition:

  https://www.obesityaction.org/education-support/learn-about-childhood-obesity/

  Offers education regarding obesity and treatment options, and links to resources for nutrition, activity, and bullying.

- Centers for Disease Control and Prevention:

  https://www.cdc.gov/healthyweight/children/index.html

  Provides recommendations and resources for helping children develop healthy habits related to eating, physical activity, sleep, and screen time.

References

Acevedo, L., Piñeres-Olave, B. E., Niño-Serna, L. F., Vega, L. M., Gómez, I. J. A., Chacón, S., Jaramillo-Bustamante, J. C., Mulett-Hoyos, H., González-Pardo, O., Zemanate, E., Izquierdo, L., Mejía, J. P., González, J. L. J., Durán, B. G., Gonzalez, C. B.,

Preciado, H., Marun, R. O., Alvarez-Olmos, M. I., Alzate, C. G., . . . Fernández-Sarmiento, J. (2021). Mortality and clinical characteristics of multisystem inflammatory syndrome in children (MIS-C) associated with COVID-19 in critically ill patients: An observational multicenter study (MISCO study). *BMC Pediatrics, 21*(1), 516. https://doi.org/10.1186/s12887-021-02974-9

Akseer, N., Mehta, S., Wigle, J., Chera, R., Brickman, Z. J., Al-Gashm, S., Sorichetti, B., Vandermorris, A., Hipgrave, D. B., Schwalbe, N., & Bhutta, Z. A. (2020). Non-communicable diseases among adolescents: Current status, determinants, interventions and policies. *BMC Public Health, 20*(1), 1908. https://doi.org/10.1186/s12889-020-09988-5

Alvarado, S. E. (2019). The indelible weight of place: Childhood neighborhood disadvantage, timing of exposure, and obesity across adulthood. *Health & Place, 58*, 102159. https://doi.org/10.1016/j.healthplace.2019.102159

Alvarado-Cruz, I., Alegría-Torres, J. A., Montes-Castro, N., Jiménez-Garza, O., & Quintanilla-Vega, B. (2018). Environmental epigenetic changes, as risk factors for the development of diseases in children: A systematic review. *Annals of Global Health, 84*(2), 212–224. https://doi.org/10.29024/aogh.909

Anda, R. F., Felitti, V. J., Bremner, J. D., Walker, J. D., Whitfield, C., Perry, B. D., Dube, S. R., & Giles, W. H. (2006). The enduring effects of abuse and related adverse experiences in childhood: A convergence of evidence from neurobiology and epidemiology. *European Archives of Psychiatry and Clinical Neuroscience, 256*(3), 174–186. https://doi.org/10.1007/s00406-005-0624-4

Anzman, S. L., Rollins, B. Y., & Birch, L. L. (2010). Parental influence on children's early eating environments and obesity risk: Implications for prevention. *International Journal of Obesity, 34*(7), 1116–1124. https://doi.org/10.1038/ijo.2010.43

Anzman-Frasca, S., Stifter, C. A., & Birch, L. L. (2012). Temperament and childhood obesity risk: A review of the literature. *Journal of Developmental and Behavioral Pediatrics, 33*(9), 732–745. https://doi.org/10.1097/DBP.0b013e31826a119f

Armitage, J. A., Poston, L., & Taylor, P. D. (2008). Developmental origins of obesity and the metabolic syndrome: The role of maternal obesity. In M. Korbonits (Ed.), *Frontiers of hormone research: Obesity and metabolism* (Vol. 36, pp. 73–84). S. Karger AG. https://doi.org/10.1159/000115355

Askie, L. M., Espinoza, D., Martin, A., Daniels, L. A., Mihrshahi, S., Taylor, R., Wen, L. M., Campbell, K., Hesketh, K. D., Rissel, C., Taylor, B., Magarey, A., Seidler, A. L., Hunter, K. E., & Baur, L. A. (2020). Interventions commenced by early infancy to prevent childhood obesity—The EPOCH Collaboration: An individual participant data prospective meta-analysis of four randomized controlled trials. *Pediatric Obesity, 15*(6), e12618. https://doi.org/10.1111/ijpo.12618

Assari, S. (2018). Family income reduces risk of obesity for White but not Black children. *Children, 5*(6), 73. https://doi.org/10.3390/children5060073

Aubert, S., Brazo-Sayavera, J., González, S. A., Janssen, I., Manyanga, T., Oyeyemi, A. L., Picard, P., Sherar, L. B., Turner, E., & Tremblay, M. S. (2021). Global prevalence of physical activity for children and adolescents; inconsistencies, research gaps, and recommendations: A narrative review. *The International Journal of Behavioral Nutrition and Physical Activity, 18*(1), 81. https://doi.org/10.1186/s12966-021-01155-2

Balantekin, K. N., Anzman-Frasca, S., Francis, L. A., Ventura, A. K., Fisher, J. O., & Johnson, S. L. (2020). Positive parenting approaches and their association with child eating and weight: A narrative review from infancy to adolescence. *Pediatric Obesity, 15*(10), e12722. https://doi.org/10.1111/ijpo.12722

Barlow, S. E., & the Expert Committee. (2007). Expert committee recommendations regarding the prevention, assessment, and treatment of child and adolescent overweight and obesity: Summary report. *Pediatrics, 120*(Suppl. 4), S164–S192. https://doi.org/10.1542/peds.2007-2329C

Bates, C. R., Buscemi, J., Nicholson, L. M., Cory, M., Jagpal, A., & Bohnert, A. M. (2018). Links between the organization of the family home environment and child obesity: A systematic review. *Obesity Reviews, 19*(5), 716–727. https://doi.org/10.1111/obr.12662

Bauer, K. W., Hearst, M. O., Escoto, K., Berge, J. M., & Neumark-Sztainer, D. (2012). Parental employment and work-family stress: Associations with family food environments. *Social Science & Medicine, 75*(3), 496–504. https://doi.org/10.1016/j.socscimed.2012.03.026

Berge, J. M., Wall, M., Larson, N., Loth, K. A., & Neumark-Sztainer, D. (2013). Family functioning: Associations with weight status, eating behaviors, and physical activity in adolescents. *Journal of Adolescent Health, 52*(3), 351–357. https://doi.org/10.1016/j.jadohealth.2012.07.006

Bohnert, A. M., Loren, D. M., & Miller, A. L. (2020). Examining childhood obesity through the lens of developmental psychopathology: Framing the issues to guide best practices in research and intervention. *American Psychologist, 75*(2), 163–177. https://doi.org/10.1037/amp0000581

Boutelle, K. N., Cafri, G., & Crow, S. J. (2011). Parent-only treatment for childhood obesity: A randomized controlled trial. *Obesity, 19*(3), 574–580. https://doi.org/10.1038/oby.2010.238

Bullock, A., Sheff, K., Moore, K., & Manson, S. (2017). Obesity and overweight in American Indian and Alaska Native children, 2006–2015. *American Journal of Public Health, 107*(9), 1502–1507. https://doi.org/10.2105/AJPH.2017.303904

Burke, N. L., & Storch, E. A. (2015). A meta-analysis of weight status and anxiety in children and adolescents. *Journal of Developmental and Behavioral Pediatrics, 36*(3), 133–145. https://doi.org/10.1097/DBP.0000000000000143

Buttitta, M., Iliescu, C., Rousseau, A., & Guerrien, A. (2014). Quality of life in overweight and obese children and adolescents: A literature review. *Quality of Life Research, 23*(4), 1117–1139. https://doi.org/10.1007/s11136-013-0568-5

Cadieux, A., Getzoff Testa, E., Baughcum, A., Shaffer, L. A., Santos, M., Sallinen Gaffka, B. J., Gray, J., Burton, E. T., & Ward, W. L. (2016). Recommendations for psychologists in Stage III pediatric obesity program. *Children's Health Care, 45*(1), 126–145. https://doi.org/10.1080/02739615.2014.979919

Caleza, C., Yañez-Vico, R. M., Mendoza, A., & Iglesias-Linares, A. (2016). Childhood obesity and delayed gratification behavior: A systematic review of experimental studies. *The Journal of Pediatrics, 169*, 201–7.e1. https://doi.org/10.1016/j.jpeds.2015.10.008

Campbell, M. K. (2016). Biological, environmental, and social influences on childhood obesity. *Pediatric Research, 79*(1–2), 205–211. https://doi.org/10.1038/pr.2015.208

Carnell, S., & Wardle, J. (2007). Measuring behavioural susceptibility to obesity: Validation of the child eating behaviour questionnaire. *Appetite, 48*(1), 104–113. https://doi.org/10.1016/j.appet.2006.07.075

Chaparro, M. P., Anderson, C. E., Crespi, C. M., Whaley, S. E., & Wang, M. C. (2019). The effect of the 2009 WIC food package change on childhood obesity varies by gender and initial weight status in Los Angeles County. *Pediatric Obesity, 14*(9), e12526. https://doi.org/10.1111/ijpo.12526

Cohen, A. K., Rai, M., Rehkopf, D. H., & Abrams, B. (2013). Educational attainment and obesity: A systematic review. *Obesity Reviews, 14*(12), 989–1005. https://doi.org/10.1111/obr.12062

Cohen, J. F., Richardson, S., Parker, E., Catalano, P. J., & Rimm, E. B. (2014). Impact of the new U.S. Department of Agriculture school meal standards on food selection, consumption, and waste. *American Journal of Preventive Medicine, 46*(4), 388–394. https://doi.org/10.1016/j.amepre.2013.11.013

Daniels, S. R., Hassink, S. G., the Committee On Nutrition, Abrams, S. A., Corkins, M. R., de Ferranti, S. D., Golden, N. H., Magge, S. N., & Schwarzenberg, S. J. (2015). The role of the pediatrician in primary prevention of obesity. *Pediatrics, 136*(1), e275–e292. https://doi.org/10.1542/peds.2015-1558

Dannlowski, U., Stuhrmann, A., Beutelmann, V., Zwanzger, P., Lenzen, T., Grotegerd, D., Domschke, K., Hohoff, C., Ohrmann, P., Bauer, J., Lindner, C., Postert, C., Konrad, C., Arolt, V., Heindel, W., Suslow, T., & Kugel, H. (2012). Limbic scars: Long-term consequences of childhood maltreatment revealed by functional and structural magnetic resonance imaging. *Biological Psychiatry, 71*(4), 286–293. https://doi.org/10.1016/j.biopsych.2011.10.021

Dietz, W. H. (1998). Health consequences of obesity in youth: Childhood predictors of adult disease. *Pediatrics, 101*(3, Pt. 2, Suppl. 2), 518–525. https://doi.org/10.1542/peds.101.S2.518

Dohle, S., Diel, K., & Hofmann, W. (2018). Executive functions and the self-regulation of eating behavior: A review. *Appetite, 124*, 4–9. https://doi.org/10.1016/j.appet.2017.05.041

Estrada, E., Eneli, I., Hampl, S., Mietus-Snyder, M., Mirza, N., Rhodes, E., Sweeney, B., Tinajero-Deck, L., Woolford, S. J., Pont, S. J., & the Children's Hospital Association. (2014). Children's Hospital Association consensus statements for comorbidities of childhood obesity. *Childhood Obesity, 10*(4), 304–317. https://doi.org/10.1089/chi.2013.0120

Fang, K., Mu, M., Liu, K., & He, Y. (2019). Screen time and childhood overweight/obesity: A systematic review and meta-analysis. *Child: Care, Health and Development, 45*(5), 744–753. https://doi.org/10.1111/cch.12701

Fiese, B. H., Hammons, A., & Grigsby-Toussaint, D. (2012). Family mealtimes: A contextual approach to understanding childhood obesity. *Economics and Human Biology, 10*(4), 365–374. https://doi.org/10.1016/j.ehb.2012.04.004

Finkelstein, E. A., Graham, W. C., & Malhotra, R. (2014). Lifetime direct medical costs of childhood obesity. *Pediatrics, 133*(5), 854–862. https://doi.org/10.1542/peds.2014-0063

Food and Nutrition Service (FNS), USDA. (2012). Nutrition standards in the national school lunch and school breakfast programs. Final rule. *Federal Register, 77*(17), 4088–4167.

Francis, L. A., & Riggs, N. R. (2018). Executive function and self-regulatory influences on children's eating.

In J. C. Lumeng & J. O. Fisher (Eds.), *Pediatric food preferences and eating behaviors* (pp. 183–206). Academic Press. https://doi.org/10.1016/B978-0-12-811716-3.00010-5

Freedman, D. S., Butte, N. F., Taveras, E. M., Lundeen, E. A., Blanck, H. M., Goodman, A. B., & Ogden, C. L. (2017). BMI z-scores are a poor indicator of adiposity among 2- to 19-year-olds with very high BMIs, NHANES 1999–2000 to 2013–2014. *Obesity, 25*(4), 739–746. https://doi.org/10.1002/oby.21782

Gariepy, G., Nitka, D., & Schmitz, N. (2010). The association between obesity and anxiety disorders in the population: A systematic review and meta-analysis. *International Journal of Obesity, 34*(3), 407–419. https://doi.org/10.1038/ijo.2009.252

Gearhardt, A. N., Yokum, S., Harris, J. L., Epstein, L. H., & Lumeng, J. C. (2020). Neural response to fast food commercials in adolescents predicts intake. *The American Journal of Clinical Nutrition, 111*(3), 493–502. https://doi.org/10.1093/ajcn/nqz305

Graziano, P. A., Calkins, S. D., & Keane, S. P. (2010). Toddler self-regulation skills predict risk for pediatric obesity. *International Journal of Obesity, 34*(4), 633–641. https://doi.org/10.1038/ijo.2009.288

Greves Grow, H. M., Cook, A. J., Arterburn, D. E., Saelens, B. E., Drewnowski, A., & Lozano, P. (2010). Child obesity associated with social disadvantage of children's neighborhoods. *Social Science & Medicine, 71*(3), 584–591. https://doi.org/10.1016/j.socscimed.2010.04.018

Guo, S. S., Wu, W., Chumlea, W. C., & Roche, A. F. (2002). Predicting overweight and obesity in adulthood from body mass index values in childhood and adolescence. *The American Journal of Clinical Nutrition, 76*(3), 653–658. https://doi.org/10.1093/ajcn/76.3.653

Hagan, J. F., Shaw, J. S., & Duncan, P. M. (Eds.). (2017). *Bright futures: Guidelines for health supervision of infants, children, and adolescents* (4th ed.). American Academy of Pediatrics. https://doi.org/10.1542/9781610020237

Halliday, J. A., Palma, C. L., Mellor, D., Green, J., & Renzaho, A. M. N. (2014). The relationship between family functioning and child and adolescent overweight and obesity: A systematic review. *International Journal of Obesity, 38*(4), 480–493. https://doi.org/10.1038/ijo.2013.213

Hampl, S., Demeule, M., Eneli, I., Frank, M., Hawkins, M. J., Kirk, S., Morris, P., Sallinen, B. J., Santos, M., Ward, W. L., & Rhodes, E. (2013). Parent perspectives on attrition from tertiary care pediatric weight management programs. *Clinical Pediatrics, 52*(6), 513–519. https://doi.org/10.1177/0009922813482515

Hampl, S. E., Carroll, C. A., Simon, S. D., & Sharma, V. (2007). Resource utilization and expenditures for overweight and obese children. *Archives of Pediatrics & Adolescent Medicine, 161*(1), 11–14. https://doi.org/10.1001/archpedi.161.1.11

Harrison, K., Bost, K. K., McBride, B. A., Donovan, S. M., Grigsby-Toussaint, D. S., Kim, J., Liechty, J. M., Wiley, A., Teran-Garcia, M., & Jacobsohn, G. C. (2011). Toward a developmental conceptualization of contributors to overweight and obesity in childhood: The six-Cs model. *Child Development Perspectives, 5*(1), 50–58. https://doi.org/10.1111/j.1750-8606.2010.00150.x

Herrera, B. M., Keildson, S., & Lindgren, C. M. (2011). Genetics and epigenetics of obesity. *Maturitas, 69*(1), 41–49. https://doi.org/10.1016/j.maturitas.2011.02.018

Hood, M. Y., Moore, L. L., Sundarajan-Ramamurti, A., Singer, M., Cupples, L. A., & Ellison, R. C. (2000). Parental eating attitudes and the development of obesity in children. The Framingham Children's Study. *International Journal of Obesity, 24*(10), 1319–1325. https://doi.org/10.1038/sj.ijo.0801396

Iob, E., Baldwin, J. R., Plomin, R., & Steptoe, A. (2021). Adverse childhood experiences, daytime salivary cortisol, and depressive symptoms in early adulthood: A longitudinal genetically informed twin study. *Translational Psychiatry, 11*(1), 420. https://doi.org/10.1038/s41398-021-01538-w

Janicke, D. M., Sallinen, B. J., Perri, M. G., Lutes, L. D., Huerta, M., Silverstein, J. H., & Brumback, B. (2008). Comparison of parent-only vs family-based interventions for overweight children in underserved rural settings: Outcomes from project STORY. *Archives of Pediatrics & Adolescent Medicine, 162*(12), 1119–1125. https://doi.org/10.1001/archpedi.162.12.1119

Janicke, D. M., Sallinen, B. J., Perri, M. G., Lutes, L. D., Silverstein, J. H., & Brumback, B. (2009). Comparison of program costs for parent-only and family-based interventions for pediatric obesity in medically underserved rural settings. *The Journal of Rural Health, 25*(3), 326–330. https://doi.org/10.1111/j.1748-0361.2009.00238.x

Janicke, D. M., Steele, R. G., Gayes, L. A., Lim, C. S., Clifford, L. M., Schneider, E. M., Carmody, J. K., & Westen, S. (2014). Systematic review and meta-analysis of comprehensive behavioral family lifestyle interventions addressing pediatric obesity. *Journal of Pediatric Psychology, 39*(8), 809–825. https://doi.org/10.1093/jpepsy/jsu023

Johnson, V. R., Acholonu, N. O., Dolan, A. C., Krishnan, A., Wang, E. H.-C., & Stanford, F. C. (2021). Racial disparities in obesity treatment among children and adolescents. *Current Obesity*

Reports, *10*(3), 342–350. https://doi.org/10.1007/s13679-021-00442-0

Kalliomäki, M., Collado, M. C., Salminen, S., & Isolauri, E. (2008). Early differences in fecal microbiota composition in children may predict overweight. *The American Journal of Clinical Nutrition*, *87*(3), 534–538. https://doi.org/10.1093/ajcn/87.3.534

Kanekar, A., & Sharma, M. (2009). Meta-analysis of school-based childhood obesity interventions in the U.K. and U.S. *International Quarterly of Community Health Education*, *29*(3), 241–256. https://doi.org/10.2190/IQ.29.3.d

Khera, A. V., Chaffin, M., Wade, K. H., Zahid, S., Brancale, J., Xia, R., Distefano, M., Senol-Cosar, O., Haas, M. E., Bick, A., Aragam, K. G., Lander, E. S., Smith, G. D., Mason-Suares, H., Fornage, M., Lebo, M., Timpson, N. J., Kaplan, L. M., & Kathiresan, S. (2019). Polygenic prediction of weight and obesity trajectories from birth to adulthood. *Cell*, *177*(3), 587–596.e9. https://doi.org/10.1016/j.cell.2019.03.028

Killedar, A., Lung, T., Petrou, S., Teixeira-Pinto, A., Tan, E. J., & Hayes, A. (2020). Weight status and health-related quality of life during childhood and adolescence: Effects of age and socioeconomic position. *International Journal of Obesity*, *44*(3), 637–645. https://doi.org/10.1038/s41366-020-0529-3

Kitzmann, K. M., Dalton, W. T., III, & Buscemi, J. (2008). Beyond parenting practices: Family context and the treatment of pediatric obesity. *Family Relations*, *57*(1), 13–23. https://doi.org/10.1111/j.1741-3729.2007.00479.x

Koleva, P. T., Bridgman, S. L., & Kozyrskyj, A. L. (2015). The infant gut microbiome: Evidence for obesity risk and dietary intervention. *Nutrients*, *7*(4), 2237–2260. https://doi.org/10.3390/nu7042237

Kumanyika, S. K. (2008). Environmental influences on childhood obesity: Ethnic and cultural influences in context. *Physiology & Behavior*, *94*(1), 61–70. https://doi.org/10.1016/j.physbeh.2007.11.019

Kumanyika, S. K. (2019). A framework for increasing equity impact in obesity prevention. *American Journal of Public Health*, *109*(10), 1350–1357. https://doi.org/10.2105/AJPH.2019.305221

Lee, J. M., Appugliese, D., Kaciroti, N., Corwyn, R. F., Bradley, R. H., & Lumeng, J. C. (2007). Weight status in young girls and the onset of puberty. *Pediatrics*, *119*(3), e624–e630. https://doi.org/10.1542/peds.2006-2188

Li, Y. (2018). Epigenetic mechanisms link maternal diets and gut microbiome to obesity in the offspring. *Frontiers in Genetics*, *9*, 342. https://doi.org/10.3389/fgene.2018.00342

Lipek, T., Igel, U., Gausche, R., Kiess, W., & Grande, G. (2015). Obesogenic environments: Environmental approaches to obesity prevention. *Journal of Pediatric Endocrinology & Metabolism*, *28*(5–6), 485–495. https://doi.org/10.1515/jpem-2015-0127

Loth, K. A. (2016). Associations between food restriction and pressure-to-eat parenting practices and dietary intake in children: A selective review of the recent literature. *Current Nutrition Reports*, *5*(1), 61–67. https://doi.org/10.1007/s13668-016-0154-x

Lumeng, J. C., & Hillman, K. H. (2007). Eating in larger groups increases food consumption. *Archives of Disease in Childhood*, *92*(5), 384–387. https://doi.org/10.1136/adc.2006.103259

Malhotra, K., Herman, A. N., Wright, G., Bruton, Y., Fisher, J. O., & Whitaker, R. C. (2013). Perceived benefits and challenges for low-income mothers of having family meals with preschool-aged children: Childhood memories matter. *Journal of the Academy of Nutrition and Dietetics*, *113*(11), 1484–1493. https://doi.org/10.1016/j.jand.2013.07.028

Mamrot, P., & Hanć, T. (2019). The association of the executive functions with overweight and obesity indicators in children and adolescents: A literature review. *Neuroscience and Biobehavioral Reviews*, *107*, 59–68. https://doi.org/10.1016/j.neubiorev.2019.08.021

Manyema, M., Norris, S. A., & Richter, L. M. (2018). Stress begets stress: The association of adverse childhood experiences with psychological distress in the presence of adult life stress. *BMC Public Health*, *18*(1), 835. https://doi.org/10.1186/s12889-018-5767-0

Martin, A., Booth, J. N., McGeown, S., Niven, A., Sproule, J., Saunders, D. H., & Reilly, J. J. (2017). Longitudinal associations between childhood obesity and academic achievement: Systematic review with focus group data. *Current Obesity Reports*, *6*(3), 297–313. https://doi.org/10.1007/s13679-017-0272-9

Martin, A., Razza, R., & Brooks-Gunn, J. (2012). Specifying the links between household chaos and preschool children's development. *Early Child Development and Care*, *182*(10), 1247–1263. https://doi.org/10.1080/03004430.2011.605522

Martin, A. M., Sun, E. W., Rogers, G. B., & Keating, D. J. (2019). The influence of the gut microbiome on host metabolism through the regulation of gut hormone release. *Frontiers in Physiology*, *10*, 446991. https://doi.org/10.3389/fphys.2019.00428

Martin-Biggers, J., Quick, V., Zhang, M., Jin, Y., & Byrd-Bredbenner, C. (2018). Relationships of family conflict, cohesion, and chaos in the home environment on maternal and child food-related behaviours. *Maternal and Child Nutrition, 14*(2), e12540. https://doi.org/10.1111/mcn.12540

Miller, A. L., & Lumeng, J. C. (2018). Pathways of association from stress to obesity in early childhood. *Obesity, 26*(7), 1117–1124. https://doi.org/10.1002/oby.22155

Miller, A. L., Rosenblum, K. L., Retzloff, L. B., & Lumeng, J. C. (2016). Observed self-regulation is associated with weight in low-income toddlers. *Appetite, 105,* 705–712. https://doi.org/10.1016/j.appet.2016.07.007

Miller, G. E., Chen, E., & Parker, K. J. (2011). Psychological stress in childhood and susceptibility to the chronic diseases of aging: Moving toward a model of behavioral and biological mechanisms. *Psychological Bulletin, 137*(6), 959–997. https://doi.org/10.1037/a0024768

Must, A., & Strauss, R. S. (1999). Risks and consequences of childhood and adolescent obesity. *International Journal of Obesity, 23*(Suppl. 2), S2–S11. https://doi.org/10.1038/sj.ijo.0800852

The NCD Risk Factor Collaboration (NCD-RisC). (2017). Worldwide trends in body-mass index, underweight, overweight, and obesity from 1975 to 2016: A pooled analysis of 2416 population-based measurement studies in 128.9 million children, adolescents, and adults. *The Lancet, 390*(10113), 2627–2642. https://doi.org/10.1016/S0140-6736(17)32129-3

Neumark-Sztainer, D., Bauer, K. W., Friend, S., Hannan, P. J., Story, M., & Berge, J. M. (2010). Family weight talk and dieting: How much do they matter for body dissatisfaction and disordered eating behaviors in adolescent girls? *Journal of Adolescent Health, 47*(3), 270–276. https://doi.org/10.1016/j.jadohealth.2010.02.001

Noar, S. M., Benac, C. N., & Harris, M. S. (2007). Does tailoring matter? Meta-analytic review of tailored print health behavior change interventions. *Psychological Bulletin, 133*(4), 673–693. https://doi.org/10.1037/0033-2909.133.4.673

O'Brien, S. H., Holubkov, R., & Reis, E. C. (2004). Identification, evaluation, and management of obesity in an academic primary care center. *Pediatrics, 114*(2), e154–e159. https://doi.org/10.1542/peds.114.2.e154

Ogden, C. L., Carroll, M. D., Lawman, H. G., Fryar, C. D., Kruszon-Moran, D., Kit, B. K., & Flegal, K. M. (2016). Trends in obesity prevalence among children and adolescents in the United States, 1988–1994 through 2013–2014. *JAMA: Journal of the American Medical Association, 315*(21), 2292–2299. https://doi.org/10.1001/jama.2016.6361

Ogden, C. L., Fryar, C. D., Hales, C. M., Carroll, M. D., Aoki, Y., & Freedman, D. S. (2018). Differences in obesity prevalence by demographics and urbanization in US children and adolescents, 2013–2016. *JAMA: Journal of the American Medical Association, 319*(23), 2410–2418. https://doi.org/10.1001/jama.2018.5158

Paul, I. M., Savage, J. S., Anzman-Frasca, S., Marini, M. E., Beiler, J. S., Hess, L. B., Loken, E., & Birch, L. L. (2018). Effect of a responsive parenting educational intervention on childhood weight outcomes at 3 years of age: The INSIGHT randomized clinical trial. *JAMA: Journal of the American Medical Association, 320*(5), 461–468. https://doi.org/10.1001/jama.2018.9432

Petraroli, M., Castellone, E., Patianna, V., & Esposito, S. (2021). Gut microbiota and obesity in adults and children: The state of the art. *Frontiers in Pediatrics, 9,* 657020. https://doi.org/10.3389/fped.2021.657020

Popkin, B. M., Du, S., Green, W. D., Beck, M. A., Algaith, T., Herbst, C. H., Alsukait, R. F., Alluhidan, M., Alazemi, N., & Shekar, M. (2020). Individuals with obesity and COVID-19: A global perspective on the epidemiology and biological relationships. *Obesity Reviews, 21*(11), e13128. https://doi.org/10.1111/obr.13128

Puhl, R. M., & Lessard, L. M. (2020). Weight stigma in youth: Prevalence, consequences, and considerations for clinical practice. *Current Obesity Reports, 9*(4), 402–411. https://doi.org/10.1007/s13679-020-00408-8

Quek, Y. H., Tam, W. W. S., Zhang, M. W. B., & Ho, R. C. M. (2017). Exploring the association between childhood and adolescent obesity and depression: A meta-analysis. *Obesity Reviews, 18*(7), 742–754. https://doi.org/10.1111/obr.12535

Rankin, J., Matthews, L., Cobley, S., Han, A., Sanders, R., Wiltshire, H. D., & Baker, J. S. (2016). Psychological consequences of childhood obesity: Psychiatric comorbidity and prevention. *Adolescent Health, Medicine and Therapeutics, 7,* 125–146. https://doi.org/10.2147/AHMT.S101631

Redsell, S. A., Edmonds, B., Swift, J. A., Siriwardena, A. N., Weng, S., Nathan, D., & Glazebrook, C. (2016). Systematic review of randomised controlled trials of interventions that aim to reduce the risk, either directly or indirectly, of overweight and obesity in infancy and early childhood. *Maternal and Child Nutrition, 12*(1), 24–38. https://doi.org/10.1111/mcn.12184

Reeves, G. M., Postolache, T. T., & Snitker, S. (2008). Childhood obesity and depression: Connection between these growing problems in growing children. *International Journal of Child Health and Human Development, 1*(2), 103–114.

Reilly, J. J., Methven, E., McDowell, Z. C., Hacking, B., Alexander, D., Stewart, L., & Kelnar, C. J. (2003).

Health consequences of obesity. *Archives of Disease in Childhood, 88*(9), 748–752. https://doi.org/10.1136/adc.88.9.748

Renehan, A. G., Tyson, M., Egger, M., Heller, R. F., & Zwahlen, M. (2008). Body-mass index and incidence of cancer: A systematic review and meta-analysis of prospective observational studies. *The Lancet, 371*(9612), 569–578. https://doi.org/10.1016/S0140-6736(08)60269-X

Riem, M. M. E., & Karreman, A. (2019). Childhood adversity and adult health: The role of developmental timing and associations with accelerated aging. *Child Maltreatment, 24*(1), 17–25. https://doi.org/10.1177/1077559518795058

Robinson, T. N., Banda, J. A., Hale, L., Lu, A. S., Fleming-Milici, F., Calvert, S. L., & Wartella, E. (2017). Screen media exposure and obesity in children and adolescents. *Pediatrics, 140*(Suppl. 2), S97–S101. https://doi.org/10.1542/peds.2016-1758K

Rupp, K., & McCoy, S. M. (2021). Flourishing and academic engagement among adolescents with overweight and obesity. *International Journal of Adolescent Medicine and Health, 33*(4), 20180180. https://doi.org/10.1515/ijamh-2018-0180

Rupp, K., & McCoy, S. M. (2019). Bullying perpetration and victimization among adolescents with overweight and obesity in a nationally representative sample. *Childhood Obesity, 15*(5), 323–330. https://doi.org/10.1089/chi.2018.0233

Russell, C. G., & Russell, A. (2019). A biopsychosocial approach to processes and pathways in the development of overweight and obesity in childhood: Insights from developmental theory and research. *Obesity Reviews, 20*(5), 725–749. https://doi.org/10.1111/obr.12838

Sallinen Gaffka, B. J., Frank, M., Hampl, S., Santos, M., & Rhodes, E. T. (2013). Parents and pediatric weight management attrition: Experiences and recommendations. *Childhood Obesity, 9*(5), 409–417. https://doi.org/10.1089/chi.2013.0069

Salvy, S.-J., & Bowker, J. C. (2014). Peers and obesity during childhood and adolescence: A review of the empirical research on peers, eating, and physical activity. *Journal of Obesity & Weight Loss Therapy, 4*(1), 207. https://doi.org/10.4172/2165-7904.1000207

Salwen, J. K., Hymowitz, G. F., Bannon, S. M., & O'Leary, K. D. (2015). Weight-related abuse: Perceived emotional impact and the effect on disordered eating. *Child Abuse & Neglect, 45*, 163–171. https://doi.org/10.1016/j.chiabu.2014.12.005

Santana, C. C. A., Hill, J. O., Azevedo, L. B., Gunnarsdottir, T., & Prado, W. L. (2017). The association between obesity and academic performance in youth: A systematic review. *Obesity Reviews, 18*(10), 1191–1199. https://doi.org/10.1111/obr.12582

Schroeder, K., Schuler, B. R., Kobulsky, J. M., & Sarwer, D. B. (2021). The association between adverse childhood experiences and childhood obesity: A systematic review. *Obesity Reviews, 22*(7), e13204. https://doi.org/10.1111/obr.13204

Segal, A. B., Huerta, M. C., Aurino, E., & Sassi, F. (2021). The impact of childhood obesity on human capital in high-income countries: A systematic review. *Obesity Reviews, 22*(1), e13104. https://doi.org/10.1111/obr.13104

Shirley, K., Rutfield, R., Hall, N., Fedor, N., McCaughey, V. K., & Zajac, K. (2015). Combinations of obesity prevention strategies in US elementary schools: A critical review. *The Journal of Primary Prevention, 36*(1), 1–20. https://doi.org/10.1007/s10935-014-0370-3

Shriver, L. H., Harrist, A. W., Page, M., Hubbs-Tait, L., Moulton, M., & Topham, G. (2013). Differences in body esteem by weight status, gender, and physical activity among young elementary school-aged children. *Body Image, 10*(1), 78–84. https://doi.org/10.1016/j.bodyim.2012.10.005

Silventoinen, K., Rokholm, B., Kaprio, J., & Sørensen, T. I. A. (2010). The genetic and environmental influences on childhood obesity: A systematic review of twin and adoption studies. *International Journal of Obesity, 34*(1), 29–40. https://doi.org/10.1038/ijo.2009.177

Skelton, J. A., Goff, D. C., Jr., Ip, E., & Beech, B. M. (2011). Attrition in a multidisciplinary pediatric weight management clinic. *Childhood Obesity, 7*(3), 185–193. https://doi.org/10.1089/chi.2011.0010

Skelton, J. A., Woolford, S. J., Skinner, A., Barlow, S. E., Hampl, S. E., Lazorick, S., & Armstrong, S. (2021). Weight management without stigma or harm: A roundtable discussion with childhood obesity experts. *Childhood Obesity, 17*(2), 79–85. https://doi.org/10.1089/chi.2021.29010.roundtable

Skinner, A. C., Ravanbakht, S. N., Skelton, J. A., Perrin, E. M., & Armstrong, S. C. (2018). Prevalence of obesity and severe obesity in US children, 1999–2016. *Pediatrics, 141*(3), e20173459. https://doi.org/10.1542/peds.2017-3459

Sleddens, E. F. C., Gerards, S. M. P. L., Thijs, C., de Vries, N. K., & Kremers, S. P. J. (2011). General parenting, childhood overweight and obesity-inducing behaviors: A review. *International Journal of Pediatric Obesity, 6*(Suppl. 3), e12–e27. https://doi.org/10.3109/17477166.2011.566339

Song, P., Zhang, Y., Yu, J., Zha, M., Zhu, Y., Rahimi, K., & Rudan, I. (2019). Global prevalence of hypertension in children. *JAMA Pediatrics, 173*(12),

1154–1163. https://doi.org/10.1001/jamapediatrics.2019.3310

Srinivasan, S. R., Bao, W., Wattigney, W. A., & Berenson, G. S. (1996). Adolescent overweight is associated with adult overweight and related multiple cardiovascular risk factors: The Bogalusa Heart Study. *Metabolism: Clinical and Experimental, 45*(2), 235–240. https://doi.org/10.1016/S0026-0495(96)90060-8

Story, M., & French, S. (2004). Food advertising and marketing directed at children and adolescents in the US. *The International Journal of Behavioral Nutrition and Physical Activity, 1*(1), 3. https://doi.org/10.1186/1479-5868-1-3

Sutter, C., Kim, J. H., & Bost, K. K. (2020). Connections between friendship quality, peer competence, and obesity in early childhood through adolescence. *Childhood Obesity, 16*(6), 393–402. https://doi.org/10.1089/chi.2019.0287

Tomiyama, A. J. (2019). Stress and Obesity. *Annual Review of Psychology, 70*(1), 703–718. https://doi.org/10.1146/annurev-psych-010418-102936

Veerman, J. L., Van Beeck, E. F., Barendregt, J. J., & Mackenbach, J. P. (2009). By how much would limiting TV food advertising reduce childhood obesity? *European Journal of Public Health, 19*(4), 365–369. https://doi.org/10.1093/eurpub/ckp039

Ventura, A. K., & Birch, L. L. (2008). Does parenting affect children's eating and weight status? *The International Journal of Behavioral Nutrition and Physical Activity, 5*(1), 15. https://doi.org/10.1186/1479-5868-5-15

Verjans-Janssen, S. R. B., van de Kolk, I., Van Kann, D. H. H., Kremers, S. P. J., & Gerards, S. M. P. L. (2018). Effectiveness of school-based physical activity and nutrition interventions with direct parental involvement on children's BMI and energy balance-related behaviors—A systematic review. *PLOS ONE, 13*(9), e0204560. https://doi.org/10.1371/journal.pone.0204560

Woo Baidal, J. A., Locks, L. M., Cheng, E. R., Blake-Lamb, T. L., Perkins, M. E., & Taveras, E. M. (2016). Risk factors for childhood obesity in the first 1,000 days: A systematic review. *American Journal of Preventive Medicine, 50*(6), 761–779. https://doi.org/10.1016/j.amepre.2015.11.012

Woolford, S. J., Gebremariam, A., Clark, S. J., & Davis, M. M. (2007). Incremental hospital charges associated with obesity as a secondary diagnosis in children. *Obesity, 15*(7), 1895–1901. https://doi.org/10.1038/oby.2007.224

World Health Organization. (n.d.). *Obesity* [Health topics]. Retrieved April 18, 2024, from https://www.who.int/westernpacific/health-topics/obesity

Wouters, E. J., Larsen, J. K., Kremers, S. P., Dagnelie, P. C., & Geenen, R. (2010). Peer influence on snacking behavior in adolescence. *Appetite, 55*(1), 11–17. https://doi.org/10.1016/j.appet.2010.03.002

Zeller, M., Kirk, S., Claytor, R., Khoury, P., Grieme, J., Santangelo, M., & Daniels, S. (2004). Predictors of attrition from a pediatric weight management program. *The Journal of Pediatrics, 144*(4), 466–470. https://doi.org/10.1016/j.jpeds.2003.12.031

Zeller, M. H., Reiter-Purtill, J., Modi, A. C., Gutzwiller, J., Vannatta, K., & Davies, W. H. (2007). Controlled study of critical parent and family factors in the obesigenic environment. *Obesity, 15*(1), 126–136. https://doi.org/10.1038/oby.2007.517

PART III

DEVELOPMENTAL-BEHAVIORAL AND MENTAL HEALTH CONDITIONS AND THE ROLE OF BEHAVIORAL HEALTH PROVIDERS

CHAPTER 16

AUTISM SPECTRUM DISORDER AND DISORDERS OF SOCIAL COGNITION ACROSS CHILDHOOD AND ADOLESCENCE

Christina Toolan, Elaine Clarke, Kathleen Campbell, Paul Carbone, and Catherine Lord

Autism spectrum disorder (ASD) is a lifelong neurodevelopmental disorder characterized by deficits in social communication as well as restricted, repetitive behaviors (American Psychiatric Association, 2013). These impairments emerge early in development and often present limitations to functioning throughout the life course. Currently, about 1 in 36 children in the United States has a diagnosis of ASD—a number that has climbed considerably since the 1990s (Maenner et al., 2023). Although ASD is typically diagnosed in childhood, a growing number of individuals are identified in adolescence or adulthood. ASD is also often accompanied by co-occurring psychiatric conditions. There are significant direct and indirect economic effects of having a child with ASD, with the lifetime cost of supporting an individual with ASD estimated at between $1 to $2 million (Buescher et al., 2014).

The model presented in Figure 16.1 illustrates our framework for conceptualizing the interplay of individual-level, family-level, and treatment and intervention factors across development in ASD. The theoretical perspective of this chapter was informed by both the developmental cascades theory (Masten & Cicchetti, 2010; see also Volume 1, Chapter 4, this handbook) and the family systems-illness model (Rolland, 1987). Developmental cascades theory asserts that competence begets competence. In ASD, symptoms arise in early childhood and may change over time but persist and cause continued challenges in later development. Treatment can play an integral role in improving the social competence of individuals with autism and promoting more positive developmental cascades.

The family systems-illness model integrates an understanding of family processes and supports as well as characteristics of a diagnosis (i.e., condition progression, duration, and onset) into broader clinical conceptualizations of a child's prognosis. ASD can be thought of as a chronic health condition, with relatively stable symptoms persisting across the lifespan. As a disorder of social development, ASD inherently alters parent–child interactions and relationships. Parents play an integral role in supporting healthy development for all children—perhaps especially children with ASD. Given the high levels of stress and economic burden associated with an ASD diagnosis, parenting skills interventions and access to both formal and informal sources of support are imperative to improving both child and family outcomes in ASD.

https://doi.org/10.1037/0000414-016
APA Handbook of Pediatric Psychology, Developmental-Behavioral Pediatrics, and Developmental Science: Vol. 2. Pediatric Psychology and Developmental-Behavioral Pediatrics: Clinical Applications of Developmental Science, P. E. Shah and M. H. Bornstein (Editors-in-Chief)
Copyright © 2025 by the American Psychological Association. All rights reserved.

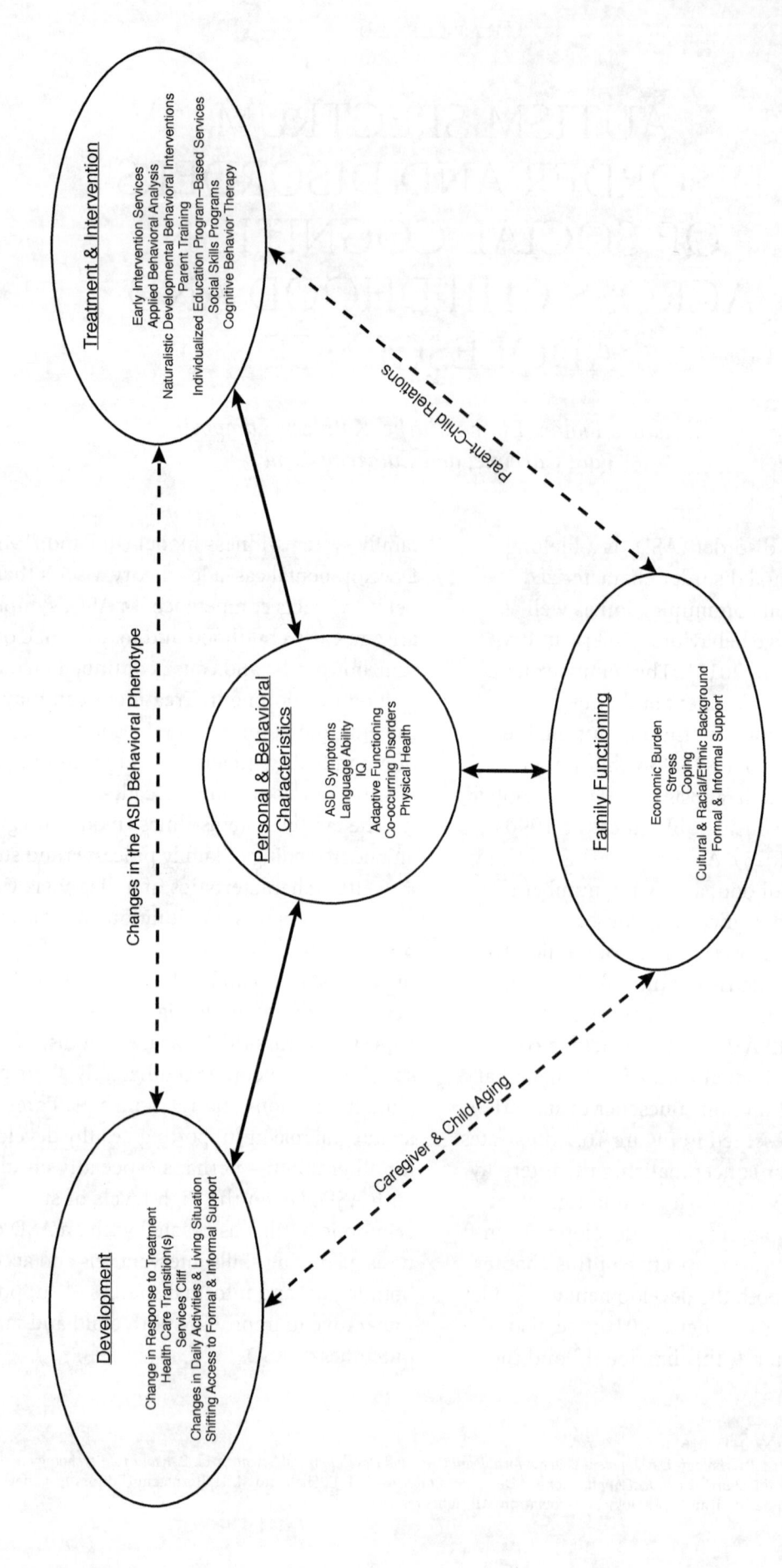

FIGURE 16.1. Conceptual framework of the interplay of individual, family, treatment, and intervention factors across development in autism spectrum disorder (ASD).

This chapter leverages these two theoretical lenses to offer a brief overview of symptomatology, epidemiology, individual and family outcomes, assessment, and treatments for ASD across the lifespan. It also highlights implications for practitioners and researchers in developmental-behavioral pediatrics, pediatric psychology, and developmental science.

SIGNS AND SYMPTOMS OF AUTISM SPECTRUM DISORDER

Diagnostic criteria for ASD in the fifth edition of the *Diagnostic and Statistical Manual of Mental Disorders* (*DSM-5*) include behaviors in two core domains: (a) difficulty with social communication, including limited eye contact or difficulty engaging socially with others, and (b) the presence of restricted and repetitive behaviors (RRBs), such as hyper- or hyposensitivity to sensory stimuli, repetitive motor movements, or resistance to changes (American Psychiatric Association, 2013, pp. 50–51). There is marked variability in the presentation of ASD symptoms across these two domains, as well as the language, cognitive, and adaptive functioning abilities of individuals with ASD, as shown in Figure 16.2. Thus, the "spectrum" in "autism spectrum disorder" captures wide-ranging phenotypic heterogeneity, exemplified in the vignettes presented in Exhibit 16.1. Symptoms must be present early in development, although for those with higher language and/or cognitive abilities, the presentation may not become clear until social demands surpass social capabilities.

Social Cognition

Many individuals with ASD demonstrate difficulty with social cognition, or the processing, understanding, and application of information in social contexts. Challenges with social cognition include impairments in executive function (EF), referring broadly to abilities facilitating the planning and execution of complex, goal-oriented behaviors. Though not a defining characteristic of ASD, EF is an area of impairment for autistic individuals. Impairments in social cognition are

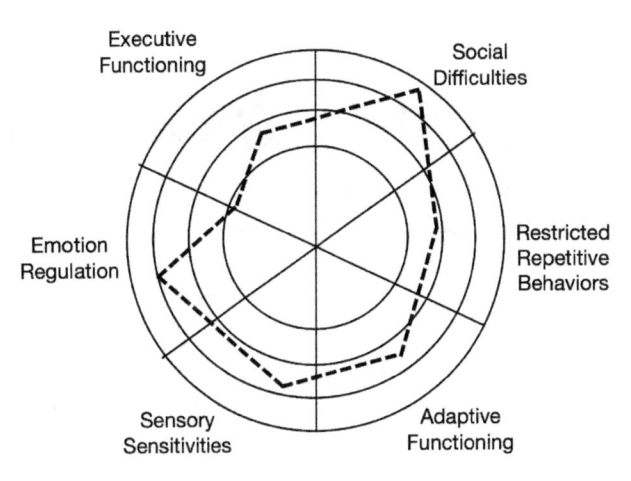

FIGURE 16.2. Heterogeneity on the autism spectrum has long been conceptualized as linear, with "low functioning" individuals on one end and "high functioning" individuals on the other. Terms such as "low functioning" and "high functioning" are now widely considered inaccurate and harmful, as support needs among those with autism spectrum disorder (ASD) are not inherently tied to IQ or language ability. Instead, heterogeneity in ASD may be more accurately described by individual profiles of symptom domains. In the individual symptom profile illustrated here, pronounced impairments exist in emotion regulation and social difficulties; in contrast, executive functioning is an area of relative strength. Symptom domains—though often related—are distinct. Weakness in one area does not preclude strengths in other areas and vice versa. The symptom domains listed here are not exhaustive but represent common areas of concern for individuals with ASD.

also seen in individuals with other conditions (e.g., attention-deficit/hyperactivity disorder [ADHD]); however, the deficits seen in ASD are thought to be more profound and generalized than those in other disorders (Kenworthy et al., 2008).

Other disorders of social cognition, such as social (pragmatic) communication disorder (SCD), are conceptually related to ASD. A diagnosis of SCD, introduced in the *DSM-5*, is intended to capture individuals with social communication deficits who do not meet the criteria for ASD. Individuals with SCD may demonstrate higher-order social pragmatic difficulties with verbal and nonverbal communication, such as following rules of conversation and understanding implied or nonliteral language. SCD and ASD are differentiated by RRBs, which are present in ASD but not in SCD.

EXHIBIT 16.1

Person Portraits Illustrating the Variability in Presentation, Strengths, and Needs of Autistic People

Adir

Adir is an 18-year-old, nonverbal young man with profound autism, intellectual disability, and epilepsy who lives in a small town. He was diagnosed with autism at age 2, and his parents enrolled him in a preschool that specialized in those with severe needs, with the hope that he could eventually participate in a mainstream classroom. There, Adir received intensive behavioral therapies (i.e., ABA), speech and language therapy, and occupational therapy, and he participated in a social skills group. Adir took medication to manage his seizures. In addition, he was given medication because his behavior could become challenging to others when he was upset or agitated. By age 16, he was over 6 feet tall, weighed 275 pounds, and his behavior was challenging for others to manage. He also never was fully toilet trained and had frequent accidents, especially when frustrated. Adir's family could not find after-school care that met his needs that they could afford, so his mother quit her job to supervise him. During outbursts, he became physically aggressive towards himself and others, creating a safety risk for him and his caregivers. Several efforts at supported employment proved unsuitable and resulted in aggressive outbursts and his being fired. His parents are currently considering residential placement where he will receive 24/7 care.

Franco

Neither Franco's parents nor his pediatrician observed any obvious early signs of autism, and Franco reached most of his developmental milestones on time. However, his parents reported that he was a very fussy baby and did not want to be cuddled or held. At around 18 months of age, he began to interact with his parents less frequently, wander off, was no longer looking at their faces, and stopped forming new words. At the time, his parents had just welcomed his sister to the family, and the pediatrician thought that his change in behavior might reflect these changes in the home. Franco spent most days walking in circles, trying to get outdoors, and sorting his toys by size and color. He insisted on eating only foods that were white and would start biting his own arm and pinching his caregiver if anyone tried to put new foods on his plate. Eventually, his parents had him assessed, and he received a formal autism diagnosis at around age 3. For the next 2 years, he received general early intervention services at home two to three times a week. By age 5, he was making enough progress to be enrolled in a mainstream kindergarten with a full-time aide. At school, he enjoyed music and was well-mannered, but spent most of his time by himself continuing to play with toys alone or in parallel with other students. Franco had little awareness of danger and would wander away from the family home. His parents had added childproof locks to all their gates and fences but with age, he became more adept at climbing them. However, he was starting to show reciprocal smiles, and his teachers and parents were pleased with his progress. He had a very strong and repetitive interest in being pushed on the swings at school and loved having his aide push him constantly during breaks. In fact, this is the one activity he clearly enjoyed and after school, he would constantly go to the door asking his mother to take him to the school playground where the "good" swings were. One afternoon, at age 7, he wandered away from his home and drowned in a nearby pond.

Sofía

Sofía lives in a large metropolitan area with her parents and sister. She received an academic scholarship to attend an elite private high school and is finishing her junior year. She is fluent in three languages, reads prolifically, and has an IQ over 125. Sofía always excelled academically but has trouble making and keeping friends. She likes to spend most of her time at the library or at home reading. Before she was diagnosed with autism, Sofía and her family saw her problems as mostly consisting of restlessness, problems concentrating, and severe sensory issues that caused her physical pain. She also had difficulty with tasks that required her to think abstractly, yet her ability to excel in most academic tasks more than made up for this relative weakness. Last year, Sofía was bullied incessantly by another student, and she became so depressed that her family considered transferring schools. Instead, Sofía's family found a therapist specializing in cognitive behavior therapy (CBT) for depression. Finally, at age 16, Sofía received an autism diagnosis from her therapist. Her depressive symptoms have steadily improved through CBT, and she intends to pursue a degree in art history after finishing high school next spring.

Note. The person portrait vignettes presented here are fictionalized composites. Adapted from "The Lancet Commission on the Future of Care and Clinical Research in Autism," by C. Lord, T. Charman, A. Havdahl, P. Carbone, E. Anagnostou, B. Boyd, T. Carr, P. J. de Vries, C. Dissanayake, G. Divan, C. M. Freitag, M. M. Gotelli, C. Kasari, M. Knapp, P. Mundy, A. Plank, L. Scahill, C. Servili, P. Shattuck, E. Simonoff, A. Tepper Singer, V. Slonims, P. P. Wang, M. Celica Ysrraelit, R. Jellett, A. Pickles, J. Cusack, P. Howlin, P. Szatmari, A. Holbrook, C. Toolan, and J. B. McCauley, 2022, *The Lancet*, 399(10321), pp. 276–277 (https://doi.org/10.1016/S0140-6736(21)01541-5). Copyright 2022 by Elsevier. Adapted with permission.

Developmental Emergence of Autism Spectrum Disorder

The median age of diagnosis for ASD in the United States is approximately 4 years (Maenner et al., 2023). However, signs typically present much earlier in development, and an ASD diagnosis can be made reliably as early as 2 years old. ASD is described from infancy to adolescence in the following sections, though it is important to note that there is variability in presentation due to the phenotypic heterogeneity characteristic of ASD.

Infancy. Much of what we know about the early emergence of ASD comes from prospective studies of high-risk (HR) infant siblings—that is, younger siblings of children with ASD. What is striking about ASD symptomatology in early development is the absence, rather than presence, of behaviors. Certain "red flag" behaviors can emerge as early as 6 months of age (e.g., no big smiles or joyful expressions), though clearer signs of ASD develop in the second year of life. HR infants who are later diagnosed with ASD demonstrate less social attunement to others when compared to typically developing (TD) children (Jones et al., 2014). Specifically, they demonstrate less and/or delayed social seeking-out behavior. These children do not lack social behavior, but rather engage in it with limited frequency and variety.

In infancy, parents and caregivers most frequently report concerns about difficulties and/or delays in communication and language, such as low frequency of babbling or delayed use of single words or phrases (Kozlowski et al., 2011). Other signs include reduced back-and-forth interaction with social partners (e.g., fewer facial expressions or gestures). Notably, the earliest signs of ASD involve social communication and joint attention, the ability to share attention and experiences with another person. Children with ASD demonstrate greater difficulty with initiation of joint attention (e.g., pointing, showing, or using language for the purpose of sharing) compared to response to joint attention (e.g., looking where another person points; Billeci et al., 2016), though response to joint attention is also impaired. Children who later receive an ASD diagnosis may also fail to respond to their name during this developmental period.

Infants and toddlers at risk for ASD may also present with RRBs, including repetitive play (e.g., pushing a car back and forth repeatedly), movements (e.g., hand flapping, spinning, hand/finger tensing), interest in parts of objects (e.g., wheels of a toy vehicle), and sensory interests or aversions (e.g., fascination with blinking lights, touching objects to lips, aversion to food textures). It should be noted that TD infants and toddlers also engage in RRBs. However, HR children demonstrate a higher frequency and greater diversity of RRBs than TD children (Harrop et al., 2014).

Many children diagnosed with ASD experience a plateau or a regression, usually in language and social skills, losing previously acquired skills for a period of at least 1 month (Boterberg et al., 2019). Most cases of regression occur gradually about halfway through the second year of life. About three-quarters of children who regress will regain some, if not all, of their lost skills (Simonoff et al., 2020).

Preschool. The preschool experience—particularly, the opportunity for extended social contact with peers—can expose social communicative impairments in children with ASD, resulting in many being first identified during the preschool years (Maenner et al., 2023). Signs may include limited pretend play, lack of interest in social interaction, and difficulty understanding others' feelings. TD preschoolers generally communicate using short sentences combined with eye contact, a range of facial expressions, and gestures (e.g., waving, pointing, descriptive gestures such as "big"). In contrast, children with ASD may have language delays or abnormalities (e.g., not speaking in sentences, echolalia) and have limited nonverbal communication.

Though very rare, some children regress around 3 to 4 years of age. Regression at these ages tends to involve loss in motor function (e.g., purposeful use of hands) and/or self-help skills (e.g., toileting) and may be related to rare genetic conditions (e.g., Landau-Kleffner syndrome; Boterberg et al., 2019). These children are less likely to regain skills (Boterberg et al., 2019).

School age and adolescence. In children and adolescents with higher cognitive and language abilities, ASD symptoms may be more subtle. Signs may not become clear until social relationships become more complex and nuanced. ASD signs and symptoms in school-aged children and adolescents may include difficulty initiating and/or sustaining engagement with peers and difficulty reading social cues. Additionally, children and adolescents may have obsessive interests and poor response to changes in routines.

Children and adolescents with ASD may present with emotion dysregulation, behavioral problems, and symptoms of depression and anxiety. They may also have other co-occurring conditions, such as intellectual disability, language delay, oppositional defiant disorder, or ADHD (Simonoff et al., 2008). Children and adolescents should receive comprehensive psychological evaluations to consider comorbidities.

Recent work suggests adolescents and adults with ASD experience gender diversity, including nonheterosexuality and gender dysphoria, at higher rates than the general population (George & Stokes, 2018). Developmental behavioral pediatricians may be among the first professionals to hear of these concerns. Providers should provide gender-affirming care (e.g., using preferred names and/or pronouns), be familiar with local educational laws, and guide families through potential conflicts and available treatment options, including recommendations for family therapy or other community resources.

EPIDEMIOLOGY

There are documented disparities in diagnosis based on sociodemographic and geographic factors. Though ASD prevalence is thought to be equal across racial and ethnic groups, on average, African American and Latin American children not only are diagnosed with ASD later than European American children (Daniels & Mandell, 2014) but also often receive other diagnoses (e.g., ADHD, conduct disorder) without appropriate ASD evaluation. Children from rural areas also tend to be diagnosed later than those from metropolitan areas (Daniels & Mandell, 2014). Disparities in diagnosis contribute to further disparities in intervention access.

Etiology and Neurobiology

Due to the heterogeneous nature of ASD, there is no single etiology underlying this complex condition. Though the full range of etiology is not yet completely understood, studies have identified genetic and environmental risk factors and neurobiological differences characterizing individuals with ASD.

Genetics. Single-gene explanations, such as those in fragile X syndrome and tuberous sclerosis complex, occur in approximately 5% of cases of ASD (de la Torre-Ubieta et al., 2016). Rare *de novo* point mutations and copy number variations in over 100 different genes have been associated with ASD, but known genetic associations are identified in only 10% to 20% of children with ASD (Lord et al., 2020). It is likely most cases of ASD are explained by the contribution of multiple common and some rare genetic variants that converge to alter brain development.

Recurrence risk and environmental factors. Certain genetic and environmental conditions may increase the risk of an ASD diagnosis. Males are diagnosed with ASD at an approximate 4:1 ratio to females (Maenner et al., 2023). Families with one child with ASD have an approximately 1 in 5 chance of having another child with ASD, with an even greater risk if there are two or more children with ASD in the family already (Palmer et al., 2017). Prenatal and perinatal environmental risk factors include maternal use of antiepileptic medications (e.g., valproate), advanced parental age (maternal >40 years, paternal >50 years), preterm birth, and neonatal hypoxia (Lord et al., 2020).

Neurobiology. The neural underpinnings of ASD have been placed at the onset in prenatal life when the brain is first developing. Genes influencing aspects of brain development that are different in ASD are expressed in the first two trimesters of prenatal brain development and impact neuron duplication and migration, dendrite growth, and synapse formation and pruning (de la Torre-Ubieta et al., 2016). Local hyperconnectivity and decreased long-distance connectivity, decreased neuron size, increased neuron density, synaptic dysfunction, imbalance of excitatory and inhibitory signals, Purkinje cell loss in the cerebellum, and microglial infiltration have all been implicated in the neural basis of ASD (de la Torre-Ubieta et al., 2016).

Abnormalities in brain growth are also associated with ASD, specifically reduced head circumference at birth, followed by accelerated brain overgrowth in the first year of life (Courchesne et al., 2011). Additionally, the early period of brain overgrowth is followed by slowed or arrested growth in later childhood in areas implicated in impaired development of social, communication, and motor abilities (Hazlett et al., 2017).

Efforts to identify other biomarkers of ASD have uncovered several promising metrics, though evidence in this field is still emerging. Preliminary but promising investigations include neurophysiological diagnostic biomarkers (e.g., N170 response to faces, gamma-band activity in response to complex visual stimuli) and abnormal visual attention to biological motion in young, presymptomatic children (Frye et al., 2019), but these strategies are not yet clinically validated.

OUTCOMES ASSOCIATED WITH AUTISM SPECTRUM DISORDER

Parents of children and adolescents diagnosed with ASD often seek a better understanding of what the future holds for their child, but there is marked heterogeneity in the outcomes of individuals with ASD. Given the range of outcomes associated with the condition, ASD is often referred to as a "diagnosis of uncertainty." This section will discuss health, developmental, and social outcomes associated with an ASD diagnosis across development.

Psychiatric Conditions

Co-occurring conditions are common in individuals with ASD. In one study of children with ASD aged 10 to 14 years, 70% of participants had at least one co-occurring psychiatric condition (Simonoff et al., 2008), including ADHD, anxiety, and oppositional defiant disorder. Intellectual disability also occurs in approximately 38% of children with ASD (Maenner et al., 2023). The presence of co-occurring psychiatric conditions can result in greater impairment than ASD alone and impact children's daily and school functioning, including academics and social relationships; however, there are more treatment options (e.g., psychotherapy, medications) for co-occurring conditions than for core symptoms of ASD.

Adolescence is a period of heightened risk for experiencing a first episode of mental health disorders in ASD, including eating disorders, depression, anxiety, suicidal ideation, and non-suicidal self-injury. Hyperactivity and irritability may decline in youth with ASD, though symptoms of withdrawal, depression, and anxiety may increase (Gotham et al., 2015).

Physical Health

Individuals with ASD are at risk for physical health issues (Byrne et al., 2022), including seizures, feeding issues, and sleep problems. Seizures occur in about 25% of people with autism across the lifespan, with an unusual onset during adolescence, and more commonly in those with co-occurring intellectual disability and slightly higher in females (Lukmanji et al., 2019). Gastrointestinal problems, including constipation, are diagnosed more commonly in children with ASD (Hyman et al., 2020). Such problems are associated with other behavioral issues, potentially due to sensory dysfunction or pain, and thus should be suspected when a behavior change is seemingly sudden or unexplained. Providers should consider underlying discomfort or medical or dental problems when children engage in new or different self-injurious behavior. It can be challenging to disentangle maladaptive behaviors from reactions to physical health problems, particularly in children with limited communication.

Sleep disruptions are common in ASD and can disrupt daytime behavior as well as family functioning. Behavioral strategies, such as setting boundaries around sleep, establishing positive bedtime routines, and cognitive behavior therapy are first-line treatments (Williams Buckley et al., 2020). Pharmacologic strategies (e.g., melatonin) may be used as an additional treatment approach in conjunction with behavioral strategies, with evidence that melatonin decreases sleep latency and increases sleep duration in children with ASD (Rossignol & Frye, 2014).

Later in childhood, youth with ASD are at elevated risk of being overweight or obese, and their risk increases with age (Byrne et al., 2022; Shedlock et al., 2016). A range of physical and behavioral factors—including lower physical activity, ASD severity, sleep problems, and family history of obesity—all contribute to risk (Hill et al., 2015), which in turn contributes to increased risk for metabolic sequelae including diabetes, hypertension, and non-alcoholic fatty liver disease (Shedlock et al., 2016). Obesity and metabolic syndrome are also made worse by the use of atypical antipsychotics to manage behavior (Byrne et al., 2022). Nutritional counseling, behavior modification, physical activity, and adjunctive metformin for children taking antipsychotics can be effective in reducing body mass index (Anagnostou et al., 2016).

Developmental Trajectories

Longitudinal studies of ASD have both reinforced what is known—that ASD is a heterogeneous disorder, with variability in individual outcomes, strengths, and challenges—and also identified developmental patterns of change and stability. One large-scale examination of California case records noted the relative stability of RRBs across childhood into adolescence, but also uncovered a group of "bloomers" who make rapid improvements in social and communication outcomes (Fountain et al., 2012). Children with less severe symptoms at diagnosis tended to make more rapid gains than those with severe symptoms. Cognitive scores increase for many people across adolescence into early adulthood, but ASD symptoms remain stable (Simonoff et al., 2020).

Analyses of language outcomes from the Early Diagnosis Study (Pickles et al., 2014), which followed toddlers who were referred at age 2 through adulthood, identified several trajectory classes, including individuals with near-typical language development, mild delay, catch-up, and marked delay. There was significant variation in language improvement across the groups before the age of 6; after age 6, however, groups maintained the rate of progress they had had. Despite the uncertainty of an ASD diagnosis, longitudinal findings highlight the malleability of the early childhood period. Providers should underscore the importance of early intervention for supporting children's language, social, and communication outcomes.

Quality of Life

Meta-analysis suggests regardless of age, IQ, and ASD symptom severity, individuals with ASD experience lower quality of life (QoL) than TD peers (van Heijst & Geurts, 2015). All individuals with ASD and their families will have different priorities for future well-being and independence. Priorities are likely to shift across development and will be informed by the individual's language ability, intellectual functioning, and other physical and mental health conditions. Due to the heterogeneity of ASD, key components for high QoL for one autistic person may not be realistic or relevant to another autistic person's QoL (McCauley et al., 2020). Providers should ask patients with ASD and their families about current and future goals, as well as steps the patient's school- and community-based providers are taking to meet those goals.

Peer Relationships and Bullying

Bullying is a concern for school-aged children and adolescents with ASD, who are more likely to be bullied than TD students (Maïano et al., 2016). As the social behaviors and expectations of peers become increasingly sophisticated, social impairments of school-aged children and adolescents with ASD may become evident, making them targets for peer victimization.

Bullying may impact the child's likelihood for success in school settings.

Older children and adolescents with ASD may also experience difficulty in forming and maintaining friendships. Many adolescents with ASD express interest in friendships and endorse feelings of loneliness; however, there is often a disparity between these adolescents' desire and ability to maintain friendships (Locke et al., 2010). The resulting feelings of peer rejection, independent of the stressors of peer victimization, can negatively impact the emotional development of children and adolescents with ASD. Such experiences may even contribute to the development of comorbid mental health conditions such as depression and anxiety, which often emerge in adolescence. Peers become an increasingly important source of knowledge and support in adolescence. Given relatively limited exposure to typical peer relationships, these missed opportunities may have cascading effects on the ability of individuals with ASD to engage in normative social experiences, such as dating and employment, in adulthood.

For patients struggling with bullying and/or social connection, social outlets relating directly to their restricted interests, such as clubs or afterschool activities, can be an effective avenue for positive connection with peers and community engagement more broadly (Volkmar et al., 2014). Social skills groups for school-aged children and adolescents with ASD can also provide a constructive social outlet and a safe space to improve social proficiency.

Executive Functioning

EF impairments have been well-characterized in children with ASD. Relatively poor EF in persons with ASD has been linked to decreased capability to care for oneself independently (Pugliese et al., 2015) and lower QoL (de Vries & Geurts, 2015). EF impairments are related to, but separate from, IQ (de Vries & Geurts, 2015) and may worsen in later childhood in those with ASD (Rosenthal et al., 2013), perhaps due to social and academic demands. There is emerging evidence that EF deficits may contribute to poor adult outcomes in ASD (Dijkhuis et al., 2020).

Providers can encourage families to pursue evidence-based EF interventions and to collaborate with school-based providers to incorporate EF supports in school. For adolescent and young adult patients with ASD assuming responsibility for their own medical care, providing additional support for scheduling appointments and refilling prescriptions (phone/email reminders, written notes) is an easy way to facilitate planning and problem-solving.

Personal Agency and Self-Determination

As children enter adolescence, they become increasingly motivated to make both big and small life decisions independently. This leads to a shift in child–caregiver dynamics, as primary decision-making responsibilities move from the parent to the adolescent. Adolescent patients may take on more active roles in treatment planning, maintaining a healthy lifestyle, and may request to conduct a portion of their medical visits without their caregiver present, particularly as they reach sexual maturity. Most individuals with ASD develop physically at the same rate as their TD peers, but their development of personal agency and autonomy may progress slowly and be limited by behavioral differences, EF deficits, and/or intellectual ability.

Additionally, many people with ASD have delayed adaptive functioning (Pugliese et al., 2015), which includes household chores, personal hygiene, and other life skills key to supporting oneself and maintaining independence in adulthood. By restricting autistic individuals' ability to live independently, deficits in adaptive functioning can also limit the development and expression of personal agency in adolescence and young adulthood. However, unlike language ability and IQ, which tend not to shift after early childhood, adaptive behaviors can be taught to individuals of various ages and abilities. Improving adaptive functioning can substantially boost autistic adolescents' independence and feelings of autonomy (Duncan et al., 2018). Providers should encourage families to target adaptive functioning in interventions.

The transition to adulthood may be an especially uncertain time for caregivers, as they simultaneously attempt to provide adequate support while scaffolding skills for their child to become more independent. There is no "one-size-fits-all" approach to balancing parent advocacy and child independence; however, families may find it helpful to transition gradually to a diverse range of supports (i.e., peer mentors, vocational counselors) as their child approaches adulthood (Anderson et al., 2018).

Providers can foster self-determination and autonomy by providing opportunities to meet with autistic patients to privately answer questions during visits. Providers can model collaborative decision-making by asking for patients' opinions of their current and/or proposed changes to treatment plans, in addition to the caregivers'. If the patient is not capable of responding to questions verbally, providers should ask if the patient uses an augmented and alternative communication device or other forms of nonverbal communication to participate to whatever extent they are able.

Transition Services and the "Services Cliff"

Although ASD is often conceptualized as a disorder of childhood, individuals with ASD spend most of their lives as adults. It is estimated that 50,000 individuals with ASD turn 18 in the United States each year (Shattuck et al., 2012). Few young adults with ASD receive ASD-specific assistance following high school exit, and families of adult children with ASD report encountering challenges in finding and accessing services related to employment, housing, and social skills, among other areas of need (Anderson et al., 2018). This so-called "services cliff" leaves youth with ASD poorly prepared to achieve positive life outcomes in adulthood.

Young adults with ASD often experience a similar "cliff" in health care services during the transition from the pediatric to adult medical home. For many families, ending their relationship with their child's pediatric health care provider(s) and shifting to the adult health care system can be a difficult experience. Additionally, many adult medical specialists feel ill-equipped to provide care for patients with ASD (P. H. White et al., 2018). Unfortunately, patients with ASD with the highest levels of need experience the longest lapses in medical care during the transition to adulthood (Enner et al., 2020).

Pediatric providers should begin discussions of transition planning with patients with ASD and their families in early adolescence, both to normalize uncertainty about the transition to adulthood and to ensure ample time for patients and their caregivers to prepare for the transition. Providers can support a smooth transition and help patients avoid lapses in medical care by discussing the transition to adult health care frequently, coordinating care with future adult providers, and if needed, connecting patients and families with specialist adult providers for physical and psychiatric co-occurring conditions.

A medical home is a centralized resource through which patients receive community-based, ongoing, comprehensive physical and mental health care and other specialty services (Carbone et al., 2010). The medical home model has been widely endorsed by the medical community and is increasingly common in pediatric practices. However, most adult providers, particularly specialists, still operate as independent hubs of medical care, with few opportunities for communication and collaboration between providers. Movement towards the medical home model of care in adult practices could lessen many of the difficulties associated with the health care transition for individuals with ASD.

Postsecondary Education and Vocational Outcomes

About one-third of youth with ASD attend college within 5 years of high school exit (Shattuck et al., 2012). Although many autistic individuals are intellectually capable of succeeding in postsecondary education, the social and personal demands of college environments may limit their likelihood of success in postsecondary settings and beyond (Elias & White, 2018). National data suggest starting in-school transition services early in adolescence (i.e., by age 14) improves vocational outcomes (Cimera et al., 2013). Providers should strive to help autistic patients find meaningful ways to remain active in their community after exiting the school system. Engaging even in less intensive vocational activities (e.g., volunteering at a church, completing supported work at a job site) is related to increased well-being for adults with ASD compared to engaging in no vocational activities (Clarke et al., 2021) Providers can support positive outcomes by encouraging families of patients with ASD to begin researching and securing adult supports and services at least several years prior to their child turning 18.

Guardianship

Many young adults with autism can make their own life decisions. However, court-appointed guardianship (typically a parent, sibling, or other caregiver) may be necessary for those who do not have the intellectual and/or language abilities to make decisions about their medical care and other important aspects of adult life and communicate those decisions to others. Guardianship is a legal relationship in which a person (the guardian) is appointed to make decisions on behalf of another person. The guardianship application process requires families to comprehensively document the extent of their child's abilities and disabilities. Families must provide forms signed by a physician or psychologist as part of their guardianship documentation. Given the length and rigor of the guardianship process, families should start preparing for guardianship in adolescence.

Residential and Adult Day Programs

Autistic adults with limited adaptive functioning, communication skills, and/or intellectual ability who cannot work and support themselves independently may require supports for some or all their adult lives, including residential support. Living program accommodations include supported/supervised living programs (community housing with built-in supports), group homes, and day programs. Availability for such programs varies widely by region, and many have long waitlists for residential and day services and thus require early planning and contacts.

FAMILY SYSTEMS APPROACH TO PROMOTE ADAPTATION AFTER AN AUTISM SPECTRUM DISORDER DIAGNOSIS

When one is diagnosed with ASD, their family's life course, as well as their own, is deeply impacted. This section explores family and contextual factors related to having a family member with ASD and includes considerations for clinicians and developmental scientists.

Caregiver Well-Being

Compared to parents of TD children and children with other disabilities, parents of children and adolescents with ASD experience higher levels of stress, depression, and anxiety (McStay et al., 2014), a trend that continues or even worsens with age (Taylor & Seltzer, 2011). Supporting a child with ASD can also negatively impact spousal and familial relationships (Thompson et al., 2018). Parents with high perceived self-efficacy report experiencing fewer psychological difficulties, while parents with an external locus of control and who engage in distancing and escape-avoidance coping strategies report experiencing more psychological difficulties (Dunn et al., 2001). Use of problem-focused and other positive coping strategies (Hastings et al., 2005) and social support from spouses and friends can also promote positive outcomes in parents of individuals with ASD (L. E. Smith et al., 2012).

Health care professionals should encourage caregivers to find formal (e.g., respite care, parent and sibling support groups, talk therapy, case management) and informal (e.g., friends, family, church groups) social supports. Providers should familiarize themselves with regional family support services and include a discussion of support services as an ongoing component of family psychoeducation. Family support services may be especially pivotal immediately following diagnosis, when caregivers may feel lost and isolated, and during the transition to adulthood, when individuals with ASD lose access to school services and family caregiving responsibilities increase. By decreasing the caregiving burden and improving caregiver QoL, formal and informal social supports can improve family well-being.

Family Relationships

Having a family member with ASD is associated with a range of challenges and stressors. However, many families also express that their relationship with their loved one with ASD is a source of great meaning and joy. Families and communities alike can be strengthened by accommodating, accepting, and supporting individuals with ASD.

There is mixed evidence regarding the impact of having a sibling with autism on the outcomes of TD siblings (Leedham et al., 2020). Some individuals report their relationship with their sibling with ASD is among the most meaningful and important of their lives. In contrast, others express feelings of ambiguity or even resentment towards their sibling with ASD. As parents and other caregivers age, siblings often play increasingly important roles in the lives of individuals with ASD. In some cases, siblings assume primary caregiving responsibilities as parents die or become too frail to continue caring for a loved one with ASD (Moss et al., 2019).

Cultural Considerations and Issues of Health Equity

Cultural factors, such as language barriers, mistrust of health care systems, beliefs about etiology, and cultural and social stigma associated with ASD may impact the diagnostic process and families' treatment choices (Mandell & Novak, 2005). Qualitative work in Asian American and Latin American communities suggests families of these backgrounds may be more likely to minimize concerns about their children's development due to negative cultural beliefs that ASD may be caused by family wrongdoings, mental illness in one or both parents, or supernatural powers such as curses and evil spirits (Kang-Yi et al., 2018; Rivera-Figueroa et al., 2022).

ASD resources specifically for culturally diverse families, though still limited, are increasing. Telehealth initiatives have greatly improved the ability to provide services to rural and families with low socioeconomic status. Autism Speaks, the Centers for Disease Control and Prevention, and many other national groups provide resources in Spanish as well as English (see the Resources box at the end of this chapter). The Color of Autism Foundation, a national nonprofit focused on supporting autistic individuals of color, is also an excellent resource for diverse families. Providers, including pediatric psychologists and developmental-behavioral pediatricians, should take special note of the intersectionality of ASD and family diversity.

Economic Considerations

There are significant direct and indirect economic effects of having a child with ASD. Insurance coverage and state financial assistance for assessments and ASD services vary widely. In addition to increased medical costs, caregiving responsibilities associated with having a child with ASD lead many parents to cut working hours or exit the workforce. Having a child with ASD is associated with an average annual loss of approximately 14% of family income (Montes & Halterman, 2008). It is important to remember ASD is a lifelong disorder. Though costs associated with ASD are often discussed in the context of diagnosis and early intervention, adulthood is a far longer phase of life than childhood. Over an individual's lifetime, adult costs far outweigh childhood costs. Providers must be mindful of, and help prepare families for, the long-term financial and personal costs associated with caring for an individual with ASD, particularly when recommending treatments to families.

SCREENING AND DIAGNOSIS OF AUTISM SPECTRUM DISORDER

Early Identification and Screening for Autism Spectrum Disorder

Early childhood health care providers should provide ongoing developmental surveillance at each medical visit, note family history of ASD and other risk factors, ask parents about their developmental or behavioral concerns, and conduct informal behavioral observations. General developmental screening can supplement parent and physician judgment and is recommended at 9-, 18-, and 30-month well-child visits (Hyman et al., 2020). The American Academy of Pediatrics recommends screening for ASD twice before age 3 years (generally at 18 and 24–30 months). Screening tools can provide a framework for conceptualizing early symptoms but have variable sensitivity, resulting in missed cases from screening with current instruments alone. Effectiveness may be limited in very young children, especially if parents do not already have developmental or behavioral concerns (Toh et al., 2018). Providers should use clinical judgment and close follow-up to ensure early detection of ASD. Figure 16.3 includes information on the screening, referral, and diagnosis process.

Screening Tools

Standardized screening tools for ASD can identify children who may be at risk for an ASD diagnosis and should be referred for diagnostic evaluation. Screening tools are designed to maximize sensitivity over specificity, capturing both children who have ASD as well as those who screen positive but do not have ASD (i.e., false positives).

One of the most commonly used ASD screeners is the Modified Checklist for Autism in Toddlers, Revised With Follow-Up (M-CHAT-R/F; Robins et al., 2014), validated for children aged 16 to 30 months. The M-CHAT-R/F consists of 20 yes/no questions and is designed to be completely quickly by a caregiver. Questions pertain to ASD symptoms thought to be present in very young children (e.g., no initiation or response to joint attention, limited eye contact, limited pretend play). Follow-up interviews are conducted with caregivers of children flagged as being "at risk" from the initial questionnaire. The M-CHAT-R/F was reported to have strong sensitivity and specificity in its validation study, though findings from other groups have been mixed.

Two other commonly used screeners are the Social Communication Questionnaire (SCQ; Rutter et al., 2003) and Social Responsiveness Scale-Second Edition (SRS-2; Constantino & Gruber, 2012). Both are designed for a broad age range (4 years to adulthood and 2.5 years to adulthood, respectively). The SCQ consists of 40 yes/no questions derived from the Autism Diagnostic Interview-Revised (ADI-R), a developmental history measure widely used as an ASD diagnostic tool. Caregivers endorse their child's current or lifetime characteristics consistent with ASD symptomatology. The SRS-2 consists of 65 items rated on a 4-point scale, with different forms across age groups and different potential informants (caregiver, teacher, or self) depending on the age of the individual being screened. The SRS-2 is designed to identify both the presence and severity of an individual's social impairment. The sensitivity and specificity of both tools range from moderate to strong. Scores from both the SCQ and SRS-2 should be interpreted by a clinician who is knowledgeable in ASD and the instruments.

Diagnostic Evaluation

Children who screen positive should be referred for clinical diagnostic evaluation. Diagnostic evaluations for ASD should be comprehensive and multidisciplinary and should consider the child within a developmental framework. Evaluations are frequently conducted by psychologists or developmental-behavioral pediatricians, although general pediatricians knowledgeable in ASD diagnostic criteria can make an initial clinical diagnosis.

A diagnosis should be informed by multiple sources of information, including a developmental history, observation, and direct assessment. The two most common diagnostic tools, used in conjunction, are the Autism Diagnostic Inventory-Revised (ADI-R; Le Couteur et al., 2003) and the Autism Diagnostic Observation Schedule, Second Edition (ADOS-2; Lord et al., 2012). Both the ADI-R and the ADOS-2 should be administered by clinicians with expertise in ASD who have undergone specific clinical training for each assessment.

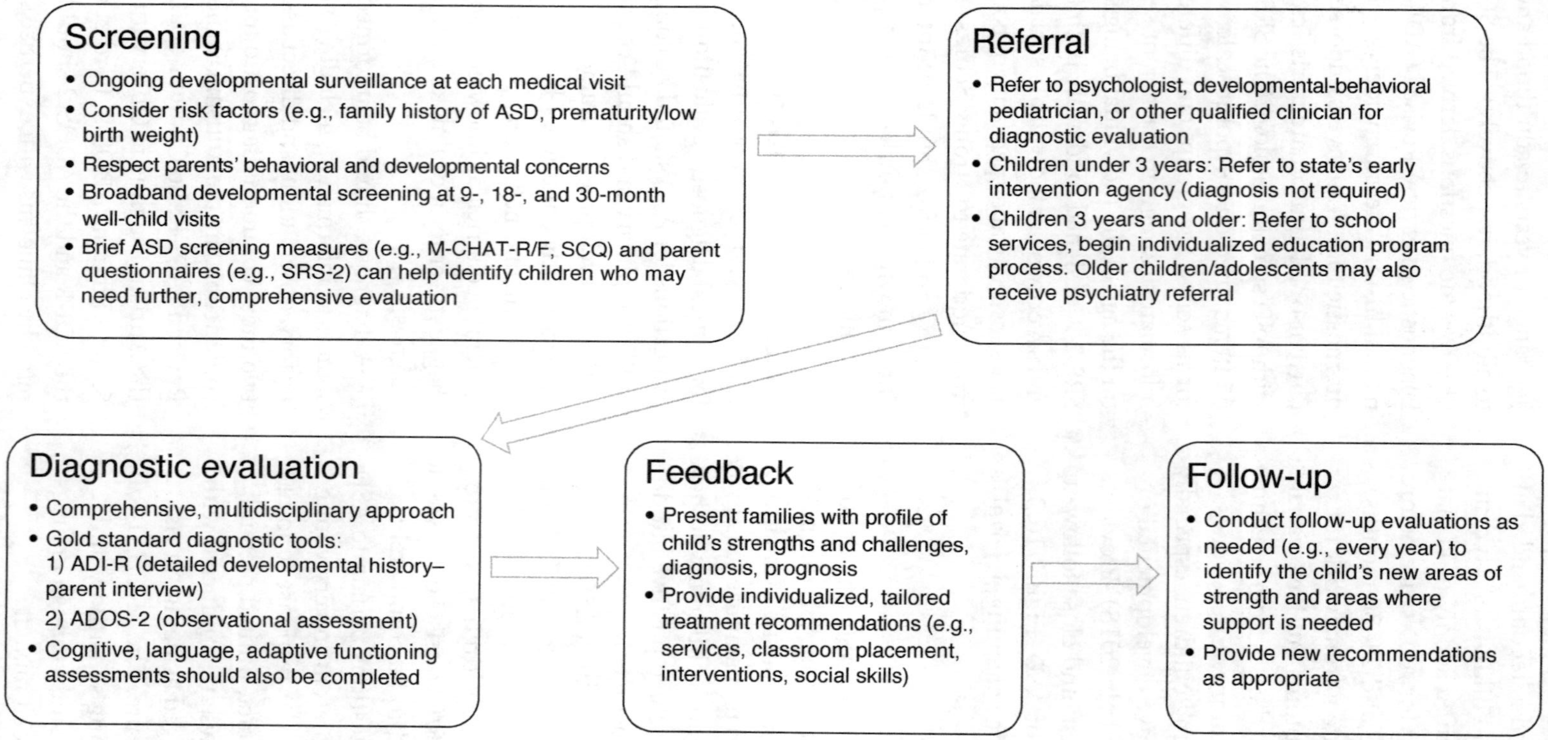

Screening
- Ongoing developmental surveillance at each medical visit
- Consider risk factors (e.g., family history of ASD, prematurity/low birth weight)
- Respect parents' behavioral and developmental concerns
- Broadband developmental screening at 9-, 18-, and 30-month well-child visits
- Brief ASD screening measures (e.g., M-CHAT-R/F, SCQ) and parent questionnaires (e.g., SRS-2) can help identify children who may need further, comprehensive evaluation

Referral
- Refer to psychologist, developmental-behavioral pediatrician, or other qualified clinician for diagnostic evaluation
- Children under 3 years: Refer to state's early intervention agency (diagnosis not required)
- Children 3 years and older: Refer to school services, begin individualized education program process. Older children/adolescents may also receive psychiatry referral

Diagnostic evaluation
- Comprehensive, multidisciplinary approach
- Gold standard diagnostic tools:
  1) ADI-R (detailed developmental history–parent interview)
  2) ADOS-2 (observational assessment)
- Cognitive, language, adaptive functioning assessments should also be completed

Feedback
- Present families with profile of child's strengths and challenges, diagnosis, prognosis
- Provide individualized, tailored treatment recommendations (e.g., services, classroom placement, interventions, social skills)

Follow-up
- Conduct follow-up evaluations as needed (e.g., every year) to identify the child's new areas of strength and areas where support is needed
- Provide new recommendations as appropriate

FIGURE 16.3. Overview of autism spectrum disorder (ASD) screening, referral, and diagnostic evaluation process. M-CHAT-R/F = Modified Checklist for Autism in Toddlers, Revised With Follow-Up; SCQ = Social Communication Questionnaire; SRS-2 = Social Responsiveness Scale–Second Edition; ADI-R = Autism Diagnostic Interview-Revised; ADOS-2 = Autism Diagnostic Observation Schedule, Second Edition.

The ADI-R is a semistructured parent interview that provides a comprehensive developmental history of the child's behaviors and is designed to obtain detailed diagnostic information associated with ASD. The ADOS-2 is a structured observational assessment, usually administered in a clinical setting, designed to elicit atypical behaviors characteristic of ASD. Different ADOS-2 modules are administered based on an individual's age and language ability, with the lowest module designed for young children <30 months who are walking independently. Each module consists of various developmentally appropriate activities—an ADOS-2 administered to a 2-year-old with minimal language is more play-based, while one administered to a verbally fluent adolescent is more conversation-based.

In addition to diagnostic assessments, testing of cognitive, language, and adaptive skills should also be completed as part of the evaluation. This additional testing is as important as the ASD evaluation itself, as it provides profiles of strengths and challenges and puts social delays in the context of other developmental delays. After the evaluation is completed, clinicians should meet with families to discuss the child's profile, diagnosis, prognosis, and individualized recommendations for treatment and support should be discussed. In most cases, follow-up evaluations in the ensuing years are crucial in noting progress and identifying new strengths and gaps in development to support the child as behavioral expectations change.

Medical/Developmental Workup

Medical professionals should evaluate children for other conditions that cause or exacerbate developmental delay. Children should be screened for hearing and vision impairment. Children who fail hearing or vision screening and those who cannot tolerate or cooperate with screening should be referred to specialists (audiology; ear, nose, and throat physicians; pediatric ophthalmology) for more extensive testing. The American Academy of Pediatrics recommends basic genetic testing, including a chromosomal microarray, fragile X testing for males, and specific testing for suspected genetic syndromes for all children with ASD (Hyman et al., 2020).

TREATMENTS AND INTERVENTIONS

Children and youth with ASD have needs that span behavioral, educational, social, and health areas, as well as family support needs. Interventions for ASD aim to reduce symptoms interfering with daily functioning and QoL. There is vast heterogeneity in ASD presentation, and no single treatment is effective for all individuals. Treatments should be individualized based on one's strengths, challenges, and developmental needs, as well as family-level and other contextual factors. This section covers the treatment of ASD, including behavioral and social skills interventions, medication management for comorbid conditions, complementary and alternative treatments, and psychoeducation.

Behavioral Interventions

Behavioral interventions are the primary method of treating core symptoms of ASD, particularly for improving social communication and reducing challenging behaviors (e.g., aggression, noncompliance, self-injury). There are many interventions and strategies for working with children with ASD, but not all have a strong base of evidence to support their effectiveness (Hume et al., 2021). Behavioral intervention efforts have largely focused on intervening during early childhood, when it is thought treatments have the most potential to improve developmental outcomes (Zwaigenbaum et al., 2015). Interventions for young children should include a combination of developmental and behavioral approaches and incorporate parents. For school-aged children and adolescents, interventions may address symptoms associated with ASD, such as anxiety, but often do not target core symptoms. Families and clinicians should work together to determine appropriate treatments based on individualized treatment priorities and goals.

Applied behavior analysis– (ABA-) based interventions apply the science of learning and behavior to real-world situations, with the goal of increasing behaviors helpful to a child (e.g., taking turns) and decreasing maladaptive behaviors (e.g., hitting). Treatment targets are individualized, focusing on areas such as communication, self-help, socialization, and academics. Skills are taught through direct teaching, modeling, reinforcement, and consequences.

Interventions vary in their approach, from more behavioral and adult-led approaches, such as discrete trial training (DTT; T. Smith, 2001), to more naturalistic, play-based interventions. DTT involves highly structured teaching of small, discrete steps via cues, prompts, and consequences from an adult. On the other hand, naturalistic developmental behavioral interventions (NDBIs) emphasize teaching in natural contexts, allowing the child to initiate and lead activities, and providing natural and contingent reinforcement (Schreibman et al., 2015). Implementation of NDBIs is often embedded within play and daily routines, promoting the development and generalization of skills across contexts. NDBIs include pivotal response treatment (PRT; Koegel et al., 2001), which targets pivotal areas in a child's development (e.g., motivation) to produce improvements in other social, communication, and behavioral areas, and the Early Start Denver Model (ESDM; Rogers & Dawson, 2010), which builds on positive adult-child relationships to encourage interaction and communication during play and everyday routines. ABA providers may use a combination of structured and naturalistic approaches depending on intervention targets, fit with family dynamics and sociocultural beliefs, developmental appropriateness and need, and cost. Some children may learn more quickly from one approach compared to the other, depending on the skill targeted.

Interventions can either be focused or comprehensive in scope; treatment targets in both approaches are individualized for each child and family. Targeted interventions focus on developing a specific set of skills (e.g., joint attention), and treatment periods may be shorter in duration (e.g., 2–4 hours/week over months). Comprehensive approaches aim to treat symptoms and teach skills across domains and require intensive long-term intervention (e.g., 15–40 hours/week over 1+ years). Greater intensity of intervention does not necessarily result in more positive outcomes for children (Rogers et al., 2021).

Providers should familiarize themselves with the evidence base for ASD interventions and evidence-based practices. Some therapies not based in ABA (e.g., DIR/Floortime) have less evidence to support their effectiveness through high-quality research designs. Clinicians should consult with families of their patients with ASD when discussing treatment options, considering family preferences, treatment needs, evidentiary support for interventions, fit, intervention availability, and health insurance coverage.

Parent-mediated therapies. Along with direct early intervention delivered by a therapist, parent training in behavioral and developmentally appropriate strategies is a key piece of early childhood ASD interventions (Hume et al., 2021; Hyman et al., 2020). Parents are ideal agents of early intervention because they can practice skills with their child throughout the day and across settings, promoting generalization. Parent-mediated treatments of ASD, often consisting of psychoeducation and coaching in intervention strategies by a clinician, support positive outcomes for young children with ASD (Nevill et al., 2018). Treatments should be tailored to the family and child. Some parents may benefit from instruction in intervention strategies and understanding ASD; others may already be familiar with basic principles of ASD intervention (e.g., ABA) and instead may require support with other practical issues (e.g., getting their child into preschool).

Psychotherapy. There are interventions for anxiety and other internalizing symptoms that have been designed or adapted specifically for individuals with ASD. For example, cognitive behavior therapy, which focuses on recognizing and reframing negative feelings, is effective in reducing anxiety in adolescents with ASD, but less effective in reducing depressive symptoms (S. W. White et al., 2018). However, we know far less than we should about how to optimize traditional talk therapy approaches across the heterogeneity of autism.

Services Through the Individuals With Disabilities Education Act (IDEA)

Early intervention and services for school-aged children are made available through the Individuals With Disabilities Education Act (IDEA), the 2004 federal law that requires all children with disabilities be provided with free and appropriate education. Part C of IDEA applies to early intervention service provision for babies and toddlers (birth through 36 months), while Part B applies to school-aged children (3–21 years).

Birth to 3 years of age.   Children under age 3 qualify for free early intervention services through state early-intervention programs (e.g., regional centers, government agencies), though eligibility criteria and services provided may vary by state. A diagnosis is not necessary for a referral, although children who already have a diagnosis of ASD or receive a diagnosis through this referral process may qualify for additional services. State early intervention programs provide free evaluations to determine children's eligibility for the program. Young children diagnosed with ASD may also require auxiliary services (e.g., speech therapy, occupational therapy, social skills), to support skill development in other areas. Families may also qualify for respite care.

School age (P-12 education and school-based services).   As children grow older, schools become the primary site where most children with ASD receive services. Once children turn 3 years old, IDEA Part B mandates children with disabilities receive free and appropriate special education and services through the public school system. Children are to receive supports that increase their access to the general education curriculum, such as behavioral supports (e.g., school aide), special education (for part or all of the day), and other related services (e.g., speech therapy, occupational therapy, adapted physical education). Services are documented in children's Individualized Education Plans (IEPs), along with individualized goals for services and classroom placement. Even if a child with ASD has a pre-existing clinical diagnosis from a health provider, a school-based evaluation must be completed to confirm eligibility under IDEA Part B.

According to IDEA, students have the right to be educated in the least restrictive environment (LRE), that is, alongside TD peers whenever possible. Classroom placement depends on the student's intellectual ability, communication, and behavior management needs, determined by evaluation by a multidisciplinary educational team. For some, education in the LRE may mean placement in a general education classroom with TD peers, which has been associated with better social and academic outcomes for students with ASD (Kim et al., 2018). For students who are more severely impacted by ASD symptoms, placement in a special-needs classroom may be more appropriate, as it allows for individualized support. Other options include partial inclusion (e.g., placement in special education with inclusion in general education classroom for part of the day), resource rooms (e.g., placement in general education with pullouts to receive individualized attention for part of the day), or individualized support from a school aide. Complex negotiations may arise between parents and school systems as appropriate placement options and potential benefits to the child are discussed and determined.

Social Skills Interventions

Social skills groups for school-aged children with ASD can provide a constructive space to improve social proficiency. Social skills interventions, including groups and deliberately created dyads, provide direct, concrete teaching of social rules, social concepts (e.g., assessing peer interest/acceptance, sarcasm), and opportunities to practice social skills (e.g., role-playing). Social outlets related directly to a child's restricted interests (e.g., clubs and afterschool activities) can also be an effective avenue for positive connection with peers (Volkmar et al., 2014). School-based interventions mediated by TD peers (Watkins et al., 2015) can also improve social skills in students with ASD.

There are also evidence-based social skills interventions for adolescents with ASD. The Program for the Education and Enrichment of Relational Skills (PEERS®), for example, is a manualized parent-assisted social skills group intervention for adolescents (Laugeson et al., 2012). It involves weekly didactic sessions on skills pertaining to making and keeping friends, role-playing exercises, and applied homework assignments. PEERS improves social skills (e.g., social responsiveness) and social skills knowledge and increases peer interactions in adolescents.

Medications

No available medications target core symptoms of ASD, but medications are frequently utilized to target co-occurring problems. When considering medication for a child with ASD, clinicians should define what symptoms they are treating, rule out other causes of symptoms, and be aware of dosing considerations specific to ASD. Symptoms of inattention and hyperactivity may warrant a diagnosis of ADHD but can also be due to decreased social attention or developmental delay. Increased irritability and aggression can be associated with rigidity and difficulty with transitions, but also may be a sign of pain or illness. The clinician's careful history and physical exam may reveal constipation, a dental abscess, or untreated gastroesophageal reflux that is causing a change in behavior. After ruling out other causes of behaviors and making a diagnosis of a co-occurring condition, the clinician must closely follow the child for symptom changes and to monitor for side effects.

Studies of children with ASD show good efficacy for medications treating ADHD, irritability and aggression, and insomnia (Table 16.1). There is less evidence for medications to treat anxiety, depression, and obsessive-compulsive disorder in children with ASD, but these medications are commonly prescribed for children with ASD based on studies of their use in children in the general population. For stimulants and serotonergic medications, starting at a low dose and slowly increasing helps limit side effects such as behavioral activation or agitation in children with ASD (Kolevzon et al., 2006). Atypical antipsychotics require baseline blood tests of liver enzymes, glucose, glycosylated hemoglobin, and lipids with repeated tests in 3 months. If blood tests remain normal, laboratory monitoring should occur annually for the duration of treatment. Additionally, antipsychotic-associated weight gain is to be expected and needs to be monitored. Metformin can be used as an adjunct with atypical antipsychotics to counteract these side effects if monitoring of weight and blood tests show signs of metabolic syndrome (Anagnostou et al., 2016). Black box warnings about increased suicidality with selective serotonin reuptake inhibitors and possible side effects such as abnormal movements with antipsychotics should be part of counseling when starting a medication.

Complementary and Alternative Medicine Approaches

Complementary and alternative medicine (CAM) refers to practices and treatments outside those typically recommended by health care professionals, used in addition to or instead of standard medical care. Approximately 50% to 75% of parents of children with ASD report using CAM treatments for their children (Höfer et al., 2017), though there is mixed evidence to support their effectiveness. Some treatments, such as melatonin, have emerging evidence to support their use (Rossignol & Frye, 2014). Others, such as gluten-free and/or casein-free diets have little to no scientific evidence to indicate they have effectiveness for improving ASD symptoms. Despite limited evidence, CAM treatments are popular with families. Providers should be prepared to discuss CAM treatments and should be knowledgeable about their potential side effects.

Psychoeducation

Psychoeducation (i.e., providing education or information about ASD to individuals and families) is an important yet often undervalued tool in helping families with children with ASD

TABLE 16.1
Commonly Used Medications in Autism Spectrum Disorder (ASD) by Target Symptom or Co-Occurring Diagnosis

Source(s)	Target symptom or diagnosis	Medication (class)	Level of evidence	Effect size*	Common adverse effects	Comments
Rodrigues et al. (2021)	Attention-deficit/ hyperactivity disorder (ADHD)	Methylphenidate (*Stimulants*)	≥2 randomized controlled trials (RCTs)	Medium to large	Insomnia, anorexia, irritability	Lower efficacy and higher rate of adverse effects seen in individuals with ASD than in those without ASD.
Patra et al. (2019)		Atomoxetine (*SNRIs*)	≥2 RCTs	Medium	Anorexia, nausea, irritability	Starting below the recommended dose and titrating slowly may prevent or ameliorate side effects.
Scahill et al. (2015); Politte et al. (2018)		Guanfacine extended release formula (*alpha agonists*)	1+ RCT	Large	Fatigue, sedation, decreased systolic blood pressure and pulse, mid-cycle insomnia	Level of evidence and expert opinion suggest guanfacine as an alternative to stimulants for the treatment of ADHD in ASD.
		Clonidine (*alpha agonists*)	No RCTs in ASD	N/A	Fatigue, sedation	Limited information on clonidine for ADHD symptoms in ASD; extended release clonidine is U.S. Food and Drug Administration (FDA)–approved for treatment of ADHD in children 6–17 years.
Fung et al. (2016); Anagnostou et al. (2016); Aman et al. (2009)	Irritability and aggression	Risperidone (*atypical antipsychotics*)	≥2 RCT	Medium to large	Sedation, weight gain, potential metabolic complications (hyperlipidemia, diabetes), hyperprolactinemia, tardive dyskinesia (low) Weight gain from atypical antipsychotics may be attenuated with concomitant use of metformin	Maladaptive behaviors may serve a purpose; assessment of the function of the behavior is warranted. If irritability and aggression are primarily due to co-occurring conditions (anxiety, ADHD, depression, discomfort due to medical conditions) consider medications/ treatments that target these conditions before atypical antipsychotics. Weight, diet and metabolic monitoring are warranted. The addition of parent training in behavioral modification may improve the response to antipsychotic medications.
Fung et al. (2016)		Aripiprazole (*atypical antipsychotics*)	≥2 RCTs	Medium to large	Sedation, weight gain, metabolic complications, akathisia	As previous
Hardan et al. (2012); Dean et al. (2017)		N-acetyl-cysteine (*antioxidant*)	1+ RCT	N/A	Gastrointestinal distress	Small studies

(*continues*)

TABLE 16.1
Commonly Used Medications in Autism Spectrum Disorder (ASD) by Target Symptom or Co-Occurring Diagnosis (*Continued*)

Source(s)	Target symptom or diagnosis	Medication (class)	Level of evidence	Effect size*	Common adverse effects	Comments
Reinblatt et al. (2009); Kolevzon et al. (2006)	Anxiety	Fluoxetine Sertraline Citalopram Escitalopram (*SSRIs*)	No RCTs in ASD	N/A	Behavioral activation (emotional lability, agitation, aggression, hyperactivity, insomnia) FDA has issued a black box warning for suicidality	There is evidence supporting the use of SSRIs in youth and adults with anxiety in the general population, but limited information in ASD.
	Depressive disorder	Fluoxetine Sertraline Citalopram Escitalopram (*SSRIs*)	No RCTs in ASD	N/A	As previous	As previous
Reddihough et al. (2019)	Obsessive-compulsive disorder	Fluoxetine Fluvoxamine Sertraline (*SSRIs*)	1 RCT for Fluoxetine in ASD, otherwise no RCTs in ASD	N/A	As previous	As previous
Rossignol & Frye (2014)	Insomnia	Melatonin (*neurohormone*)	≥2 RCTs	Large	Minimal to none in most studies. Some studies report morning drowsiness.	Expert opinion and studies showing benefit support behavioral interventions as first line intervention.

Note. SNRIs = Serotonin–norepinephrine reuptake inhibitors; SSRIs = selective serotonin reuptake inhibitors; N/A = not available. Adapted from "The Lancet Commission on the Future of Care and Clinical Research in Autism," by C. Lord, T. Charman, A. Havdahl, P. Carbone, E. Anagnostou, B. Boyd, T. Carr, P. J. de Vries, C. Dissanayake, G. Divan, C. M. Freitag, M. M. Gotelli, C. Kasari, M. Knapp, P. Mundy, A. Plank, L. Scahill, C. Servili, P. Shattuck, E. Simonoff, A. Tepper Singer, V. Slonims, P. P. Wang, M. Celica Yssraelit, R. Jellett, A. Pickles, J. Cusack, P. Howlin, P. Szatmari, A. Holbrook, C. Toolan, and J. B. McCauley, 2022, *The Lancet*, 399(10321), pp. 312–313 (https://doi.org/10.1016/S0140-6736(21)01541-5). Copyright 2022 by Elsevier. Adapted with permission.
*Effect sizes: ~0.2, small; ~0.5 medium; ~0.8 large (Cohen, 1988).

understand the diagnosis and treatment options, but to personalize and tailor this information to the realities of their everyday lives. Psychoeducation for families and individuals with ASD, as well as interventions that decrease vulnerability through knowledge, are essential components of equitable models to support family decision making. Providers should strive to address the uncertainty associated with ASD as part of psychoeducation efforts and provide families with a healthy model for effective communication about the difficult and evolving issues associated with their child's diagnosis. Psychoeducation is not simply a relaying of information, but an iterative process that continues across development. The list at the end of this chapter includes resources health care providers can use to supplement family psychoeducation efforts.

CONCLUSION

Due to the heterogeneity of the autism spectrum, ASD is inherently a diagnosis of uncertainty. There is considerable variability in individual skills, abilities, and challenges among individuals, and the quantity and quality of autism services available in each region vary widely. However, QoL for all individuals with ASD and their families can be improved via thoughtful care delivered by informed providers. Developmental-behavioral pediatricians, pediatric psychologists, and developmental scientists should value the diversity (including neurodiversity) and presume competence in individuals with ASD. Clinicians and researchers alike should understand each individual with ASD has unique strengths, needs, and outcomes, and individuals exist within complex family and community systems of support.

From initial screening and diagnosis to the transition to adulthood, informed providers can play a unique and integral role in the care of individuals with ASD and their families. Additional resources for providers and families are summarized in the Resources box. With appropriate support and coordination of care, individuals with ASD of all abilities can lead happy and healthy lives.

RESOURCES FOR PROVIDERS, FAMILIES, AND INDIVIDUALS WITH AUTISM SPECTRUM DISORDER

American Academy of Pediatrics (AAP) Autism Toolkit

A resource for health care professionals, the AAP Autism Toolkit provides a comprehensive overview from early screening to the adult transition on caring for patients with ASD in the pediatric medical home. Includes printable handouts for family members on a variety of topics in both Spanish and English.

https://publications.aap.org/toolkits/pages/Autism-Toolkit#working

A Practical Guide to Autism: What Every Parent, Family Member, and Teacher Needs to Know

This reference work for families and school providers includes an overview of ASD across the lifespan, information on common treatment approaches, and advice on obtaining and navigating school-based services.

Volkmar, F. R., & Wiesner, L. A. (2021). *A practical guide to autism: What every parent, family member, and teacher needs to know* (2nd ed.). Wiley.

Handbook of Autism and Pervasive Developmental Disorders

This two-volume reference work for researchers and health care professionals covers the state of ASD research on topics ranging from genetics and brain mechanisms to adult outcomes and psychosocial interventions.

Volkmar, F. R., Paul, R., Rogers, S. J., & Pelphrey, K. A. (Eds.). (2014). *Handbook of autism and pervasive developmental disorders* (4th ed.). Wiley. https://doi.org/10.1002/9781118911389

Autism Treatment Network

This resource for parents and families offers a searchable webpage that provides a comprehensive list of resources for individuals with ASD and their families. Searches can be customized by age, level of support (some, moderate, intensive), and geographic location.

> https://www.autismspeaks.org/taxonomy/term/2751

Autism Speaks 100-Day Kit

This resource provides an overview of autism symptoms and services for families of newly diagnosed children, as well as advice for parents on accepting their child's diagnosis. The 100-day kits are available for families of children under age 4 and school-aged children. The Autism Speaks website is also an excellent tool for resources across the lifespan.

> https://www.autismspeaks.org/tool-kit/100-day-kit-young-children

Autism Navigator

A collection of web-based tools and courses that aim to make evidence-based practices for ASD, particularly for early intervention, widely available. Their website includes a national provider directory as well as a "virtual community" for family members. Useful for health care professionals, parents, and family members.

> https://autismnavigator.com/

Centers for Disease Control Milestone Tracker

This resource encourages families to actively track their child's development from birth to age 5. Offers advice on when to contact health care providers with concerns. There is also a Milestone Tracker smartphone app that allows families to log their child's developmental progress. Materials are available in Spanish and English.

> https://www.cdc.gov/ncbddd/actearly/milestones/index.html

Got Transition

Supports a smooth transition from the pediatric to the adult medical home. Includes printable handouts on the health care transition for family members and young adults. For health care professionals, parents, and family members.

> https://www.gottransition.org/

Boyfriends and Girlfriends: A Guide to Dating for People With Disabilities

Written specifically for teens and adults with disabilities, this book explores the many practical and emotional aspects of dating and validates age-appropriate desires for romantic companionship. A great resource for individuals with ASD, family members, and providers.

> Couwenhoven, T. (2022). *Boyfriends and girlfriends: A guide to dating for people with disabilities.* Woodbine House.

References

Aman, M. G., McDougle, C. J., Scahill, L., Handen, B., Arnold, L. E., Johnson, C., Stigler, K. A., Bearss, K., Butter, E., Swiezy, N. B., Sukhodolsky, D. D., Ramadan, Y., Pozdol, S. L., Nikolov, R., Lecavalier, L., Kohn, A. E., Koenig, K., Hollway, J. A., Korzekwa, P., Gavaletz, A., . . . Research Units on Pediatric Psychopharmacology Autism Network. (2009). Medication and parent training in children with pervasive developmental disorders and serious behavior problems: results from a randomized clinical trial. *Journal of the American Academy of Child and Adolescent Psychiatry, 48*(12), 1143–1154. https://doi.org/10.1097/CHI.0b013e3181bfd669

American Psychiatric Association. (2013). *Diagnostic and statistical manual of mental disorders* (5th ed.). American Psychiatric Publishing.

Anagnostou, E., Aman, M. G., Handen, B. L., Sanders, K. B., Shui, A., Hollway, J. A., Brian, J., Arnold, L. E., Capano, L., Hellings, J. A., Butter, E., Mankad, D., Tumuluru, R., Kettel, J., Newsom, C. R., Hadjiyannakis, S., Peleg, N., Odrobina, D., McAuliffe-Bellin, S., . . . Veenstra-VanderWeele, J. (2016). Metformin for treatment of overweight induced by atypical antipsychotic medication in young people with autism spectrum disorder: A randomized clinical trial. *JAMA Psychiatry*, *73*(9), 928–937. https://doi.org/10.1001/jamapsychiatry.2016.1232

Anderson, K. A., Sosnowy, C., Kuo, A. A., & Shattuck, P. T. (2018). Transition of individuals with autism to adulthood: A review of qualitative studies. *Pediatrics*, *141*(Suppl. 4), S318–S327. https://doi.org/10.1542/peds.2016-4300I

Billeci, L., Narzisi, A., Campatelli, G., Crifaci, G., Calderoni, S., Gagliano, A., Calzone, C., Colombi, C., Pioggia, G., Muratori, F., Raso, R., Ruta, L., Rossi, I., Ballarani, A., Fulceri, F., Darini, A., Maroscia, E., Lattarulo, C., Tortorella, G., . . . Comminiello, V., & the ALERT group. (2016). Disentangling the initiation from the response in joint attention: An eye-tracking study in toddlers with autism spectrum disorders. *Translational Psychiatry*, *6*(5), e808. https://doi.org/10.1038/tp.2016.75

Boterberg, S., Charman, T., Marschik, P. B., Bölte, S., & Roeyers, H. (2019). Regression in autism spectrum disorder: A critical overview of retrospective findings and recommendations for future research. *Neuroscience and Biobehavioral Reviews*, *102*, 24–55. https://doi.org/10.1016/j.neubiorev.2019.03.013

Buescher, A. V. S., Cidav, Z., Knapp, M., & Mandell, D. S. (2014). Costs of autism spectrum disorders in the United Kingdom and the United States. *JAMA Pediatrics*, *168*(8), 721–728. https://doi.org/10.1001/jamapediatrics.2014.210

Byrne, K., Sterrett, K., Elias, R., Bal, V. H., McCauley, J. B., & Lord, C. (2022). Trajectories of seizures, medication use, and obesity status into early adulthood in autistic individuals and those with other neurodevelopmental conditions. *Autism in Adulthood: Challenges and Management*. https://doi.org/10.1089/aut.2020.0080

Carbone, P. S., Behl, D. D., Azor, V., & Murphy, N. A. (2010). The medical home for children with autism spectrum disorders: Parent and pediatrician perspectives. *Journal of Autism and Developmental Disorders*, *40*(3), 317–324. https://doi.org/10.1007/s10803-009-0874-5

Cimera, R. E., Burgess, S., & Wiley, A. (2013). Does providing transition services early enable students with ASD to achieve better vocational outcomes as adults? *Research and Practice for Persons With Severe Disabilities*, *38*(2), 88–93. https://doi.org/10.2511/027494813807714474

Clarke, E. B., Sterrett, K., & Lord, C. (2021). Work and well-being: Vocational activity trajectories in young adults with autism spectrum disorder. *Autism Research*, *14*(12), 2613–2624. https://doi.org/10.1002/aur.2606

Cohen, J. (1988). *Statistical power analysis for the behavioral sciences*. Routledge Academic.

Constantino, J. N., & Gruber, C. P. (2012). *Social Responsiveness Scale: SRS-2*. Western Psychological Services.

Courchesne, E., Campbell, K., & Solso, S. (2011). Brain growth across the life span in autism: Age-specific changes in anatomical pathology. *Brain Research*, *1380*, 138–145. https://doi.org/10.1016/j.brainres.2010.09.101

Daniels, A. M., & Mandell, D. S. (2014). Explaining differences in age at autism spectrum disorder diagnosis: A critical review. *Autism*, *18*(5), 583–597. https://doi.org/10.1177/1362361313480277

Dean, O. M., Gray, K. M., Villagonzalo, K. A., Dodd, S., Mohebbi, M., Vick, T., Tonge, B. J., & Berk, M. (2017). A randomised, double blind, placebo-controlled trial of a fixed dose of N-acetyl cysteine in children with autistic disorder. *The Australian and New Zealand Journal of Psychiatry*, *51*(3), 241–249. https://doi.org/10.1177/0004867416652735

de la Torre-Ubieta, L., Won, H., Stein, J. L., & Geschwind, D. H. (2016). Advancing the understanding of autism disease mechanisms through genetics. *Nature Medicine*, *22*(4), 345–361. https://doi.org/10.1038/nm.4071

de Vries, M., & Geurts, H. (2015). Influence of autism traits and executive functioning on quality of life in children with an autism spectrum disorder. *Journal of Autism and Developmental Disorders*, *45*(9), 2734–2743. https://doi.org/10.1007/s10803-015-2438-1

Dijkhuis, R., de Sonneville, L., Ziermans, T., Staal, W., & Swaab, H. (2020). Autism symptoms, executive functioning and academic progress in higher education students. *Journal of Autism and Developmental Disorders*, *50*(4), 1353–1363. https://doi.org/10.1007/s10803-019-04267-8

Duncan, A., Ruble, L. A., Meinzen-Derr, J., Thomas, C., & Stark, L. J. (2018). Preliminary efficacy of a daily living skills intervention for adolescents with high-functioning autism spectrum disorder. *Autism*, *22*(8), 983–994. https://doi.org/10.1177/1362361317716606

Dunn, M. E., Burbine, T., Bowers, C. A., & Tantleff-Dunn, S. (2001). Moderators of stress in parents of children with autism. *Community Mental Health Journal, 37*(1), 39–52. https://doi.org/10.1023/A:1026592305436

Elias, R., & White, S. W. (2018). Autism goes to college: Understanding the needs of a student population on the rise. *Journal of Autism and Developmental Disorders, 48*(3), 732–746. https://doi.org/10.1007/s10803-017-3075-7

Enner, S., Ahmad, S., Morse, A. M., & Kothare, S. V. (2020). Autism: Considerations for transitions of care into adulthood. *Current Opinion in Pediatrics, 32*(3), 446–452. https://doi.org/10.1097/MOP.0000000000000882

Fountain, C., Winter, A. S., & Bearman, P. S. (2012). Six developmental trajectories characterize children with autism. *Pediatrics, 129*(5), e1112–e1120. https://doi.org/10.1542/peds.2011-1601

Frye, R. E., Vassall, S., Kaur, G., Lewis, C., Karim, M., & Rossignol, D. (2019). Emerging biomarkers in autism spectrum disorder: A systematic review. *Annals of Translational Medicine, 7*(23), 792. https://doi.org/10.21037/atm.2019.11.53

Fung, L. K., Mahajan, R., Nozzolillo, A., Bernal, P., Krasner, A., Jo, B., Coury, D., Whitaker, A., Veenstra-Vanderweele, J., & Hardan, A. Y. (2016). Pharmacologic treatment of severe irritability and problem behaviors in autism: A systematic review and meta-analysis. *Pediatrics, 137*(Suppl. 2), S124–S135. https://doi.org/10.1542/peds.2015-2851K

George, R., & Stokes, M. A. (2018). Gender identity and sexual orientation in autism spectrum disorder. *Autism, 22*(8), 970–982. https://doi.org/10.1177/1362361317714587

Gotham, K., Brunwasser, S. M., & Lord, C. (2015). Depressive and anxiety symptom trajectories from school age through young adulthood in samples with autism spectrum disorder and developmental delay. *Journal of the American Academy of Child & Adolescent Psychiatry, 54*(5), 369–376.e3. https://doi.org/10.1016/j.jaac.2015.02.005

Hardan, A. Y., Fung, L. K., Libove, R. A., Obukhanych, T. V., Nair, S., Herzenberg, L. A., Frazier, T. W., & Tirouvanziam, R. (2012). A randomized controlled pilot trial of oral N-acetylcysteine in children with autism. *Biological Psychiatry, 71*(11), 956–961. https://doi.org/10.1016/j.biopsych.2012.01.014

Harrop, C., McConachie, H., Emsley, R., Leadbitter, K., Green, J., & the PACT Consortium. (2014). Restricted and repetitive behaviors in autism spectrum disorders and typical development: Cross-sectional and longitudinal comparisons. *Journal of Autism and Developmental Disorders, 44*(5), 1207–1219. https://doi.org/10.1007/s10803-013-1986-5

Hastings, R. P., Kovshoff, H., Brown, T., Ward, N. J., Espinosa, F. D., & Remington, B. (2005). Coping strategies in mothers and fathers of preschool and school-age children with autism. *Autism, 9*(4), 377–391. https://doi.org/10.1177/1362361305056078

Hazlett, H. C., Gu, H., Munsell, B. C., Kim, S. H., Styner, M., Wolff, J. J., Elison, J. T., Swanson, M. R., Zhu, H., Botteron, K. N., Collins, D. L., Constantino, J. N., Dager, S. R., Estes, A. M., Evans, A. C., Fonov, V. S., Gerig, G., Kostopoulos, P., McKinstry, R. C., . . . Piven, J., & the IBIS Network, & the Clinical Sites, & the Data Coordinating Center, & the Image Processing Core, & the Statistical Analysis. (2017). Early brain development in infants at high risk for autism spectrum disorder. *Nature, 542*(7641), 348–351. https://doi.org/10.1038/nature21369

Hill, A. P., Zuckerman, K. E., & Fombonne, E. (2015). Obesity and autism. *Pediatrics, 136*(6), 1051–1061. https://doi.org/10.1542/peds.2015-1437

Höfer, J., Hoffmann, F., & Bachmann, C. (2017). Use of complementary and alternative medicine in children and adolescents with autism spectrum disorder: A systematic review. *Autism, 21*(4), 387–402. https://doi.org/10.1177/1362361316646559

Hume, K., Steinbrenner, J. R., Odom, S. L., Morin, K. L., Nowell, S. W., Tomaszewski, B., Szendrey, S., McIntyre, N. S., Yücesoy-Özkan, S., & Savage, M. N. (2021). Evidence-based practices for children, youth, and young adults with autism: Third generation review. *Journal of Autism and Developmental Disorders, 51*(11), 4013–4032. https://doi.org/10.1007/s10803-020-04844-2

Hyman, S. L., Levy, S. E., Myers, S. M., Kuo, D. Z., Apkon, S., Davidson, L. F., Ellerbeck, K. A., Foster, J. E. A., Noritz, G. H., Leppert, M. O. C., Saunders, B. S., Stille, C., Yin, L., Weitzman, C. C., Childers, D. O., Jr., Levine, J. M., Peralta-Carcelen, A. M., Poon, J. K., Smith, P. J., . . . Bridgemohan, C., & the Council on Children With Disabilities, Section on Developmental and Behavioral Pediatrics. (2020). Identification, evaluation, and management of children with autism spectrum disorder. *Pediatrics, 145*(1), e20193447. https://doi.org/10.1542/peds.2019-3447

Jones, E. J. H., Gliga, T., Bedford, R., Charman, T., & Johnson, M. H. (2014). Developmental pathways to autism: A review of prospective studies of infants at risk. *Neuroscience and Biobehavioral Reviews, 39*(100), 1–33. https://doi.org/10.1016/j.neubiorev.2013.12.001

Kang-Yi, C. D., Grinker, R. R., Beidas, R., Agha, A., Russell, R., Shah, S. B., Shea, K., & Mandell,

D. S. (2018). Influence of community-level cultural beliefs about autism on families' and professionals' care for children. *Transcultural Psychiatry*, 55(5), 623–647. https://doi.org/10.1177/1363461518779831

Kenworthy, L., Yerys, B. E., Anthony, L. G., & Wallace, G. L. (2008). Understanding executive control in autism spectrum disorders in the lab and in the real world. *Neuropsychology Review*, 18(4), 320–338. https://doi.org/10.1007/s11065-008-9077-7

Kim, S. H., Bal, V. H., & Lord, C. (2018). Longitudinal follow-up of academic achievement in children with autism from age 2 to 18. *Journal of Child Psychology and Psychiatry*, 59(3), 258–267. https://doi.org/10.1111/jcpp.12808

Koegel, R. L., Koegel, L. K., & McNerney, E. K. (2001). Pivotal areas in intervention for autism. *Journal of Clinical Child Psychology*, 30(1), 19–32. https://doi.org/10.1207/S15374424JCCP3001_4

Kolevzon, A., Mathewson, K. A., & Hollander, E. (2006). Selective serotonin reuptake inhibitors in autism: A review of efficacy and tolerability. *The Journal of Clinical Psychiatry*, 67(3), 407–414. https://doi.org/10.4088/JCP.v67n0311

Kozlowski, A. M., Matson, J. L., Horovitz, M., Worley, J. A., & Neal, D. (2011). Parents' first concerns of their child's development in toddlers with autism spectrum disorders. *Developmental Neurorehabilitation*, 14(2), 72–78. https://doi.org/10.3109/17518423.2010.539193

Laugeson, E. A., Frankel, F., Gantman, A., Dillon, A. R., & Mogil, C. (2012). Evidence-based social skills training for adolescents with autism spectrum disorders: The UCLA PEERS program. *Journal of Autism and Developmental Disorders*, 42(6), 1025–1036. https://doi.org/10.1007/s10803-011-1339-1

Le Couteur, A., Lord, C., & Rutter, M. (2003). *The autism diagnostic interview-revised (ADI-R)*. Western Psychological Services.

Leedham, A. T., Thompson, A. R., & Freeth, M. (2020). A thematic synthesis of siblings' lived experiences of autism: Distress, responsibilities, compassion and connection. *Research in Developmental Disabilities*, 97, 103547. https://doi.org/10.1016/j.ridd.2019.103547

Locke, J., Ishijima, E. H., Kasari, C., & London, N. (2010). Loneliness, friendship quality and the social networks of adolescents with high-functioning autism in an inclusive school setting. *Journal of Research in Special Educational Needs*, 10(2), 74–81. https://doi.org/10.1111/j.1471-3802.2010.01148.x

Lord, C., Brugha, T. S., Charman, T., Cusack, J., Dumas, G., Frazier, T., Jones, E. J. H., Jones, R. M., Pickles, A., State, M. W., Taylor, J. L., & Veenstra-VanderWeele, J. (2020). Autism spectrum disorder. *Nature Reviews: Disease Primers*, 6(1), 5. https://doi.org/10.1038/s41572-019-0138-4

Lord, C., Charman, T., Havdahl, A., Carbone, P., Anagnostou, E., Boyd, B., Carr, T., de Vries, P. J., Dissanayake, C., Divan, G., Freitag, C. M., Gotelli, M. M., Kasari, C., Knapp, M., Mundy, P., Plank, A., Scahill, L., Servili, C., Shattuck, P., . . . McCauley, J. B. (2022). The Lancet Commission on the future of care and clinical research in autism. *The Lancet*, 399(10321), 271–334. https://doi.org/10.1016/S0140-6736(21)01541-5

Lord, C., Rutter, M., DiLavore, P., Risi, S., Gotham, K., & Bishop, S. (2012). *Autism Diagnostic Observation Schedule* (2nd ed.). Western Psychological Services, ADOS-2.

Lukmanji, S., Manji, S. A., Kadhim, S., Sauro, K. M., Wirrell, E. C., Kwon, C.-S., & Jetté, N. (2019). The co-occurrence of epilepsy and autism: A systematic review. *Epilepsy & Behavior*, 98(Pt. A), 238–248. https://doi.org/10.1016/j.yebeh.2019.07.037

Maenner, M. J., Warren, Z., Williams, A. R., Amoakohene, E., Bakian, A. V., Bilder, D. A., Durkin, M. S., Fitzgerald, R. T., Furnier, S. M., Hughes, M. M., Ladd-Acosta, C. M., McArthur, D., Pas, E. T., Salinas, A., Vehorn, A., Williams, S., Esler, A., Grzybowski, A., Hall-Lande, J., . . . Shaw, K. A. (2023). Prevalence and characteristics of autism spectrum disorder among children aged 8 years—Autism and Developmental Disabilities Monitoring Network, 11 sites, United States, 2020. *Morbidity and Mortality Weekly Report: Surveillance Summaries*, 72(2), 1–14. https://doi.org/10.15585/mmwr.ss7202a1

Maïano, C., Normand, C. L., Salvas, M.-C., Moullec, G., & Aimé, A. (2016). Prevalence of school bullying among youth with autism spectrum disorders: A systematic review and meta-analysis. *Autism Research*, 9(6), 601–615. https://doi.org/10.1002/aur.1568

Mandell, D. S., & Novak, M. (2005). The role of culture in families' treatment decisions for children with autism spectrum disorders. *Mental Retardation and Developmental Disabilities Research Reviews*, 11(2), 110–115. https://doi.org/10.1002/mrdd.20061

Masten, A. S., & Cicchetti, D. (2010). Developmental cascades. *Development and Psychopathology*, 22(3), 491–495. https://doi.org/10.1017/S0954579410000222

McCauley, J. B., Pickles, A., Huerta, M., & Lord, C. (2020). Defining positive outcomes in more and less cognitively able autistic adults. *Autism Research*, 13(9), 1548–1560. https://doi.org/10.1002/aur.2359

McStay, R. L., Dissanayake, C., Scheeren, A., Koot, H. M., & Begeer, S. (2014). Parenting stress and autism: The role of age, autism severity, quality of life and problem behaviour of children and adolescents with autism. *Autism, 18*(5), 502–510. https://doi.org/10.1177/1362361313485163

Montes, G., & Halterman, J. S. (2008). Association of childhood autism spectrum disorders and loss of family income. *Pediatrics, 121*(4), e821–e826. https://doi.org/10.1542/peds.2007-1594

Moss, P., Eirinaki, V., Savage, S., & Howlin, P. (2019). Growing older with autism—The experiences of adult siblings of individuals with autism. *Research in Autism Spectrum Disorders, 63*, 42–51. https://doi.org/10.1016/j.rasd.2018.10.005

Nevill, R. E., Lecavalier, L., & Stratis, E. A. (2018). Meta-analysis of parent-mediated interventions for young children with autism spectrum disorder. *Autism, 22*(2), 84–98. https://doi.org/10.1177/1362361316677838

Palmer, N., Beam, A., Agniel, D., Eran, A., Manrai, A., Spettell, C., Steinberg, G., Mandl, K., Fox, K., Nelson, S. F., & Kohane, I. (2017). Association of sex with recurrence of autism spectrum disorder among siblings. *JAMA Pediatrics, 171*(11), 1107–1112. https://doi.org/10.1001/jamapediatrics.2017.2832

Patra, S., Nebhinani, N., Viswanathan, A., & Kirubakaran, R. (2019). Atomoxetine for attention deficit hyperactivity disorder in children and adolescents with autism: A systematic review and meta-analysis. *Autism Research, 12*(4), 542–552. https://doi.org/10.1002/aur.2059

Pickles, A., Anderson, D. K., & Lord, C. (2014). Heterogeneity and plasticity in the development of language: A 17-year follow-up of children referred early for possible autism. *Journal of Child Psychology and Psychiatry, 55*(12), 1354–1362. https://doi.org/10.1111/jcpp.12269

Politte, L. C., Scahill, L., Figueroa, J., McCracken, J. T., King, B., & McDougle, C. J. (2018). A randomized, placebo-controlled trial of extended-release guanfacine in children with autism spectrum disorder and ADHD symptoms: An analysis of secondary outcome measures. *Neuropsychopharmacology, 43*(8), 1772–1778. https://doi.org/10.1038/s41386-018-0039-3

Pugliese, C. E., Anthony, L., Strang, J. F., Dudley, K., Wallace, G. L., & Kenworthy, L. (2015). Increasing adaptive behavior skill deficits from childhood to adolescence in autism spectrum disorder: Role of executive function. *Journal of Autism and Developmental Disorders, 45*(6), 1579–1587. https://doi.org/10.1007/s10803-014-2309-1

Reddihough, D. S., Marraffa, C., Mouti, A., O'Sullivan, M., Lee, K. J., Orsini, F., Hazell, P., Granich, J., Whitehouse, A. J. O., Wray, J., Dossetor, D., Santosh, P., Silove, N., & Kohn, M. (2019). Effect of fluoxetine on obsessive-compulsive behaviors in children and adolescents with autism spectrum disorders: A randomized clinical trial. *JAMA: Journal of the American Medical Association, 322*(16), 1561–1569. https://doi.org/10.1001/jama.2019.14685

Reinblatt, S. P., DosReis, S., Walkup, J. T., & Riddle, M. A. (2009). Activation adverse events induced by the selective serotonin reuptake inhibitor fluvoxamine in children and adolescents. *Journal of Child and Adolescent Psychopharmacology, 19*(2), 119–126. https://doi.org/10.1089/cap.2008.040

Rivera-Figueroa, K., Marfo, N. Y. A., & Eigsti, I.-M. (2022). Parental perceptions of autism spectrum disorder in Latinx and Black sociocultural contexts: A systematic review. *American Journal on Intellectual and Developmental Disabilities, 127*(1), 42–63. https://doi.org/10.1352/1944-7558-127.1.42

Robins, D. L., Casagrande, K., Barton, M., Chen, C.-M. A., Dumont-Mathieu, T., & Fein, D. (2014). Validation of the modified checklist for Autism in toddlers, revised with follow-up (M-CHAT-R/F). *Pediatrics, 133*(1), 37–45. https://doi.org/10.1542/peds.2013-1813

Rodrigues, R., Lai, M. C., Beswick, A., Gorman, D. A., Anagnostou, E., Szatmari, P., Anderson, K. K., & Ameis, S. H. (2021). Practitioner Review: Pharmacological treatment of attention-deficit/hyperactivity disorder symptoms in children and youth with autism spectrum disorder: A systematic review and meta-analysis. *Journal of Child Psychology and Psychiatry, 62*(6), 680–700. https://doi.org/10.1111/jcpp.13305

Rogers, S. J., & Dawson, G. (2010). *Early Start Denver Model for young children with autism: Promoting language, learning, and engagement.* Guilford Press.

Rogers, S. J., Yoder, P., Estes, A., Warren, Z., McEachin, J., Munson, J., Rocha, M., Greenson, J., Wallace, L., Gardner, E., Dawson, G., Sugar, C. A., Hellemann, G., & Whelan, F. (2021). A multisite randomized controlled trial comparing the effects of intervention intensity and intervention style on outcomes for young children with autism. *Journal of the American Academy of Child & Adolescent Psychiatry, 60*(6), 710–722. https://doi.org/10.1016/j.jaac.2020.06.013

Rolland, J. S. (1987). Chronic illness and the life cycle: A conceptual framework. *Family Process, 26*(2), 203–221. https://doi.org/10.1111/j.1545-5300.1987.00203.x

Rosenthal, M., Wallace, G. L., Lawson, R., Wills, M. C., Dixon, E., Yerys, B. E., & Kenworthy, L. (2013). Impairments in real-world executive function increase from childhood to adolescence in autism spectrum disorders. *Neuropsychology*, 27(1), 13–18. https://doi.org/10.1037/a0031299

Rossignol, D. A., & Frye, R. E. (2014). Melatonin in autism spectrum disorders. *Current Clinical Pharmacology*, 9(4), 326–334. https://doi.org/10.2174/1574884711308666072

Rutter, M., Bailey, A., & Lord, C. (2003). *The social communication questionnaire: Manual*. Western Psychological Services.

Scahill, L., McCracken, J. T., King, B. H., Rockhill, C., Shah, B., Politte, L., Sanders, R., Minjarez, M., Cowen, J., Mullett, J., Page, C., Ward, D., Deng, Y., Loo, S., Dziura, J., McDougle, C. J., & Research Units on Pediatric Psychopharmacology Autism Network. (2015). Extended-release guanfacine for hyperactivity in children with autism spectrum disorder. *The American Journal of Psychiatry*, 172(12), 1197–1206. https://doi.org/10.1176/appi.ajp.2015.15010055

Schreibman, L., Dawson, G., Stahmer, A. C., Landa, R., Rogers, S. J., McGee, G. G., Kasari, C., Ingersoll, B., Kaiser, A. P., Bruinsma, Y., McNerney, E., Wetherby, A., & Halladay, A. (2015). Naturalistic developmental behavioral interventions: Empirically validated treatments for autism spectrum disorder. *Journal of Autism and Developmental Disorders*, 45(8), 2411–2428. https://doi.org/10.1007/s10803-015-2407-8

Shattuck, P. T., Narendorf, S. C., Cooper, B., Sterzing, P. R., Wagner, M., & Taylor, J. L. (2012). Postsecondary education and employment among youth with an autism spectrum disorder. *Pediatrics*, 129(6), 1042–1049. https://doi.org/10.1542/peds.2011-2864

Shedlock, K., Susi, A., Gorman, G. H., Hisle-Gorman, E., Erdie-Lalena, C. R., & Nylund, C. M. (2016). Autism spectrum disorders and metabolic complications of obesity. *The Journal of Pediatrics*, 178, 183–187.e1. https://doi.org/10.1016/j.jpeds.2016.07.055

Simonoff, E., Kent, R., Stringer, D., Lord, C., Briskman, J., Lukito, S., Pickles, A., Charman, T., & Baird, G. (2020). Trajectories in symptoms of autism and cognitive ability in autism from childhood to adult life: Findings from a longitudinal epidemiological cohort. *Journal of the American Academy of Child & Adolescent Psychiatry*, 59(12), 1342–1352. https://doi.org/10.1016/j.jaac.2019.11.020

Simonoff, E., Pickles, A., Charman, T., Chandler, S., Loucas, T., & Baird, G. (2008). Psychiatric disorders in children with autism spectrum disorders: Prevalence, comorbidity, and associated factors in a population-derived sample. *Journal of the American Academy of Child & Adolescent Psychiatry*, 47(8), 921–929. https://doi.org/10.1097/CHI.0b013e318179964f

Smith, L. E., Greenberg, J. S., & Seltzer, M. M. (2012). Social support and well-being at mid-life among mothers of adolescents and adults with autism spectrum disorders. *Journal of Autism and Developmental Disorders*, 42(9), 1818–1826. https://doi.org/10.1007/s10803-011-1420-9

Smith, T. (2001). Discrete trial training in the treatment of autism. *Focus on Autism and Other Developmental Disabilities*, 16(2), 86–92. https://doi.org/10.1177/108835760101600204

Taylor, J. L., & Seltzer, M. M. (2011). Changes in the mother-child relationship during the transition to adulthood for youth with autism spectrum disorders. *Journal of Autism and Developmental Disorders*, 41(10), 1397–1410. https://doi.org/10.1007/s10803-010-1166-9

Thompson, C., Bölte, S., Falkmer, T., & Girdler, S. (2018). To be understood: Transitioning to adult life for people with autism spectrum disorder. *PLOS ONE*, 13(3), e0194758. https://doi.org/10.1371/journal.pone.0194758

Toh, T.-H., Tan, V. W.-Y., Lau, P. S.-T., & Kiyu, A. (2018). Accuracy of Modified Checklist for Autism in Toddlers (M-CHAT) in detecting autism and other developmental disorders in community clinics. *Journal of Autism and Developmental Disorders*, 48(1), 28–35. https://doi.org/10.1007/s10803-017-3287-x

van Heijst, B. F., & Geurts, H. M. (2015). Quality of life in autism across the lifespan: A meta-analysis. *Autism*, 19(2), 158–167. https://doi.org/10.1177/1362361313517053

Volkmar, F., Siegel, M., Woodbury-Smith, M., King, B., McCracken, J., State, M., & the American Academy of Child and Adolescent Psychiatry (AACAP) Committee on Quality Issues (CQI). (2014). Practice parameter for the assessment and treatment of children and adolescents with autism spectrum disorder. *Journal of the American Academy of Child & Adolescent Psychiatry*, 53(2), 237–257. https://doi.org/10.1016/j.jaac.2013.10.013

Watkins, L., O'Reilly, M., Kuhn, M., Gevarter, C., Lancioni, G. E., Sigafoos, J., & Lang, R. (2015). A review of peer-mediated social interaction interventions for students with autism in inclusive settings. *Journal of Autism and Developmental Disorders*, 45(4), 1070–1083. https://doi.org/10.1007/s10803-014-2264-x

White, P. H., Cooley, W. C., Transitions Clinical Report Authoring Group, The American Academy of Pediatrics, The American Academy of Family Physicians, & The American College of Physicians. (2018). Supporting the health care transition from adolescence to adulthood in the medical home. *Pediatrics*, 142(5), e20182587. https://doi.org/10.1542/peds.2018-2587

White, S. W., Simmons, G. L., Gotham, K. O., Conner, C. M., Smith, I. C., Beck, K. B., & Mazefsky, C. A. (2018). Psychosocial treatments targeting anxiety and depression in adolescents and adults on the autism spectrum: Review of the latest research and recommended future directions. *Current Psychiatry Reports, 20*(10), 82. https://doi.org/10.1007/s11920-018-0949-0

Williams Buckley, A., Hirtz, D., Oskoui, M., Armstrong, M. J., Batra, A., Bridgemohan, C., Coury, D., Dawson, G., Donley, D., Findling, R. L., Gaughan, T., Gloss, D., Gronseth, G., Kessler, R., Merillat, S., Michelson, D., Owens, J., Pringsheim, T., Sikich, L., . . . Ashwal, S. (2020). Practice guideline: Treatment for insomnia and disrupted sleep behavior in children and adolescents with autism spectrum disorder: Report of the Guideline Development, Dissemination, and Implementation Subcommittee of the American Academy of Neurology. *Neurology, 94*(9), 392–404. https://doi.org/10.1212/WNL.0000000000009033

Zwaigenbaum, L., Bauman, M. L., Choueiri, R., Kasari, C., Carter, A., Granpeesheh, D., Mailloux, Z., Smith Roley, S., Wagner, S., Fein, D., Pierce, K., Buie, T., Davis, P. A., Newschaffer, C., Robins, D., Wetherby, A., Stone, W. L., Yirmiya, N., Estes, A., . . . Natowicz, M. R. (2015). Early intervention for children with autism spectrum disorder under 3 years of age: Recommendations for practice and research. *Pediatrics, 136*(Suppl. 1), S60–S81. https://doi.org/10.1542/peds.2014-3667E

CHAPTER 17

PRETERM BIRTH: IMPLICATIONS FOR THE FAMILY SYSTEM AND CHILD AND ADOLESCENT HEALTH AND WELL-BEING

Maria Spinelli, Julie Poehlmann, and Prachi E. Shah

Preterm birth is a significant public health problem worldwide, associated with neonatal morbidity and mortality and increased risk for long-term health, neurodevelopmental, and behavioral sequelae (McCabe et al., 2014). However, there is substantial within-group variability, and many children born preterm are resilient. Although advances in obstetric and neonatal care have resulted in decreased mortality of preterm infants, the morbidities of prematurity (e.g., developmental delay, neurodevelopmental disability) remain. As a result, a growing number of families are facing the challenge of caring for vulnerable children, with caregivers experiencing racial and socioeconomic inequities disproportionately affected (Hamilton et al., 2015). The consequences of preterm birth typically affect the entire family system, resulting in long-standing impacts on the preterm child, caregivers, and caregiver–child relationships. In addition to the neurodevelopmental and behavioral sequelae of prematurity impacting the child, preterm birth can be a traumatic experience for caregivers, in which this nonnormative transition to parenthood is often associated with anxiety, grief, and trauma. Although we now know more about the antecedents and consequences of premature birth than in the past, and although the number and scope of interventions for infants born preterm have increased, the approach to caring for preterm infants remains disjointed across specialties.

To help bridge these silos of knowledge and practice, this chapter attempts to integrate research and science about preterm birth across several disciplines, including pediatrics, pediatric psychology, and developmental and family science. After a brief presentation of the definition and prevalence of preterm birth, we use a bioecological systems lens (see Bronfenbrenner & Morris, 2006) to examine the biopsychosocial antecedents, including the role of health disparities and social determinants of health, on preterm birth outcomes. We review the morbidities and developmental-behavioral outcomes of preterm birth across the childhood lifespan and the research on the impact of preterm birth on the family system, informed by a developmental science perspective. The chapter will present interdisciplinary models of care to support resilience in preterm infants and their families and will conclude with the roles of behavioral health providers, including pediatric psychologists and developmental-behavioral pediatricians in the care of children and adolescents born preterm.

https://doi.org/10.1037/0000414-017
APA Handbook of Pediatric Psychology, Developmental-Behavioral Pediatrics, and Developmental Science: Vol. 2. Pediatric Psychology and Developmental-Behavioral Pediatrics: Clinical Applications of Developmental Science, P. E. Shah and M. H. Bornstein (Editors-in-Chief)
Copyright © 2025 by the American Psychological Association. All rights reserved.

DEFINITION AND PREVALENCE

Preterm birth is defined as birth prior to 37 weeks gestation (Vogel et al., 2018). Although the degree of prematurity was previously described by variations in birthweight (e.g., low birthweight (LBW: <2,500 g), very low birthweight (VLBW: <1,500 g), and extremely low birthweight (ELBW: <1,000 g)), current conventions and the World Health Organization use gestational age cut-offs as indicators of preterm status: extreme preterm (<28 weeks gestation), very preterm (28–31$^{6/7}$ weeks gestation), moderate preterm (32–33$^{6/7}$ weeks gestation) and late preterm (34–36$^{6/7}$ weeks gestation; Kohn et al., 2000).

Prevalence estimates of preterm birth from 39 majority and minority world countries of very high health index range from 5.3% to 14.7% (Chang et al., 2013), with substantially higher prevalence rates in majority world countries. Worldwide, 14.9 million births occur prematurely, with over 60% of all preterm births occurring in sub-Saharan Africa and South Asia (Blencowe et al., 2012). In the United States, the peak prevalence of preterm birth was 12.8% in 2006, with a gradual decrease in prevalence, with an estimated prevalence of 10% in the United States and 11.1% worldwide (Vogel et al., 2018).

BIOPSYCHOSOCIAL ANTECEDENTS AND RISKS ASSOCIATED WITH PRETERM BIRTH

The etiology of preterm birth is complex, associated with multilevel ecological risk factors including individual and biological factors and societal factors associated with health disparities and social inequities. Preterm birth can be broadly classified into two groups: (a) provider-initiated or indicated preterm birth (e.g., induction of labor or elective cesarean section prior to 37 weeks for maternal or fetal indications, or nonmedical reasons), which has largely decreased due to changes in obstetric practices; and (b) spontaneous preterm birth (Blencowe et al., 2012; Frey & Klebanoff, 2016). The etiology of spontaneous preterm birth is largely unknown, but is thought to be multifactorial, associated with both maternal biological factors and psychosocial factors (Beck et al., 2020; Frey & Klebanoff, 2016).

Maternal and Obstetric Risk Factors Associated With Preterm Birth

Several maternal medical conditions have been associated with increased rates of preterm birth, including a history of diabetes, obesity, hypertension/preeclampsia, urogenital infections, chorioamnionitis, and prenatal substance exposure including tobacco, alcohol, and other illicit substances (Marchi et al., 2015). Obstetric and fetal conditions associated with an increased risk of preterm birth include a history of multiple gestation, especially with monochorionic, diamniotic pregnancies (e.g., pregnancies characterized by two amniotic sacs but one placenta), history of assisted reproductive technology, placental abnormalities (e.g., placenta previa, placental abruption), and shortened cervical length (Fuchs & Senat, 2016; Luke, 2017). Despite attempts to address and mitigate maternal and obstetric factors associated with preterm birth, the majority of all preterm births occur without an identified maternal or obstetric etiology, suggesting the possibility that environmental and psychosocial factors contribute to the pathogenesis of preterm birth.

Race/Ethnicity and Social Determinants of Health in Preterm Birth

In the United States, there is a well-documented increased risk for preterm birth and infant mortality among infants identified as African American/non-Hispanic Black compared with infants identified as having other racial–ethnic backgrounds (Reagan & Salsberry, 2005). The association of race/ethnicity and preterm birth and its outcomes likely results from complex interactive effects among structural inequities and racism, as well as maternal, paternal, genetic and sociodemographic risks, and varying by country of origin (Manuck, 2017). Although immigrant non-Hispanic Black women in the United States have experienced a lower incidence of preterm birth, genetic differences alone (e.g., variations in TNF-α levels, epigenetic- and genetic-related microbiome differences) do not explain the disparate outcomes between African Americans and immigrant Africans. Similarly, although some socioeconomic disadvantages have also been implicated as explanations for racial disparities in preterm birth, inequities in preterm birth outcomes persist even when socioeconomic factors and maternal morbidities are considered (Lu & Halfon, 2003), raising the possibility that disparities in prevalence and preterm birth outcomes among non-Hispanic Blacks may be related to a complex interaction between race/ethnicity and psychosocial and socioeconomic factors, which are amplified in systems of structural racism (Chambers et al., 2019).

The mechanisms by which structural racism contribute to disparities in preterm birth outcomes are poorly understood and are likely multifactorial. Contributing factors include segregation leading to neighborhood disadvantage, cumulative experiences of inequity related to social determinants of health, and other factors such as shorter interpregnancy intervals in non-Hispanic Black mothers compared with White mothers. Examples of societal factors underlying structural racism which have been implicated in preterm birth include an increased risk of living in poverty and use of public assistance, increased exposure to environmental toxins (e.g., lead, air pollution, phthalates), differential access to high-quality health care, educational disparities, marital status, and paternity acknowledgment (Krieger et al., 2020). The disproportionate experience of multiple stressors, including discrimination, trauma, and financial stresses, has also been implicated as contributing to racial inequities in the prevalence of preterm birth.

CONSEQUENCES OF PRETERM BIRTH: MORTALITY, MORBIDITY AND NEURODEVELOPMENTAL OUTCOMES

The outcomes of preterm birth for children and adolescents are heterogeneous and can range from neonatal mortality to a wide spectrum of morbidities involving cognition, learning, behavior, social-adaptive functioning, and health-related quality of life.

Neonatal Mortality

Preterm birth is the most common cause of death in the neonatal period (Liu et al., 2015), resulting in 1 million neonatal deaths annually, with increasing mortality and morbidity with decreasing gestational age (Harrison & Goldenberg, 2016). Prematurity is a significant cause of neonatal mortality worldwide, accounting for 35% of deaths among newborns, and 16% of all deaths in children under the age of 5 (Vogel et al., 2018), with the greatest burden of mortality seen in the majority world, particularly in low- and/or middle-income countries (LMICs).

Preterm infants in LMICs are more likely to be born at lower gestational ages and have less access to high-quality tertiary medical care compared to preterm infants born in higher-income countries (HICs; Harrison & Goldenberg, 2016). Worldwide, most preterm infants are born after 32 weeks gestation, however survival rates vary by country due to disparities in access to appropriate neonatal care. In HICs, most infants (95%) born between 28 to 32 weeks survive, with the majority (90%) surviving without significant sequelae. In contrast, only 30% of infants born in LMICs at 28 to 32 weeks survive, with most infants born at under 28 weeks dying within the first few days of life (Blencowe et al., 2013), thus reflecting a major survival gap for preterm infants depending on the country in which they were born (Lawn et al., 2013). Lower gestational ages are associated with a proportional increased risk of mortality (D'Onofrio et al., 2013), with the greatest mortality risk in infants born prior to 32 weeks (Simmons et al., 2010). Additionally, infants with the dual risk of being preterm and small for gestational age (SGA: birthweight < 10% for gestational age) have a higher likelihood of mortality (Katz et al., 2013).

Over time, advances in neonatal practices have resulted in lower mortality associated with preterm birth, although risks of short- and long-term morbidities associated with preterm birth remain. In the perinatal period, medical sequelae of prematurity include respiratory complications (e.g., respiratory distress, apnea of prematurity, chronic lung disease, bronchopulmonary dysplasia), cardiovascular sequelae (e.g., patent ductus arteriosus, hypotension), neurologic complications (e.g., intraventricular hemorrhage, periventricular leukomalacia), difficulties with temperature regulation (hypothermia), gastrointestinal complications (e.g., necrotizing enterocolitis feeding difficulties), hematologic sequelae (e.g., anemia of prematurity, hyperbilirubinemia), and difficulties with metabolism (e.g., risk for hypoglycemia; Stoll et al., 2010). Similar to mortality trends with preterm birth, the medical morbidities associated with prematurity increase with decreasing gestational age.

Long-Term Outcomes and Morbidity

Neurodevelopmental and neurosensory disabilities. Preterm infants born at earlier gestation are at increased risk for "low prevalence-high severity" neurodevelopmental disabilities including epilepsy, cerebral palsy, intellectual disability, and neurosensory impairments including blindness and deafness (Kodjebacheva & Sabo, 2016; Schieve et al., 2016). Cerebral palsy (CP) is a disorder of motor development, characterized by abnormalities of tone and reflexes, resulting in gross motor impairments. The neonatal factors most associated with an increased risk of cerebral palsy include shorter gestational age (especially <32 weeks), and patterns of neonatal brain injury (e.g., intraventricular hemorrhage, posthemorrhagic ventricular dilatation, cerebral hemorrhage, and cystic periventricular leukomalacia; Spittle et al., 2018). Intellectual disability is characterized by an IQ < 70, with statistically significant higher risks in preterm infants born at earlier gestational ages compared to those born at later gestational ages (Yin et al., 2022). Preterm infants are also at risk for neurosensory impairments including sensorineural hearing loss, which may require amplification and cochlear implants (van Dommelen et al., 2015), and visual impairments, including myopia, strabismus, and retinal detachments, which are the sequelae of retinopathy of prematurity—the leading cause of vision impairment in infants born preterm (Holmström et al., 2014). The severity of neurodevelopmental disability and neurosensory impairment increases with decreasing gestational age, with the highest prevalence associated with infants born before 26 weeks of age (Allen et al., 2011).

Cognitive and learning outcomes. Similar to the risk for neurosensory impairments, the risk for cognitive problems and learning disabilities in preterm infants increases with decreasing gestational age (Hee Chung et al., 2020; Pascoe et al., 2021; Poulsen et al., 2013; Quigley et al., 2012; Shah, Kaciroti, Richards, & Lumeng, 2016). A meta-analysis examining the relationship between gestational age and reduced IQ across 27 studies over a 30-year period found that prematurity was associated with an average 12-point reduction in IQ, with IQ decreasing for each week of decreasing gestational age (Kerr-Wilson et al., 2012). Compared to full-term infants, the greatest impairments in IQ were seen with infants born extremely preterm (<28 weeks, mean decrease = 13.9 points), followed by very preterm (28–31 weeks, mean decrease = 11.4 points), followed by infants born moderate/late preterm (32–36$^{6/7}$ weeks, mean decrease = 8.4 points). At a population level, this corresponds to intellectual deficits of 0.86 *SD* lower IQ compared with controls (95% confidence interval [−0.94, −0.78]; Twilhaar et al., 2018). Infants born preterm are also on average at increased risk for deficits in learning and academic achievement, especially in language, reading, and math academic achievement, with the highest odds of impairment in infants born very preterm and extremely preterm (Jaekel & Wolke, 2014; Putnick et al., 2017). Compared to full-term infants, on average preterm infants are more likely to require special education services, have grade retention, exhibit worse academic skills, and have lower overall educational attainment (Eryigit Madzwamuse et al., 2015; Kelly, 2016; MacKay et al., 2010).

Autism spectrum disorder. Several population-based studies have demonstrated an increased prevalence of autism spectrum disorders (ASD) in preterm infants compared with full-term infants (Brumbaugh et al., 2020; Crump et al., 2021; Guy et al., 2015; Kuzniewicz et al., 2014). Across studies, there is an increased association of autism in infants born at earlier gestational ages, with the greatest odds of autism in infants born less than 28 weeks gestation (extreme preterm). Although there is a three-fold increased risk of autism in children born less than 27 weeks (Kuzniewicz et al., 2014), there is also an elevated risk of autism in children born moderate or late preterm (32–36 weeks; Guy et al., 2015). At a population level, prevalence estimates for ASD have ranged from 6.1% for extremely preterm (22–27 weeks), to 2.6% for very to moderate preterm (28–33 weeks), to 1.9% for late preterm (34–36 weeks), and 1.4% for term infants (39–41 weeks; Crump et al., 2021).

Attention problems. At school age, children born preterm have a higher risk for attention and behavioral difficulties compared with their full-term counterparts. These difficulties include an increased risk for attention deficit/hyperactivity disorder (ADHD), and internalizing and externalizing behavior problems (Bhutta et al., 2002), with attention deficits and executive function impairments often persisting into adolescence (Rommel et al., 2017). ADHD is the most common behavioral disorder of prematurity, with preterm infants manifesting a 2.64 increased odds of ADHD compared to children born full term. Relatedly, the need for treatment for ADHD increases with decreasing gestational age, with infants born at less than 28 weeks gestation 2.1 times more likely to require treatment for ADHD compared with term-born children (Lindström et al., 2011).

Emotional outcomes: Internalizing and externalizing behaviors. Preterm children are also at increased risk for behavior problems, including anxiety disorder, obsessive-compulsive disorder, thought problems, and social difficulties (Fevang et al., 2016; Samuelsson et al., 2017), with risks sometimes persisting into adolescence or adulthood. The odds of behavioral disorders increase with decreasing gestational age and are highest for children born at less than 28 weeks gestation (Heinonen et al., 2016).

Health-related quality of life. Infants born preterm have a lower health-related quality of life compared to their full-term counterparts. Prematurity is associated with an increased risk of rehospitalization in the first 5 years of life, with worsened health outcomes for preterm children born at earlier gestational ages. Infants born very preterm have a two-fold greater risk of hospitalization compared to infants born moderately preterm, and a three-fold greater risk of hospitalization compared to infants born late preterm, suggesting a dose-response association with the degree of prematurity (Boyle et al., 2012). Self-report questionnaires have revealed a lower quality of life in adolescents born preterm (Wolke et al., 2013). Adolescents born preterm who experience health complications and disabilities (e.g., patent ductus arteriosus, ADHD, severe neurodevelopment impairment) report a lower health-related quality of life compared to healthier preterms (Natalucci et al., 2017).

Late preterm outcomes. Late preterm infants (LPIs; gestational age: 34–36$^{6/7}$ weeks) account for 75% of preterm births, translating to more than 400,000 late preterm births per year in the United States (Davidoff et al., 2006). Several studies using nationally representative data have found that LPIs have developmental deficits compared to infants born full-term (Chan & Quigley, 2014; Shah, Kaciroti, Richards, Oh, et al., 2016; Williams et al., 2013). Although compared with very preterm infants, the magnitude of academic deficits in LPIs is relatively small, these deficits remain significant at a population level. To better inform anticipatory guidance provided to LPIs, research has begun to examine patterns of heterogeneity within LPI academic outcomes to identify patterns and predictors of risk and resilience. Higher academic achievement in reading and math in LPIs is associated with protective early childhood experiences, including sensitive parenting and preschool enrollment, whereas suboptimal academic achievement is associated with biological and psychosocial risks including prenatal smoking, multiple gestation, and low maternal education (Shah et al., 2023).

Because of the population-level significance of the intellectual, learning, and behavioral deficits associated with prematurity (even mild prematurity), these data—which reveal varying patterns of development emerging over the early childhood period—speak to the importance of longitudinal surveillance of developmental functioning of preterm infants. These varying patterns of preterm development highlight the important role of clinical developmental specialists including pediatric psychologists and developmental-behavioral pediatricians in monitoring outcomes of preterm infants and implementing targeted interventions prior to school entry to mitigate academic risk and optimize later outcomes.

PRETERM BIRTH AND THE FAMILY SYSTEM: IMPACTS ON THE CAREGIVER AND DYAD

Along with the preterm birth of the infant, there is also the "preterm birth of the parent," in which caregivers are thrust into the parenting role earlier than planned. The disruption to the anticipated transition to parenthood for the parents of preterm infants can serve as a stress to the family system, increasing the risks for difficulties with parental adaptation, development of parental affective symptoms, and vulnerabilities in dyadic interaction. Drawing from theories in developmental science, including the transactional model (e.g., Sameroff, 2009) the effects of preterm birth on parental adaptation, parental affective functioning, and quality of dyadic interactions are described further in the following sections.

Preterm Birth: A Nonnormative Transition to Parenthood

The premature birth of a baby is a sudden interruption in the process of building representations of the child and the identity formation of the parent, in which parents learn to integrate new functions related to the ability to care for, protect, empathize with, and adequately respond to the newborn (Stern & Bruschweiler-Stern, 1998). The typically joyful experience of childbirth is overshadowed by preoccupations for the preterm infant's survival, forcing the parent to adjust expectations and hopes for the child in the face of medical and developmental uncertainties (Spinelli et al., 2016). These feelings of grief and loss following preterm birth are common, affecting one out of three preterm mothers even months after delivery (Shah et al., 2011), with feelings of insecurity and grief increasingly recognized in fathers of preterm infants as well (Löhr et al., 2000; O'Donovan & Nixon, 2019).

The earliest interactions between the parent and preterm infant occur in the highly technological neonatal intensive care unit (NICU) environment, where parents have limited opportunity to stay with the baby, and caregiver participation in the care of the infant is often managed by the intense involvement of the medical staff (Haward et al., 2020; Lupton & Fenwick, 2001; Obeidat et al., 2009). The milieu of the NICU is an atypical context that can interfere with the developmental process of becoming parents, contributing to caregiver stress and vulnerabilities in the mothers' and fathers' well-being, and risks to the development of the parent–child relationship, and to later infant socioemotional development. As such, optimizing outcomes of the preterm infant requires an understanding of the effects of prematurity on the caregiver and dyad (Haward et al., 2020).

Preterm birth and posttraumatic stress. Posttraumatic stress symptoms (PTSS) following preterm birth are varied and can manifest as feelings of reexperiencing aspects of the delivery experience, attempts to avoid or ignore stimuli associated with the trauma (such as child-related and hospital-related experiences), and feelings of emotional vigilance (Callahan et al., 2006). These symptoms of emotional vigilance can present as either difficulty leaving the infant's bedside, or conversely, avoidance of the NICU (Ionio et al., 2022). Although prevalence rates for posttraumatic stress disorder (PTSD) after childbirth range from 1.7% to 9% in community samples (Beck et al., 2011), prevalence rates of perinatal PTSS and acute stress disorder in mothers of preterm infants in the NICU are often much higher, with estimates of up to 33% prevalence

(Lefkowitz et al., 2010; McKeown et al., 2023; Vanderbilt et al., 2009). Perinatal posttraumatic stress appears to affect mothers more than fathers (Helle et al., 2018; Lefkowitz et al., 2010), with some estimates of acute stress disorder as high as 39.9% (Beck et al., 2022). Although symptoms of acute stress can improve as early as 1 month into the patient's NICU stay (Lefkowitz et al., 2010), symptoms of acute stress can persist after infant hospital discharge (DeMier et al., 2000), with symptoms lasting for months and even years after delivery (Åhlund et al., 2009; Brunson et al., 2021; Kersting et al., 2004).

Many factors contribute to the traumatic stress associated with preterm birth. Across studies, parental traumatic stress is related to feelings of uncertainty regarding the infant's medical condition, experiences of alienation in the medically intrusive NICU environment, and feelings of being an "outsider" in the care of the infant, all contributing to feelings of powerlessness and of being unable to protect the infant, especially from pain and painful procedures (Obeidat et al., 2009; Woodward et al., 2014). Other factors influencing the degree of PTSD after preterm delivery are related to characteristics of delivery (i.e., cesarean section), infant's medical conditions and complications, parental history of mental problems, and history of low social support (Brunson et al., 2021; Callahan et al., 2006; Helle et al., 2018; McKeown et al., 2023).

If not resolved, symptoms of perinatal PTSD may become chronic (Barthel et al., 2020) and can contribute to the development of other affective disorders including maternal postpartum depression, anxiety, and increased fears that the child might die (Brunson et al., 2021; Lefkowitz et al., 2010). Perinatal PTSD can result in negative perceptions of parenting (Suttora et al., 2014) and dysfunctional early mother-child dyadic interactions (Coppola et al., 2007; Forcada-Guex et al., 2011; Muller-Nix et al., 2004), with implications for later child academic and behavioral functioning (Cook et al., 2018; Turpin et al., 2019). Interventions focused on alleviating PTSS have been associated with more positive mother–infant interactions (Borghini et al., 2014). This suggests that addressing maternal postpartum affective symptoms and the quality of the early dyadic relationship may be potential areas of intervention that can be targeted in the perinatal period by pediatric psychologists, or other mental health providers. Additional longitudinal research is needed to further examine the effects of parental perinatal PTSD on preterm outcomes beyond the neonatal and infancy period.

Preterm birth and caregiver parenting stress. The distress associated with preterm birth can extend beyond the period of NICU hospitalization, with some parents still reporting symptoms 3 years after the delivery. Parenting stress associated with preterm birth has been reported in both mothers and fathers and has been associated with negative perceptions of parenting (Brummelte et al., 2011; Schappin et al., 2013). Levels of parental distress do not differ between caregivers of full-term and preterm infants (Gray et al., 2012; Howe et al., 2014; Treyvaud et al., 2011), but certain parent and infant characteristics can confer added risk for persistent symptoms of perinatal distress. Higher levels of parental distress following preterm birth have been associated with the presence of other risk factors, including parents' histories of depressive symptoms or other mental health problems (Gray et al., 2012, 2013; Spinelli et al., 2013; Treyvaud et al., 2011), traumatic birth experience (Suttora et al., 2014), infant feeding issues (Howe et al., 2014), infant health and developmental risks (Brummelte et al., 2011; Schappin et al., 2013), and difficult infant temperament (Gray et al., 2013). In longitudinal studies, trajectories of parenting stress have varied, with suboptimal trajectories (and persistent stress) associated with both parent and child factors, including a history of multiple births, greater neonatal medical risks, lower maternal education, and history of depressive symptoms (Chang & Fine, 2007; Spinelli et al., 2013).

High parenting stress in preterm mothers has been associated with less positive interactions (Spinelli et al., 2013; Suttora et al., 2020) and suboptimal child development outcomes including more internalizing and externalizing behaviors in early childhood (Miceli et al., 2000). Clinical interventions focused on reducing parental stress in parents of preterm infants have demonstrated positive effects (see Sabnis et al., 2019 for a meta-analysis), thus highlighting the role that NICU behavioral health specialists (e.g., pediatric psychologists, and perinatal psychiatrists) can play to identify and mitigate parental perinatal stress following preterm birth.

Preterm birth and caregiver depressive symptoms. In both mothers and fathers, feelings of depression related to preterm birth are common, with rates as high as 28% to 40% during the period of NICU hospitalization and also after hospital discharge (Cheng et al., 2016; Hawes et al., 2016; Lotterman et al., 2019). The etiology of depression in caregivers of preterm infants is likely multifactorial and is related to psychosocial elements including low education, underemployment (Moraski Mew et al., 2003), previous maternal mental health history, lack of social support, and the stresses associated with the preterm birth and NICU course (Hawes et al., 2016; Lefkowitz et al., 2010; Tahirkheli et al., 2014). Although the symptoms of depression may lessen over time, they often continue for weeks or months after NICU discharge (Miles et al., 2007; Vanderbilt et al., 2009). There are data to suggest that patterns of maternal depression in the first 2 years after preterm birth vary by family psychosocial contexts. Decreasing trajectories of maternal depression were associated with high levels of family support, in contrast to trajectories of persistent depressive symptoms, which were associated with maternal sociodemographic risks (Poehlmann et al., 2009).

Maternal depressive symptoms following a preterm birth have been associated with more negative outcomes including more negative perceptions of themselves, their preterm baby, and the parent–child relationship (Moehler et al., 2006; Trumello et al., 2018), and less positive dyadic interactions (Korja et al., 2008; Woodward et al., 2014). Maternal depressive symptoms have also been associated with suboptimal preterm outcomes including lower cognitive outcomes (Cheng et al., 2016; McManus & Poehlmann, 2012), and higher internalizing and externalizing behaviors at 36 months (Åhlund et al., 2009), and insecure attachment (Poehlmann & Fiese, 2001a), with worse outcomes associated with greater chronicity of maternal depression (Trapolini et al., 2007).

Preterm birth and caregiver anxiety symptoms. In addition to an increased risk for perinatal stress and depression, parents of preterm infants also have a heightened risk for perinatal anxiety (Obeidat et al., 2009). During the period of NICU hospitalization, 18% to 24% of mothers of preterm infants had clinically relevant anxiety scores, with anxiety symptoms persisting in 27% 6 months after hospital discharge (Lotterman et al., 2019; Matthey et al., 2003; Vanderbilt et al., 2009). Anxiety symptoms following preterm birth may persist and remain high during the first year of life (Kersting et al., 2004; Lotterman et al., 2019), with elevated levels associated with low infant gestational age (Schmücker et al., 2005), and maternal characteristics such as underemployment and low education (Doering et al., 2000). Conversely, social support and high-quality dyadic adjustment may protect against developing anxiety symptoms both in mothers and fathers of preterm infants (Zelkowitz et al., 2007). Maternal anxiety has been associated with less responsive dyadic interactions for both the caregiver and infant (Schmücker et al., 2005; Zelkowitz et al., 2007), although longitudinal studies examining the association of caregiver anxiety with preterm outcomes are largely missing.

Preterm birth and caregiver interactive behaviors. Compared to infants born full-term, preterm infants, especially in the first months of life, manifest differences in their interactive behavior. Preterm infants are less responsive to social cues (Clark et al., 2008), demonstrate lower attentional control (Bhutta et al., 2002), manifest diminished alertness and responsivity (Goldberg, 1978; Goldberg & DiVitto, 1995; Schmücker et al., 2005), less initiation (Sajaniemi et al., 1998), increased irritability (Garcia Coll et al., 1992; Hughes et al., 2002; Larroque et al., 2005), and fewer expressions of positive affect (Garcia Coll et al., 1992) compared to their full term counterparts. In addition, preterm infants have been described as less interactive, with fewer vocalizations in response to their mother (Reissland et al., 1999; Singer et al., 2003). Preterm infants' interactive behavior has been noted to vary with infants' physiological characteristics. For instance, although preterm infants with higher vagal regulation exhibit less optimal positive affect and communication at 4 months, they showed significantly greater increases in positive affect and social and communicative competence over time, so that by 24 months, their interactive skills exceeded those of infants with lower vagal regulation (Poehlmann et al., 2011). Relatedly, longitudinal studies of preterm infant interactive behavior suggest that, on average, preterm infants' quality of play, interest, and attention increase over the first 2 years, accompanied by a decrease in dysregulation and irritability (Poehlmann et al., 2011).

Preterm infants' interactive difficulties complicate their social and affective exchanges with caregivers, who may find the infant's cues and reactions difficult to understand (Loi et al., 2017). The stressful circumstances of the NICU can further contribute to difficulties in dyadic interaction. Mothers of preterm infants appear to be less responsive and less competent at coordinating their social behaviors with the infant's signals, and have been observed to look, smile, vocalize, and affectionately touch them less often compared to mothers of full-term newborns (De Schuymer et al., 2011; Feldman & Eidelman, 2007; Forcada-Guex et al., 2006; Olafsen et al., 2006; Spinelli et al., 2022). Interactional difficulties characterized by less gaze synchrony and high unresponsiveness have also been observed between fathers and their preterm infants (Feldman & Eidelman, 2007; Neri et al., 2017).

Despite evidence suggesting parent–preterm interactional difficulties, there is also variability within the pattern of parent–preterm dyadic interactions, with not all dyads manifesting challenges (Hall et al., 2015; Neri et al., 2017; Sansavini et al., 2015). The quality of caregiver–preterm interactions can vary based on the caregiver's ability to modulate their interactions, to avoid over- or underwhelming the preterm infant's communication and arousal regulation capacities (Feldman & Eidelman, 2007; Spinelli et al., 2022). The caregiver's ability to regulate their own interactive behavior with their preterm depends on specific infant and caregiver characteristics, including neonatal risks, caregiver socioeconomic status (SES), and caregiver affective symptoms. Mothers of preterm infants with greater neonatal risk have demonstrated lower sensitivity to infant cues (Agostini et al., 2009; Bilgin & Wolke, 2015), and mothers with low SES demonstrate more intrusiveness, insensitivity, and inconsistency during interactions with their preterm infants at 4 months, with effects sustained over 24 months after hospital discharge (Poehlmann et al., 2011). Preterm mothers with high PTSD symptoms were more likely to be controlling and less sensitive during dyadic interactions (Coppola et al., 2007; Forcada-Guex et al., 2011; Muller-Nix et al., 2004), and mothers who reported parenting as a more stressful experience demonstrated less attuned, less positive interactions, and more intrusive behaviors (Spinelli et al., 2013; Suttora et al., 2020). Relatedly, depression in mothers of preterm infants (but not in fathers) is associated with lower interaction synchrony (Feldman & Eidelman, 2007), and mothers with high anxiety were observed to be less facially responsive during dyadic interactions (Schmücker et al., 2005). Both mothers and fathers with high anxiety are also less interactive during feeding their preterm newborns (Zelkowitz et al., 2007).

Preterm birth and attachment. The association between preterm birth and infant attachment security has been examined in multiple studies with mixed findings reported. Although a 1992 meta-analysis (van IJzendoorn et al., 1992) and a study by Hall et al. (2015) found no association between preterm birth and insecure attachment, other studies have found lower security scores in preterm children's attachment with their mothers and fathers compared to their full-term counterparts (Ruiz et al., 2018). One explanation for these disparate findings is that it is not preterm birth *per se* that confers a risk for insecure attachment, but rather it is the *combination* of preterm birth with other risk factors (e.g., maternal depressive symptoms) that contributes to the risk for insecure infant attachment (Doering et al., 2000). Relatedly, certain populations of preterm infants are at increased risk of insecure attachment: very preterm infants, especially those with developmental delay or distressing cry appear to be at higher risk for disorganized attachment (Wolke et al., 2014). Other risk factors associated with insecure attachment in preterm infants include a history of distorted maternal representations (Hall et al., 2015) and history of unresolved grief related to preterm birth (Shah et al., 2011). Mothers of preterm infants who had "unresolved grief" at 9 months were 2.94 times more likely to have an infant with insecure attachment at 16 months, with resolution of grief and maternal interaction quality both predicting attachment security.

FAMILY-LEVEL FACTORS, PRETERM OUTCOMES, AND IMPLICATIONS FOR INTERVENTION

Many studies have examined child and parent well-being and dyadic interactions in the context of prematurity, but associations between aspects of the family context and predictors of children's long-term outcomes following preterm birth are relatively understudied. The high financial cost of preterm birth has been documented in the United States and European countries, both for families and society (Kim et al., 2022; Lambiase et al., 2023). In addition to financial challenges, studies have examined overall family burden and dysfunction following preterm birth (Lakshmanan et al., 2022). In an Australian study, compared to families of full-term infants, families with very preterm infants reported less optimal general family functioning, including greater family burden (Treyvaud et al., 2011). These differences were somewhat attenuated when economic factors and child disability were added to the models, further underscoring that the association between preterm birth and family functioning is complex and is related to multilevel contextual factors, including SES, parental affective symptoms, and child medical risk. In a related study from the United States, Lean et al. (2020) found that lower levels of family dysfunction (in addition to lower maternal distress and fewer maternal ADHD symptoms) were associated with more optimal child trajectories of psychiatric and neurodevelopmental outcomes when children were age five. Although a growing body of evidence links family characteristics with preterm outcomes, more research is still needed focusing on family well-being over time following preterm birth.

Because the family characteristics and the quality of early dyadic interactions have implications for later preterm infant development, behavioral supports, interventions to support family processes, and financial resources may be especially helpful. Specifically, the quality of parent–infant interaction has been shown to mediate the relation between neonatal risk and cognitive development, with reciprocal and engaging dyadic interactions predicting higher cognitive scores, controlling for neonatal and maternal risks (Poehlmann & Fiese, 2001b). Relatedly, a history of cooperative dyadic interactions in early infancy has been associated with fewer behavioral problems in toddlerhood (Forcada-Guex et al., 2006). Taken together, this highlights how interventions which involve parents, and which target the quality of early interactions, can have significant effects in improving preterm infants' cognitive and behavioral outcomes (Vanderveen et al., 2009).

CLINICAL CARE FOR PRETERM INFANTS AND THEIR FAMILIES: INTERDISCIPLINARY MODELS OF CARE IN THE NEONATAL PERIOD

Models of care for preterm infants have evolved to become more individualized as well as child- and family-focused. These models of care include environmental changes in the physical organization of the NICU and different approaches that have increasingly tried to foster family involvement in the care of their preterm infant. Although these models of care have not been universally implemented, they reflect a gradual transition to adopting a more inclusive, family-centered approach to the NICU care of preterm infants.

NICU Interventions to Facilitate Family Bonding

The organization of the NICU has evolved from the initial structure of large open rooms with multiple patient beds in close proximity to each other to single-family rooms (Lester et al., 2014; White et al., 2013). This transition has helped to protect the infant from intrusive environmental stimuli of the NICU and has had the added benefit of facilitating round-the-clock family presence by providing spaces where families can reside in one room for the duration of the newborn's NICU experience (Kuhn et al., 2013; Örtenstrand et al., 2010; Santos et al., 2015). In addition to this change in the physical space, NICUs have increasingly adopted a "neuroprotective" approach, emphasizing developmentally appropriate care during sensitive periods of rapid brain development. This approach has included involving families to foster supportive positioning and handling, safeguarding sleep, initiating interventions to minimize stress and pain with procedures, and optimizing nutrition to foster a "healing environment" in the NICU (Janelle Santos et al., 2015).

Evidence-Based NICU Interventions

Several NICU interventions have been developed to foster infant regulation and to support the quality of the early caregiving relationship. The most widely studied include Kangaroo Care (Charpak et al., 2001; Tessier et al., 2003), The Newborn Individualized Developmental Care and Assessment Program (NIDCAP; Als et al., 2003), and the Family Nurture Intervention (FNI; Welch et al., 2012). These models of care have adopted an interdisciplinary approach, involving a broad range of providers including nurses, social workers, parent support liaisons, and behavioral health professionals including psychologists and psychiatrists.

Kangaroo care. Kangaroo care (also referred to as skin-to-skin care) is one of the most commonly instituted NICU interventions, designed to promote early coregulation and attuned relationships between the parent and preterm infant. Kangaroo care is an evidence-based practice that has been increasingly promoted for both full term and high-risk preterm infants (Boundy et al., 2016). Kangaroo care includes three elements: (a) "kangaroo positioning" manifest by continuous skin-to-skin contact between the parent and infant, (b) exclusive breastfeeding when possible, and (c) early discharge with close follow-up. Kangaroo care has been associated with a wide range of benefits including increased survival, more optimal neurodevelopment, longer breastfeeding duration, and early maternal–infant bonding (Charpak et al., 2001; Tessier et al., 2003). Effects of kangaroo care have been observed to persist into adulthood with intergenerational social and behavioral protective effects observed (Charpak et al., 2017). Parents who experienced kangaroo care in their infancy were more protective and nurturing, and children who experienced kangaroo care manifested decreased externalizing and less socially deviant behavior in early adulthood (Charpak et al., 2017).

Neonatal individualized developmental care and assessment program. NIDCAP was developed as a holistic philosophy of care for infants in the NICU with the aims of fostering infant neurodevelopment and physiologic regulation, supporting parent–infant interactions, increasing parent involvement, and promoting early breastfeeding. NIDCAP was designed to provide individualized developmental care, tailored to the needs of the infant and family, to foster the infant's neurobehavioral organization. Numerous studies, including randomized control trials, have demonstrated numerous positive outcomes including more optimal infant neurodevelopment and greater parental involvement as a result of implementation of the NIDCAP program (Als et al., 1994, 2003; Westrup et al., 2004). Notably, the preterm infants who appeared to benefit the most from NIDCAP implementation were infants born more preterm (<29 weeks gestation) who had strong parental involvement (Örtenstrand et al., 2010).

Family nurture intervention. The Family Nurture Intervention (Welch et al., 2012) was developed to foster dyadic coregulation between the infant and parent by supporting their "early holding environment" (Hane et al., 2015; Welch et al., 2012). This intervention was designed to foster emotional attunement between the parent and child in the NICU with the aim of optimizing infant development, supporting the early dyadic relationship, and promoting caregiver emotional well-being (Welch et al., 2012). Numerous positive infant and family outcomes have been associated with the FNI including enhanced infant physiological regulation (Porges et al., 2019), more positive early dyadic interactions (Beebe et al., 2018), more optimal social, attention, and neurodevelopmental outcomes at 18 months (Welch et al., 2015), and improved theory of mind skills at school age (Firestein et al., 2022). The FNI approach has also been associated with benefits to the caregiver, manifesting in lower symptoms of anxiety and depression (Welch et al., 2013, 2014). Outcomes associated with this program have demonstrated enhanced infant, parent, and dyadic coregulation, more attuned parent–infant relationships and interactions, and better caregiver emotional well-being.

MENTAL HEALTH AND PSYCHOLOGICAL SUPPORTS IN THE NICU SETTING: THE ROLE OF PEDIATRIC PSYCHOLOGY AND PERINATAL MENTAL HEALTH PROFESSIONALS

Infants who begin their lives in the NICU often have challenges to their early regulation, and to later cognitive, social, and emotional development, but some of these risks can be mitigated through the promotion of early secure and nurturing relationships with a primary caregiver. To foster the quality of early dyadic relationships in the NICU, and to optimize parental adaptation to having a baby born preterm, neonatal care teams have expanded to include behavioral health specialists. The inclusion of perinatal mental health professionals (PMHPs) encompasses a variety of professional disciplines, including social workers, psychologists, psychotherapists, and psychiatrists. The roles of PMHPs can vary but often include providing emotional support, screening, education, psychotherapy, and potentially mental health referrals to families with the aim of fostering parental adaptation to preterm birth (Hynan et al., 2013). In addition, PMHPs can also support families by providing referrals to resources to assist with financial or other specific concerns such as food insecurity, housing insecurity, intimate partner violence, and substance issues. National standards in the United States have recommended that NICUs should have at least one full-time master's-level social worker and one full-time doctoral-level psychologist embedded in the NICU staff for the purposes of screening, counseling, providing staff education, and teaching parenting skills. In many large NICUs, this care is provided by pediatric psychologists (Hynan et al., 2015). Perinatal psychological services in the NICU can include assessment for parental perinatal psychological distress, screening for psychiatric diagnoses, and providing a variety of treatments including interpersonal therapy, cognitive behavior therapy, trauma-focused psychotherapy, couples and family therapy, mindfulness training, and infant mental health approaches. Perinatal pediatric psychologists can also provide education and support to other members of the NICU team regarding the importance of the early dyadic relationship and potential parental reactions to the NICU experience including feelings of guilt, shame, anger, distress, bereavement, and trauma, especially in the context of previous infertility or perinatal losses (Hynan et al., 2015).

The role of pediatric psychologists in supporting parental adaptation to preterm birth. Parents who unexpectedly find themselves in an intensive care unit after a high-risk birth are known to experience a myriad of stressful events which can contribute to the development of postpartum depression and symptoms of anxiety and post-traumatic stress, which can challenge the early dyadic relationship. As such, in meeting with families, the perinatal pediatric psychologist or other NICU mental health provider has an opportunity to identify parents with clinical levels of symptoms as well as parents with subclinical levels of symptoms who are at risk and who may benefit from ongoing monitoring and support during or after NICU discharge (Dempsey et al., 2022). Ideally, a family-centered NICU should include the presence of peer-to-peer support for the parent, who can work with the NICU staff, and a perinatal mental health provider to identify parents with emotional distress and perinatal mood symptoms.

Perinatal mental health providers (including perinatal pediatric psychologists and infant mental health specialists) should aim to meet with all parents in the NICU to (a) reinforce and normalize the experience of parental emotional distress, (b) reduce perceptions of stigma associated with behavioral health intervention, and (c) initiate the process of providing multilevel supports while in the NICU. These supports can include anticipatory parenting guidance to fortify the early dyadic relationship, administering and interpreting screening and assessment measures, providing basic mental health intervention to help parents in their psychological adjustment and coping with a medically fragile infant, and, when indicated, assisting with care coordination to refer parents to other mental health resources (Hall et al., 2015). Perinatal mental health providers can also help foster the development of the early relationship, by assisting parents in fostering their infant's regulation in the NICU. As the time of neonatal discharge approaches, the perinatal mental health provider can also facilitate referrals for continuing supports around these areas as the family transitions to the home.

In the NICU, the perinatal mental health provider can facilitate a parent's involvement in the care of the preterm infant while in the hospital and can identify barriers to parent engagement. The PMHP can create opportunities to ensure that the parent receives current and frequent communications about the baby and can promote opportunities to help parents feel included in decision making about their infant's care. PMHPs can also help connect families to resources to foster resilience and facilitate parental coping with the challenges of having an infant in the NICU. Parental coping strategies should be individualized according to the family's spiritual beliefs, personality traits, and particular needs for social support, with the overarching goal to foster parental engagement and involvement in their infant's care (Craig et al., 2015).

Screening for parental mental health concerns in the NICU. For behavior health providers working in the NICU (including pediatric psychologists), guidelines have been suggested regarding screening for parental emotional distress (Hynan et al., 2013, 2015). These recommendations include meeting all parents or primary caregivers within the first few days of NICU admission and screening within the first week to evaluate for symptoms of emotional distress using a validated instrument. Because parental symptoms of emotional distress can change throughout the infant's hospitalization, families should be rescreened periodically and within 48 hours of discharge. Parents/caregivers who are positive on an initial screen should be followed up with more comprehensive screening or assessment. In addition, parents should be connected to supports and services while in the NICU and after discharge to optimize their emotional well-being in transitioning home. Because symptoms of grief, trauma, and psychological distress can persist after NICU discharge, screening for emotional distress should also be considered in neonatal follow-up programs (Hynan et al., 2015). Examples of validated instruments to screen for parental psychological distress are listed in Table 17.1.

For at-risk or symptomatic parents, perinatal pediatric psychologists and other perinatal mental

TABLE 17.1

Instruments to Screen for Parental Psychological Distress

Instrument	Description	Scoring/interpretation
Depression		
Patient Health Questionnaire 2 question screener (Kroenke et al., 2003)	2-item (scores 0–3) questionnaire	Range: 0–6; scores ≥3 suggest risk of depression and need for further evaluation
Patient Health Questionnaire 9 question screener (Kroenke et al., 2001)	9-item (scores 0–3) questionnaire	Range: 0–27; scores 1–4: minimal depression; 5–9: mild depression; 10–14: moderate depression; 15–19: moderately severe depression; 20–27: severe depression
Beck Depression Inventory, 2nd edition (Beck et al., 1996)	21-item (scores 0–3) questionnaire	Range: 0–63; scores ≥20 meet clinical cutoff for depression
Center for Epidemiologic Studies-Depression Scale (Radloff, 1977)	20-item (scores 0–3) questionnaire	Range: 0–60; scores ≥16 meet clinical cutoff for depression
Edinburgh Postnatal Depression Scale (Cox et al., 1987)	10-item (scores 0–3) questionnaire	Range: 0–30; scores ≥10 suggest risk of depression and need for further evaluation
Posttraumatic stress disorder/parental stress		
Primary Care PTSD Screener for *DSM-5* (Prins et al., 1999)	5-item (scores 0–1)	Range: 0–5; scores ≥3 (in women) suggest risk of PTSD
Acute Stress Disorder Scale (Bryant et al., 2000)	19-item (scores 1–5)	Range: 19–95; scores >56 suggest acute stress disorder, and risk for developing PTSD
Posttraumatic Stress Disorder Checklist for *DSM-5* (Ashbaugh et al., 2016)	20-item (scores 0–4)	Range: 0–80; scores ≥31 suggest clinical level of PTSD
Parental Stressor Scale: Neonatal Intensive Care Unit (Miles et al., 1993)	34-item (scores 0–5)	Range: 0–170; higher scores indicate greater parent stress
Perinatal Posttraumatic Stress Disorder Questionnaire (Callahan et al., 2006)	14-item (scores 0–4)	Range: 0–56; scores ≥19 suggest clinical need for referral
Davidson Trauma Scale (Davidson, n.d.)	17-item (scores 0–4)	Range 0–68; scores ≥40 indicate clinical levels of PTSD
Anxiety		
Beck Anxiety Inventory (Beck et al., 1988)	21-item (score 0–3)	Range: 0–63; scores ≥16 suggest clinical level of anxiety
Generalized Anxiety Disorder-7 (Löwe et al., 2008)	7-item (score 0–3)	Range: 0–21; scores ≥8 suggest clinical level of anxiety

Note. Data from Bernardo et al. (2021). *DSM-5* = fifth edition of the *Diagnostic and Statistical Manual of Mental Disorders* (American Psychiatric Association, 2013).

health providers can provide relational and psychological supports to parents to focus on parental mental health and to foster the development of the early dyadic relationship. At the time of NICU discharge, perinatal pediatric psychologists can provide additional counseling or support to parents as they transition home and can help assist with care coordination to connect with supports and services in the community (e.g., infant mental health supports, peer-to-peer supports, nurse home visiting).

While having an infant in the NICU is traumatic for the parents, caring for an infant in the NICU can also be a source of trauma for the NICU providers and neonatal staff. The NICU staff may need to participate in painful procedures for the infant, and as the hospitalization course unfolds, they accompany families if complications arise. Hospital staff may observe the process of an infant dying, may witness an infant's death and often provide support to the family in their time of grieving. Over time, these experiences can lead to a secondary trauma for neonatal providers. Pediatric psychologists and perinatal mental health providers can also provide a psychological "holding environment" for the staff, helping them to reflect and process their own experiences of secondary traumatic stress, and their need for support in their professional role (Lorrain, 2016). The PMHP can create a collaborative partnership with the NICU providers to facilitate a "parallel process" to help NICU providers and staff process their own feelings and experiences which may arise in the context of their infant-parent encounters, especially in the context of stressful NICU events. By this role, the perinatal mental health provider can serve as source of support, and encouragement for the NICU team, thus helping to facilitate a culture of professional resilience in the NICU.

The role of behavioral health providers in discharge planning and transition to home. The transition from the NICU to home can result in intense and complex emotions for the family. While NICU discharge readiness for infants is reflected by the infant's physiological maturity, and evidence of stability associated with health sequelae, discharge readiness for *parents* is defined by parental comfort, confidence and skill regarding the medical care of a high risk infant at the time of discharge (Purdy et al., 2015). Discharge preparation is an opportunity to help parents develop a sense of competence and self-efficacy in the role of parenting their preterm infant, by helping them develop knowledge, skills, and confidence to successfully transition home. Recognizing that the transition home from the NICU is a potentially vulnerable and stressful time for families, NICU discharge planning should include a focus on caregiver psychosocial support, and the needs of the caregiver–child relationship (Murch & Smith, 2016). Perinatal psychologists and the perinatal care team can help facilitate the transition to home by identifying resources and facilitating referrals to appropriate community-based supports. These supports can include referrals to early intervention programs, nurse home-visiting programs, infant mental health programs, and referrals for ongoing developmental surveillance in a neonatal follow-up program for high-risk infants. Pediatric psychologists who practice in NICUs, home-visiting programs, community-based settings, and neonatal follow-up programs have an opportunity to serve as a "bridge of continuity" for families, to help support high-risk infants and their families in the transition from the neonatal ICU to home (Zeanah, 2018).

DEVELOPMENTAL SURVEILLANCE AND LONGITUDINAL MONITORING IN NEONATAL FOLLOW-UP PROGRAMS: THE ROLES OF PEDIATRIC PSYCHOLOGY AND DEVELOPMENTAL-BEHAVIORAL PEDIATRICS

After NICU discharge, follow-up care should be established with the primary care provider. For all preterm infants, periodic evaluation of developmental status is indicated to monitor for the emergence of age-expected skills, to identify deviations when they occur, and to initiate appropriate evaluations and early interventions. Most preterm infants receive this longitudinal developmental surveillance with their primary care provider, but for select populations of preterm infants (e.g., medically complex, high-risk, or extremely preterm) developmental monitoring may be provided in the context of a neonatal follow-up clinic which provides multidisciplinary care (American Academy of Pediatrics, 2008). Although the structure, composition, eligibility criteria, and developmental assessment practices of neonatal follow-up programs vary widely across centers (Kuppala et al., 2012), neonatal follow-up clinics typically include a provider skilled in developmental assessment (e.g., a pediatric psychologist, developmental-behavioral pediatrician, et al.) who can perform standardized assessments of the preterm infant for the purpose of developmental monitoring. An exhaustive review of the different models of care of neonatal follow-up programs is beyond the scope of this chapter; the reader is referred to published resources from the American Academy of Pediatrics for further information (e.g., Campbell & Imaizumi, 2020).

In the context of the neonatal follow-up clinic, the developmental provider (pediatric psychologist, developmental-behavioral pediatrician, et al.) can assess infants' developmental and behavioral skills using standardized tools validated for use in high-risk infants and can screen for parental mental health symptoms which can serve as a vulnerability for the developing parent–child dyad. When developmental risks are identified, pediatric psychologists and developmental-behavioral pediatricians can recommend necessary supports and services to help optimize the preterm infant's developmental potential. Because preterm infants are at high risk for developmental-behavioral conditions (e.g., hearing and vision impairment, intellectual disability, ADHD, autism, developmental delay, learning disabilities, emotional and behavioral disorders, etc.), pediatric psychologists and developmental-behavioral pediatricians can also monitor the child longitudinally for the emergence of symptoms for these conditions (e.g., in infancy, preschool and school-age periods) and provide diagnostic assessment for these disorders when indicated. Additional information about developmental assessment in infancy can be found in Chapter 25 of this volume. The assessment of learning and cognition in the preschool- and school-age child is further described in Chapter 26 of this volume.

In the neonatal follow-up program, additional roles of the pediatric psychologists and developmental-behavioral pediatricians are to support the family and help coordinate with community and school-based services to optimize children's long-term outcomes. Because the emergence of developmental delays can contribute to experiences of "re-grieving" in the parents of preterm children, developmental providers in the neonatal follow-up clinic are also well poised to monitor for potential affective symptoms in the parent and to provide referrals for supports and services to foster caregiver well-being when concerns are identified.

CONCLUSION AND FUTURE DIRECTIONS

Preterm birth is a complex disorder with a multifactorial etiology and multifinal sequelae. The consequences of preterm birth affect the entire family, resulting in long-standing impacts on the preterm child, caregiver, and caregiver–child relationship. Preterm infants are at increased risk for neurodevelopmental and behavioral sequelae which can persist throughout the life course. For parents, preterm birth can be a traumatic experience in which this nonnormative transition to parenthood is associated with anxiety, grief, and trauma, which can persist long beyond the infant's hospital discharge (Zeanah, 2018). Taken together, to optimize outcomes of prematurity for both the child and family, the approach to caring for preterm infants must extend beyond a purely "medical model" and must be informed by research and practice across disciplines, including pediatrics, pediatric psychology, and developmental and family science.

Despite decades of research focused on understanding the antecedents and outcomes of prematurity, many unanswered questions remain regarding what underlies the heterogeneity of predictors and sequelae associated with preterm birth. Preterm birth outcomes are not solely attributed to gestational age or level of neonatal risk but are related to multilevel, biopsychosocial-ecological factors that mutually interact. Informed by developmental science, future research should continue to examine the multilevel predictors associated with child, parent, and family outcomes, and to identify potential intervention targets to help families thrive. Recognizing that prematurity affects the family system, interdisciplinary models of care which include pediatric psychologists and developmental-behavioral pediatricians are necessary to promote family resilience following preterm birth and to mitigate the social determinants of maternal and child health underlying health disparities associated with prematurity.

RESOURCES

For Providers

- March of Dimes:

    https://www.marchofdimes.org/our-work/nicu-family-support

    NICU Family Support® (NFS) Classic and Virtual Models: NFS is offered in more than 70 neonatal intensive care units (NICUs) across the U.S. to provide family education, staff training on patient-centered care and an improved patient experience with the support of March of Dimes experts.

- The National Perinatal Association:
  https://www.nationalperinatal.org

  A community of parents and providers that takes an explicitly interdisciplinary approach to perinatal and NICU care. It promotes evidence-based practices and supports education, advocacy, and integration of care modalities.

- National Network of NICU Psychologists:
  https://www.nationalperinatal.org/psychologists

  An initiative of the National Perinatal Association, to optimize care for all infants and their families in NICU settings.

- World Health Organization (WHO). (2023). *Fact sheet: Preterm birth.* https://www.who.int/news-room/fact-sheets/detail/preterm-birth

  WHO's educational resource on preterm birth.

- Centers for Disease Control and Prevention (CDC). (2023). *Preterm birth.* https://www.cdc.gov/reproductivehealth/maternalinfant=health/pretermbirth.htm

  Educational website from the CDC's Division of Reproductive Health.

- Lauriello, N. F., & Aylward, G. P. (2023). Follow-up of the NICU patient: Overview, benefits of birth at regional centers, patient education. *Medscape.* https://emedicine.medscape.com/article/1833812-overview?form=fpf

  This article is intended to inform pediatricians, family practitioners, other health professionals, and families about the follow-up care of NICU graduates, focusing particularly on the needs of premature infants.

- Craig, J. W., Glick, C., Phillips, R., Hall, S. L., Smith, J., & Browne, J. (2015). Recommendations for involving the family in developmental care of the NICU baby. *Journal of Perinatology, 35*(Suppl. 1), S5–S8. https://doi.org/10.1038/jp.2015.142

  Recommendations for involving the family in developmental care of the NICU baby.

- Hynan, M. T., Steinberg, Z., Baker, L., Cicco, R., Geller, P. A., Lassen, S., Milford, C., Mounts, K. O., Patterson, C., Saxton, S., Segre, L., & Stuebe, A. (2015). Recommendations for mental health professionals in the NICU. *Journal of Perinatology, 35*(Suppl. 1), S14–S18. https://doi.org/10.1038/jp.2015.144.

  Recommendations for mental health professionals in the NICU.

- Dempsey, A. G., Cole, J. C. M., & Saxton, S. N. (2022). *Behavioral health services with high-risk infants and families: Meeting the needs of patients, families, and providers in fetal, neonatal intensive care unit, and neonatal follow-up settings.* Oxford University Press.

  A comprehensive, practical resource for behavioral health clinicians for multiple settings related to care of high-risk infants.

For Parents

March of Dimes:

- March of Dimes. (2017). *Coping with stress in the NICU.* https://www.marchofdimes.org/find-support/topics/neonatal-intensive-care-unit-nicu/coping-stress-nicu

  Parental resource from the March of Dimes to address parents' feelings regarding having a baby in the NICU.

- March of Dimes. (n.d.). *Unspoken stories.* https://www.marchofdimes.org/find-support/community-stories/unspoken-stories

Parental resource from the March of Dimes to find support and encouragement from other NICU parents.

HealthyChildren.org:

- HealthyChildren.org. (2019). *Your preemie's growth and developmental milestones.* https://www.healthychildren.org/English/ages-stages/baby/preemie/Pages/Preemie-Milestones.aspx

- HealthyChildren.org. (2015). *Fact sheet: Caring for a premature baby: What parents need to know.* https://www.healthychildren.org/English/ages-stages/baby/preemie/pages/Caring-For-A-Premature-Baby.aspx

Resources that give parents of a premature newborn a sense of what they can expect and advice on how to cope with stress.

Pathways.org:

- Pathways.org. (n.d.). *Premature baby.* https://pathways.org/preemie-nicu/preemie/

Parental resources to support the development of preterm infants.

Vroom.org:

- Vroom.org. (n.d.). *Sharing the science of early brain development.* https://www.vroom.org/about

Vroom is a free suite of tools that encourages parents and caregivers to play an active role in a young child's brain development.

- Tools and resources:

  https://www.vroom.org/tools-and-resources

A curated collection of evidence-informed parenting tools, tips, and resources to foster early child development for children ages 0–5 years.

References

Agostini, F., Monti, F., Fagandini, P., Duncan De Pascalis, L. L., La Sala, G. B., & Blickstein, I. (2009). Parental mental representations during late pregnancy and early parenthood following assisted reproductive technology. *Journal of Perinatal Medicine, 37*(4), 320–327. https://doi.org/10.1515/JPM.2009.062

Åhlund, S., Clarke, P., Hill, J., & Thalange, N. K. S. (2009). Post-traumatic stress symptoms in mothers of very low birth weight infants 2–3 years postpartum. *Archives of Women's Mental Health, 12*(4), 261–264. https://doi.org/10.1007/s00737-009-0067-4

Allen, M. C., Cristofalo, E. A., & Kim, C. (2011). Outcomes of preterm infants: Morbidity replaces mortality. *Clinics in Perinatology, 38*(3), 441–454. https://doi.org/10.1016/j.clp.2011.06.011

Als, H., Gilkerson, L., Duffy, F. H., McAnulty, G. B., Buehler, D. M., Vandenberg, K., Sweet, N., Sell, E., Parad, R. B., Ringer, S. A., Butler, S. C., Blickman, J. G., & Jones, K. J. (2003). A three-center, randomized, controlled trial of individualized developmental care for very low birth weight preterm infants: Medical, neurodevelopmental, parenting, and caregiving effects. *Journal of Developmental and Behavioral Pediatrics, 24*(6), 399–408. https://doi.org/10.1097/00004703-200312000-00001

Als, H., Lawhon, G., Duffy, F. H., McAnulty, G. B., Gibes-Grossman, R., & Blickman, J. G. (1994). Individualized developmental care for the very low-birth-weight preterm infant. Medical and neurofunctional effects. *JAMA: Journal of the American Medical Association, 272*(11), 853–858. https://doi.org/10.1001/jama.1994.03520110033025

American Academy of Pediatrics Committee on Fetus and Newborn. (2008). Hospital discharge of the high-risk neonate. *Pediatrics, 122*(5), 1119–1126. https://doi.org/10.1542/peds.2008-2174

American Psychiatric Association. (2013). *Diagnostic and statistical manual of mental disorders* (5th ed.). American Psychiatric Publishing.

Ashbaugh, A. R., Houle-Johnson, S., Herbert, C., El-Hage, W., & Brunet, A. (2016). Psychometric validation of the English and French versions of the posttraumatic stress disorder checklist for DSM-5 (PCL-5). *PLOS ONE, 11*(10), e0161645. https://doi.org/10.1371/journal.pone.0161645

Barthel, D., Göbel, A., Barkmann, C., Helle, N., & Bindt, C. (2020). Does birth-related trauma last? Prevalence and risk factors for posttraumatic stress in mothers and fathers of VLBW preterm and term born children 5 years after birth. [Original Research]. *Frontiers in Psychiatry, 11*, 575429. https://doi.org/10.3389/fpsyt.2020.575429

Beck, A. F., Edwards, E. M., Horbar, J. D., Howell, E. A., McCormick, M. C., & Pursley, D. M. (2020). The color of health: How racism, segregation, and inequality affect the health and well-being of preterm infants and their families. *Pediatric Research, 87*(2), 227–234. https://doi.org/10.1038/s41390-019-0513-6

Beck, A. T., Epstein, N., Brown, G., & Steer, R. A. (1988). An inventory for measuring clinical anxiety: psychometric properties. *Journal of Consulting and Clinical Psychology*, 56(6), 893–897. https://doi.org/10.1037//0022-006x.56.6.893

Beck, A. T., Steer, R. A., & Brown, G. (1996). *Beck Depression Inventory–II (BDI-II)* [Database record]. APA PsycTests. https://doi.org/10.1037/t00742-000

Beck, C. T., Gable, R. K., Sakala, C., & Declercq, E. R. (2011). Posttraumatic stress disorder in new mothers: Results from a two-stage U.S. national survey. *Birth: Issues in Perinatal Care*, 38(3), 216–227. https://doi.org/10.1111/j.1523-536X.2011.00475.x

Beck, D. C., Tabb, K. M., Tilea, A., Hall, S. V., Vance, A., Patrick, S. W., Schroeder, A., & Zivin, K. (2022). The association between NICU Admission and mental health diagnoses among commercially insured postpartum women in the US, 2010–2018. *Children*, 9(10), 1550. https://doi.org/10.3390/children9101550

Beebe, B., Myers, M. M., Lee, S. H., Lange, A., Ewing, J., Rubinchik, N., Andrews, H., Austin, J., Hane, A., Margolis, A. E., Hofer, M., Ludwig, R. J., & Welch, M. G. (2018). Family nurture intervention for preterm infants facilitates positive mother-infant face-to-face engagement at 4 months. *Developmental Psychology*, 54(11), 2016–2031. https://doi.org/10.1037/dev0000557

Bernardo, J., Rent, S., Arias-Shah, A., Hoge, M. K., & Shaw, R. J. (2021). Parental stress and mental health symptoms in the NICU: Recognition and interventions. *NeoReviews*, 22(8), e496–e505. https://doi.org/10.1542/neo.22-8-e496

Bhutta, A. T., Cleves, M. A., Casey, P. H., Cradock, M. M., & Anand, K. J. (2002). Cognitive and behavioral outcomes of school-aged children who were born preterm: A meta-analysis. *JAMA: Journal of the American Medical Association*, 288(6), 728–737. https://doi.org/10.1001/jama.288.6.728

Bilgin, A., & Wolke, D. (2015). Maternal sensitivity in parenting preterm children: a meta-analysis. *Pediatrics*, peds. 2014-3570.

Blencowe, H., Cousens, S., Chou, D., Oestergaard, M., Say, L., Moller, A.-B., Kinney, M., Lawn, J., & the Born Too Soon Preterm Birth Action Group. (2013). Born too soon: The global epidemiology of 15 million preterm births. *Reproductive Health*, 10(Suppl. 1), S2. https://doi.org/10.1186/1742-4755-10-S1-S2

Blencowe, H., Cousens, S., Oestergaard, M. Z., Chou, D., Moller, A.-B., Narwal, R., Adler, A., Vera Garcia, C., Rohde, S., Say, L., & Lawn, J. E. (2012). National, regional, and worldwide estimates of preterm birth rates in the year 2010 with time trends since 1990 for selected countries: A systematic analysis and implications. *The Lancet*, 379(9832), 2162–2172. https://doi.org/10.1016/S0140-6736(12)60820-4

Borghini, A., Habersaat, S., Forcada-Guex, M., Nessi, J., Pierrehumbert, B., Ansermet, F., & Müller-Nix, C. (2014). Effects of an early intervention on maternal post-traumatic stress symptoms and the quality of mother-infant interaction: The case of preterm birth. *Infant Behavior & Development*, 37(4), 624–631. https://doi.org/10.1016/j.infbeh.2014.08.003

Boundy, E. O., Dastjerdi, R., Spiegelman, D., Fawzi, W. W., Missmer, S. A., Lieberman, E., Kajeepeta, S., Wall, S., & Chan, G. J. (2016). Kangaroo mother care and neonatal outcomes: A meta-analysis. *Pediatrics*, 137(1), e20152238. https://doi.org/10.1542/peds.2015-2238

Boyle, E. M., Poulsen, G., Field, D. J., Kurinczuk, J. J., Wolke, D., Alfirevic, Z., & Quigley, M. A. (2012). Effects of gestational age at birth on health outcomes at 3 and 5 years of age: Population based cohort study. *BMJ: British Medical Journal*, 344, e896. https://doi.org/10.1136/bmj.e896

Bronfenbrenner, U., & Morris, P. A. (2006). The bioecological model of human development. In R. M. Lerner & W. Damon (Eds.), *Handbook of child psychology: Theoretical models of human development* (6th ed., pp. 793–828). Wiley.

Brumbaugh, J. E., Weaver, A. L., Myers, S. M., Voigt, R. G., & Katusic, S. K. (2020). Gestational age, perinatal characteristics, and autism spectrum disorder: A birth cohort study. *The Journal of Pediatrics*, 220, 175–183.e8. https://doi.org/10.1016/j.jpeds.2020.01.022

Brummelte, S., Grunau, R. E., Synnes, A. R., Whitfield, M. F., & Petrie-Thomas, J. (2011). Declining cognitive development from 8 to 18 months in preterm children predicts persisting higher parenting stress. *Early Human Development*, 87(4), 273–280. https://doi.org/10.1016/j.earlhumdev.2011.01.030

Brunson, E., Thierry, A., Ligier, F., Vulliez-Coady, L., Novo, A., Rolland, A.-C., & Eutrope, J. (2021). Prevalences and predictive factors of maternal trauma through 18 months after premature birth: A longitudinal, observational and descriptive study. *PLOS ONE*, 16(2), e0246758. https://doi.org/10.1371/journal.pone.0246758

Bryant, R. A., Moulds, M. L., & Guthrie, R. M. (2000). Acute Stress Disorder Scale: A self-report measure of acute stress disorder. *Psychological Assessment*, 12(1), 61–68. https://doi.org/10.1037/1040-3590.12.1.61

Callahan, J. L., Borja, S. E., & Hynan, M. T. (2006). Modification of the Perinatal PTSD Questionnaire to enhance clinical utility. *Journal of Perinatology*, *26*(9), 533–539. https://doi.org/10.1038/sj.jp.7211562

Campbell, D. E., & Imaizumi, S. O. (2020). Health and developmental outcomes of very preterm and very low-birth-weight infants. In D. E. Campbell (Ed.), *Neonatology for primary care* (2nd ed., pp. 1127–1170). American Academy of Pediatrics Itasca. https://doi.org/10.1542/9781610022255-41

Chambers, B. D., Baer, R. J., McLemore, M. R., & Jelliffe-Pawlowski, L. L. (2019). Using index of concentration at the extremes as indicators of structural racism to evaluate the association with preterm birth and infant mortality—California, 2011–2012. *Journal of Urban Health*, *96*(2), 159–170. https://doi.org/10.1007/s11524-018-0272-4

Chan, E., & Quigley, M. A. (2014). School performance at age 7 years in late preterm and early term birth: A cohort study. *Archives of Disease in Childhood. Fetal and Neonatal Edition*, *99*(6), F451–F457. https://doi.org/10.1136/archdischild-2014-306124

Chang, H. H., Larson, J., Blencowe, H., Spong, C. Y., Howson, C. P., Cairns-Smith, S., Lackritz, E. M., Lee, S. K., Mason, E., Serazin, A. C., Walani, S., Simpson, J. L., Lawn, J. E., & the Born Too Soon preterm prevention analysis group. (2013). Preventing preterm births: Analysis of trends and potential reductions with interventions in 39 countries with very high human development index. *The Lancet*, *381*(9862), 223–234. https://doi.org/10.1016/S0140-6736(12)61856-X

Chang, Y., & Fine, M. A. (2007). Modeling parenting stress trajectories among low-income young mothers across the child's second and third years: Factors accounting for stability and change. *Journal of Family Psychology*, *21*(4), 584–594. https://doi.org/10.1037/0893-3200.21.4.584

Charpak, N., Ruiz-Pelaez, J. G., Figueroa de C, Z., & Charpak, Y. (2001). A randomized, controlled trial of kangaroo mother care: Results of follow-up at 1 year of corrected age. *Pediatrics*, *108*(5), 1072–1079. https://doi.org/10.1542/peds.108.5.1072

Charpak, N., Tessier, R., Ruiz, J. G., Hernandez, J. T., Uriza, F., Villegas, J., Nadeau, L., Mercier, C., Maheu, F., Marin, J., Cortes, D., Gallego, J. M., & Maldonado, D. (2017). Twenty-year follow-up of kangaroo mother care versus traditional care. *Pediatrics*, *139*(1), e20162063. https://doi.org/10.1542/peds.2016-2063

Cheng, E. R., Kotelchuck, M., Gerstein, E. D., Taveras, E. M., & Poehlmann-Tynan, J. (2016). Postnatal depressive symptoms among mothers and fathers of infants born preterm: Prevalence and impacts on children's early cognitive function. *Journal of Developmental and Behavioral Pediatrics*, *37*(1), 33–42. https://doi.org/10.1097/DBP.0000000000000233

Clark, C. A., Woodward, L. J., Horwood, L. J., & Moor, S. (2008). Development of emotional and behavioral regulation in children born extremely preterm and very preterm: Biological and social influences. *Child Development*, *79*(5), 1444–1462. https://doi.org/10.1111/j.1467-8624.2008.01198.x

Cook, N., Ayers, S., & Horsch, A. (2018). Maternal posttraumatic stress disorder during the perinatal period and child outcomes: A systematic review. *Journal of Affective Disorders*, *225*, 18–31. https://doi.org/10.1016/j.jad.2017.07.045

Coppola, G., Cassibba, R., & Costantini, A. (2007). What can make the difference? Premature birth and maternal sensitivity at 3 months of age: The role of attachment organization, traumatic reaction and baby's medical risk. *Infant Behavior & Development*, *30*(4), 679–684. https://doi.org/10.1016/j.infbeh.2007.03.004

Cox, J. L., Holden, J. M., & Sagovsky, R. (1987). Detection of postnatal depression. Development of the 10-item Edinburgh Postnatal Depression Scale. *The British Journal of Psychiatry*, *150*(6), 782–786. https://doi.org/10.1192/bjp.150.6.782

Craig, J. W., Glick, C., Phillips, R., Hall, S. L., Smith, J., & Browne, J. (2015). Recommendations for involving the family in developmental care of the NICU baby. *Journal of Perinatology*, *35*(Suppl. 1), S5–S8. https://doi.org/10.1038/jp.2015.142

Crump, C., Sundquist, J., & Sundquist, K. (2021). Preterm or early term birth and risk of autism. *Pediatrics*, *148*(3), e2020032300. https://doi.org/10.1542/peds.2020-032300

D'Onofrio, B. M., Class, Q. A., Rickert, M. E., Larsson, H., Långström, N., & Lichtenstein, P. (2013). Preterm birth and mortality and morbidity: A population-based quasi-experimental study. *JAMA Psychiatry*, *70*(11), 1231–1240. https://doi.org/10.1001/jamapsychiatry.2013.2107

Davidoff, M. J., Dias, T., Damus, K., Russell, R., Bettegowda, V. R., Dolan, S., Schwarz, R. H., Green, N. S., & Petrini, J. (2006). Changes in the gestational age distribution among US singleton births: impact on rates of late preterm birth, 1992 to 2002. *Seminars in Perinatology*, *30*(1), 8–15. https://doi.org/10.1053/j.semperi.2006.01.009

Davidson, J. R. (n.d.). *Davidson Trauma Scale (DTS™)* [Database record]. APA PsycTests. https://doi.org/10.1037/t04973-000

De Schuymer, L., De Groote, I., Striano, T., Stahl, D., & Roeyers, H. (2011). Dyadic and triadic skills in preterm and full term infants: A longitudinal study in the first year. *Infant Behavior & Development*, *34*(1), 179–188. https://doi.org/10.1016/j.infbeh.2010.12.007

DeMier, R. L., Hynan, M. T., Hatfield, R. F., Varner, M. W., Harris, H. B., & Manniello, R. L. (2000). A measurement model of perinatal stressors: Identifying risk for postnatal emotional distress in mothers of high-risk infants. *Journal of Clinical Psychology*, 56(1), 89–100. https://doi.org/10.1002/(sici)1097-4679(200001)56:1%3C89::aid-jclp8%3E3.0.co;2-6

Dempsey, A. G., Cole, J. C., & Saxton, S. N. (2022). *Behavioral health services with high-risk infants and families: Meeting the needs of patients, families, and providers in fetal, neonatal intensive care unit, and neonatal follow-up settings.* Oxford University Press. https://doi.org/10.1093/med-psych/9780197545027.001.0001

Doering, L. V., Moser, D. K., & Dracup, K. (2000). Correlates of anxiety, hostility, depression, and psychosocial adjustment in parents of NICU infants. *Neonatal Network*, 19(5), 15–23. https://doi.org/10.1891/0730-0832.19.5.15

Eryigit Madzwamuse, S., Baumann, N., Jaekel, J., Bartmann, P., & Wolke, D. (2015). Neuro-cognitive performance of very preterm or very low birth weight adults at 26 years. *Journal of Child Psychology and Psychiatry*, 56(8), 857–864. https://doi.org/10.1111/jcpp.12358

Feldman, R., & Eidelman, A. I. (2007). Maternal postpartum behavior and the emergence of infant-mother and infant-father synchrony in preterm and full-term infants: The role of neonatal vagal tone. *Developmental Psychobiology*, 49(3), 290–302. https://doi.org/10.1002/dev.20220

Fevang, S. K. E., Hysing, M., Markestad, T., & Sommerfelt, K. (2016). Mental health in children born extremely preterm without severe neurodevelopmental disabilities. *Pediatrics*, 137(4), e20153002. https://doi.org/10.1542/peds.2015-3002

Firestein, M. R., Myers, M. M., Feder, K. J., Ludwig, R. J., & Welch, M. G. (2022). Effects of family nurture intervention in the nicu on theory of mind abilities in children born very preterm: A randomized controlled trial. *Children*, 9(2), 284. https://doi.org/10.3390/children9020284

Forcada-Guex, M., Borghini, A., Pierrehumbert, B., Ansermet, F., & Muller-Nix, C. (2011). Prematurity, maternal posttraumatic stress and consequences on the mother-infant relationship. *Early Human Development*, 87(1), 21–26. https://doi.org/10.1016/j.earlhumdev.2010.09.006

Forcada-Guex, M., Pierrehumbert, B., Borghini, A., Moessinger, A., & Muller-Nix, C. (2006). Early dyadic patterns of mother-infant interactions and outcomes of prematurity at 18 months. *Pediatrics*, 118(1), e107–e114. https://doi.org/10.1542/peds.2005-1145

Frey, H. A., & Klebanoff, M. A. (2016). The epidemiology, etiology, and costs of preterm birth. *Seminars in Fetal & Neonatal Medicine*, 21(2), 68–73. https://doi.org/10.1016/j.siny.2015.12.011

Fuchs, F., & Senat, M. V. (2016). Multiple gestations and preterm birth. *Seminars in Fetal & Neonatal Medicine*, 21(2), 113–120. https://doi.org/10.1016/j.siny.2015.12.010

Garcia Coll, C. T., Halpern, L. F., Vohr, B. R., Seifer, R., & Oh, W. (1992). Stability and correlates of change of early temperament in preterm and full-term infants. *Infant Behavior & Development*, 15(2), 137–153. https://doi.org/10.1016/0163-6383(92)80020-U

Goldberg, S. (1978). Prematurity: Effects on parent-infant interaction. *Journal of Pediatric Psychology*, 3(3), 137–144. https://doi.org/10.1093/jpepsy/3.3.137

Goldberg, S., & DiVitto, B. (1995). Parenting children born preterm. In M. H. Bornstein (Ed.), *Handbook of parenting, Vol. 1. Children and parenting* (pp. 209–231). Lawrence Erlbaum Associates.

Gray, P. H., Edwards, D. M., O'Callaghan, M. J., & Cuskelly, M. (2012). Parenting stress in mothers of preterm infants during early infancy. *Early Human Development*, 88(1), 45–49. https://doi.org/10.1016/j.earlhumdev.2011.06.014

Gray, P. H., Edwards, D. M., O'Callaghan, M. J., Cuskelly, M., & Gibbons, K. (2013). Parenting stress in mothers of very preterm infants—Influence of development, temperament and maternal depression. *Early Human Development*, 89(9), 625–629. https://doi.org/10.1016/j.earlhumdev.2013.04.005

Guy, A., Seaton, S. E., Boyle, E. M., Draper, E. S., Field, D. J., Manktelow, B. N., Marlow, N., Smith, L. K., & Johnson, S. (2015). Infants born late/moderately preterm are at increased risk for a positive autism screen at 2 years of age. *The Journal of Pediatrics*, 166(2), 269–275. https://doi.org/10.1016/j.jpeds.2014.10.053

Hall, R. A., Hoffenkamp, H. N., Tooten, A., Braeken, J., Vingerhoets, A. J., & van Bakel, H. J. (2015). Longitudinal associations between maternal disrupted representations, maternal interactive behavior and infant attachment: A comparison between full-term and preterm dyads. *Child Psychiatry and Human Development*, 46(2), 320–331. https://doi.org/10.1007/s10578-014-0473-3

Hamilton, B. E., Martin, J. A., Osterman, M. J., Curtin, S. C., & Mathews, T. (2015). Births: Final data for 2014. *National Vital Statistics Reports*, 64(12), 1–64. https://www.cdc.gov/nchs/data/nvsr/nvsr64/nvsr64_12.pdf

Hane, A. A., Myers, M. M., Hofer, M. A., Ludwig, R. J., Halperin, M. S., Austin, J., Glickstein, S. B., &

Welch, M. G. (2015). Family nurture intervention improves the quality of maternal caregiving in the neonatal intensive care unit: Evidence from a randomized controlled trial. *Journal of Developmental and Behavioral Pediatrics, 36*(3), 188–196. https://doi.org/10.1097/DBP.0000000000000148

Harrison, M. S., & Goldenberg, R. L. (2016). Global burden of prematurity. *Seminars in Fetal and Neonatal Medicine, 21*(2), 74–79. https://doi.org/10.1016/j.siny.2015.12.007

Haward, M. F., Lantos, J., Janvier, A., & the POST Group. (2020). Helping parents cope in the NICU. *Pediatrics, 145*(6), e20193567. https://doi.org/10.1542/peds.2019-3567

Hawes, K., McGowan, E., O'Donnell, M., Tucker, R., & Vohr, B. (2016). Social emotional factors increase risk of postpartum depression in mothers of preterm infants. *The Journal of Pediatrics, 179*, 61–67. https://doi.org/10.1016/j.jpeds.2016.07.008

Hee Chung, E., Chou, J., & Brown, K. A. (2020). Neurodevelopmental outcomes of preterm infants: A recent literature review. *Translational Pediatrics, 9*(Suppl. 1), S3–S8. https://doi.org/10.21037/tp.2019.09.10

Heinonen, K., Kajantie, E., Pesonen, A.-K., Lahti, M., Pirkola, S., Wolke, D., Lano, A., Sammallahti, S., Lahti, J., Andersson, S., Eriksson, J. G., & Raikkonen, K. (2016). Common mental disorders in young adults born late-preterm. *Psychological Medicine, 46*(10), 2227–2238. https://doi.org/10.1017/S0033291716000830

Helle, N., Barkmann, C., Ehrhardt, S., & Bindt, C. (2018). Postpartum posttraumatic and acute stress in mothers and fathers of infants with very low birth weight: Cross-sectional results from a controlled multicenter cohort study. *Journal of Affective Disorders, 235*, 467–473. https://doi.org/10.1016/j.jad.2018.04.013

Holmström, G. E., Källen, K., Hellström, A., Jakobsson, P. G., Serenius, F., Stjernqvist, K., & Tornqvist, K. (2014). Ophthalmologic outcome at 30 months' corrected age of a prospective Swedish cohort of children born before 27 weeks of gestation: The Extremely Preterm Infants in Sweden study. *JAMA Ophthalmology, 132*(2), 182–189. https://doi.org/10.1001/jamaophthalmol.2013.5812

Howe, T.-H., Sheu, C.-F., Wang, T.-N., & Hsu, Y.-W. (2014). Parenting stress in families with very low birth weight preterm infants in early infancy. *Research in Developmental Disabilities, 35*(7), 1748–1756. https://doi.org/10.1016/j.ridd.2014.02.015

Hughes, M. B., Shults, J., McGrath, J., & Medoff-Cooper, B. (2002). Temperament characteristics of premature infants in the first year of life. *Journal of Developmental and Behavioral Pediatrics, 23*(6), 430–435. https://doi.org/10.1097/00004703-200212000-00006

Hynan, M. T., Mounts, K. O., & Vanderbilt, D. L. (2013). Screening parents of high-risk infants for emotional distress: Rationale and recommendations. *Journal of Perinatology, 33*(10), 748–753. https://doi.org/10.1038/jp.2013.72

Hynan, M. T., Steinberg, Z., Baker, L., Cicco, R., Geller, P. A., Lassen, S., Milford, C., Mounts, K. O., Patterson, C., Saxton, S., Segre, L., & Stuebe, A. (2015). Recommendations for mental health professionals in the NICU. *Journal of Perinatology, 35*(Suppl. 1), S14–S18. https://doi.org/10.1038/jp.2015.144

Ionio, C., Lista, G., Veggiotti, P., Colombo, C., Ciuffo, G., Daniele, I., Landoni, M., Scelsa, B., Alfei, E., & Bova, S. (2022). Cognitive, behavioral and socioemotional development in a cohort of preterm infants at school age: A cross-sectional study. *Pediatric Reports, 14*(1), 115–126. https://doi.org/10.3390/pediatric14010017

Jaekel, J., & Wolke, D. (2014). Preterm birth and dyscalculia. *The Journal of Pediatrics, 164*(6), 1327–1332. https://doi.org/10.1016/j.jpeds.2014.01.069

Katz, J., Lee, A. C., Kozuki, N., Lawn, J. E., Cousens, S., Blencowe, H., Ezzati, M., Bhutta, Z. A., Marchant, T., Willey, B. A., Adair, L., Barros, F., Baqui, A. H., Christian, P., Fawzi, W., Gonzalez, R., Humphrey, J., Huybregts, L., Kolsteren, P., . . . Black, R. E., & the CHERG Small-for-Gestational-Age-Preterm Birth Working Group. (2013). Mortality risk in preterm and small-for-gestational-age infants in low-income and middle-income countries: A pooled country analysis. *The Lancet, 382*(9890), 417–425. https://doi.org/10.1016/S0140-6736(13)60993-9

Kelly, M. M. (2016). Educational implications of preterm birth: A national sample of 8- to 11-year-old children born prematurely and their full-term peers. *Journal of Pediatric Health Care, 30*(5), 464–470. https://doi.org/10.1016/j.pedhc.2015.11.001

Kerr-Wilson, C. O., Mackay, D. F., Smith, G. C. S., & Pell, J. P. (2012). Meta-analysis of the association between preterm delivery and intelligence. *Journal of Public Health, 34*(2), 209–216. https://doi.org/10.1093/pubmed/fdr024

Kersting, A., Dorsch, M., Wesselmann, U., Lüdorff, K., Witthaut, J., Ohrmann, P., Hörnig-Franz, I., Klockenbusch, W., Harms, E., & Arolt, V. (2004). Maternal posttraumatic stress response after the birth of a very low-birth-weight infant. *Journal of Psychosomatic Research, 57*(5), 473–476. https://doi.org/10.1016/j.jpsychores.2004.03.011

Kim, S. W., Andronis, L., Seppänen, A.-V., Aubert, A. M., Zeitlin, J., Barros, H., Draper, E. S., Petrou, S., & the SHIPS Research Group. (2022). Economic costs at age five associated with very preterm birth: Multinational European cohort study. *Pediatric Research, 92*(3), 700–711. https://doi.org/10.1038/s41390-021-01769-z

Kodjebacheva, G. D., & Sabo, T. (2016). Influence of premature birth on the health conditions, receipt of special education and sport participation of children aged 6–17 years in the USA. *Journal of Public Health, 38*(2), e47–e54. https://doi.org/10.1093/pubmed/fdv098

Kohn, M. A., Vosti, C. L., Lezotte, D., & Jones, R. H. (2000). Optimal gestational age and birth-weight cutoffs to predict neonatal morbidity. *Medical Decision Making, 20*(4), 369–376. https://doi.org/10.1177/0272989X0002000401

Korja, R., Savonlahti, E., Ahlqvist-Björkroth, S., Stolt, S., Haataja, L., Lapinleimu, H., Piha, J., Lehtonen, L., & the PIPARI study group. (2008). Maternal depression is associated with mother-infant interaction in preterm infants. *Acta Paediatrica, 97*(6), 724–730. https://doi.org/10.1111/j.1651-2227.2008.00733.x

Krieger, N., Van Wye, G., Huynh, M., Waterman, P. D., Maduro, G., Li, W., Gwynn, R. C., Barbot, O., & Bassett, M. T. (2020). Structural racism, historical redlining, and risk of preterm birth in New York City, 2013–2017. *American Journal of Public Health, 110*(7), 1046–1053. https://doi.org/10.2105/AJPH.2020.305656

Kroenke, K., Spitzer, R. L., & Williams, J. B. (2001). The PHQ-9: Validity of a brief depression severity measure. *Journal of General Internal Medicine, 16*(9), 606–613. https://doi.org/10.1046/j.1525-1497.2001.016009606.x

Kroenke, K., Spitzer, R. L., & Williams, J. B. (2003). The Patient Health Questionnaire-2: Validity of a two-item depression screener. *Medical Care, 41*(11), 1284–1292. https://doi.org/10.1097/01.MLR.0000093487.78664.3C

Kuhn, P., Zores, C., Langlet, C., Escande, B., Astruc, D., & Dufour, A. (2013). Moderate acoustic changes can disrupt the sleep of very preterm infants in their incubators. *Acta Paediatrica, 102*(10), 949–954. https://doi.org/10.1111/apa.12330

Kuppala, V. S., Tabangin, M., Haberman, B., Steichen, J., & Yolton, K. (2012). Current state of high-risk infant follow-up care in the United States: Results of a national survey of academic follow-up programs. *Journal of Perinatology, 32*(4), 293–298. https://doi.org/10.1038/jp.2011.97

Kuzniewicz, M. W., Wi, S., Qian, Y., Walsh, E. M., Armstrong, M. A., & Croen, L. A. (2014). Prevalence and neonatal factors associated with autism spectrum disorders in preterm infants. *The Journal of Pediatrics, 164*(1), 20–25. https://doi.org/10.1016/j.jpeds.2013.09.021

Lakshmanan, A., Song, A. Y., Belfort, M. B., Yieh, L., Dukhovny, D., Friedlich, P. S., & Gong, C. L. (2022). The financial burden experienced by families of preterm infants after NICU discharge. *Journal of Perinatology, 42*(2), 223–230. https://doi.org/10.1038/s41372-021-01213-4

Lambiase, C. V., Mansi, G., Salomè, S., Conelli, M. L., Vendemmia, M., Zurlo, M. C., Raimondi, F., & Capasso, L. (2023). The financial burden experienced by families during NICU hospitalization and after discharge: A single center, survey-based study. *European Journal of Pediatrics*. https://doi.org/10.1007/s00431-023-05352-y

Larroque, B., N'guyen The Tich, S., Guédeney, A., Marchand, L., Burguet, A., & the Epipage Study Group. (2005). Temperament at 9 months of very preterm infants born at less than 29 weeks' gestation: The Epipage study. *Journal of Developmental and Behavioral Pediatrics, 26*(1), 48–55.

Lawn, J. E., Davidge, R., Paul, V. K., von Xylander, S., de Graft Johnson, J., Costello, A., Kinney, M. V., Segre, J., & Molyneux, L. (2013). Born too soon: Care for the preterm baby. *Reproductive Health, 10*(Suppl. 1), S5. https://doi.org/10.1186/1742-4755-10-S1-S5

Lean, R. E., Lessov-Shlaggar, C. N., Gerstein, E. D., Smyser, T. A., Paul, R. A., Smyser, C. D., & Rogers, C. E. (2020). Maternal and family factors differentiate profiles of psychiatric impairments in very preterm children at age 5-years. *Journal of Child Psychology and Psychiatry, 61*(2), 157–166. https://doi.org/10.1111/jcpp.13116

Lefkowitz, D. S., Baxt, C., & Evans, J. R. (2010). Prevalence and correlates of posttraumatic stress and postpartum depression in parents of infants in the neonatal intensive care unit (NICU). *Journal of Clinical Psychology in Medical Settings, 17*(3), 230–237. https://doi.org/10.1007/s10880-010-9202-7

Lester, B. M., Hawes, K., Abar, B., Sullivan, M., Miller, R., Bigsby, R., Laptook, A., Salisbury, A., Taub, M., Lagasse, L. L., & Padbury, J. F. (2014). Single-family room care and neurobehavioral and medical outcomes in preterm infants. *Pediatrics, 134*(4), 754–760. https://doi.org/10.1542/peds.2013-4252

Lindström, K., Lindblad, F., & Hjern, A. (2011). Preterm birth and attention-deficit/hyperactivity disorder in schoolchildren. *Pediatrics, 127*(5), 858–865. https://doi.org/10.1542/peds.2010-1279

Liu, L., Oza, S., Hogan, D., Perin, J., Rudan, I., Lawn, J. E., Cousens, S., Mathers, C., & Black, R. E. (2015). Global, regional, and national causes of child mortality in 2000–13, with projections to inform post-2015 priorities: An updated systematic analysis. *The Lancet*, *385*(9966), 430–440. https://doi.org/10.1016/S0140-6736(14)61698-6

Löhr, T., von Gontard, A., & Roth, B. (2000). Perception of premature birth by fathers and mothers. *Archives of Women's Mental Health*, *3*(2), 41–46. https://doi.org/10.1007/s007370070004

Loi, E. C., Vaca, K. E. C., Ashland, M. D., Marchman, V. A., Fernald, A., & Feldman, H. M. (2017). Quality of caregiver-child play interactions with toddlers born preterm and full term: Antecedents and language outcome. *Early Human Development*, *115*, 110–117. https://doi.org/10.1016/j.earlhumdev.2017.10.001

Lorrain, B. (2016). Reflective peer consultation as an intervention for staff support in the NICU. *Newborn and Infant Nursing Reviews*, *16*(4), 289–292. https://doi.org/10.1053/j.nainr.2016.09.022

Lotterman, J. H., Lorenz, J. M., & Bonanno, G. A. (2019). You can't take your baby home yet: A longitudinal study of psychological symptoms in mothers of infants hospitalized in the NICU. *Journal of Clinical Psychology in Medical Settings*, *26*(1), 116–122. https://doi.org/10.1007/s10880-018-9570-y

Löwe, B., Decker, O., Müller, S., Brähler, E., Schellberg, D., Herzog, W., & Herzberg, P. Y. (2008). Validation and standardization of the Generalized Anxiety Disorder Screener (GAD-7) in the general population. *Medical Care*, *46*(3), 266–274. https://doi.org/10.1097/MLR.0b013e318160d093

Lu, M. C., & Halfon, N. (2003). Racial and ethnic disparities in birth outcomes: A life-course perspective. *Maternal and Child Health Journal*, *7*(1), 13–30. https://doi.org/10.1023/A:1022537516969

Luke, B. (2017). Pregnancy and birth outcomes in couples with infertility with and without assisted reproductive technology: With an emphasis on US population-based studies. *American Journal of Obstetrics and Gynecology*, *217*(3), 270–281. https://doi.org/10.1016/j.ajog.2017.03.012

Lupton, D., & Fenwick, J. (2001). 'They've forgotten that I'm the mum': Constructing and practising motherhood in special care nurseries. *Social Science & Medicine*, *53*(8), 1011–1021. https://doi.org/10.1016/S0277-9536(00)00396-8

MacKay, D. F., Smith, G. C. S., Dobbie, R., & Pell, J. P. (2010). Gestational age at delivery and special educational need: Retrospective cohort study of 407,503 schoolchildren. *PLOS Medicine*, *7*(6), e1000289. https://doi.org/10.1371/journal.pmed.1000289

Manuck, T. A. (2017). Racial and ethnic differences in preterm birth: A complex, multifactorial problem. *Seminars in Perinatology*, *41*(8), 511–518. https://doi.org/10.1053/j.semperi.2017.08.010

Marchi, J., Berg, M., Dencker, A., Olander, E. K., & Begley, C. (2015). Risks associated with obesity in pregnancy, for the mother and baby: A systematic review of reviews. *Obesity Reviews*, *16*(8), 621–638. https://doi.org/10.1111/obr.12288

Matthey, S., Barnett, B., Howie, P., & Kavanagh, D. J. (2003). Diagnosing postpartum depression in mothers and fathers: Whatever happened to anxiety? *Journal of Affective Disorders*, *74*(2), 139–147. https://doi.org/10.1016/S0165-0327(02)00012-5

McCabe, E. R., Carrino, G. E., Russell, R. B., & Howse, J. L. (2014). Fighting for the next generation: US prematurity in 2030. *Pediatrics*, *134*(6), 1193–1199. https://doi.org/10.1542/peds.2014-2541

McKeown, L., Burke, K., Cobham, V. E., Kimball, H., Foxcroft, K., & Callaway, L. (2023). The prevalence of PTSD of mothers and fathers of high-risk infants admitted to NICU: A systematic review. *Clinical Child and Family Psychology Review*, *26*(1), 33–49. https://doi.org/10.1007/s10567-022-00421-4

McManus, B. M., & Poehlmann, J. (2012). Parent-child interaction, maternal depressive symptoms and preterm infant cognitive function. *Infant Behavior & Development*, *35*(3), 489–498. https://doi.org/10.1016/j.infbeh.2012.04.005

Miceli, P. J., Goeke-Morey, M. C., Whitman, T. L., Kolberg, K. S., Miller-Loncar, C., & White, R. D. (2000). Brief report: birth status, medical complications, and social environment: Individual differences in development of preterm, very low birth weight infants. *Journal of Pediatric Psychology*, *25*(5), 353–358. https://doi.org/10.1093/jpepsy/25.5.353

Miles, M. S., Funk, S. G., & Carlson, J. (1993). Parental Stressor Scale: Neonatal intensive care unit. *Nursing Research*, *42*(3), 148–152. https://doi.org/10.1097/00006199-199305000-00005

Miles, M. S., Holditch-Davis, D., Schwartz, T. A., & Scher, M. (2007). Depressive symptoms in mothers of prematurely born infants. *Journal of Developmental and Behavioral Pediatrics*, *28*(1), 36–44. https://doi.org/10.1097/01.DBP.0000257517.52459.7a

Moehler, E., Brunner, R., Wiebel, A., Reck, C., & Resch, F. (2006). Maternal depressive symptoms in the postnatal period are associated with long-term impairment of mother-child bonding. *Archives of Women's Mental Health*, *9*(5), 273–278. https://doi.org/10.1007/s00737-006-0149-5

Moraski Mew, A., Holditch-Davis, D., Belyea, M., Miles, M. S., & Fishel, A. (2003). Correlates of depressive symptoms in mothers of preterm infants. *Neonatal Network, 22*(5), 51–60. https://doi.org/10.1891/0730-0832.22.5.51

Muller-Nix, C., Forcada-Guex, M., Pierrehumbert, B., Jaunin, L., Borghini, A., & Ansermet, F. (2004). Prematurity, maternal stress and mother-child interactions. *Early Human Development, 79*(2), 145–158. https://doi.org/10.1016/j.earlhumdev.2004.05.002

Murch, T. N., & Smith, V. C. (2016). Supporting families as they transition home. *Newborn and Infant Nursing Reviews, 16*(4), 298–302. https://doi.org/10.1053/j.nainr.2016.09.024

Natalucci, G., Bucher, H. U., Von Rhein, M., Borradori Tolsa, C., Latal, B., & Adams, M. (2017). Population based report on health related quality of life in adolescents born very preterm. *Early Human Development, 104*, 7–12. https://doi.org/10.1016/j.earlhumdev.2016.11.002

Neri, E., Agostini, F., Perricone, G., Morales, M. R., Biasini, A., Monti, F., & Polizzi, C. (2017). Mother- and father-infant interactions at 3 months of corrected age: The effect of severity of preterm birth. *Infant Behavior and Development, 49*, 97–103. https://doi.org/10.1016/j.infbeh.2017.08.001

Obeidat, H. M., Bond, E. A., & Callister, L. C. (2009). The parental experience of having an infant in the newborn intensive care unit. *Journal of Perinatal Education, 18*(3), 23–29. https://doi.org/10.1624/105812409X461199

O'Donovan, A., & Nixon, E. (2019). "Weathering the storm:" Mothers' and fathers' experiences of parenting a preterm infant. *Infant Mental Health Journal, 40*(4), 573–587. https://doi.org/10.1002/imhj.21788

Olafsen, K. S., Rønning, J. A., Kaaresen, P. I., Ulvund, S. E., Handegård, B. H., & Dahl, L. B. (2006). Joint attention in term and preterm infants at 12 months corrected age: The significance of gender and intervention based on a randomized controlled trial. *Infant Behavior & Development, 29*(4), 554–563. https://doi.org/10.1016/j.infbeh.2006.07.004

Örtenstrand, A., Westrup, B., Broström, E. B., Sarman, I., Akerström, S., Brune, T., Lindberg, L., & Waldenström, U. (2010). The Stockholm Neonatal Family Centered Care Study: Effects on length of stay and infant morbidity. *Pediatrics, 125*(2), e278–e285. https://doi.org/10.1542/peds.2009-1511

Pascoe, L., Burnett, A. C., & Anderson, P. J. (2021). Cognitive and academic outcomes of children born extremely preterm. *Seminars in Perinatology, 45*(8), 151480. https://doi.org/10.1016/j.semperi.2021.151480

Poehlmann, J., & Fiese, B. H. (2001a). The interaction of maternal and infant vulnerabilities on developing attachment relationships. *Development and Psychopathology, 13*(1), 1–11. https://doi.org/10.1017/S0954579401001018

Poehlmann, J., & Fiese, B. H. (2001b). Parent-infant interaction as a mediator of the relation between neonatal risk status and 12-month cognitive development. *Infant Behavior & Development, 24*(2), 171–188. https://doi.org/10.1016/S0163-6383(01)00073-X

Poehlmann, J., Schwichtenberg, A. J., Bolt, D., & Dilworth-Bart, J. (2009). Predictors of depressive symptom trajectories in mothers of preterm or low birth weight infants. *Journal of Family Psychology, 23*(5), 690–704. https://doi.org/10.1037/a0016117

Poehlmann, J., Schwichtenberg, A. J., Bolt, D. M., Hane, A., Burnson, C., & Winters, J. (2011). Infant physiological regulation and maternal risks as predictors of dyadic interaction trajectories in families with a preterm infant. *Developmental Psychology, 47*(1), 91–105. https://doi.org/10.1037/a0020719

Porges, S. W., Davila, M. I., Lewis, G. F., Kolacz, J., Okonmah-Obazee, S., Hane, A. A., Kwon, K. Y., Ludwig, R. J., Myers, M. M., & Welch, M. G. (2019). Autonomic regulation of preterm infants is enhanced by Family Nurture Intervention. *Developmental Psychobiology, 61*(6), 942–952. https://doi.org/10.1002/dev.21841

Poulsen, G., Wolke, D., Kurinczuk, J. J., Boyle, E. M., Field, D., Alfirevic, Z., & Quigley, M. A. (2013). Gestational age and cognitive ability in early childhood: A population-based cohort study. *Paediatric and Perinatal Epidemiology, 27*(4), 371–379. https://doi.org/10.1111/ppe.12058

Prins, A., Kimerling, R., Cameron, R., Oumiette, P., Shaw, J., Thrailkill, A., Sheikh, J., & Gusman, F. (1999, November 14–17). *The primary care PTSD screen (PC-PTSD)*. 15th Annual Meeting of the International Society for Traumatic Stress Studies, Miami, FL, United States.

Purdy, I. B., Craig, J. W., & Zeanah, P. (2015). NICU discharge planning and beyond: Recommendations for parent psychosocial support. *Journal of Perinatology, 35*(Suppl. 1), S24–S28. https://doi.org/10.1038/jp.2015.146

Putnick, D. L., Bornstein, M. H., Eryigit-Madzwamuse, S., & Wolke, D. (2017). Long-term stability of language performance in very preterm, moderate-late preterm, and term children. *The Journal of Pediatrics, 181*, 74–79. e73. https://doi.org/10.1016/j.jpeds.2016.09.006

Quigley, M. A., Poulsen, G., Boyle, E., Wolke, D., Field, D., Alfirevic, Z., & Kurinczuk, J. J. (2012).

Early term and late preterm birth are associated with poorer school performance at age 5 years: A cohort study. *Archives of Disease in Childhood: Fetal and Neonatal Edition, 97*(3), F167–F173. https://doi.org/10.1136/archdischild-2011-300888

Radloff, L. S. (1977). The CES-D scale: A self-report depression scale for research in the general population. *Applied Psychological Measurement, 1*(3), 385–401. https://doi.org/10.1177/014662167700100306

Reagan, P. B., & Salsberry, P. J. (2005). Race and ethnic differences in determinants of preterm birth in the USA: Broadening the social context. *Social Science & Medicine, 60*(10), 2217–2228. https://doi.org/10.1016/j.socscimed.2004.10.010

Reissland, N., Shepherd, J., & Stephenson, T. (1999). Maternal verbal interaction in different situations with infants born prematurely or at term. *Infant and Child Development, 8*(1), 39–48. https://doi.org/10.1002/(SICI)1522-7219(199903)8:1%3C39::AID-ICD189%3E3.0.CO;2-%23

Rommel, A.-S., James, S.-N., McLoughlin, G., Brandeis, D., Banaschewski, T., Asherson, P., & Kuntsi, J. (2017). Association of preterm birth with attention-deficit/hyperactivity disorder–like and wider-ranging neurophysiological impairments of attention and inhibition. *Journal of the American Academy of Child & Adolescent Psychiatry, 56*(1), 40–50. https://doi.org/10.1016/j.jaac.2016.10.006

Ruiz, N., Piskernik, B., Witting, A., Fuiko, R., & Ahnert, L. (2018). Parent-child attachment in children born preterm and at term: A multigroup analysis. *PLOS ONE, 13*(8), e0202972. https://doi.org/10.1371/journal.pone.0202972

Sabnis, A., Fojo, S., Nayak, S. S., Lopez, E., Tarn, D. M., & Zeltzer, L. (2019). Reducing parental trauma and stress in neonatal intensive care: Systematic review and meta-analysis of hospital interventions. *Journal of Perinatology, 39*(3), 375–386. https://doi.org/10.1038/s41372-018-0310-9

Sajaniemi, N., Salokorpi, T., & von Wendt, L. (1998). Temperament profiles and their role in neurodevelopmental assessed preterm children at two years of age. *European Child & Adolescent Psychiatry, 7*(3), 145–152. https://doi.org/10.1007/s007870050060

Sameroff, A. J. (2009). Conceptual issues in studying the development of self-regulation. In S. L. Olson & A. J. Sameroff (Eds.), *Biopsychosocial regulatory processes in the development of childhood behavioral problems* (pp. 1–18). Cambridge University Press. https://doi.org/10.1017/CBO9780511575877.002

Samuelsson, M., Holsti, A., Adamsson, M., Serenius, F., Hägglöf, B., & Farooqi, A. (2017). Behavioral patterns in adolescents born at 23 to 25 weeks of gestation. *Pediatrics, 140*(1), e20170199. https://doi.org/10.1542/peds.2017-0199

Sansavini, A., Zavagli, V., Guarini, A., Savini, S., Alessandroni, R., & Faldella, G. (2015). Dyadic co-regulation, affective intensity and infant's development at 12 months: A comparison among extremely preterm and full-term dyads. *Infant Behavior & Development, 40*, 29–40. https://doi.org/10.1016/j.infbeh.2015.03.005

Santos, J., Pearce, S. E., & Stroustrup, A. (2015). Impact of hospital-based environmental exposures on neurodevelopmental outcomes of preterm infants. *Current Opinion in Pediatrics, 27*(2), 254–260. https://doi.org/10.1097/MOP.0000000000000190

Schappin, R., Wijnroks, L., Uniken Venema, M. M., & Jongmans, M. J. (2013). Rethinking stress in parents of preterm infants: A meta-analysis. *PLOS ONE, 8*(2), e54992. https://doi.org/10.1371/journal.pone.0054992

Schieve, L. A., Tian, L. H., Rankin, K., Kogan, M. D., Yeargin-Allsopp, M., Visser, S., & Rosenberg, D. (2016). Population impact of preterm birth and low birth weight on developmental disabilities in US children. *Annals of Epidemiology, 26*(4), 267–274. https://doi.org/10.1016/j.annepidem.2016.02.012

Schmücker, G., Brisch, K. H., Köhntop, B., Betzler, S., Österle, M., Pohlandt, F., Pokorny, D., Laucht, M., Kächele, H., & Buchheim, A. (2005). The influence of prematurity, maternal anxiety, and infants' neurobiological risk on mother-infant interactions. *Infant Mental Health Journal, 26*(5), 423–441. https://doi.org/10.1002/imhj.20066

Shah, P., Kaciroti, N., Richards, B., Oh, W., & Lumeng, J. C. (2016). Developmental outcomes of late preterm infants from infancy to kindergarten. *Pediatrics, 138*(2), e20153496. https://doi.org/10.1542/peds.2015-3496

Shah, P. E., Clements, M., & Poehlmann, J. (2011). Maternal resolution of grief after preterm birth: Implications for infant attachment security. *Pediatrics, 127*(2), 284–292. https://doi.org/10.1542/peds.2010-1080

Shah, P. E., Kaciroti, N., Richards, B., & Lumeng, J. C. (2016). Gestational age and kindergarten school readiness in a national sample of preterm infants. *The Journal of Pediatrics, 178*, 61–67. https://doi.org/10.1016/j.jpeds.2016.06.062

Shah, P. E., Poehlmann, J., Weeks, H. M., Spinelli, M., Richards, B., Suh, J., & Kaciroti, N. (2023). Developmental trajectories of late preterm infants and predictors of academic performance. *Pediatric Research, 95*, 684–691. https://doi.org/10.1038/s41390-023-02756-2

Simmons, L. E., Rubens, C. E., Darmstadt, G. L., & Gravett, M. G. (2010). Preventing preterm birth and neonatal mortality: Exploring the epidemiology, causes, and interventions. *Seminars in Perinatology*, *34*(6), 408–415. https://doi.org/10.1053/j.semperi.2010.09.005

Singer, L. T., Fulton, S., Davillier, M., Koshy, D., Salvator, A., & Baley, J. E. (2003). Effects of infant risk status and maternal psychological distress on maternal-infant interactions during the first year of life. *Journal of Developmental and Behavioral Pediatrics*, *24*(4), 233–241. https://doi.org/10.1097/00004703-200308000-00003

Spinelli, M., Frigerio, A., Montali, L., Fasolo, M., Spada, M. S., & Mangili, G. (2016). 'I still have difficulties feeling like a mother': The transition to motherhood of preterm infants mothers. *Psychology & Health*, *31*(2), 184–204. https://doi.org/10.1080/08870446.2015.1088015

Spinelli, M., Lionetti, F., Garito, M. C., Shah, P. E., Logrieco, M. G., Ponzetti, S., Cicioni, P., Di Valerio, S., & Fasolo, M. (2022). Infant-directed speech from a multidimensional perspective: The interplay of infant birth status, maternal parenting stress, and dyadic co-regulation on infant-directed speech linguistic and pragmatic features. *Frontiers in Psychology*, *13*, 804792. https://doi.org/10.3389/fpsyg.2022.804792

Spinelli, M., Poehlmann, J., & Bolt, D. (2013). Predictors of parenting stress trajectories in premature infant–mother dyads. *Journal of Family Psychology*, *27*(6), 873–883. https://doi.org/10.1037/a0034652

Spittle, A. J., Morgan, C., Olsen, J. E., Novak, I., & Cheong, J. L. Y. (2018). Early diagnosis and treatment of cerebral palsy in children with a history of preterm birth. *Clinics in Perinatology*, *45*(3), 409–420. https://doi.org/10.1016/j.clp.2018.05.011

Stern, D. N., & Bruschweiler-Stern, N. (1998). *The birth of a mother: How the motherhood experience changes you forever*. Basic Books.

Stoll, B. J., Hansen, N. I., Bell, E. F., Shankaran, S., Laptook, A. R., Walsh, M. C., Hale, E. C., Newman, N. S., Schibler, K., Carlo, W. A., Kennedy, K. A., Poindexter, B. B., Finer, N. N., Ehrenkranz, R. A., Duara, S., Sánchez, P. J., O'Shea, T. M., Goldberg, R. N., Van Meurs, K. P., . . . Higgins, R. D. (2010). Neonatal outcomes of extremely preterm infants from the NICHD Neonatal Research Network. *Pediatrics*, *126*(3), 443–456. https://doi.org/10.1542/peds.2009-2959

Suttora, C., Spinelli, M., Aureli, T., Fasolo, M., Lionetti, F., Picciolini, O., Ravasi, M., & Salerni, N. (2020). Mind-mindedness and parenting stress: A cross-sectional study in a cohort of mothers of 3-month-old full-term and preterm infants. *International Journal of Environmental Research and Public Health*, *17*(21), 7735. https://doi.org/10.3390/ijerph17217735

Suttora, C., Spinelli, M., & Monzani, D. (2014). From prematurity to parenting stress: The mediating role of perinatal post-traumatic stress disorder. *European Journal of Developmental Psychology*, *11*(4), 478–493. https://doi.org/10.1080/17405629.2013.859574

Tahirkheli, N. N., Cherry, A. S., Tackett, A. P., McCaffree, M. A., & Gillaspy, S. R. (2014). Postpartum depression on the neonatal intensive care unit: Current perspectives. *International Journal of Women's Health*, *6*, 975–987.

Tessier, R., Cristo, M. B., Velez, S., Giron, M., Nadeau, L., Figueroa de Calume, Z., Ruiz-Paláez, J. G., & Charpak, N. (2003). Kangaroo Mother Care: A method for protecting high-risk low-birthweight and premature infants against developmental delay. *Infant Behavior & Development*, *26*(3), 384–397. https://doi.org/10.1016/S0163-6383(03)00037-7

Trapolini, T., McMahon, C. A., & Ungerer, J. A. (2007). The effect of maternal depression and marital adjustment on young children's internalizing and externalizing behaviour problems. *Child: Care, Health and Development*, *33*(6), 794–803. https://doi.org/10.1111/j.1365-2214.2007.00739.x

Treyvaud, K., Doyle, L. W., Lee, K. J., Roberts, G., Cheong, J. L., Inder, T. E., & Anderson, P. J. (2011). Family functioning, burden and parenting stress 2 years after very preterm birth. *Early Human Development*, *87*(6), 427–431. https://doi.org/10.1016/j.earlhumdev.2011.03.008

Trumello, C., Candelori, C., Cofini, M., Cimino, S., Cerniglia, L., Paciello, M., & Babore, A. (2018). Mothers' depression, anxiety, and mental representations after preterm birth: A study during the infant's hospitalization in a neonatal intensive care unit. *Frontiers in Public Health*, *6*, 359. https://doi.org/10.3389/fpubh.2018.00359

Turpin, H., Urben, S., Ansermet, F., Borghini, A., Murray, M. M., & Müller-Nix, C. (2019). The interplay between prematurity, maternal stress and children's intelligence quotient at age 11: A longitudinal study. *Scientific Reports*, *9*(1), 450. https://doi.org/10.1038/s41598-018-36465-2

Twilhaar, E. S., Wade, R. M., de Kieviet, J. F., van Goudoever, J. B., van Elburg, R. M., & Oosterlaan, J. (2018). Cognitive outcomes of children born extremely or very preterm since the 1990s and associated risk factors: A meta-analysis and meta-regression. *JAMA Pediatrics*, *172*(4), 361–367. https://doi.org/10.1001/jamapediatrics.2017.5323

Vanderbilt, D., Bushley, T., Young, R., & Frank, D. A. (2009). Acute posttraumatic stress symptoms among urban mothers with newborns in the neonatal intensive care unit: A preliminary study. *Journal of Developmental and Behavioral Pediatrics, 30*(1), 50–56. https://doi.org/10.1097/DBP.0b013e318196b0de

Vanderveen, J. A., Bassler, D., Robertson, C. M., & Kirpalani, H. (2009). Early interventions involving parents to improve neurodevelopmental outcomes of premature infants: A meta-analysis. *Journal of Perinatology, 29*(5), 343–351. https://doi.org/10.1038/jp.2008.229

van Dommelen, P., Verkerk, P. H., van Straaten, H. L., Baerts, W., Von Weissenbruch, M., Duijsters, C., van Kaam, A., Steiner, K., de Vries, L. S., & Swarte, R. (2015). Hearing loss by week of gestation and birth weight in very preterm neonates. *The Journal of Pediatrics, 166*(4), 840–843. e841.

van IJzendoorn, M. H., Goldberg, S., Kroonenberg, P. M., & Frenkel, O. J. (1992). The relative effects of maternal and child problems on the quality of attachment: A meta-analysis of attachment in clinical samples. *Child Development, 63*(4), 840–858. https://doi.org/10.1111/j.1467-8624.1992.tb01665.x

Vogel, J. P., Chawanpaiboon, S., Moller, A.-B., Watananirun, K., Bonet, M., & Lumbiganon, P. (2018). The global epidemiology of preterm birth. *Best Practice & Research Clinical Obstetrics & Gynaecology, 52*, 3–12. https://doi.org/10.1016/j.bpobgyn.2018.04.003

Welch, M. G., Firestein, M. R., Austin, J., Hane, A. A., Stark, R. I., Hofer, M. A., Garland, M., Glickstein, S. B., Brunelli, S. A., Ludwig, R. J., & Myers, M. M. (2015). Family Nurture Intervention in the neonatal intensive care unit improves social-relatedness, attention, and neurodevelopment of preterm infants at 18 months in a randomized controlled trial. *Journal of Child Psychology and Psychiatry, 56*(11), 1202–1211. https://doi.org/10.1111/jcpp.12405

Welch, M. G., Hofer, M. A., Brunelli, S. A., Stark, R. I., Andrews, H. F., Austin, J., Myers, M. M., & the Family Nurture Intervention (FNI) Trial Group. (2012). Family nurture intervention (FNI): Methods and treatment protocol of a randomized controlled trial in the NICU. *BMC Pediatrics, 12*(1), 14. https://doi.org/10.1186/1471-2431-12-14

Welch, M. G., Hofer, M. A., Stark, R. I., Andrews, H. F., Austin, J., Glickstein, S. B., Ludwig, R. J., Myers, M. M., & the FNI Trial Group. (2013). Randomized controlled trial of Family Nurture Intervention in the NICU: Assessments of length of stay, feasibility and safety. *BMC Pediatrics, 13*(1), 148. https://doi.org/10.1186/1471-2431-13-148

Welch, M. G., Myers, M. M., Grieve, P. G., Isler, J. R., Fifer, W. P., Sahni, R., Hofer, M. A., Austin, J., Ludwig, R. J., Stark, R. I., & the FNI Trial Group. (2014). Electroencephalographic activity of preterm infants is increased by Family Nurture Intervention: A randomized controlled trial in the NICU. *Clinical Neurophysiology, 125*(4), 675–684. https://doi.org/10.1016/j.clinph.2013.08.021

Westrup, B., Böhm, B., Lagercrantz, H., & Stjernqvist, K. (2004). Preschool outcome in children born very prematurely and cared for according to the Newborn Individualized Developmental Care and Assessment Program (NIDCAP). *Acta Paediatrica, 93*(4), 498–507. https://doi.org/10.1080/08035250410023548

White, R. D., Smith, J. A., & Shepley, M. M. (2013). Recommended standards for newborn ICU design, eighth edition. *Journal of Perinatology, 33*(Suppl. 1), S2–S16. https://doi.org/10.1038/jp.2013.10

Williams, B. L., Dunlop, A. L., Kramer, M., Dever, B. V., Hogue, C., & Jain, L. (2013). Perinatal origins of first-grade academic failure: Role of prematurity and maternal factors. *Pediatrics, 131*(4), 693–700. https://doi.org/10.1542/peds.2012-1408

Wolke, D., Chernova, J., Eryigit-Madzwamuse, S., Samara, M., Zwierzynska, K., & Petrou, S. (2013). Self and parent perspectives on health-related quality of life of adolescents born very preterm. *The Journal of Pediatrics, 163*(4), 1020–1026. e1022.

Wolke, D., Eryigit-Madzwamuse, S., & Gutbrod, T. (2014). Very preterm/very low birthweight infants' attachment: Infant and maternal characteristics. *Archives of Disease in Childhood—Fetal and Neonatal Edition, 99*(1), F70–F75. https://doi.org/10.1136/archdischild-2013-303788

Woodward, L. J., Bora, S., Clark, C. A., Montgomery-Hönger, A., Pritchard, V. E., Spencer, C., & Austin, N. C. (2014). Very preterm birth: Maternal experiences of the neonatal intensive care environment. *Journal of Perinatology, 34*(7), 555–561. https://doi.org/10.1038/jp.2014.43

Yin, W., Döring, N., Persson, M. S. M., Persson, M., Tedroff, K., Ådén, U., & Sandin, S. (2022). Gestational age and risk of intellectual disability: A population-based cohort study. *Archives of Disease in Childhood, 107*(9), 826–832. https://doi.org/10.1136/archdischild-2021-323308

Zeanah, C. (Ed.). (2018). *Handbook of infant mental health* (4th ed.). Guilford Press.

Zelkowitz, P., Bardin, C., & Papageorgiou, A. (2007). Anxiety affects the relationship between parents and their very low birth weight infants. *Infant Mental Health Journal, 28*(3), 296–313. https://doi.org/10.1002/imhj.20137

CHAPTER 18

NEUROSENSORY DISORDERS: HEARING, VISUAL, AND MULTISENSORY IMPAIRMENTS IN CHILDHOOD

Desmond Kelly, Anne M. Kinsman, and Erin R. Hahn

Sensory input determines our lived experience, and when sensory signals are distorted or diminished, a person's abilities to understand, interact with, and move through the world are dramatically altered. Hearing and vision are the modalities through which most learning occurs, and individual or multisensory impairments can impede navigation of the physical environment, language and social interactions, and the acquisition of learned skills necessary for a productive and fulfilling life.

This chapter provides a framework for assessment and management of individuals with neurosensory disorders (i.e., hearing, visual, and multisensory impairment) that is based on an understanding of their prevalence, underlying causes, the neuropsychological and functional impacts, and the factors that are most likely to mediate optimal outcomes. Following an overview of prognostic factors, we briefly discuss terminology, epidemiology, etiology, and neurobiology for each disorder. We also address a range of developmental outcomes, and drawing on research in developmental science, we consider how factors in the caregiving environment may foster resilience and promote optimal outcomes across the lifespan. We then offer an overview of screening, evaluation, and intervention with consideration of issues of culture, equity, and inclusion. Roles specific to developmental-behavioral pediatricians and pediatric psychologists are highlighted.

PROGNOSTIC FACTORS

Four factors should be considered regarding developmental prognosis for neurosensory disorders. First, prognosis depends on the degree of sensory impairment. A child with a mild sensory loss will be at less risk than a child with a profound impairment. Second, etiology matters. A sensory impairment that is genetic in origin might reflect disruption of a discrete neurological component of the hearing pathway or a specific component of the visual apparatus (e.g., cataracts). Those deficits will have less neurodevelopmental impact than sensory impairments secondary to a diffuse neurological insult such as infection or hypoxia. Third, prognosis is related to age of onset. Lack of exposure to language or visual input during the critical early developmental years will impart significant disadvantage compared to onset at a later age when developmental systems have already been established. Finally, the timing of identification and intervention is of critical importance. Early correction of sensory loss or efforts by parents and therapists to foster communication or alternate learning modalities will significantly improve the likelihood of successful functioning.

https://doi.org/10.1037/0000414-018
APA Handbook of Pediatric Psychology, Developmental-Behavioral Pediatrics, and Developmental Science: Vol. 2. Pediatric Psychology and Developmental-Behavioral Pediatrics: Clinical Applications of Developmental Science, P. E. Shah and M. H. Bornstein (Editors-in-Chief)
Copyright © 2025 by the American Psychological Association. All rights reserved.

HEARING IMPAIRMENT

Terminology

Health professionals should be aware of ongoing conversations in the disability community regarding preferred terminology. In the case of hearing loss, some individuals prefer person-centered terms (e.g., person with deafness or hearing loss), whereas others may favor identity-first language (e.g., deaf person). Both approaches are used in this chapter.

The term *deaf* denotes a hearing loss above a 90-decibel threshold. Those with lesser degrees of hearing loss are described as *hard of hearing*. The broad category of hearing loss includes *sensorineural* (dysfunction of the cochlea and/or its neural connections to the cortex) and *conductive* hearing loss (interruption along the conductive pathways: the pinna, external auditory canal, tympanic membrane, and middle ear structures; Kelly & Teplin, 2018). *Congenital* hearing loss is present at birth and can be genetic or acquired. *Delayed-onset* hearing loss can occur at any time after birth in association with a genetic disorder or a physical cause (see Table 18.1).

Auditory neuropathy spectrum disorder (ANSD) is a distinct condition where damage along the sensory and neural pathways is associated with fluctuating levels of hearing that impede speech discrimination (de Carvalho et al., 2016; Liu et al., 2019).

Epidemiology

The reported prevalence of hearing loss varies depending on the type and degree of impairment, as well as the age and distribution (geographic and socioeconomic) of the populations being studied. The overall rate of permanent bilateral severe to profound sensorineural hearing loss

TABLE 18.1

Causes and Clinical Features of Hearing Loss

Age of onset	Etiology	Outcomes and associated conditions
Congenital	**Genetic Syndromes**	
	Waardenburg	White hair forelock; vestibular dysfunction (balance)
	Alport	Renal disease—glomerulonephritis
	Branchio-oto-renal	Ear abnormalities; renal anomalies; mixed hearing loss
	Treacher-Collins	Facial features (ears, jaw, eyes)—conductive hearing loss
	Usher	Retinitis; vestibular dysfunction; progressive hearing loss
	Pendred	Thyroid dysfunction; progressive high-frequency loss
	Jervell and Lange-Nielsen	Motor incoordination; cardiac conduction problems
	Genetic Nonsyndromic	
	DFNB1 (*GJB2, GJB6* genes)	Mild to profound loss; autosomal recessive
	DFNB16 (*STRC* gene)	Mild to moderate loss; infertility in males
	Acquired	
	Congenital infections	Toxoplasmosis, rubella, herpes simplex, cytomegalovirus, and Zika virus—diffuse neurological injury
Perinatal	Complications of prematurity	Hyperbilirubinemia, sepsis, prolonged ventilation, ototoxic medications, exposure to loud ambient noise levels
	Hypoxic ischemic encephalopathy	Diffuse neurological injury (can include visual impairment)
Postnatal	DFNA8/12 (*TECTA* genes)	Prelingual milder high-frequency loss
	DFNB21 (*TECTA* gene)	Prelingual severe to profound hearing loss
	DFNB3 (*MYO15 A* gene)	Progressive bilateral hearing loss
	Mitochondrial hearing loss	Maternally inherited; or after exposure to aminoglycosides
	Illness; injury	Trauma, infection (including bacterial meningitis), ototoxic medications, or autoimmune disorders
	Lifestyle/environment	Prolonged exposure to loud sounds

has been reported at 1.12 per 1,000 live births. An additional 1 to 2 per 1,000 newborns have bilateral mild to moderate hearing loss or unilateral hearing loss of any degree (Lieu et al., 2020). The prevalence of hearing loss that is subsequently acquired by physical causes or due to delayed onset of genetic hearing loss is estimated to be as high as 18% by 18 years of age (Lieu et al., 2020). Up to 30% of sensorineural hearing loss is unilateral (van Wieringen et al., 2019). The implementation of universal newborn hearing screening programs has significantly increased the identification of hearing loss and lowered the age of initial diagnosis (Joint Committee on Infant Hearing, 2019).

Etiology

The most common causes of congenital sensorineural and mixed hearing loss are congenital cytomegalovirus (CMV, 5%–20% of cases), structural abnormalities of the temporal bones (30%–40%), and genetic causes (50%; Lieu et al., 2020). Only one-third of the likely genetic cases are associated with an identified syndrome (see Table 18.1). Of those children with nonsyndromic hearing loss, 80% have an autosomal-recessive pattern of inheritance, usually with no family history of hearing loss or physical manifestations of the disorder. More than 120 loci for genes associated with nonsyndromic hearing impairment have been identified.

Acquired causes of hearing loss include prenatal infections (i.e., CMV, toxoplasmosis, rubella, herpes simplex, Zika virus) and exposure to toxins such as alcohol and mercury as well as postnatal trauma, infection (meningitis and encephalitis), or autoimmune disorders. Extreme prematurity with the attendant medical challenges imparts a significantly increased risk of hearing loss. Prolonged exposure to loud noise, such as with the increasing use of personal device headphones, leads to hearing loss at the higher sound frequency range.

Auditory neuropathy spectrum disorder (ANSD) is a disorder of the inner hair cell synapse, spiral ganglion, or myelin sheath of the auditory nerve with resultant impairment of synchrony and consistency of nerve conduction. This condition accounts for up to 8% of sensorineural hearing loss; risk factors include neonatal hypoxia and hyperbilirubinemia (de Carvalho et al., 2016; Liu et al., 2019).

Neurobiology

Sensory input has a profound impact on early development and subsequent structure of the brain. *Sensitive periods* are windows during brain development in which lack of stimulation can impair synaptogenesis and brain maturation (Bornstein, 1989). Animal studies have suggested that those reared with a conductive hearing loss had a slower rate of amplitude modulation discrimination, raising the prospect of conductive hearing loss being associated with delays in auditory learning and poor performance on temporal discrimination tasks. In clinical reports hearing loss at an early age has also been associated with later hyperacusis and tinnitus (Sun et al., 2017).

Outcomes

In this section, we present key findings regarding developmental outcomes for deaf and hard of hearing (DHH) children and offer insights into the factors that appear to confer resilience.

Language and cognitive development. More than 90% of DHH children are born to hearing parents, the vast majority of whom are not fluent in sign language (Mitchell & Karchmer, 2004). These children are thus deprived of early opportunities for communication and have limited ability to communicate their thoughts and needs or readily acquire information verbally.

Unilateral hearing loss also increases the risk of language and learning difficulties with a reported negative impact on preverbal vocalization of infants and impeded sound localization and perception of speech in both quiet and noisy environments such as classrooms (Huttunen et al., 2019; van Wieringen et al., 2019).

Longitudinal research indicates that children with hearing loss are more likely to experience receptive and expressive language delays relative to their hearing peers (Tomblin et al., 2015). However, language outcomes improve substantially with assistive-hearing devices (Svirsky et al., 2000; Tomblin et al., 2015). Language skills are critically important, not only for their communicative value but also because of the ways in which they impact other aspects of cognitive development. "Inner language" development is impeded. For example, language skills in DHH children mediate the development of theory of mind (Yu et al., 2021) and executive function (Botting et al., 2017; Goodwin et al., 2022; Jones et al., 2020).

For many DHH children, pragmatic language skills, or the effective and appropriate use of language in social contexts, present a special set of challenges (Goberis et al., 2012; Paul et al., 2020). Specifically, children with hearing loss may dominate conversations, use language imprecisely, and repair conversational breakdowns less often. In a mainstream classroom setting, pragmatic deficits have the potential to negatively impact both peer relationships and academic achievement (Paatsch & Toe, 2020). Relational factors between children and their caregivers have been shown to influence the development of pragmatic skills in DHH children, including whether the child has opportunities for interaction with adequate visual supports and whether the child understands the context of the communication and others' understanding (Mood et al., 2020).

Other areas of cognitive development are unimpaired by hearing deficits. Young children engage in similar forms of symbolic play irrespective of their hearing status (Bornstein et al., 1999). In the context of word learning, both DHH and hearing children assume that an unfamiliar label refers to an unnamed object, a heuristic known as the novel mapping strategy (Lederberg et al., 2000). Further, DHH second-grade students demonstrate similar levels of reading achievement to their hearing peers, an achievement that belies relatively lower levels of prereading performance at age five (Tomblin et al., 2020).

Social development. The communication challenges that DHH children experience set the stage for obstacles in the formation and maintenance of peer relationships. Children who are DHH have diminished social status (Nunes et al., 2005), report higher levels of loneliness (Most, 2007), and are judged by teachers to have more psychosocial difficulties compared to hearing children (Dammeyer, 2010). The research on DHH children's perceptions of their social acceptance, however, is mixed. Some studies have found that DHH youth report having trouble fitting in with their hearing peers (e.g., Punch & Hyde, 2011), whereas other studies have concluded that this group of young people have positive, supportive relationships (Terlektsi et al., 2020).

With respect to social competence, two primary factors emerge from the research. First, DHH children with corrected hearing appear to do better in one-on-one interactions with hearing peers than in group settings (Martin et al., 2011; Punch & Hyde, 2011). Group interactions may present special challenges for DHH children because of acoustic interference, as well as the visual-attentional demands of having multiple conversational partners. Second, access to sign language among children with corrected hearing may provide opportunities to identify with the Deaf community and thus foster a sense of belonging that DHH children may struggle to establish elsewhere. Moreover, some DHH adolescents may be self-conscious of how their hearing peers perceive their deafness and whether the visible hearing technologies that they use, such as cochlear implants, will be accepted (Punch & Hyde, 2011)—concerns that are less relevant when interacting with other DHH individuals. The prevalence of autism spectrum disorder in children with neurosensory disorders is discussed later in the chapter.

Quality of life. Although it has long been suspected that children who are DHH have a lower quality of life compared to their peers without a disability, the empirical evidence is mixed. Some studies have found the expected pattern (e.g.,

Roland et al., 2016), whereas others have found no systematic differences in quality of life (e.g., Qi et al., 2020). The identity of the reporter also seems to matter. Parents' estimates of their children's quality of life tend to be more positive than their children's reports (Fellinger et al., 2008). Higher levels of quality of life are related to emotional intelligence (Ashori & Jalil-Abkenar, 2021) and comprehension of parents' communication (Kushalnagar et al., 2011), but the degree of deafness does not predict qualify of life scores (Fellinger et al., 2008). Generally, adolescence appears to be a developmental point at which DHH children may experience lower quality of life (Loy et al., 2010).

Protective factors associated with resilience in children who are deaf and hard of hearing. Despite the developmental risks associated with hearing impairments, some children will go on to flourish. Resilience is a dynamic process that operates on multiple contextual levels. At the level of the individual, personal abilities such as a sense of humor, a willingness to embrace challenges, and self-advocacy skills confer broad advantages (Eichengreen et al., 2022). Aspects of one's identity may also act as protective factors, but in ways that vary across development. Young DHH children may benefit from minimizing the centrality of deafness in their identity to feel accepted by and similar to others. Later in development, however, integrating a hearing impairment into one's identity and connecting with the Deaf community may offer a degree of protection.

Resilience is also strengthened through meaningful social interactions. One of the most notable protective factors in this respect is simply having access to information, language, and communication that DHH individuals might be deprived of inadvertently in a social environment that is hearing-dominant (Johnson et al., 2018). Supportive relationships within the family and at school with both teachers and peers also confer resilience (Freitas et al., 2022). Within the family system in particular, a sense of togetherness and commitment to shared routines and activities, including family chores, are hallmarks of adaptive families (Ahlert & Greeff, 2012).

ASSESSMENT, TESTING, AND DIAGNOSIS

Figure 18.1 provides an overview of the approach to assessing and managing a child with neurosensory disorder.

Screening

With the implementation of universal newborn hearing screening in the United States, the average age at which hearing loss is detected has dropped significantly. For other children, whose hearing loss is not detected until later ages (e.g., progressive or delayed onset of hearing loss, inadequate or inconsistent health care access) there are typically early warning signs, most notably language delays. Subtle indicators can be missed, and hearing screening should be a routine component of health checks and assessments in the school setting.

Objective measures of hearing are the most reliable means of assessing hearing in infants and younger children who cannot provide consistent behavioral responses. *Auditory evoked potentials* are electrophysiological responses that assess auditory function and neurologic integrity. *Otoacoustic emissions* (OAE) testing measures the function of the cochlea by detecting the acoustic energy produced by active movements of the outer hair cells of the cochlea in response to sound.

Hearing tests that elicit behavioral responses allow for more frequency-specific testing and confirmation that sound is being perceived by the child. *Visual reinforcement audiometry* measures the child's response by conditioning a turn to a lighted toy when the sound is presented, then presenting the sound before the visual stimulus. *Pure tone and speech audiometry* allows for more accurate measurement of older children's responses to calibrated sounds (Kelly & Teplin, 2018). Ear-specific assessment is possible when the child is old enough to tolerate headphones. The results of hearing tests are represented graphically on an audiogram, that displays

Assessment and Management of Neurosensory Disorders

Early Indicators/Screening and Identification

Hearing Loss
Medical risk factors;
Family history;
Behavioral patterns (nonresponse);
Universal newborn hearing screening;
Delayed language development

Visual Impairment
Medical risk factors; Family history;
Behavioral patterns (atypical gaze);
Abnormal eye movements or position;
Cataracts; Leukocoria (white pupil);
Automated photo-screening

Medical Evaluation and Specialized Testing

Hearing Loss
Viral testing;
Auditory brainstem responses;
Otoacoustic emissions testing;
Audiometry;
CT temporal bone;
MRI (3D);
(ECG; Thyroid function)

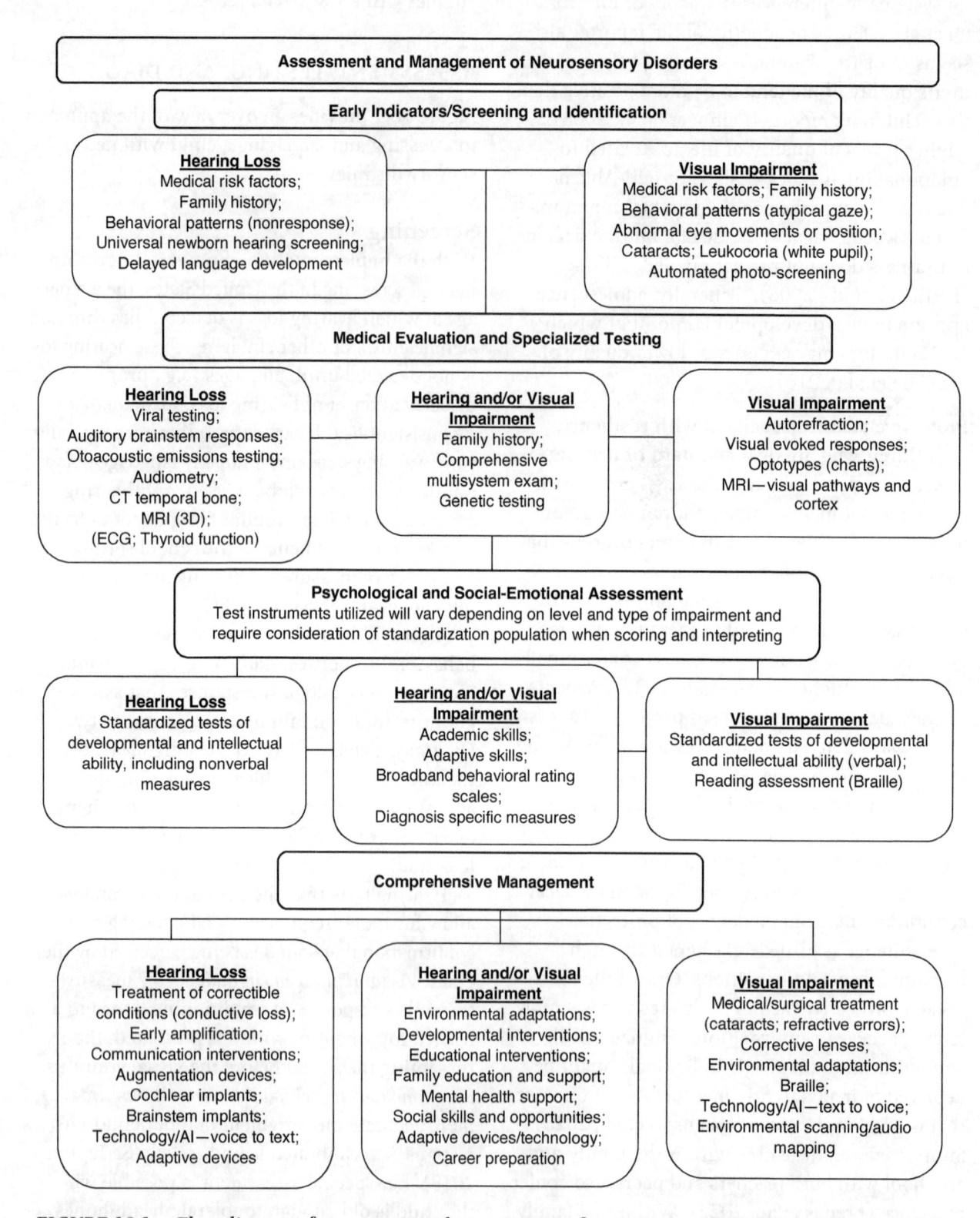

Hearing and/or Visual Impairment
Family history;
Comprehensive multisystem exam;
Genetic testing

Visual Impairment
Autorefraction;
Visual evoked responses;
Optotypes (charts);
MRI—visual pathways and cortex

Psychological and Social-Emotional Assessment
Test instruments utilized will vary depending on level and type of impairment and require consideration of standardization population when scoring and interpreting

Hearing Loss
Standardized tests of developmental and intellectual ability, including nonverbal measures

Hearing and/or Visual Impairment
Academic skills;
Adaptive skills;
Broadband behavioral rating scales;
Diagnosis specific measures

Visual Impairment
Standardized tests of developmental and intellectual ability (verbal);
Reading assessment (Braille)

Comprehensive Management

Hearing Loss
Treatment of correctible conditions (conductive loss);
Early amplification;
Communication interventions;
Augmentation devices;
Cochlear implants;
Brainstem implants;
Technology/AI—voice to text;
Adaptive devices

Hearing and/or Visual Impairment
Environmental adaptations;
Developmental interventions;
Educational interventions;
Family education and support;
Mental health support;
Social skills and opportunities;
Adaptive devices/technology;
Career preparation

Visual Impairment
Medical/surgical treatment (cataracts; refractive errors);
Corrective lenses;
Environmental adaptations;
Braille;
Technology/AI—text to voice;
Environmental scanning/audio mapping

FIGURE 18.1. Flow diagram of assessment and management of neurosensory disorders. CT = computed tomography; MRI = magnetic resonance imaging; ECG = electrocardiogram; AI = artificial intelligence.

auditory threshold in decibels across the range of frequency in hertz.

Medical Evaluation

Medical assessment of DHH children should rule out associated conditions seen in syndromic deafness such as cardiac conduction defects of Jervell and Lange-Nielsen syndrome or retinitis pigmentosa with progressive loss of vision in children with Usher syndrome. Routine vision testing assumes even more importance in DHH children, who are much more reliant on visual input than non-DHH children for learning and social communication.

All children with sensorineural hearing loss should have a high-resolution computed tomography (CT) scan of the temporal bone to rule out abnormalities of the vestibular aqueduct, cochlea, and semicircular canals. Magnetic resonance imaging scans can identify anatomic abnormalities (such as cochlear anomalies that might preclude cochlear implantation) or neoplasms (Liu et al., 2019). Rapid advances in genetic testing such as next-generation sequencing (whole exome and whole genome sequencing) will eventually enable definitive diagnosis of most genetic causes of hearing loss.

Psychological and Social Assessment

A wide range of tests has been used to assess developmental skills, cognitive functioning, and language in DHH children (e.g., Reesman et al., 2014; Udholm et al., 2017). However, due to the range of measures used, it is often difficult to make comparisons across groups (e.g., type of hearing loss; see Udholm et al., 2017). Another challenge is that many tests do not describe the population of children in the standardization or clinical sample, nor do they offer specific information as to the use of translation or its impact on task demands (Reesman et al., 2014). Many measures do offer guidance for accommodating or modifying the measure to adapt to the child's needs, or guidance for interpreting the measure and specific information regarding inclusion of DHH children in studies of the measure such as assessment of intellectual abilities (Reesman et al., 2014). The Wechsler Intelligence Scale for Children, Fifth Edition, offers specific guidance when testing DHH children, including administration guidance dependent on mode of communication (Day et al., 2015). Roid et al. (2013) conducted a clinical validity study of The Leiter International Performance Scale, Third Edition, concluding that the results for DHH individuals did not significantly vary compared to the normative sample. The variability in presentation of DHH children and in assessment measures thus must be taken into consideration when selecting and interpreting measures. Whitaker and Thomas-Presswood (2017) outlined best practices for the assessment of DHH children that include training the individual administering the assessment in how to properly adapt a test, select instruments, interpret results, and understand the domain being assessed as it relates to the individual's disability as well as factors related to the test design (e.g., language demands, materials used), analysis and interpretation (e.g., normative data, sample size, reliability of the measure if it is adapted or accommodations made), and applicability of even specialized norms identified with a specific measure. Nevertheless, assessment of skills is usually necessary to recommend interventions. A process or domain-based approach that utilizes a detailed history, multiple informants, and a variety of tests to examine patterns of strengths and challenges may better allow for understanding the specific intervention needs of the child (Lueck et al., 2019; Whitaker & Thomas-Presswood, 2017).

Children and adolescents who are DHH are more likely to have a comorbid mental health diagnosis compared to those without hearing loss (Hindley et al., 1994). Some research has, however, found no evidence of a greater risk of mental health disorders (Crowe, 2019; Niclasen & Dammeyer, 2016; Theunissen et al., 2014)

Emotional and Behavioral Functioning

A range of measures has been utilized to assess psychopathology, although these are often broadband measures rather than specific to a diagnosis and were not developed or validated specifically to children and adolescents with hearing loss (Theunissen et al., 2014). Some measures, such as the Strengths and Difficulties Questionnaire, have specific recommendations for use with DHH children (Niclasen & Dammeyer, 2016). Similarly, the Autism Diagnostic Observation Schedule, Second Edition, and the Autism Diagnostic Interview-R have been specifically adapted to use with DHH individuals, with specific recommendations for administration and scoring (ADOS-2 Deaf Adaptation). Allgar et al. (2021) offer guidance on using the two measures in combination.

MANAGEMENT AND INTERVENTIONS: THE IMPORTANCE OF MULTIDISCIPLINARY CARE

Treatment and management interventions for children who are DHH should start as early as possible, be interdisciplinary, and adhere to a lifespan approach.

Developmental-Behavioral Pediatrics

The role of the developmental-behavioral pediatrician is to ensure that all necessary medical testing and treatment have been addressed and that appropriate and effective management and interventions are implemented. In addition, because DHH children are at increased risk of developmental and behavioral vulnerabilities, evaluation and longitudinal monitoring by developmental-behavioral pediatricians and pediatric psychologists with expertise in school assessment can help guide interventions and educational planning across the childhood lifespan.

Audiology and Otolaryngology

The management of hearing loss is predicated on early identification and intervention. The Joint Committee on Infant Hearing (2019) reaffirmed the Centers for Disease Control and Prevention's 1-3-6 Early Hearing Detection and Intervention goals (Centers for Disease Control and Prevention, 2023): screening completed by 1 month of age, audiologic diagnosis completed by 3 months of age, and early intervention initiated no later than 6 months of age. Early treatment of any medical causes of hearing loss can be beneficial. In children with hearing loss due to CMV infection, studies have suggested improved hearing after long-term antiviral therapy with valganciclovir (Liu et al., 2019).

When significant hearing loss has been discovered, the child should be fitted with a hearing aid as soon as possible. Once a child is old enough to participate in behavioral hearing tests, the results can be used to calibrate hearing aids. The goal of amplification is to make speech and other environmental sounds audible while also avoiding high-intensity sound levels that are aversive or that could damage residual hearing. A variety of forms of amplification is available, including behind-the-ear or ear-level hearing aids. Bone conduction devices are used for children with certain types of conductive hearing loss who cannot be fitted with conventional hearing aids.

Cochlear implants are the treatment of choice for profound hearing loss. These devices consist of a microphone, a speech processor that converts the sound into an electric code, and an external coil that then transmits the signal across the skin to the internal receiver system implanted in the temporal bone. This is connected to multichannel electrodes within the cochlea that impart electrical inputs across the frequency range. Cochlear implants enable the perception of environmental sounds as well as recognition and understanding of speech. Advances in technology and surgical technique have enabled implantation before 12 months of age with a low risk of complications and positive functional impact. In general, children who receive implants before 2 years of age have the best outcomes regarding speech perception and language development and can enter school with typical language abilities.

Children who use any form of amplification device, and especially those who have cochlear implants, need intensive follow-up with specialized speech and language therapy and auditory training (aural rehabilitation) to learn the meaning of the newly amplified sounds and to optimize their language development (Kelly & Teplin, 2018).

For children who have anatomic conditions that preclude cochlear implantation auditory brainstem implantation can provide direct electric stimulation to the cochlear nucleus in the brainstem. Early outcome studies suggest improvement in sound detection with slow progress in speech perception over 5 years or more (Liu et al., 2019).

Assistive devices and advances in information technology have increased opportunities for communication for DHH individuals. Devices such as flashing doorbells and alarms enhance safety, and closed captioning is pervasive in videos and tele-videoconferencing. Wireless and Bluetooth systems can link amplification devices directly to smartphones or a microphone worn by a classroom teacher or instructor. Text messaging and social media are now primary forms of communication among older children and young adults, which has mitigated many disparities and previous barriers to communication.

Pediatric Psychology, Neuropsychology, and Clinical Psychology

Psychologists offer important contributions in the assessment, management, and provision of intervention. As part of the assessment team, psychologists—including pediatric psychologists and pediatric neuropsychologists—should utilize assessment tools (e.g., assessing cognitive skills, neuropsychological assessments) with careful consideration of necessary measures and modifications to identify strengths and areas of need for intervention. As part of an interdisciplinary team, the psychologist will play an important role in integrating results, observations, and other information gathered by all those involved in the assessment process to develop intervention programming across developmental, educational, and social-emotional domains that meets the individualized needs of the individual. Psychologists are also resources for assisting families in identifying, accessing, and utilizing resources to promote continued development and monitoring progress over time (e.g., Spellun et al., 2022). Behavioral health strategies may include providing support to families in maintaining the integrity of the intervention programming and navigating the complex dynamics of a familial relationship such as in behavioral intervention or psychotherapy.

Several factors must be considered in the context of behavioral intervention and psychotherapy/counseling. The provider must understand and incorporate the child's strengths, needs, and skills to facilitate participation, including necessary environmental modifications or structures. A culturally affirmative and disability perspective is also important in DHH individuals' mental health (Glickman & Hall, 2019). If the provider is not fluent in the child's language, it is important to consider whether intervention is more appropriate or available with a practitioner who is fluent in the child's language. In instances in which it is determined that an interpreter is necessary, care must be taken to ensure accurate communication. The potential effects of the interpreter on the relationship between the provider and child should also be considered. It is also important to note that caregivers may or may not use the same primary language as their child, and the professional may need to be fluent in multiple languages or have access to interpreters if the caregiver(s) and child use different means of primary communication.

Speech and Language Pathology

Intervention focused on the development of pragmatic language skills has been increasingly identified as needed for DHH children (Paatsch & Toe, 2020; Yoshinaga-Itano et al., 2020). Therapies provided by a speech and language pathologist can include naturalistic interventions such as increasing child-directed parent talk with young children (Yoshinaga-Itano et al., 2020), a conversational model of intervention (including providing opportunities for interaction and conversation), the use of nonverbal cues to support understanding of the context/meaning of verbal information, use of language with correct semantics, syntax, and phonology to promote others' understanding, and strategies to maintain and sustain conversation (Paatsch & Toe, 2020; Paatsch et al., 2017), and attention to relational factors that promote pragmatic language development (Mood et al., 2020).

Early Literacy Supports

Focused attention should also be given to promoting reading skills and outcomes through specific early literacy instruction and intervention (Runnion & Gray, 2019). This includes interventions focused on alphabet knowledge, print concept knowledge, phonological awareness, and oral language skills (Lederberg et al., 2014; Runnion & Gray, 2019).

VISUAL IMPAIRMENT

Terminology

Low vision is defined by the World Health Organization (WHO) as a best-corrected visual acuity (BCVA) in the better-seeing eye of less than 20/60. *Legal blindness*, a term used exclusively in the United States, is defined as a BCVA of 20/200 or less by the U.S. Social Security Administration. The WHO defines *blindness* as a BCVA of 20/400 or worse with no light perception. The term *monocular blindness* denotes loss of vision in one eye with accompanying increased risk of subsequent visual impairment (Solebo et al., 2017). The logMar (Logarithm of the Minimum Angle of Resolution) chart is also used internationally as a measure of vision with logMar 0.00 equating to 20/20 vision and 1.00 equating to 20/200 vision.

Epidemiology

It has been estimated that up to 14 million children in the world are blind, with socioeconomic deprivation as a major determinant of prevalence. Visual impairment (VI) is quite likely underestimated. The prevalence of blindness in children under 16 years of age has been estimated at 12 to 15 per 10,000 in low- and/or middle-income countries and 3 to 4 per 10,000 in more economically affluent countries (Solebo et al., 2017).

Etiology

In affluent countries, childhood VI most commonly results from underlying conditions of the central nervous system. In more impoverished developing countries, VI is more frequently caused by infections, nutritional deficiencies (vitamin A deficiency), and inadequate access to ophthalmologic treatments (Solebo et al., 2017).

Prenatal causes of VI include genetic conditions, fetal malformations, prenatal infections, and hypoxia. In some cases, congenital abnormalities of the brain and/or eye may be localized to a specific structure, whereas in other cases, they might affect multiple parts of the visual system. In the perinatal period, VI may result from central nervous system (CNS) hypoxia/ischemia (prenatally or during labor and delivery), retinopathy of prematurity, and/or infection. Postnatal etiologies include amblyopia, tumors, nutritional deficiencies, trauma (including nonaccidental injury secondary to child abuse), infection, increased intracranial pressure, and systemic conditions (Kelly & Teplin, 2018; see Table 18.2).

Cerebral (or cortical) visual impairment (CVI) occurs when visual signals received from the retinas and optic nerves are not accurately or consistently interpreted by the brain's posterior visual pathways, either temporarily (e.g., in delayed visual maturation) or permanently. CVI is most often associated with hypoxic-ischemic encephalopathy (HIE). Diagnosis is often difficult because the classic signs and symptoms of eye disorders are absent (e.g., normal pupillary responses, eye movements, and eye examination), and visual symptoms associated with CVI are often subtle. The most common difficulty is in distinguishing objects against patterned backgrounds (Chang & Borchert, 2020).

Neurobiology

The impact of sensory deprivation has been extensively studied in vision where the absence of visual experience disrupts the creation of neural networks and subsequent normal function. The visual system becomes progressively less responsive after about 8 years of age, after which time amblyopia (developmental VI) becomes permanent (Solebo & Rahi, 2014).

Outcomes

Visual impairment can have broad-reaching effects across the domains of communication, cognitive development, social and emotional

TABLE 18.2

Causes and Outcomes of Visual Impairment

Condition	Etiology	Outcomes and associated conditions
Retinopathy of prematurity	Extreme prematurity—mechanical ventilation—new vessel formation in retina	Difficulties with spatial awareness; motor coordination; behavioral challenges
Optic nerve hypoplasia	Maternal diabetes; fetal alcohol; chromosomal abnormalities	Variable acuity—can have severe impairment; learning problems; increased risk of autism
Cortical visual impairment	CNS injury (hypoxia-ischemia); infections; tumors disruption of optic radiations	Variable impairment—can improve; difficulty with cluttered visual background
Cataract	Often unknown etiology; congenital rubella	Requires prompt treatment; can cause permanent vision loss
Corneal opacity	Vitamin A deficiency or infection (developing countries)	Blindness; only treatment is corneal transplant
Retinal photoreceptor dystrophies; retinitis pigmentosa	Inherited—Leber's amarosis; gene mutations	Variable outcomes; can have progressive vision loss

Note. CNS = central nervous system.

functioning, and overall quality of life (Chokron & Dutton, 2016; Keil et al., 2017; Lieu et al., 2020; Lueck et al., 2019).

In this section, we highlight some of the most notable outcomes of VI from the developmental science literature and consider some of the key factors associated with resilience.

Motor development. In children with VI, motor skills such as sitting and standing progress at typical rates. However, skills that require awareness of surroundings, such as walking, running, and kicking, are delayed (Wagner et al., 2013). Fine motor coordination also lags (Houwen et al., 2009).

Language and cognitive development. Vision serves a unique role in enabling the rapid synthesis of multisensory information, automatically boosting the efficiency of the brain's associative and executive functions.

Both blind infants and those with visual impairments eventually develop joint attention, but typically later than sighted infants (Bigelow, 2003; Urqueta Alfaro et al., 2018). Research has also documented an increased risk of errors in speech sound production (Gordon-Pershey et al., 2019). Structural language appears to develop relatively intact in VI children, but pragmatic language skills may represent an area of special concern for this population (Tadić et al., 2010).

With respect to cognitive development, the bulk of the available research indicates a great deal of overlap between VI and sighted children. For the most part, the documented differences tend to be both small and temporary. They include limited deficits in attentional processes (Tadić et al., 2009) and delays in theory of mind (Bartoli et al., 2019) and symbolic and functional play (Lewis et al., 2000). School-age children with VI may develop literacy skills several years later than their sighted counterparts, but once established, no differences in reading or listening comprehension exist (Edmonds & Pring, 2006). There is some evidence that children with VI may possess enhanced memory (Swanson & Luxenberg, 2009; Withagen et al., 2013).

Social development. Social interactions rely heavily on visual information, and to the extent that VI children lack access to this input, their opportunities to engage effectively with peers may be limited.

Social communication deficits emerge as early as the first year (Dale et al., 2014). Based on parental surveys, toddlers with VI lag sighted peers in their social-emotional development, including the expression of empathy and peer relations (Lang et al., 2017). Further, the degree of VI predicts social-emotional competency, with more profound VI linked to lower levels of performance. As social demands increase with age, children with VI continue to face challenges when interacting with peers. In general, they are more likely to engage in solitary than cooperative play (Roe, 2008), but this pattern is marked by substantial variation that can be at least partly attributed to individual characteristics of the child, such as language ability and temperament (Verver et al., 2020). Children with VI who receive social support from peers in the form of cooperation, empathetic behavior, and practical assistance report higher levels of self-esteem and social acceptance (Manitsa & Doikou, 2022).

Peer relationships continue to challenge young people with VI in adolescence, a time when social interactions take on increasing significance. Compared to sighted teens, those with VI report having fewer friends (Pinquart & Pfeiffer, 2011) and spending more time alone (Jessup et al., 2018). Limited interactions with peers may further compound deficits in social skills. VI appears to have the most pronounced effects on the size of a friend group rather than the ability to establish a close friendship (Pinquart & Pfeiffer, 2011). Moreover, teens who attend specialized schools for students with VI experience less peer rejection than VI adolescents in mainstream classrooms.

The co-occurrence of autism spectrum disorder (ASD) has been specifically examined in children with VI and/or DHH (Do et al., 2017). ASD co-occurs with VI or hearing loss at rates higher than the population prevalence of ASD, with risk ratios in one study greater than 31.0 times in VI children and 14.1 times in DHH children (Kancherla et al., 2013). VI children were diagnosed with ASD significantly later (median age 79 months) than those without VI (median age 56 months) despite similarities in the initial age of evaluation for ASD. In contrast, DHH children were initially evaluated at a younger age than those without hearing loss although the age of diagnosis was comparable (Kancherla et al., 2013).

Quality of life. Few studies have examined quality of life in children and youth with VI. One study found that school-age children with VI have a lower quality of life compared to sighted peers according to parental report (Bathelt et al., 2019). Further, the relationship between VI and quality of life is mediated by adaptive behavior. That is, children who had more profound VI had fewer adaptive behaviors, which then predicted lower levels of quality of life. Other research has found that parents may not be reliable reporters of children's quality of life. Children and adolescents with VI reported higher quality of life scores compared to their parents (Oliveira et al., 2018)—a finding that echoes a similar pattern found with DHH youth (Fellinger et al., 2008). Quality of life among children and adolescents with VI also varies depending on individual characteristics. Specifically, better quality of life has been reported among males compared to females, younger children compared to adolescents, and youth with low vision compared to those with profound vision loss (Oliveira et al., 2018). Age of vision loss is also related to quality of life, such that youth with congenital or early-onset VI fare better than those who lost vision after the age of 2 years (Robertson et al., 2021).

Protective factors associated with resilience in children with visual impairment. Leisure activities contribute to resilience in VI youth by promoting social relationships, strengthening identity formation, and establishing a sense of agency (Jessup et al., 2010). Meaningful social relationships with age-mates confer resilience in children and adolescents with VI (Kef & Deković, 2004) and may even facilitate the healthy formation of self (Robertson et al., 2021). Parental overprotection has been found to be inversely related to the size of VI adolescents' friend networks (Pinquart & Pfeiffer, 2011). Other parenting behaviors have been identified in the research as key protective factors for children with VI. Specifically, maternal responsivity and sensitivity have been correlated with positive developmental outcomes (Dote-Kwan, 1995; Sakkalou et al., 2021; see also Grumi et al., 2021, for a review). In contrast, negative outcomes have been linked to maternal control and directiveness (Hughes et al., 1999). It is worth noting that mothers of infants with VI report substantial parenting stress and are at high risk of developing anxiety and depression (Sakkalou et al., 2018) which may reduce the likelihood of being able to engage in protective parenting behaviors.

Assessment

Screening. Professionals working with infants and young children should be vigilant in screening for any signs that might suggest loss of vision, such as persisting wandering eye movements and lack of visual tracking (such as following movement of a caregiver's face) by age 3 to 6 months of age or other abnormalities of the eye, including tearing and redness, lack of alignment (strabismus), or the appearance of a white pupil (a sign of retinoblastoma). However, many forms of visual impairment, such as decreased vision in one eye (amblyopia), could be missed without the routine, systematic screening that should occur at health visits or in schools (Kelly & Teplin, 2018).

Testing. Visual ability is best assessed in young preverbal children by assessing their ability to visually fixate on and track an object. Vision screening and testing technologies include automated photoscreening and autorefraction that can identify risk for amblyopia in children as young as 12 months, or those with developmental disabilities (Donahue et al., 2016). By 3 to 4 years of age, visual acuity can be tested directly using validated instruments such as LEA symbols and HOTV letter charts. Sloan or Snellen letter charts are recommended for school-aged children, with the logMar charts used internationally. For children with CVI, The CVI Range assessment of visual functioning is utilized (Roman-Lantzy, 2018).

Medical evaluation: The role of developmental-behavioral pediatricians. Developmental-behavioral pediatricians should evaluate children for medical and neurological complications that could accompany syndromes associated with VI and ensure that they are being appropriately addressed (see Table 18.2). The medical evaluation team could incorporate a teacher of the visually impaired (TVI) and certified orientation and mobility specialist (COMS) to comprehensively evaluate the child's functional profile, including strengths as well as VI-related limitations (Kelly & Teplin, 2018).

Psychological and social assessment: The role of psychologists. Psychological assessment of VI children requires consideration of the child's means of perception and how that may impact skill acquisition and performance. Thus, when conducting an assessment, psychologists (e.g., pediatric psychologists and neuropsychologists) must determine the most appropriate methods of assessment and the goal for the assessment.

Developmental measures such as the Oregon Project for Preschool Children Who Are Blind or Visually Impaired (Anderson et al., 2007) and Reynell-Zinkin Developmental Scales (Reynell, 1979; Vervloed et al., 2000) are specifically developed for use with VI children. Such measures may be used to assist in examining skills across a range of domains over time (initial assessment and progress) and in developing intervention programming.

In assessing intellectual and cognitive skills, verbal scales of standardized measures may often be utilized (e.g., Wechsler Scales; Chen et al., 2021). The Woodcock Johnson-IV offers both large print and Braille editions (Schrank et al., 2014). However, with these modifications and adaptations, consideration must be given to whether the measures are assessing the same underlying competencies (Atkins, 2012). Haptic assessments have been developed to assess a VI child's skills a VI child's skills (Ballesteros et al., 2005; Withagen et al., 2013). However, many of the measures are not developed for children and often lack psychometric properties (Mazella et al., 2014).

When conducting assessments, it is important to consider the consistency of skills across the varied environments in which the child interacts and factors that may impact the implementation of a particular skill. Information gathered from multiple sources, including across environments and informants that can then be integrated with information gained from assessment measures will provide a more comprehensive profile of the child.

Emotional and behavioral functioning. As with DHH children, the commonly used screening inventories have not been normed or validated for children with VI, and they should be interpreted with caution. Interviews and observations of behavioral responses and changes from baseline mood and behavior will provide indicators of the need for further evaluation or treatment.

Interventions

Management interventions should focus on learning necessary compensatory skills (e.g., reading Braille, safe and independent mobility with a COMS, efficient use of residual vision, listening skills, and adaptive low-vision devices such as magnifiers).

Intervention strategies vary widely based on the specifics of the VI. Furthermore, as there may be changes in the child's sight over time, interventions need to be carefully monitored for appropriateness and effectiveness. Consideration needs to be given to how to modify many frequently used curriculum and intervention programs as they often incorporate pictorial or gestural supports (e.g., pictures can be replaced with touch, objects, or auditory input). Environmental modifications may also be recommended, including lighting, visual contrast, and the amount of visual and auditory material (Chang & Borchert, 2020; Jayaraman et al., 2021). Advances in digital technology also hold much promise for VI such as scanning devices and screen reading software programs that convert text to voice. Smartphones and wearable devices with GPS capabilities and camera applications can facilitate independent mobility by building audio maps or describing the color, size, and shape of objects in the immediate environment. Other artificial intelligence capabilities are being incorporated into "smart glasses" that can use AI to provide navigation information and potentially identify faces.

MULTISENSORY IMPAIRMENT

Deaf-Blindness (DB) denotes multisensory impairment with varying levels of impairment of each sensory modality.

Etiology

Conditions associated with diffuse neurological injury such as extreme prematurity, hypoxia and ischemia, and inherited conditions such as Usher syndrome can impair both vision and hearing.

Developmental Outcomes

Approximately 85% of children with this dual sensory impairment have additional disabilities, particularly intellectual disability, speech/language disorders, and orthopedic conditions.

Without unimpeded access to the distant senses, children with DB face extraordinary challenges in connecting with the physical and social world. Developmental research on this population of children is woefully scarce, but it is reasonable to assume that the condition has widespread developmental consequences. Notable challenges include orientation and mobility, communication, social isolation, and conceptual development (Miles & Riggio, 1999). DB individuals must be carefully, patiently, and consistently trained so that their hands become their primary sensory organs as well as the primary means of communication.

Assessment

Few measures exist that are specifically developed for assessing the cognitive skills of DB children. Many adaptations of measures for DHH children or VI children or traditionally used measures cannot be utilized as described for children and adolescents with multisensory impairment, as these adaptations often emphasize utilization of either auditory or visual assessment strategies or measures that do not include DB children in their samples.

A careful assessment is critical to provide information necessary for identifying learning needs and promoting development. The Callier-Azusa Scale (Stillman, 1974) has been a long-standing rating scale used to assess the competencies of DB children. However, the use of a multiple assessment pathways approach offers a means of gaining a more comprehensive picture of a child's strengths and weaknesses (Nicholas, 2020). Included in this is a multimethod, multi-informant assessment; an assessment of the environments and systems that influence cognitive skills; and adynamic assessment integrating instruction and learning (Nicholas, 2020). If standardized testing measures are used, specific and detailed documentation of testing accommodations and/or modifications should be outlined (Nicholas, 2020).

Intervention

Children with multisensory impairment present with unique needs in the home, school, and community. The modalities of presentation, materials utilized, and all aspects of the environment must be developed with consideration of not just the child's visual and auditory needs (both individually and in combination), but also how the child most effectively perceives and responds to the environment. An interdisciplinary team that represents expertise in all domains, including communication, education, and vision impairment, hearing impairment, is imperative to creating and meeting the diverse needs of the child. The National Center on Deaf-Blindness (https://www.nationaldb.org) has published guidelines for components of intervention, including interacting with the child, structuring the environment, and assessing/monitoring skills to assist those in developing intervention programming.

Equity and Inclusion and Rights and Advocacy

Educational and other legal entitlements, accommodations, and protections are provided to children with visual and/or hearing impairments under three federal laws: the 1973 Rehabilitation Act, specifically Section 504 (U.S. Congress, 1973); the Americans with Disabilities Act (ADA; U.S. Congress, 1990); and the Individuals With Disabilities Education Act (IDEA; U.S. Congress, 2004). Under IDEA, within the public educational setting, the child, the child's family, caregivers, or guardians and designated educational personnel are part of a team that participates in a formalized process of evaluation and determination of eligibility for educational services (see the Resources box for more information). As part of the evaluation process, the educational team, which is mandated to evaluate the child, is also able to, and can be requested to, review and utilize information (e.g., assessments, observations) from other sources outside of the educational environment. If a child is determined eligible for educational services, an Individualized Education Plan (IEP) is then developed, identifying goals, measurable objectives, and required supports for promoting educational progress. The IEP is used to guide educational planning and the child's educational team meets regularly to assess progress and determine if alterations to the IEP may be necessary.

The Rehabilitation Act and the ADA also have implications for a child's access to educational services (e.g., a Section 504 plan) as well as broader reach. The ADA guides rights across systems including within the community (e.g., housing), health care, and employment. Implementation and interpretation of the ADA are guided by regulations as well as legal decisions. As such, the landscape of how the ADA is applied is evolving. See the Resources box for more information.

As with other vulnerable populations, including those with intellectual disabilities, individuals with neurosensory disorders are at increased risk for the consequences of disparities in health care. These disparities include not only access to primary and preventive medical services but also to interventions and assistive devices specific to their impairment. Women, racial/ethnic minorities, and low-income beneficiaries of medical services with self-reported hearing impairment are less likely to report using hearing aids than their peers (Willink et al., 2021). In addition to advocacy for legislative change in health care reimbursement, developmental pediatricians and pediatric psychologists should be at the forefront of researching and developing alternate models of care that address these inequities.

SUMMARY AND IMPLICATIONS FOR CLINICAL PRACTICE AND FUTURE RESEARCH

Neurosensory disorders pose complex challenges, both to the individuals with the disorder and to the professionals who test and treat them. There have been significant advances in understanding etiology and underlying pathophysiology, but there is much interindividual variation with multiple factors mediating functional outcomes and responses to intervention.

A comprehensive, individualized approach to both assessment and treatment is essential. Drawing from research in developmental science, identifying opportunities to mitigate risk and foster resilience can help children with neurosensory conditions achieve optimal outcomes across the childhood lifespan. Multidisciplinary longitudinal care from developmental-behavioral pediatricians and pediatric psychologists can help individualize treatment and interventions across home, school, medical, and community settings, with the aim of helping foster independence, functionality, and maximal inclusion for children with neurosensory disorders.

There remains a paucity of research regarding optimal methods of assessing children with neurosensory disorders (including those utilizing augmentative technologies) and a dearth of professionals with the requisite background and training for developmental and educational interventions for these children. Rapid advances in technology have contributed to increased opportunities for independent functioning for individuals with neurosensory disorders. However, longstanding barriers to access to advanced treatments and technologies threaten the ability of many of the most underserved, who are already at increased risk for neurosensory disorders, to benefit from these advances. There is an urgent need for advocacy.

Research is needed to better define demographic disparities and to identify optimal approaches to prevention, early identification, testing, and management along with delineation of prognostic factors. Further advances in artificial intelligence and machine learning technology and the prospect of brain augmentation techniques hold almost limitless promise for increased functional abilities for those facing neurosensory disorders.

RESOURCES

Deaf and Hard of Hearing

American Academy of Pediatrics (https://www.aap.org)

- Recommendations on early hearing detection and intervention:

  https://www.aap.org/en/patient-care/early-hearing-detection-and-intervention/

- Recommendations on hearing assessment and intervention beyond infancy (2023):

  https://publications.aap.org/pediatrics/article/152/3/e2023063288/193755/Hearing-Assessment-in-Infants-Children-and

Centers for Disease Control and Prevention (https://www.cdc.gov)

Educational resources for individuals who are deaf or hard of hearing, and their caregivers.

- CDC resource guide: *A Parent's Guide to Hearing Loss*:

  https://www.cdc.gov/ncbddd/hearingloss/parentsguide/index.html

- CDC's Hearing Loss in Children online resource portal:

  https://www.cdc.gov/ncbddd/hearingloss/

Hands and Voices (https://handsandvoices.org)

Advocacy and support for parents and caregivers of children who are deaf or hard of hearing.

National Association of the Deaf (https://www.nad.org)

A civil rights group of, by, and for individuals who are deaf and hard of hearing with advocacy focused in the areas of early intervention, education, employment, health care, technology, and telecommunications. Also focuses on the promotion of American Sign Language.

Visual Impairment

American Academy of Pediatrics (https://www.aap.org)

- Recommendations on procedures for assessing vision loss in children:

  https://publications.aap.org/pediatrics/article/137/1/e20153597/52806/Procedures-for-the-Evaluation-of-the-Visual-System

- Recommendations for screening premature infants for retinopathy:

  https://publications.aap.org/pediatrics/article/142/6/e20183061/37478/Screening-Examination-of-Premature-Infants-for

Centers for Disease Control and Prevention (https://www.cdc.gov)

Basic resources on vision loss in children.

- Keep an eye on your child's vision:

  https://www.cdc.gov/visionhealth/resources/features/vision-health-children.html

- Facts about vision loss in children:

  https://www.cdc.gov/vision-health/prevention/youth-vision-problems.html

The Oregon Project

A curricular resource for visually impaired children ages 0 to 6 years:

https://www.soesd.k12.or.us/or-project/

Perkins School for the Blind (https://www.perkins.org)

Resource Center:

https://www.perkins.org/resource-center/

National Federation for the Blind (https://nfb.org/)

- Programs and services for persons with vision impairment:

  https://nfb.org/programs-services

- Resources for individuals who are deaf-blind:

  https://nfb.org/resources/deafblind-resources

WonderBaby (https://www.wonderbaby.org/)

Resources for children who have visual impairment and those with multiple disabilities.

Education of Children With Disabilities

- **Rehabilitation Act of 1973, Section 504**

  https://www.hhs.gov/sites/default/files/ocr/civilrights/resources/factsheets/504.pdf

  Section 504 of the Rehabilitation Act of 1973 requires publicly funded schools to accommodate children's disabilities in the school setting.

- **Americans With Disabilities Act of 1990**

  https://www.ada.gov/

  Comprehensive information about the rights of parents of children with disabilities is available via the Department of Justice, Civil Rights Division website (https://www.ada.gov/topics/parental-rights/).

- **Individuals With Disabilities Education Act (IDEA)**

  https://sites.ed.gov/idea/

  Comprehensive information about the right to education services under the IDEA.

References

Ahlert, I. A., & Greeff, A. P. (2012). Resilience factors associated with adaptation in families with deaf and hard of hearing children. *American Annals of the Deaf*, 157(4), 391–404. https://doi.org/10.1353/aad.2012.1629

Allgar, V., Wright, B., Taylor, A., Couter, A. L., & Phillips, H. (2021). Diagnosing autism spectrum disorders in deaf children using two standardized assessment instruments: The ADIR-deaf adaptation and the ADOS-2 deaf adaptation. *Journal of Clinical Medicine, 10*(19), 4374–4388. https://doi.org/10.3390/jcm10194374

Anderson, S., Boigon, S., Davis, K., DeWaard, C., & Southern Oregon Education Service District. (2007). *The Oregon Project for preschool children who are blind or visually impaired* (6th ed.). Southern Oregon Education Service District.

Ashori, M., & Jalil-Abkenar, S. S. (2021). Emotional intelligence: Quality of life and cognitive emotion regulation of deaf and hard-of-hearing adolescents. *Deafness & Education International, 23*(2), 84–102. https://doi.org/10.1080/14643154.2020.1766754

Atkins, S. (2012). *Assessing the ability of blind and partially sighted people: Are psychometric tests fair?* RNIB Centre for Accessible Information.

Ballesteros, S., Bardisa, D., Millar, S., & Reales, J. M. (2005). The haptic test battery: A new instrument to test tactual abilities in blind and visually impaired and sighted children. *British Journal of Visual Impairment, 23*(1), 11–24. https://doi.org/10.1177/0264619605051717

Bartoli, G., Bulgarelli, D., & Molina, P. (2019). Theory of mind development in children with visual impairment: The contribution of the adapted comprehension test ToM storybooks. *Journal of Autism and Developmental Disorders, 49*(9), 3494–3503. https://doi.org/10.1007/s10803-019-04064-3

Bathelt, J., de Haan, M., & Dale, N. J. (2019). Adaptive behaviour and quality of life in school-age children with congenital visual disorders and different levels of visual impairment. *Research in Developmental Disabilities, 85*, 154–162. https://doi.org/10.1016/j.ridd.2018.12.003

Bigelow, A. E. (2003). The development of joint attention in blind infants. *Development and Psychopathology, 15*(2), 259–275. https://doi.org/10.1017/S0954579403000142

Bornstein, M. H. (1989). Sensitive periods in development: Structural characteristics and causal interpretations. *Psychological Bulletin, 105*(2), 179–197. https://doi.org/10.1037/0033-2909.105.2.179

Bornstein, M. H., Selmi, A. M., Haynes, O. M., Painter, K. M., & Marx, E. S. (1999). Representational abilities and the hearing status of child/mother dyads. *Child Development, 70*(4), 833–852. https://doi.org/10.1111/1467-8624.00060

Botting, N., Jones, A., Marshall, C., Denmark, T., Atkinson, J., & Morgan, G. (2017). Nonverbal executive function is mediated by language: A study of deaf and hard of hearing children. *Child Development, 88*(5), 1689–1700. https://doi.org/10.1111/cdev.12659

Centers for Disease Control and Prevention. (2023). *Screening and diagnosis of hearing loss*. National Center on Birth Defects and Developmental Disabilities, Centers for Disease Control and Prevention. https://www.cdc.gov/ncbddd/hearingloss/screening.html

Chang, M. Y., & Borchert, M. S. (2020). Advances in the evaluation and management of cortical/cerebral visual impairment in children. *Survey of Ophthalmology, 65*(6), 708–724. https://doi.org/10.1016/j.survophthal.2020.03.001

Chen, X., Lu, M., Bu, W., Wang, L., Wang, Y., Xu, Y., & Zhong, M. (2021). Psychometric properties of WISC-IV verbal scales: A study of students in China who are blind. *Journal of Visual Impairment & Blindness, 115*(3), 228–241. https://doi.org/10.1177/0145482X211018520

Chokron, S., & Dutton, G. N. (2016). Impact of cerebral visual impairments on motor skills: Implications for developmental coordination disorders. *Frontiers in Psychology, 7*, 1471. https://doi.org/10.3389/fpsyg.2016.01471

Crowe, T. V. (2019). Deaf child and adolescent consumers of public behavioral health services. *Journal of Deaf Studies and Deaf Education, 24*(2), 57–64. https://doi.org/10.1093/deafed/eny036

Dale, N. J., Tadić, V., & Sonksen, P. (2014). Social communicative variation in 1–3-year-olds with severe visual impairment. *Child: Care, Health and Development, 40*(2), 158–164. https://doi.org/10.1111/cch.12065

Dammeyer, J. (2010). Psychosocial development in a Danish population of children with cochlear implants and deaf and hard-of-hearing children. *Journal of Deaf Studies and Deaf Education, 15*(1), 50–58. https://doi.org/10.1093/deafed/enp024

Day, L. A., Adams Costa, E. B., & Raiford, S. E. (2015). *Testing children who are deaf or hard of hearing*. Wechsler Intelligence Scale for Children, Fifth Edition [Technical report #2]. Pearson Assessments. https://www.pearsonassessments.com/content/dam/school/global/clinical/us/assets/wisc-v/wisc-v-technical-report-2.pdf

de Carvalho, G. M., Ramos, P., Arthur, C., Guimarães, A., & Sartorato, E. (2016). Performance of cochlear implants in pediatric patients with auditory neuropathy spectrum disorder. *The Journal of International Advanced Otology, 12*(1), 8–15. https://doi.org/10.5152/iao.2016.2232

Do, B., Lynch, P., Macris, E. M., Smyth, B., Stavrinakis, S., Quinn, S., & Constable, P. A.

(2017). Systematic review and meta-analysis of the association of Autism Spectrum Disorder in visually or hearing impaired children. *Ophthalmic & Physiological Optics, 37*(2), 212–224. https://doi.org/10.1111/opo.12350

Donahue, S. P., Baker, C. N., Simon, G. R., Boudreau, A. D. A., Baker, C. N., Barden, G. A., III, Hackell, J. M., Hardin, A. P., Meade, K. E., Moore, S. B., Richerson, J., Lehman, S. S., Granet, D. B., Bradford, G. E., Rubin, S. E., Siatkowski, R. M., Suh, D. W., Granet, D. B., & the Committee on Practice and Ambulatory Medicine, American Academy of Pediatrics, & the Section on Ophthalmology, American Academy of Pediatrics, & the American Association of Certified Orthoptists, & the American Association for Pediatric Ophthalmology and Strabismus, & the American Academy of Ophthalmology. (2016). Procedures for the evaluation of the visual system by pediatricians. *Pediatrics, 137*(1), e20153597. https://doi.org/10.1542/peds.2015-3597

Dote-Kwan, J. (1995). Impact of mothers' interactions on the development of their young visually impaired children. *Journal of Visual Impairment & Blindness, 89*(1), 46–58. https://doi.org/10.1177/0145482X9508900109

Edmonds, C. J., & Pring, L. (2006). Generating inferences from written and spoken language: A comparison of children with visual impairment and children with sight. *British Journal of Developmental Psychology, 24*(2), 337–351. https://doi.org/10.1348/026151005X35994

Eichengreen, A., Zaidman-Zait, A., Most, T., & Golik, G. (2022). Resilience from childhood to young adulthood: Retrospective perspectives of deaf and hard of hearing people who studied in regular schools. *Psychology & Health, 37*(3), 331–349. https://doi.org/10.1080/08870446.2021.1905161

Fellinger, J., Holzinger, D., Sattel, H., & Laucht, M. (2008). Mental health and quality of life in deaf pupils. *European Child & Adolescent Psychiatry, 17*(7), 414–423. https://doi.org/10.1007/s00787-008-0683-y

Freitas, E., Simões, C., Santos, A. C., & Mineiro, A. (2022). Resilience in deaf children: A comprehensive literature review and applications for school staff. *Journal of Community Psychology, 50*(2), 1198–1223. https://doi.org/10.1002/jcop.22730

Glickman, N. S., & Hall, W. C. (2019). *Language deprivation and deaf mental health*. Routledge.

Goberis, D., Beams, D., Dalpes, M., Abrisch, A., Baca, R., & Yoshinaga-Itano, C. (2012). The missing link in language development of deaf and hard of hearing children: Pragmatic language development. *Seminars in Speech and Language, 33*(4), 297–309. https://doi.org/10.1055/s-0032-1326916

Goodwin, C., Carrigan, E., Walker, K., & Coppola, M. (2022). Language not auditory experience is related to parent-reported executive functioning in preschool-aged deaf and hard-of-hearing children. *Child Development, 93*(1), 209–224. https://doi.org/10.1111/cdev.13677

Gordon-Pershey, M., Zeszut, S., & Brouwer, K. (2019). A survey of speech sound productions in children with visual impairments. *Communication Disorders Quarterly, 40*(4), 206–219. https://doi.org/10.1177/1525740118789101

Grumi, S., Cappagli, G., Aprile, G., Mascherpa, E., Gori, M., Provenzi, L., & Signorini, S. (2021). Togetherness, beyond the eyes: A systematic review on the interaction between visually impaired children and their parents. *Infant Behavior and Development, 64*, 101590. https://doi.org/10.1016/j.infbeh.2021.101590

Hindley, P. A., Hill, P. D., McGuigan, S., & Kitson, N. (1994). Psychiatric disorder in deaf and hearing impaired children and young people: A prevalence study. *Journal of Child Psychology and Psychiatry, 35*(5), 917–934. https://doi.org/10.1111/j.1469-7610.1994.tb02302.x

Houwen, S., Visscher, C., Lemmink, K. A. P. M., & Hartman, E. (2009). Motor skill performance of children and adolescents with visual impairments: A review. *Exceptional Children, 75*(4), 464–492. https://doi.org/10.1177/001440290907500405

Hughes, M., Dote-Kwan, J., & Dolendo, J. (1999). Characteristics of maternal directiveness and responsiveness with young children with visual impairments. *Child: Care, Health, and Development, 25*(4), 285–298. https://doi.org/10.1046/j.1365-2214.1999.00118.x

Huttunen, K., Erixon, E., Löfkvist, U., & Mäki-Torkko, E. (2019). The impact of permanent early-onset unilateral hearing impairment in children—A systematic review. *International Journal of Pediatric Otorhinolaryngology, 120*, 173–183. https://doi.org/10.1016/j.ijporl.2019.02.029

Jayaraman, D., Jacob, N., & Swaminathan, M. (2021). Visual function assessment, ocular examination, and intervention in children with developmental delay: A systematic approach—Part 2. *Indian Journal of Ophthalmology, 69*(8), 2012–2017. https://doi.org/10.4103/ijo.IJO_2396_20

Jessup, G., Bundy, A. C., Broom, A., & Hancock, N. (2018). Fitting in or feeling excluded: The experiences of high school students with visual impairments. *Journal of Visual Impairment & Blindness, 112*(3), 261–273. https://doi.org/10.1177/0145482X1811200305

Jessup, G. M., Cornell, E., & Bundy, A. C. (2010). The treasure in leisure activities: Fostering resilience in young people who are blind. *Journal of*

Visual Impairment & Blindness, 104(7), 419–430. https://doi.org/10.1177/0145482X101040070

Johnson, P., Cawthon, S., Fink, B., Wendel, E., & Schoffstall, S. (2018). Trauma and resilience among deaf individuals. *Journal of Deaf Studies and Deaf Education, 23*(4), 317–330. https://doi.org/10.1093/deafed/eny024

Joint Committee on Infant Hearing. (2019). Year 2019 position statement: Principles and guidelines for early hearing detection and intervention programs. *Journal of Early Hearing Detection and Intervention, 4*(2), 1–44. https://doi.org/10.15142/fptk-b748

Jones, A., Atkinson, J., Marshall, C., Botting, N., St Clair, M. C., & Morgan, G. (2020). Expressive vocabulary predicts nonverbal executive function: A 2-year longitudinal study of deaf and hearing children. *Child Development, 91*(2), e400–e414. https://doi.org/10.1111/cdev.13226

Kancherla, V., Van Naarden Braun, K., & Yeargin-Allsopp, M. (2013). Childhood vision impairment, hearing loss and co-occurring autism spectrum disorder. *Disability and Health Journal, 6*(4), 333–342. https://doi.org/10.1016/j.dhjo.2013.05.003

Kef, S., & Deković, M. (2004). The role of parental and peer support in adolescents well-being: A comparison of adolescents with and without a visual impairment. *Journal of Adolescence, 27*(4), 453–466. https://doi.org/10.1016/j.adolescence.2003.12.005

Keil, S., Fielder, A., & Sargent, J. (2017). Management of children and young people with vision impairment: Diagnosis, developmental challenges and outcomes. *Archives of Disease in Childhood, 102*(6), 566–571. https://doi.org/10.1136/archdischild-2016-311775

Kelly, D. P., & Teplin, S. (2018). Sensory impairments: Hearing and vision. In R. G. Voigt, M. M. Macias, & S. M. Myers (Eds.), *Developmental and behavioral pediatrics* (2nd ed., pp. 467–493). American Academy of Pediatrics. https://doi.org/10.1542/9781610021357-13

Kushalnagar, P., Topolski, T. D., Schick, B., Edwards, T. C., Skalicky, A. M., & Patrick, D. L. (2011). Mode of communication, perceived level of understanding, and perceived quality of life in youth who are deaf or hard of hearing. *Journal of Deaf Studies and Deaf Education, 16*(4), 512–523. https://doi.org/10.1093/deafed/enr015

Lang, M., Hintermair, M., & Sarimski, K. (2017). Social-emotional competences in very young visually impaired children. *British Journal of Visual Impairment, 35*(1), 29–43. https://doi.org/10.1177/0264619616677171

Lederberg, A. R., Miller, E. M., Easterbrooks, S. R., & Connor, C. M. (2014). Foundations for literacy: An early literacy intervention for deaf and hard-of-hearing children. *Journal of Deaf Studies and Deaf Education, 19*(4), 438–455. https://doi.org/10.1093/deafed/enu022

Lederberg, A. R., Prezbindowski, A. K., & Spencer, P. E. (2000). Word-learning skills of deaf preschoolers: The development of novel mapping and rapid word-learning strategies. *Child Development, 71*(6), 1571–1585. https://doi.org/10.1111/1467-8624.00249

Lewis, V., Norgate, S., Collis, G., & Reynolds, R. (2000). The consequences of visual impairment for children's symbolic and functional play. *British Journal of Developmental Psychology, 18*(3), 449–464. https://doi.org/10.1348/026151000165797

Lieu, J. E. C., Kenna, M., Anne, S., & Davidson, L. (2020). Hearing loss in children: A review. *JAMA: Journal of the American Medical Association, 324*(21), 2195–2205. https://doi.org/10.1001/jama.2020.17647

Liu, C. C., Anne, S., & Horn, D. L. (2019). Advances in management of pediatric sensorineural hearing loss. *Otolaryngologic Clinics of North America, 52*(5), 847–861. https://doi.org/10.1016/j.otc.2019.05.004

Loy, B., Warner-Czyz, A. D., Tong, L., Tobey, E. A., & Roland, P. S. (2010). The children speak: An examination of the quality of life of pediatric cochlear implant users. *Otolaryngology—Head and Neck Surgery, 142*(2), 247–253. https://doi.org/10.1016/j.otohns.2009.10.045

Lueck, A. H., Dutton, G. N., & Chokron, S. (2019). Profiling children with cerebral visual impairment using multiple methods of assessment to aid in differential diagnosis. *Seminars in Pediatric Neurology, 31*, 5–14. https://doi.org/10.1016/j.spen.2019.05.003

Manitsa, I., & Doikou, M. (2022). Social support for students with visual impairments in educational institutions: An integrative literature review. *British Journal of Visual Impairment, 40*(1), 29–47. https://doi.org/10.1177/0264619620941885

Martin, D., Bat-Chava, Y., Lalwani, A., & Waltzman, S. B. (2011). Peer relationships of deaf children with cochlear implants: Predictors of peer entry and peer interaction success. *Journal of Deaf Studies and Deaf Education, 16*(1), 108–120. https://doi.org/10.1093/deafed/enq037

Mazella, A., Albaret, J.-M., & Picard, D. (2014). Haptic tests for use with children and adults with visual impairments: A literature review. *Journal of Visual Impairment & Blindness, 108*(3), 227–237. https://doi.org/10.1177/0145482X1410800306

Miles, B., & Riggio, M. (1999). Understanding deafblindness. In B. Miles & M. Riggio (Eds.),

Remarkable conversations: A guide to developing meaningful communication with children and young adults who are deafblind (pp. 21–37). Perkins School for the Blind.

Mitchell, R. E., & Karchmer, M. A. (2004). Chasing the mythical ten percent: Parental hearing status of deaf and hard of hearing students in the United States. *Sign Language Studies, 4*(2), 138–163. https://doi.org/10.1353/sls.2004.0005

Mood, D., Szarkowski, A., Brice, P. J., & Wiley, S. (2020). Relational factors in pragmatic skill development: Deaf and hard of hearing infants and toddlers. *Pediatrics, 146*(Suppl. 3), S246–S261. https://doi.org/10.1542/peds.2020-0242D

Most, T. (2007). Speech intelligibility, loneliness, and sense of coherence among deaf and hard-of-hearing children in individual inclusion and group inclusion. *Journal of Deaf Studies and Deaf Education, 12*(4), 495–503. https://doi.org/10.1093/deafed/enm015

Nicholas, J. (2020). Cognitive assessment of young children who are deafblind: Perspectives and suggestions for assessments. *Frontiers in Psychology, 11*, 571358. https://doi.org/10.3389/fpsyg.2020.571358

Niclasen, J., & Dammeyer, J. (2016). Psychometric properties of the strengths and difficulties questionnaire and mental health problems among children with hearing loss. *Journal of Deaf Studies and Deaf Education, 21*(2), 129–140. https://doi.org/10.1093/deafed/env067

Nunes, T., Pretzlik, U., & Ilicak, S. (2005). Validation of a parent outcome questionnaire from pediatric cochlear implantation. *Journal of Deaf Studies and Deaf Education, 10*(4), 330–356. https://doi.org/10.1093/deafed/eni027

Oliveira, O., Ribeiro, C., Simões, C., & Pereira, P. (2018). Quality of life of children and adolescents with visual impairments. *British Journal of Visual Impairment, 36*(1), 42–56. https://doi.org/10.1177/0264619617737123

Paatsch, L., & Toe, D. (2020). The impact of pragmatic delays for deaf and hard of hearing students in mainstream classrooms. *Pediatrics, 146*(Suppl. 3), S292–S297. https://doi.org/10.1542/peds.2020-0242I

Paatsch, L., Toe, D., & Church, A. (2017). Hearing loss and cochlear implantation. In L. Cummings (Ed.), *Research in clinical pragmatics* (pp. 411–439). Springer International. https://doi.org/10.1007/978-3-319-47489-2_16

Paul, R., Paatsch, L., Caselli, N., Garberoglio, C. L., Goldin-Meadow, S., & Lederberg, A. (2020). Current research in pragmatic language use among deaf and hard of hearing children. *Pediatrics, 146*(Suppl. 3), S237–S245. https://doi.org/10.1542/peds.2020-0242C

Pinquart, M., & Pfeiffer, J. P. (2011). Associations of extroversion and parental overprotection with forming relationships with peers among adolescents with and without visual impairments. *Journal of Visual Impairment & Blindness, 105*(2), 96–107. https://doi.org/10.1177/0145482X1110500207

Punch, R., & Hyde, M. (2011). Social participation of children and adolescents with cochlear implants: A qualitative analysis of parent, teacher, and child interviews. *Journal of Deaf Studies and Deaf Education, 16*(4), 474–493. https://doi.org/10.1093/deafed/enr001

Qi, L., Zhang, H., Nie, R., Xiao, A., Wang, J., & Du, Y. (2020). Quality of life of hearing-impaired middle school students: A cross-sectional study in Hubei Province, China. *Journal of Developmental and Physical Disabilities, 32*(5), 821–837. https://doi.org/10.1007/s10882-019-09722-z

Reesman, J. H., Day, L. A., Szymanski, C. A., Hughes-Wheatland, R., Witkin, G. A., Kalback, S. R., & Brice, P. J. (2014). Review of intellectual assessment measures for children who are deaf or hard of hearing. *Rehabilitation Psychology, 59*(1), 99–106. https://doi.org/10.1037/a0035829

Reynell, J. (1979). *Manual for the Reynell-Zinkin Developmental Scales for young visually handicapped children—Part 1. Mental development*. NFER-Nelson.

Robertson, A. O., Tadić, V., & Rahi, J. S. (2021). This is me: A qualitative investigation of young people's experience of growing up with visual impairment. *PLOS ONE, 16*(7), e0254009. https://doi.org/10.1371/journal.pone.0254009

Roe, J. (2008). Social inclusion: Meeting the socio-emotional needs of children with vision needs. *British Journal of Visual Impairment, 26*(2), 147–158. https://doi.org/10.1177/0264619607088277

Roid, G. H., Miller, L. J., Pomplun, M., & Koch, C. (2013). *Leiter International Performance Scale* (3rd ed.). Stoelting.

Roland, L., Fischer, C., Tran, K., Rachakonda, T., Kallogjeri, D., & Lieu, J. E. C. (2016). Quality of life in children with hearing impairment: Systematic review and meta-analysis. *Otolaryngology—Head and Neck Surgery, 155*(2), 208–219. https://doi.org/10.1177/0194599816640485

Roman-Lantzy, C. (2018). *Cortical visual impairment: An approach to assessment and intervention* (2nd ed.). American Foundation for the Blind.

Runnion, E., & Gray, S. (2019). What clinicians need to know about early literacy development in children with hearing loss. *Language, Speech,* and Hearing Services in Schools, 50(1), 16–33. https://doi.org/10.1044/2018_LSHSS-18-0015

Sakkalou, E., O'Reilly, M. A., Sakki, H., Springall, C., de Haan, M., Salt, A. T., & Dale, N. J. (2021). Mother-infant interactions with infants with congenital visual impairment and associations with longitudinal outcomes in cognition and language. Journal of Child Psychology and Psychiatry, 62(6), 742–750. https://doi.org/10.1111/jcpp.13308

Sakkalou, E., Sakki, H., O'reilly, M. A., Salt, A. T., & Dale, N. J. (2018). Parenting stress, anxiety, and depression in mothers with visually impaired infants: A cross-sectional and longitudinal cohort analysis. Developmental Medicine & Child Neurology, 60(3), 290–298. https://doi.org/10.1111/dmcn.13633

Schrank, F. A., McGrew, K. S., & Mather, N. (2014). Woodcock-Johnson IV. Riverside.

Solebo, A. L., & Rahi, J. (2014). Epidemiology, aetiology and management of visual impairment in children. Archives of Disease in Childhood, 99(4), 375–379. https://doi.org/10.1136/archdischild-2012-303002

Solebo, A. L., Teoh, L., & Rahi, J. (2017). Epidemiology of blindness in children. Archives of Disease in Childhood, 102(9), 853–857. https://doi.org/10.1136/archdischild-2016-310532

Spellun, A., Shearer, E., Fitzpatrick, K., Salamy, N., Landsman, R., Wiley, S., & Augustyn, M. (2022). The importance of accessible language for development in deaf and hard of hearing children. Journal of Developmental and Behavioral Pediatrics, 43(4), 240–244. https://doi.org/10.1097/DBP.0000000000001078

Stillman, R. D. (Ed.). (1974). The Callier-Azusa Scale (ED102796). Callier Center for Communication Disorders, University of Texas at Dallas. Bureau of Education for the Handicapped. https://eric.ed.gov/?id=ED102796

Sun, W., Yang, S., Liu, K., & Salvi, R. J. (2017). Hearing loss and auditory plasticity. Hearing Research, 347, 1–2. https://doi.org/10.1016/j.heares.2017.03.010

Svirsky, M. A., Robbins, A. M., Kirk, K. I., Pisoni, D. B., & Miyamoto, R. T. (2000). Language development in profoundly deaf children with cochlear implants. Psychological Science, 11(2), 153–158. https://doi.org/10.1111/1467-9280.00231

Swanson, H. L., & Luxenberg, D. (2009). Short-term memory and working memory in children with blindness: Support for a domain general or domain specific system? Child Neuropsychology, 15(3), 280–294. https://doi.org/10.1080/09297040802524206

Tadić, V., Pring, L., & Dale, N. (2009). Attentional processes in young children with congenital visual impairment. British Journal of Developmental Psychology, 27(2), 311–330. https://doi.org/10.1348/026151008X310210

Tadić, V., Pring, L., & Dale, N. (2010). Are language and social communication intact in children with congenital visual impairment at school age? Journal of Child Psychology and Psychiatry, 51(6), 696–705. https://doi.org/10.1111/j.1469-7610.2009.02200.x

Terlektsi, E., Kreppner, J., Mahon, M., Worsfold, S., & Kennedy, C. R. (2020). Peer relationship experiences of deaf and hard-of-hearing adolescents. Journal of Deaf Studies and Deaf Education, 25(2), 153–166. https://doi.org/10.1093/deafed/enz048

Theunissen, S. C. P. M., Rieffe, C., Netten, A. P., Briaire, J. J., Soede, W., Schoones, J. W., & Frijns, J. H. M. (2014). Psychopathology and its risk and protective factors in hearing-impaired children and adolescents: A systematic review. JAMA Pediatrics, 168(2), 170–177. https://doi.org/10.1001/jamapediatrics.2013.3974

Tomblin, J. B., Harrison, M., Ambrose, S. E., Walker, E. A., Oleson, J. J., & Moeller, M. P. (2015). Language outcomes in young children with mild to severe hearing loss. Ear and Hearing, 36(Suppl. 1), 76S–91S. https://doi.org/10.1097/AUD.0000000000000219

Tomblin, J. B., Oleson, J., Ambrose, S. E., Walker, E. A., & Moeller, M. P. (2020). Early literacy predictors and second-grade outcomes in children who are hard of hearing. Child Development, 91(1), e179–e197. https://doi.org/10.1111/cdev.13158

Udholm, N., Jørgensen, A. W., & Ovesen, T. (2017). Cognitive skills affect outcome of CI in children: A systematic review. Cochlear Implants International, 18(2), 63–75. https://doi.org/10.1080/14670100.2016.1273434

United States Congress. (1973). Rehabilitation Act of 1973, 29 U.S.C. § 701 et seq.

United States Congress. (1990). Americans With Disabilities Act of 1990, 42 U.S.C. § 12101 et seq.

United States Congress. (2004). Individuals With Disabilities Education Act, 20 U.S.C. § 1400.

Urqueta Alfaro, A., Morash, V. S., Lei, D., & Orel-Bixler, D. (2018). Joint engagement in infants and its relationship to their visual impairment measurements. Infant Behavior & Development, 50, 311–323. https://doi.org/10.1016/j.infbeh.2017.05.010

van Wieringen, A., Boudewyns, A., Sangen, A., Wouters, J., & Desloovere, C. (2019). Unilateral congenital hearing loss in children: Challenges and potentials. Hearing Research, 372, 29–41. https://doi.org/10.1016/j.heares.2018.01.010

Verver, S. H., Vervloed, M. P. J., & Steenbergen, B. (2020). Characteristics of peer play in children with visual impairments. *Research in Developmental Disabilities, 105*, 103714. https://doi.org/10.1016/j.ridd.2020.103714

Vervloed, M. P. J., Hamers, J. H. M., van Mens-Weisz, M. M., & and Timmer-Van de Vosse, H. (2000). New age levels of the Reynell-Zinkin developmental scales for young children with visual impairments. *Journal of Visual Impairment & Blindness, 94*(10), 613–624. https://doi.org/10.1177/0145482X0009401002

Wagner, M. O., Haibach, P. S., & Lieberman, L. J. (2013). Gross motor skill performance in children with and without visual impairments—Research to practice. *Research in Developmental Disabilities, 34*(10), 3246–3252. https://doi.org/10.1016/j.ridd.2013.06.030

Whitaker, R., & Thomas-Presswood, T. (2017). School psychological evaluation reports for deaf and hard of hearing children: Best practices. *Journal of Social Work in Disability & Rehabilitation, 16*(3–4), 276–297. https://doi.org/10.1080/1536710X.2017.1372242

Willink, A., Assi, L., Nieman, C., McMahon, C., Lin, F. R., & Reed, N.S. (2021). Alternative pathways for hearing care may address disparities in access. *Frontiers in Digital Health, 25*(3), 740323. https://doi.org/10.3389/fdgth.2021.740323

Withagen, A., Kappers, A. M. L., Vervloed, M. P. J., Knoors, H., & Verhoeven, L. (2013). Short term memory and working memory in blind versus sighted children. *Research in Developmental Disabilities, 34*(7), 2161–2172. https://doi.org/10.1016/j.ridd.2013.03.028

Yoshinaga-Itano, C., Sedey, A. L., Mason, C. A., Wiggin, M., & Chung, W. (2020). Early intervention, parent talk, and pragmatic language in children with hearing loss. *Pediatrics, 146*(Suppl. 3), S270–S277. https://doi.org/10.1542/peds.2020-0242F

Yu, C.-L., Stanzione, C. M., Wellman, H. M., & Lederberg, A. R. (2021). Theory-of-mind development in young deaf children with early hearing provisions. *Psychological Science, 32*(1), 109–119. https://doi.org/10.1177/0956797620960389

CHAPTER 19

SLEEP AND SLEEP DISORDERS IN CHILDREN

Judith A. Owens

For pediatric psychologists, developmental-behavioral pediatricians and developmental scientists, basic knowledge of and appreciation for the contribution of poor sleep (including insufficient quantity for sleep needs, quality, and circadian misalignment) to a myriad of detrimental outcomes in the pediatric population are imperative. Disordered sleep can contribute to the presentation of diverse clinical conditions including inattention and impulsivity, depressed mood, substance use, and school failure and should therefore be considered as a contributing etiology to these diagnoses. Failure to recognize the contribution of sleep problems to these presenting symptoms can lead to treatment failures, which can have long-term repercussions on mental health, cognitive and emotional development, self-regulation, and overall quality of life. Mental health and development professionals including pediatric psychologists and developmental-behavioral pediatricians have responsibilities to regularly screen for sleep issues, as well as to provide basic sleep health education to patients, including recommendations for age and developmentally appropriate sleep duration and timing (Paruthi et al., 2016). In addition, providers can encourage healthy sleep-related behaviors such as bedtime routines, restricted electronic device use, and avoidance of caffeinated beverages as preventative measures (Kira et al., 2014; Short et al., 2011).

Sleep disturbances in children and adolescents can present with a broad constellation of concerns, resulting from multifactorial etiologies. Evaluating sleep concerns in children and adolescents often requires the expertise of groups of professionals involved in the application of developmental science across childhood, who utilize a collaborative and multidisciplinary approach with patients and families. Etiologies contributing to sleep disorders are manifest in many clinical situations and many ecological contexts from developmental science including the following:

- the biology and homeostatic circadian regulation of sleep; environmental factors such as home and neighborhood characteristics;
- family system factors such as parenting styles, family values, and caregiver stressors;
- cultural considerations;
- child factors such as temperament, developmental level, comorbid medical, and neurodevelopmental and mental health disorders; and
- socioeconomic factors including poverty and racial and ethnic disparities.

The last set of issues has been increasingly recognized as a major contributor to sleep health disparities, an important emerging field in sleep medicine (Buckhalt, 2011; Guglielmo et al., 2018; Wang & Yip, 2020).

Using a developmental framework, this chapter will present an interdisciplinary approach to understanding sleep and sleep disorders across the pediatric age spectrum. It will begin with a description of the public health significance of sleep in children and adolescents. This will be followed by an overview of "normal sleep" across childhood and adolescence, including key "sleep milestones"; the basics of sleep neurobiology and sleep regulation; the normative patterns of sleep from a neurodevelopmental perspective; the consequences of deficient sleep and a framework for diagnosing sleep disorders; and diagnostic tools and assessment paradigms for elucidating and quantifying sleep issues in clinical settings. The prevalence, key features, diagnostic criteria, evaluation and treatment of common sleep disorders—insomnia, sleep disordered breathing, parasomnias, circadian rhythm disorders, restless legs syndrome, and central hypersomnias—will also be discussed. Finally, the chapter will conclude with implications for the roles of pediatric psychologists and developmental-behavioral pediatricians in the interdisciplinary care of children with sleep disorders.

SCOPE AND PUBLIC HEALTH SIGNIFICANCE OF SLEEP IN CHILDREN AND ADOLESCENTS

Sleep is a biological foundation underlying optimal brain and body functioning. Sufficient amounts of key sleep stages in particular (i.e., slow-wave sleep [SWS], rapid eye movement [REM] sleep) are fundamental prerequisites for optimal cognitive, emotional, and behavioral functioning and the development of self-regulation. Sleep disturbances can arise when there is a "mismatch" between an individual's intrinsic circadian rhythms and sleep needs, with extrinsic time-related expectations (e.g., demands due to shift work schedules and early school start times). When prolonged, this imbalance between sleep needs and work/school expectations can result in alterations in both *amount* and *timing* of sleep, resulting in deficient sleep.

Prolonged deficiencies in sleep can contribute to a range of adverse outcomes including suboptimal cognitive function, impaired self-regulation, increased emotional and behavioral problems, greater risk-taking behaviors, and negative health outcomes. There is a dose-response relationship between the degree of sleep deficiency and cognitive functioning, especially in tasks requiring sustained attention and higher level cognitive skills, with worse performance associated with greater cumulative sleep deprivation (Groen & Pabilonia, 2019). Although the economic and long-term public health implications of sleep disorders including sleep-disordered breathing have been examined in adults, there remains much work to be done to assess similar outcomes in the pediatric population. One area of growing public health interest considers the economic impact and other potential benefits of changing school start times to align with the normal sleep patterns of adolescents, who are at increased risk for deficient sleep (Hafner et al., 2017).

NEUROBIOLOGY AND REGULATION OF SLEEP

Sleep is a complex, highly regulated, neurobiological system that is impacted by multiple factors. These factors include all the physiologic systems in the body; multiple ecological factors in the microenvironment (e.g., sleeping surface, position) and macroenvironment (e.g., sleeping space, noise level); and sociocultural practices such as bed sharing, napping patterns, and bedtime routines (see Figure 19.1).

Sleep Stages

There are four sleep stages:

1. Awake
2. Non-REM sleep (consisting of light sleep, N1 [transitional], and N2 sleep)
3. N3 (deep/slow-wave/delta sleep)
4. REM sleep

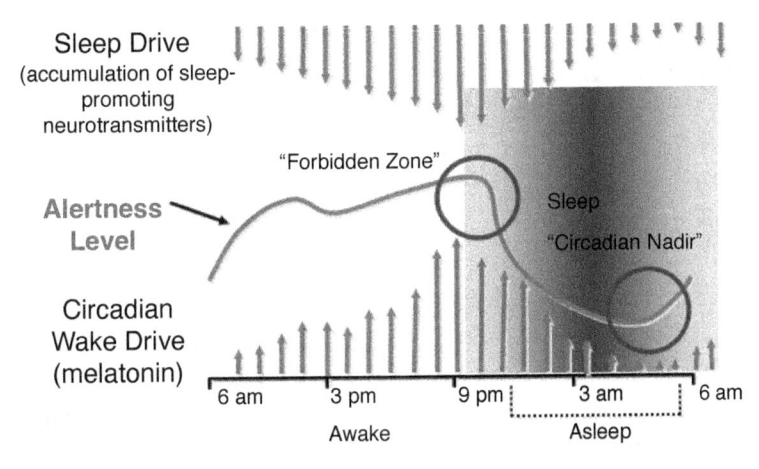

FIGURE 19.1. The two-process model of sleep regulation. From *A Clinical Guide to Pediatric Sleep: Diagnosis and Management of Sleep Problems in Children and Adolescents* (2nd ed.), by J. A. Mindell and J. A. Owens, 2010, Wolters Kluwer. Copyright 2010 by Wolters Kluwer Health. Reprinted with permission.

In a typical night, the sleep stages progress in cycles. Slow-wave sleep (N3), which is believed to be the most restorative form of sleep, is entered into relatively quickly after sleep onset. Slow-wave sleep is preserved in the face of reduced total sleep time and can increase (rebound) after a night of deficient sleep. The restorative properties of sleep are thought to be related to the glymphatic system, which is believed to orchestrate efficient clearance of neurotoxic "waste products" (soluble proteins and metabolites) produced by neural activity in the awake brain. This eliminative process is largely relegated to the sleeping brain. Failures of this system are believed to contribute to the pathogenesis of neurodegenerative disorders such as Alzheimer's disease.

REM sleep (i.e., stage R or "dream" sleep) contributes to several critical brain processes, including the consolidation of memory, promoting central nervous system (CNS) plasticity, and protecting the brain from injury (Nguyen et al., 2022). In response to sleep debt, the homeostatic system responds by increasing the percentage of SWS and REM sleep as a compensatory mechanism.

Sleep Regulation

The sleep and wake cycles are regulated through the simultaneous operation of two highly coupled processes (see Figure 19.1). The homeostatic process (process S), regulates the length and depth of sleep through the accumulation of sleep-promoting chemicals (somnogens) during extended periods of wakefulness. The strength of this sleep drive is partially dependent upon the duration and quality of previous sleep and the duration of wakefulness since the last sleep period. In infants and young children, the drive for sleep builds, resulting in an increasing need for periods of daytime sleep (i.e., naps) and shorter duration of daytime wakefulness.

The internal organization of sleep and the timing and duration of daily sleep–wake cycles are driven by endogenous circadian rhythms (process C). These rhythms help govern predictable patterns (relative peaks and troughs) of alertness throughout the 24-hour day. Within a 24-hour period there are two periods of maximum sleepiness: late afternoon (e.g., from 3:00 to 5:00 p.m.) and middle to end of the night (e.g., from 3:00 to 5:00 a.m.). The periods of maximum alertness are in the midmorning and later evening, just before the onset of natural sleep. These periods have been called the "forbidden zone," which has been associated with maintenance of wakefulness in the face of an accumulated sleep drive, sometimes described the "second-wind phenomenon" (Owens, 2019).

There is a master circadian "clock," which is regulated by melatonin secretion from the hypothalamus, that serves as a circadian "pacemaker" to control sleep–wake patterns. Circadian clocks are present in almost every cell throughout the body and thus play a role in the physiological regulation of other biological systems including the cardiovascular, endocrine, renal, and pulmonary systems. Environmental cues (i.e., zeitgebers), especially the dark–light cycle, and timing of meals and clock time help to synchronize or "entrain" the circadian rhythms to follow a 24-hour/day cycle.

NORMATIVE DEVELOPMENTAL PATTERNS OF PEDIATRIC SLEEP

Several basic trends in sleep emerge across the transition from infancy to adolescence that are likely reflective of physiologic/chronobiologic, developmental, and social-environmental changes. As children mature from infancy to adolescence, they develop a more adult sleep pattern. Table 19.1 provides a detailed list of normative sleep parameters and behaviors.

From infancy to adolescence, there are severable notable sleep changes:

1. In early development, sleep is the primary activity of the brain, with children spending, on average, 9,500 hours (approximately 13 months) asleep versus 8,000 hours awake by age 2. Between 2 and 5 years, the time asleep diminishes and becomes more equal to the time spent awake.
2. From infancy through adolescence, there is a gradual decline in average sleep duration in a 24-hour period due to decreases in the amount of time spent in diurnal and nocturnal sleep. The reduction in daytime sleep (i.e., scheduled naps) often results in the cessation of naps by age 5, although the age at which children stop napping can vary considerably.
3. Across the infancy to school-age transition, the length of the within-sleep ultradian cycle of sleep stages increases from about 50 minutes in infancy to 90 to 110 minutes by school age. At the termination of each ultradian cycle, brief arousals (i.e., night awakenings) can occur. As the length of the ultradian cycles increases with age, there is an associated decrease in the number of these end-of-cycle night wakings.
4. With pubertal onset in middle childhood, there is a gradual shift in the circadian sleep–wake rhythm to a delayed (later) sleep onset, which accelerates in early to mid-adolescence. Concomitant environmental factors (e.g., evening exposure to electronic screens [television, computers], social networking, academic and extracurricular demands), which further delay bedtime, and early high school start times (e.g., before 8:30 a.m.) can also result in insufficient sleep duration and cumulative sleep deprivation. In addition, the accumulation of the homeostatic sleep drive across the day slows, and both sensitivity and exposure to evening light increases (especially blue spectrum light from electronic devices) during adolescence, conspiring to further delay sleep onset. These changes have profound effects on adolescent brain development of particular interest to developmental scientists (Fontanellaz-Castiglione et al., 2020).
5. From childhood to adolescence, irregularities in sleep–wake patterns can increase as a result of greater differences between school night and non–school-night bedtimes and morning wake times and an increased need to "sleep in" on weekends to compensate for chronic weekday sleep insufficiency. This phenomenon, often referred to as "social jet lag," not only fails to mitigate the performance deficits associated with insufficient sleep on school nights, but also exacerbates the normal adolescent phase delay, resulting in additional disruptions to circadian physiology (Malone et al., 2016).

Table 19.2 provides an overview of the principles of healthy sleep habits.

TABLE 19.1
Normative and Developmental Considerations in Children's Sleep

Age	Sleep duration (total sleep/24 hrs)	Sleep behaviors	Developmental considerations
Newborn (0–2 months)	Total sleep: 9–18 (average about 14 hrs) Sleep duration may be higher in premature infants	Wide range of total sleep time No established nocturnal-diurnal pattern in 1st few weeks Sleep is evenly distributed throughout the day and night, averaging 8.5 hrs at night and 5.75 hrs during the day Bottle-fed infants generally sleep for longer periods (2- to 5-hr bouts) than breastfed infants (1–3 hr) Sleep periods are separated by 1–2 hrs of wake	American Academy of Pediatrics advocates against bed sharing in the first year of life. Instead, it encourages proximate but separate sleeping surfaces for the caregiver and infant. Place infants on their back on a flat surface to sleep at night and during nap times. Infants should not sleep in an inclined position. Place the infant on a firm mattress with well-fitting sheet in safety-approved crib. Do not use pillows or comforters. Standards require crib bars to be no farther apart than 2.5 inches. Infant's face and head stay uncovered and clear of blankets and other coverings.
Infant (2–12 months)	Total sleep: 12–16 hrs; wide individual variability in sleep duration	Infants develop the ability to consolidate sleep (sleep throughout the night) between 6 weeks and 3 months	The capacity to self-soothe develops in the first 3 months of life and is a reflection of learning and neurodevelopmental maturation. Sleep regulation or self-soothing involves the infant's ability to negotiate the sleep–wake transition, both at sleep onset and following normal awakenings throughout the night.
Toddler (1–2 years)	Total sleep: 11–14 hrs (including naps)	Daytime naps decrease from two to one around 18 months of age	Cognitive, motor, language, and social-emotional ability may impact sleep. Nighttime fears develop; transitional objects and bedtime routines are important.
Preschool (3–5 years)	Total sleep: 10–13 hrs (including naps)	Decline in napping, and eventual cessation of daytime naps About 26% of 4-year-old and 15% of 5-year-old children nap	Persistent cosleeping tends to be highly associated with sleep problems at this age. Sleep problems may become chronic.
Middle childhood (6–12 years)	Total sleep: 9–12 hrs	Irregularity of sleep–wake schedules reflects increasing discrepancy between school and non-school-night bedtimes and wake times	School and behavior problems may be attributed to sleep problems. Environmental competing influences from media (electronics, television, computer, video games) are associated with later bedtimes.
Adolescence (13–18 years)	Total sleep: 8–10 hrs	Later bedtimes increase the discrepancy between sleep patterns during the weekday and weekend	Puberty-mediated phase delay (later sleep onset and wake times) relative to sleep–wake cycles in adolescents. Earlier required wake times. Environmental competing priorities for sleep.

Note. Data from Mindell and Owens (2015).

TABLE 19.2
Principles of Healthy Sleep Habits

Practices promoting sleep regulation (circadian and sleep drive)
- Maintain an organized and consistent sleep–wake cycle
- Set and enforce a consistent bedtime weekdays and weekends
- Set and enforce a consistent wake time weekdays and weekends
- Keep a regular daily schedule of activities, including meals
- Avoid bright light in the bedroom at bedtime and during the night
- Increase light exposure in the morning
- Establish an appropriate napping schedule

Practices promoting sleep conditioning
- Establish a regular and consistent bedtime routine
- Limit activities that promote wakefulness while in bed (watching TV, using a cell phone); use the bed for sleep only
- Don't use the bed for punishment (time out)
- Avoid using staying up late as a reward for good behavior and going to bed as a punishment for undesired behavior
- Avoid sleeping in environments other than the bedroom (couch, car)

Practices reducing arousal and promoting relaxation
- Keep electronics out of the bedroom and limit use of electronics before bedtime
- Reduce stimulating play at bedtime
- Avoid heavy meals and vigorous exercise close to bedtime
- Reduce cognitive and emotional stimulation before bedtime
- Eliminate caffeine
- Include activities in the bedtime routine that are relaxing and calming

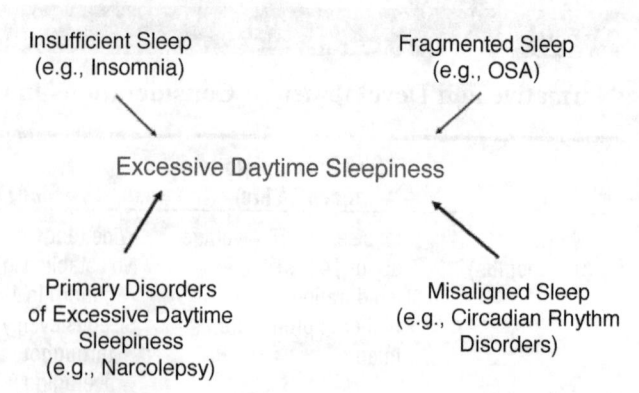

FIGURE 19.2. Sleep dysfunction in children. OSA = obstructive sleep apnea. Adapted from *A Clinical Guide to Pediatric Sleep: Diagnosis and Management of Sleep Problems in Children and Adolescents* (3rd ed., p. 38), by J. A. Mindell and J. A. Owens, 2015, Wolters Kluwer. Copyright 2015 by Wolters Kluwer Health. Adapted with permission.

CONCEPTUAL FRAMEWORK OF SLEEP DISORDERS

Sleep problems in children and adolescents can be related to an insufficient quantity of sleep, poor quality of sleep, or poor timing of sleep and can manifest as excessive daytime sleepiness (EDS) and decreased daytime alertness levels (see Figure 19.2). Symptoms of sleepiness in children can present as drowsiness, yawning, and other classic sleepy behaviors: a need to nap in older children and a desire to extend sleep on weekends when given the opportunity (if you can sleep more, you need more sleep). Excessive daytime sleepiness can also manifest with symptoms of mood disturbance, such as irritability, emotional lability, low frustration tolerance, and depressed or negative mood. It can present with physical symptoms including fatigue and somatic complaints (e.g., headaches, gastrointestinal disturbances). Other manifestations of EDS include neurocognitive and behavioral deficits such as cognitive impairment; problems with memory, attention, concentration, decision making, and problem solving; daytime behavior problems (e.g., hyperactivity, impulsivity, noncompliance); and academic problems including chronic tardiness/school absences, and school failure resulting from insufficient sleep. Because children with EDS/chronic sleep deprivation can present with deficits in learning, behavior, and emotion (Liu et al., 2019), providers who assess children for school failure (e.g., pediatric psychologists, developmental-behavioral pediatricians, and neuropsychologists) should consider the role of sleep and EDS in a child's academic functioning.

Sleepiness and fatigue may overlap in their clinical presentation, but sleepiness is characterized by the propensity to fall asleep, particularly under conditions of low stimulation (e.g., riding in the car) whereas fatigue is characterized by a state of low energy, decreased motivation, and exhaustion. Using a developmental science framework, Figure 19.3 presents a schematic

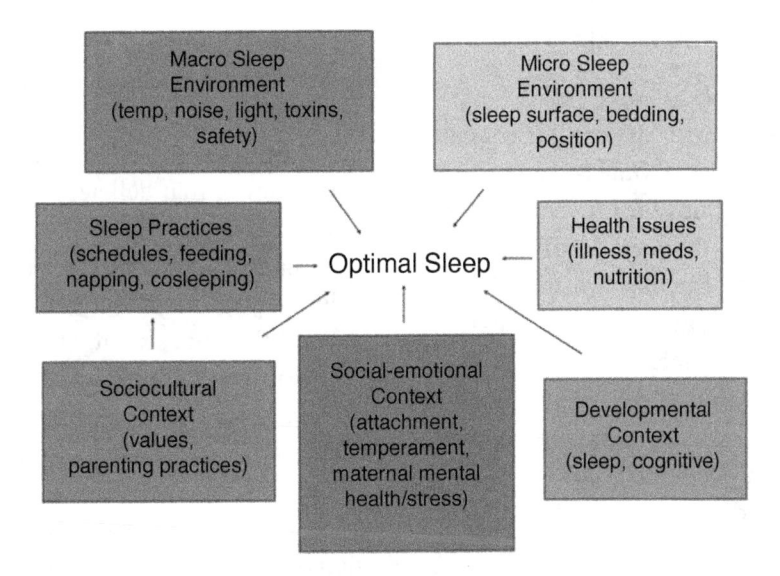

FIGURE 19.3. Contributors to optimal sleep in children. From *A Clinical Guide to Pediatric Sleep: Diagnosis and Management of Sleep Problems in Children and Adolescents* (3rd ed., p. 27), by J. A. Mindell and J. A. Owens, 2015, Wolters Kluwer. Copyright 2015 by Wolters Kluwer Health. Reprinted with permission.

representation of the multilevel factors (e.g., individual, parent–child, family, home, cultural, societal) that are necessary for optimal sleep, and that, if disrupted, can result in EDS.

PREVALENCE OF SLEEP PROBLEMS

Although estimates can vary significantly by age, the presence or absence of comorbidities and the type of sleep disorder, the overall prevalence of sleep problems in children is estimated to be as high as 25% (Owens, 2007). However, within the pediatric population, certain subgroups of children are at higher risk for the development of acute or chronic sleep problems, such as children with medical problems (e.g., chronic illnesses, pain conditions), children with psychiatric disorders (e.g., attention-deficit/hyperactivity disorder [ADHD], depression, bipolar disorder, anxiety disorders), and children taking wake-promoting medications (e.g., stimulants), sleep-disrupting medications (e.g., corticosteroids), or daytime-sedating medications. In addition, children with neurodevelopmental disorders such as autism, intellectual disability, blindness, fetal alcohol spectrum disorders, and some genetic disorders (e.g., Smith-Magenis, Fragile X) have especially high rates of sleep disturbances. These children may also have multiple risk factors for disordered sleep including medical comorbidities, the use of sleep-disrupting medications, a history of nocturnal seizures, an increased susceptibility to environmental cues contributing to vulnerabilities in circadian disruption, or other psychiatric and behavioral comorbidities that further predispose them to disrupted sleep (Owens, 2019).

An emerging literature is beginning to identify additional factors associated with sleep health disparities. For example, children from low socioeconomic households, children of ethnic minorities, and children in alternative care (e.g., foster placement) are more likely to experience sleep problems, are less likely to be diagnosed and treated, and are more vulnerable to the negative impact of sleep disorders (Hash et al., 2022). Because specialists in the developmental sciences are more likely to encounter these children in clinical practice, it is imperative that they are aware of the high prevalence and presentation of sleep disorders in these populations in order to have a systematic approach to screening.

CONSEQUENCES ASSOCIATED WITH SLEEP PROBLEMS

Disordered sleep can contribute to adverse health, safety, and performance outcomes due to the failure to meet the basic need for sufficient sleep. For an individual child, the level of impairment due to inadequate sleep can vary by the child's age, developmental level, and to a certain extent, individual variability in sleep need. Chronic, partial sleep loss (i.e., due to sleep restriction) can lead to a cumulative sleep debt, which, over several days, can produce deficits equivalent to those seen under conditions of one night of total sleep deprivation (Maski & Kothare, 2013). The effects of disordered sleep are multifocal, associated with multiple impacts to physical health, emotional and behavioral functioning, and academic achievement.

Physical Health

Direct consequences of deficient sleep on physical health pose a considerable public health challenge. Deficient sleep has been associated with negative impacts to cardiovascular health, metabolic function, and systemic inflammation, contributing to an increased risk of obesity, hypertension, and Type 2 diabetes (Tambalis et al., 2018). There are complex bidirectional associations between sleep and immune function, with insufficient sleep associated with increased susceptibility to and slower recovery from infection, as well as a poorer antibody response to vaccines (Donners et al., 2015). Recovery from acute injury, such as sports-related injury (Gao et al., 2019) and mild traumatic brain injury (concussions; Wickwire et al., 2018), is also impaired by deficient sleep. In addition, there is a bidirectional relation between poor sleep and pain, with insufficient sleep associated with increased pain perception and intensity and a decreased threshold for and tolerance to pain (Evans et al., 2017).

Health Behaviors

Deficient sleep has been associated with impairments in health and safety, in part because of its impact on health risk behaviors. Multiple cross-sectional and longitudinal prospective studies link deficient sleep with increased risk behaviors (Hasler & Clark, 2013; Meldrum et al., 2015; Miller et al., 2017; Winsler et al., 2015). It is believed that deficient sleep can contribute to executive function deficits, potentially leading to impairments in decision making and problem solving, poor judgment, and reduced impulse and inhibitory control. Disordered sleep also contributes to emotional dysregulation and altered reward-related decision-making behavior, manifesting in greater risk-taking behavior, likely related to perceptions of lesser consequences associated with the risky behavior. This combination of factors can result in increased motor vehicle crashes and pedestrian injuries coupled with reduced vigilance and reaction time (Bin-Hasan et al., 2020). The association between obesity and poor sleep is not only due to altered metabolism and biologic changes in appetite regulation, but is also believed to be related to changes in behavioral control and mood leading to maladaptive eating patterns (Franckle et al., 2015).

Mental Health Outcomes

Poor sleep and a history of sleep disorders have been linked with symptoms of depression, anxiety, and suicidal behavior, particularly in adolescents (Berger et al., 2019; Chiu et al., 2018; Johnson et al., 2006). Sleep-disordered effects on mood and emotional regulation contribute to impairments in social relationships (Foley & Weinraub, 2017) and increased risk-taking behaviors including substance use, alcohol consumption (Weaver et al., 2018) and aggressive and bullying behavior (O'Brien et al., 2011). Although sleep loss promotes emotional reactivity, the restoration of sleep mitigates limbic reactivity to prior emotional memories (Gujar et al., 2011), thus reinforcing the idea that improving sleep quantity and timing can contribute to more optimal mood and mental health (Freeman et al., 2017).

Academic Achievement

Across studies, deficient sleep has been associated with impairment in numerous cognitive functions including attention, memory, self-regulation, and processing speed, contributing to poor school performance (Baert et al., 2015; Beebe, 2011; Shochat et al., 2014; Vriend et al., 2013). One of the major contributors to insufficient and misaligned sleep in middle and high school students is earlier school start times. Numerous studies have demonstrated the negative impact of deficient sleep on grade point averages, performance on standardized tests, school attendance, and even graduation rates (Dunster et al., 2018; Groen & Pabilonia, 2019; Heissel & Norris, 2018; Lenard et al., 2020) as well as the corresponding benefits of delaying start times and improving sleep (Wheaton et al., 2016; Widome et al., 2020).

Special pediatric populations, including children with ADHD, already struggle with learning and performance challenges in the school setting (as well as social skills and emotional regulation), all of which may be exacerbated by chronic sleep deficient. It is well known that children with ADHD have a high prevalence of sleep problems, including shortened sleep duration and disrupted sleep compared to neurotypical peers despite a lack of evidence suggesting differences in sleep architecture. In addition, children with ADHD have a higher prevalence of sleep disorders including obstructive sleep apnea and restless legs syndrome/periodic limb movement disorder compared with typically developing peers (Cortese et al., 2009; Lunsford-Avery et al., 2016). As a result, the presence of a concomitant sleep disorder should be considered in a child with ADHD who presents with learning and academic difficulties.

CLINICAL ASSESSMENT OF SLEEP PROBLEMS IN CHILDREN AND ADOLESCENTS

The clinical interview remains the most important tool for the assessment of sleep complaints. In addition to a thorough medical, developmental/school, psychiatric, and social history, a systematic evaluation and thorough history should include the following elements:

- complete history of sleep problem(s) including detailed presenting complaint (symptoms, duration, identified triggers, level of disruption to family);
- any additional sleep complaints such as snoring or restless sleep;
- evening (dinnertime and beyond) and bedtime routines, including electronics use;
- sleeping environment (own/shared room; caregiver room/bed; quiet, dark, and caregiver presence at bedtime);
- frequency (per night and per week), timing, duration, and character of night awakenings (e.g., need for caregiver presence, transition to caregiver/other bed, caregiver response, level of child's associated anxiety, awake vs. asleep);
- sleep patterns (average/range of bedtimes, wake time on weekdays/weekends) and average/range duration of sleep (over 24 hours in younger children);
- resistance to bedtime and latency to sleep onset (average and range);
- sleep-related morning and daytime behavior (difficulty waking, daytime sleepiness, perceived sleep-related impairments in functioning);
- sleep quality (physical discomfort, restlessness, unusual movements);
- family's level of concern and response to sleep problems and current and prior management strategies (including prescription and over the counter medications);
- patient's previous sleep patterns; and
- family history of sleep problems (particularly relevant for sleep disorders with a genetic component such as sleep-disordered breathing, restless legs syndrome, parasomnias).

In addition to these sleep-related questions, the clinical interview and history should include an exploration of other environmental/familial factors that are potential contributors to sleep disorders, such as a family history of mental health issues including anxiety/depression and social-environmental and cultural issues potentially impacting sleep.

Screening Tools

Several brief sleep screening tools are available, including the BEARS, a five-item screening tool that examines the five basic categories of sleep problems most commonly encountered in pediatric clinical practice (see Table 19.3). Other screening instruments include

- the Brief Infant Sleep Questionnaire for ages 0 to 2 years;
- the Children's Sleep Habits Questionnaire for children aged 4 to 12 years, available in over 25 languages (a preschool version, a 23-item abbreviated form for behavioral sleep problems, and a version for children with autism spectrum disorder are also available);
- the Pediatric Sleep Questionnaire for ages 2 to 18 years;
- the PROMIS Pediatric Sleep Disturbances and the Pediatric Sleep-Related Impairments surveys; and
- the Adolescent Sleep-Wake Scale for ages 12 to 18 years.

The modified version of the Epworth Sleepiness Scale is also useful for quantifying subjective daytime sleepiness.

Sleep Diagnostic Tools

Considerations for employing specific sleep diagnostic tools are largely based on the clinical data obtained during the initial evaluation. In general, a 2-week sleep diary (downloadable from the American Academy of Sleep Medicine website at https://sleepeducation.org) is useful in most circumstances to clarify and document sleep patterns. The sleep diary may also reveal additional sleep concerns as a substantial percentage of referred children diagnosed with obstructive sleep apnea have at least one additional sleep disorder (Owens et al., 2008).

Actigraphy is a validated technology that uses a computerized algorithm to quantify

TABLE 19.3

The BEARS Sleep Screening Tool

	Preschool (2–5 years)	School-aged (6–12 years)	Adolescent (13–18 years)
Bedtime problems	Does your child have any problems going to bed? Falling asleep? (P)	Does your child have any problems at bedtime? (P) Do you have any problems going to bed? (C)	Do you have any problems falling asleep at bedtime? (C)
Excessive daytime sleepiness	Does your child often seem overtired or sleepy? a lot during the day? Does he/she still take naps?	Does your child have difficulty waking in the morning, seem sleepy during the day, or take naps? (P) Do you feel tired a lot? (C)	Do you feel sleepy a lot during the day? in school? while driving? (C)
Awakenings during the night	Does your child wake up a lot at night? (P)	Does your child seem to wake up a lot at night? Any sleepwalking or nightmares? (P) Do you wake up a lot at night? Do you have trouble getting back to sleep? (C)	Do you wake up a lot at night? Have trouble getting back to sleep? (C)
Regularity and duration of sleep	Does your child have a regular bedtime and wake time? What are they? (P)	What time does your child go to bed and get up on school days? Weekends? Do you think he/she is getting enough sleep? (P)	What time do you usually go to bed on school nights? Weekends? How much sleep do you usually get? (C)
Sleep-disordered breathing	Does your child snore a lot or have difficulty breathing at night? (P)	Does your child have loud or nightly snoring or any breathing difficulties at night? (P)	Does your teenager snore loudly or nightly? (P)

Note. P = parent; C = child. From "Use of the 'BEARS' Sleep Screening Tool in a Pediatric Residents' Continuity Clinic: A Pilot Study," by J. A. Owens and V. Dalzell, 2005, *Sleep Medicine*, 6(1), p. 68 (https://doi.org/10.1016/j.sleep.2004.07.015). Copyright 2005 by Elsevier. Reprinted with permission.

body movements. Actigraphs are collected with a wristwatch-like device to approximate sleep–wake patterns, are used in sleep centers, and are more accurate than commercial wearable devices.

Overnight attended polysomnography (PSG) measures specific sleep parameters, including sleep architecture (i.e., sleep onset latency, awakenings after sleep onset, sleep efficiency in time asleep/time in bed, total sleep time, arousals during sleep, sleep stages); respiratory parameters (i.e., oxygen and carbon dioxide levels, respiratory rate and effort, obstructive and central events); cardiac status; and body/leg movements. Polysomnography is also used for the diagnosis and assessment of the severity of obstructive sleep apnea and periodic limb movements, and is required for interpretation of the multiple sleep latency test (MSLT). The MSLT consists of five 20-minute nap opportunities two hours apart on the day following a PSG, and is the best available measure for objective assessment of daytime sleepiness, including EDS associated with central hypersomnias. Evaluation of parasomnias, such as sleep terrors and sleepwalking, usually does not require an overnight sleep study but is more reliably captured with home video. Evaluation of specific sleep disorders are included in the following sections.

BEHAVIORAL SLEEP DISORDERS— DEVELOPMENTAL CONSIDERATIONS FROM INFANCY TO ADOLESCENCE

Insomnia is defined as difficulty initiating and/or maintaining sleep, which occurs despite initiating sleep at the age-appropriate time and having adequate opportunity for sleep. Insomnia can impact daytime functioning with varying degrees of impairment, with symptoms ranging from fatigue, lack of energy, and sleepiness to dysregulated mood, impaired school performance, and lower quality of life. Insomnia may be transient and short lived (usually related to an acute event) or it may be characterized as long term and chronic (defined as ≥3×/week for ≥3 months in duration). In young children, insomnia is often identified through caregiver concerns, and therefore evaluation for insomnia should examine the ecological context of family and consider the contribution of parental factors (e.g., parental depression, stress), child factors (e.g., temperament, child developmental level), and environmental factors (e.g., cultural practices, sleeping space; Owens, 2019).

Behavioral Insomnia of Childhood

Although most insomnia in children and adults is categorized as chronic insomnia disorder in the *Diagnostic and Statistical Manual of Mental Disorders* (American Psychiatric Association, 2013), behavioral insomnia of childhood and its subtypes (sleep onset association and limit setting) are a helpful framework for the clinical evaluation of sleep concerns in young children (0 to 5 years). Behavioral insomnia of childhood presents differently by developmental age.

Infancy through toddlerhood. Behavioral insomnia typically presents as the sleep-onset association type, in which the child typically falls asleep only if specific conditions or bedtime associations are provided (e.g., the caregiver presence, being rocked or fed). With these sleep conditions, the child does not learn the strategies to soothe themselves, is unable to fall asleep alone, and if awakened in the middle of the night (e.g., if the child experiences brief arousals that occur at the end of a sleep cycle), cannot fall back asleep without the accustomed bedtime associations (Calhoun et al., 2017). The child may elicit the caregiver's help to return to sleep by vocalizing (e.g., calling, crying) or by seeking the parents' presence (e.g., by going into the parents' room). The clinical history is often described by episodes of prolonged night waking that require the parent's presence and intervention. Over time, this can contribute to deficient sleep for both the parent and child (Corkum et al., 2018).

Treatment of night wakings and sleep onset association disorders should emphasize establishing a regular bedtime routine and consistent sleep schedule and the implementation of behavioral interventions. Because the first line treatment of insomnia in children focuses on behavioral strategies, the role of pediatric psychologists in managing childhood insomnia is particularly pertinent. The treatment typically involves a program of extinction (i.e., rapid withdrawal) or graduated extinction (i.e., stepwise/gradual withdrawal) of caregiver assistance at the beginning of sleep and during times of nighttime awakenings. Extinction/rapid withdrawal (e.g., cry it out, the cold turkey approach) involves putting the child to bed while drowsy but still awake at a desired bedtime to optimize their propensity for sleep. The parent is advised to consistently ignore the child's protests throughout the night and until a designated time the following morning. Despite support for its efficacy, extinction is often difficult for parents to implement consistently and successfully. Graduated extinction/withdrawal (also known as check-ins, Ferber method, sleep training) requires the child to learn to fall asleep without the presence of the caregiver. This approach typically requires the parent to leave the room at the desired bedtime, and to periodically return or check in at fixed or successively longer time intervals to briefly reassure the child until the child falls asleep. The time interval between check-ins can vary and is individualized to the child's temperament and the parents' tolerance for the child's distress. The goal of graduated extinction is to allow enough time between checks for the child to fall asleep independently while avoiding extended time intervals that result in continued escalation of protest behaviors (e.g., screaming, gagging, vomiting).

In older infants and toddlers, the introduction of transitional objects (e.g., a blanket, toy), can provide an alternate sleep association that will be available to the child during the night to help them return to sleep. Other strategies can include positive reinforcement (e.g., stickers for remaining in bed). For healthy, normally growing, full-term infants who have become accustomed to waking for nighttime feedings (learned hunger), these feedings should be eliminated (either cold turkey or by gradually decreasing the volume or the milk to water ratio) as night feedings are not needed for nutrition. Importantly, parents must apply behavioral interventions consistently to avoid inadvertent negative reinforcement of night wakings. They should also be counseled that crying or protest behavior typically escalates at the beginning of treatment (i.e., postextinction burst) before subsiding.

The goal of treatment is to encourage the infant or child to develop the skills to self-soothe at bedtime, which then generalizes to wakings during the night. Although sleep training is typically not instituted until about 6 months of age, the practice of putting the infant to sleep "drowsy but awake" starting at 3 to 4 months can help encourage self-soothing, potentially avoiding the need for later intervention.

Preschool through school age. In preschool- and school-aged children, behavioral insomnia of childhood is related to difficulties in limit setting, often characterized by parental difficulties in setting consistent bedtime rules and enforcing a regular bedtime. Bedtime problems can manifest as stalling (i.e., "curtain calls"), refusal to go to bed, and refusal to return to their own room after night wakings. In some cases, caregivers adopt an inconsistent approach to night wakings that involves intermittently allowing the child to share their bed. The conditions contributing to limit-setting behavioral insomnia of childhood are varied and can include child behavior problems (e.g., oppositionality), underlying medical problems contributing to sleep difficulties (e.g., medical conditions such as asthma or medication use, an underlying sleep disorder such as restless legs syndrome, anxiety) or a mismatch between the child's intrinsic fall asleep time and parental expectations regarding an appropriate bedtime (Mindell & Owens, 2015).

Successful treatment of limit-setting sleep problems typically includes a variety of parent management strategies including (a) establishing regular bedtime routines, (b) appropriate and consistent limit setting, (c) decreased parental attention to bedtime-delaying behavior (i.e., curtain calls), and (d) positive reinforcement (e.g., sticker charts) for appropriate behavior at bedtime and during the night. These behavioral interventions highlight the importance of utilizing a family systems framework and the integral role the pediatric psychologist plays in ongoing management. For problematic night wakings, it is essential for caregivers to have a consistent response (e.g., returning the child to their bedroom after every night waking).

Other behavioral management strategies that have been empirically supported include bedtime fading (i.e., temporarily setting the bedtime closer to the actual sleep-onset time, with gradual advancement of the bedtime by 15-minute increments once the child is consistently falling asleep close to the later bedtime). The sweet spot is an appropriate bedtime, but moving to an earlier bedtime than the sweet spot results in delayed sleep onset. For older children, relaxation techniques may be taught to help them fall asleep or back to sleep more readily.

A third type of childhood behaviorally based insomnia is manifest as a mismatch between parental expectations regarding amount of time in bed and the child's intrinsic sleep needs. For example, if the sleep window is set for 12 hours (7 p.m. to 7 a.m.) but the child's typical sleep time (i.e., need for sleep) is only 10 hours, the likely result is a prolonged sleep onset of 2 hours, one or more extended periods of wakefulness during the night, and/or early morning waking (Figure 19.4). These night wakings are caused by non-distressed behavior as the child is simply not sleepy. For this type of behavioral insomnia of childhood, management is simple and often effective and involves reducing the time in bed to the actual sleep time.

Primary, Psychophysiologic, or Learned Insomnia

Insomnia presenting in older children and adolescents has often been described as primary, psychophysiologic, or learned insomnia. This type of insomnia is characterized by a combination of learned sleep-preventing associations and heightened physiologic arousal, resulting in symptoms of sleeplessness at night and decreased daytime functioning. Primary insomnia often presents with a comorbid anxiety disorder; symptoms include excessive worry about sleep and heightened concerns about potential daytime consequences of sleeplessness. Primary insomnia can present with physiologic arousal and cognitive hypervigilance, with the baseline level of arousal exacerbated by a secondary anxiety about sleeplessness (American Academy of Sleep Medicine, 2023).

Treatment for primary insomnia usually involves a multistep behavioral program called cognitive behavior therapy for insomnia (CBT-I), which includes the following:

- education regarding the principles of healthy sleep practices,

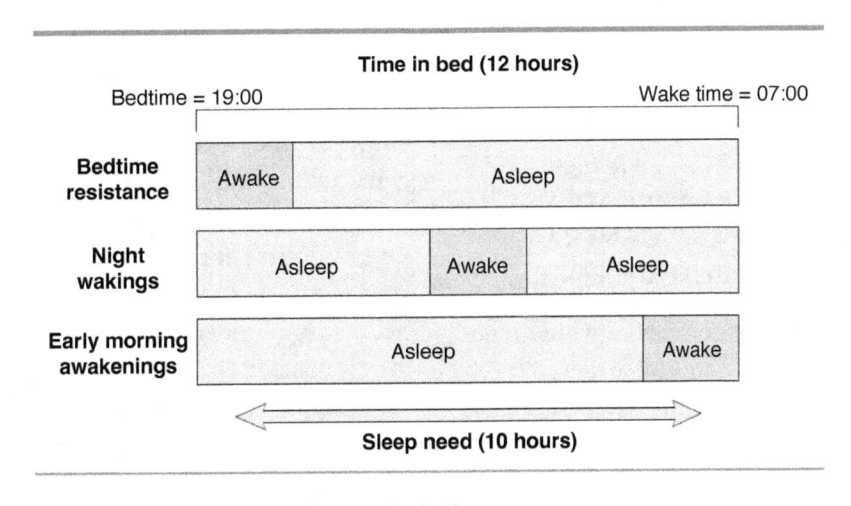

FIGURE 19.4. Too much time in bed.

- implementation of a consistent sleep–wake schedule,
- instruction to avoid daytime napping,
- directions to use the bed only for sleeping and to get out of bed if unable to fall asleep (stimulus control),
- restricting time in bed to the actual time asleep (sleep restriction),
- addressing maladaptive cognitions about sleep, and
- teaching relaxation and mindfulness techniques to reduce anxiety (de Bruin et al., 2015).

Treatment is ideally managed by a pediatric psychologist with specialized training in CBT-I implementation and tracking outcomes.

For all types of insomnia that impact children and adolescents, successful behavioral sleep interventions require forming an alliance with the family, negotiating tailored solutions that the family can successfully implement, and setting appropriate agreed upon treatment goals with planned follow-up. Behavioral treatments for insomnia, even in young children, appear to be highly effective and well tolerated. Behavioral strategies for insomnia have been associated with benefits to family functioning including the quality of parent–child relationship, attachment, psychosocial-emotional functioning, and chronic stress (Bilgin & Wolke, 2020; Price et al., 2012). In typically developing children, behavioral interventions for insomnia should be considered the first-line treatment, with hypnotic medications (e.g., melatonin) used infrequently as an adjunct to behavioral therapy.

OTHER SLEEP DISORDERS: SLEEP-DISORDERED BREATHING, PARASOMNIAS, MOVEMENT DISORDERS, CIRCADIAN RHYTHM DISORDERS, AND CENTRAL DISORDERS OF HYPERSOMNOLENCE

Primary sleep disorders encompass a wide range of diagnoses and include sleep-disordered breathing, parasomnias, movement disorders, circadian rhythm disorders, and central disorders of somnolence. Each condition will be described in greater detail in the following subsections.

Sleep-Disordered Breathing

Sleep-disordered breathing (SDB) in children describes a constellation of respiratory disorders occurring in or exacerbated by sleep. Obstructive sleep apnea (OSA), the most important clinical entity within the SDB spectrum, is characterized by repeated episodes of prolonged upper airway obstruction during sleep despite continued or increased respiratory effort. It can cause complete (apnea) or partial (hypopnea) cessation of airflow at the nose and/or mouth. These obstructive events can result in multiple nocturnal arousals, intermittent hypoxia, and disrupted sleep. Obstructive sleep apnea has also been linked with metabolic, cardiovascular, and neurocognitive-neurobehavioral morbidity. Primary snoring is characterized by snoring without associated abnormalities in oxygenation, ventilation, or sleep continuity. While considered non-pathologic, primary snoring in children may be associated with subtle sleep-related breathing abnormalities (e.g., increased respiratory effort) that may in turn be associated with adverse neurodevelopmental outcomes similar to those associated with OSA (Yu et al., 2022).

Etiology. Obstructive sleep apnea results from an anatomically or functionally narrowed upper airway due to upper airway obstruction and/or decreased upper airway diameter or to low upper airway tone/increased upper airway collapsibility, combined with a decreased drive to breathe in the face of this reduced upper airway patency (i.e., reduced central respiratory drive). In the pediatric population, upper airway obstruction is largely due to enlarged tonsils and adenoids, although the degree and level of obstruction can vary. Other etiologies associated with airway obstruction include nasal congestion secondary to environmental allergies, laryngomalacia, and craniofacial abnormalities (e.g., a small or recessed jaw, deviated nasal septum, asymmetry or elongation of the face) suggestive of an underlying congenital syndrome. Conditions contributing to low upper airway tone include neuromuscular diseases or hypothyroidism (Mindell & Owens, 2015). Reduced central respiratory drive may be seen in children with neurological disorders involving the control of breathing.

In other situations, the etiology is mixed; for example, children with Down syndrome are at increased risk for OSA due to multiple factors including generalized hypotonia, craniofacial structure, large tongue, obesity, and risk for comorbid hypothyroidism, resulting in prevalence rates of OSA as high as 70% in this population (Mindell & Owens, 2015). There is a significant association between weight and SDB, with an increasingly large percentage of children with SDB/OSA being overweight or obese. In addition to enlarged tonsils and adenoids, which are often seen in overweight/obese children with OSA, mechanical factors secondary to increased fat tissue in the throat, neck, chest, and abdominal wall can also contribute to upper airway obstruction. The metabolic consequences of SDB and obesity are significant, including insulin resistance and systemic hypertension, with obese children also at increased risk for postoperative complications, and residual OSA after adenotonsillectomy.

Prevalence. The pediatric prevalence rate for OSA is 1% to 4% overall (Tsukada et al., 2018) but prevalence rates can vary by demographic characteristics such as age (increased prevalence in children aged 2 to 8 years), sex (higher prevalence in boys, especially after puberty), ethnicity (increased prevalence in African American and Asian children), medical history (increased prevalence in preterm infants), and family history (higher prevalence with a positive family history of OSA).

Pathophysiology. The consequences of OSA are related to increased systemic inflammation, affecting blood vessels throughout the brain and body and leading to metabolic dysfunction, increased cardiovascular risk (e.g., hypertension), and cognitive impairments. Obstructive sleep apnea is believed to negatively impact cognitive function through repeated episodic arousals from sleep, resulting in sleep fragmentation and increasing sleepiness (Mindell & Owens, 2015). This, combined with intermittent hypoxia due to periodic apneas and hypopneas, is thought to contribute to systemic inflammatory changes in cerebral blood vessels. Elucidation of these multiple mechanisms also raises concerns regarding the irreversibility of changes, particularly in the developing brain.

Clinical symptoms. Children with OSA typically present with loud, disruptive, and frequent snoring; pauses in breathing; nocturnal arousals associated with choking and gasping; and restless sleep. Although many children who snore do not have OSA (and not all children with OSA are observed to snore). Notably, parents may not always be aware that their child is snoring, (especially in older children), although children with OSA may manifest other symptoms including mouth breathing, restless sleep, and diaphoresis during sleep. Children who have OSA may also sleep in unusual positions (e.g., keeping their necks hyperextended to maintain an open airway, avoiding supine sleeping position) and may have symptoms of nighttime enuresis or bedwetting. Children with OSA often present with a constellation of symptoms including difficulty waking up in the morning, daytime somnolence, drowsiness throughout the day, and dozing off or desire to nap during activities. Although hypersomnolence is present in children, it is less common than in adults (Mindell & Owens, 2015).

Neurobehavioral comorbidities. An often overlooked but important sequelae of OSA relates to its impact on mood, behavior, learning, and academic functioning. Affective changes associated with OSA are varied and can include increased irritability, mood lability, dysregulated emotions, lower frustration tolerance, and symptoms of anxiety or depression. Children with OSA can also present with behavioral disturbances with internalizing symptoms (i.e., increased somatic complaints and social withdrawal) and externalizing symptoms including aggressive behavior, hyperactivity, impulsivity, oppositional behavior, and conduct problems (Beebe et al., 2004; Biggs et al., 2014; Crabtree et al., 2004; Isaiah et al., 2021b; Landau et al., 2012). As mentioned earlier, there is notable overlap between the neurobehavioral impairments seen in OSA and ADHD, with children with OSA also manifesting signs of inattention, poor concentration, and distractibility. As a result, children who present for evaluation of these neurobehavioral complaints should also be screened for signs, symptoms, and risk factors for SDB. Mounting evidence also suggests that children with SDB symptoms (e.g., loud, frequent snoring) who do not meet polysomnographic criteria for OSA may experience neurobehavioral and cognitive consequences similar to those in children with diagnosed OSA (Bourke et al., 2011; Isaiah et al., 2021).

Evaluation. The 2012 revised American Academy of Pediatrics Clinical Practice Guidelines provide a framework for evaluating and managing uncomplicated childhood OSA (Marcus et al., 2012). Physical examination features suggestive of OSA include abnormal growth parameters (obesity or, less frequently, failure to thrive), signs of chronic nasal obstruction (adenoidal facies), signs of atopic disease (i.e., "allergic shiners"), enlarged tonsils, teeth crowding (suggesting a narrowed oropharyngeal space), and high arched palate.

The most reliable test to diagnose OSA is an overnight polysomnogram (PSG) performed in the hospital or sleep center. Sleep-disordered breathing is identified on a PSG by the apnea-hypopnea index (AHI), which captures the number of apneic and hypopneic (i.e., obstructive, central) events during each hour of sleep. Although there is no standard cutoff score on the PSG that is universally accepted for the diagnosis of OSA in children, normal preschool and school-age children generally have an obstructive AHI (OAHI) that is less than 1 per hour. This value (OAHI < 1/hour) is considered as the threshold to diagnose OSA in children younger than 12 years old. An OAHI of 1–5/hour is generally considered mild OSA, > 5–10 moderate, and > 10/hour severe OSA (Mindell & Owens, 2015).

Treatment. There are no universally accepted guidelines indicating when to treat primary snoring, pediatric SDB, and OSA. The decision to treat OSA in children depends on several parameters, including the severity of symptoms (e.g., presence of nocturnal symptoms, daytime symptoms and signs of impairment, sleep study results); duration of disease; and individual patient characteristics such as age of child, presence of comorbidities, and other underlying factors (Mindell & Owens, 2015). Most pediatric sleep specialists recommend that children with moderate and severe disease (characterized by AHI > 5) should be treated. In addition, children with habitual snoring (>3×/week) but without polysomnographic evidence of OSA may experience adverse neurobehavioral and neurocognitive outcomes and should therefore be treated. Ongoing studies are examining whether these children may benefit from more aggressive treatment (e.g., adenotonsillectomy; Redline et al., 2023).

In most cases of pediatric OSA, surgical adenotonsillectomy is the first-line treatment in any child with significant adenotonsillar hypertrophy, even in the presence of additional risk factors such as obesity. In uncomplicated cases (70%–90% of children), adenotonsillectomy results in complete resolution of symptoms, although regrowth of adenoidal tissue after surgical removal occurs in some cases. Although some evidence suggests that neuropsychologic functioning in children and impairments in mood, behavior, academics, and quality of life improve significantly following adenotonsillectomy for OSA (Mitchell & Kelly, 2005, 2007), results have been mixed, with other studies demonstrating variable improvement in neurocognitive deficits following surgical treatment. This suggests that other multifactorial concerns may influence these outcomes, including individual factors such as genetic susceptibility and ethnic background and proximal and distal environmental influences (e.g., passive smoking exposure, pollution), and comorbid conditions, such as obesity, shortened sleep duration, and other sleep disorders, as well as duration of sleep-disordered breathing (Chervin et al., 2015; Marcus et al., 2013). High risk groups that require special consideration include young children

(<3 years old), children with severe OSA, and children with significant clinical sequelae of OSA or associated medical conditions (e.g., craniofacial syndromes, Down syndrome, obesity). Following adenotonsillectomy, patients should be reevaluated to determine if a repeat PSG or additional treatment is indicated.

In addition to surgical management for OSA, other interventions may include recommendations for weight loss, positional therapy (e.g., having a child sleep with a tennis ball in a fanny pack to prevent supine sleeping), and aggressive treatment of potential risk factors (e.g., asthma, seasonal allergies). Medications including intranasal corticosteroids (fluticasone) and leukotriene inhibitors (monteleukast) may help reduce upper airway inflammation associated with mild OSA. Continuous or bilevel positive airway pressure (PAP) can also be used successfully in children and adolescents. Positive airway pressure may be suggested if adenotonsillectomy is not indicated, if symptoms persist following adenotonsillectomy, or if surgery is contraindicated. Because compliance with PAP therapy is often suboptimal, education of the child and family, including initiation of desensitization protocols, can help foster adherence to treatment.

Parasomnias (Sleepwalking, Sleep Terrors, Confusional Arousals)

Parasomnias are episodic behaviors during sleep characterized by a dissociation of the sleep and wake state, which typically present with confusion, disorientation, and autonomic/skeletal muscle disturbance. These episodic events are more common in young children because of the higher percentage of SWS in this age group. Partial arousal parasomnias typically occur in the first third of the night, when SWS predominates. In contrast, nightmares (although more common than and often confused with partial arousal parasomnias) are concentrated in the last third of the night, when REM sleep predominates. Factors that increase in the relative percentage of SWS (e.g., medications, previous sleep restriction) can increase the frequency of parasomnias. Because genetics may play a role in both sleepwalking and night terrors, evaluation for these concerns should also include questions about a family history of parasomnias (Mindell & Owens, 2015). Partial arousal parasomnias can also be confused with nocturnal seizures. Table 19.4 summarizes similarities and differences among these nocturnal arousal events.

TABLE 19.4

Similarities and Differentiating Features of Non-REM and REM Parasomnias and Nocturnal Seizures

	Confusion arousal	Sleep terrors	Sleepwalking	Nightmares	Nocturnal seizures
Timing (night)	Early	Early	Early–mid	Late	Any
Sleep stage	SWS	SWS	SWS	REM	Any
Distress and autonomic activation	+	++++	+	+	+
Motor activity	−	+	+++	+	++++
Duration (min.)	0.5–10; more gradual offset	1–10; more gradual offset	2–30; more gradual offset	3–20	5–15; abrupt onset and offset
Post-event confusion	+	+	+	−	+
Age	Child	Child	Child	Child, young adult	Adolescent, young adult
Genetics	+	+	+	−	±

Note. SWS = slow wave sleep; REM = rapid eye movement; − = none; ± = in some cases; + = mild; +++ = moderate; ++++ = marked. Adapted from *A Clinical Guide to Pediatric Sleep: Diagnosis and Management of Sleep Problems in Children and Adolescents* (3rd ed., p. 108), by J. A. Mindell and J. A. Owens, 2015, Wolters Kluwer. Copyright 2015 by Wolters Kluwer Health. Adapted with permission.

Prevalence. The lifetime prevalence of sleepwalking (somnambulism) by age 10 is 13%, with a tenfold greater prevalence in children with a family history of sleepwalking (Maski & Owens, 2016). Although sleep terrors are less common (1%–3%), children with sleep terrors have a 2 times higher risk of developing sleepwalking after age 5 (Ohayon et al., 2012; Petit et al., 2015). Sleep terrors usually emerge between 4 and 12 years of age, with most individuals outgrowing this condition by adolescence, although sleepwalking may persist into adulthood. Prevalence rates for confusional arousals are approximately >15% in children aged 3 to 13 years and may be associated with sleepwalking and sleep terrors (Mindell & Owens, 2015).

Clinical symptoms. Partial arousal parasomnias are characterized by symptoms associated with wakefulness (e.g., ambulation, vocalizations) and sleep (e.g., high arousal threshold, unresponsiveness to the environment and caregivers, amnesia for the events). Partial arousal parasomnias are also characterized by the child's avoidance of or increased agitation with comforting by parents or prolongation of events by attempts to awaken the child.

Parasomnias may be triggered by external factors (noise) or internal factors (sleep fragmentation from a variety of causes). Although the duration of sleep terrors is usually a few minutes, confusional arousals can persist for up to 30 to 40 minutes. Sleep terrors are characterized by a sudden onset and a high degree of autonomic arousal (e.g., increased heart rate, sweating, dilated pupils; Mindell & Owens, 2015). In contrast, confusional arousals emerge more gradually and may present with thrashing in bed, mumbling and other vocalizations, slow mentation, disorientation, and confusion, but they do not usually result in displacement of the child from bed. Sleepwalking raises concern for risks to safety (e.g., falling downstairs, leaving the house and wandering in the neighborhood).

Treatment. Treatment of partial arousal parasomnias includes several strategies: (a) parental education and reassurance, (b) guidance on healthy sleep routines, and (c) avoidance of potential triggers (e.g., insufficient sleep, which can result in an increase in SWS; environmental noise; caffeine; Owens & Mohan, 2016). Evaluation should include an assessment for conditions such as OSA that may lead to fragmented sleep. For children with a history of sleepwalking, treatment should include implementation of safety precautions, including gates at the top of staircases and in doorways, locks on outside windows and doors, and caregiver notification systems such as bedroom door alarms. Caregivers should also be advised that parasomnias may be more likely to occur when sleeping in an unfamiliar environment. If partial arousals occur nightly, at a regular time, scheduled awakening, in which the caregiver awakens the child about 30 minutes before the time of typical night arousal, is often a successful behavioral intervention.

Pharmacotherapy is often not necessary, but may be indicated if the episodes are frequent or severe or if there is an elevated risk of injury or violent behavior or concerns about significant familial disruptions. The main pharmacologic agents to treat parasomnias include benzodiazepines and tricyclic antidepressants, which can help suppress SWS.

Movement Disorders: Restless Leg and Periodic Limb Movement

Restless legs syndrome (RLS) is characterized by a constant urge to move the legs during sleep, often with feelings of discomfort in the lower extremities. The drive to move and the lower leg sensations are typically worse when resting and in the evening and are partially mitigated with continuous movement (e.g., walking, stretching, rubbing). Restless legs syndrome is a disorder of the CNS sensorimotor network, and diagnosis is based on the presence of the clinical symptoms described previously (Durmer & Quraishi, 2011).

Periodic limb movement disorder (PLMD) is characterized by periodic, repetitive, brief leg jerks during sleep. Although clinical history may include complaints of kicking movements in sleep or restless sleep, the diagnosis of periodic limb movements (PLMs) is made after overnight PSG showing evidence of the characteristic limb movements. Because symptoms of PLMs can vary considerably from night to night in children, a single-night PSG may not accurately reflect the severity of symptoms (Durmer & Quraishi, 2011).

Prevalence, etiology, and pathophysiology. There is a strong genetic predisposition with RLS, with a sixfold to sevenfold increase in the prevalence in patients who have first-degree relatives with a history of RLS. Prevalence rates of RLS in the pediatric population range from 1% to 6% (Picchietti et al., 2007), although prevalence rates of significant PLMs (more than five per hour) in the general pediatric population are more difficult to ascertain because of the need for a PSG to make the diagnosis. Low serum iron levels (even without anemia) contribute to the presence and severity of RLS symptoms and PLMs. Laboratory analysis in children with RLS often reveals low serum ferritin levels (<50 ng/ml), reflective of decreased iron stores. Restless legs syndrome is thought to be related to dopaminergic dysfunction in the brain and can be impacted by low iron stores as iron is a cofactor in the rate-limiting step in dopamine synthesis (Dosman et al., 2012). RLS/PLMD can be exacerbated by certain medications including antidepressants (e.g., tricyclic antidepressants and selective serotonin reuptake inhibitors [SSRIs], first-generation antihistamines, dopamine receptor antagonists [e.g., Compazine], caffeine).

Clinical symptoms and evaluation. Children typically present with an urge to move their legs and may endorse sensory symptoms such as growing pains, a "funny feeling," tickling, pain, or a sensation of bugs on the legs. A helpful clinical question in eliciting RLS complaints from a child is "If I asked you to lie perfectly still on your bed at bedtime, could you be able to do it?" Because symptoms can be worse in the evening, common presenting complaints of RLS often include a history of bedtime struggles and difficulty falling asleep (Mindell & Owens, 2015). As opposed to patients with RLS, who are aware of the urge to move their legs, individuals with PLMs are usually unaware of these movements, although children with PLM may endorse morning muscle pain or fatigue. As with RLS, PLM may cause arousals during sleep, contributing to significant sleep disruption (Mindell & Owens, 2015). Because in clinical samples up to 26% of patients with RLS have ADHD or ADHD symptoms, and up to 44% of individuals with ADHD have RLS or RLS symptoms, a dual diagnosis of ADHD should be considered in children who present with RLS symptoms.

Treatment. The decision to treat RLS and PLMD varies, based on the severity of symptoms, presence of sleep disturbances, and effect on daytime functioning. The management approach for RLS/PLMD in children is described by the acronym **AIMS** (Mindell & Owens, 2015):

- *Avoidance:* Avoid drugs and substances that may exacerbate RLS/PLMD (e.g., caffeine, medications such as SSRIs).
- *Iron:* Provide iron supplementation to replete deficient iron stores.
- *Muscles:* Address myalgias with increased physical activity, massage, application of heat/cold, muscle relaxation, and biofeedback.
- *Sleep:* Encourage regular and adequate sleep.

Treatment with iron supplementation is indicated for serum ferritin levels < 50 ng/ml, with a recommended dose of 3 to 6 mg kg/day of elemental iron with vitamin C for 3 months. Serum ferritin levels are monitored to assess response. In rare cases, if ferritin levels do not improve after treatment with iron, hematology consultation may be indicated for consideration of IV infusion. For children with moderate-severe RLS symptoms and PLMD whose symptoms do not improve with these measures, pharmacological management may be indicated, although there are no medications approved by the U.S. Food and Drug Administration (FDA) for children. Although dopaminergic medications are considered the first line of treatment for RLS in adults, data on children are limited. Other classes of medications used to treat PLS/PLMD include alpha agonists, opiates, and benzodiazepines (Mindell & Owens, 2015).

Circadian Rhythm Disorders: Delayed Sleep–Wake Phase Disorder

Delayed sleep–wake phase disorder (DSWPD) is characterized by a significant and persistent phase shift in an individual's sleep–wake schedule and is evidenced by later sleep onset and wake times. This later wake time can conflict with the child's regular school and work schedule and can serve as a challenge to daily functioning. Although DSWPD can occur at any age, is most common in adolescents and young adults (Gradisar & Crowley, 2013). Individuals with DSWPD have an underlying biological predisposition/circadian-based "eveningness" chronotype, characterized by a preference for staying up relatively late at night and sleeping in until late in the morning. These night owls can struggle to get up in time for school or work during weekdays, but they usually revert to their preferred (later) sleep schedule on weekends, holidays, and summer vacations. In extreme cases, this sleep–wake pattern can result in a complete day-night reversal. The prevalence of DSWPD is estimated at 7% to 16% in adolescents and young adults (Sivertsen et al., 2013).

Clinical symptoms and evaluation. DSWPD presents clinically with sleep-initiation insomnia in which the patient tries to fall asleep at a desired or socially acceptable bedtime, but experiences very delayed sleep onset (often after 1 to 2 a.m.). This results in daytime sleepiness due to a combination of insufficient sleep and circadian misalignment. Patients often report extreme difficulty with morning waking, even for preferred activities, and can manifest confusion on waking (i.e., sleep inertia). Caregivers may often complain of the need for multiple reminders or even the complete failure to awaken the adolescent in time to attend school. Sleep maintenance is typically intact, without symptoms of sleep-onset insomnia if the individual's bedtime coincides with the preferred sleep-onset time (e.g., on weekends, school vacations). If the individual spends a prolonged time in bed attempting to fall asleep, they are at risk of developing a secondary insomnia.

DSWPD can contribute to difficulties in school performance as a result of school tardiness, frequent absenteeism, and a decline in academic performance (Mindell & Owens, 2015). In extreme cases, patients may experience school-related disciplinary action (i.e., suspension, truancy label) or a need to justify home-based schooling/tutoring, which motivates families to seek help. It is important to recognize that there may also be issues related to family dynamics and psychological factors at play. For example, some patients may have comorbid anxiety, depression, or learning disabilities that motivate school avoidance. Taken together, these issues highlight how difficulties in school performance can also originate from a disturbance in sleep. Therefore, in the evaluation of adolescents who present with school difficulties, behavioral providers (e.g. pediatric psychologists and developmental-behavioral pediatricians) should consider the possible contribution of DSWPD to the patient's symptoms.

Treatment. The goal of treatment of DSWPD is to shift the sleep–wake schedule to an earlier, preferable time and to maintain the earlier schedule (Sletten et al., 2018). Treatment begins by gradually advancing the sleep–wake schedule, often by alternating the start of an earlier morning waking time and an earlier evening bedtime. If there are more significant phase delays (i.e., if there is a larger difference between the time of current sleep onset and the preferred bedtime) chronotherapy may be required. Chronotherapy involves prolonging the child's bedtime and awakening time by 2 to 3 hours every 24 hours to "forward around the clock" until the desired bedtime is achieved. Because the secretion of melatonin is inhibited by light, exposure to light in the daytime (either in sunlight or by using a light box, which typically emits light at approximately 10,000 lux) and avoiding light exposure in the evening (especially blue light exposure from screens) may be beneficial. In addition, supplemental melatonin may be helpful. Administration of oral melatonin at physiological doses (i.e., 0.3 to 0.5 mg) in the afternoon or early evening (5 to 7 hours prior to the habitual sleep-onset time or 2 hours before the desired bedtime) has demonstrated efficacy in advancing the sleep phase (Mindell & Owens, 2015).

In general, because the treatment of DSWPD is multipronged, referral to a sleep specialist is often the best option for success. Collaboration with a mental health professional (e.g., pediatric psychologist) in complex, treatment-resistant cases that involve comorbid conditions such as depression, anxiety, and school avoidance may also be indicated.

Central Disorders of Hypersomnolence

Hypersomnia describes a constellation of sleep disorders characterized by (a) recurring bouts of EDS, (b) diminished alertness at baseline, and/or (c) prolonged periods of sleep at night which interfere with typical daily functioning. The causes of EDS are broadly described as extrinsic (e.g., insufficient and/or disrupted sleep) or intrinsic (e.g., a centrally mediated drive for increased sleep, of which the most clinically important are narcolepsy types 1 and 2). In adolescents presenting with daytime sleepiness, the most common extrinsic etiology for EDS is inadequate sleep secondary to early rising to accommodate earlier school start times. Extrinsic causes of EDS should be evaluated before considering a work-up for a central hypersomnia (Liu et al., 2019).

Narcolepsy.

Definition and etiology. Narcolepsy is a chronic lifelong CNS disorder manifest in extreme daytime sleepiness that contributes to significant functional impairment (Babiker & Prasad, 2015; Maski et al., 2017). Most patients with narcolepsy (>50%) have cataplexy (type 1 narcolepsy), characterized by the sudden brief onset of partial or complete loss of muscle tone while retaining consciousness. Narcolepsy is often triggered by strong emotion, with resumption of normal tone and function after the event. Other symptoms of narcolepsy include hypnogogic/hypnopompic hallucinations (which occur just prior to falling asleep/awakening) and sleep paralysis, which reflects an intrusion of REM-related phenomena (e.g., dream mentation, loss of motor tone) into the awake state (Mindell & Owens, 2015). Other REM-related symptoms of narcolepsy include the presence of eye movements or twitches at the beginning of sleep, related to shortened REM onset latency; a history of vivid dreams; and increased sleep fragmentation. Rapid weight gain (especially at the time of onset of symptoms) and the development of precocious puberty, due to alterations in the hypocretin/orexin system, has been observed in young children with narcolepsy (Mindell & Owens, 2015).

Pathophysiology. The pathophysiology underlying narcolepsy with cataplexy (type 1) has been attributed to a select deficit in the hypothalamic orexin/hypocretin neurotransmitter system, resulting in the loss of cells that produce hypocretin/orexin in the hypothalamus (Scammell, 2015). Hypocretin neurons produce neurochemicals that sustain the state of wakefulness, thus preventing lapses into sleep. These cells are also believed to play a role in appetite regulation. The etiology of narcolepsy with cataplexy is most likely multifactorial, involving autoimmune mechanisms (possibly triggered by viral infections including influenza and H1N1), in combination with a genetic predisposition and environmental factors (Mindell & Owens, 2015).

Narcolepsy without cataplexy (type 2) is believed to have a markedly different underlying pathophysiology. For example, although patients with type 1 narcolepsy have low hypocretin levels, the hypocretin levels are typically normal in patients with type 2 narcolepsy (Maski & Owens, 2016). Secondary narcolepsy has been attributed to several etiologies including traumatic brain injury involving the hypothalamus; neuro-inflammatory processes, such as pediatric autoimmune neuropsychiatric disorders associated with streptococcal infections; and neurogenetic diseases such as Prader-Willi syndrome.

Prevalence. Narcolepsy is a rare disorder. Prevalence has been estimated at approximately 1 in 2,000, with equal sex distribution. Some geographic populations (e.g., Japan) appear to have relatively higher prevalence rates than the general population. In families with a history of narcolepsy in a first-degree relative, the risk of developing narcolepsy with cataplexy is only slightly higher than in the general population (Mindell & Owens, 2015).

Clinical symptoms. Narcolepsy typically presents in adolescence and early adulthood, although the onset of symptoms may occur in school-aged or younger children. The onset may be abrupt or slowly progressive. Of note, the initial presenting symptoms of narcolepsy are often under-identified, misinterpreted, or attributed to other medical, neurologic, or psychiatric conditions. As a result, the initial diagnosis of narcolepsy can be delayed for years (Maski et al., 2017). Narcolepsy is characterized by EDS and repeated episodes of "sleep attacks" demonstrated by sudden, unpredictable, and irresistible sleep episodes. Other symptoms of narcolepsy include an increased sleep requirement at night and extreme difficulty in waking up (either in the morning or after a nap). Cataplexy is pathognomonic for a diagnosis of narcolepsy, although cataplexy may not develop until several years after the initial symptoms of EDS appear. Manifestations of cataplexy are often triggered by strong emotions, both positive (e.g., joy, emotions that elicit laughter) or negative (e.g., anger, frustration, fear). Symptoms of cataplexy may appear as facial relaxation, head nodding, jaw dropping, or infrequently, with knees giving way or total bodily collapse and falling to the ground. Cataplectic facies (unique to children) manifests with prolonged tongue protrusion, ptosis (eyelid droop), relaxed jaw, slurred speech, grimacing, and gait instability. These symptoms can persist for prolonged periods (e.g., lasting hours or days in a condition known as status cataplecticus). Other symptoms include hypnogogic/hypnopompic hallucinations (characterized by vivid visual hallucinations, auditory hallucinations, or tactile sensory experiences) during the period between sleeping and waking. These symptoms can present at the onset of sleep (hypnogogic) or at the termination of sleep (hypnopompic). Sleep paralysis (the brief inability to move or speak at the beginning or end of sleep) can often accompany the hallucinations. Other symptoms associated with narcolepsy include impairments in cognition; symptoms similar to ADHD (e.g., inattention); and dysregulation of mood, affect, and behavior (Blackwell et al., 2017).

Evaluation. Evaluation should begin with a detailed neurologic examination and assessment of typical sleep patterns with a sleep diary or actigraphy. A patient who presents with severe unexplained daytime sleepiness or with concerns for narcolepsy should also receive an overnight PSG and MSLT. Relatedly, a diagnosis of type 1 narcolepsy can be made by an analysis of hypocretin-1 levels in the cerebrospinal fluid (Mindell & Owens, 2015).

Treatment. In general, pediatric narcolepsy is best managed in conjunction with a sleep specialist. The therapeutic aim for the child with narcolepsy should be symptom management to facilitate a return to normal functioning in home, school, and social settings. Treatment for narcolepsy should be individualized. It usually involves a combination of education; guidance around sleep hygiene; behavioral/psychological interventions to address cognitive, mood, and lifestyle challenges; and at times medication. Scheduled daytime naps may be helpful, and medications that promote wakefulness, such as psychostimulants, modafinil, or armodafinil, may also be prescribed to mitigate EDS. Antidepressants (SSRIs, tricyclic antidepressants, venlafaxine) may also be prescribed to decrease cataplexy. Sodium oxybate is now FDA approved for use in children older than 7 years with narcolepsy for cataplexy and/or EDS (Lecendreux, 2014).

MEDICAL COMORBIDITIES, AND CONSIDERATIONS IN THE EVALUATION OF SLEEP DISORDERS

In the evaluation of children with sleep disorders, the overlap among mood, behavior, and sleep disorders should be kept in mind. For example, there is a well-established bidirectional relationship between effective treatment of anxiety and mood disorders and successful resolution of insomnia symptoms (and vice versa), and relatedly persistent insomnia symptoms may predict depression relapse (Kennard et al., 2006). Children with an ADHD profile may have an underlying sleep disorder, such as OSA or RLS/PLMD, that mimics ADHD symptoms. For children presenting with ADHD symptoms, a detailed evaluation to screen for symptoms and risks related to a primary sleep disorder is mandatory. Of note, medications used to treat ADHD symptoms, as well as comorbid conditions such as anxiety or oppositional defiant disorder, may be important contributory factors to the development of insomnia in some patients (Accardo et al., 2012; Cortese et al., 2009).

Children with autism spectrum disorders (ASD) often present with atypical sleep patterns including highly irregular sleep–wake cycles, extended bedtime routines characterized by repetitive and stereotypic behaviors, prolonged periods of waking during the night characterized by wandering, very early morning waking, short sleep duration, and complaints of insomnia (Hodge et al., 2014; Moore et al., 2017). A myriad of factors contributes to risk for sleeplessness in children with autism spectrum disorders, including medical (gastrointestinal issues, seizure disorders, medication-related effects), mental health (comorbid anxiety), and cognitive and psychosocial issues (learned maladaptive sleep behaviors). Challenges posed by core symptoms of ASD, such as poor response to social cues, limited communication skills, self-stimulatory and self-injurious behaviors, emotional dysregulation and sensory integration deficits, need to be considered when developing a comprehensive treatment plan. In addition, caregiver stress and exhaustion can hinder management of sleep issues. Although modifications to standard behavioral interventions may e necessary in special populations, such as children with ASD, ADHD, or other neurodevelopmental disabilities (Esposito et al., 2020), and although pharmacologic treatments are indicated for some patients (van der Heijden et al., 2018), many of the same basic management principles apply to neurotypical children. Two excellent resources that address the management of sleep concerns in neurodiverse populations are the 2020 American Academy of Neurology's guidelines for practitioners (Buckley et al., 2020) and the Autism Speaks Autism Treatment Network website for families (https://www.autismspeaks.org/taxonomy/term/2751).

PHARMACOLOGICAL MANAGEMENT OF SLEEP DISORDERS

A comprehensive discussion of medications used to treat insomnia in children is beyond the scope of this chapter; however, some basic principles are important to review. First, there are no medications approved by the FDA for the treatment of insomnia in children, and only one sleep medication has been approved for the treatment of pediatric sleep disorders (sodium oxybate [XYREM] for narcolepsy). Medication use should *not* be first line and should always be combined with a behavioral plan, highlighting the importance of collaboration between medical and behavioral specialists (e.g., between pediatricians and pediatric psychologists) in the management of sleep disorders (Mindell & Owens, 2015). Treatment goals should be realistic, clearly defined, and measurable. The medication type should be based on clinical assessment of the best possible match between the clinical situation and drug properties. Possible interactions with concomitant psychotropic medications should be carefully considered, and providers should avoid adding sedating/hypnotic drugs to offset side effects of other prescribed medications. Potential dosing modifications should be addressed up front with families, including dose escalation, middle of the night dosing, and nightly versus intermittent use. Despite the overall lack of clinical trial data, there are a number of hypnotic medications that are used off-label in clinical practice with the pediatric population. Table 19.5 summarizes selected drugs with important caveats included.

A few additional comments regarding additional categories of drugs that are not included in Table 19.5 but may be prescribed off-label for sleep by developmental-behavioral practitioners: First, in general, antidepressants are potent REM suppressants that may result in rebound REM on discontinuation and may mask REM-related symptoms of narcolepsy such as cataplexy. They may also exacerbate RLS and PLM (as discussed later in this chapter), and their use should be considered largely in patients with comorbid mood disorders or anxiety. Secondly, unless there

TABLE 19.5
Properties of Selected Medications Used for Pediatric Insomnia

Medications	Mechanism of action	Suggested dosage (mg/day)*	Common side effects	Comments
Benzodiazepine receptor agonists (BzDRA): Clonazepam (Klonopin)**	Bind to central GABA receptors	0.5–2.0	Residual daytime sedation, rebound insomnia on discontinuation; psycho-motor impairment; anterograde amnesia (dose dependent); potential respiratory depression; anti-convulsant, anxiolytic, myorelaxant properties	Also used to reduce partial arousal parasomnias (sleep terrors, sleepwalking) Limited use in pediatrics due to abuse/dependence potential
Nonbenzodiazepine receptor agonists (BzDRA): Zolpidem (Ambien)** Zaleplon (Sonata)**	Bind to α_1 subunits, GABA receptors	5–10	Headache, retrograde amnesia; morning grogginess; reports of complex sleep-related behaviors raise safety concerns (black box warning)	Clinical trial data shows little efficacy; limited clinical experience in children
α Agonists: Clonidine (Catapres) Guanfacine (Tenex)	α adrenergic receptor agonists (guanfacine more selective); decrease norepinephrine release	0.05–0.3 0.5–2	Dry mouth, bradycardia, hypotension, possible rebound hypertension on discontinuation; may cause midsleep awakenings and exacerbate partial arousal parasomnias; narrow therapeutic index	Also used in daytime treatment of ADHD
Atypical antidepressants (e.g., Trazadone)	5-HT$_{2A/C}$ antagonist	25–50	Dizziness, CNS over-stimulation. cardiac arrhythmias, hypotension, priapism	Main use with comorbid depression
Novel mechanism hypnotics: Selective histamine receptor antagonist Doxepin (Silenor)**	Selective antagonism of the histamine H1 receptor	3–6	Daytime somnolence and residual next-day effect	Used for sleep maintenance insomnia
OTC medications: Antihistamines Diphenhydramine (Benadryl) Cyproheptadine (Periactin) Hydroxyzine (Atarax)	Competitive histamine (H1) receptor blocker in the central nervous system	25–50 4–8 25–100	Daytime drowsiness, gastrointestinal symptoms (appetite loss, vomiting, constipation, dry mouth), paradoxical excitation	Weak soporifics despite high-level parental/practitioner acceptance; short-term use only
Hormone analog: Melatonin	Main effect suprachiasmatic nucleus; non-selective action at MT$_1$ and MT$_2$ receptors	1–6 (usual range in typically developing children) Reported doses (up to 10 mg in children with neurodevelopmental disorders) Low dose (0.3–0.5 mg) 1–2 hrs before desired bedtime in DSWPD	Headache, nightmares, morning grogginess; possible exacerbation of comorbid autoimmune diseases	Robust empirical evidence for use in children with developmental disabilities, autism, neurologic impairment, blindness, jet lag, DSWPD OTC preparations may be highly variable in actual melatonin content

Note. DSWPD = delayed sleep–wake phase disorder. Adapted from *A Clinical Guide to Pediatric Sleep: Diagnosis and Management of Sleep Problems in Children and Adolescents* (3rd ed., pp. 217–222), by J. A. Mindell and J. A. Owens, 2015, Wolters Kluwer. Copyright 2015 by Wolters Kluwer Health. Adapted with permission.
*Largely based on extrapolation of adult data and clinical experience. **U.S. Food and Drug Administration–approved medications in adults.

is an indication in addition to insomnia, antipsychotics (e.g., risperidone, anticonvulsants, mood stabilizers) have limited use in children due to side effects. Gabapentin has some limited empirical evidence for use in treating insomnia or for pediatric pain management in children with neurodevelopmental and psychiatric disorders.

Finally, melatonin is increasingly used to treat sleep onset insomnia. In several clinical trials evaluating its use in children with ADHD and ASD, there is some empirical support demonstrating efficacy (Parvataneni et al., 2020). Short-term side effects of melatonin are mild; however, data regarding long-term consequences (e.g., pubertal development and psychological dependency) are limited. Because clinical guidelines regarding its use are largely lacking, melatonin should be used with caution, and only when indicated (Bruni et al., 2015; Skrzelowski et al., 2021). Melatonin in a larger dose (e.g., 3 to 5 mg) is sedating when given at bedtime, but can also advance sleep onset when administered in small doses (e.g., 0.5 mg) 1 to 3 hours before the desired time of sleep onset. Melatonin is primarily indicated for sleep onset and not sleep maintenance insomnia, although a few studies of extended-release formulation have shown efficacy for the latter. Because melatonin is not regulated by the FDA in the United States, products may vary regarding actual melatonin content, and the use of pharmaceutical grade melatonin is recommended (Erland & Saxena, 2017).

IMPLICATIONS FOR PEDIATRIC PSYCHOLOGISTS AND DEVELOPMENTAL-BEHAVIORAL PEDIATRICIANS

An interdisciplinary approach that reinforces the connections among developmental-behavioral pediatrics, pediatric psychology, and developmental science is imperative in the clinical identification and management of sleep disorders across childhood. The causes and consequences of sleep problems in children and adolescents are multifactorial and impact multiple levels of the family system. Identification and evaluation of sleep concerns, development of a management plan, and subsequent monitoring for the efficacy of interventions targeting sleep, daytime function, and family well-being need to consider a number of factors. These considerations include developmental aspects of sleep and circadian biology across the lifespan; family systems strengths and vulnerabilities, including caregiver education, socioeconomic status, race/ethnicity, and social support (Billings et al., 2021); cultural variables such as parenting practices and priorities regarding sleep; and medical, mental health, and neurodevelopmental comorbidities. The role of the pediatric psychologist in management of sleep disorders is underscored by the predominance of behavioral interventions, particularly for pediatric insomnia. Furthermore, a collaborative approach between physicians and psychologists is highlighted to foster acceptance of and adherence to pharmacologic and other medical treatments in disorders such as OSA, delayed sleep-wake phase disorder, and narcolepsy. Future development of novel treatment paradigms for pediatric sleep disorders that include medical, psychological, and family systems approaches represents an opportunity for merging the expertise and skill sets of all three disciplines.

RESOURCES

General Resources

- American Academy of Sleep Medicine
  https://aasm.org; https://sleepeducation.org

- National Sleep Foundation
  https://www.sleepfoundation.org

- Narcolepsy Network
  https://narcolepsynetwork.org

- Wake Up Narcolepsy
  https://www.wakeupnarcolepsy.org

- Autism Speaks Autism Treatment Network
  https://www.autismspeaks.org/taxonomy/term/2751

- Start School Later Healthy Hours
  https://www.startschoollater.net/

Resources and Guidelines for Providers

- American Academy of Child and Adolescent Psychiatry. (2021). *Sleep disorders: Parents' medication guide.* American Psychiatric Association. https://www.aacap.org/App_Themes/AACAP/Docs/families_and_youth/med_guides/SleepDisorders_Parents-Medication-Guideweb.pdf
- BRIQ-R (Brief Infant Sleep Questionnaire—Revised)

  https://www.babysleep.com/bisq/
- Buckley, W. A., Hirtz, D., Oskoui, M., Armstrong, M. J., Batra, A., Bridgemohan, C., Coury, D., Dawson, G., Donley, D., Findling, R. L., Gaughan, T., Gloss, D., Gronseth, G., Kessler, R., Merillat, S., Michelson, D., Owens, J., Pringsheim, T., Sikich, L., Stahmer, A., Thurm, A., Tuchman, R., Warren, Z., Wetherby, A., Wiznitzer, M., & Ashwal, S. (2020). Practice guideline: Treatment for insomnia and disrupted sleep behavior in children and adolescents with autism spectrum disorder: Report of the Guideline Development, Dissemination, and Implementation Subcommittee of the American Academy of Neurology. *Neurology, 94*(9), 392–404. https://doi.org/10.1212/WNL.0000000000009033
- Marcus, C. L., Brooks, L. J., Draper, K. A., Gozal, D., Halbower, C. A., Jones, J., Schechter, M. S, Sheldon, S. C., Spruyt, K., Davidson Ward, S., Lehmann, C., & Shiffman, R. N. (2012). Diagnosis and management of childhood obstructive sleep apnea syndrome [Clinical practice guidelines]. *Pediatrics, 130*(3), 576–584. https://doi.org/10.1542/peds.2012-1671
- Mindell, J. A., & Owens, J. A. (2015). Evaluation of pediatric sleep disorders. In *A clinical guide to pediatric sleep: Diagnosis and management of sleep problems* (3rd ed., pp. 37–47). Wolters Kluwer.

References

Accardo, J. A., Marcus, C. L., Leonard, M. B., Shults, J., Meltzer, L. J., & Elia, J. (2012). Associations between psychiatric comorbidities and sleep disturbances in children with attention-deficit/hyperactivity disorder. *Journal of Developmental and Behavioral Pediatrics, 33*(2), 97–105. https://doi.org/10.1097/DBP.0b013e31823f6853

American Academy of Sleep Medicine. (2023). *International classification of sleep disorders* (3rd ed., text rev.). https://aasm.org/clinical-resources/international-classification-sleep-disorders/

American Psychiatric Association. (2013). *Diagnostic and statistical manual of mental disorders* (5th ed.). https://doi.org/10.1176/appi.books.9780890425596

Babiker, M. O., & Prasad, M. (2015). Narcolepsy in children: A diagnostic and management approach. *Pediatric Neurology, 52*(6), 557–65. https://doi.org/10.1016/j.pediatrneurol.2015.02.020

Baert, S., Omey, E., Verhaest, D., & Vermeir, A. (2015). Mister Sandman, bring me good marks! On the relationship between sleep quality and academic achievement. *Social Science & Medicine, 130*, 91–98. https://doi.org/10.1016/j.socscimed.2015.02.011

Beebe, D. W. (2011). Cognitive, behavioral, and functional consequences of inadequate sleep in children and adolescents. *Pediatric Clinics of North America, 58*(3), 649–665. https://doi.org/10.1016/j.pcl.2011.03.002

Beebe, D. W., Wells, C. T., Jeffries, J., Chini, B., Kalra, M., & Amin, R. (2004). Neuropsychological effects of pediatric obstructive sleep apnea. *Journal of the International Neuropsychological Society, 10*(7), 962–975. https://doi.org/10.1017/S135561770410708X

Berger, A. T., Wahlstrom, K. L., & Widome, R. (2019). Relationships between sleep duration and adolescent depression: A conceptual replication. *Sleep Health, 5*(2), 175–179. https://doi.org/10.1016/j.sleh.2018.12.003

Biggs, S. N., Vlahandonis, A., Anderson, V., Bourke, R., Nixon, G. M., Davey, M. J., & Horne, R. S. (2014). Long-term changes in neurocognition and behavior following treatment of sleep disordered breathing in school-aged children. *Sleep, 37*(1), 77–84. https://doi.org/10.5665/sleep.3312

Bilgin, A., & Wolke, D. (2020). Parental use of "cry it out" in infants: No adverse effects on attachment and behavioural development at 18 months. *Journal of Child Psychology and Psychiatry, 61*(11), 1184–1193. https://doi.org/10.1111/jcpp.13223

Billings, M. E., Cohen, R. T., Baldwin, C. M., Johnson, D. A., Palen, B. N., Parthasarathy, S., Patel, S. R., Russell, M., Tapia, I. E., Williamson, A. A., & Sharma, S. (2021). Disparities in sleep health and potential intervention models: A focused review. *Chest, 159*(3), 1232–1240. https://doi.org/10.1016/j.chest.2020.09.249

Bin-Hasan, S., Kapur, K., Rakesh, K., & Owens, J. (2020). School start time change and motor vehicle crashes in adolescent drivers. *Journal of Clinical Sleep Medicine, 16*(3), 371–376. https://doi.org/10.5664/jcsm.8208

Blackwell, J. E., Alammar, H. A., Weighall, A. R., Kellar, I., & Nash, H. M. (2017). A systematic review of cognitive function and psychosocial well-being in school-age children with narcolepsy. *Sleep Medicine Reviews, 34*, 82–93. https://doi.org/10.1016/j.smrv.2016.07.003

Bourke, R. S., Anderson, V., Yang, J. S., Jackman, A. R., Killedar, A., Nixon, G. M., Davey, M. J., Walker, A. M., Trinder, J., & Horne, R. S. (2011). Neurobehavioral function is impaired in children with all severities of sleep disordered breathing. *Sleep Medicine, 12*(3), 222–229. https://doi.org/10.1016/j.sleep.2010.08.011

Bruni, O., Alonso-Alcondada, D., Besag, F., Biran, V., Braam, W., Cortese, S., Moavero, R., Parisi, P., Smits, M., van der Heijden, K., & Curatolo, P. (2015). Current role of melatonin in pediatric neurology: Clinical recommendations. *European Journal of Paediatric Neurology, 19*(2), 122–133. https://doi.org/10.1016/j.ejpn.2014.12.007

Buckhalt, J. A. (2011). Insufficient sleep and the socioeconomic status achievement gap. *Child Development Perspectives, 5*(1), 59–65. https://doi.org/10.1111/j.1750-8606.2010.00151.x

Buckley, A. W., Hirtz, D., Oskoui, M., Armstrong, M. J., Batra, A., Bridgemohan, C., Coury, D., Dawson, G., Donley, D., Findling, R. L., Gaughan, T., Gloss, D., Gronseth, G., Kessler, R., Merillat, S., Michelson, D., Owens, J., Pringsheim, T., Sikich, L., . . . Ashwal, S. (2020). Practice guideline: Treatment for insomnia and disrupted sleep behavior in children and adolescents with autism spectrum disorder: Report of the Guideline Development, Dissemination, and Implementation Subcommittee of the American Academy of Neurology. *Neurology, 94*(9), 392–404. https://doi.org/10.1212/WNL.0000000000009033

Calhoun, S. L., Fernandez-Mendoza, J., Vgontzas, A. N., Mayes, S. D., Liao, D., & Bixler, E. O. (2017). Behavioral profiles associated with objective sleep duration in young children with insomnia symptoms. *Journal of Abnormal Child Psychology, 45*(2), 337–344. https://doi.org/10.1007/s10802-016-0166-4

Chervin, R. D., Ellenberg, S. S., Hou, X., Marcus, C. L., Garetz, S. L., Katz, E. S., Hodges, E. K., Mitchell, R. B., Jones, D. T., Arens, R., Amin, R., Redline, S., Rosen, C. L., & the Childhood Adenotonsillectomy Trial. (2015). Prognosis for spontaneous resolution of OSA in children. *Chest, 148*(5), 1204–1213. https://doi.org/10.1378/chest.14-2873

Chiu, H.-Y., Lee, H.-C., Chen, P.-Y., Lai, Y.-F., & Tu, Y.-K. (2018). Associations between sleep duration and suicidality in adolescents: A systematic review and dose-response meta-analysis. *Sleep Medicine Reviews, 42*, 119–126. https://doi.org/10.1016/j.smrv.2018.07.003

Corkum, P. V., Reid, G. J., Hall, W. A., Godbout, R., Stremler, R., Weiss, S. K., Gruber, R., Witmans, M., Chambers, C. T., Begum, E. A., Andreou, P., & Rigney, G. (2018). Evaluation of an internet-based behavioral intervention to improve psychosocial health outcomes in children with insomnia (better nights, better days): Protocol for a randomized controlled trial. *JMIR Research Protocols, 7*(3), e76. https://doi.org/10.2196/resprot.8348

Cortese, S., Faraone, S. V., Konofal, E., & Lecendreux, M. (2009). Sleep in children with attention-deficit/hyperactivity disorder: Meta-analysis of subjective and objective studies. *Journal of the American Academy of Child & Adolescent Psychiatry, 48*(9), 894–908. https://doi.org/10.1097/CHI.0b013e3181ae09c9

Crabtree, V. M., Varni, J. W., & Gozal, D. (2004). Health-related quality of life and depressive symptoms in children with suspected sleep-disordered breathing. *Sleep, 27*(6), 1131–1138. https://doi.org/10.1093/sleep/27.6.1131

de Bruin, E. J., Bögels, S. M., Oort, F. J., & Meijer, A. M. (2015). Efficacy of cognitive behavioral therapy for insomnia in adolescents: A randomized controlled trial with internet therapy, group therapy and a waiting list condition. *Sleep, 38*(12), 1913–1926. https://doi.org/10.5665/sleep.5240

Donners, A. A., Tromp, M. D., Garssen, J., Roth, T., & Verster, J. C. (2015). Perceived immune status and sleep: A survey among Dutch students. *Sleep Disorders, 2015*, 721607. https://doi.org/10.1155/2015/721607

Dosman, C., Witmans, M., & Zwaigenbaum, L. (2012). Iron's role in paediatric restless legs syndrome—A review. *Paediatrics & Child Health, 17*(4), 193–197. https://doi.org/10.1093/pch/17.4.193

Dunster, G. P., de la Iglesia, L., Ben-Hamo, M., Nave, C., Fleischer, J. G., Panda, S., & de la Iglesia, H. O. (2018). Sleepmore in Seattle: Later school start times are associated with more sleep and better performance in high school students. *Science Advances, 4*(12), eaau6200. https://doi.org/10.1126/sciadv.aau6200

Durmer, J. S., & Quraishi, G. H. (2011). Restless legs syndrome, periodic leg movements, and periodic limb movement disorder in children. *Pediatric Clinics of North America*, 58(3), 591–620. https://doi.org/10.1016/j.pcl.2011.03.005

Erland, L. A., & Saxena, P. K. (2017). Melatonin natural health products and supplements: Presence of serotonin and significant variability of melatonin content. *Journal of Clinical Sleep Medicine*, 13(2), 275–281. https://doi.org/10.5664/jcsm.6462

Esposito, D., Belli, A., Ferri, R., & Bruni, O. (2020). Sleeping without prescription: Management of sleep disorders in children with autism with non-pharmacological interventions and over-the-counter treatments. *Brain Sciences*, 10(7), 441. https://doi.org/10.3390/brainsci10070441

Evans, S., Djilas, V., Seidman, L. C., Zeltzer, L. K., & Tsao, J. C. I. (2017). Sleep quality, affect, pain, and disability in children with chronic pain: Is affect a mediator or moderator? *The Journal of Pain*, 18(9), 1087–1095. https://doi.org/10.1016/j.jpain.2017.04.007

Foley, J. E., & Weinraub, M. (2017). Sleep, affect, and social competence from preschool to preadolescence: Distinct pathways to emotional and social adjustment for boys and for girls. *Frontiers in Psychology*, 8, 711. https://doi.org/10.3389/fpsyg.2017.00711

Fontanellaz-Castiglione, C. E., Markovic, A., & Tarokh, L. (2020). Sleep and the adolescent brain. *Current Opinion in Physiology*, 15, 167–171. https://doi.org/10.1016/j.cophys.2020.01.008

Franckle, R. L., Falbe, J., Gortmaker, S., Ganter, C., Taveras, E. M., Land, T., & Davison, K. K. (2015). Insufficient sleep among elementary and middle school students is linked with elevated soda consumption and other unhealthy dietary behaviors. *Preventive Medicine*, 74, 36–41. https://doi.org/10.1016/j.ypmed.2015.02.007

Freeman, D., Sheaves, B., Goodwin, G. M., Yu, L.-M., Nickless, A., Harrison, P. J., Emsley, R., Luik, A. I., Foster, R. G., Wadekar, V., Hinds, C., Gumley, A., Jones, R., Lightman, S., Jones, S., Bentall, R., Kinderman, P., Rowse, G., Brugha, T., . . . Espie, C. A. (2017). The effects of improving sleep on mental health (OASIS): A randomised controlled trial with mediation analysis. *The Lancet Psychiatry*, 4(10), 749–758. https://doi.org/10.1016/S2215-0366(17)30328-0

Gao, B., Dwivedi, S., Milewski, M. D., & Cruz, A. I., Jr. (2019). Lack of sleep and sports injuries in adolescents: A systematic review and meta-analysis. *Journal of Pediatric Orthopedics*, 39(5), e324–e333. https://doi.org/10.1097/BPO.0000000000001306

Gradisar, M., & Crowley, S. J. (2013). Delayed sleep phase disorder in youth. *Current Opinion in Psychiatry*, 26(6), 580–585. https://doi.org/10.1097/YCO.0b013e328365a1d4

Groen, J. A., & Pabilonia, S. W. (2019). Snooze or lose: High school start times and academic achievement. *Economics of Education Review*, 72, 204–218. https://doi.org/10.1016/j.econedurev.2019.05.011

Guglielmo, D., Gazmararian, J. A., Chung, J., Rogers, A. E., & Hale, L. (2018). Racial/ethnic sleep disparities in US school-aged children and adolescents: A review of the literature. *Sleep Health*, 4(1), 68–80. https://doi.org/10.1016/j.sleh.2017.09.005

Gujar, N., McDonald, S. A., Nishida, M., & Walker, M. P. (2011). A role for REM sleep in recalibrating the sensitivity of the human brain to specific emotions. *Cerebral Cortex*, 21(1), 115–123. https://doi.org/10.1093/cercor/bhq064

Hafner, M., Stepanek, M., & Troxel, W. M. (2017). *Later school start times in the U.S.: An economic analysis*. Rand Corporation.

Hash, J. B., Alfano, C. A., Owens, J., Littlewood, K., Day, A., Pandey, A., Ordway, M. R., & Ward, T. M. (2022). Call to action: Prioritizing sleep health among US children and youth residing in alternative care settings. *Sleep Health*, 8(1), 23–27. https://doi.org/10.1016/j.sleh.2021.10.002

Hasler, B. P., & Clark, D. B. (2013). Circadian misalignment, reward-related brain function, and adolescent alcohol involvement. *Alcohol: Clinical and Experimental Research*, 37(4), 558–565. https://doi.org/10.1111/acer.12003

Heissel, J. A., & Norris, S. (2018). Rise and shine the effect of school start times on academic performance from childhood through puberty. *The Journal of Human Resources*, 53(4), 957–992. https://doi.org/10.3368/jhr.53.4.0815-7346R1

Hodge, D., Carollo, T. M., Lewin, M., Hoffman, C. D., & Sweeney, D. P. (2014). Sleep patterns in children with and without autism spectrum disorders: Developmental comparisons. *Research in Developmental Disabilities*, 35(7), 1631–1638. https://doi.org/10.1016/j.ridd.2014.03.037

Isaiah, A., Ernst, T., Cloak, C. C., Clark, D. B., & Chang, L. (2021a). Association between habitual snoring and cognitive performance among a large sample of preadolescent children. *JAMA Otolaryngology—Head & Neck Surgery*, 147(5), 426–433. https://doi.org/10.1001/jamaoto.2020.5712

Isaiah, A., Ernst, T., Cloak, C. C., Clark, D. B., & Chang, L. (2021b). Associations between frontal lobe structure, parent-reported obstructive sleep disordered breathing and childhood behavior in the ABCD dataset. *Nature Communications*, 12(1), 2205. https://doi.org/10.1038/s41467-021-22534-0

Johnson, E. O., Roth, T., & Breslau, N. (2006). The association of insomnia with anxiety disorders and depression: Exploration of the direction of risk. *Journal of Psychiatric Research, 40*(8), 700–708. https://doi.org/10.1016/j.jpsychires.2006.07.008

Kennard, B., Silva, S., Vitiello, B., Curry, J., Kratochvil, C., Simons, A., Hughes, J., Feeny, N., Weller, E., Sweeney, M., Reinecke, M., Pathak, S., Ginsburg, G., Emslie, G., March, J., & the TADS Team. (2006). Remission and residual symptoms after short-term treatment in the Treatment of Adolescents with Depression Study (TADS). *Journal of the American Academy of Child & Adolescent Psychiatry, 45*(12), 1404–1411. https://doi.org/10.1097/01.chi.0000242228.75516.21

Kira, G., Maddison, R., Hull, M., Blunden, S., & Olds, T. (2014). Sleep education improves the sleep duration of adolescents: A randomized controlled pilot study. *Journal of Clinical Sleep Medicine, 10*(7), 787–792. https://doi.org/10.5664/jcsm.3874

Landau, Y. E., Bar-Yishay, O., Greenberg-Dotan, S., Goldbart, A. D., Tarasiuk, A., & Tal, A. (2012). Impaired behavioral and neurocognitive function in preschool children with obstructive sleep apnea. *Pediatric Pulmonology, 47*(2), 180–188. https://doi.org/10.1002/ppul.21534

Lecendreux, M. (2014). Pharmacological management of narcolepsy and cataplexy in pediatric patients. *Paediatric Drugs, 16*(5), 363–372. https://doi.org/10.1007/s40272-014-0083-3

Lenard, M., Morrill, M. S., & Westall, J. (2020). High school start times and student achievement: Looking beyond test scores. *Economics of Education Review, 76*, 101975. https://doi.org/10.1016/j.econedurev.2020.101975

Liu, Y., Zhang, J., Li, S. X., Chan, N. Y., Yu, M. W. M., Lam, S. P., Chan, J. W. Y., Li, A. M., & Wing, Y. K. (2019). Excessive daytime sleepiness among children and adolescents: Prevalence, correlates, and pubertal effects. *Sleep Medicine, 53*, 1–8. https://doi.org/10.1016/j.sleep.2018.08.028

Lunsford-Avery, J. R., Krystal, A. D., & Kollins, S. H. (2016). Sleep disturbances in adolescents with ADHD: A systematic review and framework for future research. *Clinical Psychology Review, 50*, 159–174. https://doi.org/10.1016/j.cpr.2016.10.004

Malone, S. K., Zemel, B., Compher, C., Souders, M., Chittams, J., Thompson, A. L., & Lipman, T. H. (2016). Characteristics associated with sleep duration, chronotype, and social jet lag in adolescents. *The Journal of School Nursing, 32*(2), 120–131. https://doi.org/10.1177/1059840515603454

Marcus, C. L., Brooks, L. J., Draper, K. A., Gozal, D., Halbower, A. C., Jones, J., Schechter, M. S., Ward, S. D., Sheldon, S. H., Shiffman, R. N., Lehmann, C., Spruyt, K., & the American Academy of Pediatrics. (2012). Diagnosis and management of childhood obstructive sleep apnea syndrome. *Pediatrics, 130*(3), e714–e755. https://doi.org/10.1542/peds.2012-1672

Marcus, C. L., Moore, R. H., Rosen, C. L., Giordani, B., Garetz, S. L., Taylor, H. G., Mitchell, R. B., Amin, R., Katz, E. S., Arens, R., Paruthi, S., Muzumdar, H., Gozal, D., Thomas, N. H., Ware, J., Beebe, D., Snyder, K., Elden, L., Sprecher, R. C., . . . the Childhood Adenotonsillectomy Trial (CHAT). (2013). A randomized trial of adenotonsillectomy for childhood sleep apnea. *The New England Journal of Medicine, 368*(25), 2366–2376. https://doi.org/10.1056/NEJMoa1215881

Maski, K., & Owens, J. A. (2016). Insomnia, parasomnias, and narcolepsy in children: Clinical features, diagnosis, and management. *The Lancet Neurology, 15*(11), 1170–1181. https://doi.org/10.1016/S1474-4422(16)30204-6

Maski, K., Steinhart, E., Williams, D., Scammell, T., Flygare, J., McCleary, K., & Gow, M. (2017). Listening to the patient voice in narcolepsy: Diagnostic delay, disease burden, and treatment efficacy. *Journal of Clinical Sleep Medicine, 13*(3), 419–425. https://doi.org/10.5664/jcsm.6494

Maski, K., Trotti, L. M., Kotagal, S., Auger, R. R., Rowley, J. A., Hashmi, S. D., & Watson, N. F. (2021). Treatment of central disorders of hypersomnolence: An American Academy of Sleep Medicine clinical practice guideline. *Journal of Clinical Sleep Medicine, 17*(9), 1881–1893. https://doi.org/10.5664/jcsm.9328

Maski, K. P., & Kothare, S. V. (2013). Sleep deprivation and neurobehavioral functioning in children. *International Journal of Psychophysiology, 89*(2), 259–264. https://doi.org/10.1016/j.ijpsycho.2013.06.019

Meldrum, R. C., Barnes, J. C., & Hay, C. (2015). Sleep deprivation, low self-control, and delinquency: A test of the strength model of self-control. *Journal of Youth and Adolescence, 44*(2), 465–477. https://doi.org/10.1007/s10964-013-0024-4

Miller, M. B., Janssen, T., & Jackson, K. M. (2017). The prospective association between sleep and initiation of substance use in young adolescents. *Journal of Adolescent Health, 60*(2), 154–160. https://doi.org/10.1016/j.jadohealth.2016.08.019

Mindell, J. A., & Owens, J. A. (2010). *A clinical guide to pediatric sleep: Diagnosis and management of sleep problems* (2nd ed.). Wolters Kluwer.

Mindell, J. A., & Owens, J. A. (2015). *A clinical guide to pediatric sleep: Diagnosis and management of sleep problems* (3rd ed.). Wolters Kluwer.

Mitchell, R. B., & Kelly, J. (2005). Quality of life after adenotonsillectomy for SDB in children. *Otolaryngology—Head and Neck Surgery*, 133(4), 569–572. https://doi.org/10.1016/j.otohns.2005.05.040

Mitchell, R. B., & Kelly, J. (2007). Behavioral changes in children with mild sleep-disordered breathing or obstructive sleep apnea after adenotonsillectomy. *The Laryngoscope*, 117(9), 1685–1688. https://doi.org/10.1097/MLG.0b013e318093edd7

Moore, M., Evans, V., Hanvey, G., & Johnson, C. (2017). Assessment of sleep in children with autism spectrum disorder. *Children*, 4(8), 72. https://doi.org/10.3390/children4080072

Nguyen, J., Zhang, B., Hanson, E., Mylonas, D., & Maski, K. (2022). Neurobehavioral associations with NREM and REM sleep architecture in children with autism spectrum disorder. *Children*, 9(9), 1322. https://doi.org/10.3390/children9091322

O'Brien, L. M., Lucas, N. H., Felt, B. T., Hoban, T. F., Ruzicka, D. L., Jordan, R., Guire, K., & Chervin, R. D. (2011). Aggressive behavior, bullying, snoring, and sleepiness in schoolchildren. *Sleep Medicine*, 12(7), 652–658. https://doi.org/10.1016/j.sleep.2010.11.012

Ohayon, M. M., Mahowald, M. W., Dauvilliers, Y., Krystal, A. D., & Léger, D. (2012). Prevalence and comorbidity of nocturnal wandering in the U.S. adult general population. *Neurology*, 78(20), 1583–1589. https://doi.org/10.1212/WNL.0b013e3182563be5

Owens, J. (2007). Classification and epidemiology of childhood sleep disorders. *Sleep Medicine Clinics*, 2(3), 353–361. https://doi.org/10.1016/j.jsmc.2007.05.009

Owens, J., & Mohan, M. (2016). Behavioral interventions for parasomnias. *Current Sleep Medicine Reports*, 2(2), 81–86. https://doi.org/10.1007/s40675-016-0046-z

Owens, J. A. (2019). Sleep medicine. In R. M. Kliegman & J. W. St. Geme III (Eds.), *Nelson textbook of pediatrics* (21st ed., Chap. 31). Elsevier.

Owens, J. A., & Dalzell, V. (2005). Use of the 'BEARS' sleep screening tool in a pediatric residents' continuity clinic: A pilot study. *Sleep Medicine*, 6(1), 63–69. https://doi.org/10.1016/j.sleep.2004.07.015

Owens, J. A., Mehlenbeck, R., Lee, J., & King, M. M. (2008). Effect of weight, sleep duration, and comorbid sleep disorders on behavioral outcomes in children with sleep-disordered breathing. *Archives of Pediatrics & Adolescent Medicine*, 162(4), 313–321. https://doi.org/10.1001/archpedi.162.4.313

Paruthi, S., Brooks, L. J., D'Ambrosio, C., Hall, W. A., Kotagal, S., Lloyd, R. M., Malow, B. A., Maski, K., Nichols, C., Quan, S. F., Rosen, C. L., Troester, M. M., & Wise, M. S. (2016). Recommended amount of sleep for pediatric populations: A consensus statement of the American Academy of Sleep Medicine. *Journal of Clinical Sleep Medicine*, 12(6), 785–786. https://doi.org/10.5664/jcsm.5866

Parvataneni, T., Srinivas, S., Shah, K., & Patel, R. S. (2020). Perspective on melatonin use for sleep problems in autism and attention-deficit hyperactivity disorder: A systematic review of randomized clinical trials. *Cureus*, 12(5), e8335. https://doi.org/10.7759/cureus.8335

Petit, D., Pennestri, M.-H., Paquet, J., Desautels, A., Zadra, A., Vitaro, F., Tremblay, R. E., Boivin, M., & Montplaisir, J. (2015). Childhood sleepwalking and sleep terrors: A longitudinal study of prevalence and familial aggregation. *JAMA Pediatrics*, 169(7), 653–658. https://doi.org/10.1001/jamapediatrics.2015.127

Picchietti, D., Allen, R. P., Walters, A. S., Davidson, J. E., Myers, A., & Ferini-Strambi, L. (2007). Restless legs syndrome: Prevalence and impact in children and adolescents—The Peds REST study. *Pediatrics*, 120(2), 253–266. https://doi.org/10.1542/peds.2006-2767

Pizza, F., Franceschini, C., Peltola, H., Vandi, S., Finotti, E., Ingravallo, F., Nobili, L., Bruni, O., Lin, L., Edwards, M. J., Partinen, M., Dauvilliers, Y., Mignot, E., Bhatia, K. P., & Plazzi, G. (2013). Clinical and polysomnographic course of childhood narcolepsy with cataplexy. *Brain: A Journal of Neurology*, 136(12), 3787–3795. https://doi.org/10.1093/brain/awt277

Price, A. M., Wake, M., Ukoumunne, O. C., & Hiscock, H. (2012). Five-year follow-up of harms and benefits of behavioral infant sleep intervention: Randomized trial. *Pediatrics*, 130(4), 643–651. https://doi.org/10.1542/peds.2011-3467

Redline, S., Cook, K., Chervin, R. D., Ishman, S., Baldassari, C. M., Mitchell, R. B., Tapia, I. E., Amin, R., Hassan, F., Ibrahim, S., Ross, K., Elden, L. M., Kirkham, E. M., Zopf, D., Shah, J., Otteson, T., Naqvi, K., Owens, J., Young, L., . . . Wang, R. (2023). Adenotonsillectomy for snoring and mild sleep apnea in children: A randomized clinical trial. *JAMA: Journal of the American Medical Association*, 330(21), 2084–2095. https://doi.org/10.1001/jama.2023.22114

Scammell, T. E. (2015). Narcolepsy. *The New England Journal of Medicine*, 373(27), 2654–2662. https://doi.org/10.1056/NEJMra1500587

Shochat, T., Cohen-Zion, M., & Tzischinsky, O. (2014). Functional consequences of inadequate sleep in adolescents: A systematic review. *Sleep Medicine*

Reviews, 18(1), 75–87. https://doi.org/10.1016/j.smrv.2013.03.005

Short, M. A., Gradisar, M., Wright, H., Lack, L. C., Dohnt, H., & Carskadon, M. A. (2011). Time for bed: Parent-set bedtimes associated with improved sleep and daytime functioning in adolescents. *Sleep, 34*(6), 797–800. https://doi.org/10.5665/SLEEP.1052

Sivertsen, B., Pallesen, S., Stormark, K. M., Bøe, T., Lundervold, A. J., & Hysing, M. (2013). Delayed sleep phase syndrome in adolescents: Prevalence and correlates in a large population based study. *BMC Public Health, 13*(1), 1163. https://doi.org/10.1186/1471-2458-13-1163

Skrzelowski, M., Brookhaus, A., Shea, L. A., & Berlau, D. J. (2021). Melatonin use in pediatrics: Evaluating the discrepancy in evidence based on country and regulations regarding production. *The Journal of Pediatric Pharmacology and Therapeutics, 26*(1), 4–20. https://doi.org/10.5863/1551-6776-26.1.4

Sletten, T. L., Magee, M., Murray, J. M., Gordon, C. J., Lovato, N., Kennaway, D. J., Gwini, S. M., Bartlett, D. J., Lockley, S. W., Lack, L. C., Grunstein, R. R., Rajaratnam, S. M. W., & the Delayed Sleep on Melatonin (DelSoM) Study Group. (2018). Efficacy of melatonin with behavioural sleep-wake scheduling for delayed sleep-wake phase disorder: A double-blind, randomised clinical trial. *PLOS Medicine, 15*(6), e1002587. https://doi.org/10.1371/journal.pmed.1002587

Tambalis, K. D., Panagiotakos, D. B., Psarra, G., & Sidossis, L. S. (2018). Insufficient sleep duration is associated with dietary habits, screen time, and obesity in children. *Journal of Clinical Sleep Medicine, 14*(10), 1689–1696. https://doi.org/10.5664/jcsm.7374

Tsukada, E., Kitamura, S., Enomoto, M., Moriwaki, A., Kamio, Y., Asada, T., Arai, T., & Mishima, K. (2018). Prevalence of childhood obstructive sleep apnea syndrome and its role in daytime sleepiness. *PLOS ONE, 13*(10), e0204409. https://doi.org/10.1371/journal.pone.0204409

van der Heijden, K. B., Stoffelsen, R. J., Popma, A., & Swaab, H. (2018). Sleep, chronotype, and sleep hygiene in children with attention-deficit/hyperactivity disorder, autism spectrum disorder, and controls. *European Child & Adolescent Psychiatry, 27*(1), 99–111. https://doi.org/10.1007/s00787-017-1025-8

Vriend, J. L., Davidson, F. D., Corkum, P. V., Rusak, B., Chambers, C. T., & McLaughlin, E. N. (2013). Manipulating sleep duration alters emotional functioning and cognitive performance in children. *Journal of Pediatric Psychology, 38*(10), 1058–1069. https://doi.org/10.1093/jpepsy/jst033

Wang, Y., & Yip, T. (2020). Sleep facilitates coping: Moderated mediation of daily sleep, ethnic/racial discrimination, stress responses, and adolescent well-being. *Child Development, 91*(4), e833–e852. https://doi.org/10.1111/cdev.13324

Weaver, M. D., Barger, L. K., Malone, S. K., Anderson, L. S., & Klerman, E. B. (2018). Dose-dependent associations between sleep duration and unsafe behaviors among US high school students. *JAMA Pediatrics, 172*(12), 1187–1189. https://doi.org/10.1001/jamapediatrics.2018.2777

Wheaton, A. G., Chapman, D. P., & Croft, J. B. (2016). School start times, sleep, behavioral, health, and academic outcomes: A review of the literature. *The Journal of School Health, 86*(5), 363–381. https://doi.org/10.1111/josh.12388

Wickwire, E. M., Schnyer, D. M., Germain, A., Williams, S. G., Lettieri, C. J., McKeon, A. B., Scharf, S. M., Stocker, R., Albrecht, J., Badjatia, N., Markowitz, A. J., Manley, G. T. (2018). Sleep, sleep disorders, and circadian health following mild traumatic brain injury in adults: Review and research agenda. *Journal of Neurotrauma, 35*(22), 2615–2631. https://doi.org/10.1089/neu.2017.5243

Widome, R., Berger, A. T., Iber, C., Wahlstrom, K., Laska, M. N., Kilian, G., Redline, S., & Erickson, D. J. (2020). Association of delaying school start time with sleep duration, timing, and quality among adolescents. *JAMA Pediatrics, 174*(7), 697–704. https://doi.org/10.1001/jamapediatrics.2020.0344

Winsler, A., Deutsch, A., Vorona, R. D., Payne, P. A., & Szklo-Coxe, M. (2015). Sleepless in Fairfax: The difference one more hour of sleep can make for teen hopelessness, suicidal ideation, and substance use. *Journal of Youth and Adolescence, 44*(2), 362–378. https://doi.org/10.1007/s10964-014-0170-3

Yu, P. K., Radcliffe, J., Taylor, H. G., Amin, R. S., Baldassari, C. M., Boswick, T., Chervin, R. D., Elden, L. M., Furth, S. L., Garetz, S. L., George, A., Ishman, S. L., Kirkham, E. M., Liu, C., Mitchell, R. B., Kamal Naqvi, S., Rosen, C. L., Ross, K. R., Shah, J. R., . . . Redline, S. (2022). Neurobehavioral morbidity of pediatric mild sleep-disordered breathing and obstructive sleep apnea. *Sleep, 45*(5), zsac035. https://doi.org/10.1093/sleep/zsac035

CHAPTER 20

ELIMINATION DISORDERS IN CHILDREN AND ADOLESCENTS

Dawn Dore-Stites and Barbara T. Felt

The goal of toilet training is relatively simple: placement of urine and feces in a socially appropriate place (e.g., toilet). Most children attain continence within relatively restricted age ranges, with 80% to 90% of children across cultures successfully toilet trained within the first few years of life (Fischel & Wallis, 2014).

Delays in attaining continence are diagnosed as a disorder after the age of 4 to 5 years old. Elimination disorders are common, affecting more than 5% of children (Mohammadi et al., 2021). Conceptualization of elimination disorders has evolved from "arcane, speculative and nonproductive perspectives" to developmental science models that inform current evidence-based assessment and treatments (Christophersen & Friman, 2010). The current biopsychosocial model views the development of continence for urine and stool as shaped by anatomical, physiological, developmental, cognitive, behavioral, family, and cultural factors.

Factors impeding progression towards continence mirror barriers to acquisition of skills in many other areas, including academic progress, self-care activities, and gross motor abilities. In contrast to many of those skills, the importance of attaining continence at an "appropriate" age has been described as "among the most basic and universal targets of socialization everywhere" (Fischel & Wallis, 2014). This underlies the urgency and intensity that families and children may feel when they do not successfully toilet train within the toddler/preschool years.

Given the multiple factors that can delay continence, as well as the impact of an individual child's development on the toilet training course, elimination disorders provide a rich area for collaboration among developmental-behavioral pediatricians, developmental scientists, and pediatric psychologists. Clinically, pediatric psychologists and developmental-behavioral pediatricians often work together in interdisciplinary settings serving children with elimination disorders. An interdisciplinary approach to disorders of incontinence reflects the biopsychosocial model underlying the etiology of elimination disorders by considering the influence of medical, behavioral, and social factors on the presentation and course of treatment. Elimination disorders do not remit spontaneously and can persist into adolescence and adulthood, highlighting the need for effective management informed by multiple perspectives.

In research, the developmental science underlying theoretical models for these disorders continues to emerge. Given the importance across cultures of attaining continence, the lack of large-scale treatment studies is striking and provides opportunities for collaboration with experts in

https://doi.org/10.1037/0000414-020
APA Handbook of Pediatric Psychology, Developmental-Behavioral Pediatrics, and Developmental Science: Vol. 2. Pediatric Psychology and Developmental-Behavioral Pediatrics: Clinical Applications of Developmental Science, P. E. Shah and M. H. Bornstein (Editors-in-Chief)
Copyright © 2025 by the American Psychological Association. All rights reserved.

developmental science, clinical/pediatric psychology, and developmental-behavioral pediatrics.

The primary goal of this chapter is to illuminate the significant impact elimination disorders have on children and families and to provide the groundwork for management and for understanding both clinical and research areas in need of further data. The chapter begins with an overview of the normal course of toilet training. It then provides definitions of disorders of incontinence, followed by the epidemiology, risk/protective factors, and outcomes. An approach to comprehensive evaluation and management is outlined along with recommendations for future research. This chapter reviews what is known and what is under exploration related to the multiple factors influencing disorders of incontinence. As this area lacks large-scale treatment studies, we also rely on expert opinion and clinical experience of the authors.

DEVELOPMENT OF CONTINENCE: TOILET TRAINING

Toilet training includes several behaviors that evolve over time leading to independently initiated voids in the toilet for urine and stool. The strategies described below are more common in Western cultures and constitute the foci of this chapter; however, other strategies (e.g., assisted infant toilet training) are used in other countries, with increasing (although still low) adoption in Western cultures (see Bender et al., 2021).

Toilet training is best initiated when a child demonstrates signs of physiological/anatomical maturity and basic behavioral skills (e.g., can follow parental requests) in the absence of medical comorbidities such as constipation or urinary tract infections (UTIs). As parents/caregivers are usually the primary coaches in this process, stability in the home environment (e.g., consistent routines) is also necessary. These four areas—maturity of bladder/bowel, age-appropriate behavior regulation, absence of medical comorbidities, and stable environment—can be viewed as individually necessary but likely insufficient in a vacuum. The need for all factors to coalesce likely results from the complexity of the behavioral skills needed, ranging from recognition of subtle somatic cues to executive functioning skills (e.g., shifting attention from preferred activities to body signals and getting to the bathroom).

Anatomically and physiologically, typically developing children with no underlying medical conditions generally attain maturity of the lower urinary tract between the ages of 2.5 to 4 years old (Bakker et al., 2002). There has been a trend toward older age initiation of toilet training over the past century (Kaerts et al., 2014; Schum et al., 2001). This implies that, although physiological/anatomical maturity is necessary for development of continence, it is not the exclusive factor contributing to toilet training.

Initiating Toilet Training: Identifying Signs of Readiness

Kaerts et al. (2012) reviewed the literature on toilet training readiness signs in typically developing children and identified 21 different sequential signals. Selected signs are listed in Table 20.1 (Kaerts et al., 2012; Schum et al., 2002). Significant variability in age of attaining some signs of readiness (up to 1 to 2 years difference between children) makes it difficult to determine a right age to begin toilet training. However, as the sequence of behaviors observed in the literature was more consistent from child to child, this may

TABLE 20.1

Sample of Toilet Training Readiness Signs

Physiological signs	Behavioral signs	Motor development
Bowel movements only passed during wake times	Imitates others' behaviors	Child can sit without assistance
Bowel movements are regular and predictable	Shows interest in using potty	Child can take on/off clothing
Stays dry for 2 hours/ dry after naps	Follows simple instructions	
	Reports when wet/soiled and requests clean diaper	

provide guidance on initiating toilet training for individual children.

Toilet Training Methods

There are several different methods of toilet training with most sharing common elements. Strategies discuss initiating training when cues suggest that the child is ready, emphasizing parent education about readiness signs and normalizing that it is often a lengthy (several-month) process with accidents commonly observed. Studies suggest an association between less positive strategies (e.g., prompts to strain; punishment for accidents) and negative outcomes, including bladder dysfunction (Bakker et al., 2002) or hiding soiled clothing (Christophersen & Friman, 2010). As a result, positive praise for cooperation with using the toilet and avoiding punishment or shame around accidents are common elements of several successful methods.

The intensity of the intervention varies more widely from method to method. As an example, the parent-directed approach outlined by Azrin and Foxx (1989) uses intensive training over the course of 2 to 3 days. Child-directed methods, such as those outlined by T Berry Brazelton or Benjamin Spock, focus on gradual instruction spread out over time. Data suggest that continence is attained more quickly when using a more intensive method although longer term outcomes are less known. More intensive strategies are less frequently recommended by pediatricians than child-directed approaches (Choby & George, 2008). Data on acceptability of approaches are limited, leading to limited understanding of factors contributing to medical recommendations around toilet training.

Course of Toilet Training

Data are limited, but toilet training is often initiated between 18 and 36 months (Kaerts et al., 2014; Yang et al., 2011). Earlier initiation is often seen in girls (Kaerts et al., 2014; Yang et al., 2011), non-White (Schum et al., 2001), and in children of mothers with lower education levels (Kaerts et al., 2014).

Age at completion. Reporting the age at completion of toilet training is complicated by varying definitions of continence. Using parent report, Schum et al. (2001) found that 50% of their sample were classified as completed with toilet training at 35 months (girls) and 39 months (boys). Completion was determined by caregivers and did not specify whether it was for urine, feces, or both. However, in other analyses, they found that 67% of parents described completed as continent for both urine and feces, both day and night. In these data, factors associated with completion of toilet training included older age at initiation, non-White race, female sex, and single-parent household. They did not find that maternal employment or use of day care were associated with attainment of continence. There were differences between African American and White parents' rating of the importance of a child being toilet trained by age 2, with African American parents placing higher importance (50% vs. 4%).

There are limited data regarding the optimal age of initiating toilet training. Some studies suggest that earlier age of initiation of toilet training is associated with earlier attainment of continence for urine (Yang et al., 2011). Others found that intensive training (direction to sit more than three times a day) at a younger age (<27 months) led to training lasting longer (Blum et al., 2003).

Complications considered normative over the course of toilet training include stool toileting refusal (voiding stools exclusively in a diaper) or withholding behaviors. The frequency of the behaviors (e.g., occurring on one to two occasions versus over the course of weeks) and consequences (e.g., stool back-ups, stress in family) should be considered when determining whether and how to intervene. Parents should be educated on normal complications to ensure that they continue to implement training in a calm and consistent manner. In addition, as constipation can be associated with higher frequency of complications in toilet training (Blum et al., 2004), education around signs of constipation should be discussed.

Definitions of continence vary widely, leading to limitations in identifying conclusions; however, two trends have been observed. First, taking parent/family and child readiness into account is critical. This lessens the probability that demands are placed on a child before they are ready. This likely leads to fewer opportunities for negative interactions around toilet training. Second, positive strategies are not likely to cause long-term medical or behavioral complications, especially in the context of realistic parental expectations regarding the toilet training process.

DEFINITIONS OF DISORDERS OF INCONTINENCE

Historically, psychological and medical criteria for disorders of incontinence developed independently, leading to differences in terms and definitions today. In the *Diagnostic and Statistical Manual of Mental Disorders* (*DSM*; American Psychiatric Association, 2013), the term "elimination disorders" leads the section on enuresis and encopresis. Regarding medical criteria, there are individual diagnostic systems for urinary (Austin et al., 2016) and fecal incontinence/constipation (Hyams et al., 2016). The definitions for enuresis and urine incontinence are compared in Table 20.2, and the definitions for encopresis and fecal incontinence/constipation in Table 20.3. In this chapter, we use the medical terms (i.e., urinary or fecal incontinence, enuresis for bedwetting) to foster clarity in recommendations related to clinical care and future research in these areas.

Urinary Incontinence

In the *DSM*, enuresis describes daytime urine incontinence and bedwetting. Criticisms exist about a single term capturing both conditions (von Gontard, 2013). The International Children's Continence Society defines urinary incontinence as any "uncontrollable leakage of urine" (Austin et al., 2016); however, it differentiates between daytime incontinence and enuresis (night-time incontinence; see Table 20.2). Urine incontinence exclusively at night is considered monosymptomatic. Urine incontinence day and night would be labeled as non-monosymptomatic. Urine

TABLE 20.2

Definitions of Urinary Incontinence

	Diagnostic and Statistical Manual of Mental Disorders (5th ed.)	International Children's Continence Society	
	Enuresis	**Daytime incontinence**	**Enuresis**
Description	Involuntary or intentional voiding into clothes or bed repeatedly	Intermittent urine incontinence daytime	Intermittent urine incontinence at night
Frequency	≥2×/week	>1×/month	>1×/month
Duration	≥3 consecutive months	≥3×/3 months	≥3×/3 months
Age	≥5 years (or equivalent developmental age)	>5 years	≥5 years
Other	Incontinence not exclusive to: • medications • medical condition	Comorbidity: • Medical conditions • Behavioral issues	Comorbidity: • Medical conditions • Behavioral issues
Types	Diurnal: day only Nocturnal: night only Nocturnal and diurnal	Several examples include: overactive or underactive bladder, voiding postponement, dysfunctional voiding, stress incontinence	Monosymptomatic: No lower urinary tract (LUT) symptoms* Non-monosymptomatic: LUT symptoms* present

Note. Data from the American Psychiatric Association (2013) and Austin et al. (2016). *LUT symptoms: Daytime urine incontinence, urgency, weak stream, abnormal frequency of voiding during day (high or low).

TABLE 20.3

Definitions of Fecal Incontinence

	Diagnostic and Statistical Manual of Mental Disorders (5th ed.)*	**Functional gastrointestinal disorders****	
Description	Encopresis: repeated passage and inappropriate placement of feces	Fecal incontinence: involuntary passage of feces in inappropriate places after toilet training	
Frequency	1×/month	≥1×/week	
Duration	≥3 months	≥1 month	
Age	≥4 years (or equivalent developmental age)	≥4 years	
Types	With constipation and overflow incontinence	Retentive; associated with constipation and withholding	Nonretentive: no symptoms of constipation or withholding
	Without constipation and overflow incontinence		
Other	Involuntary or intentional; not due to medications or a medical condition (except constipation)	Functional constipation at ≥4 years of age±	Congenital anorectal malformations

Note. Data from *American Psychiatric Association (2013), **Hyams et al. (2016), and Tabbers et al. (2014). ±Functional constipation is defined as presenting with two or more of the following conditions at least 1× per week for at least 1 month: ≤ 2 stools in the toilet/week; ≥ 1 fecal incontinence/week; history of stool retention; history of painful or hard stools; history of large caliber stools that can obstruct toilet.

incontinence is considered primary if there is no preceding period of dryness that is greater than 6 months. A child experiencing urine incontinence after being dry for more than 6 months has secondary urine incontinence. Diagnosis of secondary urine incontinence suggests that an evaluation for other problems (e.g., constipation, obstructive sleep apnea) is needed. Daytime urine incontinence is typically intermittent, but if it is continuous, referral for urology evaluation is recommended.

Fecal Incontinence

The criteria for fecal incontinence based on *DSM* and medical guidelines are compared in Table 20.3. In both guidelines, stool passage into inappropriate places after 4 years of age defines a problem. The *DSM* uses the term "encopresis," whereas medical sources use "fecal incontinence." The definitions differ in terms of problem duration and frequency. Both systems acknowledge the role of constipation (see Table 20.3). Neither system includes elements to assess toileting refusal behaviors (e.g., escaping toileting times) apart from retentive/withholding behaviors.

Urine or fecal incontinence rarely occurs volitionally apart from underlying developmental and/or mental health concerns. Data guiding etiology (Joinson et al., 2019b) and intervention are limited (Stark, 2000); however, more thorough assessment of psychiatric and behavioral factors is generally supported.

EPIDEMIOLOGY OF DISORDERS OF INCONTINENCE

Disorders of incontinence include both lack of control of either the bladder or bowel. The percentage of children affected by daytime urine incontinence ranges from 0.5% to 2% (Christophersen & Friman, 2010) to 17% (Deshpande et al., 2012). Girls have higher rates of daytime incontinence than boys (Christophersen & Friman, 2010). Variability in prevalence rates often results from differing definitions of urinary incontinence or varying age groups. As all disorders of incontinence decrease with age, it is difficult to compare one study assessing a wide range of ages with smaller studies and/or younger age ranges. In the absence of medical comorbidities (e.g., constipation), daytime urine incontinence is rare after the age of 9 (American Psychiatric Association, 2013).

Enuresis (bedwetting) is more common than daytime urinary incontinence and is more frequent in boys (Christophersen & Friman, 2010).

Estimates of enuresis range from 5% to 10% of 5- to 6-year-olds (American Psychiatric Association, 2013) or 7-year-olds (Nevéus et al., 2020) By age 15, 1% to 3% of pediatric patients experience enuresis (American Psychiatric Association, 2013; Nevéus et al., 2020). Resolution of enuresis can occur in the absence of intervention with spontaneous remission rates of 15% per year (Christophersen & Friman, 2010) or lower rates if enuresis is more frequent (Nevéus et al., 2020). By adulthood, 0.5% to 1% still wet the bed (Nevéus et al., 2020).

Fecal incontinence affects 1% to 3% of children aged 5 years or older (American Psychiatric Association, 2013; Kuhn et al., 1999). Recent meta-analyses report no difference in prevalence by sex (Koppen et al., 2018). The majority (80–95%) of children who have fecal incontinence have concurrent constipation (Christophersen & Friman, 2010; Kuhn et al., 1999), a common condition affecting 9.5% of individuals aged 0 to 18 years worldwide (Koppen et al., 2018). Fecal incontinence in adulthood affects about 8% (Ditah et al., 2014); however, the underlying factors are more complicated (e.g., side effects of medications, chronic illness) than for most cases of childhood constipation. About 25% of individuals with constipation onset in childhood continue to have constipation symptoms as adults (Vriesman et al., 2020); however, rates of fecal incontinence for this specific group are not known.

THEORETICAL MODELS OF ELIMINATION DISORDERS

Historically, models discussing the etiology of elimination disorders have included medical and behavioral factors although the individual contribution of each has varied over time. The first recorded description of elimination disorders occurred in 1550 B.C. with dietary changes (a concoction of juniper berries, cypress and beer) as the primary recommendation (Riddle, 1989). Medications (e.g., chloral hydrate, strychnine, belladonna) and behavioral strategies (e.g., restriction of fluids, bedtime alarms) have been used to reduce incontinence since the 19th century.

This implies acknowledgment of both biological and behavioral factors contributing to incontinence even hundreds of years ago.

There have also been explanations of incontinence that have dismissed biological contributors, leading to potentially higher emotional reactivity around these disorders. A Freudian approach, that incontinence relates to psychopathology, does not promote targeting modifiable behavioral factors to decrease incontinence (Christophersen & Friman, 2010).

Currently, most evidence-based providers at the front line of managing elimination disorders adhere to a biopsychosocial model explaining the etiology and maintenance of incontinence. This model stems from maturation of both the medical and behavioral fields as well as increased focus on evidence-based interventions and interdisciplinary care. It also leads to viewing the attainment of continence as an acquisition of skills, with protective and risk factors similar to those influencing learning in other areas of childhood.

RISK AND COMORBIDITIES IN DISORDERS OF INCONTINENCE

Elevated risks for incontinence may be related to developmental/behavioral, ecological/psychosocial, and medical factors. Overall, these factors play multiple and changing roles in the development and maintenance of disorders of incontinence. For instance, a history of diaper rashes may predict a greater likelihood of early stool withholding behaviors. Such withholding may result in constipation that is associated with increased risk for both urine and fecal incontinence. Similarly, UTIs may be a risk factor that predicts more urine withholding but may also be a consequence of incomplete bladder emptying due to rushing through toilet sits. Having a neurodevelopmental disorder (such as autism spectrum disorder) may also predict greater risks for problems with toilet training leading to development of incontinence (Peeters et al., 2013). This section will review common factors related to child and family context; however, references provide more complete reviews.

Developmental/Behavioral Factors

Bowel and bladder dysfunction is more common in individuals with neurodevelopmental disorders, particularly those with moderate to severe intellectual disabilities (Saral & Ulke-Kurkcuoglu, 2020). Considering how their skills align with proposed sequences in typically developing children (see Kaerts et al., 2012) can be helpful in promoting toilet training when children with neurodevelopmental disorders show signs of readiness.

Mental health factors may increase the risk of a bladder and/or bowel problem developing and/or influence the time to successful management. Some research suggests no or small differences in rates of behavioral health diagnoses in children with incontinence whereas other research suggests elevated rates of specific disorders (Christophersen & VanScoyoc, 2013). Two diagnoses, autism spectrum disorder (ASD) and attention-deficit/hyperactivity disorder (ADHD), warrant specific discussion in this population.

Children with ASD have higher rates of all elimination disorders although reported prevalence ranges vary widely (von Gontard et al., 2022) and there may be several risk factors. Children with ASD have higher constipation rates, which raise risk for urine and fecal incontinence (Peeters et al., 2013; von Gontard et al., 2022). Medication for behavioral management may cause risks, especially for urinary incontinence (von Gontard et al., 2022). Impairments in sensory processing may influence the interpretation of or attention to urge sensations (Peeters et al., 2013). Finally, behavioral challenges including rigidity and limited responses to common behavioral methods (e.g., positive reinforcement), may make treatment planning and child/family adherence to the treatment plan more difficult (Peeters et al., 2013).

In children with ADHD, the enuresis rate is approximately 30%. Some studies suggest higher rates of fecal incontinence as well (McKeown et al., 2013); however, less is known about the association with other incontinence disorders overall (von Gontard et al., 2022). Children with ADHD may be as inattentive to bodily signals (e.g., sensation of full bladder) as they are to external ones and/or impulsively leave the toilet before completely emptying.

Ecological/Psychosocial Factors

Despite caregivers' critical roles in toilet training, data on risk or protective factors are limited. Available data suggest that maternal postpartum depression (Joinson et al., 2019a) is correlated with persistent urinary incontinence in offspring. Single parenthood has been associated with improved outcomes in toilet training relative to dual-parent households (Schum et al., 2001). Authors posit that better outcomes in single parent households may be related to financial factors (ridding diapers more quickly) or increased consistency in implementation of toilet training strategies (one parent conducting treatment).

Urine or stool accidents may result from sexual abuse (Mellon et al., 2006), especially if the onset of incontinence appears sudden. Much of the research in this area uses small and psychiatrically complex samples. Using a larger sample including both clinical and nonclinical populations, Mellon et al. assessed the clinical utility of fecal incontinence as a specific predictor of sexual abuse. Findings suggested that occasional fecal incontinence was not useful in solely identifying sexual abuse, especially relative to sexualized behavior. The authors noted that "suspicion of abuse should have no more relevance in the assessment of soiling symptoms than it does for a child referred for most other behavior problems" (Mellon et al., 2006, p. 31).

Data on higher frequency stressors (e.g., transition to school, divorce of parents) are limited. Clinical experiences support that many families report some stressors during the toilet training period (e.g., birth of sibling, job loss, moves) that may amplify preexisting problems (e.g., constipation) or disrupt the implementation of toilet training strategies.

Medical Conditions

Common medical risk factors for urine and fecal incontinence are reviewed in Table 20.4. In general, it is important to recognize that the longer stool

TABLE 20.4

Medical Risk Factors for Urine and Fecal Incontinence and Underlying Constipation

Factor	Description	Reference
Urinary tract infection	Painful urine passage (dysuria), urgency and foul-smelling urine	Austin et al., 2016
Other bladder conditions	Underactive/overactive bladder	Bauer, 2002
	Dyssynergy of bladder contraction and relaxation; holding behaviors	Austin et al., 2016
Discomfort leading to withholding	Painful stool passage early in life	Partin et al., 1992
	Hard stools as a toddler	Heron et al., 2018
	Diaper rash*	
Medical conditions with increased risk for constipation	Anorectal abnormalities (e.g., anteriorly displaced anus)	Vriesman et al., 2020
	Cerebral palsy—constipation affects 60%–70%	Veugelers et al., 2010
	Others: dehydration, eating disorders, Hirschsprung disease, hypothyroidism, immobilization due to surgery, low muscle tone (e.g., trisomy 21), medications (e.g., opiates), pelvic floor dyssynergy	
Medical conditions with increased risk of incontinence	Tethered cord	Bauer, 2002
	Neural tube defects (e.g., spina bifida)	Smith et al., 2016
Genetics	Family bowel patterns suggest predispositions for constipation	Vriesman et al., 2020

Note. *Denotes clinical observation by authors.

is held in the colon, the firmer it becomes as water is absorbed. Constipation can underlie both urine and fecal incontinence and is crucial to identify and address early in treatment. In addition, interrelations between the lower urinary tract and gastrointestinal systems have been proposed and termed bladder-bowel disfunction (Austin et al., 2016; Burgers et al., 2013; see also Table 20.3). In simple terms, a rectum full of stool may impinge on the bladder and increase risks for urine incontinence through incomplete bladder emptying and bladder muscle overactivity. Chronic contraction of the anal sphincter muscle and a large burden of stool in the rectum may influence and contribute to dyssynergy between bladder muscle contraction and urinary sphincter muscle relaxation (Burgers et al., 2013).

In clinical care, underlying constipation affects from 30% to nearly 90% of children with urine incontinence and 80% of children with fecal incontinence (Mugie et al., 2011; O'Regan & Yazbeck, 1985). Effective management of constipation relieves urine and fecal incontinence and the risks for UTIs for a majority of children (O'Regan et al., 1986; Partin et al., 1992; Sureshkumar et al., 2000).

IMPACT AND OUTCOMES RELATED TO DISORDERS OF INCONTINENCE

Potential consequences of absent or suboptimal management of an incontinence disorder are hypothetically numerous; however, determining a temporal association between the incontinence and impact is limited by the available data.

Psychological/Behavioral Impact

Incontinence has been associated with behavioral and mental health concerns (von Gontard et al., 2011), but relationship or directionality are not conclusive (Christophersen & VanScoyoc, 2013). It does appear that many maladaptive behaviors including fecal retention (withholding) are shaped over time as the child avoids stooling due to history of discomfort due to defecation (Christophersen & Friman, 2010).

Behavioral health symptoms. Several studies support elevated frequency of behavioral health symptoms in children with incontinence (Cox et al., 2002; Shepard et al., 2017); however, they are not always at clinically significant levels (Cox et al., 2002). In a large epidemiological study (Joinson et al., 2006), rates of psychological problems were compared in 7- to 8-year-old children who soil frequently (once per week or more; 1.4%) to those who occasionally soiled (less than once per week; 5.4%) and those with no soiling (controls). Overall, children with any soiling had more emotional and behavioral problems than children without. Children with frequent soiling met diagnostic criteria for ADHD, oppositional defiant disorder, and anxiety, although still at relatively small percentages (1.7% to 11.9%, depending on disorder). The rate of psychological problems associated with urine incontinence was also assessed in this cohort for 7- to 9-year-old children. Comparing these children with those without daytime wetting, the following concerns were observed at statistically significant ($p < .001$) elevations: separation anxiety (11.4% vs 6.8%), attention deficit (24.8% vs 11.8%), oppositional behavior (10.9% vs 5.8%), and conduct problems (11.8% vs 6.2%; Joinson et al., 2006).

Most data come from parent-reports, but children also express frustrations over continued incontinence. One study reported that more than 30% of children with enuresis rated bedwetting as "really difficult," ranked eighth among stressful life events (Butler & Heron, 2008).

Limited data exist on potentially mediating factors (e.g., peer teasing) on the presentation of behavioral health symptoms as well as the directionality of the interaction. Limited data have demonstrated that problems at toddler age (e.g., difficult temperament) predicted later problems with constipation (Joinson et al., 2019b).

Negative social interactions. Using child reports in a large epidemiological sample, Joinson et al. (2006) described increased rates of bullying among children with soiling (both as the victim and as the perpetrator). Teasing and rejection are also correlated with fecal soiling (Shepard et al., 2017). There are limited numbers of prospective studies identifying relationships between parent factors and incontinence risk.

Health-related quality of life. A multicenter study looked at constipation with or without fecal incontinence and effects on quality of life (QoL) and family functioning (Kovacic et al., 2015). Children with incontinence in addition to constipation reported lower QoL, and family functioning was reported as worse than that of children with constipation alone. Children with fecal incontinence in addition to constipation had lower QoL on the PedsQL Total Score. Comparing older to younger children, older children with incontinence had worse QoL, family functioning, parental stress and poorer psychosocial functioning. The between-age-subgroup analysis did not find significant interactions for incontinence frequency or severity and family impact ($p = 0.064$; Kovacic et al., 2015).

Caregiver/family stress. Stress around toileting is clinically evident; however, systematic data are limited, and measures and definitions of stress vary. In toilet training, pressure to train at earlier ages was not a predictor of bladder dysfunction (abnormal urine flow pattern or elevated post-void residual; Yang et al., 2011). However, Bakker et al. (2002) found later initiation of toilet training accompanied by punishment or directives to strain increased risk of later problems with urine continence.

Once the delayed acquisition of toilet training has led to diagnosis of an elimination disorder, management is similar to other chronic conditions (e.g., asthma or diabetes). Managing chronic conditions, whether medical (Cousino & Hazen, 2013) or behavioral (Victor et al., 2007), results in stress for the family. Specific to elimination disorders, parents of children with urinary incontinence (Roccella et al., 2019) and fecal incontinence (Shepard et al., 2017) report increased stress related to managing the medical, behavioral, and social aspects of the disorders. Shepard et al. discussed that stress is amplified especially if there is dishonesty around fecal accidents and the demands of cleaning up soils. Other factors that can increase stress (e.g., conflict with schools on managing incontinence, financial costs related to incontinence supplies) are numerous but understudied. The burdens are often hidden; for instance, emergency room visits and over-the-counter medication use are increased for families managing constipation (Liem et al., 2009; Sommers et al., 2015), leading to potential for increased financial burden and/or loss of work days.

Medical Impact

The duration and severity of bladder dysfunction can increase the risk of a thickened bladder wall, which can further worsen bladder function and require more and longer medical treatments. The duration and severity of constipation may increase risk for physiological changes such as "capacious" or "tortuous" colon. These terms describe a stretched and dysfunctional colon musculature that will require more medical intervention to move stool effectively. It is important to have a strong suspicion of underlying bladder or bowel pathology if concerns have been chronic and to refer for subspecialty medical evaluation as early as possible.

ASSESSMENT OF DISORDERS OF INCONTINENCE

A team approach involving a pediatric psychologist and developmental-behavioral pediatrician aligns well with the biopsychosocial model of elimination problems. This team approach fosters patient and family understanding that it is equally important to address behavioral/psychosocial and medical factors in order to attain effective treatment. Depending on the initial presentation and course over time, one team member may take the lead early in treatment; subsequently, the balance of care between providers may shift in a flexible manner.

There are a number of ways in which the initial interview can set the stage for effective engagement with the family, and assessment/treatment of the disorders, including:

- Starting the interview by asking about the primary concerns of the family/child establishes collaboration as the norm.
- Providing education about disorders of incontinence often starts as early as the initial clinical interview and can facilitate patient and family communication and understanding.
- Normalizing stress and dysfunction related to disorders of incontinence can allow the family to share variables (e.g., yelling on occasion) that they may not typically discuss.
- Asking details about school and preferred interests elucidates how incontinence may affect all aspects of family life.

These items would likely be included in any clinical interview; however, here are additional issues that are unique to assessment of disorders of incontinence, as described in the following subsections.

History of Continence/Incontinence

A thorough assessment of medical/behavioral and psychosocial factors (see Table 20.5) helps providers (ideally a medical and separate behavioral provider) understand the scope of the problem, including the consequences for patient and family QoL and medical needs.

Current status of continence and incontinence. Understanding the current patterns of disorders of incontinence is critical for informing relevant interventions. Table 20.6 presents the key parts of assessing current status of incontinence. It can be helpful to give the family a time frame (e.g., the preceding month) on which to base the answers to lessen the probability of recency bias. In addition, asking these questions at every visit helps to promote family recognition of symptoms and track subjective outcomes.

Elimination log. A log of the location, frequency, volume, and character of urine and stool outputs for two weeks prior to the clinical assessment provides helpful information to differentially diagnosis disorders of incontinence as well as for initial treatment planning. Regular urine output volumes and stool output consistency and volume provide reassurance that risks for withholding and intermittent stool back-ups are low. The timing and location of outputs (e.g., in vs. outside the toilet) also provide clues regarding child comfort across settings.

Symptom/behavioral screening. Given the elevated rates of behavioral symptoms and

TABLE 20.5
Clinical Interview for Disorders of Incontinence

Question–Domain	Association	
	Urine incontinence* problem	**Fecal incontinence** problem**
Perinatal observations	Urine passed and stream strong	Delay/absence of meconium stool
Discomfort during passage of urine and/or stool before toilet training	Diaper rashes; painful urination; history of UTI; passing large/hard stools; blood in urine; urine withholding	Diaper rashes; passage of large/hard stools; blood and/or mucous on stool; straining during bowel movement; stool withholding

	Urine* or fecal incontinence** problem
Past continence	Continence attained for >6 months
	Regression in continence and any associations (family/life change or stressor, medical problem)
Past treatments	Behavioral interventions (frequent sit times, rewards, punishment)
	Consultation with subspecialists (e.g., urology; gastrointestinal)
	Emergency department or hospitalization for incontinence problem
	Use of oral or rectally administered medications for incontinence problem
Other history	Family history of disorder of incontinence
	Family history of disorders with risk for constipation (e.g., hypothyroidism)
	Family history of disorders affecting behavior (e.g., ADHD)
Patient behavioral variables	Discern if any of the following occur primarily in the context of toileting or with other triggers/settings as well: difficulties with cooperation/adherence, anxiety, selective eating, sensory concern, attention deficits, speech/language difficulties
Patient and family psychosocial variables	Family life events (e.g., birth of sibling, parental divorce)
	Pressure from others (e.g., day care, grandparents)
	Parental conflict due to different perspectives on toileting concerns
	Parental stress (job, separation, divorce)

Note. For a complete review of the medical considerations for evaluation and management of incontinence, see relevant society guidelines. UTI = urinary tract infection; ADHD = attention-deficit/hyperactivity disorder. Data from *Austin et al. (2016) and **Tabbers et al. (2014).

diminished QoL it can be helpful to include normed rating scales to identify risk factors for these problems. Such ratings may also inform why complications have occurred in treatment (Van Herzeele et al., 2015).

Broadband measures of behaviors. The Child Behavior Checklist is frequently recommended (Christophersen & Friman, 2010; Van Herzeele et al., 2015). For older children and adolescents, collecting self-report measures of behavioral symptoms and QoL may capture underreported or unrecognized symptoms by caregivers (Wolfe-Christensen et al., 2016).

Medical evaluation. The physical exam for disorders of incontinence includes assessment for abdominal distention, location and appearance of the urethra and anus, back exam for tuft or dimple and lower spinal cord reflexes (indications of an underlying spinal cord abnormality), and possibly a digital rectal exam to assess for anal sphincter tone and integrity and stool impaction. Other procedures that may inform treatment include abdominal x-rays and urinalysis.

INTERVENTION FOR DISORDERS OF INCONTINENCE

Timely and effective management of incontinence and associated risk factors is important for recovery. For instance, a delay of effective interventions for constipation of more than 3 months from the onset of concerns is associated with a prolonged recovery (Bongers et al., 2010).

Interventions in Elimination Disorders

Across all incontinence conditions, systematic reviews of interventions are complicated by the

TABLE 20.6

Current Patterns of Urine and Fecal Incontinence and Constipation

Domain	Questions
Urine patterns	■ Frequency of urinating in toilet vs. elsewhere ■ Estimate of volume passed in toilet vs. elsewhere ■ Strength of stream
Bowel patterns	■ Frequency of stools passed in toilet vs. elsewhere ■ Size: volume of outputs in toilet vs. elsewhere ■ Consistency of size and stool quality between outputs ■ Stools passed large enough to clog a toilet ■ Stool quality (hard vs. soft): Bristol Scale (Lewis & Heaton, 1997)
Other factors	■ Timing of incontinence: day vs. night ■ Child recognition of incontinence ■ Adherence for medications and behavioral recommendations ■ Factors related to adherence
Toileting patterns	■ Voiding urine/stool only during scheduled sit times ■ Parents monitor toileting behaviors ■ Hiding soiled/wet clothing
Medication regimen	■ Medications used ■ Supplements used
Signs of discomfort	■ Dysuria ■ Straining at stool passage ■ Other complaint of pain in perianal area ■ Complaints of abdominal pain ■ Blood in urine or on stool ■ Decreased appetite ■ Rashes in perianal area
Impact	■ Bullying/teasing ■ Absences from school or day care ■ Time lost at work due to managing toileting of child ■ Family/parent stress

lack of scientifically rigorous research. In addition, varying definitions of incontinence and treatment strategies complicate the ability to compare interventions. Finally, strategies commonly recommended (e.g., components of parent education; sit time frequency) have never been individually researched, leading to difficulties identifying the critical elements to treatment.

This chapter provides a summary of commonly studied incontinence interventions. Specific evidence-based intervention strategies used to direct clinical care for individual patients are beyond the scope of this chapter. For this information, readers are directed to Christophersen and Friman (2010) and Christophersen and VanScoyoc (2013).

Education about the common occurrence of disorders of incontinence and their common underlying developmental, behavioral, and medical factors (Christophersen & Friman, 2010) serves as a foundation for treatment elements. A goal of education is to help the child and family be on the same team and ready to tackle the intervention together.

Medical Interventions Across Conditions

Initial treatment in disorders of incontinence includes assessment of whether constipation is a factor and, if so, whether a clean-out is needed. Current recommendations suggest using high-dose polyethylene glycol and enemas for clean-out (Tabbers et al., 2014). After that, a maintenance regimen is recommended to support regular comfortable passage of soft stool. In addition to stool softeners, recent reports support the use of sennosides to move the stool and avoid back-up of stool (Vilanova-Sanchez et al., 2018).

Dyssynergia of the pelvic floor muscles contributes to urine or stool withholding and pelvic floor physical therapy may be a helpful addition to the treatment plan. Pelvic floor physical therapy helps the child learn about muscle coordination that will facilitate urine and/or stool outputs (Zar-Kessler et al., 2019). Other considerations for urinary incontinence include antibiotic management of co-occurring UTIs and the use of medications to reduce bladder muscle overactivity (e.g., anticholinergic agents). For enuresis, desmopressin or tricyclic antidepressants may be recommended although efficacy rates are lower than those of behavioral treatments. In addition, these medications have potentially significant side effects (e.g., electrolyte abnormalities with desmopressin, cardiac abnormalities with tricyclic antidepressants; Nevéus et al., 2020).

Urinary incontinence. Considering daytime incontinence first, one review (Sureshkumar et al., 2003) assessed results from randomized controlled trials of medications (terodiline; imipramine), daytime urine alarms, and a combined treatment (biofeedback/oxybutynin). No randomized controlled trial demonstrated benefits with an adequate safety profile. Specifically, terodiline demonstrated benefits, but links between the drug and cardiac complications gave it an inadequate safety profile. Other strategies did not demonstrate significant impact on urine incontinence.

Behavioral strategies for daytime incontinence are understudied despite it being a common condition (Christophersen & Friman, 2010). Behavioral targets generally focus on increasing frequency (and possibly duration) of sit times as well as increasing recognition of the sensation of a full bladder.

Sit times can be prompted with parental requests or multiple-alarm watches; however, a urine alarm both targets cues to sit and alerts the child when urine is passing. A urine alarm uses a sensor placed on the underwear that detects small volumes of urine. The urine triggers an auditory and/or vibratory alarm that is designed to prompt the child to use the toilet. The alarm is used more commonly in bedwetting (described further in the following subsection). Modest data suggest that the urine alarm may be beneficial in decreasing episodes of daytime incontinence; however, this should be viewed in the context of all data on elimination disorders: they are limited due to study size and methods (Christophersen & Friman, 2010).

For nighttime urine incontinence (enuresis), the use of the urine alarm (described above), either alone or combined with other elements, is evaluated as an effective treatment for management (Mellon & McGrath, 2000). The urine alarm is 65% to 80% effective with a relapse rate of 15% to 30% over 6 months (Christophersen & Friman, 2010) The urine alarm in conjunction with medication (desmopressin) may lead to elevated rates of effectiveness. Other behavioral strategies (retention control training, Kegel exercises, scheduled wakings) can be used independently; however, there are other strategies (e.g., reward systems, overlearning, cleanliness training) that should be used only adjunctively (Christophersen & Friman, 2010).

Fecal incontinence. Given the high rates of constipation associated with fecal soiling, medical management is a critical first step. Behavioral strategies are often used to reinforce behaviors associated with the medical management (e.g., targeting adherence to medications) as well as to increase cooperation around dietary changes and scheduled sit times.

Reviews of behavioral interventions for fecal incontinence are written from both psychological (Freeman et al., 2014; McGrath et al., 2000) and medical (Tabbers et al., 2014; Vriesman et al., 2020) perspectives. An array of strategies for fecal incontinence has been assessed, including biofeedback, play therapy, parent management training, awareness techniques (e.g., pants checks), skill building, acupuncture, clear fluid intake, increased fiber intake, psychoeducation, response cost/punishment, scheduled toilet sits, and defecation skills training. Behavioral or biofeedback therapy has not been empirically supported as stand-alone treatment (Tabbers et al., 2014) and use of medication alone leads to only 40% of children being cured of fecal incontinence (Freeman et al., 2014). Combined treatment (medication and behavioral strategies) appears to decrease fecal soiling but does not necessarily positively impact other outcomes related to constipation (e.g., number of stools in the toilet), although data available for meta-analysis are limited.

Overall, most evidence-based combined treatments for fecal incontinence use positive reinforcement or other behavioral techniques (McGrath et al., 2000). Package interventions including several treatment components have been studied. Group-based treatment for constipation/fecal incontinence directed by a pediatric psychologist and pediatric gastroenterologist using a standardized protocol including medical and behavioral management strategies demonstrated improvement in dietary factors and incontinence

(Stark et al., 1990, 1997). Borowitz et al. (2002) compared intensive medical treatment alone to medical treatment plus enhance toilet training, and the latter plus external anal biofeedback. The enhanced toilet training approach showed benefits to reduce fecal incontinence. While limited in number, such studies suggest improved management when medical and behavioral strategies are combined.

OUTCOME MEASURES

Assessment of medical and behavioral factors concurrently is important both in identification of treatment targets and outcomes.

Behavioral/Psychological

At the time of assessment, tools to monitor associated mental health symptoms and the impact of care on child and family QoL can be helpful in guiding interventions (Bower et al., 2006; Silverman et al., 2015). In clinical care, the target outcome measures are often individualized to the child/family but monitoring impacts treatment progress. Factors may include QoL (Bower et al., 2006; Silverman et al., 2015), adherence (Quittner et al., 2008), or functional morbidity (e.g., missed days of school/work).

Medical

A goal of incontinence treatment is to increase the child's comfort in eliminating urine or stool in the appropriate place. The guidance of the International Children's Continence Society for daytime incontinence suggests documenting symptom frequency at baseline and after treatment (Austin et al., 2016). As the child's comfort improves, withholding behaviors are reduced and more complete emptying for urine or stool occurs. On a urine and/or stool log, early in treatment, withholding may be evidenced by frequent small urine or stool outputs interspersed with larger ones and widely variable stool consistency (hard to liquid). Progress toward effective management can be seen on logs as less frequent outputs and better regularity of volume and character. Logs can also be used when weaning medication support to help ensure that the child is staying on track.

Delivery of Care

No guidance exists regarding the frequency of visits to treat disorders of incontinence. In general, it is helpful to have at least monthly visits with both pediatric psychology and developmental-behavioral pediatrician providers early in treatment. An important benefit of the pediatric psychology/developmental-behavioral pediatrician team approach is the ability to identify if and what interventions are getting off track early enough to avoid significant regression. In our experience, repeated periods of regression discourage families from reengaging in treatment.

Initial behavioral support often focuses on increasing adherence, decreasing maladaptive communication around incontinence problems, and normalizing that recovery takes time and steady progress is our goal. After output comfort and regularity are improved through medication management, behavioral treatment increases in scope. Continued medical support includes check-in visits about quarterly. However, each child's and family's course of care is individual. In our experience, most children in treatment for incontinence do well with the combined behavioral and medical approach but are referred for individual or family therapy if indicated on close follow-up and monitoring.

Other treatment team members. Other team members may include a physical therapist to evaluate muscle strength/integrity and coordination and provide pelvic floor muscle training/retaining if needed. Common physical therapy strategies include biofeedback, prompted contraction/relaxation and home-based activities (e.g., colon massage, scheduled sit times). Many of the techniques align well with behavioral strategies directed by a pediatric psychologist. Nursing calls are made between visits to check on patient and family adherence to behavioral and medical components of treatment and the pattern (frequency, volume, character, and place) of outputs. Social work can define financial sources of support for over-the-counter medications and costs related to incontinence supplies (e.g., diapers; Liem et al., 2009). School personnel can partner with the parent and psychology/medical team to develop a plan for sits, medication taking, and methods to support clean-up and privacy at school through a 504 plan, which provides accommodations for students with a disability or medical need that affects availability for learning.

Treatment Course

As noted previously, symptoms of disorders of incontinence may continue to affect individuals into teen and adult years; however, research studies to date often do not clarify if the course of treatment was complicated by a medical or mental health factor. Thus, it is possible that outcomes could improve if collaborative care were implemented with psychology and medical providers throughout the course of care (Van Herzeele et al., 2015).

DIRECTIONS IN RESEARCH

Throughout much of the chapter, limitations in available research were outlined in all areas of elimination disorders. There are opportunities for pediatric psychologists, developmental-behavioral pediatricians, and developmental scientists to work collaboratively to advance the field. Questions to be addressed are numerous, with the following areas in most critical need from a clinical perspective:

- directionality between early child and parent factors and influence on development of disorders of elimination;
- directionality between elimination disorders and mental health factors;
- variance by diagnosis (urine or bowel primarily vs. bladder-bowel dysfunction);
- effect of psychosocial-ecological resources available to promote optimal interventions depending on child age and child diagnoses;
- influence of regressions during treatment and effect on outcomes;
- long-term outcomes for incontinence and whether specific factors (e.g., age, genetic predisposition, adherence to treatment) mediate or moderate these outcomes;
- the influence of the sequence of treatment elements on outcomes; and
- the brain–gut connections relevant to constipation, and as a corollary, urine incontinence.

CONCLUSION

Toilet training is a skill acquired by many children within relatively consistent ages across cultures. It occurs most easily when development across several systems—biological, behavioral, and ecological—align. When this alignment does not occur, failing to attain continence can lead to deleterious outcomes across several domains for the child and their family.

Given this involvement and influence of several systems, elimination disorders provide a rich opportunity for collaboration across developmental science, developmental-behavioral pediatrics, and pediatric psychology. The diverse perspectives of clinicians and researchers can inform care within a biopsychosocial model and drive research agendas to address gaps in the current literature.

RESOURCES

For Children and Families

Books

- Harbison, J., & Sulgit, N. (2020). *We Poop on the Potty*. Little Grasshopper Books.
- *We Poop on the Potty* (Brain Games Sticker Activity Book). (2021). Publications International.
- Bennett, H. J. (2007). *It Hurts When I Poop! A Story for Children Who Are Scared to Use the Potty*. Magination Press.
- Gehringer, L., & Gehringer, N. (2019). *From Chewing to Pooing: Food's Journey Through Your Body to the Potty*.
- DuHamel, T. (2015). *Softy the Poop: Helping Families Talk About Poop*. Maret Publishing.

- Gomi, T. (2020). *Everyone Poops*. Chronical Books.
- Vessillo, T., & Motz, M. (2011). *I Can't, I Won't, No Way! A Book for Children Who Refuse to Poop*. CreateSpace Publishing.
- Hayden, W. (2020). *Dash's Potty Accidents: A Book for Children Who Have Pee or Poop Accidents*.
- Hayden, W. (2019). *Dash's Belly Ache: A Book for Children Who Can't or Won't Poop*.

Apps and Videos

- Daniel Tiger's Stop & Go Potty:

  https://pbskids.org/apps/daniel-tigers-stop--go-potty.html

- Daniel Tiger: Games in My Bathroom:

  https://pbskids.org/daniel/games/in-my-bathroom

- Daniel's Tummy Hurts:

  https://video.aptv.org/video/daniels-tummy-hurts-poz2m6/

- See Me Go Potty [App] by AvaKid Productions:

  https://apps.apple.com/us/app/see-me-go-potty-english/id450495594

For Parents

Books and Fact Sheets

- DuHamel, T. (2012). *Ins and Outs of Poop: A Guide to Treating Childhood Constipation*. Maret Publishing.
- Society of Pediatric Psychology Fact Sheet: Encopresis in Children and Adolescents:

  https://pedpsych.org/fact_sheets/encopresis/

- Cincinnati Children's Hospital, Encopresis in Children:

  https://www.cincinnatichildrens.org/health/e/encopresis

- Boston Children's Hospital, Encopresis:

  https://www.childrenshospital.org/conditions/encopresis

Information on Behavioral Treatments

Society of Clinical Child & Adolescent Psychology, Effective Child Therapy: Elimination Disorders:

  https://effectivechildtherapy.org/concerns-symptoms-disorders/disorders/elimination-disorders/

Video

Colorado Pediatric Gastroenterology: The Poo in You—Constipation & Encopresis Educational Video:

  https://coloradopediatricgastroenterology.com/poo-constipation-encopresis-educational-video/

For Providers

- Borowitz, S. M., Cox, D. J., Sutphen, J. L., & Kovatchev, B. (2002). Treatment of childhood encopresis: A randomized trial comparing three treatment protocols. *Journal of Pediatric Gastroenterology and Nutrition*, 34(4), 378–384.
- Christophersen, E. R., & Friman, P. C. (2010). *Elimination disorders in children and adolescents*. Hogrefe.

References

American Psychiatric Association. (2013). *Diagnostic and statistical manual of mental disorders* (5th ed.). https://doi.org/10.1176/appi.books.9780890425596

Azrin, N., & Foxx, R. (1989). *Toilet training in less than a day: A tested method for teaching your child quickly and happily!* Pocket Books.

Austin, P. F., Bauer, S. B., Bower, W., Chase, J., Franco, I., Hoebeke, P., Rittig, S., Walle, J. V., von Gontard, A., Wright, A., Yang, S. S., & Nevéus, T. (2016). The standardization of terminology of lower urinary tract function in children and adolescents: Update report from the standardization committee of the International Children's Continence Society. *Neurology and Urodynamics*, 35(4), 471–481. https://doi.org/10.1002/nau.22751

Bakker, E., Van Gool, J. D., Van Sprundel, M., Van Der Auwera, C., & Wyndaele, J. J. (2002).

Results of a questionnaire evaluating the effects of different methods of toilet training on achieving bladder control. *BJU International, 90*(4), 456–461. https://doi.org/10.1046/j.1464-410X.2002.02903.x

Bauer, S. (2002). Special considerations of the overactive bladder in children. *Urology, 60,* 43–49.

Bender, J. M., Lee, Y., Ryoo, J. H., Boucke, L., Sun, M., Ball, T. S., Rugolotto, S., & She, R. C. (2021). A longitudinal study of assisted infant toilet training during the first year of life. *Journal of Developmental and Behavioral Pediatrics, 42*(8), 648–655. https://doi.org/10.1097/DBP.0000000000000936

Blum, N. J., Taubman, B., & Nemeth, N. (2003). Relationship between age at initiation of toilet training and duration of training: A prospective study. *Pediatrics, 111*(4), 810–814. https://doi.org/10.1542/peds.111.4.810

Blum, N. J., Taubman, B., & Nemeth, N. (2004). During toilet training, constipation occurs before stool toileting refusal. *Pediatrics, 113*(6), e520–e522. https://doi.org/10.1542/peds.113.6.e520

Bongers, M. E. J., van Wijk, M. P., Reitsma, J. B., & Benninga, M. A. (2010). Long-term prognosis for childhood constipation: Clinical outcomes in adulthood. *Pediatrics, 126*(1), e156–e162. https://doi.org/10.1542/peds.2009-1009

Borowitz, S. M., Cox, D. J., Sutphen, J. L., & Kovatchev, B. (2002). Treatment of childhood encopresis: A randomized trial comparing three treatment protocols. *Journal of Pediatric Gastroenterology and Nutrition, 34*(4), 378–384. https://doi.org/10.1097/00005176-200204000-00012

Bower, W. F., Wong, E. M. C., & Yeung, C. K. (2006). Development of a validated quality of life tool specific to children with bladder dysfunction. *Neurology and Urodynamics, 25*(3), 221–227. https://doi.org/10.1002/nau.20171

Burgers, R. E., Mugie, S. M., Chase, J., Cooper, C. S., von Gontard, A., Rittig, C. S., Homsy, Y., Bauer, S. B., & Benninga, M. A. (2013). Management of functional constipation in children with lower urinary tract symptoms: Report from the Standardization Committee of the International Children's Continence Society. *The Journal of Urology, 190*(1), 29–36. https://doi.org/10.1016/j.juro.2013.01.001

Butler, R., & Heron, J. (2008). An exploration of children's views of bed-wetting at 9 years. *Child: Care, Health, and Development, 34*(1), 65–70. https://doi.org/10.1111/j.1365-2214.2007.00781.x

Choby, B., & George, S. (2008). Toilet training. *American Family Physician, 78*(9), 1059–1064. https://pubmed.ncbi.nlm.nih.gov/19007052/

Christophersen, E. R., & Friman, P. C. (2010). *Elimination disorders in children and adolescents. Vol. 16. Advances in psychotherapy—Evidence-based practice.* Hogrefe.

Christophersen, E. R., & VanScoyoc, S. M. (2013). Diagnosis and management of encopresis. In E. R. Christophersen & S. M. VanScoyoc (Eds.), *Treatments that work with children: Empirically supported strategies for managing childhood problems* (2nd ed., pp. 109–128). American Psychological Association. https://doi.org/10.1037/14137-006

Cousino, M. K., & Hazen, R. A. (2013). Parenting stress among caregivers of children with chronic illness: A systematic review. *Journal of Pediatric Psychology, 38*(8), 809–828. https://doi.org/10.1093/jpepsy/jst049

Cox, D. J., Morris, J. B., Jr., Borowitz, S. M., & Sutphen, J. L. (2002). Psychological differences between children with and without chronic encopresis. *Journal of Pediatric Psychology, 27*(7), 585–591. https://doi.org/10.1093/jpepsy/27.7.585

Deshpande, A. V., Craig, J. C., Smith, G. H. H., & Caldwell, P. H. Y. (2012). Management of daytime urinary incontinence and lower urinary tract symptoms in children. *Journal of Paediatrics and Child Health, 48*(2), E44–E52. https://doi.org/10.1111/j.1440-1754.2011.02216.x

Ditah, I., Devaki, P., Luma, H. N., Ditah, C., Njei, B., Jaiyeoba, C., Salami, A., Ditah, C., Ewelukwa, O., & Szarka, L. (2014). Prevalence, trends, and risk factors for fecal incontinence in United States adults, 2005–2010. *Clinical Gastroenterology and Hepatology, 12*(4), 636–643.e2. https://doi.org/10.1016/j.cgh.2013.07.020

Fischel, J. E., & Wallis, K. E. (2014). Enuresis and encopresis: The elimination disorders. In M. Lewis & K. Rudolph (Eds.), *Handbook of developmental psychopathology* (3rd ed., pp. 631–648). Springer. https://doi.org/10.1007/978-1-4614-9608-3_32

Freeman, K. A., Riley, A., Duke, D. C., & Fu, R. (2014). Systematic review and meta-analysis of behavioral interventions for fecal incontinence with constipation. *Journal of Pediatric Psychology, 39*(8), 887–902. https://doi.org/10.1093/jpepsy/jsu039

Heron, J., Grzeda, M., Tappin, D., von Gontard, A., & Joinson, C. (2018). Early childhood risk factors for constipation and soiling at school age: An observational cohort study. *BMJ Paediatric Open, 2*(1), e000230. https://doi.org/10.1136/bmjpo-2017-000230

Hyams, J. S., Di Lorenzo, C., Saps, M., Shulman, R. J., Staiano, A., & van Tilburg, M. (2016). Childhood functional gastrointestinal disorders: Child/adolescent. *Gastroenterology, 150*(6), 1456–1468.e2. https://doi.org/10.1053/j.gastro.2016.02.015

Joinson, C., Grzeda, M. T., von Gontard, A., & Heron, J. (2019a). A prospective cohort study of biopsychosocial factors associated with childhood urinary incontinence. *European Child & Adolescent Psychiatry, 28*(1), 123–130. https://doi.org/10.1007/s00787-018-1193-1

Joinson, C., Grzeda, M. T., von Gontard, A., & Heron, J. (2019b). Psychosocial risks for constipation and soiling in primary school children. *European Child & Adolescent Psychiatry, 28*(2), 203–210. https://doi.org/10.1007/s00787-018-1162-8

Joinson, C., Heron, J., Butler, U., von Gontard, A., & the Avon Longitudinal Study of Parents and Children Study Team. (2006). Psychological differences between children with and without soiling problems. *Pediatrics, 117*(5), 1575–1584. https://doi.org/10.1542/peds.2005-1773

Kaerts, N., Van Hal, G., Vermandel, A., & Wyndaele, J.-J. (2012). Readiness signs used to define the proper moment to start toilet training: A review of the literature. *Neurology and Urodynamics, 31*(4), 437–440. https://doi.org/10.1002/nau.21211

Kaerts, N., Vermandel, A., Van Hal, G., & Wyndaele, J.-J. (2014). Toilet training in healthy children: Results of a questionnaire study involving parents who make use of day-care at least once a week. *Neurology and Urodynamics, 33*(3), 316–323. https://doi.org/10.1002/nau.22392

Koppen, I. J. N., Vriesman, M. H., Saps, M., Rajindrajith, S., Shi, X., van Etten-Jamaludin, F. S., Di Lorenzo, C., Benninga, M. A., & Tabbers, M. M. (2018). Prevalence of functional defecation disorders in children: A systematic review and meta-analysis. *The Journal of Pediatrics, 198,* 121–130.e6. https://doi.org/10.1016/j.jpeds.2018.02.029

Kovacic, K., Sood, M. R., Mugie, S., Di Lorenzo, C., Nurko, S., Heinz, N., Ponnambalam, A., Beesley, C., Sanghavi, R., & Silverman, A. H. (2015). A multicenter study on childhood constipation and fecal incontinence: Effects on quality of life. *The Journal of Pediatrics, 166*(6), 1482–1487.E1. https://doi.org/10.1016/j.jpeds.2015.03.016

Kuhn, B. R., Marcus, B. A., & Pitner, S. L. (1999). Treatment guidelines for primary nonretentive encopresis and stool toileting refusal. *American Family Physician, 59*(8), 2171–2178, 2184–2186. https://pubmed.ncbi.nlm.nih.gov/10221303/

Lewis, S. J., & Heaton, K. W. (1997). Stool form scale as a useful guide to intestinal transit time. *Scandinavian Journal of Gastroenterology, 32*(9), 920–924. https://doi.org/10.3109/00365529709011203

Liem, O., Harman, J., Benninga, M., Kelleher, K., Mousa, H., & Di Lorenzo, C. (2009). Health utilization and cost impact of childhood constipation in the United States. *The Journal of Pediatrics, 154*(2), 258–262. https://doi.org/10.1016/j.jpeds.2008.07.060

McGrath, M. L., Mellon, M. W., & Murphy, L. (2000). Empirically supported treatments in pediatric psychology: Constipation and encopresis. *Journal of Pediatric Psychology, 25*(4), 225–254. https://doi.org/10.1093/jpepsy/25.4.225

McKeown, C., Hisle-Gorman, E., Eide, M., Gorman, G. H., & Nylund, C. M. (2013). Association of constipation and fecal incontinence with attention-deficit/hyperactivity disorder. *Pediatrics, 132*(5), e1210–e1215. https://doi.org/10.1542/peds.2013-1580

Mellon, M. W., & McGrath, M. L. (2000). Empirically supported treatments in pediatric psychology: Nocturnal enuresis. *Journal of Pediatric Psychology, 25*(4), 193–214. https://doi.org/10.1093/jpepsy/25.4.193

Mellon, M. W., Whiteside, S. P., & Friedrich, W. N. (2006). The relevance of fecal soiling as an indicator of child sexual abuse: A preliminary analysis. *Journal of Developmental and Behavioral Pediatrics, 27*(1), 25–32. https://doi.org/10.1097/00004703-200602000-00004

Mohammadi, M. R., Hojjat, S. K., Ahmadi, N., Alavi, S. S., Hooshyari, Z., Khaleghi, A., Ahmadi, A., Hesari, M. J., Shakiba, A., Amiri, S., Molavi, P., Arman, S., Mohammadzadeh, S., Kousha, M., Golbon, A., Hosseini, S. H., Delpisheh, A., Mojahed, A., ArmaniKian, A., . . . Khalili, M. N. (2021). Prevalence of elimination disorders and comorbid psychiatric disorders in Iranian children and adolescents. *Journal of Pediatric Rehabilitation Medicine, 14*(1), 19–29. https://doi.org/10.3233/PRM-190628

Mugie, S. M., Benninga, M. A., & Di Lorenzo, C. (2011). Epidemiology of constipation in children and adults: A systematic review. *Best Practice & Research Clinical Gastroenterology, 25*(1), 3–18. https://doi.org/10.1016/j.bpg.2010.12.010

Nevéus, T., Fonseca, E., Franco, I., Kawauchi, A., Kovacevic, L., Nieuwhof-Leppink, A., Raes, A., Tekgül, S., Yang, S. S., & Rittig, S. (2020). Management and treatment of nocturnal enuresis—An updated standardization document from the International Children's Continence Society. *Journal of Pediatric Urology, 16*(1), 10–19. https://doi.org/10.1016/j.jpurol.2019.12.020

O'Regan, S., & Yazbeck, S. (1985). Constipation: A cause of enuresis, urinary tract infection and vesico-ureteral reflux in children. *Medical Hypotheses, 17*(4), 409–413. https://doi.org/10.1016/0306-9877(85)90100-8

O'Regan, S., Yazbeck, S., Hamberger, B., & Schick, E. (1986). Constipation a commonly unrecognized cause of enuresis. *American Journal of Diseases of*

Children, 140(3), 260–261. https://doi.org/10.1001/archpedi.1986.02140170086039

Partin, J. C., Hamill, S. K., Fischel, J. E., & Partin, J. S. (1992). Painful defecation and fecal soiling in children. *Pediatrics, 89*(6), 1007–1009. https://doi.org/10.1542/peds.89.6.1007

Peeters, B., Noens, I., Philips, E. M., Kuppens, S., & Benninga, M. A. (2013). Autism spectrum disorders in children with functional defecation disorders. *The Journal of Pediatrics, 163*(3), 873–878. https://doi.org/10.1016/j.jpeds.2013.02.028

Quittner, A. L., Modi, A. C., Lemanek, K. L., Ievers-Landis, C. E., & Rapoff, M. A. (2008). Evidence-based assessment of adherence to medical treatments in pediatric psychology. *Journal of Pediatric Psychology, 33*(9), 916–936. https://doi.org/10.1093/jpepsy/jsm064

Riddle, M. (1989). Elimination disorders. In G. O. Gabbard (Ed.), *Treatments of psychiatric disorders* (Vol. 1, pp. 717–730). American Psychiatric Association.

Roccella, M., Smirni, D., Smirni, P., Precenzano, F., Operto, F. F., Lanzara, V., Quatrosi, G., & Carotenuto, M. (2019). Parental stress and parental ratings of behavioral problems of enuretic children. *Frontiers in Neurology, 10*(October), 1054. https://doi.org/10.3389/fneur.2019.01054

Saral, D., & Ulke-Kurkcuoglu, B. (2020). Toilet training individuals with developmental delays: A comprehensive review. *International Journal of Early Childhood Special Education, 12*(1), 120–137. https://doi.org/10.20489/intjecse.728240

Schum, T. R., Kolb, T. M., McAuliffe, T. L., Simms, M. D., Underhill, R. L., & Lewis, M. (2002). Sequential acquisition of toilet-training skills: A descriptive study of gender and age differences in normal children. *Pediatrics, 109*(3), e48. https://doi.org/10.1542/peds.109.3.e48

Schum, T. R., McAuliffe, T. L., Simms, M. D., Walter, J. A., Lewis, M., & Pupp, R. (2001). Factors associated with toilet training in the 1990s. *Ambulatory Pediatrics, 1*(2), 79–86. https://doi.org/10.1367/1539-4409(2001)001<0079:FAWTTI>2.0.CO;2

Shepard, J. A., Poler, J. E., Jr., & Grabman, J. H. (2017). Evidence-based psychosocial treatments for pediatric elimination disorders. *Journal of Clinical Child and Adolescent Psychology, 46*(6), 767–797. https://doi.org/10.1080/15374416.2016.1247356

Silverman, A. H., Berlin, K. S., Di Lorenzo, C., Nurko, S., Kamody, R. C., Ponnambalam, A., Mugie, S., Gorges, C., Sanghavi, R., & Sood, M. R. (2015). Measuring health-related quality of life with the parental opinions of pediatric constipation questionnaire. *Journal of Pediatric Psychology, 40*(8), 814–824. https://doi.org/10.1093/jpepsy/jsv028

Smith, K., Neville-Jan, A., Freeman, K. A., Adams, E., Mizokawa, S., Dudgeon, B. J., Merkens, M. J., & Walker, W. O. (2016). The effectiveness of bowel and bladder interventions in children with spina bifida. *Developmental Medicine & Child Neurology 58*(9), 979–988. https://doi.org/10.1111/dmcn.13095

Sommers, T., Corban, C., Sengupta, N., Jones, M., Cheng, V., Bollom, A., Nurko, S., Kelley, J., & Lembo, A. (2015). Emergency department burden of constipation in the United States from 2006 to 2011. *The American Journal of Gastroenterology, 110*(4), 572–579. https://doi.org/10.1038/ajg.2015.64

Stark, L. J. (2000). Commentary: Treatment of encopresis: Where do we go from here? *Journal of Pediatric Psychology, 25*(4), 255–256. https://doi.org/10.1093/jpepsy/25.4.255

Stark, L., Opipari, L., Donaldson, D., Donovsky, M., Rasile, D., & DelSanto, A. (1997). Treatment of childhood encopresis: A randomized trial comparing three treatment protocols. *Journal of Pediatric Psychology, 22*(5), 619–633.

Stark, L., Owens-Stively, J., Spirito, A., Lewis, A., & Guevremont, D. (1990). Group behavioral treatment of retentive encopresis. *Journal of Pediatric Psychology, 15*(5), 659–671.

Sureshkumar, P., Bower, W., Craig, J. C., & Knight, J. F. (2003). Treatment of daytime urinary incontinence in children: A systematic review of randomized controlled trials. *The Journal of Urology, 170*(1), 196–200. https://doi.org/10.1097/01.ju.0000072341.34333.43

Sureshkumar, P., Craig, J. C., Roy, L. P., & Knight, J. F. (2000). Daytime urinary incontinence in primary school children: A population-based survey. *The Journal of Pediatrics, 137*(6), 814–818. https://doi.org/10.1067/mpd.2000.109196

Tabbers, M. M., DiLorenzo, C., Berger, M. Y., Faure, C., Langendam, M. W., Nurko, S., Staiano, A., Vandenplas, Y., Benninga, M. A. (2014). Evaluation and treatment of functional constipation in infants and children: Evidence-based recommendations from ESPGHAN and NASPGHAN. *Journal of Pediatric Gastroenterology and Nutrition, 58*(2), 258–274. https://doi.org/10.1097/MPG.0000000000000266

van Dijk, M., de Vries, G. J., Last, B. F., Benninga, M. A., & Grootenhuis, M. A. (2015). Parental child-rearing attitudes are associated with functional constipation in childhood. *Archives of Disease in Childhood, 100*(4), 329–333. https://doi.org/10.1136/archdischild-2014-305941

Van Herzeele, C., De Bruyne, P., De Bruyne, E., & Walle, J. V. (2015). Challenging factors for enuresis treatment: Psychological problems and non-adherence. *Journal of Pediatric Urology, 11*(6), 308–313. https://doi.org/10.1016/j.jpurol.2015.04.035

Veugelers, R., Benninga, M. A., Calis, E. A., Willemsen, S. P., Evenhuis, H., Tibboel, D., & Penning, C. (2010). Prevalence and clinical presentation of constipation in children with severe generalized cerebral palsy. *Developmental Medicine & Child Neurology, 52*(9), e216–221. https://doi.org/10.1111/j.1469-8749.2010.03701.x

Victor, A. M., Bernat, D. H., Bernstein, G. A., & Layne, A. E. (2007). Effects of parent and family characteristics on treatment outcome of anxious children. *Journal of Anxiety Disorders, 21*(6), 835–848. https://doi.org/10.1016/j.janxdis.2006.11.005

Vilanova-Sanchez, A., Gasior, A. C., Toocheck, N., Weaver, L., Wood, R. J., Reck, C. A., Wagner, A., Hoover, E., Gagnon, R., Jaggers, J., Maloof, T., Nash, O., Williams, C., & Levitt, M. A. (2018). Are *Senna* based laxatives safe when used as long term treatment for constipation in children? *Journal of Pediatric Surgery, 53*(4), 722–727. https://doi.org/10.1016/j.jpedsurg.2018.01.002

von Gontard, A. (2013). The impact of *DSM-5* and guidelines for assessment and treatment of elimination disorders. *European Child & Adolescent Psychiatry, 22*(Suppl. 1), 61–67. https://doi.org/10.1007/s00787-012-0363-9

von Gontard, A., Baeyens, D., Van Hoecke, E., Warzak, W. J., & Bachmann, C. (2011). Psychological and psychiatric issues in urinary and fecal incontinence. *The Journal of Urology, 185*(4), 1432–1436. https://doi.org/10.1016/j.juro.2010.11.051

von Gontard, A., Hussong, J., Yang, S. S., Chase, J., Franco, I., & Wright, A. (2022). Neurodevelopmental disorders and incontinence in children and adolescents: Attention-deficit/hyperactivity disorder, autism spectrum disorder, and intellectual disability—A consensus document of the International Children's Continence Society. *Neurology and Urodynamics, 41*(1), 102–114. https://doi.org/10.1002/nau.24798

Vriesman, M. H., Koppen, I. J. N., Camilleri, M., Di Lorenzo, C., & Benninga, M. A. (2020). Management of functional constipation in children and adults. *Nature Reviews Gastroenterology & Hepatology, 17*(1), 21–39. https://doi.org/10.1038/s41575-019-0222-y

Wolfe-Christensen, C., Guy, W. C., Mancini, M., Kovacevic, L. G., & Lakshmanan, Y. (2016). Evidence of need to use self-report measures of psychosocial functioning in older children and adolescents with voiding dysfunction. *The Journal of Urology, 195*(5), 1570–1574. https://doi.org/10.1016/j.juro.2015.11.045

Yang, S. S. D., Zhao, L. L., & Chang, S. J. (2011). Early initiation of toilet training for urine was associated with early urinary continence and does not appear to be associated with bladder dysfunction. *Neurology and Urodynamics, 30*(7), 1253–1257. https://doi.org/10.1002/nau.20982

Zar-Kessler, C., Kuo, B., Cole, E., Benedix, A., & Belkind-Gerson, J. (2019). Benefit of pelvic floor physical therapy in pediatric patients with dyssynergic defecation constipation. *Digestive Diseases, 37*(6), 478–485. https://doi.org/10.1159/000500121

CHAPTER 21

ATTENTION AND ATTENTION-DEFICIT/ HYPERACTIVITY DISORDER IN CHILDHOOD

Tanya E. Froehlich and Stephen P. Becker

As children grow, their ability to regulate their attention, activity level, and impulses is key to success in family and peer relationships, daily living skills, academic endeavors, and later employment efforts. However, for some, regulation of these domains does not follow a typical developmental pattern. In these cases, individuals may meet criteria for attention-deficit/hyperactivity disorder (ADHD), which is present in approximately 7% of youth and among the most common pediatric neurobehavioral disorders. Given its adverse effects on social relationships, self-concept, and school and job functioning, as well as serious long-term negative outcomes such as criminal activity, substance use disorders, and death due to accidents and suicide, ADHD is a critical disorder to recognize and treat. In this chapter, we provide the developmental science foundation through an overview of the typical development of processes regulating attention, activity, and impulse control; conceptual models of dysfunction and neural pathways in attention/ADHD; ADHD genetic, environmental, and medical risk factors; ADHD epidemiology; and multilevel (ecological) factors that contribute to resilience as well as poor prognosis. Informed by this foundation, we then review methodological and practical issues in diagnosis and treatment to guide the pediatric psychologist and developmental-behavioral pediatrician in the care of children with ADHD.

DEVELOPMENTAL SCIENCE FOUNDATIONS FOR ADHD CARE: NORMATIVE DEVELOPMENT AND CLINICALLY SIGNIFICANT DEVIATIONS OF ATTENTION AND MOTOR ACTIVITY

An understanding of the typical development of attention, activity, and impulse control processes is needed to contextualize and identify differences in children with ADHD.

Attention Processes

Attention processes undergo rapid development in infancy and early childhood (Ruff & Rothbart, 2001). Around age 2, attention transitions from being primarily governed by external stimuli to being primarily governed by cognitive factors including planning and goals. As self-regulatory skills advance through age 4 via developmental cascades and interactions involving environmental factors (e.g., caregiving) and brain maturation (e.g., growth of brain gray and white matter; Vink et al., 2020), focused attention increases and distractibility decreases (Ruff & Capozzoli, 2003). After age 4, related but separable attention processes emerge (Breckenridge et al., 2013), such that by ages 6 to 11 years distinct component processes of attention are in place, including selective attention (attending to relevant stimuli while ignoring irrelevant stimuli), sustained attention (maintaining attention over time), and attention control (also referred to or closely related to executive or effortful control or the ability to resolve conflict; Breckenridge et al., 2013; Manly et al., 2001; Nigg, 2017). Of note, individuals with ADHD may be more likely to have difficulties in sustained attention and attentional control than in selective attention (Manly et al., 2001), although exceptions have also been reported (Wilding, 2005).

Activity and Impulse Control Processes

Surgency, which includes both activity level and sociability during or in anticipation of reward or high-intensity activity, is a higher order factor in temperament (Shiner et al., 2012). Like the more narrow domain of activity level, surgency is apparent early in infancy and highly stable into toddlerhood (Putnam et al., 2008). Overactivity generally decreases across toddlerhood, although there is much interindividual variability (Gray et al., 2014). Inhibitory control, a component of effortful control involving the ability to inhibit a dominant response, also develops rapidly in early childhood. By middle childhood, impulsivity usually starts to decline (Olson et al., 1999), as 61% of boys and 31% of girls have decreasing impulsivity levels from ages 6 to 12 (Côté et al., 2002).

Clinical Definition of ADHD

Diagnostic criteria for ADHD are defined in the *Diagnostic and Statistical Manual of Mental Disorders* (*DSM*; American Psychiatric Association, 2013). The fifth edition of the *DSM* (*DSM-5*), published in 2013, sets forth the current criteria. It lists the 18 ADHD symptoms, which are split between two dimensions: inattention and hyperactivity–impulsivity. To meet criteria for ADHD, six symptoms of inattention and/or hyperactivity–impulsivity must be present for individuals ages 16 and younger or five symptoms for individuals ages 17 and older (criterion A).

These symptoms must have been present prior to age 12 (criterion B), be present in two or more settings (criterion C), be inconsistent with developmental level, and interfere with or reduce the quality of functioning (criterion D). Finally, the symptoms cannot occur exclusively during the course of schizophrenia or another psychotic disorder or be better explained by another mental disorder (criterion E).

Domain-specific presentations. Hyperactive–impulsive symptoms of ADHD emerge early in development (by age 19 months; Leblanc et al., 2008), followed by a group mean-level decrease across childhood and adolescence, whereas ADHD inattentive symptoms may manifest later (often as school demands increase) and then show group mean-level continuity over time (Larsson et al., 2011). Given the varied trajectories of ADHD symptoms across development, individuals with ADHD often present with different symptom profiles at different points in time. For example, a preschool-aged child may present with primarily hyperactive–impulsive behaviors, transition to displaying both hyperactive–impulsive and inattentive behaviors in middle childhood, and then in adolescence display primarily inattentive behaviors. Accordingly, the *DSM-5* refers to ADHD "presentations," acknowledging that the underlying disorder's symptom presentation often changes across development. There are currently three ADHD presentations: combined (presence of both hyperactive–impulsive and inattentive symptoms), predominantly inattentive (clinically significant inattentive but not hyperactive–impulsive symptoms), and predominantly hyperactive–impulsive (clinically significant hyperactive–impulsive but not inattentive symptoms). Of note, the predominantly hyperactive–impulsive presentation is uncommon after early childhood, and evidence for the validity of this presentation after approximately age 6 is weak. The ADHD predominantly inattentive presentation is the most common in the general population, whereas the combined presentation is more likely in clinical referral populations (Willcutt, 2012).

CONCEPTUAL MODELS OF DYSFUNCTION IN ADHD AND INATTENTION

There are numerous prominent and emerging conceptual models of ADHD and inattention (Sonuga-Barke et al., 2023), several of which are briefly reviewed in this section.

Dual Pathway Model

Recognizing that single core deficit models were unlikely to explain ADHD's vast heterogeneity, Sonuga-Barke (2002) proposed a dual pathway model integrating executive dysfunction and delay aversion (a motivational style to escape or avoid delay) as two largely independent deficits that each contribute to ADHD. We briefly describe these two pathways, noting that more research is needed to fully test this model, and consider the possibility of a third pathway characterized by temporal processing deficits (Sonuga-Barke et al., 2010).

Executive dysfunction. Executive function refers to higher cognitive control processes involving optimal problem solving to attain a future goal (Pennington & Ozonoff, 1996). It is well established that, as a group, individuals with ADHD have greater executive dysfunction than those without ADHD, including across executive function domains of response inhibition (inhibiting a prepotent response), working memory (holding and updating information), set shifting (being able to switch between tasks), and planning (the ability to create a program of action to accomplish a goal; Willcutt et al., 2005). The dual pathway model emphasizes the role of inhibitory deficits underpinned by dysregulation in the fronto- and dorsal-stratal circuits and associated dopaminergic branches (e.g., mesocortical pathway involving the ventral tegmentum and prefrontal cortex) involved in executive processes. Inhibitory deficits manifested by an inability to stop a prepotent or ongoing response precede broader executive functioning deficits such as working memory, which in turn lead to the emergence of ADHD behaviors (Barkley, 1997; Sonuga-Barke, 2003).

Delay aversion. Individuals with ADHD show a bias toward small immediate rather than larger delayed rewards (Marx et al., 2021), driving models of ADHD that focus on motivational processes. In the dual pathway model, dysfunction in the ventral fronto-striatal circuits involved in a range of brain functions including reinforcement leads to altered signaling of delayed rewards and delay aversion, in turn contributing to ADHD behaviors. Proximal culturally based factors are also highlighted in this pathway, particularly parent responses to children's impulsive behaviors, although this is a key component of the model in need of further empirical testing (Sonuga-Barke, 2003).

Default Mode Network

The default mode network (DMN) is a large-scale brain network that is strongly implicated in mind wandering and task-unrelated thought (Fox et al., 2015). It increases its activity during passive states and has three subsystems: a midline core subsystem (consisting of the anterior medial prefrontal cortex, posterior cingulate cortex, and portions of the inferior parietal lobule), a dorsal medial prefrontal cortex subsystem (dorsal medial prefrontal cortex, lateral temporal cortex, temporal parietal junction, and temporal pole), and a medial temporal lobe subsystem (including hippocampal formation, parahippocampal cortex, ventromedial prefrontal cortex, posterior inferior parietal lobule, and retrosplenial cortex; Andrews-Hanna et al., 2010). There is increasing attention to the role of the DMN in ADHD because ADHD is associated with reduced connectivity within the DMN core subsystem during resting state (Sutcubasi et al., 2020). Although the neurotransmitters involved in the DMN are not clearly established, DMN core subsystem hypoconnectivity has been shown to mediate the association between ADHD and delay aversion in adolescents with ADHD, suggesting that the DMN may play an important role in how individuals with ADHD regulate negative affective responses to waiting or the imposing of delay (Broulidakis et al., 2022).

Cognitive Disengagement Syndrome

Cognitive disengagement syndrome (CDS), previously referred to as "sluggish cognitive tempo," refers to a set of behaviors including excessive daydreaming, hypoactivity, and mental confusion (Becker et al., 2023). These behaviors are strongly associated with but also distinct from ADHD and other psychopathologies. Symptoms of CDS are independently associated with poorer social, academic, and occupational functioning (Becker et al., 2016, 2023). Cognitive disengagement syndrome may represent a type of pathological mind wandering (Becker & Barkley, 2021). Although it is not yet clear how to best conceptualize CDS (e.g., as a diagnostic specifier across disorders, ADHD subtype, or distinct disorder), there is growing interest in understanding its negative and positive impacts as well as its importance in prevention and interventions for children and adolescents with ADHD (Becker, Fredrick, et al., 2022).

ADHD EPIDEMIOLOGY AND RISK FACTORS

A meta-analysis of 175 studies from 1977 to 2013 estimated ADHD's pooled worldwide prevalence in children and youth to be 7.2% (Thomas et al., 2015). This study reported that using criteria from later *DSM* editions (e.g., *DSM-IV* compared to earlier editions) was linked to higher prevalence estimates. Despite concern about widely varying ADHD rates by region of the world, one meta-analysis did not find prevalence to differ between regions worldwide (Willcutt, 2012), whereas another found that North American studies had higher rates than European studies (but were not different from other regions; Thomas et al., 2015). Worldwide studies have reported higher ADHD rates in boys than girls (ratio of 2:1 to 3:1 in the general population; American Psychiatric Association, 2013). Studies around the world have also noted differences in ADHD rates by racial or ethnic group. European studies have reported lower rates among immigrant versus non-immigrant groups (Slobodin & Masalha, 2020). Black children are more likely to be diagnosed with ADHD than White children, whereas Latinx children are less likely to be diagnosed with ADHD than non-Latinx White or non-Latinx Black children (Danielson et al., 2018; Zablotsky & Alford, 2020). Rates of ADHD also vary by socioeconomic status. Higher ADHD rates have been observed in children of lower socioeconomic status, possibly due to their higher exposure to ADHD risk factors (e.g., environmental toxicants such as lead, prenatal and perinatal complications; Froehlich et al., 2007; Willcutt, 2012).

Genetic Risk Factors

Attention-deficit/hyperactivity disorder has high heritability, with studies of twins and adopted children yielding ADHD heritability estimates of ~75%. Hence, there is much interest in identifying ADHD-related genes, although these efforts have proven challenging because ADHD is a complex genetic disorder with many genes of small effect and gene–environment interactions likely involved (Palladino et al., 2019). Investigators have pursued genome-wide association studies, which analyze single-nucleotide polymorphisms across the entire genome. One such study found associations between ADHD and 12 independent loci, with associations enriched in loss-of-function intolerant genes and around brain-expressed regulatory marks (Demontis et al., 2019). Although most cases of ADHD appear to be multifactorial and polygenic in etiology, there are also a number of uncommon neurodevelopmental genetic syndromes (e.g., Turner, Williams, Down, Fragile X, Klinefelter, and velocardiofacial syndromes, neurofibromatosis Type I) for which ADHD and its phenotypic features appear at higher rates than in the general population (Thapar & Cooper, 2016).

Environmental Risk Factors

Although ADHD is highly familial, links to environmental risk factors include associations with prenatal exposures, such as in utero alcohol, tobacco, cannabis, opiate, bisphenol A, and per- and polyfluoroalkyl exposures (Ayonrinde et al., 2021; Nygaard et al., 2016; Vuong et al., 2021). Childhood toxicant exposures linked to increased ADHD risk include lead, organophosphates, pyrethroid pesticides, phthalates, bisphenol A, secondhand smoke, and air pollution (Huang et al., 2021; Minatoya & Kishi, 2021; Yuchi et al., 2022), with evidence emerging for mercury and manganese (Nilsen & Tulve, 2020). A growing literature also suggests that having low levels of certain micronutrients (such as iron and magnesium; Degremont et al., 2021; Effatpanah et al., 2019) may be linked to ADHD. In addition, there is evidence that child maltreatment and severe early social deprivation are associated with ADHD (Hunt et al., 2017). However, it is unclear whether the links between environmental exposures and ADHD are causal or related to unmeasured confounding factors or reverse causation (i.e., the ADHD phenotype influences the environmental exposure). Of note, multiple studies have not implicated poor parenting as a cause of ADHD, but instead have shown that child ADHD symptoms can spur or exacerbate negative parent–child interactions (Banaschewski et al., 2017).

Medical Risk Factors

Offspring ADHD has been linked to prenatal and perinatal risk factors (e.g., prematurity, low birthweight, preeclampsia, in utero substance exposures; Serati et al., 2017). Traumatic brain injury (Bolikal et al., 2021) and childhood stroke or CNS infections (e.g., meningitis or encephalitis) also increase ADHD risk (Langberg et al., 2008).

NATURAL HISTORY OF ADHD

Although the average age of diagnosis for pediatric ADHD is 6, age of diagnosis does depend on parent-reported severity, with the median age of diagnosis for severe ADHD being 4 years, for moderate ADHD being 6 years, and for mild ADHD being 7 years (Visser et al., 2014). During preschool, the major manifestation of ADHD is motor hyperactivity; symptoms of inattention may be difficult to discern given the limited demands for sustained attention in this age group. In elementary school, inattention (for those with predominantly inattentive or combined presentation) becomes more prominent and impairing. As individuals enter puberty, symptoms of overt hyperactivity (climbing, difficulties staying seated when expected) are less pronounced, and may be replaced by inner feelings of restlessness whereas symptoms of inattention and impulsivity are more persistent during adolescence (American Psychiatric Association, 2013).

OUTCOMES ASSOCIATED WITH ADHD

In the preschool age group, ADHD is linked to numerous adverse outcomes, including negative parent–child relationships, elevated family stress, peer interaction difficulties, impaired pre-academic skills (Harpin, 2005), expulsion from preschool/child care settings (Gilliam, 2005), and increased accidents/injuries (Childress & Stark, 2018). In school-age children ADHD continues to be associated with intrafamily conflict and poor peer relationships, including portending higher risk for being a victim *and* perpetrator of bullying, (e.g., verbal, physical, cyber, relational bullying). In addition, school-age ADHD has been linked to poor academic achievement and school failure, higher rates of psychiatric comorbidity (e.g., anxiety, depression), and increased rates of injury and accidents (Barkley, 2015). Furthermore, studies have shown that children with ADHD have difficulties with self-care tasks, including having poorer oral hygiene and dental health compared to their typically developing peers. Additional adverse outcomes experienced by adolescents with ADHD include increased rates of pregnancy, risky sexual behavior, smoking, substance abuse, internet/gaming addiction, poor self-esteem, suicidality, and unsafe driving behavior/motor vehicle accidents (Barkley, 2015; Becker, 2020). Children and adolescents with ADHD followed into adulthood are also noted to have lower total years of education and lower occupational achievement as well as higher rates of antisocial behavior, criminality, and death (Barbaresi et al., 2013; Di Lorenzo et al., 2021).

PROGNOSTIC FACTORS

A number of factors have been shown to predict ADHD symptom prognosis (i.e., having increasing, persistently high, or declining symptoms over time). For example, factors such as early aggression/conduct problems and hyperactivity in school and emotion dysregulation at home have been shown to distinguish children with a persistently high versus a declining symptom trajectory (Sasser et al., 2016). Other factors linked to worsening symptoms over time (as opposed to stable or declining symptoms) include lower IQ, more impaired spatial working memory, and more impaired visual motor integration skills (Sudre et al., 2021). Additional poor pediatric ADHD prognostic indicators include caregiver psychopathology, family conflict, and caregiver–child hostility. Of note, negative parental cognitions such as child-blaming attributions have been linked to increased disruptive behavior over time in children with ADHD, even when accounting for initial levels of ADHD and disruptive symptomatology (Barkley, 2015).

Factors linked to favorable prognosis include higher socioeconomic status, greater child intelligence, and positive peer relationships (Barkley, 2015). Additionally, positive parenting practices, such as the setting of consistent and reasonable limits on behavior, have been shown to protect against the development of oppositional–defiant behavior in young children with ADHD (Harvey et al., 2011). Protective effects of firm limit setting by parents has also been shown in studies of adolescents with ADHD; consistent parental monitoring has been linked to reductions in delinquency and substance use in teens with ADHD (Molina et al., 2012; Walther et al., 2012).

PRACTICAL ISSUES IN ADHD DIAGNOSIS FOR PEDIATRIC PSYCHOLOGISTS AND DEVELOPMENTAL-BEHAVIORAL PEDIATRICIANS

Informed by a developmental science foundation, pediatric psychologists and developmental-behavioral pediatricians collaborate to provide evidence-based diagnosis and treatment for pediatric ADHD, often providing complementary expertise as highlighted in the following subsections.

ADHD Diagnostic Evaluation

A diagnosis of ADHD requires a thorough evaluation integrating reports of behaviors across settings from multiple observers (which is in the purview of both the pediatric psychologist and developmental-behavioral pediatrician) coupled with a complete physical examination (which requires input from a medical doctor such as a developmental-behavioral pediatrician). The three principal means of gathering the necessary information are reviewed: behavior rating scales, caregiver and patient interview, and physical examination. The role of objective diagnostic testing is also covered, along with the key diagnostic considerations across development that are informed by developmental science.

Collection and interpretation of standardized rating scales. The clinician must document that the child meets ADHD *DSM-5* criteria (reviewed previously). The Vanderbilt ADHD Rating Scales (Wolraich et al., 1998, 2003), the ADHD Rating Scale-5 (DuPaul et al., 2016), and the Conners Rating Scale (Conners, 2008) are psychometrically valid measures that include all 18 *DSM-5* symptoms (Wolraich et al., 2019). Having both caregivers and teachers complete these scales provides information about child behaviors across settings to determine if the requisite number of *DSM-5* symptoms are present and pervasive. If the caregiver and teacher reports disagree, with one but not both reporting a high level of ADHD symptomatology on ADHD rating scales, the clinician should take a careful history and use clinical judgment to determine if reported problematic behaviors are indeed present across settings or instead reflect one reporter's distinctive reporting standards (i.e., one rater has an unusually high threshold for reporting; conversely, one rater is an overreporter with an unusually low threshold for endorsing symptoms). To assess impairment (which should also be queried in the clinical interview), performance-rated items on the Vanderbilt scales or the Impairment Rating Scale (Fabiano et al., 2006) can be helpful. It is also critical to screen for coexisting or mimicking conditions, including disruptive behavior (oppositional defiant and conduct disorders) and internalizing disorders (anxiety and depression), which can be done by having caregivers and teachers complete broadband rating scales such as the Child Behavior Checklist and Teacher's Report Form (Achenbach & Rescorla, 2001) or the Behavior Assessment System for Children (Reynolds & Kamphaus, 2015). Additional information regarding assessing coexisting or mimicking conditions appears in the Differential Diagnoses/Comorbidities of ADHD section of this chapter.

Key elements of the clinical history. Behavior rating scales alone are insufficient to diagnose ADHD as they do not include information related to *DSM*-5 criteria for symptom age of onset, duration, persistence, and discrepancy from developmental level. Rather, this information must be gleaned from the family interview, during which the clinician must also verify presence and degree of impairment, probing key areas including social relationships, self-care, leisure activities, self-esteem, and school achievement. The interview also allows for assessment of whether endorsed difficulties are ADHD related or are better attributed to another condition. The clinician should evaluate discrepancies between family and teacher reports, paying particular attention to differential expectations and structure between settings. In addition, the clinician must take a careful history regarding use of medications or supplements that can produce ADHD-like symptoms and rule out physical conditions that can mimic ADHD symptoms or represent coexisting or predisposing conditions (such as sleep, including apnea) and endocrine, neurologic (including absence seizures and tics), genetic, post-infectious, sensory, developmental (including learning, intellectual and autism spectrum), mental health, and substance use disorders (Langberg et al., 2008).

Developmental Science Perspective: Diagnostic Considerations by Age in Typically Developing Children/Youth

It is important for clinicians to approach the assessment of ADHD with a firm understanding of developmental science and related considerations.

Preschool. In the preschool age group, ADHD often presents as excessive motor activity, which can be difficult to distinguish from typical behavior. Red flags include hyperactivity or impulsivity that causes impairment to the extent that children are unable to maintain placements with babysitters, day cares, or preschools; caregivers have difficulty taking children to stores, restaurants, or other family-friendly settings; or safety concerns arise. Attentional problems in preschool children are often hard to identify due to the generally limited demands placed on this cohort and the potential that a shorter than typical attention span is related to developmental or language delays rather than to ADHD, underscoring the importance of obtaining standardized language and developmental evaluations if these concerns are present (Wolraich et al., 2019). Assessing ADHD symptoms in preschool children can also be complicated by a lack of easily applicable measures and/or suitable raters of behavior. Although general ADHD rating scales, such as the Vanderbilt, can be employed for preschoolers because the same 18 *DSM*-5 ADHD symptoms are used for this and older age groups, caregivers and teachers may have difficulty understanding how some items manifest in young children. Hence, it is worth noting that the Conners Early Childhood Rating Scale and the ADHD Rating Scale-IV Preschool Version have been adapted and validated for use in children 5 years of age and under (Wolraich et al., 2019). If teacher ratings are unavailable because a child is not enrolled in preschool, another out-of-home adult who knows the child well can be asked to complete behavior ratings (e.g., babysitter, speech or occupational therapist, out-of-home family member). Finally, if there is insufficient evidence to support an ADHD diagnosis in a preschool child, the clinician can consider recommending parent behavior management training. In fact, clinical practice guidelines encourage clinicians to recommend behavior training for parents of preschool children before assigning an ADHD diagnosis (Wolraich et al., 2019).

School age. During elementary school, children with hyperactive–impulsive or combined presentation ADHD manifest motor overactivity (e.g., being in constant motion, being overly fidgety even when quiet) as well as impulsivity (e.g., acting without thinking, interrupting, engaging in dangerous activities without a sense of fear). For children with inattentive or combined presentation ADHD, symptoms of inattention (e.g., difficulty completing tasks due to distractibility or forgetting, difficulty sustaining attention to boring and more effortful activities) become increasingly apparent and impairing during elementary school. During the ADHD evaluation of school-age children (as with other age groups), it is important to consider the patient's age relative to their classroom cohort because individuals who are relatively younger than their classmates have an increased risk of being diagnosed with ADHD. Hence, as directed by *DSM-5*, clinicians must carefully consider the child's developmental level relative to the expectations placed upon the child (Caye et al., 2020).

Adolescence. During the adolescent evaluation, clinicians should be aware that some ADHD-related problems may be less obvious than in younger children because overt motor hyperactivity typically wanes during puberty, with challenges due to internal restlessness, impatience, impulsivity (including risk-taking behaviors), inattention, poor planning, and disorganization persisting (American Psychiatric Association, 2013). For this reason, many individuals who were diagnosed with combined presentation ADHD earlier in childhood may shift to meeting criteria for inattentive presentation after entering adolescence (Biederman et al., 2000). For adolescent evaluations, it is crucial to verify (per *DSM-5* criteria) that some ADHD symptoms were present before age 12, either via clinical history or documentation from past report cards or school records. Of note, the requirement to document symptoms and impairment in two or more settings can be complicated in adolescent evaluations because high school teachers often spend relatively little time with each student. In the adolescent age group, guidelines recommend that clinicians obtain ADHD rating scales from at least two non-family sources, which can include teachers or other adults who know the teen well (e.g., coaches, extracurricular activity leaders; Wolraich et al., 2019). Some variability in ratings is expected because adolescent behaviors often differ by setting; identifying reasons for variability can yield important insights into the youth's issues and functioning. Obtaining adolescents' behavior self-ratings is also critical to understand how they view their own functioning, with the knowledge that the diagnostic formulation cannot rest on these self-reports because adolescents (particularly those with ADHD) often minimize their own problematic behaviors (Sibley et al., 2012). Rating scales that offer self-report versions include the Conners-3 and the Adult ADHD Self-Report Scale (Conners, 2008; Ustun et al., 2017). An additional need in the adolescent evaluation is to identify cases for which the ADHD diagnosis is sought for secondary gain (e.g., school or standardized test accommodations, stimulant medication prescriptions; Wolraich et al., 2019). Conditions that can either mimic or coexist with ADHD in adolescence and are therefore important to rule out include anxiety and depressive and substance use disorders (American Psychiatric Association, 2013).

Key Elements of the Physical Examination and Observation

A comprehensive physical examination is a crucial part of the ADHD evaluation. Physical examination elements needed to evaluate for mimicking and/or coexisting medical conditions include growth parameters (height, weight, and head circumference), vital signs, hearing and vision screening, dysmorphic features, skin stigmata, and neurologic signs. A mental status examination is needed to exclude an emerging thought or psychiatric disorder than may mimic ADHD. Clinicians should determine the presence or absence of paranoid ideation, delusions, or hallucinations, which could indicate an emerging psychosis, as well as pressured speech, flight of ideas, or grandiosity, which could suggest emerging mania. Attention should be paid to interpersonal, language, and developmental skills to determine need for further assessment for coexisting developmental disorders. The clinician must also conduct a behavioral observation, focusing on attention span, impulse control, and activity level. Observation of dysfunction in these areas (e.g., attending to irrelevant environmental cues, verbal interruptions or impulsive responding, out-of-seat behaviors, excessive fidgetiness) can corroborate an ADHD diagnosis. However, absence of these behaviors does not exclude the disorder as individuals with ADHD may not demonstrate them in novel settings with one-on-one interactions (Wolraich et al., 2019).

Role of Ancillary Data and Objective Diagnostic Testing

Prior school records such as report cards (which frequently contain comments about or ratings of behavior), cognitive or academic standardized test results, other behavior assessments, and discipline records are helpful to assess ADHD symptoms and impairment in the school setting. Psychoeducational and cognitive testing are not a standard part of the ADHD evaluation, but are indicated if academic problems are significant and suggest a comorbid learning disorder. Although individuals with ADHD may have deficits on attention, executive function, or memory tests, computer-based studies of sustained attention (e.g., the "continuous performance task") are not routinely recommended because their sensitivity and specificity are insufficient to reliably indicate the diagnosis. Objective diagnostic testing is indicated only if suggested by the history and physical examination (e.g., laboratory tests for thyroid function or lead exposure, electroencephalogram [commonly known as EEG] or neuroimaging when unexpected or focal neurological findings or symptoms are present; Wolraich et al., 2019).

Sociodemographic Considerations in Diagnosis

Compared with boys, girls are less likely to present with easily observable hyperactivity symptoms and more likely to exhibit inattention. Hence, it is critical to consider a diagnosis of ADHD-inattentive presentation when female patients and their families express concerns about focus, organization, and forgetfulness (American Psychiatric Association, 2013).

Disparity in ADHD diagnosis by racial and ethnic group is an area of increasing concern. Numerous factors may influence these disparities, including caregiver perceptions of ADHD (and explanatory models of child behavior) as well as implicit bias by teachers and clinicians. For example, studies suggest that White parents have lower thresholds for ADHD-related problem recognition and treatment seeking than parents from other groups (Slobodin & Masalha, 2020). This may be due to stigma around the ADHD diagnosis in some minoritized groups. Differing child behavior explanatory models may also play a role. Some studies have found that Latinx caregivers attribute child behavior to fate (and believe that problems will remit on their own), whereas Chinese parents are apt to blame themselves for child behavior and believe that a child is "bad" as opposed to having a mental health concern (Dong et al., 2020). Black parents have expressed concerns that ADHD is due to inappropriate parenting practices, that ADHD is a label applied to exert social control, and that clinicians are too quick to diagnose ADHD (Olaniyan et al., 2007). Teachers' implicit bias may also decrease their likelihood of alerting caregivers about ADHD-related concerns, as prior studies have shown that teachers label non-White, and particularly Black children, as "problem" or "bad" students more frequently than White children (Riddle & Sinclair, 2019; Staats, 2014), potentially obscuring their recognition of ADHD or related conditions as a driver of behavior. Clinician implicit bias may play a similar role because emerging evidence indicates that ethnic minority youth, compared with non-Latinx White youth, may be more likely to be diagnosed with a disruptive behavior disorder than with ADHD (Fadus et al., 2020).

Differential Diagnoses/Comorbidities of ADHD

Given that the diagnosis of ADHD depends on excluding other conditions that can produce similar symptoms, and that the majority of children with ADHD have co-existing neurobehavioral conditions, clinicians must carefully consider differential diagnoses and evaluation for comorbid conditions during patient visits.

Learning disorders. Depending on the assessment means and criteria, studies suggest that ~50% of children with ADHD may have coexisting learning disorders, with written expression disorders being the most common (DuPaul et al., 2013). Learning disorders can mimic ADHD; this scenario should be considered when ADHD symptoms manifest solely in school or when performing academic tasks but otherwise children show typical ability to focus, plan, organize, and stay on task. One key differential diagnostic question in children who appear to have typical development (i.e., are not concerning for global developmental delay/intellectual disability) is whether academic problems are pervasive across subjects. If performance issues are mainly present or significantly more severe during a particular class for which there is difficulty understanding concepts, a specific learning disorder may be present. Children with academic impairment linked solely to ADHD have age-appropriate conceptual understanding across academic subjects, but their grades are below their potential in a range of classes because they fail to execute a sound study plan and to carefully complete and turn in schoolwork. In addition, when children receive effective treatment for their ADHD symptoms, yet their pervasive issues across academic subjects persist, psychoeducational evaluation is warranted to rule out more global learning difficulties or intellectual disability (Langberg et al., 2008).

When psychoeducational testing is conducted, note that a substantial number of studies have found that children with ADHD perform worse on both verbal working memory (such as the digit span task on IQ testing) and visual–spatial working memory than non-ADHD peers (Barkley, 2015). Group-level comparisons in research studies have also been shown that individuals with ADHD perform more poorly on other executive functioning tasks, such as response inhibition and planning, compared with typically developing peers, although only a minority of children with ADHD score in the impaired range on traditional executive functioning tests (Barkley, 2015).

Intellectual disability. Children with intellectual disability or borderline intellectual disability (IQ < 85) have a greater than sixfold risk for ADHD compared with the general population. For these evaluations, the clinician must determine if the inattention, overactivity, and impulsivity are consistent with mental rather than chronological age, in which case the diagnosis would be intellectual disability only, or if the symptoms are beyond what is typical for those of the same mental age, suggesting comorbid ADHD. Hence, assessment by teachers or professionals who are able to benchmark the ADHD symptoms against the child's developmental level are critical (Rosen et al., 2011).

Autism spectrum disorder. Studies suggest that more than half of children with autism spectrum disorder (ASD) have coexisting ADHD. Children with ADHD often have issues with social interaction, communication, and reciprocal behavior even without coexisting ASD, frequently leading clinicians to wonder when an ASD evaluation is warranted (Rosen et al., 2011). Some social-communication and behavioral patterns qualitatively differentiate ADHD and ASD. Mulligan et al. (2009) found that children with ADHD only, unlike those with ASD, had relatively intact nonverbal communication skill development (e.g., use of eye gaze and head nods) and social intent (e.g., spontaneously pointing, seeking to share enjoyment with others), as well as low rates of unusual sensory interests and preoccupations. Anckarsäter et al. (2006) found that children with ADHD only tended to display high novelty seeking, whereas children with ASD exhibited the unusual preoccupations and predilection for sameness associated with low novelty seeking.

Internalizing disorders. Among children with ADHD, 25% to 35% have a coexisting anxiety disorder and 20% to 30% have a coexisting depressive disorder (Rosen et al., 2011). The *DSM-5* diagnostic criteria for generalized anxiety disorder and depression include difficulty concentrating and restless/overactivity (American Psychiatric Association, 2013) so that these conditions are considered to mimic rather than be comorbid with ADHD. It is therefore important to recognize that internalizing disorders and ADHD often show different patterns in symptom onset and setting. Symptoms due to ADHD have onset early in childhood, whereas concentration difficulties and restlessness due solely to anxiety or depression do not manifest until the onset of the anxiety or mood disorder and may be specific to anxiety-provoking situations or periods of low mood (Rosen et al., 2011).

Trauma and maltreatment. Children who have experienced maltreatment and/or trauma are at higher risk for a range of mental health and behavioral disorders, including ADHD. Trauma and ADHD can be coexisting conditions, but they can also mimic one another as posttraumatic hyperarousal symptoms can appear similar to ADHD symptoms. Taking a history of the temporal relation between the trauma and the ADHD-like symptom onset is important for diagnostic clarification because symptoms that began abruptly after the trauma, particularly if not present prior to age 12, would suggest trauma as the etiology (Keeshin et al., 2020).

Disruptive behavior disorders. Studies suggest that more than 45% of children with ADHD have a coexisting disruptive behavior disorder (DBD), with oppositional defiant disorder more commonly present than conduct disorder. Shared aspects of ADHD and DBD, including failure to follow directions, complete tasks, and conform to environmental rules, can make these diagnoses difficult to disentangle. Nonetheless, ADHD and DBDs can be differentiated by their core symptoms and the etiology of their behavioral difficulties. First, children with DBDs but not ADHD do not usually manifest inattention or hyperactivity (American Psychiatric Association, 2013). Similarly, core features of ADHD only do not include the chronic oppositionality and defiance that characterize oppositional defiant disorder or the pattern of chronic violation of social norms and the rights of others that characterizes conduct disorder. The driver of the behavioral difficulties can also distinguish ADHD from DBD. Both disorders often involve failure to follow directions and rules, but in ADHD only these behavioral challenges tend to be driven by impulsivity or inattention to/forgetting instructions rather than intentional defiance. Children with DBD have a pattern of willful oppositionality, defiance, and resistance to authority (Langberg et al., 2008).

PRACTICAL ISSUES IN ADHD TREATMENT FOR PEDIATRIC PSYCHOLOGISTS AND DEVELOPMENTAL-BEHAVIORAL PEDIATRICIANS

A large body of research has examined nonpharmacological and pharmacological interventions for managing pediatric ADHD, with numerous empirically supported treatments currently available.

Nonpharmacological Interventions

The pediatric psychologist has special training and expertise in the implementation of ADHD non-pharmacological interventions, which enable the family (caregivers in concert with children and adolescents) and teachers to modify the environment and manage behaviors in ways that set youth up for success and foster adaptations that compensate for areas of challenge. Given that behavioral interventions are foundational in the treatment of ADHD (Barbaresi et al., 2020a), the developmental-behavioral pediatrician must be knowledgeable of the principles of pediatric psychology that inform these interventions to provide evidence-based counsel and referrals to partnering psychologists.

Well-established nonpharmacological interventions. Behavior management interventions focus on changing contingencies in the environment so that the child is likely to increase the rate, frequency, or intensity of desired behaviors while reducing undesired behaviors. Behavior management approaches for ADHD include behavioral parent training and behavioral peer interventions, which are considered well-established interventions for preschool and elementary-age ADHD (S. W. Evans, Owens, et al., 2018; Wolraich et al., 2019). Behavioral parent training is considered possibly efficacious for adolescent ADHD (S. W. Evans, Owens, et al., 2018). Although there are numerous behavioral parent training programs, they share many similarities, including psychoeducation; praise, positive attending, and positive caregiver–child quality time; planned ignoring; using effective commands; incentive systems (e.g., token economies); and time out from positive reinforcement (Barkley, 2015). Behavioral management approaches may have less impact on ADHD symptoms but instead are likely to improve the functional impairments (Daley et al., 2014; S. W. Evans, Owens, et al., 2018).

Behavioral classroom management is another efficacious intervention for preschool and elementary-age ADHD (S. W. Evans, Owens, et al., 2018). The daily report card is the most commonly recommended ADHD behavioral intervention in the school setting (Pfiffner & DuPaul, 2015). This contingency-based intervention first identifies clearly defined target behaviors for the student. The teacher then monitors these behaviors and gives quantitative feedback ratings to the student over the course of the day. A critical component of a successful daily report card is having the student bring the report card home each day so that the parent can implement positive and negative consequences.

Organizational skills training, which teaches organization and homework skills with repeated practice and feedback, may be delivered in the clinic or in schools by school mental health professionals (S. W. Evans, Owens, et al., 2018). The benefits are greatest when this training is continued over an extended time period and includes frequent constructive feedback. It is effective in the 9- to 18-year-old age group but may not be appropriate or helpful for younger children (Wolraich et al., 2019).

Less well-established nonpharmacological interventions. Given ADHD's pervasive peer problems, there is much interest in social skills intervention (SSI; Mikami et al., 2017). However, SSIs, at least as delivered in traditional clinic settings, have questionable efficacy (S. W. Evans, Owens et al., 2018). Accordingly, work has focused on training parents as friendship coaches (Mikami et al., 2020) or showing teachers how to create socially inclusive classrooms that challenge the negative reputations many children with ADHD have in their peer group (Mikami et al., 2022). Although trials have not shown improvement in the primary outcomes, SSI may have positive effects on other functional domains and/or be especially beneficial for certain subgroups of children with ADHD, particularly those with primarily inattentive symptoms and/or withdrawn social behaviors (Mikami et al., 2020, 2022). Peer coaching, either by same-age or older peers, is another possible avenue to improve social functioning in children with ADHD, although to date randomized controlled trials (RCTs) are lacking (Mikami et al., 2017).

Given the central role of attention (dys)regulation in ADHD, it is not surprising that mindfulness meditation therapies have been trialed for this population. A meta-analysis found that mindfulness meditation interventions reduce both inattentive and hyperactive–impulsive symptoms in individuals with ADHD (Cairncross & Miller, 2020). However, the current evidence base is small and largely composed of lower quality studies (S. Evans, Ling, et al., 2018). Accordingly, mindfulness meditation is not currently recommended for treating children with ADHD (Wolraich et al., 2019).

Cognitive training interventions are based on the premise that key ADHD brain networks can be strengthened by improving cognitive processes through repeated exposure to information processing tasks. These interventions have primarily been tested in school-aged children and adolescents and appear to improve the cognitive domain being trained (e.g., working memory), but do not generally reduce ADHD symptoms or functional impairments (Cortese et al., 2015). Hence, cognitive training is currently considered an experimental treatment for youth with ADHD (S. W. Evans, Owens, et al., 2018).

Neurofeedback (also termed EEG biofeedback) applies operant conditioning principles to brain electrical signals to train self-regulation via real-time feedback. Evidence for neurofeedback has been mixed, and the clinical guideline (Wolraich et al., 2019) of the American Academy of Pediatrics (AAP), a meta-analysis (Rahmani et al., 2022), and a multisite double-blind placebo RCT (Arnold et al., 2021) do not support it as an effective ADHD treatment, although one review concluded that it may possibly be efficacious (S. W. Evans, Owens, et al., 2018).

Although families often ask clinicians about the use of play therapy, vision or interactive metronome training, and sensory processing therapy, these interventions have not been rigorously tested in randomized control trials and are not considered evidence-based treatments for ADHD (Wolraich et al., 2019).

Medication Interventions Approved by the U.S. Food and Drug Administration

Medication management for ADHD has been the special purview of medical specialists such as developmental-behavioral pediatricians, who collaborate with pediatric psychologists to ensure that children whose ADHD is not adequately managed with behavioral interventions can receive evidence-based pharmacological treatment. However, it should be noted that currently psychologists can obtain prescribing privileges in five states following additional training. At this time, there are three classes of medication approved by the U.S. Food and Drug Administration (FDA) for treating ADHD in children and youth: psychostimulants, selective norepinephrine reuptake inhibitors, and the alpha agonists. The AAP clinical guideline (Wolraich et al., 2019) includes a detailed discussion of these medication classes in its main text and process of care algorithms. A free and updated list of currently available FDA-approved ADHD medications, along with their characteristics (availability of generics, prescribed doses, and modality [tablet, capsule, liquid]) is also available (https://www.ADHDMedicationGuide.com). A broad overview of these medication classes and considerations in their management is provided in this chapter.

Stimulant medications. This family, which includes the methylphenidate (MPH) and amphetamine (AMPH)/dextroamphetamine (DEX) families, is first-line ADHD pharmacotherapy because it has the highest response rate (>90% of patients have a positive response if both the MPH and AMPH/DEX families are tried) and effect size (amount of symptom change) of any ADHD medication class. The stimulants work primarily by increasing synaptic dopamine and norepinephrine levels through dopamine and norepinephrine transporter blockade. Both the MPH and AMPH/DEX families can be effective, but ~25% of patients may respond to only one family. The most common stimulant side effects include decreased appetite, sleep difficulties, headache, and stomachache (Wolraich et al., 2019). Emotional symptoms (irritability and anxiety) can also be seen but are sometimes improved, rather than worsened, by stimulant treatment. Meta-analyses have documented some subtle group-level differences in MPH and AMPH/DEX adverse effects. One meta-analysis found that overall adverse effects (including sleep and emotional side effects) were more prominent with AMPH/DEX than with MPH (Cortese et al., 2018). Another reported that AMPH/DEX increased emotional lability compared with premedication baseline, whereas MPH tended to reduce irritability and anxiety compared with premedication ratings (Pozzi et al., 2018). However, responses among individual patients can and do vary from these averages.

Norepinephrine reuptake inhibitors. The norepinephrine reuptake inhibitors atomoxetine and viloxazine are also approved for treating pediatric ADHD, although they are considered second-line treatments because their response rates and effect sizes lag behind those of the stimulants. Atomoxetine has been linked to lower rates of sleep difficulties compared with stimulants and may also have mild beneficial effects on anxiety so it is a reasonable option when stimulants worsen insomnia or anxiety. Common atomoxetine and viloxazine adverse effects include sedation/fatigue, upset stomach, nausea/vomiting, reduced appetite, headache, and irritability. It is also important to inform families that both atomoxetine and viloxazine have FDA black box warnings for suicide risk, because suicidal ideation is a rarely reported adverse effect of both (Edinoff et al., 2021; Garnock-Jones & Keating, 2009).

Alpha agonists. Like the norephinephrine reuptake inhibitors, the alpha agonists extended release guanfacine (GUA) and extended release clonidine are considered second line due to their lower response rates and effect sizes compared with the stimulants Both work by stimulating α_2 adrenergic receptors, which control norepinephrine release and cell firing rate. Their most common adverse effect is drowsiness (which is more prominent with clonidine than with guanfacine); other common adverse effects include dizziness, irritability, headaches, and stomachaches (Froehlich et al., 2013).

Medical tests and clinical monitoring. Current clinical guidelines do not recommend any laboratory tests as standard procedures before starting or for monitoring any FDA-approved ADHD medications. However, medical tests should be ordered as needed based on the clinical history and physical examination (e.g., thyroid function tests to rule out thyroid function if indicated by history and examination). According to existing guidelines, ADHD pharmacogenetic testing should not be standard practice due to a consensus that no genetic variants are known to reliably predict ADHD medication response (Wolraich et al., 2019).

Before beginning any of the FDA-approved ADHD medication classes, clinicians should measure vital signs and conduct cardiac risk factor screening. All three classes are associated with heart rate and blood pressure variations that are generally not clinically significant but warrant baseline measurement and ongoing monitoring, as changes can be more substantial in a subset of patients. Large studies indicate that the risk of severe cardiovascular outcomes (e.g., sudden cardiac death, long QT syndrome, and stroke) are not higher in children receiving ADHD medications than for the general population. However, due to rare reports of significant cardiovascular events in patients taking stimulants and nonstimulants before starting these medications, clinicians should also screen for personal and family cardiac risk factors (e.g., personal history of unexplained shortness of breath with exercise or heart palpitations, family history of a sudden cardiac death at <35 years of age, long QT syndrome). A full list of screening questions is provided in Vetter et al., 2008. If there are pertinent positive responses to screening questions, it is advisable to obtain an ECG and/or input from a cardiologist (Cortese et al., 2013; Perrin et al., 2008).

Follow-up monitoring should take place within a month of starting ADHD medications and occur frequently in the first year to review side effects and overall progress until consistent optimal response (ideally, functioning in the range of a typically developing child) is achieved. Subsequently, monitoring should occur at least twice yearly, including obtaining parent and teacher ADHD rating scales, as an increased frequency of obtaining rating scales has been linked to improved outcomes (Barbaresi et al., 2020a; Wolraich et al., 2019). With the rise of telehealth, clinicians, families, and teachers may find electronic systems helpful for collecting behavior rating scales and other information (Wolraich et al., 2019). In addition to regularly measuring heart rate and blood pressure, height and weight should be monitored throughout treatment as many ADHD medications can depress appetite. In addition, some but not all studies suggest that children treated with psychostimulants or atomoxetine may show mild linear growth suppression, underscoring the importance of tracking height (Froehlich et al., 2013).

Medication treatment outcomes. Pharmacological treatment for ADHD has been shown to improve current core symptoms and to some extent functioning (e.g., peer interactions, academic test performance and achievement). Medication treatment reduces the risk of important adverse coexisting conditions or circumstances such as criminality, antisocial behavior, depression, suicidality, substance use disorder, motor vehicle accidents, and other physical injuries (Barbaresi et al., 2020a; Chang et al., 2020).

Additional Intervention Considerations

Research has increasingly examined combined nonpharmacological and pharmacological approaches, as well as new areas for intervention.

Role of combined behavioral and medication therapy. For many highly salient outcomes—including oppositional, aggressive, and anxiety symptoms; parent–child conflict; academic difficulties; and social skills—combined behavioral and medication management (rather than either in isolation) achieves the best results. Combining medication and behavior treatment may also allow for optimal symptom control with lower medication doses (MTA Cooperative Group, 1999).

Role of lifestyle modifications. Individuals with ADHD frequently have sleep problems (Cortese et al., 2009), and shortened sleep duration is causally linked to greater inattentive symptoms and daytime impairments in adolescents with ADHD (Becker et al., 2019). There has thus been much interest in using behavioral sleep interventions to target sleep as well as ADHD symptoms and impairments. A large RCT found that a brief behavioral intervention improved sleep and daily functioning in pediatric ADHD (Hiscock et al., 2015), although a subsequent cluster-randomized translational trial with community clinicians found improvements in sleep but not child functioning (Hiscock et al., 2019). An open trial found a behavioral sleep intervention to improve sleep, ADHD symptoms, and other functional outcomes in adolescents with ADHD and co-occurring sleep problems (Becker, Duraccio, et al., 2022). Additional studies are needed to evaluate the role of sleep in the evidence-based treatment of ADHD.

Physical exercise may improve ADHD symptoms (Neudecker et al., 2019) and ADHD-related outcomes such as executive functions (Vysniauske et al., 2020). An RCT also found aerobic physical activity to reduce inattention and moodiness in the home setting as well as to improve some peer-directed behaviors among young children at risk for ADHD (Hoza et al., 2015). Nevertheless, given the limited research and design differences across studies, physical activity interventions may be useful as adjunctive treatment for pediatric ADHD (Hoza et al., 2016) but have questionable efficacy as a stand-alone treatment (S. W. Evans, Owens, et al., 2018).

A meta-analysis found small but significant effects for omega-3 supplements in reducing ADHD symptoms and larger effects for artificial food color exclusion, although often in individuals selected for food sensitivities (Sonuga-Barke et al., 2013). There is some evidence that supplementing zinc, iron, and magnesium may reduce ADHD symptoms in children with deficiencies in these minerals, although results across studies are inconsistent (Lange et al., 2017). Some children may benefit, but dietary and nutrition interventions lack support as frontline evidence-based ADHD treatments (Abdullah et al., 2019).

Developmental Science and Sociodemographic Considerations in Treatment

The appropriateness and effectiveness of evidence-based ADHD interventions vary according to many factors, including the developmental level, sex, race and ethnicity, and coexisting conditions of the pediatric patient.

Age. For preschool children, evidence-based parent and/or teacher-administered behavioral therapy are first-line treatment. The AAP ADHD guideline recommends medication treatment with MPH (which has a stronger evidence base than AMPH/DEX or GUA in this age group) only if there is moderate to severe continued impairment despite behavioral treatment. In preschool-aged children, MPH may be somewhat less effective and adverse effects more common than in older children (Wolraich et al., 2019). Based on clinical consensus and evidence from a large retrospective chart review study (Harstad et al., 2021), the Society for Developmental and Behavioral Pediatrics (SDBP) Complex ADHD guideline differs somewhat from that of the AAP in its preschool ADHD medication recommendations. The SDBP guideline advises that children with ADHD in this age group who have significant baseline irritability or mood disturbance use GUA and that those whose principal issue is hyperactivity be treated with MPH (Barbaresi et al., 2020a).

For 6- to 11-year-old children, first-line ADHD therapy includes FDA-approved ADHD medications, along with parent behavioral management training and behavioral classroom interventions (often including an individualized education program or 504 plan). In this age group, the evidence for ADHD medication efficacy is particularly strong for stimulant medications (both the MPH and AMPH/DEX families); it is adequate, but not as robust, for atomoxetine, extended-release GUA, and extended-release clonidine in that order (Wolraich et al., 2019).

For 12- to 18-year-old youth, treatment recommendations include FDA-approved ADHD medications, prescribed with the adolescent's consent, in addition to educational interventions and classroom supports (including direct instruction in use of a planner, study skills, note taking, and summarizing notes; Wolraich et al., 2019). Evidence-based training interventions (e.g., organization skills training) and/or behavioral interventions are encouraged to target academic and behavioral impairments respectively. However, clinicians should be aware that evidence for parent behavior training and behavioral classroom interventions is much stronger for children younger than 12 years of age than for older youth, and organizational skills training has stronger evidence for 9- to 18-year-olds than for younger children (Wolraich et al., 2019). Adolescents also differ from younger children in that they have lower adherence to ADHD treatment regimens, likely due to this age group's developmental drive for autonomy. Hence, for adolescents, strategies to promote engagement and motivation (e.g., motivational interviewing) may be helpful (Barbaresi et al., 2020a). In addition, use of long-acting ADHD medication formulations with once daily dosing can improve adherence and are also less likely to be misused or diverted (Mattingly et al., 2021).

Sex. Rates of ADHD treatment initiation and adherence/continuity are lower in girls than in boys with ADHD (Wolraich et al., 2019). This disparity may be due to girls typically presenting with fewer externalizing behaviors (i.e., hyperactivity–impulsivity and comorbid DBD symptoms) than boys, which is a strong predictor of ADHD medication use (Wolraich et al., 2019). It is important for ADHD treatment to be considered in girls, especially given evidence that adolescent girls with ADHD have elevated rates of self-injurious and suicidal behavior (Hinshaw et al., 2012), and ADHD medication treatment may decrease risk for suicidality (Chang et al., 2020).

Race and ethnicity. Medication treatment rates for ADHD are lower and attrition from ADHD psychosocial treatments is higher for ethnic minority children compared with non-Latinx White children. Reasons for these disparities may include that ethnic minority caregivers often view ADHD medication treatment as less acceptable, expect less benefit from treatment, and have reduced access to general health care services as well as to psychosocial treatments utilizing culturally sensitive approaches. Hence, clinicians should be cognizant that caregivers from different racial and ethnic backgrounds may have differing experiences with and perceptions about ADHD treatment, as well as differential access to health care services. Strategies such as motivational interviewing, efforts to reduce barriers to care, family navigator approaches (which offer social support and problem solving among peers), and enhanced coaching during behavior therapy have been proposed to improve family engagement in ADHD treatment for racial and ethnic minority groups (Barbaresi et al., 2020a; Slobodin & Masalha, 2020).

Role of coexisting conditions in treatment. Efficacy, adverse effects, and the strength of the evidence base for ADHD treatments can vary by coexisting conditions. Detailed recommendations for treating ADHD in the setting of co-occurring conditions are available in the SDBP Complex ADHD guideline and its process of care algorithms (Barbaresi et al., 2020a, 2020b), as well as in the

Texas Children's medication algorithms (Pliszka et al., 2006) and a review by Mattingly et al. (2021).

CONCLUSION

Due to its high prevalence and negative effects on a broad range of domains across the lifespan (including serious adverse effects on mental health, functioning within society, and even mortality risk), it is crucial that pediatric psychologists, developmental-behavioral practitioners, and allied professionals have the developmental-science-informed skills and knowledge needed to appropriately diagnose and treat ADHD and that developmental scientists continue to advance an understanding of its causes and manifestations. Importantly, ADHD is heterogeneous in its presentation and outcomes, and care is likewise not a one-size-fits-all proposition. Clinicians must adapt the diagnostic and treatment plan to each patient's unique circumstances, including their developmental stage, psychosocial context, and possible coexisting conditions. In addition, clinicians must address ADHD in a multipronged and interdisciplinary fashion that evaluates for and addresses co-occurring mental health and medical conditions, integrates behavioral interventions at home and school, and considers the role of medication treatments if appropriate and acceptable to the family.

RESOURCES

- Society for Developmental and Behavioral Pediatrics Clinical Practice Guideline

  https://sdbp.org/adhd-guideline/cag-guidelines/

- American Academy of Pediatrics Clinical Practice Guideline, Recommendations, and Quality Improvement Tools

  https://www.aap.org/en/patient-care/attention-deficit-hyperactivity-disorder-adhd/

- American Academy of Child and Adolescent Psychiatry ADHD [Attention-Deficit/Hyperactivity Disorder] Resource Center

  https://www.aacap.org/AACAP/Families_and_Youth/Resource_Centers/ADHD_Resource_Center/Home.aspx

- Society of Clinical Child and Adolescent Psychology Effective (nonpharmacological) Therapies for ADHD

  https://effectivechildtherapy.org/concerns-symptoms-disorders/disorders/inattention-and-hyperactivity-adhd/#effective-treatments

- Children and Adults With Attention-Deficit/Hyperactivity Disorder (CHADD)

  https://chadd.org/

- American Professional Society of ADHD and Related Disorders

  https://apsard.org/

- ADDitude (also includes webinars and other resources)

  https://www.additudemag.com/

- Attention (published by CHADD)

  https://chadd.org/get-attention-magazine/

- Podcasts (by CHADD)

  https://chadd.org/podcasts/

References

Abdullah, M., Jowett, B., Whittaker, P. J., & Patterson, L. (2019). The effectiveness of omega-3 supplementation in reducing ADHD associated symptoms in children as measured by the Conners' rating scales: A systematic review of randomized controlled trials. *Journal of Psychiatric Research*, *110*, 64–73. https://doi.org/10.1016/j.jpsychires.2018.12.002

Achenbach, T. M., & Rescorla, L. A. (2001). *Manual for the ASEBA school-age forms and profiles*. University of Vermont, Research Center for Children, Youth, and Families.

American Psychiatric Association. (2013). *Diagnostic and statistical manual of mental disorders* (5th ed.).

Anckarsäter, H., Stahlberg, O., Larson, T., Hakansson, C., Jutblad, S. B., Niklasson, L., Nydén, A., Wentz, E., Westergren, S., Cloninger, C. R., Gillberg, C., & Rastam, M. (2006). The impact of ADHD and autism spectrum disorders on temperament, character, and personality development. *The American Journal of Psychiatry*, *163*(7), 1239–1244. https://doi.org/10.1176/ajp.2006.163.7.1239

Andrews-Hanna, J. R., Reidler, J. S., Sepulcre, J., Poulin, R., & Buckner, R. L. (2010). Functional-anatomic fractionation of the brain's default network. *Neuron, 65*(4), 550–562. https://doi.org/10.1016/j.neuron.2010.02.005

Arnold, L. E., Arns, M., Barterian, J., Bergman, R., Black, S., Conners, C. K., Connor, S., Dasgupta, S., deBeus, R., Higgins, T., Hirshbeg, L., Hollway, J. A., Kerson, C., Lightstone, H., Lofthouse, N., Lubar, J., McBurnett, K., Monastra, V., Buchan-Page, K., . . . William, C. E. (2021). Double-blind placebo-controlled randomized clinical trial of neurofeedback for attention-deficit/hyperactivity disorder with 13-month follow-up. *Journal of the American Academy of Child & Adolescent Psychiatry, 60*(7), 841–855. https://doi.org/10.1016/j.jaac.2020.07.906

Ayonrinde, O. T., Ayonrinde, O. A., Van Rooyen, D., Tait, R., Dunn, M., Mehta, S., White, S., & Ayonrinde, O. K. (2021). Association between gestational cannabis exposure and maternal, perinatal, placental, and childhood outcomes. *Journal of Developmental Origins of Health and Disease, 12*(5), 694–703. https://doi.org/10.1017/S2040174420001166

Banaschewski, T., Becker, K., Döpfner, M., Holtmann, M., Rösler, M., & Romanos, M. (2017). Attention-deficit/hyperactivity disorder. *Deutsches Ärzteblatt International, 114*(9), 149–159. https://doi.org/10.3238/arztebl.2017.0149

Barbaresi, W. J., Campbell, L., Diekroger, E. A., Froehlich, T. E., Liu, Y. H., O'Malley, E., Pelham, W. E., Jr., Power, T. J., Zinner, S. H., & Chan, E. (2020a). Society for Developmental and Behavioral Pediatrics clinical practice guideline for the assessment and treatment of children and adolescents with complex attention-deficit/hyperactivity disorder. *Journal of Developmental and Behavioral Pediatrics, 41*(Suppl. 2), S35–S57. https://doi.org/10.1097/DBP.0000000000000770

Barbaresi, W. J., Campbell, L., Diekroger, E. A., Froehlich, T. E., Liu, Y. H., O'Malley, E., Pelham, W. E., Jr., Power, T. J., Zinner, S. H., & Chan, E. (2020b). The Society for Developmental and Behavioral Pediatrics clinical practice guideline for the assessment and treatment of children and adolescents with complex attention-deficit/hyperactivity disorder: Process of care algorithms. *Journal of Developmental and Behavioral Pediatrics, 41*(Suppl. 2), S58–S74. https://doi.org/10.1097/DBP.0000000000000781

Barbaresi, W. J., Colligan, R. C., Weaver, A. L., Voigt, R. G., Killian, J. M., & Katusic, S. K. (2013). Mortality, ADHD, and psychosocial adversity in adults with childhood ADHD: A prospective study. *Pediatrics, 131*(4), 637–644. https://doi.org/10.1542/peds.2012-2354

Barkley, R. A. (1997). Behavioral inhibition, sustained attention, and executive functions: Constructing a unifying theory of ADHD. *Psychological Bulletin, 121*(1), 65–94. https://doi.org/10.1037/0033-2909.121.1.65

Barkley, R. A. (2015). *Attention-deficit hyperactivity disorder: A handbook for diagnosis and treatment* (4th ed.). Guilford Press.

Becker, S. P. (Ed.). (2020). *ADHD in adolescents: Development, assessment, and treatment*. Guilford Press.

Becker, S. P., & Barkley, R. A. (2021). Field of daydreams? Integrating mind wandering in the study of sluggish cognitive tempo and ADHD. *JCPP Advances, 1*(1), e12002. https://doi.org/10.1111/jcv2.12002

Becker, S. P., Duraccio, K. M., Sidol, C. A., Fershtman, C. E. M., Byars, K. C., & Harvey, A. G. (2022). Impact of a behavioral sleep intervention in adolescents with ADHD: Feasibility, acceptability, and preliminary effectiveness from a pilot open trial. *Journal of Attention Disorders, 26*(7), 1051–1066. https://doi.org/10.1177/10870547211056965

Becker, S. P., Epstein, J. N., Tamm, L., Tilford, A. A., Tischner, C. M., Isaacson, P. A., Simon, J. O., & Beebe, D. W. (2019). Shortened sleep duration causes sleepiness, inattention, and oppositionality in adolescents with attention-deficit/hyperactivity disorder: Findings from a crossover sleep restriction/extension study. *Journal of the American Academy of Child & Adolescent Psychiatry, 58*(4), 433–442. https://doi.org/10.1016/j.jaac.2018.09.439

Becker, S. P., Fredrick, J. W., Foster, J. A., Yeaman, K. M., Epstein, J. N., Froehlich, T. E., & Mitchell, J. T. (2022). "My mom calls it Annaland": A qualitative study of phenomenology, daily life impacts, and treatment considerations of sluggish cognitive tempo. *Journal of Attention Disorders, 26*(6), 915–931. https://doi.org/10.1177/10870547211050946

Becker, S. P., Leopold, D. R., Burns, G. L., Jarrett, M. A., Langberg, J. M., Marshall, S. A., McBurnett, K., Waschbusch, D. A., & Willcutt, E. G. (2016). The internal, external, and diagnostic validity of sluggish cognitive tempo: A meta-analysis and critical review. *Journal of the American Academy of Child & Adolescent Psychiatry, 55*(3), 163–178. https://doi.org/10.1016/j.jaac.2015.12.006

Becker, S. P., Willcutt, E. G., Leopold, D. R., Fredrick, J. W., Smith, Z. R., Jacobson, L. A., Burns, G. L., Mayes, S. D., Waschbusch, D. A., Froehlich, T. E., McBurnett, K., Servera, M., & Barkley, R. A. (2023). Report of a work group on sluggish cognitive tempo: Key research directions and a consensus change in terminology to cognitive disengagement syndrome. *Journal of the American Academy of Child & Adolescent Psychiatry, 62*(6), 630–645. https://doi.org/10.1016/j.jaac.2022.07.821

Biederman, J., Mick, E., & Faraone, S. V. (2000). Age-dependent decline of symptoms of attention deficit hyperactivity disorder: Impact of remission definition and symptom type. *The American Journal of Psychiatry*, 157(5), 816–818. https://doi.org/10.1176/appi.ajp.157.5.816

Bolikal, P. D., Narad, M., Raj, S., Kennelly, M., & Kurowski, B. G. (2021). Biopsychosocial factors associated with attention problems in children after traumatic brain injury: A systematic review. *American Journal of Physical Medicine & Rehabilitation*, 100(3), 215–228. https://doi.org/10.1097/PHM.0000000000001643

Breckenridge, K., Braddick, O., & Atkinson, J. (2013). The organization of attention in typical development: A new preschool attention test battery. *British Journal of Developmental Psychology*, 31(3), 271–288. https://doi.org/10.1111/bjdp.12004

Broulidakis, M. J., Golm, D., Cortese, S., Fairchild, G., & Sonuga-Barke, E. (2022). Default mode network connectivity and attention-deficit/hyperactivity disorder in adolescence: Associations with delay aversion and temporal discounting, but not mind wandering. *International Journal of Psychophysiology*, 173, 38–44. https://doi.org/10.1016/j.ijpsycho.2022.01.007

Cairncross, M., & Miller, C. J. (2020). The effectiveness of mindfulness-based therapies for ADHD: A meta-analytic review. *Journal of Attention Disorders*, 24(5), 627–643. https://doi.org/10.1177/1087054715625301

Caye, A., Petresco, S., de Barros, A. J. D., Bressan, R. A., Gadelha, A., Gonçalves, H., Manfro, A. G., Matijasevich, A., Menezes, A. M. B., Miguel, E. C., Munhoz, T. N., Pan, P. M., Salum, G. A., Santos, I. S., Kieling, C., & Rohde, L. A. (2020). Relative age and attention-deficit/hyperactivity disorder: Data from three epidemiological cohorts and a meta-analysis. *Journal of the American Academy of Child & Adolescent Psychiatry*, 59(8), 990–997. https://doi.org/10.1016/j.jaac.2019.07.939

Chang, Z., Quinn, P. D., O'Reilly, L., Sjölander, A., Hur, K., Gibbons, R., Larsson, H., & D'Onofrio, B. M. (2020). Medication for attention-deficit/hyperactivity disorder and risk for suicide attempts. *Biological Psychiatry*, 88(6), 452–458. https://doi.org/10.1016/j.biopsych.2019.12.003

Childress, A. C., & Stark, J. G. (2018). Diagnosis and treatment of attention-deficit/hyperactivity disorder in preschool-aged children. *Journal of Child and Adolescent Psychopharmacology*, 28(9), 606–614. https://doi.org/10.1089/cap.2018.0057

Conners, K. C. (2008). *Conners 3rd edition manual*. Pearson. https://www.pearsonassessments.com/store/usassessments/en/Store/Professional-Assessments/Behavior/Comprehensive/Conners-3rd-Edition/p/100000523.html

Cortese, S., Adamo, N., Del Giovane, C., Mohr-Jensen, C., Hayes, A. J., Carucci, S., Atkinson, L. Z., Tessari, L., Banaschewski, T., Coghill, D., Hollis, C., Simonoff, E., Zuddas, A., Barbui, C., Purgato, M., Steinhausen, H. C., Shokraneh, F., Xia, J., & Cipriani, A. (2018). Comparative efficacy and tolerability of medications for attention-deficit hyperactivity disorder in children, adolescents, and adults: A systematic review and network meta-analysis. *The Lancet Psychiatry*, 5(9), 727–738. https://doi.org/10.1016/S2215-0366(18)30269-4

Cortese, S., Faraone, S. V., Konofal, E., & Lecendreux, M. (2009). Sleep in children with attention-deficit/hyperactivity disorder: Meta-analysis of subjective and objective studies. *Journal of the American Academy of Child & Adolescent Psychiatry*, 48(9), 894–908. https://doi.org/10.1097/CHI.0b013e3181ae09c9

Cortese, S., Ferrin, M., Brandeis, D., Buitelaar, J., Daley, D., Dittmann, R. W., Holtmann, M., Santosh, P., Stevenson, J., Stringaris, A., Zuddas, A., & Sonuga-Barke, E. J. (2015). Cognitive training for attention-deficit/hyperactivity disorder: Meta-analysis of clinical and neuropsychological outcomes from randomized controlled trials. *Journal of the American Academy of Child & Adolescent Psychiatry*, 54(3), 164–174. https://doi.org/10.1016/j.jaac.2014.12.010

Cortese, S., Holtmann, M., Banaschewski, T., Buitelaar, J., Coghill, D., Danckaerts, M., Dittmann, R. W., Graham, J., Taylor, E., & Sergeant, J. (2013). Practitioner review: Current best practice in the management of adverse events during treatment with ADHD medications in children and adolescents. *Journal of Child Psychology and Psychiatry*, 54(3), 227–246. https://doi.org/10.1111/jcpp.12036

Côté, S., Tremblay, R. E., Nagin, D., Zoccolillo, M., & Vitaro, F. (2002). The development of impulsivity, fearfulness, and helpfulness during childhood: Patterns of consistency and change in the trajectories of boys and girls. *Journal of Child Psychology and Psychiatry*, 43(5), 609–618. https://doi.org/10.1111/1469-7610.00050

Daley, D., van der Oord, S., Ferrin, M., Danckaerts, M., Doepfner, M., Cortese, S., Sonuga-Barke, E. J. S., & the European ADHD Guidelines Group. (2014). Behavioral interventions in attention-deficit/hyperactivity disorder: A meta-analysis of randomized controlled trials across multiple outcome domains. *Journal of the American Academy of Child & Adolescent Psychiatry*, 53(8), 835–847.e5. https://doi.org/10.1016/j.jaac.2014.05.013

Danielson, M. L., Bitsko, R. H., Ghandour, R. M., Holbrook, J. R., Kogan, M. D., & Blumberg, S. J.

(2018). Prevalence of parent-reported ADHD diagnosis and associated treatment among U.S. children and adolescents, 2016. *Journal of Clinical Child and Adolescent Psychology, 47*(2), 199–212. https://doi.org/10.1080/15374416.2017.1417860

Degremont, A., Jain, R., Philippou, E., & Latunde-Dada, G. O. (2021). Brain iron concentrations in the pathophysiology of children with attention deficit/hyperactivity disorder: A systematic review. *Nutrition Reviews, 79*(5), 615–626. https://doi.org/10.1093/nutrit/nuaa065

Demontis, D., Walters, R. K., Martin, J., Mattheisen, M., Als, T. D., Agerbo, E., Baldursson, G., Belliveau, R., Bybjerg-Grauholm, J., Bækvad-Hansen, M., Cerrato, F., Chambert, K., Churchhouse, C., Dumont, A., Eriksson, N., Gandal, M., Goldstein, J. I., Grasby, K. L., Grove, J., . . . Neale, B. M. (2019). Discovery of the first genome-wide significant risk loci for attention deficit/hyperactivity disorder. *Nature Genetics, 51*(1), 63–75. https://doi.org/10.1038/s41588-018-0269-7

Di Lorenzo, R., Balducci, J., Poppi, C., Arcolin, E., Cutino, A., Ferri, P., D'Amico, R., & Filippini, T. (2021). Children and adolescents with ADHD followed up to adulthood: A systematic review of long-term outcomes. *Acta Neuropsychiatrica, 33*(6), 283–298. https://doi.org/10.1017/neu.2021.23

Dong, Q., Garcia, B., Pham, A. V., & Cumming, M. (2020). Culturally responsive approaches for addressing ADHD within multi-tiered systems of support. *Current Psychiatry Reports, 22*(6), 27. https://doi.org/10.1007/s11920-020-01154-3

DuPaul, G. J., Gormley, M. J., & Laracy, S. D. (2013). Comorbidity of LD and ADHD: Implications of *DSM-5* for assessment and treatment. *Journal of Learning Disabilities, 46*(1), 43–51. https://doi.org/10.1177/0022219412464351

DuPaul, G. J., Power, T. J., Anastopoulos, A. D., & Reid, R. (2016). *ADHD Rating Scale-5 for children and adolescents: Checklists, norms, and clinical interpretation.* Guilford Press.

Edinoff, A. N., Akuly, H. A., Wagner, J. H., Boudreaux, M. A., Kaplan, L. A., Yusuf, S., Neuchat, E. E., Cornett, E. M., Boyer, A. G., Kaye, A. M., & Kaye, A. D. (2021). Viloxazine in the treatment of attention deficit hyperactivity disorder. *Frontiers in Psychiatry, 12*, 789982. https://doi.org/10.3389/fpsyt.2021.789982

Effatpanah, M., Rezaei, M., Effatpanah, H., Effatpanah, Z., Varkaneh, H. K., Mousavi, S. M., Fatahi, S., Rinaldi, G., & Hashemi, R. (2019). Magnesium status and attention deficit hyperactivity disorder (ADHD): A meta-analysis. *Psychiatry Research, 274*, 228–234. https://doi.org/10.1016/j.psychres.2019.02.043

Evans, S., Ling, M., Hill, B., Rinehart, N., Austin, D., & Sciberras, E. (2018). Systematic review of meditation-based interventions for children with ADHD. *European Child & Adolescent Psychiatry, 27*(1), 9–27. https://doi.org/10.1007/s00787-017-1008-9

Evans, S. W., Owens, J. S., Wymbs, B. T., & Ray, A. R. (2018). Evidence-based psychosocial treatments for children and adolescents with attention deficit/hyperactivity disorder. *Journal of Clinical Child and Adolescent Psychology, 47*(2), 157–198. https://doi.org/10.1080/15374416.2017.1390757

Fabiano, G. A., Pelham, W. E., Jr., Waschbusch, D. A., Gnagy, E. M., Lahey, B. B., Chronis, A. M., Onyango, A. N., Kipp, H., Lopez-Williams, A., & Burrows-Maclean, L. (2006). A practical measure of impairment: Psychometric properties of the impairment rating scale in samples of children with attention deficit hyperactivity disorder and two school-based samples. *Journal of Clinical Child and Adolescent Psychology, 35*(3), 369–385. https://doi.org/10.1207/s15374424jccp3503_3

Fadus, M. C., Ginsburg, K. R., Sobowale, K., Halliday-Boykins, C. A., Bryant, B. E., Gray, K. M., & Squeglia, L. M. (2020). Unconscious bias and the diagnosis of disruptive behavior disorders and ADHD in African American and Hispanic youth. *Academic Psychiatry, 44*(1), 95–102. https://doi.org/10.1007/s40596-019-01127-6

Fox, K. C., Spreng, R. N., Ellamil, M., Andrews-Hanna, J. R., & Christoff, K. (2015). The wandering brain: Meta-analysis of functional neuroimaging studies of mind-wandering and related spontaneous thought processes. *NeuroImage, 111*, 611–621. https://doi.org/10.1016/j.neuroimage.2015.02.039

Froehlich, T. E., Delgado, S. V., & Anixt, J. S. (2013). Expanding medication options for pediatric ADHD. *Current Psychiatry, 12*(12), 20–29. https://www.ncbi.nlm.nih.gov/pmc/articles/PMC4296564/

Froehlich, T. E., Lanphear, B. P., Epstein, J. N., Barbaresi, W. J., Katusic, S. K., & Kahn, R. S. (2007). Prevalence, recognition, and treatment of attention-deficit/hyperactivity disorder in a national sample of US children. *Archives of Pediatrics & Adolescent Medicine, 161*(9), 857–864. https://doi.org/10.1001/archpedi.161.9.857

Garnock-Jones, K. P., & Keating, G. M. (2009). Atomoxetine: A review of its use in attention-deficit hyperactivity disorder in children and adolescents. *Paediatric Drugs, 11*(3), 203–226. https://doi.org/10.2165/00148581-200911030-00005

Gilliam, W. S. (2005). *Pre-kindergarteners left behind: Expulsion rates in state pre-kindergarten systems.* Yale University Child Study Center. https://www.fcd-us.org/wp-content/uploads/2016/04/ExpulsionCompleteReport.pdf

Gray, S. A. O., Carter, A. S., Briggs-Gowan, M. J., Jones, S. M., & Wagmiller, R. L. (2014). Growth trajectories of early aggression, overactivity, and inattention: Relations to second-grade reading. *Developmental Psychology*, *50*(9), 2255–2263. https://doi.org/10.1037/a0037367

Harpin, V. A. (2005). The effect of ADHD on the life of an individual, their family, and community from preschool to adult life. *Archives of Disease in Childhood*, *90*, i2–i7. https://doi.org/10.1136/adc.2004.059006

Harstad, E., Shults, J., Barbaresi, W., Bax, A., Cacia, J., Deavenport-Saman, A., Friedman, S., LaRosa, A., Loe, I. M., Mittal, S., Tulio, S., Vanderbilt, D., & Blum, N. J. (2021). α$_2$-adrenergic agonists or stimulants for preschool-age children with attention-deficit/hyperactivity disorder. *JAMA: Journal of the American Medical Association*, *325*(20), 2067–2075. https://doi.org/10.1001/jama.2021.6118

Harvey, E. A., Metcalfe, L. A., Herbert, S. D., & Fanton, J. H. (2011). The role of family experiences and ADHD in the early development of oppositional defiant disorder. *Journal of Consulting and Clinical Psychology*, *79*(6), 784–795. https://doi.org/10.1037/a0025672

Hinshaw, S. P., Owens, E. B., Zalecki, C., Huggins, S. P., Montenegro-Nevado, A. J., Schrodek, E., & Swanson, E. N. (2012). Prospective follow-up of girls with attention-deficit/hyperactivity disorder into early adulthood: Continuing impairment includes elevated risk for suicide attempts and self-injury. *Journal of Consulting and Clinical Psychology*, *80*(6), 1041–1051. https://doi.org/10.1037/a0029451

Hiscock, H., Mulraney, M., Heussler, H., Rinehart, N., Schuster, T., Grobler, A. C., Gold, L., Bohingamu Mudiyanselage, S., Hayes, N., & Sciberras, E. (2019). Impact of a behavioral intervention, delivered by pediatricians or psychologists, on sleep problems in children with ADHD: A cluster-randomized, translational trial. *Journal of Child Psychology and Psychiatry*, *60*(11), 1230–1241. https://doi.org/10.1111/jcpp.13083

Hiscock, H., Sciberras, E., Mensah, F., Gerner, B., Efron, D., Khano, S., & Oberklaid, F. (2015). Impact of a behavioural sleep intervention on symptoms and sleep in children with attention deficit hyperactivity disorder, and parental mental health: Randomised controlled trial. *BMJ: British Medical Journal*, *350*, h68. https://doi.org/10.1136/bmj.h68

Hoza, B., Martin, C. P., Pirog, A., & Shoulberg, E. K. (2016). Using physical activity to manage ADHD symptoms: The state of the evidence. *Current Psychiatry Reports*, *18*(12), 113. https://doi.org/10.1007/s11920-016-0749-3

Hoza, B., Smith, A. L., Shoulberg, E. K., Linnea, K. S., Dorsch, T. E., Blazo, J. A., Alerding, C. M., & McCabe, G. P. (2015). A randomized trial examining the effects of aerobic physical activity on attention-deficit/hyperactivity disorder symptoms in young children. *Journal of Abnormal Child Psychology*, *43*(4), 655–667. https://doi.org/10.1007/s10802-014-9929-y

Huang, A., Wu, K., Cai, Z., Lin, Y., Zhang, X., & Huang, Y. (2021). Association between postnatal second-hand smoke exposure and ADHD in children: A systematic review and meta-analysis. *Environmental Science and Pollution Research International*, *28*(2), 1370–1380. https://doi.org/10.1007/s11356-020-11269-y

Hunt, T. K. A., Slack, K. S., & Berger, L. M. (2017). Adverse childhood experiences and behavioral problems in middle childhood. *Child Abuse & Neglect*, *67*, 391–402. https://doi.org/10.1016/j.chiabu.2016.11.005

Keeshin, B., Forkey, H. C., Fouras, G., MacMillan, H. L., American Academy of Pediatrics, Council on Child Abuse and Neglect, Council on Foster Care, Adoption, and Kinship Care, American Academy of Child and Adolescent Psychiatry, Committee on Child Maltreatment and Violence, & Committee on Adoption and Foster Care. (2020). Children exposed to maltreatment: Assessment and the role of psychotropic medication. *Pediatrics*, *145*(2), e20193751. https://doi.org/10.1542/peds.2019-3751

Langberg, J. M., Froehlich, T. E., Loren, R. E., Martin, J. E., & Epstein, J. N. (2008). Assessing children with ADHD in primary care settings. *Expert Review of Neurotherapeutics*, *8*(4), 627–641. https://doi.org/10.1586/14737175.8.4.627

Lange, K. W., Hauser, J., Lange, K. M., Makulska-Gertruda, E., Nakamura, Y., Reissmann, A., Sakaue, Y., Takano, T., & Takeuchi, Y. (2017). The role of nutritional supplements in the treatment of ADHD: What the evidence says. *Current Psychiatry Reports*, *19*(2), 8. https://doi.org/10.1007/s11920-017-0762-1

Larsson, H., Dilshad, R., Lichtenstein, P., & Barker, E. D. (2011). Developmental trajectories of *DSM-IV* symptoms of attention-deficit/hyperactivity disorder: Genetic effects, family risk and associated psychopathology. *Journal of Child Psychology and Psychiatry* *52*(9), 954–963. https://doi.org/10.1111/j.1469-7610.2011.02379.x

Leblanc, N., Boivin, M., Dionne, G., Brendgen, M., Vitaro, F., Tremblay, R. E., & Pérusse, D. (2008). The development of hyperactive–impulsive behaviors during the preschool years: The predictive validity of parental assessments. *Journal of Abnormal Child Psychology*, *36*(7), 977–987. https://doi.org/10.1007/s10802-008-9227-7

Manly, T., Anderson, V., Nimmo-Smith, I., Turner, A., Watson, P., & Robertson, I. H. (2001). The differential assessment of children's attention: The Test of Everyday Attention for Children (TEA-Ch), normative sample and ADHD performance. *Journal of Child Psychology and Psychiatry, and Allied Disciplines*, 42(8), 1065–1081. https://doi.org/10.1111/1469-7610.00806

Marx, I., Hacker, T., Yu, X., Cortese, S., & Sonuga-Barke, E. (2021). ADHD and the choice of small immediate over larger delayed rewards: A comparative meta-analysis of performance on simple choice-delay and temporal discounting paradigms. *Journal of Attention Disorders*, 25(2), 171–187. https://doi.org/10.1177/1087054718772138

Mattingly, G. W., Wilson, J., Ugarte, L., & Glaser, P. (2021). Individualization of attention-deficit/hyperactivity disorder treatment: Pharmacotherapy considerations by age and co-occurring conditions. *CNS Spectrums*, 26(3), 202–221. https://doi.org/10.1017/S1092852919001822

Mikami, A. Y., Normand, S., Hudec, K. L., Guiet, J., Na, J. J., Smit, S., Khalis, A., & Maisonneuve, M.-F. (2020). Treatment of friendship problems in children with attention-deficit/hyperactivity disorder: Initial results from a randomized clinical trial. *Journal of Consulting and Clinical Psychology*, 88(10), 871–885. https://doi.org/10.1037/ccp0000607

Mikami, A. Y., Owens, J. S., Evans, S. W., Hudec, K. L., Kassab, H., Smit, S., & Khalis, A. (2022). Promoting classroom social and academic functioning among children at risk for ADHD: The MOSAIC program. *Journal of Clinical Child and Adolescent Psychology*, 1(6), 1039–1052.

Mikami, A. Y., Smit, S., & Khalis, A. (2017). Social skills training and ADHD—What works? *Current Psychiatry Reports*, 19(12), 93. https://doi.org/10.1007/s11920-017-0850-2

Minatoya, M., & Kishi, R. (2021). A review of recent studies on bisphenol A and phthalate exposures and child neurodevelopment. *International Journal of Environmental Research and Public Health*, 18(7), 3585. https://doi.org/10.3390/ijerph18073585

Molina, B. S. G., Pelham, W. E., Cheong, J., Marshal, M. P., Gnagy, E. M., & Curran, P. J. (2012). Childhood attention-deficit/hyperactivity disorder (ADHD) and growth in adolescent alcohol use: The roles of functional impairments, ADHD symptom persistence, and parental knowledge. *Journal of Abnormal Psychology*, 121(4), 922–935. https://doi.org/10.1037/a0028260

MTA Cooperative Group. (1999). A 14-month randomized clinical trial of treatment strategies for attention-deficit/hyperactivity disorder. *Archives of General Psychiatry*, 56(12), 1073–1086. https://doi.org/10.1001/archpsyc.56.12.1073

Mulligan, A., Anney, R. J., O'Regan, M., Chen, W., Butler, L., Fitzgerald, M., Buitelaar, J., Steinhausen, H. C., Rothenberger, A., Minderaa, R., Nijmeijer, J., Hoekstra, P. J., Oades, R. D., Roeyers, H., Buschgens, C., Christiansen, H., Franke, B., Gabriels, I., Hartman, C., . . . Gill, M. (2009). Autism symptoms in attention-deficit/hyperactivity disorder: A familial trait which correlates with conduct, oppositional defiant, language and motor disorders. *Journal of Autism and Developmental Disorders*, 39(2), 197–209. https://doi.org/10.1007/s10803-008-0621-3

Neudecker, C., Mewes, N., Reimers, A. K., & Woll, A. (2019). Exercise interventions in children and adolescents with ADHD: A systematic review. *Journal of Attention Disorders*, 23(4), 307–324. https://doi.org/10.1177/1087054715584053

Nigg, J. T. (2017). Annual Research Review: On the relations among self-regulation, self-control, executive functioning, effortful control, cognitive control, impulsivity, risk-taking, and inhibition for developmental psychopathology. *Journal of Child Psychology and Psychiatry*, 58(4), 361–383. https://doi.org/10.1111/jcpp.12675

Nilsen, F. M., & Tulve, N. S. (2020). A systematic review and meta-analysis examining the interrelationships between chemical and non-chemical stressors and inherent characteristics in children with ADHD. *Environmental Research*, 180, 108884. https://doi.org/10.1016/j.envres.2019.108884

Nygaard, E., Slinning, K., Moe, V., & Walhovd, K. B. (2016). Behavior and attention problems in eight-year-old children with prenatal opiate and poly-substance exposure: A longitudinal study. *PLOS ONE*, 11(6), e0158054. https://doi.org/10.1371/journal.pone.0158054

Olaniyan, O., dosReis, S., Garriett, V., Mychailyszyn, M. P., Anixt, J., Rowe, P. C., & Cheng, T. L. (2007). Community perspectives of childhood behavioral problems and ADHD among African American parents. *Ambulatory Pediatrics*, 7(3), 226–231. https://doi.org/10.1016/j.ambp.2007.02.002

Olson, S. L., Schilling, E. M., & Bates, J. E. (1999). Measurement of impulsivity: Construct coherence, longitudinal stability, and relationship with externalizing problems in middle childhood and adolescence. *Journal of Abnormal Child Psychology*, 27(2), 151–165. https://doi.org/10.1023/A:1021915615677

Palladino, V. S., McNeill, R., Reif, A., & Kittel-Schneider, S. (2019). Genetic risk factors and gene-environment interactions in adult and childhood attention-deficit/hyperactivity disorder. *Psychiatric Genetics, 29*(3), 63–78. https://doi.org/10.1097/YPG.0000000000000220

Pennington, B. F., & Ozonoff, S. (1996). Executive functions and developmental psychopathology. *Journal of Child Psychology and Psychiatry, 37*(1), 51–87. https://doi.org/10.1111/j.1469-7610.1996.tb01380.x

Perrin, J. M., Friedman, R. A., Knilans, T. K., the Black Box Working Group, & the Section on Cardiology and Cardiac Surgery. (2008). Cardiovascular monitoring and stimulant drugs for attention-deficit/hyperactivity disorder. *Pediatrics, 122*(2), 451–453. https://doi.org/10.1542/peds.2008-1573

Pfiffner, L. J., & DuPaul, G. J. (2015). Treatment of ADHD in school settings. In R. A. Barkley (Ed.), *Attention-deficit hyperactivity disorder: A handbook for diagnosis and treatment* (4th ed., pp. 596–629). Guilford Press.

Pliszka, S. R., Crismon, M. L., Hughes, C. W., Corners, C. K., Emslie, G. J., Jensen, P. S., McCracken, J. T., Swanson, J. M., Lopez, M., & the Texas Consensus Conference Panel on Pharmacotherapy of Childhood Attention Deficit Hyperactivity Disorder. (2006). The Texas Children's Medication Algorithm Project: Revision of the algorithm for pharmacotherapy of attention-deficit/hyperactivity disorder. *Journal of the American Academy of Child & Adolescent Psychiatry, 45*(6), 642–657. https://doi.org/10.1097/01.chi.0000215326.51175.eb

Pozzi, M., Carnovale, C., Peeters, G. G. A. M., Gentili, M., Antoniazzi, S., Radice, S., Clementi, E., & Nobile, M. (2018). Adverse drug events related to mood and emotion in paediatric patients treated for ADHD: A meta-analysis. *Journal of Affective Disorders, 238,* 161–178. https://doi.org/10.1016/j.jad.2018.05.021

Putnam, S. P., Rothbart, M. K., & Gartstein, M. A. (2008). Homotypic and heterotypic continuity of fine-grained temperament during infancy, toddlerhood, and early childhood. *Infant and Child Development, 17*(4), 387–405. https://doi.org/10.1002/icd.582

Rahmani, E., Mahvelati, A., Alizadeh, A., Mokhayeri, Y., Rahmani, M., Zarabi, H., & Hassanvandi, S. (2022). Is neurofeedback effective in children with ADHD? A systematic review and meta-analysis. *Neurocase, 28*(1), 84–95. https://doi.org/10.1080/13554794.2022.2027456

Reynolds, C. R., & Kamphaus, R. W. (2015). *Behavioral assessment system for children* (3rd ed.). Pearson.

Riddle, T., & Sinclair, S. (2019). Racial disparities in school-based disciplinary actions are associated with county-level rates of racial bias. *Proceedings of the National Academy of Sciences of the United States of America, 116*(17), 8255–8260. https://doi.org/10.1073/pnas.1808307116

Rosen, P. J., Froehlich, T. E., Langberg, J. M., & Epstein, J. N. (2011). Assessment of comorbid conditions. In B. Hoza & S. Evans (Eds.), *Attention deficit hyperactivity disorder: State of the science and best practices* (Vol. 2, pp. 1–19). Civic Research Institute.

Ruff, H. A., & Capozzoli, M. C. (2003). Development of attention and distractibility in the first 4 years of life. *Developmental Psychology, 39*(5), 877–890. https://doi.org/10.1037/0012-1649.39.5.877

Ruff, H. A., & Rothbart, M. K. (2001). *Attention in early development: Themes and variations.* Oxford University Press. https://doi.org/10.1093/acprof:oso/9780195136326.001.0001

Sasser, T. R., Kalvin, C. B., & Bierman, K. L. (2016). Developmental trajectories of clinically significant attention-deficit/hyperactivity disorder (ADHD) symptoms from grade 3 through 12 in a high-risk sample: Predictors and outcomes. *Journal of Abnormal Psychology, 125*(2), 207–219. https://doi.org/10.1037/abn0000112

Serati, M., Barkin, J. L., Orsenigo, G., Altamura, A. C., & Buoli, M. (2017). Research Review: The role of obstetric and neonatal complications in childhood attention deficit and hyperactivity disorder—A systematic review. *Journal of Child Psychology and Psychiatry, 58*(12), 1290–1300. https://doi.org/10.1111/jcpp.12779

Shiner, R. L., Buss, K. A., McClowry, S. G., Putnam, S. P., Saudino, K. J., & Zentner, M. (2012). What is temperament now? Assessing progress in temperament research on the twenty-fifth anniversary of Goldsmith et al. *Child Development Perspectives, 6*(4), 436–444. https://doi.org/10.1111/j.1750-8606.2012.00254.x

Sibley, M. H., Pelham, W. E., Molina, B. S. G., Gnagy, E. M., Waschbusch, D. A., Garefino, A. C., Kuriyan, A. B., Babinski, D. E., & Karch, K. M. (2012). Diagnosing ADHD in adolescence. *Journal of Consulting and Clinical Psychology, 80*(1), 139–150. https://doi.org/10.1037/a0026577

Slobodin, O., & Masalha, R. (2020). Challenges in ADHD care for ethnic minority children: A review of the current literature. *Transcultural Psychiatry, 57*(3), 468–483. https://doi.org/10.1177/1363461520902885

Sonuga-Barke, E., Bitsakou, P., & Thompson, M. (2010). Beyond the dual pathway model: Evidence for the dissociation of timing, inhibitory, and delay-related impairments in attention-deficit/hyperactivity disorder. *Journal of the American Academy of Child & Adolescent Psychiatry, 49*(4), 345–355. https://doi.org/10.1016/j.jaac.2009.12.018

Sonuga-Barke, E. J. S. (2002). Psychological heterogeneity in AD/HD—A dual pathway model of behaviour and cognition. *Behavioural Brain Research, 130*(1–2), 29–36. https://doi.org/10.1016/S0166-4328(01)00432-6

Sonuga-Barke, E. J. S. (2003). The dual pathway model of AD/HD: An elaboration of neuro-developmental characteristics. *Neuroscience and Biobehavioral Reviews, 27*(7), 593–604. https://doi.org/10.1016/j.neubiorev.2003.08.005

Sonuga-Barke, E. J. S., Becker, S. P., Bölte, S., Castellanos, F. X., Franke, B., Newcorn, J. H., Nigg, J. T., Rohde, L. A., & Simonoff, E. (2023). Annual Research Review: Perspectives on progress in ADHD science—From characterization to cause. *Journal of Child Psychology and Psychiatry, 64*(4), 506–532. https://doi.org/10.1111/jcpp.13696

Sonuga-Barke, E. J. S., Brandeis, D., Cortese, S., Daley, D., Ferrin, M., Holtmann, M., Stevenson, J., Danckaerts, M., van der Oord, S., Döpfner, M., Dittmann, R. W., Simonoff, E., Zuddas, A., Banaschewski, T., Buitelaar, J., Coghill, D., Hollis, C., Konofal, E., Lecendreux, M., . . . the European ADHD Guidelines Group. (2013). Nonpharmacological interventions for ADHD: Systematic review and meta-analyses of randomized controlled trials of dietary and psychological treatments. *The American Journal of Psychiatry, 170*(3), 275–289. https://doi.org/10.1176/appi.ajp.2012.12070991

Staats, C. (2014). *Implicit racial bias and school discipline disparities: Exploring the connection.* Kirwan Institute. https://kirwaninstitute.osu.edu/sites/default/files/documents/ki-ib-argument-piece03.pdf

Sudre, G., Sharp, W., Kundzicz, P., Bouyssi-Kobar, M., Norman, L., Choudhury, S., & Shaw, P. (2021). Predicting the course of ADHD symptoms through the integration of childhood genomic, neural, and cognitive features. *Molecular Psychiatry, 26*(8), 4046–4054. https://doi.org/10.1038/s41380-020-00941-x

Sutcubasi, B., Metin, B., Kurban, M. K., Metin, Z. E., Beser, B., & Sonuga-Barke, E. (2020). Resting-state network dysconnectivity in ADHD: A system-neuroscience-based meta-analysis. *The World Journal of Biological Psychiatry, 21*(9), 662–672. https://doi.org/10.1080/15622975.2020.1775889

Thapar, A., & Cooper, M. (2016). Attention deficit hyperactivity disorder. *The Lancet, 387*(10024), 1240–1250. https://doi.org/10.1016/S0140-6736(15)00238-X

Thomas, R., Sanders, S., Doust, J., Beller, E., & Glasziou, P. (2015). Prevalence of attention-deficit/hyperactivity disorder: A systematic review and meta-analysis. *Pediatrics, 135*(4), e994–e1001. https://doi.org/10.1542/peds.2014-3482

Ustun, B., Adler, L. A., Rudin, C., Faraone, S. V., Spencer, T. J., Berglund, P., Gruber, M. J., & Kessler, R. C. (2017). The World Health Organization Adult Attention-Deficit/Hyperactivity Disorder Self-Report Screening Scale for *DSM-5. JAMA Psychiatry, 74*(5), 520–527. https://doi.org/10.1001/jamapsychiatry.2017.0298

Vetter, V. L., Elia, J., Erickson, C., Berger, S., Blum, N., Uzark, K., & Webb, C. L. (2008). Cardiovascular monitoring of children and adolescents with heart disease receiving medications for attention deficit/hyperactivity disorder [corrected]: A scientific statement from the American Heart Association Council on Cardiovascular Disease in the Young Congenital Cardiac Defects Committee and the Council on Cardiovascular Nursing. *Circulation, 117*(18), 2407–2423. https://doi.org/10.1161/CIRCULATIONAHA.107.189473

Vink, M., Gladwin, T. E., Geeraerts, S., Pas, P., Bos, D., Hofstee, M., Durston, S., & Vollebergh, W. (2020). Towards an integrated account of the development of self-regulation from a neurocognitive perspective: A framework for current and future longitudinal multi-modal investigations. *Developmental Cognitive Neuroscience, 45*, 100829. https://doi.org/10.1016/j.dcn.2020.100829

Visser, S. N., Danielson, M. L., Bitsko, R. H., Holbrook, J. R., Kogan, M. D., Ghandour, R. M., Perou, R., & Blumberg, S. J. (2014). Trends in the parent-report of health care provider-diagnosed and medicated attention-deficit/hyperactivity disorder: United States, 2003–2011. *Journal of the American Academy of Child & Adolescent Psychiatry, 53*(1), 34–46.e2. https://doi.org/10.1016/j.jaac.2013.09.001

Vuong, A. M., Webster, G. M., Yolton, K., Calafat, A. M., Muckle, G., Lanphear, B. P., & Chen, A. (2021). Prenatal exposure to per- and polyfluoroalkyl substances (PFAS) and neurobehavior in US children through 8 years of age: The HOME study. *Environmental Research, 195*, 110825. https://doi.org/10.1016/j.envres.2021.110825

Vysniauske, R., Verburgh, L., Oosterlaan, J., & Molendijk, M. L. (2020). The effects of physical exercise on functional outcomes in the treatment of ADHD: A meta-analysis. *Journal of Attention Disorders, 24*(5), 644–654. https://doi.org/10.1177/1087054715627489

Walther, B., Morgenstern, M., & Hanewinkel, R. (2012). Co-occurrence of addictive behaviours: Personality factors related to substance use, gambling and computer gaming. *European Addiction Research, 18*(4), 167–174. https://doi.org/10.1159/000335662

Wilding, J. (2005). Is attention impaired in ADHD? *British Journal of Developmental Psychology, 23*(4), 487–505. https://doi.org/10.1348/026151005X48972

Willcutt, E. G. (2012). The prevalence of *DSM-IV* attention-deficit/hyperactivity disorder: A meta-analytic review. *Neurotherapeutics, 9*(3), 490–499. https://doi.org/10.1007/s13311-012-0135-8

Willcutt, E. G., Doyle, A. E., Nigg, J. T., Faraone, S. V., & Pennington, B. F. (2005). Validity of the executive function theory of attention-deficit/hyperactivity disorder: A meta-analytic review. *Biological Psychiatry, 57*(11), 1336–1346. https://doi.org/10.1016/j.biopsych.2005.02.006

Wolraich, M. L., Feurer, I. D., Hannah, J. N., Baumgaertel, A., & Pinnock, T. Y. (1998). Obtaining systematic teacher reports of disruptive behavior disorders utilizing *DSM-IV*. *Journal of Abnormal Child Psychology, 26*(2), 141–152. https://doi.org/10.1023/A:1022673906401

Wolraich, M. L., Hagan, J. F., Jr., Allan, C., Chan, E., Davison, D., Earls, M., Evans, S. W., Flinn, S. K., Froehlich, T., Frost, J., Holbrook, J. R., Lehmann, C. U., Lessin, H. R., Okechukwu, K., Pierce, K. L., Winner, J. D., Zurhellen, W., & the Subcommittee on Children and Adolescents With Attention-Deficit/Hyperactive Disorder. (2019). Clinical practice guideline for the diagnosis, evaluation, and treatment of attention-deficit/hyperactivity disorder in children and adolescents. *Pediatrics, 144*(4), e20192528. https://doi.org/10.1542/peds.2019-2528

Wolraich, M. L., Lambert, W., Doffing, M. A., Bickman, L., Simmons, T., & Worley, K. (2003). Psychometric properties of the Vanderbilt ADHD diagnostic parent rating scale in a referred population. *Journal of Pediatric Psychology, 28*(8), 559–568. https://doi.org/10.1093/jpepsy/jsg046

Yuchi, W., Brauer, M., Czekajlo, A., Davies, H. W., Davis, Z., Guhn, M., Jarvis, I., Jerrett, M., Nesbitt, L., Oberlander, T. F., Sbihi, H., Su, J., & van den Bosch, M. (2022). Neighborhood environmental exposures and incidence of attention deficit/hyperactivity disorder: A population-based cohort study. *Environment International, 161*, 107120. https://doi.org/10.1016/j.envint.2022.107120

Zablotsky, B., & Alford, J. M. (2020). Racial and ethnic differences in the prevalence of attention-deficit/hyperactivity disorder and learning disabilities among U.S. children aged 3–17 years. *NCHS Data Brief*, (358), 1–8. National Center for Health Statistics.

CHAPTER 22

INTERNALIZING AND EXTERNALIZING PROBLEMS IN CHILDREN AND YOUTH

Lana Mahgoub, David Meyer, and Mary Margaret Gleason

Across the disciplines of developmental-behavioral pediatrics, psychiatry, pediatric psychology, and developmental psychology, children's emotional, behavioral, and social problems are often clustered into two broad groups: internalizing and externalizing. In internalizing problems, a child experiences negative internal emotional experiences such as excessive fears, anxiety, or depressive symptoms that cause distress to child. This internal distress presents itself with observable behavioral patterns including facial expressions, avoidance of fear-inducing experiences, social withdrawal, emotional reactivity, and hypervigilance to potential threat.

Although fears are adaptive and necessary for survival, these adaptive reactions become pathologic when their intensity and persistence are developmentally atypical and when they interfere with functioning or cause child or family distress (American Psychiatric Association, 2013; Zero to Three, 2016). Anxiety symptoms represent a generalized response to a perceived threat and can include avoidance, hypervigilance, hyper-reactivity to benign stimuli, heightened sensitivity to threat, somatic complaints, and catastrophic reactions (Chiu et al., 2016). Similarly, depression is characterized by excessive or inappropriate sadness or irritability. It is associated with low energy, changes in thinking, somatic changes like sleep and eating, and it may include excessive guilt and thoughts of suicide. This constellation of symptoms is considered a disorder when it interferes with a child's functioning.

In externalizing problems, a child's observable (external) behavior patterns are the symptoms and often include impulsivity, emotional explosions, and rule breaking. These externalizing symptoms and their consequences can be disruptive to the people and environment around the child and also cause distress to the child. Although internalizing and externalizing problems are often described as distinct, it is not uncommon for children to experience difficulties with both internalizing and externalizing symptoms, both concurrently and over time (Hentges et al., 2019).

In clinical settings, general pediatricians, developmental-behavioral pediatricians, and child mental health professionals including pediatric psychologists and child psychiatrists commonly evaluate children presenting with internalizing or externalizing problems. These conditions frequently co-occur with physical health conditions and developmental delays so they very commonly present to the care of a pediatric psychologist or developmental-behavioral pediatrician. Pediatric psychologists and other mental health professionals, as well as developmental-behavioral pediatricians, may be involved in offering therapy

https://doi.org/10.1037/0000414-022
APA Handbook of Pediatric Psychology, Developmental-Behavioral Pediatrics, and Developmental Science: Vol. 2. Pediatric Psychology and Developmental-Behavioral Pediatrics: Clinical Applications of Developmental Science, P. E. Shah and M. H. Bornstein (Editors-in-Chief)
Copyright © 2025 by the American Psychological Association. All rights reserved.

for these conditions. The developmental science literature related to internalizing and externalizing problems informs our understanding of etiology, contexts, and course of these problems, with attention to the multilevel factors that influence these conditions across generations and communities.

Most fundamentally, internalizing and externalizing problems are relevant to child behavioral health providers, including pediatric psychologists and developmental-behavioral pediatricians, because they are associated with suffering, functional impairment, and adverse outcomes. The most important cost is the suffering of the child, family, and peers. Children with internalizing problems are impaired by their anxiety or depression across their ability to function in social or culturally typical activities, cognitive impairment, sleep and eating problems, and disordered thoughts, including suicidal thoughts. Children with externalizing problems often suffer because of exclusion from school or peer activities, consequences for disruptive behaviors, being characterized as "bad" in some settings, and in some cases, feeling remorse related to the behavioral patterns.

Children with both internalizing and externalizing problems are at higher than typical risk of dying from suicide, the second leading cause of death among youth older than 10 years in the United States, and the third leading cause for youth 15 to 19 globally (World Health Organization [WHO], 2019). Given the significant public health impact of the consequences of these conditions, their identification and treatment by child-serving clinicians is critical to fostering child emotional well-being.

This chapter provides an overview of the clinical presentation of the most common types of internalizing and externalizing problems, with focus on presentation in children and adolescents. We discuss the classification and epidemiology of each category of problem, risk and protective factors, cultural considerations and developmental variations in the presentation of each disorder, and screenings and clinical assessment tools, as well as evidence-based interventions that can guide treatment of each disorder.

CLASSIFICATION OF INTERNALIZING AND EXTERNALIZING PROBLEMS

Although the concept of internalizing and externalizing problems is consistent across clinical and academic disciplines, their descriptions and classification vary. For example, these problems can be examined and described as categorical problems or disorders or as continuous processes. Even when these conditions are described by their intensity or severity on a continuous scale, describing them as "problems" or "disorders" creates a categorical construct distinguishing them from a state that is healthy or without problematic behaviors. Categorical approaches, often used in clinical settings, explicitly distinguish between typical and pathologic patterns and diagnostic criteria to define specific clinical syndromes like major depressive disorder or attention-deficit/hyperactivity disorder.

The *Diagnostic and Statistical Manual of Mental Disorders*, fifth edition (*DSM-5*; American Psychiatric Association, 2013) and the *International Classification of Diseases*, 11th revision (WHO, 2017) each provide criteria for categorically defined clinical disorders, with significant overlap across the two nosologies. Each authoring agency periodically reviews and updates the criteria based on advancing empirical research. Therefore, the small differences in diagnostic criteria and nomenclature between the two nosologies represent different timing of the reviews and usually slight differences in interpretations of the strengths or implications of the evidence base. Each disorder is defined by specific criteria, which include internal and external experiences or behaviors (symptoms), timing and duration. In most cases, the criteria also require that the symptoms cause impairment in the life of the individual and/or their family. For example, mood symptoms may interfere with a child's ability to function in the family, school, with peers, or in extracurricular activities. Internalizing problems are represented in the *DSM-5* in anxiety and depressive disorders, and externalizing problems are represented in attention-deficit/hyperactivity disorder, oppositional defiant disorder, and conduct disorder (see Table 22.1).

TABLE 22.1

Overview of Internalizing and Externalizing Disorders

Internalizing	Externalizing
Anxiety	Attention-deficit/hyperactivity disorder
Depression	
Separation anxiety disorder	Oppositional defiant disorder
Social mutism	Conduct disorder
Social phobia	
Generalized anxiety disorder	

First they separate symptoms into clinical versus subclinical thresholds, which can facilitate communication among clinicians and help differentiate emotions and behaviors from those seen in healthy individuals not in need of clinical care. Additionally, because the diagnostic criteria are used in intervention research, rigorous application allows study of distinct interventions for different disorders. From a practical perspective, meeting criteria for a specific diagnosis is often required in the United States and other settings to justify billing for clinical care.

Categorical approaches to internalizing and externalizing problems also offer some challenges. For example, a child may have impairing and distressing anxiety or disruptive behavior patterns that do not fully meet the specific criteria for any disorder. Additionally, most diagnostic criteria do not specify how to assess the severity of internalizing and externalizing disorders, with the striking exception of autism spectrum disorder.

By definition, continuous approaches to describing internalizing and externalizing disorders offer insight into the intensity, frequency, or number of signs of the problem. Continuous measures of these conditions are often calculated using a combination of frequency and number of signs of the problem in both research and clinical practice. Continuous measures are especially valuable for assessing severity, comparing symptoms across children and reporters and tracking symptom trajectory over time. In clinical practice, it is most useful to combine continuous and categorical approaches to internalizing and externalizing problems. Specifically, a clinician will apply diagnostic criteria to describe the condition as a clinical disorder. The clinician may use a continuous measure with a clinical cutoff score as one piece of the data supporting a diagnosis and track the trajectory of the disorder using continuous measurements in the form of child or caregiver reports on standardized measures.

In research settings, continuous measurements offer the ability to look for more nuanced relationships between the internalizing or externalizing problem and other factors. When continuous measures are used, "problems" are differentiated from typical emotions and behaviors using da defined cutoff such as standard deviations from representative norms or other statistical approaches. For the purposes of this chapter, we will use internalizing and externalizing problems to describe broad clusters of emotional and behavioral patterns. Internalizing and externalizing disorders refer to the clusters of mental health problems defined in the *DSM-5*. Symptoms represent the individual internal or external experiences that contribute to the definition of the problem or disorder.

EPIDEMIOLOGY AND SOCIETAL COSTS OF CLINICALLY SIGNIFICANT INTERNALIZING AND EXTERNALIZING PROBLEMS

Rates of internalizing and externalizing problems vary by population, but overall global rates are strikingly similar, with estimates of around 10% to 20% across low-, middle-, and high-income countries (Kieling et al., 2011; Whitney & Peterson, 2019). This means that 220 to 440 million children globally experience internalizing or externalizing problems (Kieling et al., 2011). Although broad prevalence estimates are similar among countries, intra-country variability is high. The variability across populations is notable. In four distinct U.S. communities, the 12-month prevalence of an internalizing or externalizing disorder ranged from 8.7% to 14.7% and from

10.1% to 24.3%, respectively (Danielson et al., 2021) with no differences in prevalence by age, gender, or parent education.

Internalizing and externalizing disorders share more similarities than differences by age. Epidemiological studies of preschoolers in the United States and Europe show rates of internalizing disorders around 5.8% to 20.3% and externalizing disorders around 3.5% to 10.2%, similar to rates for school age children (Bufferd et al., 2011; Egger & Angold, 2006; Wichstrøm et al., 2012). The stability of prevalence over time reinforces that mental health concerns, in the form of internalizing and externalizing disorders, are not only present in older children, but that impairing differences in emotional and behavioral regulation can begin early in life.

Although the overall prevalence of internalizing and externalizing disorders is similar across ages, children may experience complex developmental trajectories, including both homotypic and heterotypic continuity. For example, although homotypic continuity of externalizing symptoms and disorders from toddlerhood to pre-adolescence is well-established, early onset externalizing problems also predict later internalizing disorders (e.g., Côté et al., 2006; Finsaas et al., 2018; Mesman et al., 2001). To date, prediction of homotypic versus heterotypic continuity of early externalizing problems has not been established. Homotypic continuity has also been shown for anxiety and depression (Finsaas et al., 2018). Continuity is stronger later in life than earlier in life, consistent with our understanding of neuroplasticity (Oldehinkel & Ormel, 2022). Although the factors related to the differential trajectories of symptoms in children are not fully understood, biological, psychological, and social factors likely play moderating roles. Specifically, hypothalamic–pituitary–adrenal (HPA) axis functioning appears to be associated with the course (homotypic or heterotypic) of internalizing/externalizing problems from preschool to adolescence (Frost et al., 2019). Patterns of homotypic or heterotypic continuity are likely influenced by and influence social and relational factors, especially caregiving environment, peer relationships, educational attainment, and stressful life experience (Oldehinkel & Ormel, 2022).

Gender patterns related to internalizing and externalizing problems are emerging and complex. In preschoolers, studies examining gender differences for internalizing disorders are mixed, but taken together, a number of studies indicate that boys are more likely to have attention-deficit/hyperactivity disorder (ADHD) than girls and one study indicates a higher rate of depressive disorders in boys than girls (e.g., Bufferd et al., 2011; Egger & Angold, 2006; Wichstrøm et al., 2012). In school-age and adolescent youth, patterns are more established. Generally, girls show higher rates of anxiety but not depression in school age (Gutman & Codiroli McMaster, 2020). Although both girls and boys demonstrate an increase in rates of both anxiety and depression in adolescence, the gender gap increases, with higher rates of both depression and anxiety in girls compared with boys (Crockett et al., 2013; Gutman & Codiroli McMaster, 2020).

There is more variation by geography and culture within countries than between cultures and countries. In the United States, where 16.5% of children 6 to 18 years old had been told that they have a mental health concern, not specifically internalizing/externalizing problems, prevalence ranged from 7.6% (Hawai'i) to 27.6% (Maine; Whitney & Peterson, 2019). Similarly, in parent report measures across 45 countries, nearly 90% of the variance of a validated measure of child symptoms scores could not be explained by specific community or cultural factors (Rescorla et al., 2019). Broadly speaking, children in the highest income countries had lower rates of internalizing symptoms compared with children from lower income countries. Nonclinical factors like distance to treatment facilities, density of treatment providers, cultural generalizations about communities, educational patterns, and socioeconomic disadvantage also contribute to variability of diagnoses, although equitable access to clinical care does not eliminate variability (Fulton et al., 2009; Kumar & Gleason, 2019; Madsen et al., 2015; Mykletun et al., 2021; Upadhyay et al., 2019).

Internalizing and externalizing disorders also carry direct costs of clinical care as well as indirect costs including lost days of school, lost parental workdays, and societal and community costs of addressing educational and legal issues. In the United States, annual clinical and family costs for anxiety disorders are estimated at more than $6,000 per child (Mandell et al., 2003; Pella et al., 2020), not including the societal impact of educational costs and legal system costs. Worldwide, the societal costs for internalizing and externalizing problems are also significant. In Britain, 3-year costs for hyperkinetic problems were more than £9,000, and nearly £6,000 for conduct problems; costs for internalizing problems were just over £3,000, with mental health care and school accommodations representing the largest proportions of the costs (WHO, 2019). Costs for internalizing and externalizing problems accumulate over time, with one estimate for the cumulative cost of externalizing problems at £16,435 over 25 years in health, education, crimes, and social support.

IDENTIFICATION OF INTERNALIZING/ EXTERNALIZING PROBLEMS

Many factors likely influence identification and interpretation of internalizing and externalizing problems in children. Generalizations about cultural belief patterns should be made with caution, as research into explanatory models of child internalizing and externalizing patterns is not robust. Children's behavioral patterns have meanings at the family and cultural levels, although most cultural groups in the United States at least partially endorse a biopsychosocial model of disruptive behaviors. This model ascribes symptom patterns to a combination of biology (genetics, physical health status), psychological patterns (relational patterns, world view, temperamental patterns), and social factors (family, peer, school, community, environment; Lawton et al., 2014). In the United States, European American caregivers of young children are more likely to use a medical (biological) model to explain externalizing patterns, whereas African American caregivers tend to attribute externalizing patterns to behavioral or personality descriptors (Bussing et al., 1998). In older children, European American parents are more likely to endorse physical, personality, familial, or trauma causes for their child's difficulties, whereas African American parents identify prejudice as a foundation for their child's symptoms, and Latina American mothers as a group endorse spiritual explanations (Yeh et al., 2004). Outside of high-income countries, exploration of the meaning of child mental health symptoms is limited. One study in Ethiopia reported a wide scope of explanatory models, with 80% of parents describing possible genetic underpinnings for child mental health concerns and 93%, 82%, and 74%, respectively endorsing the roles of magic, curses, and sin (Abera et al., 2015). These different attributional models have importance in building rapport with families and developing culturally respectful treatment plans, and so clinicians should explore the family's explanatory model with curiosity and humility, acknowledging what they don't know.

Attributions and implicit biases of adults outside the family also play a role in understanding internalizing and externalizing patterns. For example, both Black and White preschool teachers are likely to identify Black boys (compared with White boys or any girls) as requiring extra behavioral attention (Gilliam et al., 2016). Experiences shape this assessment, as teachers in this study rated a child's behavior concerns more severely if they were told a child of a different ethnicity had faced adversity. Taken together, these findings emphasize the importance of understanding the lens through which behaviors are interpreted and the critical role that implicit biases play in interpreting behavioral patterns as problems.

Implicit biases and racially specific attributions may contribute to disparities in treatment patterns and must be monitored in clinical settings. For example, European American boys are treated for ADHD at higher rates than African American boys, although epidemiologic studies do not reveal differences in prevalence (Coker et al., 2016). This difference may be because the symptoms in European American boys are seen as clinical concerns whereas the symptoms in African

American boys may be seen as behavior problems. Attributions of the observer influence how children's behavioral patterns are experienced, labeled, and addressed.

RISK AND PROTECTIVE FACTORS ASSOCIATED WITH INTERNALIZING AND EXTERNALIZING PROBLEMS

Risk and protective factors for internalizing and externalizing problems tend to be opposite ends of the same spectrum, with significant overlap between risk factors for each pattern (see Figure 22.1). Drawing from research in developmental science, risk factors can contribute to the development and perpetuation of the internalizing or externalizing problem, and similarly most protective factors can serve as resilience factors that allow resolution of the internalizing or externalizing problem. It is almost universally true that a child's individual risk for internalizing or externalizing problems is due to interactions between their inherited and acquired biology and their experiences; it is almost never just a representation of only biology or experience. Although the following subsections highlight specific factors, the complex interactions among genetic and epigenetic factors, experiences, and environment influence the risk development of internalizing and externalizing problems.

Risk and Resilience

Genetic predisposition
Prenatal context
Temperament
Age
Developmental status
Physical health status
Caregiving
Educational context
Home and community

Resilience Factors — Development — Risk Factors
Prevention

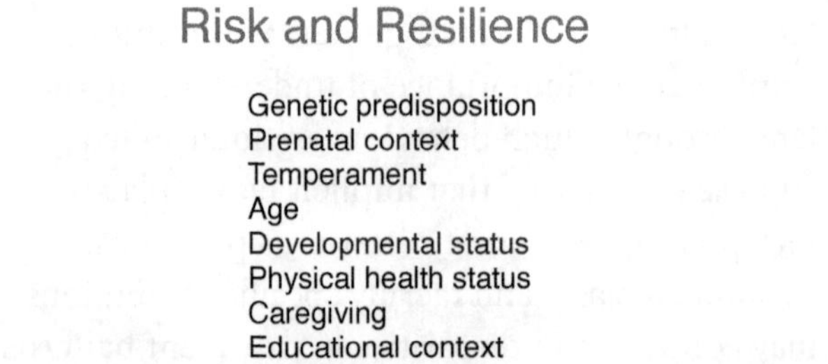

FIGURE 22.1. Risk and resilience factors.

Genetics

Children enter the world with biological risks related to their prenatal course and their inherited genetic and epigenetic predispositions to mental health problems. The heritable risk for internalizing and externalizing disorders is high, with 30% of variance being explained by inherited factors (Nikstat & Riemann, 2020). After extensive searches for single "candidate genes" to explain the development of mental health problems including these conditions, there is a growing awareness that combinations of genetic risk factors (polygenetic) likely contribute to a common factor that puts an individual at risk of developing a range of mental health problems including internalizing or externalizing problems. This common factor is denoted the p factor and is thought to interact with the environment to result in clinical presentations (Caspi & Moffitt, 2018). The p factor may be a consistent underlying factor for children with apparent heterotypic continuity of their early onset internalizing or externalizing problems, meaning that the underlying problem persists over time with the addition of new manifestations.

Prenatal Context

Many studies suggest that prenatal stress is associated with increased risk of both internalizing and externalizing problems during childhood and adolescence (Hentges et al., 2019; Madigan et al., 2018; Van den Bergh et al., 2008). Similar patterns have been seen in low- and middle-income countries, where women may be at higher risk of being exposed to physical and emotional stresses during pregnancy than in higher resource countries (Herba et al., 2016). Prenatal stresses that are associated with internalizing or externalizing problems may include maternal depression and to a lesser extent anxiety, as well as interpersonal violence exposure. Perinatal health factors including maternal overweight status, maternal infection or inflammation, and exposure to toxins through substance use or environmental exposure also contribute to both internalizing and externalizing disorders in children and adolescents (Tien et al., 2020). Of particular note is the consistent association between prenatal smoking exposure, illicit substance use, and alcohol with externalizing problems, especially hyperactivity and inattention, as well as developmental delays.

The mechanisms by which perinatal factors influence child mental health risk are complex. It is thought that prenatal exposures influence the development of child internalizing or externalizing problems through a number of mechanisms including fetal programming (direct impact on brain development) and the interpersonal transmission of prenatal stress to the infant and developing child through caregiving patterns, as well as through continued stress into the postnatal period. Each of these hypotheses explains some of the association between prenatal stress and child internalizing and externalizing problems (Hentges et al., 2019). Specific elements of fetal programming likely involve the HPA functioning, immune functioning, and white matter organization, especially in the corpus callosum (Borchers et al., 2021; Stein et al., 2014).

Child Factors

Temperamental traits (like adaptability or high frustration) in infancy and early childhood are strongly associated with the risk of future internalizing or externalizing problems. Other traits, like high fear, are associated only with internalizing patterns, and low effortful control is associated only with externalizing patterns (e.g., Ormel et al., 2005). Like other factors, temperament interacts in complex ways with other risk and protective factors, including familial psychopathology, cognitive processes, biology, or caregiving quality in contributing to internalizing and externalizing problems (e.g., Fox et al., 2021; Hoyniak & Petersen, 2019). A child also brings their inherited predispositions for internalizing or externalizing problems, which may protect or confer risk.

Age

In considering the developmental trajectories of internalizing and externalizing problems, it is useful to consider at what age these problems can present. The long-term trajectories of internalizing and externalizing behaviors begin as early as 18 months (Côté et al., 2009; Teymoori et al., 2018). For internalizing problems, caregiver-reported rates increase from 18 months to 5 years (Côté et al., 2009). For both girls and boys, there is a group of children, representing about 9% overall, who display the highest rates of internalizing symptoms that persist through adolescence (Gutman & Codiroli McMaster, 2020). There is a separate group whose symptoms are consistently low in childhood through adolescence, with a modest increase in early childhood, and a third group whose symptoms increase beginning around age 8 with a persistent rise in girls and a plateau in adolescence. The trajectories of externalizing behaviors show a peak for all children around age 4. For both boys and girls, and overall, there is a group with the highest and most persistent aggressive behaviors, which represents 6% of boys and 20% of girls, with girls displaying fewer aggressive behaviors than boys at every age except 18 months (Teymoori et al., 2018). Importantly, the specific factors associated with these trajectories, which include family, community, and caregiving factors, differ somewhat between girls and boys. These developmental trajectory studies examine behavior counts rather than impairment or problems.

Rates of clinical problems are fairly consistent across two longitudinal studies from preschool to school age (7% to 22%), with an increase in rates in adolescence, mostly explained by internalizing disorders in girls (Bufferd et al., 2011; Wichstrøm et al., 2012, 2017). The patterns within specific internalizing and externalizing disorders are more complex. Specifically, rates of ADHD (an externalizing problem) increase, rates of disruptive behaviors decrease, and anxiety remains fairly consistent during the school-age period and depression increases in adolescence (Finsaas et al., 2018). The changes in overall rates by age reflect heterotypic continuity, meaning that young children with mental health problems often continue to experience a clinical problem but it has a different manifestation over time (e.g., Finsaas et al., 2018; Lavigne et al., 2014; Wichstrøm et al., 2017). For example, preschool children with externalizing problems may grow into elementary school-age children with both externalizing and internalizing problems (heterotypic continuity) or continue to have externalizing problems (homotypic continuity).

Developmental Status

Typical development is a protective factor against the development of internalizing or externalizing problems. By contrast, children with developmental delays have higher rates of all internalizing and externalizing disorders, with rates at least two to three times that of the general population (Baker et al., 2010; De Ruiter et al., 2007). Children with autism spectrum disorder are at higher risk for developing internalizing and externalizing problem than neurotypical children as well. A number of genetic syndromes confer unique behavioral phenotypes. For example, children with trisomy 21 are at higher risk of most internalizing and externalizing problems, including anxiety, mood symptoms, ADHD, and disruptive behavior (Visootsak & Sherman, 2007). Although externalizing problems are most prominent in children with Fragile X, these children may also experience elevated rates of internalizing problems. Similarly, prenatal alcohol exposure is associated with elevated rates of internalizing and externalizing problems in a dose-dependent manner, even when controlling for other prenatal exposures and postnatal experiences and exposures (Lees et al., 2020). A robust literature demonstrates an association between illicit prenatal substance exposures and externalizing problems, and a smaller literature reveals an association with internalizing problems, recognizing that the prenatal exposure is best characterized as an "intergenerational cascade of events" rather than a solitary exposure (Conradt et al., 2023; Lin et al., 2018). Although findings are somewhat inconsistent, studies that include familial comparisons suggest that there is a direct link between externalizing problems and prenatal smoking (Palmer et al., 2016; Sutin et al., 2017). By contrast, healthy pregnancies without prenatal exposures are associated with healthier mental health in preschoolers and beyond.

Physical Health

Physical health is a protective factor against internalizing and externalizing problems, possibly because it confers the ability to fully participate in developmentally and culturally appropriate activities without pain or limitations. In a large meta-analysis, children and adolescents with chronic illness are at higher risk of both internalizing and externalizing problems, with chronic fatigue syndrome having highest rates of internalizing problems and epilepsy and headaches showing highest rates of externalizing problems (Pinquart & Shen, 2011). There is significant variability among internalizing and externalizing problems among children with chronic illnesses because the family, school, and community context of the illness, the direct and indirect impact of the illness on the child, and developmental variations all may play a role in adaptation to chronic illness. Other aspects of physical health are also related to internalizing and externalizing problems. For example, children with higher levels of physical activity and movement have lower risk for internalizing and externalizing disorders than their more sedentary counterparts (Zahl et al., 2017).

Caregiving Factors

The caregiving context is powerfully associated with children's development of internalizing and externalizing problems. The quality of early attachment relationships is associated with early internalizing and externalizing symptoms, and the quality of caregiver–child relationships continues to be associated with these symptoms throughout development (Groh et al., 2017; Sroufe, 2005). This association makes caregiver–child relationships a critical target of assessment and intervention for clinicians. Caregiver–child interactions that are sensitive, nurturing, and consistent are most likely to support healthy emotional and behavioral regulation (Zeanah et al., 2011). Conversely, harsh, overly strict, or inconsistent parenting is associated with internalizing and externalizing problems in children. It is critical to note that these quality relationships can involve any important adult in a child's life, not just the child's biological parents. The quality of attachment relationships with early care and education professionals can be protective for healthy emotional and behavioral development (Gallagher & Mayer, 2008).

Caregiver mental health is a clinically relevant factor in child mental health, likely because adult psychopathology can interfere with optimal caregiving and consistent emotional availability and because of the potential for genetic heritability (Ormel et al., 2005; Suchman et al., 2019; Weissman et al., 2006). Like other risks highlighted here, adverse caregiver mental health that is presenting as a risk factor can be modifiable and a focus of intervention.

Educational Contexts

Educational settings also offer opportunities for both risk and protection. Powerful risk factors in school center around unsupportive or unsafe relationships with teachers, staff, or peers, with bullying being an especially important context. Contrariwise, schools can create healthy cultures to support and mitigate these risks (Paulus et al., 2016).

Home/Community Factors

Child safety in the home and community is protective, whereas exposures to maltreatment, interpersonal violence, and community violence contribute to the development of internalizing and externalizing symptoms. Neighborhood factors, including neighborhood cohesion can also serve as protective factors to children. Overall, exposure to adversity is associated with increased risk of developing internalizing and externalizing symptoms in a linear (dose–response) association. The traditional adverse childhood experiences, which include caregiving abuse, impairment, and disruptions, have been expanded in the pediatric literature to include exposure to community violence and discrimination, which contribute to internalizing and externalizing disorders. Violence, whether directed toward a child or experienced indirectly through the community or other relationships, including war, is associated with higher than usual rates of internalizing and especially externalizing patterns (Fleckman et al., 2016; Foster & Brooks-Gunn, 2015).

Resilience and the Interactive Effects Among Risk and Protective Factors

The overall balance of positive and adverse experiences also influences the development of internalizing and externalizing disorders in children. The number of protective factors—individual, personal, and social—can protect children against exposure to adverse risk factors. A recent meta-analysis identified 13 unique individual factors that serve as resilience factors, categorized into cognitive (mental flexibility), emotional regulation patterns, attachment and relationship, and positive view of self (Fritz et al., 2018). Family factors include support, cohesion, and a positive family climate, as well as parental support and involvement in a child's life. At the community level, social support is similarly a well-supported resilience factor. Although different studies show slightly different specific factors, the most consistent findings are that healthy relationships and support at every level of relationship are associated with lower risk of internalizing and externalizing disorders. The overall cumulative burden of adverse experiences or risk factors influences the development and severity of internalizing and externalizing disorders more than specific risk factors differentially shape specific disorders (Murray et al., 2020; Patalay et al., 2017; Sameroff, 2009; Speyer et al., 2022). For example, in a large population study in the United Kingdom, male sex, lower maternal age, maternal mental health problems, maternal smoking during pregnancy, as well as polygenic factors, distinguished children with and without symptoms, but not the different clusters of internalizing or externalizing symptoms (Speyer et al., 2022). At the family level, lack of access to basic needs, especially food insecurity, is also an important modifiable factor associated with internalizing and externalizing disorders (Slopen et al., 2010). Physical and emotional safety are also significant factors the development of internalizing and externalizing disorders.

CLINICAL PRESENTATIONS OF INTERNALIZING AND EXTERNALIZING PROBLEMS

Internalizing and externalizing disorders have a range of clinical presentations that can be differentiated by the symptoms the child and family endorse as well as the observations in the assessments.

Internalizing Disorders: Anxiety Disorders

Anxiety problems are the most common form of internalizing problems, with specific disorders defined by the trigger of the anxiety (American Psychiatric Association, 2013). Common specific child anxiety disorders are characterized by exaggerated or misplaced fears—of separation from a caregiver, of social interactions and evaluation, of speaking in public, or of discrete benign objects or events—or by anxiety without a specific source. Children with any anxiety disorder may present with obvious fears, avoidance, sleep, and somatic and cognitive symptoms, and the avoidance and distress may also appear as defiant behaviors and/or extreme mood and behavioral dysregulation. Importantly, there is significant heterotypic continuity among the anxiety disorders, meaning that a young child may present with separation anxiety and grow into an adolescent with generalized anxiety.

Separation anxiety disorder. Healthy children develop distress upon separation from their caregivers concurrently with focused attachment behaviors at around 7 to 9 months. This typical developmental process does not interfere with typical functioning, and the distress resolves over time. However, some toddlers, preschoolers, and older children show a developmentally and culturally atypical intensity or duration of separation distress symptoms that should raise concerns about separation anxiety disorder (Beesdo et al., 2009).

Separation anxiety disorder (SAD; Strawn et al., 2021) presents at a mean age of 8 years. Children and adolescents with SAD experience recurrent excessive distress related to actual or anticipated separation from their major attachment figure. They often worry about losing their attachment figure or that either they or their attachment figure will experience harm during a separation. This anxiety often manifests in persistent reluctance or refusal to be alone or away from the major attachment figure (including to sleep), repeated nightmares involving the theme of separation, and/or repeated complaints of physical symptoms when separating from the major attachment figure. Young children may be described as clingy, and the inability to sleep alone may be prominent. School-age children and teenagers may experience fear of kidnapping, catastrophic accidents (e.g., a car accident that causes them to lose their caregiver), or other situations that could lead to danger. Adolescents may also avoid sleepovers with peers and show frequent checking behaviors (e.g., frequently texting caregivers for their location). Across childhood, school refusal related to SAD is common and can interfere with peer relationships and academic success. Behavioral inhibition in toddlers is associated with later development of SAD, and early SAD is associated with generalized anxiety disorder later (Beesdo et al., 2009; Calkins & Fox, 1992).

Selective mutism. Selective mutism is characterized by an inability to speak, for at least one month, in specific social situations in which there is an expectation of speaking (e.g., school) despite being able to speak in other situations (e.g., home). The disturbance is often associated with high social anxiety and can cause academic or educational challenges. Onset typically occurs before the age of 5 but may not become apparent until a child enters school with its requirement to speak in new settings.

Social anxiety disorder. Social anxiety disorder involves excessive and impairing anxiety and avoidance of social situations that may involve social evaluation (e.g., meeting new people), being observed (e.g., eating in public), and/or performing in front of other children as well as adults. Social anxiety generally presents by age 12, although there is a wide range of onsets. Young children may express fear by crying, freezing, clinging, tantrums, or failure to speak in social situations. Older children or adolescents may express fear of embarrassment, humiliation, or rejection by others. It is notable that, in the wake of school closures to mitigate the spread of COVID-19, youth with social anxiety might have experienced a temporary decrease in distress as the social expectations diminished (Morrissette, 2021).

Like separation anxiety, social anxiety disorder is strongly associated with subsequent other anxiety disorders (Strawn et al., 2021).

Specific phobias. Specific phobias are irrational persistent fears of a specific object, activity, or situation. Developmentally, typical fears shift across ages. Separation anxiety tends to predominate before age 2, followed by fear of natural events (e.g., thunderstorms) and animals in older toddlers (Beesdo et al., 2009). In children 3 to 6 years old, a predominance of fears of death may be evident. As children get older, they may demonstrate fears of real or pretend objects (monsters), or illnesses or school anxiety, and by adolescence, rejection by peers may predominate. Most clinically impairing specific phobias develop prior to age 10. In young children, symptoms related to specific phobias may manifest as crying, tantrums, clinging, extreme avoidance, and freezing.

Generalized anxiety. Generalized anxiety is one of the most common forms of anxiety disorders peaking in onset in adolescence. Generalized anxiety disorder (GAD) a diffuse anxiety that happens in almost any setting and without a stable, specific trigger. Accompanying the anxiety, children with GAD may experience irritability, concentration difficulties, muscle tension, and/or sleep disturbance (American Psychiatric Association, 2013). Children with GAD may seek frequent reassurance about their performance and worries and may present with irritability that may contribute to disruptive behaviors.

Depressive disorders. Depressive disorders represent the other major component of internalizing disorders. Early mood dysregulation can present in toddlers with prevailing sadness or irritability. Major depressive disorder can be validly diagnosed in children as young as 3, although it typically presents later, with a female predominance beginning in adolescence (Luby et al., 2003; Wang et al., 2016). In clinical settings, major depressive disorder is characterized by predominantly sad or irritable mood that lasts at least 2 weeks (American Psychiatric Association, 2013). Associated symptoms include decreased interest or joy in pleasurable activities; changes in sleep, energy, appetite, concentration, and memory; excessive guilt; and/or suicidal symptoms. Clinical presentation of depression in younger children may be associated with more irritability and the potential for regression with regard to recently acquired milestones. In children, the first presentation of depression may be weight loss, withdrawal from extracurricular activities, academic difficulties, discord in peer or family relationships, suicidal symptoms, or diminished interest in play.

Externalizing Problems

Externalizing problems represent an exaggerated and developmentally atypical behavioral pattern that causes disruption, distress, and/or impairment. In the *DSM* nosology, the main categories of externalizing disorders are oppositional defiant disorder and conduct disorder (American Psychiatric Association, 2013). The problematic hyperactivity, impulsivity, and inattention of ADHD is also sometimes included in externalizing problems (see Chapter 21, this volume). Oppositional defiant disorder (ODD) describes a disorder of impairing and age atypical arguing, defiance, and irritability. In the diagnostic criteria 0–5, this constellation of symptoms is characterized as a disorder of dysregulated anger and aggression in very young children, recognizing that mood dysregulation (internalizing problem) is often at the core of what appear to be externalizing patterns in preschoolers (Zeanah et al., 2016). To date, there are no data indicating the developmental trajectory of dysregulated anger and aggression beyond age 6, although the expectation is that, like ODD, some children will persist with externalizing problems and some will have internalizing problems when they start school. The more severe types of externalizing patterns are described as conduct disorder in the *DSM* 5. These behaviors include major theft, severe aggression, and significant rule breaking. In the *DSM*, conduct disorder can be associated with limited prosocial emotion, which has been characterized as a callous–unemotional trait in empirical research (Frick et al., 2014). These traits are associated with a more persistent form of externalizing as well as physiologic hyporeactivity to stress. Externalizing disorders commonly co-occur with other externalizing disorders, especially ADHD. Oppositional defiant disorder and conduct disorder both co-occur with anxiety, and ODD often presents concurrently with mood disorders (Rowe et al., 2010).

SCREENING AND CLINICAL ASSESSMENT

Identification of concerns for internalizing and externalizing patterns in children and youth often occurs in primary care settings or schools. In 2015, the American Academy of Pediatrics (AAP) published a clinical guideline promoting use of structured validated measures of mental health in primary care (Weitzman et al., 2015). Without systematic use of validated measures (described in the following) to identify internalizing and externalizing problems, most children with clinically significant problems are not identified (Sheldrick et al., 2011). Cases of missed identification are not distributed equally across ethnic groups, with rates of missing a clinically significant problem higher for youth of color than White youth (Brown & Wissow, 2010). As of 2022, the AAP recommends universal behavioral/social/emotional screening at every well child visit, which can include validated screening for internalizing and externalizing problems (AAP, 2022).

Universal screening for depression in adolescents is the standard of care in the United States, often using the Patient Health Questionnaire-Adolescents (AAP, 2021b; Johnson et al., 2002). The AAP's 2021 national quality improvement initiative addressing social health and early childhood wellness focused on screening for internalizing and externalizing disorders in the preschool period (AAP, 2021a). Screening resources are available for primary care or other clinicians, including the AAP's Screening Technical Assistance and Resource Center website (AAP, 2021c). Because of the co-occurrence of internalizing and externalizing disorders, in pediatric settings, child care facilities, and schools, it may be more appropriate as a first-line approach to implement a general screening tool, followed by a symptom-specific measure if the history suggests a specific symptom cluster (see the Resource box for more information).

In specialty mental health settings and developmental-behavioral pediatric settings, global mental health measures are commonly used as part of the initial evaluation. For example, the American Psychiatric Association parent- and self-rated Level 1 Cross-Cutting Symptoms Measures screen for several mental health disorders (American Psychiatric Association, 2013). This measure includes broad stem questions about depression, anxiety, anger, and irritability, as well as other domains and defined thresholds that trigger use of second-level measures. The Child Behavior Checklist (CBCL) and the Behavioral Assessment System for Children (BASC) are also commonly used proprietary global measures (Achenbach, 1991; Reynolds & Kamphaus, 2015). Symptom-specific measures continue to have value in all settings to track the trajectory of symptoms with interventions. For example, the best-researched anxiety scales for youth over 8 include the Multidimensional Anxiety Scale for Children (March et al., 1997), the Spence Children's Anxiety Scale, and the Screen for Child Anxiety-Related Emotional Disorders (Birmaher et al., 1999). The Revised Children's Manifest Anxiety Scale and the State-Trait Anxiety Inventory for Children are also commonly used for children as young as 6. All have parent and child versions, show strong internal reliability in terms of total scores, and have good test–retest reliability (Spence, 2018; see the Resources box).

In all settings, a positive screen or clinical concern should trigger a clinical history exploring the symptoms, context, and level of impairment with the child as well as the caregiver. For all chief complaints, it is helpful to gather information over multiple appointments to provide multiple time points and to create a trusting relationship with the child and family, which is likely to facilitate obtaining valid information. Throughout the assessment, clear structure and effective boundaries support the clinical process, as does providing reinforcement for positive behavior to support the relationship. Engaging with toys or games can facilitate rapport building with the child and allow expression through play and nonverbal communication.

Clinical assessment includes identifying symptoms and their frequency, severity, onset, and duration; degree of associated distress and functional impairment; developmental deviations; and signs of physical health concerns that may be related to the internalizing or externalizing problems (e.g., facial dysmorphic features suggestive of Fragile X; Walter et al., 2020). Beginning with broad stem questions, followed by a review of disorder-specific symptoms, is a useful way of organizing history taking for/from the child and caregiver (see Figure 22.2). Stem questions for internalizing and externalizing symptoms may begin broadly with "does your child have a hard time with managing emotions or behaviors?" Broad-based questions about anxiety may include "Does your child worry a lot? Get nervous? Or scared?" If symptoms are endorsed, the next set of questions will explore the focus or trigger of the anxiety. For depressive symptoms, a clinician may ask "does your child get sad more than you expect? Cry? Get more irritable or angry?" For externalizing symptoms, a clinician may ask "does your child have a hard time with managing frustration, following rules, or staying safe?" Follow-up questions focus on the detailed manifestations of temper dysregulation (verbal frustration, yelling, aggression), including context, duration, timing, exacerbating factors, and how the events end.

Similarly, an exploration of defiance and rule breaking patterns must include the specifics of context and behaviors. Attention to the ABCs of behaviors—**a**ntecedents, **b**ehavior specifics, and **c**onsequences—is a useful paradigm for considering anxiety as well as externalizing patterns (e.g., Spence, 2018; Steiner et al., 2007). In developmental-behavioral pediatrics and mental

All chief complaints	Social history	Observations

• Sleep
• Appetite
• Memory/concentration
• Thoughts of self-harm
	• Household members
	• Quality of relationships with
	  • Caregivers and siblings
	  • Peers
	  • Other important adults
	• School (grade and performance)
	• Extracurricular activities
	• Faith practices and community
	• Major life events
	• History of adverse childhood experiences and/or traumatic experiences
		• Caregiver–child interactions
		  • Mutual engagement
		  • Warmth
		  • Familiarity with each other
		  • Ability to show perspective taking and self-reflective skills
		• Child
		  • Physical appearance
		  • Behaviors (activity level, rule following, engagement)
		  • Rate, rhythm, volume, prosody of speech
		  • Self-reported mood
		  • Observed affective range and content
		  • Organization of thought process
		  • Themes of thought content (including suicidal thoughts)
		  • Evidence of response to internal stimuli
		  • Understanding of clinical issue
		  • Judgment
		  • Cognitive level

Medical and developmental history		
• Preterm birth • Prenatal exposures • Central nervous system problems (e.g., seizures) • Chronic illness • Serious acute illness or injury • Growth trajectory • Milestones (on time or delayed) • Medications		

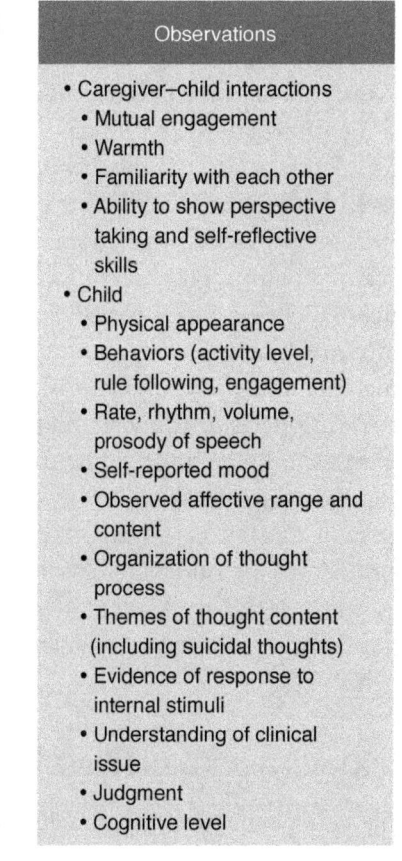

FIGURE 22.2. Elements of an assessment.

health settings including pediatric psychology, more extended formal assessments of behavior may be indicated.

Follow-up questions about the additional criteria for each disorder, including attention to neurovegetative symptoms, cognitive patterns, and safety risks, are helpful. Careful review of symptoms that may indicate a different or concurrent diagnosis is critical. As with any clinical assessment, the child's past medical, developmental, family, and social histories and the cultural context of the child and family should be explored. The history taking should focus on the factors that may either predispose to or protect from internalizing or externalizing problems.

Direct clinical observations provide valuable information during assessments. Observations of children with internalizing and externalizing disorders may appear typical in a brief visit, whereas multiple or extended visits may provide opportunities to observe more symptoms. Signs of anxiety may include fidgety behaviors, shyness, reticence to respond to questions, or limited eye contact (Spence, 2018). Level of distress with separation from a caregiver may provide useful information as well. Behavioral observations provide information about response to a child's fears. Children and youth with depression may present with lower levels of engagement, sad or irritable expressions, and slowness of speech and movement, although observations may not raise concerns. Observations focused on externalizing symptoms may include tracking responses to adults (including adult limit setting) to potentially frustrating parts of the visit, and differential responses to limits imposed by the caregiver or the clinician. Monitoring for observations suggestive of ADHD is also important. Collateral information from other sources can be especially important in the assessment of externalizing symptoms, which may vary across settings (Spence, 2018).

TREATMENT AND INTERVENTION

Some nonspecific intervention approaches are relevant to consider for all youth with internalizing or externalizing disorders, regardless of clinical setting. First, the health care professional who identifies a concern should review modifiable risk or protective factors and implement strategies to mitigate risk or enhance protection. Nonspecific approaches can include addressing unmet basic or clinical needs, expanding caregiving supports, addressing developmental and educational needs, supporting family wellness, and optimizing wellness (see Figures 22.3 and 22.4). It is critical for any health care facility to have a list of the most commonly used local resources available. Increasingly, local services may be accessed by free shared data platforms, such as local 411 numbers or the https://www.findhelp.org site.

Psychoeducation about symptoms can be valuable to reduce unwarranted fears or misconceptions and optimize ongoing engagement in care (Lindsey et al., 2014; Martinez et al., 2017). Including realistic reasons for hopefulness and empathy in psychoeducational conversations is likely to support ongoing engagement and reduce child and family distress (Brown et al., 2013; Foy et al., 2010).

A medical health professional may also partner with nonprescribing mental health clinicians to provide first-line psychopharmacologic treatment while a child is engaged in therapy. In combined care, bidirectional interdisciplinary communication between the professionals facilitates effective treatment. Tracking symptoms with validated measures can help to monitor treatment effectiveness and determine when higher levels of care may be needed.

Evidence-based therapies are critical elements of care for many children (Weisz & Kazdin, 2010). The psychotherapist may collaborate with primary care clinician, psychiatrist, or developmental-behavioral pediatrician to evaluate the appropriateness of medication as part of the treatment plan or recommend psychiatric care. A psychologist may offer formal testing including cognitive testing and caregiver and youth self-report measures to further clarify diagnosis as needed.

In the psychiatric or developmental-behavioral pediatrics setting, a patient may receive psychopharmacologic treatment and/or evidence-based psychotherapies. The doctoral level clinician may

Internalizing and Externalizing Problems in Children and Youth

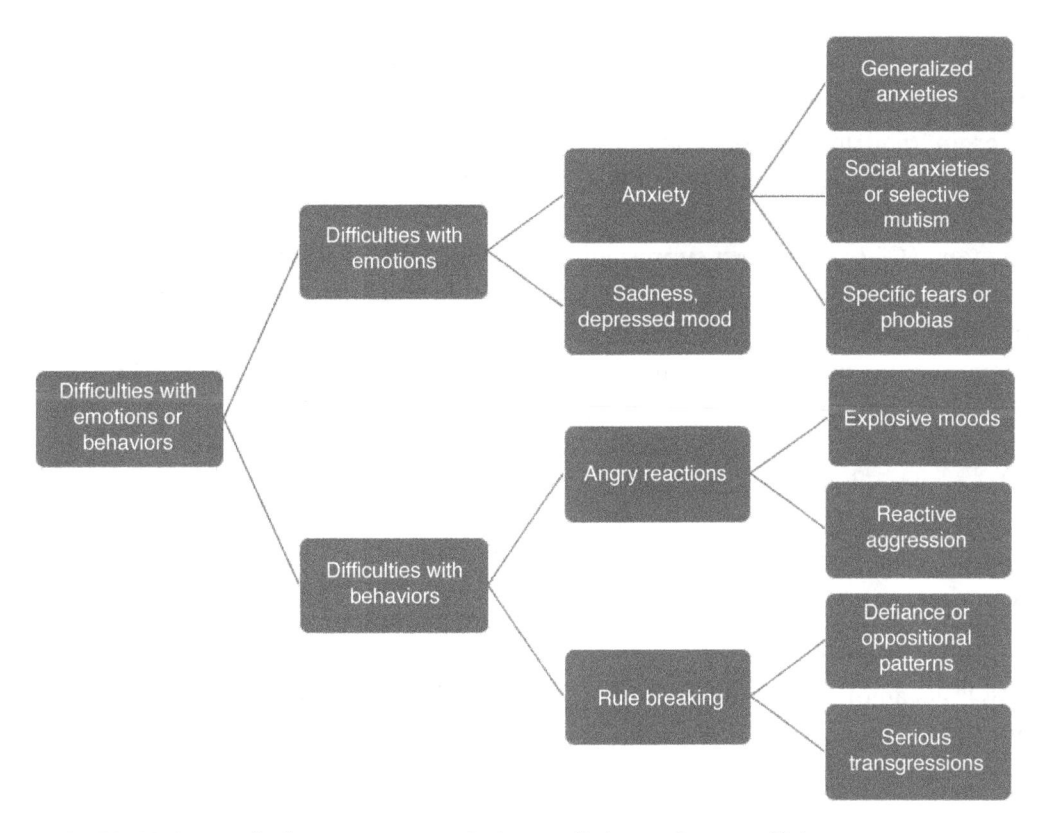

FIGURE 22.3. Underlying constructs in internalizing and externalizing symptoms, excluding developmental, physical, and stressor-related pattern.

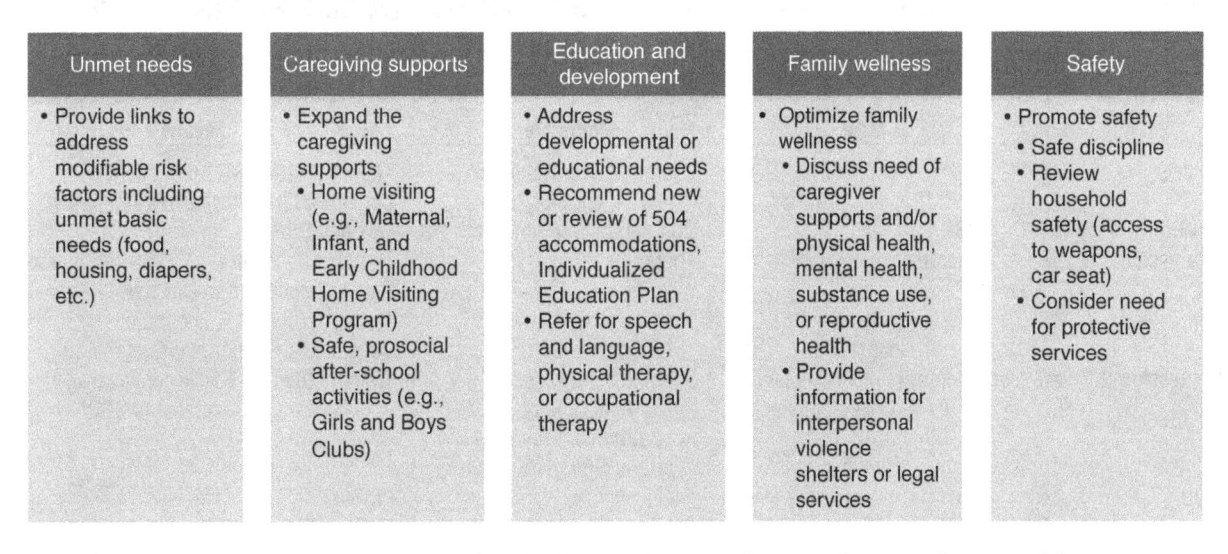

Unmet needs	Caregiving supports	Education and development	Family wellness	Safety
• Provide links to address modifiable risk factors including unmet basic needs (food, housing, diapers, etc.)	• Expand the caregiving supports • Home visiting (e.g., Maternal, Infant, and Early Childhood Home Visiting Program) • Safe, prosocial after-school activities (e.g., Girls and Boys Clubs)	• Address developmental or educational needs • Recommend new or review of 504 accommodations, Individualized Education Plan • Refer for speech and language, physical therapy, or occupational therapy	• Optimize family wellness • Discuss need of caregiver supports and/or physical health, mental health, substance use, or reproductive health • Provide information for interpersonal violence shelters or legal services	• Promote safety • Safe discipline • Review household safety (access to weapons, car seat) • Consider need for protective services

FIGURE 22.4. Universal interventions for children with internalizing and externalizing problems.

also serve as the treatment team lead to coordinate the additional services including educational advocacy, links with other medical providers, and mobilizing community resources.

Internalizing Disorders

Treatment for internalizing disorders generally begins with psychotherapy for mild symptoms. For both anxiety and depression, cognitive behavior therapy (CBT) is the best supported psychotherapy, although for mild depression a range of treatments can be effective (Table 22.2). For children as young as 3 and throughout adulthood, CBT adaptations have demonstrated effect (Banneyer et al., 2018; Hirshfeld-Becker et al., 2011). For older children and adolescents with moderate to severe depression, either therapy or antidepressants can be a first-line treatment for anxiety or depression.

Psychotherapy. CBT supports patients in appreciating links among thoughts, feelings, and behaviors. It entails psychoeducation, cognitive skills development (including thought evaluation and restructuring), problem solving, and behavioral approaches (e.g., goal-setting, relaxation techniques). It encourages a collaborative therapeutic relationship and includes in-session and homework assignments (Walter et al., 2020). Treatment for preschoolers with internalizing disorders is centered around the nonspecific interventions described previously and psychotherapy. CBT can help address anxiety in children as young as 3, with family-based CBT, parent group CBT, and group CBT for both parents and children all effective modalities (Comer et al., 2019). In very young children individual CBT without family involvement is not effective. Nonspecific play therapy and attachment-focused treatments have not been shown empirically to reduce preschool anxiety, although they may have a role in supporting expression of internal experiences. For preschool depressive symptoms, parent–child interaction therapy, especially the child-directed interaction portion and the novel emotional development interaction (EDI) portion, is effective (Luby et al., 2020). The EDI module teaches the caregiver to validate and label children's emotions and support emotional regulation skill

TABLE 22.2

Overview of Evidence-Based Treatments for Internalizing and Externalizing Symptoms

	Age	Mild	Moderate	Severe
Anxiety	≤6	Therapy (supportive, CBT, PMT adaptation)	Therapy (supportive, CBT, PMT adaptation)	Therapy (CBT, PMT adaptation) Consider SSRI after failure of therapy
Anxiety	≥6	CBT	CBT and/or SSRI	CBT and SSRI
Depression	≤6	Therapy	Therapy	Therapy; consideration of SSRI if therapy is ineffective or unavailable
Depression	≤6	Therapy (supportive, CBT, PMT adaptation)	Therapy (supportive, CBT, PMT adaptation)	Therapy (CBT, PMT adaptation) Consider SSRI after failure of therapy
Depression	≥6	Therapy (supportive, CBT, IPT-A, close follow-up with primary care)	Specific therapy (CBT, IPT-A, acceptance and commitment therapy) and/or SSRI	Therapy (CBT, IPT-A, acceptance and commitment therapy) and SSRI
ODD	<6	PMT	PMT	PMT
	≥6	PMT	PMT or CBT or family-focused wraparound	PMT or CBT or family-focused wraparound Consider medication for severe aggression (stimulant, alpha agonist, atypical antipsychotic agent, anti-epileptic agent)

Note. CBT = cognitive behavior therapy; IPT-A = Interpersonal psychotherapy for depressed adolescents; ODD = oppositional defiant disorder; PMT = parent management training; SSRI = selective serotonin reuptake inhibitors.

development. Only the EDI portion has been associated with changes in neural network activity on evoked potential responses. When parent–child interaction therapy is not available, family-focused play-based interventions may reduce preschool depression (Gleason et al., 2007). Although limited data support the use of medications to treat internalizing disorders in children under 6, clinical guidelines suggest that selective serotonin reuptake inhibitors could be considered to treat internalizing disorders in this age group for children whose moderate to severe symptoms have not responded to therapy or if therapy is not available (Gleason et al., 2007, 2016).

For older children and adolescents, CBT is an effective approach to address anxiety disorders (Apolinário-Hagen et al., 2020; Walter et al., 2020). Exposure to anxiety is an especially salient behavioral technique in CBT for desensitizing clients to feared stimuli, a finding supported by a meta-analysis showing that in vivo and lack of focus on relaxation strategies is associated with CBT efficacy (Whiteside et al., 2020). A growing evidence base supports mindfulness-based stress reduction, and mindfulness-based CBT has shown promise in treatment of anxiety disorders (Apolinário-Hagen et al., 2020; Wehry et al., 2015). Because child anxiety develops in the context of relationships, family-directed interventions that support family communication and help parents "avoid avoidance" (face fears) can play important roles in addressing anxiety (O'Connor et al., 2020). As in the case of preschoolers, there is a range of effective delivery mechanisms for child and adolescent anxiety including individual, group, parent coaching, and internet-based treatments (James et al., 2020; Vigerland et al., 2016). Evidence supports use of CBT for children and adolescents and interpersonal therapy and dialectical behavioral therapy for adolescents (as reviewed in Cheung et al., 2018). Mindfulness-based treatments and acceptance-commitment therapy also offer promise. Importantly, a range of modalities is effective for depression, including telehealth, group, and individual. App-based CBT approaches are not yet supported by robust research, although they are widely available and many have face validity (Horsch et al., 2017).

Pharmacologic treatment. Selective serotonin reuptake inhibitors (SSRIs) are the first-line and mainstay of pharmacotherapy for pediatric internalizing disorders in children older than 6, especially those with moderate to severe symptoms. Rigorous research supports fluoxetine, fluvoxamine, paroxetine, and sertraline in treating pediatric anxiety (Walter et al., 2020). Beyond the SSRIs, duloxetine, venlafaxine, and atomoxetine are superior to placebos in addressing pediatric anxiety. Benzodiazepines and eye movement desensitization and reprocessing do not have empirical support in pediatrics to date (Wang et al., 2017). For depression, fluoxetine has the strongest efficacy and safety evidence for depression in children older than 8 and is the only SSRI with an indication for children with depression (Bridge et al., 2007). In adolescents, some evidence supports escitalopram and sertraline, and to a lesser extent, citalopram, for use in depression (as reviewed in Cheung et al., 2018).

Externalizing Disorders

The presentation of externalizing disorders varies by age.

Preschool age/children under 6. The primary interventions for externalizing disorders in children under 6 are parent management training (PMT) approaches (Hautmann et al., 2018; Weber et al., 2019). In PMT, the focus is on supporting parental skills to promote positive behaviors and use consistent safe strategies to address misbehaviors. The foundation of these interventions is selective attention, which promotes positive attention for positive behaviors, withdrawing attention for low-level provocative behaviors, and implementing safe consistent consequences for inappropriate or unsafe behaviors. Attention to both the positive relationship enhancement and consistent consequences contributes to the treatment outcomes (Leijten et al., 2018). Examples of evidence-based PMT include parent–child interaction therapy, Incredible Years Series, New Forrest Program, Parent Management Training: the Oregon Model, and Triple P (as reviewed in Gleason et al., 2016). Self-directed, group, and online treatment methods have similar effectiveness (Thongseiratch et al., 2020). Established treatment guidelines recommend psychosocial interventions as first-line interventions for externalizing problems among preschoolers (Gleason et al., 2016). When PMT or other therapy is not effective in reducing impairment or safety concerns related to disruptive behavior problems, medication treatments can be considered, first by addressing concurrent disorders like ADHD. In the rare situation in which there are no other co-occurring disorders, stimulants, alpha agonists, and judicious use of atypical antipsychotic agents can be considered.

School age/children older than 6. One of the best studied child-focused approaches to disruptive behavior disorders in children older than 6 is CBT, which can enhance the effects of PMT (Nystrand et al., 2021; Riise et al., 2021). CBT focuses on problem-solving strategies and adopting a reflective stance, especially related to interpersonal stressors. Wraparound services like functional family therapy and multisystemic therapy apply family- and child-focused therapies focused on effective communication skills and problem-solving skills as well as community-based approaches like coaching in community or educational settings (McCart & Sheidow, 2016). Collaborative problem solving is another model of care based on the premise that "children do well if they can" in which caregivers are taught tools to support children's emerging self-regulation skill sets (Wang et al., 2022).

Pharmacologic treatment. There are no evidence-based medications treatments for ODD or conduct disorder. Several medication classes reduce non-specific aggressive symptoms, including stimulants (especially in youth with ADHD), antipsychotic agents, antidepressants, and anti-epileptic agents, particularly divalproex. Alpha agonists are commonly used to address aggression, although with limited data to support their use. When antipsychotic agents are used, the lowest possible dose is recommended, with a planned duration limited to 6 months before considering a discontinuation trial, limiting the number of concurrent medications. Medication is never the primary treatment modality for externalizing disorders.

CONCLUSION

Internalizing and externalizing problems in children and youth are prevalent, impairing, and treatable. They develop in the context of complex interactions of biological, psychological, developmental, and environmental factors. Of these factors, healthy caregivers and caregiving relationships, home and community safety, and access to basic needs are modifiable and powerful in shaping children's internalizing and externalizing. Although these problems are most often first identified in primary care settings, specialists including developmental-behavioral pediatricians, psychiatrists, and pediatric and clinical psychologists all may play an important role in diagnostic assessment and in team-based treatment. Effective interventions include addressing modifiable risk factors, evidence-based psychotherapies, and medications. Future developments will focus on strengthening preventive efforts at the individual, family, and community levels and developing effective population-based systems of care to ensure timely delivery of services to children and adolescents with internalizing or externalizing problems and their families.

RESOURCES

For Providers

Free validated measures to identify internalizing and externalizing problems in primary care, developmental-behavioral pediatrics, pediatric psychology, and other mental health settings. These include:

- Early Childhood Screening Assessment, for ages 18–60 months (40 items)

  https://www.aap.org/en/patient-care/screening-technical-assistance-and-resource-center/screening-tool-finder/early-childhood-screening-assessment-ecsa/

- Preschool Pediatric Checklist, for ages 2–5 years (17 items)

  https://www.aap.org/en/patient-care/screening-technical-assistance-and-resource-center/screening-tool-finder/pediatric-symptom-checklist-baby--preschool/

- Pediatric Symptom Checklist for ages 5–17 years (17 items)

  https://www.massgeneral.org/psychiatry/treatments-and-services/pediatric-symptom-checklist

- Screen for Anxiety Related Emotional Disorders, for ages 8–18 (41 items)

  https://pediatricbipolar.pitt.edu/clinical-services/clinical-tools

- Pediatric Symptom Checklist for Adolescents (PSC-A)

- Mood and Feelings Questionnaire, for ages 8–16 years (34 items; 13 items in the short form)

  https://psychiatry.duke.edu/research/research-programs-areas/assessment-intervention/developmental-epidemiology-instruments-0

- Strengths and Difficulties Questionnaires, for ages 2–8 (25 items)

  https://www.sdqinfo.org/a0.html

  with additional language options at

  https://www.sdqinfo.org/py/sdqinfo/b0.py

- The General Anxiety Disorder-7, for ages 13–adult (seven items)

  https://adaa.org/sites/default/files/GAD-7_Anxiety-updated_0.pdf

- American Academy of Pediatrics' PSQ-A depression questionnaire

  https://downloads.aap.org/AAP/PDF/Mental_Health_Tools_for_Pediatrics.pdf

For Parents

Resources for internalizing disorders include:

- Anxiety and Depression Association of America. (2023). *Children and teens—Anxiety and depression.* https://adaa.org/find-help/by-demographics/children/children-teens
- The American Academy of Child and Adolescent Psychiatry. (2018). *Depression: Parents medication guide.* American Psychiatric Association. https://www.aacap.org/App_Themes/AACAP/docs/resource_centers/resources/med_guides/DepressionGuide-web.pdf
- The Society of Clinical Child and Adolescent Psychology. (2024). *What is interpersonal psychotherapy?* https://effectivechildtherapy.org/therapies/what-is-interpersonal-psychotherapy/

Resources for externalizing disorders include:

- Disruptive Behavior Disorders, including ODD and CD

  https://www.healthychildren.org/English/health-issues/conditions/emotional-problems/Pages/Disruptive-Behavior-Disorders.aspx

- American Academy of Child and Adolescent Psychiatry. (2009). *ODD: A guide for families.* https://www.aacap.org/App_Themes/AACAP/docs/resource_centers/odd/odd_resource_center_odd_guide.pdf
- The Agency for Healthcare Research and Quality. (2016). *Treating disruptive behavior disorders in children and teens.* https://effectivehealthcare.ahrq.gov/products/disruptive-behavior-disorder/consumer

- Parent Training in Behavior Management for ADHD

    https://www.cdc.gov/adhd/treatment/behavior-therapy.html

- Parent–Child Interaction Therapy (PCIT) parent resources

    https://www.pcit.org/for-parents.html

- Pocket PCIT, a free resource for parents available 24 hours a day, 7 days a week

    https://www.pocketpcit.com/

- Think:Kids. (n.d.). *Collaborative Problem Solving®*. Massachusetts General Hospital. https://thinkkids.org/cps-overview/

References

Abera, M., Robbins, J. M., & Tesfaye, M. (2015). Parents' perception of child and adolescent mental health problems and their choice of treatment option in southwest Ethiopia. *Child and Adolescent Psychiatry and Mental Health, 9*(1), 40–48. https://doi.org/10.1186/s13034-015-0072-5

Achenbach, T. M. (1991). *Manual for the child behavior checklist and revised child behavior profile*. University of Vermont, Department of Psychiatry.

American Academy of Pediatrics. (2021a). *Addressing social health and early childhood wellness*. https://www.aap.org/en/patient-care/screening-technical-assistance-and-resource-center/screening-office-systems-for-practice-transformation/addressing-social-health-and-early-childhood-wellness-in-your-practice/

American Academy of Pediatrics. (2021b). *Recommendations for preventive pediatric health care*. https://downloads.aap.org/AAP/PDF/periodicity_schedule.pdf

American Academy of Pediatrics. (2021c). *Screening technical assistance and resource*. https://www.aap.org/en/patient-care/screening-technical-assistance-and-resource-center/

American Academy of Pediatrics. (2022). *Bright futures: Recommendations for preventative pediatric health care* [Periodicity schedule]. https://downloads.aap.org/AAP/PDF/periodicity_schedule.pdf?_ga=2.58869165.1487283860.1672536753-2059318530.1667669076

American Psychiatric Association. (2013). *Diagnostic and statistical manual of mental disorders* (5th ed.).

Apolinário-Hagen, J., Drüge, M., & Fritsche, L. (2020). Cognitive behavioral therapy, mindfulness-based cognitive therapy and acceptance commitment therapy for anxiety disorders: Integrating traditional with digital treatment approaches. In Y.-K. Kim (Ed.), *Anxiety disorders: Rethinking and understanding recent discoveries* (pp. 291–329). Springer Nature Singapore. https://doi.org/10.1007/978-981-32-9705-0_17

Baker, B. L., Neece, C. L., Fenning, R. M., Crnic, K. A., & Blacher, J. (2010). Mental disorders in five-year-old children with or without developmental delay: Focus on ADHD. *Journal of Clinical Child and Adolescent Psychology, 39*(4), 492–505. https://doi.org/10.1080/15374416.2010.486321

Banneyer, K. N., Bonin, L., Price, K., Goodman, W. K., & Storch, E. A. (2018). Cognitive behavioral therapy for childhood anxiety disorders: A review of recent advances. *Current Psychiatry Reports, 20*(8), 65–73. https://doi.org/10.1007/s11920-018-0924-9

Beesdo, K., Knappe, S., & Pine, D. S. (2009). Anxiety and anxiety disorders in children and adolescents: Developmental issues and implications for *DSM-V*. *Psychiatric Clinics of North America, 32*(3), 483–524. https://doi.org/10.1016/j.psc.2009.06.002

Birmaher, B., Brent, D. A., Chiappetta, L., Bridge, J., Monga, S., & Baugher, M. (1999). Psychometric properties of the Screen for Child Anxiety Related Emotional Disorders (SCARED): A replication study. *Journal of the American Academy of Child & Adolescent Psychiatry, 38*(10), 1230–1236. https://doi.org/10.1097/00004583-199910000-00011

Borchers, L. R., Dennis, E. L., King, L. S., Humphreys, K. L., & Gotlib, I. H. (2021). Prenatal and postnatal depressive symptoms, infant white matter, and toddler behavioral problems. *Journal of Affective Disorders, 282*, 465–471. https://doi.org/10.1016/j.jad.2020.12.075

Bridge, J. A., Iyengar, S., Salary, C. B., Barbe, R. P., Birmaher, B., Pincus, H. A., Ren, L., & Brent, D. A. (2007). Clinical response and risk for reported suicidal ideation and suicide attempts in pediatric antidepressant treatment: A meta-analysis of randomized controlled trials. *JAMA: Journal of the American Medical Association, 297*(15), 1683–1696. https://doi.org/10.1001/jama.297.15.1683

Brown, J. D., & Wissow, L. S. (2010). Screening to identify mental health problems in pediatric primary care: Considerations for practice. *International Journal of Psychiatry in Medicine, 40*(1), 1–19. https://doi.org/10.2190/PM.40.1.a

Brown, J. D., Wissow, L. S., Cook, B. L., Longway, S., Caffery, E., & Pefaure, C. (2013). Mental health communications skills training for medical assistants in pediatric primary care. *The Journal of Behavioral Health Services & Research, 40*(1), 20–35. https://doi.org/10.1007/s11414-012-9292-0

Bufferd, S. J., Dougherty, L. R., Carlson, G. A., & Klein, D. N. (2011). Parent-reported mental health in preschoolers: Findings using a diagnostic interview. *Comprehensive Psychiatry, 52*(4), 359–369. https://doi.org/10.1016/j.comppsych.2010.08.006

Bussing, R., Schoenberg, N. E., Rogers, K. M., Zima, B. T., & Angus, S. (1998). Explanatory models of ADHD: Do they differ by ethnicity, child gender, or treatment status? *Journal of Emotional and Behavioral Disorders, 6*(4), 233–242. https://doi.org/10.1177/106342669800600405

Calkins, S. D., & Fox, N. A. (1992). The relations among infant temperament, security of attachment, and behavioral inhibition at twenty-four months. *Child Development, 63*(6), 1456–1472. https://doi.org/10.2307/1131568

Caspi, A., & Moffitt, T. E. (2018). All for one and one for all: Mental disorders in one dimension. *The American Journal of Psychiatry, 175*(9), 831–844. https://doi.org/10.1176/appi.ajp.2018.17121383

Cheung, A. H., Zuckerbrot, R. A., Jensen, P. S., Laraque, D., Stein, R. E. K., & GLAD-PC Steering Group. (2018). Guidelines for adolescent depression in primary care (GLAD-PC): Part II. Treatment and ongoing management. *Pediatrics, 141*(3), e20174082. https://doi.org/10.1542/peds.2017-4082

Chiu, A., Falk, A., & Walkup, J. T. (2016). Anxiety disorders among children and adolescents. *Focus, 14*(1), 26–33. https://doi.org/10.1176/appi.focus.20150029

Coker, T. R., Elliott, M. N., Toomey, S. L., Schwebel, D. C., Cuccaro, P., Tortolero Emery, S., Davies, S. L., Visser, S. N., & Schuster, M. A. (2016). Racial and ethnic disparities in ADHD diagnosis and treatment. *Pediatrics, 138*(3), e20160407. https://doi.org/10.1542/peds.2016-0407

Comer, J. S., Hong, N., Poznanski, B., Silva, K., & Wilson, M. (2019). Evidence base update on the treatment of early childhood anxiety and related problems. *Journal of Clinical Child and Adolescent Psychology, 48*(1), 1–15. https://doi.org/10.1080/15374416.2018.1534208

Conradt, E., Camerota, M., Maylott, S., & Lester, B. M. (2023). Annual Research Review: Prenatal opioid exposure—A two-generation approach to conceptualizing neurodevelopmental outcomes. *Journal of Child Psychology and Psychiatry, 64*(4), 566–578. https://doi.org/10.1111/jcpp.13761

Côté, S. M., Boivin, M., Liu, X., Nagin, D. S., Zoccolillo, M., & Tremblay, R. E. (2009). Depression and anxiety symptoms: Onset, developmental course and risk factors during early childhood. *Journal of Child Psychology and Psychiatry, 50*(10), 1201–1208. https://doi.org/10.1111/j.1469-7610.2009.02099.x

Côté, S. M., Vaillancourt, T., LeBlanc, J. C., Nagin, D. S., & Tremblay, R. E. (2006). The development of physical aggression from toddlerhood to pre-adolescence: A nation wide longitudinal study of Canadian children. *Journal of Abnormal Child Psychology, 34*(1), 71–85. https://doi.org/10.1007/s10802-005-9001-z

Crockett, L. J., Carlo, G., Wolff, J. M., & Hope, M. O. (2013). The role of pubertal timing and temperamental vulnerability in adolescents' internalizing symptoms. *Development and Psychopathology, 25*(2), 377–389. https://doi.org/10.1017/S0954579412001125

Danielson, M. L., Bitsko, R. H., Holbrook, J. R., Charania, S. N., Claussen, A. H., McKeown, R. E., Cuffe, S. P., Owens, J. S., Evans, S. W., Kubicek, L., & Flory, K. (2021). Community-based prevalence of externalizing and internalizing disorders among school-aged children and adolescents in four geographically dispersed school districts in the United States. *Child Psychiatry and Human Development, 52*(3), 500–514. https://doi.org/10.1007/s10578-020-01027-z

De Ruiter, K. P., Dekker, M. C., Verhulst, F. C., & Koot, H. M. (2007). Developmental course of psychopathology in youths with and without intellectual disabilities. *Journal of Child Psychology and Psychiatry, 48*(5), 498–507. https://doi.org/10.1111/j.1469-7610.2006.01712.x

Egger, H. L., & Angold, A. (2006). Common emotional and behavioral disorders in preschool children: Presentation, nosology, and epidemiology. *Journal of Child Psychology and Psychiatry, 47*(3–4), 313–337. https://doi.org/10.1111/j.1469-7610.2006.01618.x

Finsaas, M. C., Bufferd, S. J., Dougherty, L. R., Carlson, G. A., & Klein, D. N. (2018). Preschool psychiatric disorders: Homotypic and heterotypic continuity through middle childhood and early adolescence. *Psychological Medicine, 48*(13), 2159–2168. https://doi.org/10.1017/S0033291717003646

Fleckman, J. M., Drury, S. S., Taylor, C. A., & Theall, K. P. (2016). Role of direct and indirect violence exposure on externalizing behavior in children. *Journal of Urban Health, 93*(3), 479–492. https://doi.org/10.1007/s11524-016-0052-y

Foster, H., & Brooks-Gunn, J. (2015). Children's exposure to community and war violence and mental health in four African countries. *Social Science & Medicine, 146*, 292–299. https://doi.org/10.1016/j.socscimed.2015.10.020

Fox, N. A., Buzzell, G. A., Morales, S., Valadez, E. A., Wilson, M., & Henderson, H. A. (2021). Understanding the emergence of social anxiety in children with behavioral inhibition. *Biological Psychiatry*, *89*(7), 681–689. https://doi.org/10.1016/j.biopsych.2020.10.004

Foy, J. M., Kelleher, K. J., Laraque, D., & the American Academy of Pediatrics Task Force on Mental Health. (2010). Enhancing pediatric mental health care: Strategies for preparing a primary care practice. *Pediatrics*, *125*(Suppl. 3), S87–S108. https://doi.org/10.1542/peds.2010-0788E

Frick, P. J., Ray, J. V., Thornton, L. C., & Kahn, R. E. (2014). Annual research review: A developmental psychopathology approach to understanding callous-unemotional traits in children and adolescents with serious conduct problems. *Journal of Child Psychology and Psychiatry*, *55*(6), 532–548. https://doi.org/10.1111/jcpp.12152

Fritz, J., de Graaff, A. M., Caisley, H., van Harmelen, A.-L., & Wilkinson, P. O. (2018). A systematic review of amenable resilience factors that moderate and/or mediate the relationship between childhood adversity and mental health in young people. *Frontiers in Psychiatry*, *9*, 230–247. https://doi.org/10.3389/fpsyt.2018.00230

Frost, A., Kessel, E., Black, S., Goldstein, B., Bernard, K., & Klein, D. N. (2019). Homotypic and heterotypic continuity of internalizing and externalizing symptoms from ages 3 to 12: The moderating role of diurnal cortisol. *Development and Psychopathology*, *31*(2), 789–798. https://doi.org/10.1017/S0954579418000573

Fulton, B. D., Scheffler, R. M., Hinshaw, S. P., Levine, P., Stone, S., Brown, T. T., & Modrek, S. (2009). National variation of ADHD diagnostic prevalence and medication use: Health care providers and education policies. *Psychiatric Services*, *60*(8), 1075–1083. https://doi.org/10.1176/ps.2009.60.8.1075

Gallagher, K. C., & Mayer, K. (2008). Enhancing development and learning through teacher-child relationships. *Young Children*, *63*(6), 80–87. https://eric.ed.gov/?id=EJ819346

Gilliam, W. S., Maupin, A. N., Reyes, C. R., Accavitti, M., & Shic, F. (2016). *Do early educators' implicit biases regarding sex and race relate to behavior expectations and recommendations of preschool expulsions and suspensions?* Yale University Child Study Center.

Gleason, M. M., Egger, H. L., Emslie, G. J., Greenhill, L. L., Kowatch, R. A., Lieberman, A. F., Luby, J. L., Owens, J., Scahill, L. D., Scheeringa, M. S., Stafford, B., Wise, B., & Zeanah, C. H. (2007). Psychopharmacological treatment for very young children: Contexts and guidelines. *Journal of the American Academy of Child & Adolescent Psychiatry*, *46*(12), 1532–1572. https://doi.org/10.1097/chi.0b013e3181570d9e

Gleason, M. M., Goldson, E., Yogman, M. W., Council on Early Childhood, Committee on Psychosocial Aspects of Child and Family Health, Section on Developmental and Behavioral Pediatrics, Lieser, D., DelConte, B., Donoghue, E., Earls, M., Glassy, D., McFadden, T., Mendelsohn, A., Scholer, S., Takagishi, J., Vanderbilt, D., Williams, P. G., Yogman, M., Bauer, N., . . . Voigt, R. G. (2016). Addressing early childhood emotional and behavioral problems [Technical report]. *Pediatrics*, *138*(6), e20163025. https://doi.org/10.1542/peds.2016-3025

Groh, A. M., Fearon, R. P., van IJzendoorn, M. H., Bakermans-Kranenburg, M. J., & Roisman, G. I. (2017). Attachment in the early life course: Meta-analytic evidence for its role in socioemotional development. *Child Development Perspectives*, *11*(1), 70–76. https://doi.org/10.1111/cdep.12213

Gutman, L. M., & Codiroli McMaster, N. (2020). Gendered pathways of internalizing problems from early childhood to adolescence and associated adolescent outcomes. *Journal of Abnormal Child Psychology*, *48*(5), 703–718. https://doi.org/10.1007/s10802-020-00623-w

Hautmann, C., Dose, C., Duda-Kirchhof, K., Greimel, L., Hellmich, M., Imort, S., Katzmann, J., Pinior, J., Scholz, K., Schürmann, S., Wolff Metternich-Kaizman, T., & Döpfner, M. (2018). Behavioral versus nonbehavioral guided self-help for parents of children with externalizing disorders in a randomized controlled trial. *Behavior Therapy*, *49*(6), 951–965. https://doi.org/10.1016/j.beth.2018.02.002

Hentges, R. F., Graham, S. A., Plamondon, A., Tough, S., & Madigan, S. (2019). A developmental cascade from prenatal stress to child internalizing and externalizing problems. *Journal of Pediatric Psychology*, *44*(9), 1057–1067. https://doi.org/10.1093/jpepsy/jsz044

Herba, C. M., Glover, V., Ramchandani, P. G., & Rondon, M. B. (2016). Maternal depression and mental health in early childhood: An examination of underlying mechanisms in low-income and middle-income countries. *The Lancet Psychiatry*, *3*(10), 983–992. https://doi.org/10.1016/S2215-0366(16)30148-1

Hirshfeld-Becker, D. R., Micco, J. A., Mazursky, H., Bruett, L., & Henin, A. (2011). Applying cognitive-behavioral therapy for anxiety to the younger child. *Child and Adolescent Psychiatric Clinics of North America*, *20*(2), 349–368. https://doi.org/10.1016/j.chc.2011.01.008

Horsch, C. H. G., Lancee, J., Griffioen-Both, F., Spruit, S., Fitrianie, S., Neerincx, M. A., Beun, R. J., & Brinkman, W. P. (2017). Mobile phone-delivered cognitive behavioral therapy for insomnia: A randomized waitlist-controlled trial. *Journal of Medical Internet Research*, 19(4), e70. https://doi.org/10.2196/jmir.6524

Hoyniak, C. P., & Petersen, I. T. (2019). A meta-analytic evaluation of the N2 component as an endophenotype of response inhibition and externalizing psychopathology in childhood. *Neuroscience and Biobehavioral Reviews*, 103, 200–215. https://doi.org/10.1016/j.neubiorev.2019.06.011

James, A. C., Reardon, T., Soler, A., James, G., & Creswell, C. (2020). Cognitive behavioural therapy for anxiety disorders in children and adolescents. *Cochrane Database of Systematic Reviews*, 2020(11), CD013162. https://doi.org/10.1002/14651858.CD013162.pub2

Johnson, J. G., Harris, E. S., Spitzer, R. L., & Williams, J. B. (2002). The patient health questionnaire for adolescents: Validation of an instrument for the assessment of mental disorders among adolescent primary care patients. *Journal of Adolescent Health*, 30(3), 196–204. https://doi.org/10.1016/S1054-139X(01)00333-0

Kieling, C., Baker-Henningham, H., Belfer, M., Conti, G., Ertem, I., Omigbodun, O., Rohde, L. A., Srinath, S., Ulkuer, N., & Rahman, A. (2011). Child and adolescent mental health worldwide: Evidence for action. *The Lancet*, 378(9801), 1515–1525. https://doi.org/10.1016/S0140-6736(11)60827-1

Kumar, R., & Gleason, M. M. (2019). Pediatric attention-deficit/hyperactivity disorder in Louisiana: Trends, challenges, and opportunities for enhanced quality of care. *The Ochsner Journal*, 19(4), 357–368. https://doi.org/10.31486/toj.18.0103

Lavigne, J. V., Gouze, K. R., Bryant, F. B., & Hopkins, J. (2014). Dimensions of oppositional defiant disorder in young children: Heterotypic continuity with anxiety and depression. *Journal of Abnormal Child Psychology*, 42(6), 937–951. https://doi.org/10.1007/s10802-014-9853-1

Lawton, K. E., Gerdes, A. C., Haack, L. M., & Schneider, B. (2014). Acculturation, cultural values, and Latino parental beliefs about the etiology of ADHD. *Administration and Policy in Mental Health and Mental Health Services Research*, 41(2), 189–204. https://doi.org/10.1007/s10488-012-0447-3

Lees, B., Mewton, L., Jacobus, J., Valadez, E. A., Stapinski, L. A., Teesson, M., Tapert, S. F., & Squeglia, L. M. (2020). Association of prenatal alcohol exposure with psychological, behavioral, and neurodevelopmental outcomes in children from the adolescent brain cognitive development study. *The American Journal of Psychiatry*, 177(11), 1060–1072. https://doi.org/10.1176/appi.ajp.2020.20010086

Leijten, P., Melendez-Torres, G. J., Gardner, F., van Aar, J., Schulz, S., & Overbeek, G. (2018). Are relationship enhancement and behavior management "the golden couple" for disruptive child behavior? Two meta-analyses. *Child Development*, 89(6), 1970–1982. https://doi.org/10.1111/cdev.13051

Lin, B., Ostlund, B. D., Conradt, E., Lagasse, L. L., & Lester, B. M. (2018). Testing the programming of temperament and psychopathology in two independent samples of children with prenatal substance exposure. *Development and Psychopathology*, 30(3), 1023–1040. https://doi.org/10.1017/S0954579418000391

Lindsey, M. A., Brandt, N. E., Becker, K. D., Lee, B. R., Barth, R. P., Daleiden, E. L., & Chorpita, B. F. (2014). Identifying the common elements of treatment engagement interventions in children's mental health services. *Clinical Child and Family Psychology Review*, 17(3), 283–298. https://doi.org/10.1007/s10567-013-0163-x

Luby, J. L., Gilbert, K., Whalen, D., Tillman, R., & Barch, D. M. (2020). The differential contribution of the components of parent-child interaction therapy emotion development for treatment of preschool depression. *Journal of the American Academy of Child & Adolescent Psychiatry*, 59(7), 868–879. https://doi.org/10.1016/j.jaac.2019.07.937

Luby, J. L., Heffelfinger, A. K., Mrakotsky, C., Brown, K. M., Hessler, M. J., Wallis, J. M., & Spitznagel, E. L. (2003). The clinical picture of depression in preschool children. *Journal of the American Academy of Child & Adolescent Psychiatry*, 42(3), 340–348. https://doi.org/10.1097/00004583-200303000-00015

Madigan, S., Oatley, H., Racine, N., Fearon, R. P., Schumacher, L., Akbari, E., Cooke, J. E., & Tarabulsy, G. M. (2018). A meta-analysis of maternal prenatal depression and anxiety on child socioemotional development. *Journal of the American Academy of Child & Adolescent Psychiatry*, 57(9), 645–657.e648.

Madsen, K. B., Ersbøll, A. K., Olsen, J., Parner, E., & Obel, C. (2015). Geographic analysis of the variation in the incidence of ADHD in a country with free access to healthcare: A Danish cohort study. *International Journal of Health Geographics*, 14(1), 24. https://doi.org/10.1186/s12942-015-0018-4

Mandell, D. S., Guevara, J. P., Rostain, A. L., & Hadley, T. R. (2003). Economic grand rounds: Medical expenditures among children with psychiatric disorders in a Medicaid population. *Psychiatric*

Services, 54(4), 465–467. https://doi.org/10.1176/appi.ps.54.4.465

March, J. S., Parker, J. D., Sullivan, K., Stallings, P., & Conners, C. K. (1997). The Multidimensional Anxiety Scale for Children (MASC): Factor structure, reliability, and validity. *Journal of the American Academy of Child & Adolescent Psychiatry*, 36(4), 554–565.

Martinez, J. I., Lau, A. S., Chorpita, B. F., Weisz, J. R., & the Research Network on Youth Mental Health. (2017). Psychoeducation as a mediator of treatment approach on parent engagement in child psychotherapy for disruptive behavior. *Journal of Clinical Child and Adolescent Psychology*, 46(4), 573–587. https://doi.org/10.1080/15374416.2015.1038826

McCart, M. R., & Sheidow, A. J. (2016). Evidence-based psychosocial treatments for adolescents with disruptive behavior. *Journal of Clinical Child and Adolescent Psychology*, 45(5), 529–563. https://doi.org/10.1080/15374416.2016.1146990

Mesman, J., Bongers, I. L., & Koot, H. M. (2001). Preschool developmental pathways to preadolescent internalizing and externalizing problems. *Journal of Child Psychology and Psychiatry*, 42(5), 679–689. https://doi.org/10.1111/1469-7610.00763

Morrissette, M. (2021). School closures and social anxiety during the COVID-19 pandemic. *Journal of the American Academy of Child & Adolescent Psychiatry*, 60(1), 6–7. https://doi.org/10.1016/j.jaac.2020.08.436

Murray, A. L., Eisner, M., Nagin, D., & Ribeaud, D. (2020). A multi-trajectory analysis of commonly co-occurring mental health issues across childhood and adolescence. *European Child & Adolescent Psychiatry*, 31(1), 145–159.

Mykletun, A., Widding-Havneraas, T., Chaulagain, A., Lyhmann, I., Bjelland, I., Halmøy, A., Elwert, F., Butterworth, P., Markussen, S., Zachrisson, H. D., & Rypdal, K. (2021). Causal modelling of variation in clinical practice and long-term outcomes of ADHD using Norwegian registry data: The ADHD controversy project. *BMJ Open*, 11(1), e041698. https://doi.org/10.1136/bmjopen-2020-041698

Nikstat, A., & Riemann, R. (2020). On the etiology of internalizing and externalizing problem behavior: A twin-family study. *PLOS ONE*, 15(3), e0230626. https://doi.org/10.1371/journal.pone.0230626

Nystrand, C., Helander, M., Enebrink, P., Feldman, I., & Sampaio, F. (2021). Adding the Coping Power Programme to parent management training: The cost-effectiveness of stacking interventions for children with disruptive behaviour disorders. *European Child & Adolescent Psychiatry*, 30(10), 1603–1614. https://doi.org/10.1007/s00787-020-01638-w

O'Connor, E. E., Holly, L. E., Chevalier, L. L., Pincus, D. B., & Langer, D. A. (2020). Parent and child emotion and distress responses associated with parental accommodation of child anxiety symptoms. *Journal of Clinical Psychology*, 76(7), 1390–1407. https://doi.org/10.1002/jclp.22941

Oldehinkel, A. J., & Ormel, J. (2022). Annual research review: Stability of psychopathology: Lessons learned from longitudinal population surveys. *Journal of Child Psychology and Psychiatry*, 64(4), 489–502. https://doi.org/10.1111/jcpp.13737

Ormel, J., Oldehinkel, A. J., Ferdinand, R. F., Hartman, C. A., De Winter, A. F., Veenstra, R., Vollebergh, W., Minderaa, R. B., Buitelaar, J. K., & Verhulst, F. C. (2005). Internalizing and externalizing problems in adolescence: General and dimension-specific effects of familial loadings and preadolescent temperament traits. *Psychological Medicine*, 35(12), 1825–1835. https://doi.org/10.1017/S0033291705005829

Palmer, R. H., Bidwell, L. C., Heath, A. C., Brick, L. A., Madden, P. A., & Knopik, V. S. (2016). Effects of maternal smoking during pregnancy on offspring externalizing problems: Contextual effects in a sample of female twins. *Behavior Genetics*, 46(3), 403–415. https://doi.org/10.1007/s10519-016-9779-1

Patalay, P., Moulton, V., Goodman, A., & Ploubidis, G. B. (2017). Cross-domain symptom development typologies and their antecedents: Results from the UK millennium cohort study. *Journal of the American Academy of Child & Adolescent Psychiatry*, 56(9), 765–776.e2. https://doi.org/10.1016/j.jaac.2017.06.009

Paulus, F. W., Ohmann, S., & Popow, C. (2016). Practitioner Review: School-based interventions in child mental health. *Journal of Child Psychology and Psychiatry*, 57(12), 1337–1359. https://doi.org/10.1111/jcpp.12584

Pella, J. E., Slade, E. P., Pikulski, P. J., & Ginsburg, G. S. (2020). Pediatric anxiety disorders: A cost of illness analysis. *Journal of Abnormal Child Psychology*, 48(4), 551–559. https://doi.org/10.1007/s10802-020-00626-7

Pinquart, M., & Shen, Y. (2011). Depressive symptoms in children and adolescents with chronic physical illness: An updated meta-analysis. *Journal of Pediatric Psychology*, 36(4), 375–384. https://doi.org/10.1093/jpepsy/jsq104

Rescorla, L. A., Althoff, R. R., Ivanova, M. Y., & Achenbach, T. M. (2019). Effects of society and culture on parents' ratings of children's mental health problems in 45 societies. *European Child*

& *Adolescent Psychiatry, 28*(8), 1107–1115. https://doi.org/10.1007/s00787-018-01268-3

Reynolds, C., & Richmond, B. O. (1985). Revised children's manifest anxiety scale. *Psychological Assessment*. Western Psychological Service. https://doi.org/10.1177/073428298700500110

Reynolds, C. R., & Kamphaus, R. W. (2015). *Behavior assessment for children* (3rd ed.). Pearson.

Riise, E. N., Wergeland, G. J. H., Njardvik, U., & Öst, L.-G. (2021). Cognitive behavior therapy for externalizing disorders in children and adolescents in routine clinical care: A systematic review and meta-analysis. *Clinical Psychology Review, 83*, e101954. https://doi.org/10.1016/j.cpr.2020.101954

Rowe, R., Costello, E. J., Angold, A., Copeland, W. E., & Maughan, B. (2010). Developmental pathways in oppositional defiant disorder and conduct disorder. *Journal of Abnormal Psychology, 119*(4), 726–738. https://doi.org/10.1037/a0020798

Sameroff, A. (Ed.). (2009). *The Transactional model of development: How children and contexts shape each other*. American Psychological Association. https://doi.org/10.1037/11877-000

Sheldrick, R. C., Merchant, S., & Perrin, E. C. (2011). Identification of developmental-behavioral problems in primary care: A systematic review. *Pediatrics, 128*(2), 356–363. https://doi.org/10.1542/peds.2010-3261

Slopen, N., Fitzmaurice, G., Williams, D. R., & Gilman, S. E. (2010). Poverty, food insecurity, and the behavior for childhood internalizing and externalizing disorders. *Journal of the American Academy of Child & Adolescent Psychiatry, 49*(5), 444–452.

Spence, S. H. (1998). A measure of anxiety symptoms among children. *Behaviour Research and Therapy, 36*(5), 545–566. https://doi.org/10.1016/S0005-7967(98)00034-5

Spence, S. H. (2018). Assessing anxiety disorders in children and adolescents. *Child and Adolescent Mental Health, 23*(3), 266–282. https://doi.org/10.1111/camh.12251

Speyer, L. G., Neaves, S., Hall, H. A., Hemani, G., Lombardo, M. V., Murray, A. L., Auyeung, B., & Luciano, M. (2022). Polygenic risks for joint developmental trajectories of internalizing and externalizing problems: Findings from the ALSPAC cohort. *Journal of Child Psychology and Psychiatry, 63*(8), 948–956. https://doi.org/10.1111/jcpp.13549

Spielberger, C. D., Edwards, C. D., Montouri, J., & Lushene, R. (1973). *State-Trait Anxiety Inventory for Children (STAI-CH)* [Database record]. APA PsycTests. https://doi.org/10.1037/t06497-000

Sroufe, L. A. (2005). Attachment and development: A prospective, longitudinal study from birth to adulthood. *Attachment & Human Development, 7*(4), 349–367. https://doi.org/10.1080/14616730500365928

Stein, A., Pearson, R. M., Goodman, S. H., Rapa, E., Rahman, A., McCallum, M., Howard, L. M., & Pariante, C. M. (2014). Effects of perinatal mental disorders on the fetus and child. *The Lancet, 384*(9956), 1800–1819. https://doi.org/10.1016/S0140-6736(14)61277-0

Steiner, H., Remsing, L., & the Work Group on Quality Issues. (2007). Practice parameter for the assessment and treatment of children and adolescents with oppositional defiant disorder. *Journal of the American Academy of Child & Adolescent Psychiatry, 46*(1), 126–141. https://doi.org/10.1097/01.chi.0000246060.62706.af

Strawn, J. R., Lu, L., Peris, T. S., Levine, A., & Walkup, J. T. (2021). Research review: Pediatric anxiety disorders—What have we learnt in the last 10 years? *Journal of Child Psychology and Psychiatry, 62*(2), 114–139. https://doi.org/10.1111/jcpp.13262

Suchman, N. E., DeCoste, C., & Dias, H. E. (2019). Parental psychopathology. In M. H. Bornstein (Ed.), *Handbook of parenting: Vol. 4. Social conditions and applied parenting* (pp. 517–555). Routledge. https://doi.org/10.4324/9780429398995-17

Sutin, A. R., Flynn, H. A., & Terracciano, A. (2017). Maternal cigarette smoking during pregnancy and the trajectory of externalizing and internalizing symptoms across childhood: Similarities and differences across parent, teacher, and self reports. *Journal of Psychiatric Research, 91*, 145–148. https://doi.org/10.1016/j.jpsychires.2017.03.003

Teymoori, A., Côté, S. M., Jones, B. L., Nagin, D. S., Boivin, M., Vitaro, F., Orri, M., & Tremblay, R. E. (2018). Risk factors associated with boys' and girls' developmental trajectories of physical aggression from early childhood through early adolescence. *JAMA Network Open, 1*(8), e186364. https://doi.org/10.1001/jamanetworkopen.2018.6364

Thongseiratch, T., Leijten, P., & Melendez-Torres, G. J. (2020). Online parent programs for children's behavioral problems: A meta-analytic review. *European Child & Adolescent Psychiatry, 29*(11), 1555–1568. https://doi.org/10.1007/s00787-020-01472-0

Tien, J., Lewis, G. D., & Liu, J. (2020). Prenatal risk factors for internalizing and externalizing problems in childhood. *World Journal of Pediatrics, 16*(4), 341–355. https://doi.org/10.1007/s12519-019-00319-2

Upadhyay, N., Aparasu, R., Rowan, P. J., Fleming, M. L., Balkrishnan, R., & Chen, H. (2019). The association between geographic access to providers and the treatment quality of pediatric depression.

Van den Bergh, B. R., Van Calster, B., Smits, T., Van Huffel, S., & Lagae, L. (2008). Antenatal maternal anxiety is related to HPA-axis dysregulation and self-reported depressive symptoms in adolescence: A prospective study on the fetal origins of depressed mood. *Neuropsychopharmacology, 33*(3), 536–545. https://doi.org/10.1038/sj.npp.1301450

Vigerland, S., Lenhard, F., Bonnert, M., Lalouni, M., Hedman, E., Ahlen, J., Olén, O., Serlachius, E., & Ljótsson, B. (2016). Internet-delivered cognitive behavior therapy for children and adolescents: A systematic review and meta-analysis. *Clinical Psychology Review, 50*, 1–10. https://doi.org/10.1016/j.cpr.2016.09.005

Visootsak, J., & Sherman, S. (2007). Neuropsychiatric and behavioral aspects of trisomy 21. *Current Psychiatry Reports, 9*(2), 135–140. https://doi.org/10.1007/s11920-007-0083-x

Walter, H. J., Bukstein, O. G., Abright, A. R., Keable, H., Ramtekkar, U., Ripperger-Suhler, J., & Rockhill, C. (2020). Clinical practice guideline for the assessment and treatment of children and adolescents with anxiety disorders. *Journal of the American Academy of Child & Adolescent Psychiatry, 59*(10), 1107–1124. https://doi.org/10.1016/j.jaac.2020.05.005

Wang, H., Lin, S. L., Leung, G. M., & Schooling, C. M. (2016). Age at onset of puberty and adolescent depression: "Children of 1997" birth cohort. *Pediatrics, 137*(6), e20153231. https://doi.org/10.1542/peds.2015-3231

Wang, L., Stoll, S., Hone, M., Ablon, J. S., & Pollastri, A. R. (2022). Effects of a collaborative problem solving parent group on parent and child outcomes. *Child & Family Behavior Therapy, 44*(4), 241–258. https://doi.org/10.1080/07317107.2022.2117464

Wang, Z., Whiteside, S. P. H., Sim, L., Farah, W., Morrow, A. S., Alsawas, M., Barrionuevo, P., Tello, M., Asi, N., Beuschel, B., Daraz, L., Almasri, J., Zaiem, F., Larrea-Mantilla, L., Ponce, O. J., LeBlanc, A., Prokop, L. J., & Murad, M. H. (2017). Comparative effectiveness and safety of cognitive behavioral therapy and pharmacotherapy for childhood anxiety disorders: A systematic review and meta-analysis. *JAMA Pediatrics, 171*(11), 1049–1056. https://doi.org/10.1001/jamapediatrics.2017.3036

Weber, L., Kamp-Becker, I., Christiansen, H., & Mingebach, T. (2019). Treatment of child externalizing behavior problems: A comprehensive review and meta-meta-analysis on effects of parent-based interventions on parental characteristics. *European Child & Adolescent Psychiatry, 28*(8), 1025–1036. https://doi.org/10.1007/s00787-018-1175-3

Wehry, A. M., Beesdo-Baum, K., Hennelly, M. M., Connolly, S. D., & Strawn, J. R. (2015). Assessment and treatment of anxiety disorders in children and adolescents. *Current Psychiatry Reports, 17*(7), 52. https://doi.org/10.1007/s11920-015-0591-z

Weissman, M. M., Pilowsky, D. J., Wickramaratne, P. J., Talati, A., Wisniewski, S. R., Fava, M., Hughes, C. W., Garber, J., Malloy, E., King, C. A., Cerda, G., Sood, A. B., Alpert, J. E., Trivedi, M. H., & Rush, A. J. (2006). Remissions in maternal depression and child psychopathology: A STAR*D-child report. *JAMA: Journal of the American Medical Association, 295*(12), 1389–1398. https://doi.org/10.1001/jama.295.12.1389

Weisz, J. R., & Kazdin, A. E. (2010). *Evidence-based psychotherapies for children and adolescents*. Guilford Press.

Weitzman, C., Wegner, L., the Section on Developmental and Behavioral Pediatrics, Committee on Psychosocial Aspects of Child and Family Health, Council on Early Childhood, & Society for Developmental and Behavioral Pediatrics. (2015). Promoting optimal development: Screening for behavioral and emotional problems. *Pediatrics, 135*(2), 384–395. https://doi.org/10.1542/peds.2014-3716

Whiteside, S. P. H., Sim, L. A., Morrow, A. S., Farah, W. H., Hilliker, D. R., Murad, M. H., & Wang, Z. (2020). A meta-analysis to guide the enhancement of CBT for childhood anxiety: Exposure over anxiety management. *Clinical Child and Family Psychology Review, 23*(1), 102–121. https://doi.org/10.1007/s10567-019-00303-2

Whitney, D. G., & Peterson, M. D. (2019). US national and state-level prevalence of mental health disorders and disparities of mental health care use in children. *JAMA Pediatrics, 173*(4), 389–391. https://doi.org/10.1001/jamapediatrics.2018.5399

World Health Organization. (2017). *The IDC-11 classification of mental and behavioural disorders: Clinical descriptions and diagnostic guidelines*. https://www.who.int/publications/i/item/9789240077263

World Health Organization. (2019). *Suicide worldwide in 2019: Global health estimates*. WHO. https://www.who.int/publications/i/item/9789240026643

Wichstrøm, L., Belsky, J., & Steinsbekk, S. (2017). Homotypic and heterotypic continuity of symptoms of psychiatric disorders from age 4 to 10 years: A dynamic panel model. *Journal of Child Psychology and Psychiatry, 58*(11), 1239–1247. https://doi.org/10.1111/jcpp.12754

Wichstrøm, L., Berg-Nielsen, T. S., Angold, A., Egger, H. L., Solheim, E., & Sveen, T. H. (2012). Prevalence of psychiatric disorders in preschoolers. *Journal of Child Psychology and Psychiatry, and Allied Disciplines, 53*(6), 695–705. https://doi.org/10.1111/j.1469-7610.2011.02514.x

Yeh, M., Hough, R. L., McCabe, K., Lau, A., & Garland, A. (2004). Parental beliefs about the causes of child problems: Exploring racial/ethnic patterns. *Journal of the American Academy of Child & Adolescent Psychiatry, 43*(5), 605–612. https://doi.org/10.1097/00004583-200405000-00014

Zahl, T., Steinsbekk, S., & Wichstrøm, L. (2017). Physical activity, sedentary behavior, and symptoms of major depression in middle childhood. *Pediatrics, 139*(2), e20161711. https://doi.org/10.1542/peds.2016-1711

Zeanah, C. H., Berlin, L. J., & Boris, N. W. (2011). Practitioner review: Clinical applications of attachment theory and research for infants and young children. *Journal of Child Psychology and Psychiatry, 52*(8), 819–833. https://doi.org/10.1111/j.1469-7610.2011.02399.x

Zeanah, C. H., Carter, A. S., Cohen, J., Egger, H., Gleason, M. M., Keren, M., Lieberman, A., Mulrooney, K., & Oser, C. (2016). *The Diagnostic Classification of Mental Health and Developmental Disorders of Infancy and Early Childhood DC:0–5:* Selective reviews from a new nosology for early childhood psychopathology. *Infant Mental Health Journal, 37*(5), 471–475.

Zero to Three. (2016). *DC:0–5: Diagnostic classification of mental health and developmental disorders of infancy and early childhood* (Rev. ed.).

CHAPTER 23

EATING DISORDERS IN CHILDREN AND ADOLESCENTS

Terrill Bravender, Natalie Prohaska, and Jessica Van Huysse

The term "eating disorder" encompasses a wide variety of unhealthy and maladaptive behaviors, perceptions, and emotions related to food, eating, and body image. The common perception of an individual with an eating disorder is an adolescent or young adult female with anorexia nervosa (AN): impossibly thin, chronically dieting, driven to extreme weight loss, and believing herself to be overweight despite her malnourished appearance. This characterization fits some individuals with AN, but the term eating disorder encompasses a much broader range of unhealthy behaviors (see Table 23.1) and includes individuals of all body sizes, genders, and ethnicities from all socioeconomic strata. Over the course of a lifetime, almost 1 in 20 people will develop a diagnosable eating disorder; the risk rises to 1 in 10 when subthreshold disordered eating behaviors are considered (Hudson et al., 2007).

Although eating disorders can occur at any age, the highest risk of onset is during adolescence (Frank et al., 2019), meaning that all pediatric health care providers are likely to encounter patients with eating disorders frequently. Families and patients often do not present seeking care for an eating disorder; the comorbid physical and mental health conditions described in detail later in this chapter are often the chief complaint. Hence, those in general pediatrics, developmental-behavioral pediatrics, and pediatric psychology should be alert for eating disorders when evaluating weight loss, chronic abdominal pain, anxiety, depression, and other concerns.

This chapter will provide an overview of the historical context and diagnostic criteria for eating disorders, the epidemiology, and the genetic and physiologic factors (shaped by cultural and ecological contexts) that play strong roles in the development of eating disorders. Additionally, we will provide an overview of evidence-based medical, psychological, and psychiatric treatments and prevention efforts. The key to all of these interventions is the involvement of a multidisciplinary team that includes professionals from medicine, psychiatry, nursing, psychology, and clinical nutrition. As will be described in the sections that follow, the most important member of the treatment team is often the patient's family.

HISTORICAL OVERVIEW

Cultural influences are illustrated by the earliest descriptions of behaviors that we now view as eating disorders. In the Middle Ages, there were numerous reports of *anorexia mirabilis*, young women who abstained from food, denying themselves the pleasures of the world to focus on ideals of perfection and purity (Harris, 2014). One of

TABLE 23.1

DSM-5 Eating Disorders

Anorexia nervosa
Atypical anorexia nervosa
Bulimia nervosa
Avoidant/restrictive food intake disorder
Binge eating disorder
Rumination disorder
Pica
Other specified feeding and eating disorder
Unspecified feeding and eating disorder

Note. DSM-5 = Fifth edition of the *Diagnostic and Statistical Manual of Mental Disorders* (American Psychiatric Association, 2013).

the most famous and earliest of these women was Saint Catherine of Siena, the patron saint of Italy. She, like many of those who followed her, claimed to abstain from all food aside from the consecrated Host. Living for years in this emaciated state was seen as divine, causing her fame to spread and other women to exhibit similar behaviors. Extreme starvation and self-denial are similar to the modern illness anorexia nervosa, but there are some important differences. Body image distortion and cultural ideals of beauty were irrelevant in the Middle Ages; the driving force for these fasting saints was self-abnegation to destroy an untrustworthy and sinful body (Bell, 1985). Eventually, the Catholic Church no longer recognized extreme fasting as saintly and instead emphasized good works. By the Renaissance, these behaviors had largely faded from view.

The late 1800s saw another wave of reports regarding young women who refused to eat to the point of starvation. In 1868, Dr. William Gull delivered a lecture to the British Medical Association describing the condition that, 5 years later, he would describe in a paper entitled "Anorexia Nervosa (Apepsia Hysterica, Anorexia Hysterica)" (Moncrieff-Boyd, 2016). This paper marked the first conceptualization of our modern concept of AN, and so-called "fasting girls" were frequently featured in the popular press.

Although media attention to AN faded at the beginning of the 20th century, the 1970s saw renewed attention to "the starving disease" (Brumberg, 1989). In 1978, the psychiatrist Hilda Bruch published a widely read book about AN for the general public, *The Golden Cage: The Enigma of Anorexia Nervosa*. This book was a milestone in Western society's understanding of AN, although it may have perpetuated a stereotype that eating disorders affect only wealthy White females. It is worth noting that our knowledge of the scope of eating disorders is relatively new, with the first case reports of the bingeing and purging behaviors that we now recognize as bulimia nervosa (BN) appearing in the medical literature in 1979 (Russell).

MAJOR TYPES OF EATING DISORDERS

The fifth edition of the *Diagnostic and Statistical Manual of Mental Disorders* (DSM-5; American Psychiatric Association, 2013) defines feeding and eating disorders as disturbances of eating or eating-related behaviors that are persistent and impair physical health and/or psychosocial functioning.

Anorexia nervosa must include three key diagnostic components: intentional and persistent restrictive energy intake leading to an abnormally low weight or failure to gain expected weight, intense fear of gaining weight or becoming fat, and a disturbance in the self-perception of one's weight or shape. Although patients may present with dramatic weight loss and malnutrition, there is no specific weight threshold required for the diagnosis, and pediatric patients may begin to dramatically deviate from their prior growth trajectory simply by failure to gain over time with relatively little weight loss.

Anorexia nervosa is subdivided into two categories: restricting type and binge-eating/purging type. Those with restricting type AN have not engaged in recurrent episodes of binge eating or purging behavior in the past three months, whereas those with binge-eating/purging type AN have had at least one episode. Weight loss is typically achieved through severely limited dietary intake and may also include excessive exercise and episodes of fasting. Some patients experience most of the criteria for AN, including significant weight loss, yet still have a weight that is in the normal range and are thus classified as having atypical AN. Because of their normal-appearing weight, patients with atypical AN may have a delay in diagnosis despite having physical and mental health impairments as severe as those with AN (Garber et al., 2019).

Bulimia nervosa is characterized by recurrent episodes of binge eating followed by compensatory behavior(s) intended to prevent weight gain. Compensatory behaviors may include self-induced vomiting as well as misuse of laxatives or diuretics, prolonged fasting, or excessive exercise. On average episodes occur weekly for at least 3 months. Patients with BN also have self-evaluations that are unduly influenced by body shape and weight. That is, the reason for the purging behaviors is related to weight management rather than, for example, to contamination fears or obsessive compulsive disorder. Elements of a binge episode can be difficult to determine because some individuals with eating disorders perceive a normal quantity of food intake as a binge. Clinically, a binge is defined as eating, in a discrete time period, a quantity of food that is unambiguously larger than most individuals would consume under similar circumstances combined with a lack of control around eating (Wolfe et al., 2009).

Avoidant/restrictive food intake disorder (ARFID) is new to the *DSM-5* and is characterized by avoidance or restriction of food intake that is severe enough to cause nutritional deficiencies or impact psychosocial development (Mammel & Ornstein, 2017). Weight loss is not necessarily present; children and adolescents may develop malnutrition due to inadequate weight gain for their developmental trajectory. Individuals who depend on nutritional supplements or enteral tube feedings rather than consuming food may also fit criteria for ARFID. The psychosocial impact of ARFID often includes the inability to participate in normal social activities related to food, such as eating in the presence of others or the ability to eat only a small select, set of foods. Avoidant/restrictive food intake disorder should be differentiated from picky eating or food neophobia, both of which are common and may be developmentally normal during the toddler years. Rates of picky eating are highest at about age 3 years and then likely fall by age 6 years (Cardona Cano et al., 2015). Although there is no lower age limit for ARFID, the impairments that are necessary to make the diagnosis are typically not seen until early school age. (Bryant-Waugh, 2019) Some individuals with ARFID have extreme sensitivities to food textures, smells, colors, and tastes that often appear during childhood and may persist through the lifespan (Harer et al., 2018). Others may develop food avoidance following an adverse food-related experience, such as choking or vomiting (Fisher et al., 2014). Lack of food availability or fasting due to religious or cultural practices do not represent ARFID, nor do developmentally appropriate behaviors such as picky eating in toddlers. Importantly, if restrictive eating is related to excessive concern about body weight or shape, even in young children, the diagnosis is more likely to be AN.

Binge eating disorder (BED) is also new to the *DSM-5* and is characterized by binge episodes that occur at least weekly for 3 months. The diagnosis also requires at least three of the following: eating more rapidly than normal; eating until feeling uncomfortably full; eating large amounts when not hungry; eating alone due to embarrassment or feeling disgusted, guilty, or depressed after a binge. Finally, the binges must result in significant distress (Hilbert, 2019), and do not occur within the context of BN or AN.

Rumination disorder is the repeated and frequent regurgitation of food that occurs for at least 1 month. Regurgitation is usually involuntary and occurs without nausea, retching, or disgust. Symptoms can appear similar to BN, but the rumination disorder diagnosis cannot be made in the presence of another eating disorder diagnosis. Rumination disorder can occur across the lifespan, from infants through adults (Murray et al., 2019). Pica is a disorder characterized by the consumption of nonnutritive and nonfood substances (e.g., paper, ice) for at least 1 month in a manner that is developmentally inappropriate, not culturally sanctioned, and significant enough to require clinical attention. Pica may occur in those with

AN who consume non-nutritive items to quell their appetite (Delaney et al., 2015).

Disorders that cause significant clinical impairment in physical, social, or emotional functioning yet do not fit criteria for the diagnoses described in the preceding paragraphs may be classified as other specified feeding and eating disorder (OSFEDs). This category includes atypical AN as well as low-frequency BN and BED of shorter duration and purging disorder, which is similar to BN without binge eating (Krug et al., 2020). Also in this category, night eating syndrome involves recurrent episodes of waking up at night to eat or eating excessively after the evening meal in a manner that causes significant distress or impairment and is not better explained by a primary sleep disturbance or BED (Latzer et al., 2020). Last, in situations in which an eating disorder is diagnosed but there is insufficient information to identify a specific disorder, the diagnosis of unspecified feeding or eating disorder can be given.

EPIDEMIOLOGY OF EATING DISORDERS

Eating disorders can occur at any age; however, the risk of developing AN peaks at age 15. The lifetime prevalence for AN is as high as 4% in females and 0.3% in males. Bulimia nervosa has a lifetime prevalence of 3% in females and 1% in males (van Eeden et al., 2021). Despite otherwise stable overall incidence rates over the past 10 to 20 years, AN has increased among females aged 10 to 14 years (Petkova et al., 2019). It is unclear why more younger patients are developing AN, but some have theorized that younger children are being exposed to the sociocultural factors that facilitate its development (Favaro et al., 2009). Anorexia nervosa has one of the highest mortality risks among psychiatric illnesses, with a standardized mortality rate of about 6, meaning that those with anorexia nervosa are six times as likely to die of any cause as compared with age-matched controls. Approximately 20% of AN deaths are due to suicide (Arcelus et al., 2011).

Eating disorders are frequently perceived to mostly affect wealthy, White adolescents and young adult females in Western countries, but eating disorders affect all genders in diverse ethnic, socioeconomic, and geographic populations. In the United States, there are no statistically significant differences in the lifetime prevalence of AN, BN, and BED among European American, Latin American, African American, or Asian American women. Only Latin American men are more likely to report a lifetime history of BN than European American men (Marques et al., 2011). In this same study, service utilization between groups was significantly different. Of those reporting an eating disorder history, more European Americans reported accessing mental health services for their conditions (76%) than Latin Americans (62%), African Americans (62%), and Asian Americans (63%).

Disparities in diagnosis and poor access to treatment may be even more prominent in U.S. college students. In a recent study of 1,747 college students, all of whom reported eating disorder symptoms, only 11% had ever received a formal eating disorder diagnosis, 14% had received treatment in the past year, and only 31% perceived that they had a need for treatment. (Sonneville & Lipson, 2018) In the same study, women were 1.6 times as likely to have received treatment, almost twice as likely to perceive a need for treatment, and more than four times as likely to be diagnosed with an eating disorder than men despite having similar symptoms. European American students and students of color were just as likely to perceive a need for treatment, yet European American students were 1.8 times as likely to be diagnosed with an eating disorder and 1.6 times as likely to receive treatment. Even when controlling for ethnicity, affluent students were more likely than non-affluent students to perceive a need for treatment, be diagnosed with an eating disorder, and receive treatment.

Etiology and Maintaining Mechanisms

Eating disorders are serious illnesses with complex etiologies that include the interplay among biological, psychological, and sociocultural risk factors (Culbert et al., 2015). Understanding common etiological influences on eating disorders can aid in case conceptualization and treatment planning. However, despite the importance of understanding the etiology underlying eating disorders, current evidence-based treatments for eating disorders in youth focus on interrupting ongoing eating disorder behaviors and cognitions because, once these behaviors are established, their psychological and biological effects become maintaining mechanisms of the illness that need to be interrupted in treatment (Fairburn et al., 2003).

RISK FACTORS FOR EATING DISORDERS: CONSIDERATIONS FROM DEVELOPMENTAL SCIENCE

Non-modifiable risk factors for eating disorders can be classified by age, sex, ethnicity, sexual orientation, and gender identity.

Age
Although people of all ages can be affected by any eating disorder, peak periods of risk differ depending on the specific eating disorder. The most common onsets of AN and BN occur during adolescence, with the average age of onset for AN slightly lower than that for BN. The peak incidence for AN is age 15, whereas for BN it ranges between ages 15 and 29 years (van Eeden et al., 2021) Full-threshold BED is often not diagnosed until late adolescence or adulthood (Keski-Rahkonen, 2021). Avoidant/restrictive food intake disorder can occur at any time across the lifespan, although onset is often at younger ages than for other eating disorders (Strand et al., 2019).

Sex
Sex differences in eating disorders are important to acknowledge. The proportions of BED and ARFID cases occurring in males tend to be higher than the proportion of AN and BN cases, although all eating disorders are more common in females overall (Keski-Rahkonen, 2021; Strand et al., 2019). Sexual minority status is likely associated with increased risk for a range of eating disorder behaviors, especially in sexual minority men (Calzo et al., 2017). Eating disorder symptoms and diagnoses also appear to be elevated in youth who are transgender or nonbinary, which may be related to attempts to suppress secondary sex characteristics during puberty or otherwise align one's body with gender identity (Coelho et al., 2019). Consistent with this hypothesis, some studies suggest that gender-affirming medical treatments lead to a reduction in eating disorder behaviors in transgender or nonbinary people (Testa et al., 2017).

Genetic Risk Factors
Twin and adoption studies suggest moderate to high heritability of AN, BN, BED, and disordered eating symptoms with average heritability estimates around 50% (Culbert et al., 2015). These findings suggest that individual genetic differences may explain differences in susceptibility to eating disorders. The specific nature of genetic risk remains largely unknown, as many molecular genetic and genome-wide association studies (GWAS) have been underpowered to consistently detect effects. However, accumulating evidence suggests involvement of serotonergic and dopaminergic systems, and some studies have identified specific interactions between environmental risk factors and serotonin or dopamine genes (Culbert et al., 2015). The largest GWAS completed to date (Watson et al., 2019) examined 16,992 AN cases and 55,525 controls and identified eight significant genetic loci on chromosomes 1, 2, 3, 5, 10, and 11. The significant loci were genetically correlated with other psychiatric disorders, including obsessive compulsive disorder (genetic correlation $[r_g] = 0.45$), major depressive disorder ($r_g = 0.28$), anxiety disorders ($r_g = 0.25$), and schizophrenia ($r_g = 0.25$), as well as metabolic variables, such as fasting insulin ($r_g = -0.24$) and leptin ($r_g = -0.26$). The authors suggested that underlying metabolic dysregulation may contribute to risk and maintenance for weight loss/low body mass index in individuals with anorexia nervosa. Future research is needed to identify the specific neurobiological mechanisms that may underlie these genetic correlations.

Psychological and Personality Risk Factors
Several personality risk factors for eating disorders have been identified. Negative

emotionality/neuroticism (i.e., tendency to experience negative emotions such as anxiety, depression, or anger) prospectively predicts AN and BN diagnoses. Similarly, perfectionism is prospectively linked to eating disorder symptoms. Impulsivity is another personality variable that prospectively predicts binge eating and purging behaviors (rather than eating disorder diagnoses more broadly). One form of impulsivity, negative urgency (i.e., tendency to engage in rash action when distressed), is a strong predictor of binge eating and purging symptoms (Culbert et al., 2015). The specific mechanisms that link personality variables to eating disorder onset are the subject of ongoing investigation.

Because personality characteristics such as those noted previously are themselves heritable, it may be that the same genes confer risk to both certain personality traits and disordered eating symptoms. Early evidence from twin studies has supported this hypothesis (Culbert et al., 2015). For example, in the case of associations between impulsivity (specifically, negative urgency) and binge eating, it has been theorized that the combination of elevated dopamine and low serotonin levels may confer shared risk and explain the high overlap in genetic risk between negative urgency and binge eating (Racine et al., 2017). Given that high dopamine has been associated with the approach to rewarding stimuli, and serotonin is involved in emotion-guided planning, the combination of elevated dopamine and low serotonin is thought to increase biological risk for behaviors that are risky and poorer regulation of planning and pursuit of long-term goals.

Environmental and Sociocultural Influences

Etiological models of eating disorders often include variables related to the idealization of thinness in Westernized cultures. Such influences, including media exposure, perceived pressures to achieve thinness, thin-ideal internalization (i.e., extent of buy-in to the thin ideal), and thinness expectancies (i.e., expectation that thinness will result in life improvement), have been identified as risk factors for disordered eating (Culbert et al., 2015).

However, consistent with the biopsychosocial model, it is likely that exposure to the thin ideal may not universally confer risk for disordered eating. Instead, risk appears to result from the interaction of exposure to these variables and other individual differences related to biological, psychological, family, and environmental risks. Although exposure to the idealization of thinness is largely unavoidable in Western cultures, eating disorder prevention and interventions often aim to modify patient and family perceptions and understanding by identifying problems with the thin ideal and developing strategies to challenge these internalized beliefs (Kroon Van Diest & Perez, 2013).

Childhood maltreatment, including emotional, physical, and sexual abuse, is an additional environmental risk factor for eating disorders (Molendijk et al., 2017). Rates of childhood maltreatment in patients with eating disorders have been reported to be high (21% to 59%) relative to individuals with other psychiatric diagnoses (5% to 46%) and healthy controls (1% to 35%; Molendijk et al., 2017). Trauma-related risk factors are often conceptualized as nonspecific risk factors for eating disorders, as these events increase risk for psychopathology in general. The precise pathways between trauma exposure and development of an eating disorder are unclear but are assumed to be related to interactions with other biological, genetic, personality, family, and environmental factors.

IMPACTS OF DISEASE AND MAINTAINING MECHANISMS

In addition to the risk factors for the development of disordered eating symptoms, several factors contribute to maintaining symptoms once they have begun. Many of these maintaining mechanisms were initially identified in studies of human starvation. For example, in the 1940s, the Minnesota Starvation Study recruited 36 healthy men to undergo 6 months of "semi-starvation" (i.e., limit to about 1,500 kcal per day), followed by a period or renourishment, to study the psychological and biological impacts of starvation, both during the period of starvation and during the period of renourishment (Kalm & Semba, 2005). Many behavioral and psychological changes seen in the participants in the Minnesota Starvation Study are also apparent in individuals with eating disorders. Individuals who are undereating and malnourished become more rigid and inflexible in decisions and routines and often withdraw socially. They experience increases in food preoccupation; decreases in concentration; and increases in depression, anxiety, and irritability (Fairburn, 2008). Additionally, periods of restrictive eating predict the onset of binge eating, and thus dieting is thought to maintain binge eating. These behavioral and psychological changes are reversible with adequate nutrition, regular eating patterns, and appropriate weight restoration (Kalm & Semba, 2005).

NEUROBIOLOGY OF EATING DISORDERS

Studies of brain structure and function in individuals with eating disorders have pointed to neurologic dysfunction during the disease state. Many biological differences resolve fully or partially during recovery, leading some researchers to conceptualize these impacts as likely effects of the illness rather than premorbid risk factors (Kappou et al., 2021), although the issue of risk versus illness effect remains unresolved.

Altered decision making and reward processing in individuals with AN is an important area of interest (Haynos et al., 2021). Those with AN appear to have decision-making deficits (e.g., inflexibility) that impair responsiveness to experiences that are usually rewarding (e.g., social interactions). Simultaneously, people with AN have a heightened reward response to eating-disorder behaviors such as restrictive eating and exercising. This pattern likely maintains eating disorder behaviors because they provide rewards that are not obtainable from more typical rewarding experiences (Haynos et al., 2021). The specific biological mechanisms underlying altered reward responsivity in anorexia are under investigation and may be related to individual differences in dopamine responsivity. Reward processing differences have also been implicated in neuroimaging studies of BN and BED (Wonderlich et al., 2021). People with binge eating behaviors demonstrate hyper reward responsivity to food cues, such as images of highly palatable foods (i.e., likely binge foods; high in fat, sugar, sodium, and/or carbohydrates).

Structural and functional neuroimaging studies in AN also suggest neurological changes during illness. Reduced grey and white matter volume, sometimes referred to as pseudoatrophy, has been observed during the acute period of illness when individuals are underweight. This reduction in brain volume appears to resolve with weight restoration, suggesting that these brain alterations may reflect malnourishment. However, research suggests that more nuanced approaches may be needed to understand specific impacts on various brain structures, including controlling for state of starvation (King et al., 2018). Other structural and functional neuroimaging studies have implicated involvement of the orbitofrontal cortex, with the larger volume observed in AN thought to be implicated in the ability to restrict food intake, as well as alternations in the insula, which is implicated in the taste and reward system (Frank, 2015). There have also been findings in those with AN and BN implicating alterations in limbic pathways that are important in both emotion and food intake regulation.

CLINICAL PRESENTATIONS

Although eating disorders may present at any age, as noted previously, health care providers should be particularly alert for ARFID in children aged 8 to 12, AN in children aged 12 to 18, and BN in children and adults aged 15 to 29 years. Given that the physical health effects of eating disorders can involve virtually every organ system, patients with eating disorders may present with a variety of health concerns. (Bravender, 2011) Some patients or their parents may present seeking care specifically for eating problems, and providers should maintain a high index of suspicion for eating disorders related to a variety of other concerns. Those with AN may present concerned about amenorrhea, fatigue, constipation, difficulty concentrating, or cold intolerance. Additionally, their parents may be concerned about their child being agitated, irritable, or exhibiting other behavioral changes. The physical examination of those with AN will be notable for a low body mass index or a substantial decrease from their prior growth curve, as well as significant bradycardia, hypotension, hypothermia, hair loss, peripheral edema, or lanugo (a fine downy hair often seen on the chest, abdomen, and back).

Those with BN may have no signs or symptoms but will sometimes present for syncope, fatigue, swollen cheeks, and abdominal discomfort or heartburn. One unusual concern that should raise suspicion for BN is a subconjunctival hemorrhage that, while benign, will appear dramatic to the patient and family and may be related to recurrent forceful vomiting. The physical examination of those with BN may be normal, but providers should be alert to parotid gland enlargement, peripheral edema, dental enamel erosion, angular stomatitis, or Russell's sign (an abrasion or callous on the knuckles of the dominant hand related to recurrent self-induced vomiting).

It is important to note that those with ARFID may or may not develop malnutrition. They may have normal growth and development, severe malnutrition, or a slow loss of growth percentiles due to their eating difficulties. Those with atypical AN, particularly those who were previously overweight or obese, may present with a normal body mass index but still exhibit other signs of malnutrition such as profound bradycardia, hypotension, and amenorrhea (Garber et al., 2019).

MEDICAL COMPLICATIONS

Given the wide range of medical complications related to eating disorders, it is useful to consider complications by organ system and to examine those issues related to malnutrition versus those related to recurrent vomiting (Hornberger et al., 2021). Table 23.2 provides a summary of such complications. Malnutrition may result in both acute and chronic dehydration states. Whereas acute dehydration may manifest as dizziness,

TABLE 23.2
Physical Health Complications of Eating Disorders

Associated with inadequate calorie intake

Fluids, electrolytes	Acute and chronic dehydration
	Hyponatremia
	Hypokalemia
	Peripheral edema
Cardiovascular	Bradycardia
	Hypotension
	Myocardial atrophy
	Dysrhythmias
	Pericardial effusion
	Congestive heart failure
Gastrointestinal	Delayed gastric emptying
	Impaired gastric accommodation
	Slow intestinal motility
	Constipation
	Transaminitis
	Superior mesenteric artery syndrome
Endocrine	Amenorrhea
	Hypogonadotropic hypogonadism
	Low bone mineral density
	Hypoglycemia, hyperglycemia
	Nonthyroidal illness syndrome
Skin, hair, nails	Acrocyanosis
	Xerosis
	Lanugo
	Telogen effluvium
Hematologic	Leukopenia
	Anemia
	Thrombocytopenia
	Low erythrocyte sedimentation rate
Dental	Xerostomia
	Caries
Neurologic	Cortical pseudoatrophy
	Cognitive slowing
	Compression neuropathy
Psychiatric	Depressed mood
	Obsessive thoughts and behaviors
	Anxiety
	Suicide

Associated with vomiting

Fluids, electrolytes	Hypokalemia
	Hypochloremia
	Metabolic alkalosis
	Acute and chronic dehydration
	Peripheral edema
Gastrointestinal	Parotid gland enlargement
	Elevated serum amylase
	Gastroesophageal reflux
	Esophagitis
	Mallory-Weiss tear
Dental	Enamel erosions
	Caries

Note. Data from Bravender (2011) and Hornberger et al. (2021).

light-headedness, or syncope, chronic dehydration may result in activation of the renin-aldosterone system with subsequent hypokalemia and peripheral edema. Malnutrition may also result in decreased glomerular filtration rate and kidney injury (Stheneur et al., 2019), likely due this chronic dehydration.

The low heart rate (<40 beats/minute) seen in AN can be profound. The etiology of this bradycardia is thought to be related to high resting vagal tone and may be an appropriate adaptation to a low-energy state (Sachs et al., 2016). Most patients tolerate the bradycardia, but many providers use bradycardia as a marker for metabolic impairment indicative of the need for inpatient medical management. Bradycardia is often related to hypotension, which may be symptomatic, particularly with exercise. Severe bradycardia may also result in dysrhythmias such as junctional rhythms. Myocardial atrophy is frequently seen in association with severe malnutrition. Patients with myocardial atrophy are unable to increase stroke volume and so are dependent on increases in heart rate to increase cardiac output. Thus, the simple demands of standing upright may result in a relative tachycardia (increased heart rate) as compared to a recumbent heart rate regardless of hydration status, making interpretation of orthostatic assessments challenging. In severe malnutrition, patients may develop pericardial effusion and congestive heart failure; thus providers should be very cautious about use of intravenous fluid resuscitation for hypotension.

The gastrointestinal system is often slowed, and patients often experience delayed gastric emptying, slow intestinal transit time, and chronic constipation as well as impaired gastric accommodation (Perez et al., 2013). The endocrine system is also affected by malnutrition, most obviously by a hypogonadotropic hypogonadism resulting in amenorrhea. A combination of severe malnutrition and amenorrhea increases the risk of low bone mineral density and future risk for pathological fractures (Fazeli & Klibanski, 2018). This hypogonadal state is also seen in young men with AN, increasing the risk for low bone mineral density and testicular atrophy. Patients often have hypoglycemia that they perceive as asymptomatic despite cognitive impairments. Although this condition is understudied in AN, it is likely similar to that seen in diabetics with hypoglycemia unawareness who, despite having no subjective low blood sugar symptoms, exhibit delayed reaction time and poor working memory (Sejling et al., 2015). Hyperglycemia is less frequently seen, but may occur, during the initial refeeding period of treatment.

Many of the symptoms experienced by malnourished patients mimic hypothyroidism, and laboratory testing may show low triiodothyronine (T3), elevated reverse T3, normal or slightly low thyroxine (T4), and thyroid-stimulating hormone levels, all consistent with non-thyroidal illness syndrome. However, treatment with thyroid hormone is not indicated because exogenous thyroid hormone may exacerbate weight loss and worsen symptoms (Schorr & Miller, 2017).

Patients often have acrocyanosis and poor skin perfusion, resulting in chronically dry skin and atopic dermatitis. Lanugo and scalp hair thinning may also be seen. Xerostomia, or dry mouth, is frequently seen and is likely the reason for a heightened risk of caries, even in the absence of recurrent vomiting (Miller et al., 2022). The peripheral nervous system may also be affected due to the loss of subcutaneous fat and skeletal muscle atrophy resulting in nerve compression and subsequent motor and sensory impairments.

In some patients, self-induced vomiting may be asymptomatic for years, but others may develop medical complications quickly. Laboratory findings of low potassium, low chloride, and high bicarbonate levels are consistent with gastric acid loss, and recurrent vomiting must be considered regardless of the patient's stated history. Recurrent vomiting may also result in acute and chronic dehydration and peripheral edema; gastroesophageal reflux; esophagitis; and in extreme cases, severe gastric distention, gastric or esophageal rupture, or Mallory-Weiss tear (Bravender & Story, 2007). Some patients may develop parotid gland hypertrophy with attendant increases in serum amylase. Complications of BED are most frequently related to weight gain and obesity, although more severe cases have resulted in gastric rupture and oral/esophageal injuries due to rapid ingestion of food.

PSYCHIATRIC COMPLICATIONS

For patients with eating disorders, psychiatric comorbidities are common: 55% of youth with AN, 88% of youth with BN, and 83% of youth with BED have at least one other lifetime comorbid psychiatric disorder (Swanson et al., 2011). The most common comorbidities include mood, anxiety, and substance use disorders (Hudson et al., 2007; Udo & Grilo, 2019; Ulfvebrand et al., 2015). Given the high levels of comorbidity, it should come as no surprise that adolescents with eating disorders are at a much higher risk for non-suicidal self-injury and suicide attempts (Svirko & Hawton, 2007; Udo et al., 2019). College students with eating disorder symptoms have been found to be 11 times more likely to attempt suicide than students without symptoms (Lipson & Sonneville, 2020) emphasizing the need for regular and careful safety assessments with this population. Prevalence of comorbidities in ARFID seem to differ from those of eating disorders with body image disturbance. In a retrospective study adolescents seeking treatment for ARFID were more likely to have anxiety or a medical comorbidity and less likely to have a mood disorder than those with AN or BN (Fisher et al., 2014).

Interestingly, despite the significant effects of malnutrition on an adolescent's brain and body, they typically continue to be successful in both academic and athletic pursuits (Lock et al., 2015). However, as malnutrition progresses the patient can become more compulsive and driven to the detriment of social connections, as seen in the Minnesota Starvation Study (Kalm & Semba, 2005).

DETERMINING APPROPRIATE LEVEL OF CARE

The initial clinical evaluation of a patient with an eating disorder should focus on determining the appropriate diagnosis as well as providing treatment recommendations. The proper level of care is based on the presence of medical complications and risk factors, social and family support, and the degree of cognitive and behavioral impairment. Available levels of care include inpatient medical or psychiatric care, residential care, partial hospitalization/day treatment programs, intensive outpatient programs, and outpatient care.

The need for inpatient medical stabilization should be discussed early in treatment and should be framed as a safety net, not as a punishment. Many patients and their families view hospitalization as a wake-up call, and this may enhance motivation to continue treatment (Bravender et al., 2017). Those needing medical stabilization should be admitted urgently, not as planned admissions that occur with residential treatment. There are no absolute requirements for inpatient medical admission, but the American Academy of Pediatrics (Hornberger et al., 2021) and the Society for Adolescent Health and Medicine (Golden et al., 2015) have developed best practice criteria (see Table 23.3). The primary focus of medical admission should be nutritional stabilization, and treatment teams should focus on the concept of food as medicine. Medical admission, if necessary, should be framed as a brief nutritional

TABLE 23.3

Indications for Inpatient Medical Stabilization for Eating Disorders

Symptoms that may merit hospitalization
Severe malnutrition
Dehydration
Abnormal electrolytes
Cardia dysrhythmias
Physiologic instability
   Severe bradycardia (<45 beats/minute), hypotension
   Hypotension (<90/45 mm Hg)
   Hypothermia (<35.6 C)
   Orthostatic blood pressure changes (>20 mm Hg systolic or >10 mm Hg diastolic)
Uncontrollable bingeing and purging
Acute food refusal (especially >24 hours)
Acute psychiatric emergencies if medical management cannot be assured
Other severe complications of malnutrition as noted in Table 23.2

Note. Data from Golden et al. (2015).

rescue, with the interdisciplinary eating disorder treatment primarily occurring in the outpatient, partial hospital, or residential treatment setting.

Psychotherapeutic Treatment

Evidence-based psychotherapies for eating disorders are specific protocols that typically require specialized training and are often delivered within eating disorder specialty clinics. Given the specialized training involved in eating disorder care, pediatric psychologists may find that they are likely to refer many cases to a specialized setting. However, the general skills offered by a pediatric psychologist in terms of assessment, differential diagnosis, motivational interviewing, and psychoeducation can aid families in initiating care while they await longer term treatment within a specialized eating disorder setting.

Additionally, it is important to note that research on eating disorder treatments generally under-represents people who are non-White, from sexual or gender minority groups, of lower socioeconomic status, or fail to assess or report on these variables (Burnette et al., 2022), and relatively little is known about specific modifying variables that may increase treatment responsibility or effectiveness. Thus, pediatric psychologists can use a clinical skill set to consider culturally informed formulations and modifications to existing treatments. Additionally, pediatric psychologists may be asked to assess for multiple co-occurring diagnoses when they receive a referral for a possible eating disorder.

In patients who are under-eating or underweight, it is important to consider the role of starvation in symptom presentation. For example, in a patient who reports attention difficulties in school that have co-occurred with the eating disorder, the likely etiology may be cognitive changes related to starvation rather than attention/deficit hyperactivity disorder (ADHD). However, even if ADHD symptoms predated the eating disorder, neuropsychological evaluation should be delayed until weight restoration has occurred to reduce the impact of starvation on test performance. After identifying an eating disorder, pediatric psychologists can assist in referral to appropriate treatment and provide psychoeducation and support to the family until specialized care is initiated. Some of the principles of two evidence-based eating disorder psychotherapies, family-based treatment (FBT) and enhanced cognitive behavior therapy will be outlined in the following sections.

Family-based treatment. Family-based treatment (FBT) is considered a first-line treatment for youth with AN (Academy for Eating Disorders [AED], 2020), may also be implemented for those with BN, and is likely indicated for ARFID (Lock et al., 2019). Family-based treatment is an outpatient treatment designed to use family members to assist with interruption of eating disorder behaviors (Lock & Le Grange, 2015). Parents/caregivers are highly involved in every psychotherapy session and in day-to-day management of the eating disorder.

At the start of treatment, the psychotherapist meets with the family to provide psychoeducation and convey the seriousness of the illness. The family is taught to conceptualize the eating disorder as a separate entity from the patient, and the therapist highlights that the patient has been unable to interrupt the eating disorder on their own. Eating disorder symptoms are further complicated by ambivalence that characterizes many adolescent eating disorders, especially AN, limiting motivation to reduce eating disorder behaviors. Thus, in phase 1 of FBT, parents/caregivers are tasked with managing all eating-related decisions on behalf of the patient, as well as providing supervision and support to reduce other eating disorder behaviors, such as excessive exercise, purging, and binge eating.

Practically, parents of an adolescent with AN are encouraged to immediately begin choosing, portioning, and supervising all of their child's meals and snacks. They are asked to choose foods according to what they know their adolescent needs given the child's state of starvation and informed by their eating preferences prior to the onset of the eating disorder rather than accommodating the food choices and portions that are dictated by the eating disorder. For example, if the patient has been making a separate dinner of mostly vegetables, parents would be asked to no longer allow this and instead to begin preparing normal dishes that their adolescent previously ate, provided in portions that will promote weight restoration, and sit with the child to provide support while the child completes the meal.

Phase 2 begins when eating disorder behaviors are minimal, underweight individuals are nearly weight restored, and there is little resistance to eating. At this point, developmentally appropriate decisions about eating are gradually returned to the patient while caregivers remain closely involved to prevent reemergence of eating disorder symptoms. The final phase 3 of FBT focuses on returning the adolescent and family to normative adolescent development. Family-based treatment is typically delivered in 20 psychotherapy sessions over the course of 6 to 12 months, with sessions initially occurring at weekly intervals and gradually spaced to biweekly and then monthly sessions over the course of phases 2 and 3 (Lock & Le Grange, 2015).

Most clinical trials of FBT have used adolescent-focused therapy as the comparison intervention. Adolescent-focused therapy is an individual psychotherapy approach in which the therapist works with the adolescent to encourage change in eating disorder behaviors using self-exploration and identification of problematic developmental and emotional concerns (Fitzpatrick et al., 2010). Family-based treatment results in rapid weight increases, higher rates of remission, and lower hospitalization rates (Agras et al., 2014; Lock et al., 2010). A parent-focused version of FBT that does not involve the adolescent in sessions is also effective when compared with regular conjoint FBT (Le Grange et al., 2016). Despite these promising findings, end-of-treatment remission rates are around 40%, leading to explorations of augmentations to FBT to further enhance outcomes. For example, ongoing studies are investigating various adaptations of FBT including implementation in higher levels of care, multi-family therapy, exposure-based FBT, FBT with supplemental parent interventions, and short-term intensive FBT (Richards et al., 2018).

Cognitive behavior therapy for eating disorders. Cognitive behavior therapy for eating disorders (CBT-ED) is a first-line recommended treatment for youth with BN (AED, 2020). It is considered a second-line treatment for BED, and there are ongoing investigations of applications of CBT-ED for youth with AN (Dalle Grave et al., 2019) and ARFID (Thomas et al., 2020). A primary difference between FBT and CBT-ED is the nature of parent/caregiver involvement. Rather than parents being the primary agents of change, in CBT-ED the patient is responsible for making changes to their eating behaviors and cognitions, with guidance from the therapist and with support, as indicated, from parents (Dalle Grave & Calugi, 2020).

Patients are initially provided with psycho-education on their eating disorder symptoms, and in collaboration with the therapist they develop a visual formulation of the eating disorder, which demonstrates the maintaining mechanisms of their illness. For example, in a patient with BN, the formulation would demonstrate the cyclical relation between overevaluation of shape and weight, extreme dieting behaviors, binge eating, and purging. This formulation highlights for the patient the ways in which eating disorder behaviors reinforce one another as well as unhelpful thinking patterns related to their body shape and weight. CBT-ED then proceeds to systematically interrupt these maintaining factors by working toward regular eating (e.g., typically eating three meals and two snacks per day or three snacks if underweight) and eventually challenging the patient's food rules and fears. The initial eating interventions typically reduce episodes of binge eating and purging, and residual episodes are managed by teaching the patient skills to resist these urges. Once progress is being made on behavioral symptoms, several specific cognitive interventions are used to challenge eating disorder cognitions.

Although no specific randomized clinical trials have examined CBT-ED for BED in youth, transdiagnostic samples including a portion of participants with BED have shown promising outcomes (Dalle Grave et al., 2015), and this treatment is well-established in adults with BED (Atwood & Friedman, 2020). CBT-ED may result in improvement in weight and cognitive symptoms of AN (Dalle Grave et al., 2019; Le Grange et al., 2020) and may be considered for those patients for whom FBT is not an option.

Treatment approaches for ARFID remain in the early stages of empirical testing, yet CBT for ARFID (CBT-AR) shows promise (Thomas & Eddy, 2019). Cognitive behavior therapy for ARFID is designed to increase the volume and variety of food consumed and is adaptable to various patient ages, maturities, and motivation. For example, in family-supported and individual treatment versions of CBT-AR parents are involved to differing degrees. Cognitive therapy for ARFID is an outpatient treatment composed of 20 to 30 weekly sessions. Interventions include psychoeducation, developing an individualized formulation of the maintaining mechanisms of ARFID, self (or parent) monitoring of food intake, increasing volume of preferred foods, and increasing variety of foods. The treatment then involves systematically challenging the maintaining mechanisms of ARFID using exposure-based strategies. Early studies of treatment outcomes for CBT-AR in youth are promising, with 70% of adolescent patients no longer meeting criteria for ARFID on treatment completion (Thomas et al., 2020).

Psychiatric medication management. To date there are no medications approved by the U.S. Food and Drug Administration for the treatment of children and adolescents with eating disorders. However, the use of psychotropics in clinical settings for eating disorders is very common and seen more often in patients with a longer duration of illness, need for higher levels of care, and psychiatric comorbidity (Mizusaki et al., 2018; Monge et al., 2015).

The medication with the largest body of evidence for the treatment of AN in children and adolescents is olanzapine. Although the empirical data have shown mixed results, clinically it is used at low doses (average dose of 5 mg daily) to improve weight gain and decrease cognitive rigidity (Couturier et al., 2019). Olanzapine's side effect profile of weight gain has been a commonly cited reason for its use. Although metabolic-syndrome-like side effects are not commonly seen in patients with AN (Attia et al., 2019), risks should be monitored (Academy of Child and Adolescent Psychiatry, 2011). Given that olanzapine has the potential for prolonging the QT interval corrected for heart rate (QTc), patients should have a screening electrocardiogram prior to initiating treatment, as electrolyte disturbances and low body weight can exacerbate QTc prolongation (Peebles & Sieke, 2019). Given the side effect profile and inconclusive outcomes studies, olanzapine should only be used in combination with psychotherapy and nutritional restoration and reserved for patients who are struggling to make clinical progress with evidence-based behavioral interventions.

The core symptoms of AN do not respond well to antidepressants (Holtkamp et al., 2005). However, many patients experience comorbid mood and anxiety disorders that may benefit from treatment with a psychotropic, such as a selective serotonin reuptake inhibitor (SSRI). Providers should be aware that malnutrition reduces the amount of available serotonin, which makes SSRIs less effective when body weight is low. Some levels of obsessional and depressive symptoms are seen in starvation and improve with weight restoration alone (Kalm & Semba, 2005). Therefore, it is beneficial to wait for some level of weight restoration prior to the start of an antidepressant.

Limited studies of SSRIs have shown improvement in symptoms of BN in children and adolescents. One open label study of fluoxetine (maximum dose of 60 mg) showed improvement in both bingeing and purging behaviors (Kotler et al., 2003). Because fluoxetine has a listed indication for treatment of BN in adults, it is frequently recommended for youth with BN. However, it is likely that any of the SSRIs could provide similar benefits. Providers should avoid the use of bupropion in patients with AN or BN due to the increased risk of seizures.

To date no studies regarding medication management for children or adolescents with BED exist. Lisdexamfetamine has a listed indication for BED in adults, but no studies have been completed with younger populations. The only currently available data for psychotropic use in patients with ARFID come from case reports and series. Many reports describe a combination of medications, but it appears that low doses of olanzapine may be helpful for weight gain if the patient is malnourished (Brewerton & D'Agostino, 2017; Spettigue et al., 2018). Selective serotonin reuptake inhibitors also help specifically with the phobic or post-traumatic type of ARFID (Couturier et al., 2019).

Treatment Outcomes and Prevention

Despite the significant impact of eating disorders on affected individuals and their families, there is much to be learned to improve treatment outcomes. Unfortunately, the current treatment landscape for eating disorders, and especially AN, has been described as a "crisis in care" due to poor access to evidence-based treatments combined with inadequate rates of recovery even with the best available treatments (Kaye & Bulik, 2021). Compared with the standardized mortality rate of about 6 for AN, the mortality rates of BN and eating disorder not otherwise specified are also elevated at 1.93 and 1.92, respectively (Arcelus et al., 2011). In general, less than 50% of those with AN will reach full recovery, 33% will have some improvement, and about 20% will go on to have a chronic and severe course. Similar outcomes are seen in BN, with 47.5% reaching recovery, 26% showing improvement, and 26% having a chronic and enduring illness (Steinhausen, 2009). Given that people with eating disorders are often ambivalent about recovery, rates of treatment dropout can be high. Even in intensive, randomized controlled trials, as many as 1 in 4 patients drop out of treatment (Linardon et al., 2018).

Younger age at onset, shorter duration of illness, fewer psychiatric comorbidities, low parental expressed emotion, and early symptom improvement in treatment are predictive of better outcomes for both AN and BN (Steinhausen, 2009). Further, research has not adequately considered socioeconomic factors that may impact treatment recommendations such as cultural background, sexual minority status, and socioeconomic status (Burnette et al., 2022), although it is often suggested that these variables could impact treatment outcomes. For example, given the substantial parental involvement required in FBT, families often elect to have one parent take time away from work to dedicate to supervising and supporting their child; progress may be slower in families that do not have access to or financial resources for time out of work. Adjustments to the treatment have been suggested, such as more flexible and creative planning to identify an adequate support systems, such as including extended family members (Accurso et al., 2021).

Although most of the medical consequences of eating disorders improve with treatment, some effects endure long after recovery. Endocrine disturbances associated with AN and BN alter reproduction with delayed first birth and lower parity in patients with a history of these diagnoses (Tabler et al., 2018). Adolescents with eating disorders can have low bone mineral density, which can lead to fractures and osteoporosis later in life. Growth retardation can also occur in patients with early adolescent AN, likely due to the growth hormone resistance and decreased insulin-like growth factor 1 (Peebles & Sieke, 2019). A Canadian study followed women for 12 years following medical hospitalization for BN. Investigators found a higher incidence of cardiovascular disease including ischemic heart disease, atherosclerosis, and cardiac conduction defects and recommended that women with a history of BN be regular screened for cardiovascular disease (Tith et al., 2020). Many long-term medical consequences of BED, including hyperlipidemia, diabetes, and hypertension, are felt secondary to be secondary to obesity, which frequently coexists with BED (Voderholzer et al., 2020).

The high morbidity and mortality associated with eating disorders have given rise to a push for preventative strategies (Pearson et al., 2002). Studies have looked at universal prevention for whole populations and selective prevention targeting high-risk individuals (e.g., those with body image distress) and have indicated prevention strategies for people with eating disorder symptoms who have not yet met diagnostic criteria. Media literacy, cognitive dissonance education, and CBT are efficacious at decreasing risk factors for eating disorders (Le et al., 2017). Universal interventions have started to be incorporated into school curricula and can be used with children as young as 5 years old (Chua et al., 2020). However, further research is needed to improve the implementation and uptake of these interventions. It is important to note that interventions to increase awareness of eating disorders should be evidence based with well-trained presenters. Poorly designed prevention programs may normalize and thus encourage disordered eating behaviors. (Doley et al., 2017).

CONCLUSION

Rigorous development of evidence-based treatments remains in its infancy, but a few general statements are clear. Eating disorders continue to impact the health of adolescents, particularly in industrialized countries. Pediatric providers should be alert to signs and symptoms of eating disorders, particularly as younger and younger patients are affected. Patients with a higher percent estimated body weight and shorter duration of illness when presenting for treatment are more likely to recover (Forman et al., 2011), and adolescents are more likely to recover than adults (Ackard et al., 2014). Once in treatment, early weight restoration increases the likelihood for recovery (Van Huysse et al., 2020). Thus, it is critical that patients and families access evidence-based treatment as quickly as possible. With proper intervention, eating disorders can be treated successfully, and adolescents can move on from these culture-bound yet deadly illnesses.

RESOURCES

For Families

Organizations and websites:

- National Eating Disorders Association

  https://www.nationaleatingdisorders.org

- ARFID Collaborative

  https://www.arfidcollaborative.com/welcome

- F.E.A.S.T.

  https://www.feast-ed.org

Books:

- Lock, J., & Le Grange, D. (2015). *Help your teenager beat an eating disorder* (2nd ed.). Guilford Press.
- Mulheim, L. (2018). *When your teenager has an eating disorder: Practical strategies to help your teen recover from anorexia, bulimia, and binge eating.* New Harbinger Publications.

For Clinicians

- Academy for Eating Disorders

  https://www.aedweb.org

- Society for Adolescent Health and Medicine

  https://www.adolescenthealth.org

References

Academy for Eating Disorders. (2020). *A guide to selecting evidence-based psychological therapies for eating disorders.* https://higherlogicdownload.s3.amazonaws.com/AEDWEB/27a3b69a-8aae-45b2-a04c-2a078d02145d/UploadedImages/Publications_Slider/FINAL_AED_Psycholohgical_book.pdf

Accurso, E. C., Mu, K. J., Landsverk, J., & Guydish, J. (2021). Adaptation to family-based treatment for Medicaid-insured youth with anorexia nervosa in publicly-funded settings: Protocol for a mixed methods implementation scale-out pilot study. *Journal of Eating Disorders, 9*(1), 99. https://doi.org/10.1186/s40337-021-00454-0

Ackard, D. M., Richter, S., Egan, A., & Cronemeyer, C. (2014). Poor outcome and death among youth, young adults, and midlife adults with eating disorders: An investigation of risk factors by age at assessment. *International Journal of Eating Disorders, 47*(7), 825–835. https://doi.org/10.1002/eat.22346

Agras, W. S., Lock, J., Brandt, H., Bryson, S. W., Dodge, E., Halmi, K. A., Booil, J., Johnson, C., Kaye, W., Wilfley, D., & Woodside, B. (2014). Comparison of 2 family therapies for adolescent anorexia nervosa: A randomized parallel trial. *JAMA Psychiatry, 71*(11), 1279–1286. https://doi.org/10.1001/jamapsychiatry.2014.1025

American Academy of Child and Adolescent Psychiatry. (2011). *AACAP practice parameter for the use of atypical antipsychotic medications in children and adolescents*. https://www.aacap.org/App_Themes/AACAP/docs/practice_parameters/Atypical_Antipsychotic_Medications_Web.pdf

American Psychiatric Association. (2013). *Diagnostic and statistical manual of mental disorders* (5th ed.). https://doi.org/10.1176/appi.books.9780890425596

Arcelus, J., Mitchell, A. J., Wales, J., & Nielsen, S. (2011). Mortality rates in patients with anorexia nervosa and other eating disorders. A meta-analysis of 36 studies. *Archives of General Psychiatry, 68*(7), 724–731. https://doi.org/10.1001/archgenpsychiatry.2011.74

Attia, E., Steinglass, J. E., Walsh, B. T., Wang, Y., Wu, P., Schreyer, C., Wildes, J., Yilmaz, Z., Guarda, A. S., Kaplan, A. S., & Marcus, M. D. (2019). Olanzapine versus placebo in adult outpatients with anorexia nervosa: A randomized clinical trial. *The American Journal of Psychiatry, 176*(6), 449–456. https://doi.org/10.1176/appi.ajp.2018.18101125

Atwood, M. E., & Friedman, A. (2020). A systematic review of enhanced cognitive behavioral therapy (CBT-E) for eating disorders. *International Journal of Eating Disorders, 53*(3), 311–330. https://doi.org/10.1002/eat.23206

Austin, A., Flynn, M., Richards, K., Hodsoll, J., Duarte, T. A., Robinson, P., Kelly, J., & Schmidt, U. (2021). Duration of untreated eating disorder and relationship to outcomes: A systematic review of the literature. *European Eating Disorders Review, 29*(3), 329–345. https://doi.org/10.1002/erv.2745

Becker, P., Carney, L. N., Corkins, M. R., Monczka, J., Smith, E., Smith, S. E., Spear, B. A., White, J. V., the Academy of Nutrition and Dietetics, & the American Society for Parenteral and Enteral Nutrition. (2015). Consensus statement of the Academy of Nutrition and Dietetics/American Society for Parenteral and Enteral Nutrition: Indicators recommended for the identification and documentation of pediatric malnutrition (undernutrition). *Nutrition in Clinical Practice, 30*(1), 147–161. https://doi.org/10.1177/0884533614557642

Bell, R. M. (1985). *Holy anorexia*. University of Chicago Press. https://doi.org/10.7208/chicago/9780226169743.001.0001

Bravender, T. (2011). Eating disorders. In E. B. Berlan & T. Bravender (Eds.), *Adolescent medicine today: A guide to care for the adolescent patient* (pp. 269–290). World Scientific Publishing. https://doi.org/10.1142/9789814324496_0016

Bravender, T., Elkus, H., & Lange, H. (2017). Inpatient medical stabilization for adolescents with eating disorders: Patient and parent perspectives. *Eating and Weight Disorders, 22*(3), 483–489. https://doi.org/10.1007/s40519-016-0270-z

Bravender, T., & Story, L. (2007). Massive binge eating, gastric dilatation and unsuccessful purging in a young woman with bulimia nervosa. *Journal of Adolescent Health, 41*(5), 516–518. https://doi.org/10.1016/j.jadohealth.2007.06.018

Brewerton, T. D., & D'Agostino, M. (2017). Adjunctive use of olanzapine in the treatment of avoidant restrictive food intake disorder in children and adolescents in an eating disorders program. *Journal of Child and Adolescent Psychopharmacology, 27*(10), 920–922. https://doi.org/10.1089/cap.2017.0133

Bruch, H. (1978). *The golden cage: The enigma of anorexia nervosa*. Harvard University Press.

Brumberg, J. J. (1989). *Fasting girls: The history of anorexia nervosa*. Penguin Books.

Bryant-Waugh, R. (2019). Feeding and eating disorders in children. *The Psychiatric Clinics of North America, 42*(1), 157–167. https://doi.org/10.1016/j.psc.2018.10.005

Burnette, C. B., Luzier, J. L., Weisenmuller, C. M., & Boutté, R. L. (2022). A systematic review of sociodemographic reporting and representation in eating disorder psychotherapy treatment trials in the United States. *International Journal of Eating Disorders, 55*(4), 423–454. https://doi.org/10.1002/eat.23699

Calzo, J. P., Blashill, A. J., Brown, T. A., & Argenal, R. L. (2017). Eating disorders and disordered weight and shape control behaviors in sexual minority populations. *Current Psychiatry Reports, 19*(8), 49. https://doi.org/10.1007/s11920-017-0801-y

Cardona Cano, S. C., Tiemeier, H., Van Hoeken, D., Tharner, A., Jaddoe, V. W., Hofman, A., Verhulst, F. C., & Hoek, H. W. (2015). Trajectories of picky eating during childhood: A general population study. *International Journal of Eating Disorders, 48*(6), 570–579. https://doi.org/10.1002/eat.22384

Chua, J. Y. X., Tam, W., & Shorey, S. (2020). Research Review: Effectiveness of universal eating disorder prevention interventions in improving body image among children: A systematic review and meta-analysis. *Journal of Child Psychology and Psychiatry*, 61(5), 522–535. https://doi.org/10.1111/jcpp.13164

Coelho, J. S., Suen, J., Clark, B. A., Marshall, S. K., Geller, J., & Lam, P. Y. (2019). Eating disorder diagnoses and symptom presentation in transgender youth: A scoping review. *Current Psychiatry Reports*, 21(11), 107. https://doi.org/10.1007/s11920-019-1097-x

Couturier, J., Isserlin, L., Spettigue, W., & Norris, M. (2019). Psychotropic medication for children and adolescents with eating disorders. *Child and Adolescent Psychiatric Clinics of North America*, 28(4), 583–592. https://doi.org/10.1016/j.chc.2019.05.005

Culbert, K. M., Racine, S. E., & Klump, K. L. (2015). Research review: What we have learned about the causes of eating disorders—A synthesis of sociocultural, psychological, and biological research. *Journal of Child Psychology and Psychiatry, and Allied Disciplines*, 56(11), 1141–1164. https://doi.org/10.1111/jcpp.12441

Dalle Grave, R., & Calugi, S. (2020). *Cognitive behavioral therapy for adolescents with eating disorders*. Guilford Press.

Dalle Grave, R., Calugi, S., Sartirana, M., & Fairburn, C. G. (2015). Transdiagnostic cognitive behaviour therapy for adolescents with an eating disorder who are not underweight. *Behaviour Research and Therapy*, 73, 79–82. https://doi.org/10.1016/j.brat.2015.07.014

Dalle Grave, R., Sartirana, M., & Calugi, S. (2019). Enhanced cognitive behavioral therapy for adolescents with anorexia nervosa: Outcomes and predictors of change in a real-world setting. *International Journal of Eating Disorders*, 52(9), 1042–1046. https://doi.org/10.1002/eat.23122

Delaney, C. B., Eddy, K. T., Hartmann, A. S., Becker, A. E., Murray, H. B., & Thomas, J. J. (2015). Pica and rumination behavior among individuals seeking treatment for eating disorders or obesity. *International Journal of Eating Disorders*, 48(2), 238–248. https://doi.org/10.1002/eat.22279

Doley, J. R., Hart, L. M., Stukas, A. A., Morgan, A. J., Rowlands, D. L., & Paxton, S. J. (2017). Development of guidelines for giving community presentations about eating disorders: A Delphi study. *Journal of Eating Disorders*, 5(1), 54. https://doi.org/10.1186/s40337-017-0183-x

Fairburn, C. G. (2008). *Cognitive behavior therapy and eating disorders*. Guilford Press.

Fairburn, C. G., Cooper, Z., & Shafran, R. (2003). Cognitive behaviour therapy for eating disorders: A "transdiagnostic" theory and treatment. *Behaviour Research and Therapy*, 41(5), 509–528. https://doi.org/10.1016/S0005-7967(02)00088-8

Favaro, A., Caregaro, L., Tenconi, E., Bosello, R., & Santonastaso, P. (2009). Time trends in age at onset of anorexia nervosa and bulimia nervosa. *The Journal of Clinical Psychiatry*, 70(12), 1715–1721. https://doi.org/10.4088/JCP.09m05176blu

Fazeli, P. K., & Klibanski, A. (2018). Effects of anorexia nervosa on bone metabolism. *Endocrine Reviews*, 39(6), 895–910. https://doi.org/10.1210/er.2018-00063

Fisher, M. M., Rosen, D. S., Ornstein, R. M., Mammel, K. A., Katzman, D. K., Rome, E. S., Callahan, S. T., Malizio, J., Kearney, S., & Walsh, B. T. (2014). Characteristics of avoidant/restrictive food intake disorder in children and adolescents: A "new disorder" in *DSM-5*. *Journal of Adolescent Health*, 55(1), 49–52. https://doi.org/10.1016/j.jadohealth.2013.11.013

Fitzpatrick, K. K., Moye, A., Hoste, R., Lock, J., & Le Grange, D. (2010). Adolescent focused psychotherapy for adolescents with anorexia nervosa. *Journal of Contemporary Psychotherapy*, 40(1), 31–39. https://doi.org/10.1007/s10879-009-9123-7

Forman, S. F., Grodin, L. F., Graham, D. A., Sylvester, C. J., Rosen, D. S., Kapphahn, C. J., Callahan, S. T., Sigel, E. J., Bravender, T., Peebles, R., Romano, M., Rome, E. S., Fisher, M., Malizio, J. B., Mammel, K. A., Hergenroeder, A. C., Buckelew, S. M., Golden, N. H., Woods, E. R., & the National Eating Disorder QI Collaborative. (2011). An eleven site national quality improvement evaluation of adolescent medicine-based eating disorder programs: Predictors of weight outcomes at one year and risk adjustment analyses. *The Journal of Adolescent Health*, 49(6), 594–600. https://doi.org/10.1016/j.jadohealth.2011.04.023

Frank, G. K. W. (2015). Advances from neuroimaging studies in eating disorders. *CNS Spectrums*, 20(4), 391–400. https://doi.org/10.1017/S1092852915000012

Frank, G. K. W., Shott, M. E., & DeGuzman, M. C. (2019). The neurobiology of eating disorders. *Child and Adolescent Psychiatric Clinics of North America*, 28(4), 629–640. https://doi.org/10.1016/j.chc.2019.05.007

Friedli, N., Stanga, Z., Sobotka, L., Culkin, A., Kondrup, J., Laviano, A., Mueller, B., & Schuetz, P. (2017). Revisiting the refeeding syndrome: Results of a systematic review. *Nutrition*, 35, 151–160. https://doi.org/10.1016/j.nut.2016.05.016

Garber, A. K., Cheng, J., Accurso, E. C., Adams, S. H., Buckelew, S. M., Kapphahn, C. J., Kreiter, A.,

Le Grange, D., Machen, V. I., Moscicki, A. B., Saffran, K., Sy, A. F., Wilson, L., & Golden, N. H. (2019). Weight loss and illness severity in adolescents with atypical anorexia nervosa. *Pediatrics*, *144*(6), e20192339. https://doi.org/10.1542/peds.2019-2339

Garber, A. K., Sawyer, S. M., Golden, N. H., Guarda, A. S., Katzman, D. K., Kohn, M. R., Le Grange, D., Madden, S., Whitelaw, M., & Redgrave, G. W. (2016). A systematic review of approaches to refeeding in patients with anorexia nervosa. *International Journal of Eating Disorders*, *49*(3), 293–310. https://doi.org/10.1002/eat.22482

Golden, N. H., Katzman, D. K., Sawyer, S. M., Ornstein, R. M., Rome, E. S., Garber, A. K., Kohn, M., & Kreipe, R. E. (2015). Update on the medical management of eating disorders in adolescents. *Journal of Adolescent Health*, *56*(4), 370–375. https://doi.org/10.1016/j.jadohealth.2014.11.020

Harer, K., Baker, J., Reister, N., Collins, K., Watts, L., Phillips, C., & Chey, W. D. (2018). Avoidant/restrictive food intake disorder in the adult gastroenterology population: An under-recognized diagnosis? *The American Journal of Gastroenterology*, *113*(Suppl.), S247–S248. https://doi.org/10.14309/00000434-201810001-00417

Harris, J. C. (2014). Anorexia nervosa and anorexia mirabilis: Miss K. R—and St Catherine of Siena. *JAMA Psychiatry*, *71*(11), 1212–1213. https://doi.org/10.1001/jamapsychiatry.2013.2765

Haynos, A. F., Anderson, L. M., Askew, A. J., Craske, M. G., & Peterson, C. B. (2021). Adapting a neuroscience-informed intervention to alter reward mechanisms of anorexia nervosa: A novel direction for future research. *Journal of Eating Disorders*, *9*(1), 63. https://doi.org/10.1186/s40337-021-00417-5

Hilbert, A. (2019). Binge-eating disorder. *Psychiatric Clinics of North America*, *42*(1), 33–43. https://doi.org/10.1016/j.psc.2018.10.011

Holtkamp, K., Konrad, K., Kaiser, N., Ploenes, Y., Heussen, N., Grzella, I., & Herpertz-Dahlmann, B. (2005). A retrospective study of SSRI treatment in adolescent anorexia nervosa: Insufficient evidence for efficacy. *Journal of Psychiatric Research*, *39*(3), 303–310. https://doi.org/10.1016/j.jpsychires.2004.08.001

Hornberger, L. L., Lane, M. A., & the Committee on Adolescence. (2021). Identification and management of eating disorders in children and adolescents. *Pediatrics*, *147*(1), e2020040279. https://doi.org/10.1542/peds.2020-040279

Hudson, J. I., Hiripi, E., Pope, H. G., Jr., & Kessler, R. C. (2007). The prevalence and correlates of eating disorders in the National Comorbidity Survey Replication. *Biological Psychiatry*, *61*(3), 348–358. https://doi.org/10.1016/j.biopsych.2006.03.040

Kalm, L. M., & Semba, R. D. (2005). They starved so that others be better fed: Remembering Ancel Keys and the Minnesota experiment. *The Journal of Nutrition*, *135*(6), 1347–1352. https://doi.org/10.1093/jn/135.6.1347

Kappou, K., Ntougia, M., Kourtesi, A., Panagouli, E., Vlachopapadopoulou, E., Michalacos, S., Gonidakis, F., Mastorakos, G., Psaltopoulou, T., Tsolia, M., Bacopoulou, F., Sergentanis, T. N., & Tsitsika, A. (2021). Neuroimaging findings in adolescents and young adults with anorexia nervosa: A systematic review. *Children*, *8*(2), 137. https://doi.org/10.3390/children8020137

Kaye, W. H., & Bulik, C. M. (2021). Treatment of patients with anorexia nervosa in the US—A crisis in care. *JAMA Psychiatry*, *78*(6), 591–592. https://doi.org/10.1001/jamapsychiatry.2020.4796

Keski-Rahkonen, A. (2021). Epidemiology of binge eating disorder: Prevalence, course, comorbidity, and risk factors. *Current Opinion in Psychiatry*, *34*(6), 525–531. https://doi.org/10.1097/YCO.0000000000000750

King, J. A., Frank, G. K. W., Thompson, P. M., & Ehrlich, S. (2018). Structural neuroimaging of anorexia nervosa: Future direction in the quest of mechanisms underlying dynamic alterations. *Biological Psychiatry*, *83*(3), 224–234. https://doi.org/10.1016/j.biopsych.2017.08.011

Kotler, L. A., Devlin, M. J., Davies, M., & Walsh, B. T. (2003). An open trial of fluoxetine for adolescents with bulimia nervosa. *Journal of Child and Adolescent Psychopharmacology*, *13*(3), 329–335. https://doi.org/10.1089/104454603322572660

Kroon Van Diest, A. M., & Perez, M. (2013). Exploring the integration of thin-ideal internalization and self-objectification in the prevention of eating disorders. *Body Image*, *10*(1), 16–25. https://doi.org/10.1016/j.bodyim.2012.10.004

Krug, I., Granero, R., Giles, S., Riesco, N., Agüera, Z., Sánchez, I., Jiménez-Murcia, S., Del Pino-Gutierrez, A., Codina, E., Baenas, I., Valenciano-Mendoza, E., Menchón, J. M., & Fernández-Aranda, F. (2020). A cluster analysis of purging disorder: Validation analyses with eating disorder symptoms, general psychopathology and personality. *European Eating Disorders Review*, *28*(6), 643–656. https://doi.org/10.1002/erv.2769

Latzer, Y., Yutal, A. E., Givon, M., Kabakov, O., Alon, S., Zuckerman-Levin, N., Rozenstain-Hason, M., & Tzischinsky, O. (2020). Dietary patterns of patients with binge eating disorders with and without night eating. *Eating and Weight Disorders*,

25(2), 321–328. https://doi.org/10.1007/s40519-018-0590-2

Le, L. K., Barendregt, J. J., Hay, P., & Mihalopoulos, C. (2017). Prevention of eating disorders: A systematic review and meta-analysis. *Clinical Psychology Review*, 53, 46–58. https://doi.org/10.1016/j.cpr.2017.02.001

Le Grange, D., Eckhardt, S., Dalle Grave, R., Crosby, R. D., Peterson, C. B., Keery, H., Lesser, J., & Martell, C. (2020). Enhanced cognitive-behavior therapy and family-based treatment for adolescents with an eating disorder: A non-randomized effectiveness trial. *Psychological Medicine*, 52(13), 1–11. https://doi.org/10.1017/S0033291720004407

Le Grange, D., Hughes, E. K., Court, A., Yeo, M., Crosby, R. D., & Sawyer, S. M. (2016). Randomized clinical trial of parent-focused treatment and family-based treatment for adolescent anorexia nervosa. *Journal of the American Academy of Child & Adolescent Psychiatry*, 55(8), 683–692. https://doi.org/10.1016/j.jaac.2016.05.007

Linardon, J., Hindle, A., & Brennan, L. (2018). Dropout from cognitive-behavioral therapy for eating disorders: A meta-analysis of randomized, controlled trials. *International Journal of Eating Disorders*, 51(5), 381–391. https://doi.org/10.1002/eat.22850

Lipson, S. K., & Sonneville, K. R. (2020). Understanding suicide risk and eating disorders in college student populations: Results from a National Study. *International Journal of Eating Disorders*, 53(2), 229–238. https://doi.org/10.1002/eat.23188

Lock, J., La Via, M. C., & the American Academy of Child and Adolescent Psychiatry (AACAP) Committee on Quality Issues (CQI). (2015). Practice parameter for the assessment and treatment of children and adolescents with eating disorders. *Journal of the American Academy of Child & Adolescent Psychiatry*, 54(5), 412–425. https://doi.org/10.1016/j.jaac.2015.01.018

Lock, J., & Le Grange, D. (2015). *Treatment manual for anorexia nervosa: A family-based approach* (2nd ed.). Guilford Press.

Lock, J., Le Grange, D., Agras, W. S., Moye, A., Bryson, S. W., & Jo, B. (2010). Randomized clinical trial comparing family-based treatment with adolescent-focused individual therapy for adolescents with anorexia nervosa. *Archives of General Psychiatry*, 67(10), 1025–1032. https://doi.org/10.1001/archgenpsychiatry.2010.128

Lock, J., Sadeh-Sharvit, S., & L'Insalata, A. (2019). Feasibility of conducting a randomized clinical trial using family-based treatment for avoidant/restrictive food intake disorder. *International Journal of Eating Disorders*, 52(6), 746–751. https://doi.org/10.1002/eat.23077

Mammel, K. A., & Ornstein, R. M. (2017). Avoidant/restrictive food intake disorder: A new eating disorder diagnosis in the diagnostic and statistical manual 5. *Current Opinion in Pediatrics*, 29(4), 407–413. https://doi.org/10.1097/MOP.0000000000000507

Marques, L., Alegria, M., Becker, A. E., Chen, C. N., Fang, A., Chosak, A., & Diniz, J. B. (2011). Comparative prevalence, correlates of impairment, and service utilization for eating disorders across US ethnic groups: Implications for reducing ethnic disparities in health care access for eating disorders. *International Journal of Eating Disorders*, 44(5), 412–420. https://doi.org/10.1002/eat.20787

Miller, C. T., Boynton, J. R., & Bravender, T. (2022). Eating disorders in adolescents: Facts and recommendations for the oral health care team. *The Journal of the Michigan Dental Association*, 104(1), 38–45.

Mizusaki, K., Gih, D., LaRosa, C., Richmond, R., & Rienecke, R. D. (2018). Psychotropic usage by patients presenting to an academic eating disorders program. *Eating and Weight Disorders*, 23(6), 769–774. https://doi.org/10.1007/s40519-018-0520-3

Molendijk, M. L., Hoek, H. W., Brewerton, T. D., & Elzinga, B. M. (2017). Childhood maltreatment and eating disorder pathology: A systematic review and dose-response meta-analysis. *Psychological Medicine*, 47(8), 1402–1416. https://doi.org/10.1017/S0033291716003561

Moncrieff-Boyd, J. (2016). Anorexia nervosa (apepsia hysterica, anorexia hysterica), Sir William Gull, 1873. *Advances in Eating Disorders*, 4(1), 112–117. https://doi.org/10.1080/21662630.2015.1079694

Monge, M. C., Forman, S. F., McKenzie, N. M., Rosen, D. S., Mammel, K. A., Callahan, S. T., Hehn, R., Rome, E. S., Kapphahn, C. J., Carlson, J. L., Romano, M. E., Malizio, J. B., Bravender, T. D., Sigel, E. J., Rouse, M. R., Graham, D. A., Jay, M. S., Hergenroeder, A. C., Fisher, M. M., . . . Woods, E. R. (2015). Use of psychopharmacologic medications in adolescents with restrictive eating disorders: Analysis of data from the National Eating Disorder Quality Improvement Collaborative. *Journal of Adolescent Health*, 57(1), 66–72. https://doi.org/10.1016/j.jadohealth.2015.03.021

Murray, H. B., Juarascio, A. S., Di Lorenzo, C., Drossman, D. A., & Thomas, J. J. (2019). Diagnosis and treatment of rumination syndrome: A critical review. *The American Journal of Gastroenterology*, 114(4), 562–578. https://doi.org/10.14309/ajg.0000000000000060

Pearson, J., Goldklang, D., & Striegel-Moore, R. H. (2002). Prevention of eating disorders: Challenges and opportunities. *International Journal of Eating*

Disorders, 31(3), 233–239. https://doi.org/10.1002/eat.10014

Peebles, R., & Sieke, E. H. (2019). Medical complications of eating disorders in youth. *Child and Adolescent Psychiatric Clinics of North America, 28*(4), 593–615. https://doi.org/10.1016/j.chc.2019.05.009

Perez, M. E., Coley, B., Crandall, W., Di Lorenzo, C., & Bravender, T. (2013). Effect of nutritional rehabilitation on gastric motility and somatization in adolescents with anorexia. *The Journal of Pediatrics, 163*(3), 867–72.e1. https://doi.org/10.1016/j.jpeds.2013.03.011

Petkova, H., Simic, M., Nicholls, D., Ford, T., Prina, A. M., Stuart, R., Livingstone, N., Kelly, G., Macdonald, G., Eisler, I., Gowers, S., Barrett, B. M., & Byford, S. (2019). Incidence of anorexia nervosa in young people in the UK and Ireland: A national surveillance study. *BMJ Open, 9*(10), e027339. https://doi.org/10.1136/bmjopen-2018-027339

Racine, S. E., VanHuysse, J. L., Keel, P. K., Burt, S. A., Neale, M. C., Boker, S., & Klump, K. L. (2017). Eating disorder-specific risk factors moderate the relationship between negative urgency and binge eating: A behavioral genetic investigation. *Journal of Abnormal Psychology, 126*(5), 481–494. https://doi.org/10.1037/abn0000204

Richards, I. L., Subar, A., Touyz, S., & Rhodes, P. (2018). Augmentative approaches in family-based treatment for adolescents with restrictive eating disorders: A systematic review. *European Eating Disorders Review, 26*(2), 92–111. https://doi.org/10.1002/erv.2577

Russell, G. (1979). Bulimia nervosa: An ominous variant of anorexia nervosa. *Psychological Medicine, 9*(3), 429–448. https://doi.org/10.1017/S0033291700031974

Sachs, K. V., Harnke, B., Mehler, P. S., & Krantz, M. J. (2016). Cardiovascular complications of anorexia nervosa: A systematic review. *International Journal of Eating Disorders, 49*(3), 238–248. https://doi.org/10.1002/eat.22481

Schorr, M., & Miller, K. K. (2017). The endocrine manifestations of anorexia nervosa: Mechanisms and management. *Nature Reviews Endocrinology, 13*(3), 174–186. https://doi.org/10.1038/nrendo.2016.175

Sejling, A. S., Kjær, T. W., Pedersen-Bjergaard, U., Diemar, S. S., Frandsen, C. S. S., Hilsted, L., Faber, J., Holst, J. J., Tarnow, L., Nielsen, M. N., Remvig, L. S., Thorsteinsson, B., & Juhl, C. B. (2015). Hypoglycemia-associated changes in the electroencephalogram in patients with Type 1 diabetes and normal hypoglycemia awareness or unawareness. *Diabetes, 64*(5), 1760–1769. https://doi.org/10.2337/db14-1359

Sonneville, K. R., & Lipson, S. K. (2018). Disparities in eating disorder diagnosis and treatment according to weight status, race/ethnicity, socioeconomic background, and sex among college students. *International Journal of Eating Disorders, 51*(6), 518–526. https://doi.org/10.1002/eat.22846

Spettigue, W., Norris, M. L., Santos, A., & Obeid, N. (2018). Treatment of children and adolescents with avoidant/restrictive food intake disorder: A case series examining the feasibility of family therapy and adjunctive treatments. *Journal of Eating Disorders, 6*(1), 20. https://doi.org/10.1186/s40337-018-0205-3

Steinhausen, H. C. (2009). Outcome of eating disorders. *Child and Adolescent Psychiatric Clinics of North America, 18*(1), 225–242. https://doi.org/10.1016/j.chc.2008.07.013

Stheneur, C., Bergeron, S. J., Frappier, J. Y., Jamoulle, O., Taddeo, D., Sznajder, M., & Lapeyraque, A. L. (2019). Renal injury in pediatric anorexia nervosa: A retrospective study. *Eating and Weight Disorders, 24*(2), 323–327. https://doi.org/10.1007/s40519-017-0401-1

Strand, M., von Hausswolff-Juhlin, Y., & Welch, E. (2019). A systematic scoping review of diagnostic validity in avoidant/restrictive food intake disorder. *International Journal of Eating Disorders, 52*(4), 331–360. https://doi.org/10.1002/eat.22962

Svirko, E., & Hawton, K. (2007). Self-injurious behavior and eating disorders: The extent and nature of the association. *Suicide & Life-Threatening Behavior, 37*(4), 409–421. https://doi.org/10.1521/suli.2007.37.4.409

Swanson, S. A., Crow, S. J., Le Grange, D., Swendsen, J., & Merikangas, K. R. (2011). Prevalence and correlates of eating disorders in adolescents. Results from the national comorbidity survey replication adolescent supplement. *Archives of General Psychiatry, 68*(7), 714–723. https://doi.org/10.1001/archgenpsychiatry.2011.22

Tabler, J., Utz, R. L., Smith, K. R., Hanson, H. A., & Geist, C. (2018). Variation in reproductive outcomes of women with histories of bulimia nervosa, anorexia nervosa, or eating disorder not otherwise specified relative to the general population and closest-aged sisters. *International Journal of Eating Disorders, 51*(2), 102–111. https://doi.org/10.1002/eat.22827

Testa, R. J., Rider, G. N., Haug, N. A., & Balsam, K. F. (2017). Gender confirming medical interventions and eating disorder symptoms among transgender individuals. *Health Psychology, 36*(10), 927–936. https://doi.org/10.1037/hea0000497

Thomas, J. J., Becker, K. R., Kuhnle, M. C., Jo, J. H., Harshman, S. G., Wons, O. B., Keshishian, A. C., Hauser, K., Breithaupt, L., Liebman, R. E., Misra, M., Wilhelm, S., Lawson, E. A., & Eddy, K. T. (2020). Cognitive-behavioral therapy for avoidant/restrictive food intake disorder: Feasibility, acceptability, and proof-of-concept for children and adolescents. *International Journal of Eating Disorders, 53*(10), 1636–1646. https://doi.org/10.1002/eat.23355

Thomas, J. J., & Eddy, K. (2019). *Cognitive-behavioral therapy for avoidant/restrictive food intake disorder: Children, adolescents, and adults.* Cambridge University Press.

Tith, R. M., Paradis, G., Potter, B. J., Low, N., Healy-Profitós, J., He, S., & Auger, N. (2020). Association of bulimia nervosa with long-term risk of cardiovascular disease and mortality among women. *JAMA Psychiatry, 77*(1), 44–51. https://doi.org/10.1001/jamapsychiatry.2019.2914

Udo, T., Bitley, S., & Grilo, C. M. (2019). Suicide attempts in US adults with lifetime *DSM-5* eating disorders. *BMC Medicine, 17*(1), 120. https://doi.org/10.1186/s12916-019-1352-3

Udo, T., & Grilo, C. M. (2019). Psychiatric and medical correlates of *DSM-5* eating disorders in a nationally representative sample of adults in the United States. *International Journal of Eating Disorders, 52*(1), 42–50. https://doi.org/10.1002/eat.23004

Ulfvebrand, S., Birgegård, A., Norring, C., Högdahl, L., & von Hausswolff-Juhlin, Y. (2015). Psychiatric comorbidity in women and men with eating disorders results from a large clinical database. *Psychiatry Research, 230*(2), 294–299. https://doi.org/10.1016/j.psychres.2015.09.008

van Eeden, A. E., van Hoeken, D., & Hoek, H. W. (2021). Incidence, prevalence and mortality of anorexia nervosa and bulimia nervosa. *Current Opinion in Psychiatry, 34*(6), 515–524. https://doi.org/10.1097/YCO.0000000000000739

Van Huysse, J. L., Smith, K., Mammel, K. A., Prohaska, N., & Rienecke, R. D. (2020). Early weight gain predicts treatment response in adolescents with anorexia nervosa enrolled in a family-based partial hospitalization program. *International Journal of Eating Disorders, 53*(4), 606–610. https://doi.org/10.1002/eat.23248

Voderholzer, U., Haas, V., Correll, C. U., & Körner, T. (2020). Medical management of eating disorders: An update. *Current Opinion in Psychiatry, 33*(6), 542–553. https://doi.org/10.1097/YCO.0000000000000653

Watson, H. J., Yilmaz, Z., Thornton, L. M., Hübel, C., Coleman, J. R. I., Gaspar, H. A., Bryois, J., Hinney, A., Leppä, V. M., Mattheisen, M., Medland, S. E., Ripke, S., Yao, S., Giusti-Rodríguez, P., Anorexia Nervosa Genetics Initiative, Hanscombe, K. B., Purves, K. L., Eating Disorders Working Group of the Psychiatric Genomics Consortium, Adan, R. A. H., . . . Bulik, C. M. (2019). Genome-wide association study identifies eight risk loci and implicates metabo-psychiatric origins for anorexia nervosa. *Nature Genetics, 51*(8), 1207–1214. https://doi.org/10.1038/s41588-019-0439-2

Wolfe, B. E., Baker, C. W., Smith, A. T., & Kelly-Weeder, S. (2009). Validity and utility of the current definition of binge eating. *International Journal of Eating Disorders, 42*(8), 674–686. https://doi.org/10.1002/eat.20728

Wonderlich, J. A., Bershad, M., & Steinglass, J. E. (2021). Exploring neural mechanisms related to cognitive control, reward, and affect in eating disorders: A narrative review of FMRI studies. *Neuropsychiatric Disease and Treatment, 17,* 2053–2062. https://doi.org/10.2147/NDT.S282554

CHAPTER 24

SUICIDAL THINKING AND BEHAVIOR IN YOUTH: PREVENTION, INTERVENTION, AND IMPLICATIONS FOR CHILD AND ADOLESCENT HEALTH

Cynthia Ewell Foster, Seth Finkelstein, Daniel Epstein, and Cheryl A. King

Suicide is the second leading cause of death (after unintentional injuries, such as motor vehicle accidents) among youth ages 10 to 14 years, and it is the third leading cause of death (after unintentional injuries and homicide) for youth and young adults ages 15 to 24 in the United States (Centers for Disease Control and Prevention [CDC] National Center for Health Statistics, 2021). Every life lost to suicide is a tragedy. With rates of youth suicide in the United States increasing by 54% from 2007 to 2020 (CDC, 2021) and with 700,000 lives lost to suicide across the world each year (World Health Organization, 2021), the prevention of death by suicide is a global imperative.

Suicide is a complex phenomenon with multiple contributing factors at the individual, family, and community levels and as such, comprehensive efforts to reduce suicide mortality require a multidisciplinary, multifaceted approach. The National Strategy for Suicide Prevention (U.S. Surgeon General & National Action Alliance for Suicide Prevention, 2012) offers a comprehensive roadmap for national prevention efforts. It incorporates key aspects of developmental science and provides guidance for child-serving medical and behavioral health professionals, including pediatric psychologists, developmental-behavioral pediatricians, and primary care physicians, regarding key evidence-based suicide prevention clinical practices. The National Strategy focuses on four strategic priorities: (a) healthy and empowered individuals, families, and communities; (b) clinical and community preventive services; (c) treatment and support services; and (d) surveillance, research, and evaluation. To address these priorities, the National Strategy calls for science-based prevention and health promotion in youth prior to the onset of suicidal behavior, use of an ecological framework to understand risk and tailor interventions, and use of health care contacts as an opportunity to screen and provide supports for youth with elevated risk for suicide and their families.

In this chapter, we begin with a review of the definitions of suicidal thinking and behavior, describe surveillance data documenting the prevalence of suicide morbidity and mortality and its variability across different populations, and detail several theoretical models of suicidal behavior. We then turn to developmental considerations in the emergence of suicide risk and review relevant risk and protective factors, with a particular focus on the role of medical and behavioral health providers in preventing suicide. Finally, we review several promising public health

https://doi.org/10.1037/0000414-024
APA Handbook of Pediatric Psychology, Developmental-Behavioral Pediatrics, and Developmental Science: Vol. 2. Pediatric Psychology and Developmental-Behavioral Pediatrics: Clinical Applications of Developmental Science, P. E. Shah and M. H. Bornstein (Editors-in-Chief)
Copyright © 2025 by the American Psychological Association. All rights reserved.

suicide prevention strategies, as well as research challenges and future directions. At the conclusion of the chapter, we provide a list of accessible resources to support ongoing learning about this critical topic.

DEFINITIONS AND TERMINOLOGY

The use of uniform terminology to describe suicide-related thinking and behavior has led to improved surveillance, clinical care, and research. As defined by the CDC, *suicide* is "a death caused by self-injurious behavior with any intent to die as a result of the behavior" (Crosby et al., 2011, p. 23). A *suicide attempt* is a "non-fatal self-directed potentially injurious behavior with any intent to die" (p. 21); suicide attempts may include actions that are interrupted by others, aborted by oneself, or that result in mild or no medical complications (Crosby et al., 2011). *Suicidal ideation* (SI) is thinking about ending one's life and may range from a passive wish to be dead to more active thoughts about how, when, and where to engage in self-harming behaviors. *Nonsuicidal self-injury* (*NSSI*) is behavior that is "self-directed and deliberately results in injury or the potential for injury" with no evidence of suicidal intent (Crosby et al., 2011, p. 21). Common presentations of NSSI among youth include cutting, scratching, and burning (Cipriano et al., 2017).

The National Violent Death Reporting System (NVDRS; Blair et al., 2016) utilizes these standard terms to collect data on the circumstances of suicide deaths in the United States, integrating medical examiner, law enforcement, and death certificate data. Unfortunately, standard definitions for international surveillance are lacking, which may contribute to the wide variability in youth suicide rates across nations (Cha et al., 2018).

Use of Respectful Language

Based on input from survivors regarding stigma that can be inadvertently conveyed with language (Padmanathan et al., 2019), the term "committed suicide" is discouraged due to its association with committing a sin or a crime. Similarly, language such as a "failed suicide attempt" or "manipulative gesture" reflects an inappropriate value judgment, which can negatively impact clinical care. Use of such terms should be avoided (Crosby et al., 2011).

EPIDEMIOLOGY AND PREVALENCE

In 2020, there were 45,979 deaths by suicide in the United States; 20 (0.04%) of these deaths were suicides of children under 10 years of age; 581 (1.26%) were of youth ages 10 to 14; and 2,216 were of youth ages 15 to 19 (4.82%). Despite concern that the social isolation, stress, and economic impact of the COVID-19 pandemic would increase suicide rates, there were no significant differences in the youth suicide rate between 2019 (prior to the pandemic) and 2020 (the latest year for which complete data are available; CDC, 2020; Ehlman et al., 2022), although selected demographic subgroups demonstrated concerning increases.

Suicide Surveillance Data

Suicide deaths represent only a fraction of the number of individuals who experience suicide-related thinking or behavior. The Youth Risk Behavior Surveillance System (YRBS; CDC, 2020), which is administered biannually to a representative U.S. sample of high school students in 9th through 12th grades (approximate ages of 14–18 years), suggests that, within a 12-month period, 18.8% of youth seriously considered suicide, 15.7% made a plan for ending their lives, and 8.9% reported they attempted suicide at least once, with 2.5% reporting that their attempt required medical treatment (Ivey-Stephenson et al., 2020).

Suicide mortality, thinking, and behavior vary by demographic subgroup. Although surveillance data are critical to drive the allocation of prevention resources, they should be used cautiously for clinical decision making, as suicide can and does occur, although in varying degrees, across all demographic groups.

Gender. Across most Western countries, males are more likely to die by suicide than females, although this gender gap is narrowing because mortality rates are increasing at a faster rate in females (Ruch et al., 2019). In 2020, 72% of youth suicides in the United States were male (CDC WISQARS, 2020). Paradoxically, females report higher rates of suicidal thinking and attempts (CDC, 2021; Ivey-Stephenson et al., 2020). According to the YRBS, 24% of female high school respondents endorsed serious SI compared to 13% of males, with 11% of females reporting a suicide attempt versus 6.6% of males (Ivey-Stephenson et al., 2020). A critical implication of this gender paradox is to refrain from relying on the endorsement of SI as the primary indicator of suicide risk, especially among males.

Demographic and cultural subgroups. Across the world, Indigenous youth have the highest rates of suicide mortality (CDC WISQARS, 2020; Cha et al., 2018). Data show alarming increases in suicide among Black/African American youth (from 2.55 per 100,000 in 2007 to 5.58 per 100,000 in 2020), with Black/African American children ages 5 to 12 now twice as likely to die by suicide as European American children (CDC, 2021), spurring a report by the Congressional Black Caucus (2019): *Ring the Alarm: The Crisis of Black Youth Suicide in America.* Suicide deaths among Asian American/Pacific Islander and Hispanic youth are also demonstrating concerning increases, suggesting that minority youth in the United States are an emerging high-risk demographic (CDC, 2021). Figure 24.1 illustrates youth suicide mortality by gender in the United States, using population categories established by the CDC.

Sexual and gender minority status. Youth who identify as lesbian, gay, bisexual, transgender, or queer/questioning (LGBTQ) are four times more likely to report suicidal ideation and attempts relative to their non-LGBTQ peers (Johns et al., 2020). Although sexual minority (but not gender minority) status has been added to the YRBS survey, neither is collected consistently via NVDRS, resulting in limited suicide mortality data for LGBTQ youth. Unique risk factors associated with suicide risk in LGBTQ youth include internalized self-stigma, distress around coming out, family conflict and rejection, and LGBTQ-related victimization and discrimination (Green et al., 2021).

Geography. Residents of rural areas are at increased risk for suicide relative to individuals in urban or suburban regions of the United States. This circumstance may reflect economic factors, disparities in access to care, and higher rates of firearm ownership (Ivey-Stephenson et al., 2017).

Means of Suicide and Suicide Attempts

Firearms account for over half of all suicide deaths in the United States, and 91% of attempts with a firearm are fatal (Conner et al., 2019). Of all youth suicides occurring in the United States in 2020, 46% were firearm-related, 40% were due to hanging/suffocation, and 7% to poisoning (CDC WISQARS, 2020). An analysis of youth firearm suicides in five states indicated that in 79% of deaths, the firearm belonged to a family member, highlighting the critical role of reducing access to highly lethal means as a prevention strategy (Barber et al., 2022). Among very young suicide decedents, ages 5 to 11 years, hanging or strangulation accounted for 78% of deaths, which frequently occurred in the child's home (Ruch et al., 2021), pointing to the need to carefully supervise and monitor young children with elevated risk as a safety strategy. The most common method of suicide attempt among youth is poisoning, reflecting almost 43% of nonfatal self-harm injuries among youth (CDC WISQARS, 2020), followed by cutting or piercing, which is responsible for 39% of nonfatal self-harm injuries.

THEORY

Theories provide useful conceptual frameworks that can inform both research and clinical risk formulation, and can help guide screening, risk assessment, and treatment planning (Joiner et al., 2021). The Interpersonal Theory of Suicide (IPTS; Joiner et al., 2021) posits that desire to die by suicide arises from the interaction of three main constructs: (a) *thwarted belongingness*, which may include loneliness or a lack of reciprocal

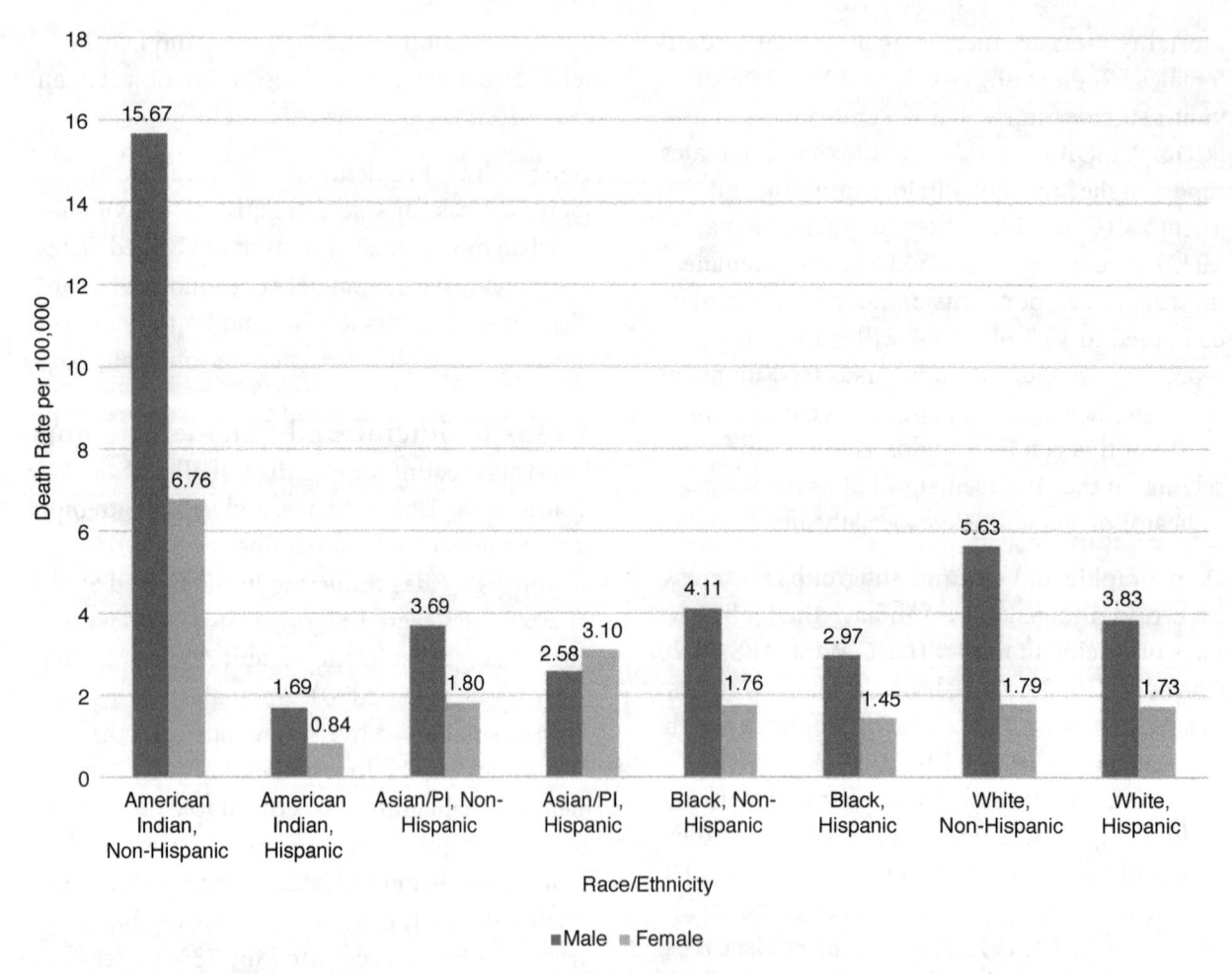

FIGURE 24.1. Surveillance data for suicide mortality in the United States in 2020, ages 19 and under, illustrating gender and ethnicity differences. Ethnicity categories are consistent with the Centers for Disease Control and Prevention (CDC) WISQARS database (CDC, 2020). PI = Pacific Islander. Data from CDC, National Center for Injury Prevention and Control (2020). Use of these data does not imply endorsement by the CDC. Additionally, the data are available on the website for no charge through the WISQARS database (https://www.cdc.gov/injury/wisqars/).

relationships; (b) *perceived burdensomeness*, the often-distorted view that one's death would benefit loved ones; and (c) *acquired capability* for suicide, which may include experiences such as abuse, combat exposure, or previous suicidal behaviors that reduce fear of death or injury, making suicidal behavior more acceptable. A meta-analysis of 122 published and unpublished studies (Chu et al., 2017) supported univariate relations between IPTS constructs and both suicidal ideation (SI) and suicide attempt (SA); however, the hypothesized three-way interaction was no better at predicting SA than the interaction of burdensomeness and belongingness. Other theories that attempt to explain the transition from thinking about suicide to acting on those thoughts, such as the Three Step Theory (3ST; Klonsky & May, 2015) have received less empirical examination. The 3ST asserts that a combination of pain and hopelessness leads to SI (step 1); SI escalates from passive to active when pain exceeds feelings of connectedness (step 2); and strong/active SI progresses to action when one has the capacity to attempt suicide (step 3). Contributors to the capacity for self-harm can include dispositional, genetic, or acquired factors (e.g., high pain threshold, occupational expertise with lethal means). Although the 3ST has not been validated in adolescents, a study with adults supports the importance of pain and hopelessness as predictors of suicidal thoughts as well as the protective role of connectedness (Klonsky & May, 2015). A key future direction for theories of suicidal behavior is the incorporation of developmental science to further specify the onset, progression, and course of suicidal thinking and behavior (Oppenheimer et al., 2022).

DEVELOPMENTAL CONSIDERATIONS IN THE ONSET OF SUICIDAL THINKING AND BEHAVIOR

The National Strategy for Suicide Prevention advocates an "upstream" prevention approach (Wyman, 2014) that focuses on identifying and changing developmental precursors to suicidal thinking and behavior (as opposed to an approach that focuses on "pulling people out of the river," once suicidal thinking and behavior have emerged). With the majority of studies still conducted in adults and most studies of youth being cross-sectional or retrospective in nature, prospective longitudinal studies that document developmental trajectories of suicide risk in youth are sorely needed. Nevertheless, childhood and adolescence are likely to be key windows of opportunity for prevention (Cha et al., 2018; Oppenheimer et al., 2022), highlighting the critical role that pediatric health professionals and developmental science researchers can play to better understand and interrupt a child's path toward risk. In the following discussion, we summarize the extent of our current understanding regarding the emergence of suicidal thinking and behavior in youth, with clinical implications for assessing and monitoring risk.

Suicide deaths are rare in young children, yet the greatest acceleration in the numbers of suicide deaths across the entire lifespan occurs during the early adolescent to young adult period (Cha et al., 2018). Both SI and SAs become increasingly prevalent as youth enter adolescence, with community surveillance data suggesting that almost 20% of teens experience serious thoughts of ending their lives (CDC, 2020) and approximately 9% report an attempt within the last year (CDC, 2020). Emerging data among clinical samples of children under 9 years old suggest rates of SI between 11% and 19% and rates of suicide attempt about 3% (Oppenheimer et al., 2022), with some suggesting that early onset of SI and behavior may be associated with a particularly persistent and recurrent course of suicide risk over time (Oppenheimer et al., 2022).

Adolescents who experience SI are 12 times more likely to make a SA by age 30 relative to those who do not (Reinherz et al., 2006), yet only one-third of adolescents who experience SI go on to either plan or attempt suicide (Nock et al., 2013). Youth with more frequent, severe, and persistent SI and those who feel less able to control their thoughts tend to be most likely to attempt in the future (Horwitz et al., 2015). In a study of over 10,000 teens aged 13 to 17, 60% of those who made a plan went on to make a SA, with most reporting that the transition from thinking to planning to attempt occurred within a one-year time frame (Nock et al., 2013).

From a clinical standpoint, disclosure of suicidal ideation in youth warrants risk assessment and support but does not automatically constitute an emergency, as many youth with suicidal thoughts can be managed safely with added family, school, and behavioral health supports. Youth who endorse suicidal intent or have a plan to end their lives should be carefully assessed for acuity and level of risk, which often involves a comprehensive evaluation conducted by a trained behavioral health professional. It is also important to remember that not all suicide attempts are preceded by suicidal thinking, with 20% to 40% of adolescents who attempt suicide describing their SA as unplanned (Cha et al., 2018).

RISK AND PROTECTIVE FACTORS

Suicide risk is multifactorial; there is no one developmental pathway or constellation of risk factors that leads to suicidal thinking and behavior. Using an ecological model framework, individual, family, and community-level risk factors are considered in the following sections. Much of this research has focused on the identification of univariate risk factors; developmental science approaches that consider bidirectional and transactional influences of risk and protection on youth trajectories are needed (Oppenheimer et al., 2022).

Individual Level Risk Factors

The best predictor of future death by suicide is a previous SA (Cha et al., 2018; Nock et al., 2013). Other behaviors, such as preparatory actions (researching methods of suicide, writing a suicide note) or self-injurious behaviors, are also key behavioral risk indicators for SA and death by suicide (Posner et al., 2011). Among adolescent inpatients, the number of lifetime SA has been associated with the number of years engaged in NSSI and number of NSSI methods (Nock et al., 2006), highlighting the importance of assessing current and historical NSSI behaviors. In the ED STARS multisite study of youth seeking emergency services for psychiatric or nonpsychiatric complaints, 104 of 2,104 (5%) youths made a suicide attempt between their emergency department (ED) visit and 3-month follow-up. A multivariate prediction model identified four prospective predictors of SA: SI within the past week, lifetime severity of SI, lifetime history of suicidal behavior, and school connectedness (King, Grupp-Phelan, et al., 2019). Nearly one-third of the youths who made a SA at 3 months had denied SI during their ED visit, making it extremely challenging to identify them for preventive care. For those youth, predictors of SA included lifetime SI severity and social connectedness. Clinically, this study suggests that the identification of suicide risk should extend beyond the assessment of current SI and should consider protective factors such as social connectedness.

Psychopathology is also a primary risk factor for suicide attempts and death by suicide (Cha et al., 2018), yet a significant proportion of youth who make a suicide attempt or die by suicide have not received mental health services prior to their initial attempt (McKean et al., 2018), highlighting the need to screen youth at risk in other settings, such as primary care, emergency departments, and other community settings. Mood disorders and associated symptoms such as hopelessness, negative self-worth, and anhedonia have been associated with suicidal ideation, suicide attempts, and suicide deaths in youth (Cha et al., 2018). Alcohol is present at the time of death in 51% of teen deaths by suicide (Marttunen et al., 1991). In a pediatric ED sample, alcohol and cannabis use, anxiety, agitation, sleep problems, impulsivity, and a history of physical fighting/aggressive behavior were associated at the univariate level with 3-month risk of SA (King, Grupp-Phelan, et al., 2019). In a large community sample, depression emerged as the strongest predictor of SI (Nock et al., 2013), with a variety of diagnoses predicting transition from SI to SA: major depressive disorder, eating disorders, ADHD, conduct disorder, and intermittent explosive disorder. These data suggest the importance of screening for psychopathology, substance use, and behavioral discontrol, which can convey potential risk for suicide.

Family- and Community-Level Risk Factors

Within the family, risk factors for youth suicidal behavior include parental suicide attempt or death by suicide (Geulayov et al., 2012), other parental separation or loss (Hughes et al., 2017), parental psychopathology (Goodday et al., 2019), insecure attachment, parenting style, and high levels of family conflict (Diamond et al., 2022). Conversely, positive parent–child relationships and family environment are also potential protective factors (Diamond et al., 2022; King, Grupp-Phelan, et al., 2019), and the important role of parents in facilitating treatment linkage and outcomes for high-risk youth is increasingly recognized (Asarnow et al., 2011; Diamond et al., 2022; Ewell Foster et al., 2022).

Trauma and adverse child experiences. History of trauma, including abuse, neglect, and other types of interpersonal violence or adverse childhood experiences (ACEs), increases the likelihood of suicidal thinking and behavior in youth (Castellví et al., 2017; Hughes et al., 2017). A population-based case control study found that among children and adolescents who died by suicide, 56.5% had a history of abuse/neglect allegations, and those with any Child Protective Services (CPS) involvement had three times the odds of suicide compared to children with no CPS history (Palmer et al., 2021). Peer victimization has also been shown to relate to suicidal thinking and behavior in youth, and this relation holds whether the youth is the victim, the perpetrator, or has played both roles and whether the bullying is done in person or as cyber-bullying (Cha et al., 2018). Youth who have experienced trauma in their homes or communities are a key high-risk group for suicide prevention efforts.

Disparities, marginalized populations, and social determinants of health. Disparities among groups in access to quality mental health care and in the experience of life stressors may be important factors in understanding differences in suicidal thinking and behavior across demographic groups. For example, African American youth are more likely than other ethnic groups to receive short-term, crisis-focused services (Bruckner et al., 2020), and data suggest that the stress and discrimination faced by marginalized groups may increase the risk for suicide (Cha et al., 2018; Congressional Black Caucus, 2019; Johns et al., 2020). LGBTQ youth in communities coded as "unsupportive" (e.g., limited LGBTQ support groups or protective policies in schools) have been found to be at 20% greater risk of suicide attempts relative to youth in more supportive communities (Hatzenbuehler, 2011). Yet investment in access to care may yield benefits; a 10% increase in a state's mental health workforce was found to be associated with a 1.35% relative reduction in nonfirearm suicides in youth ages 10 to 24 years (Goldstein et al., 2022). A key future research direction is to move beyond documenting risk factors among particular subgroups, to studying the mechanisms by which these community-level risk factors may enhance suicidal processes over time for marginalized youth.

Multilevel Protective Factors

Although less is known about factors that protect against or reduce risk for suicide, several key factors that may be modifiable therapeutically or via prevention strategies have been identified. These include social support and connectedness to family, peers, schools, and other social structures (King, Grupp-Phelan, et al., 2019). In addition, religiosity, defined as private spiritual practices as well as involvement in a religious community, has been associated with reduced levels of SI and SA (Kim et al., 2020). Youth with strong coping or problem-solving skills, who are focused on the future, or who can articulate their "reasons for living" have lower rates of suicidal thinking and behavior (Breton et al., 2015). Taken together, factors such as family cohesion, family and peer support, social connectedness, and "upstream factors," such as coping skills, self-regulation, and a "future-oriented" viewpoint, appear to be important protections and potential targets for intervention.

SUICIDE PREVENTION IN SPECIAL CLINICAL POPULATIONS: RELEVANCE FOR DEVELOPMENTAL-BEHAVIORAL PEDIATRICIANS AND PEDIATRIC PSYCHOLOGY

Developmental-behavioral pediatricians and pediatric psychologists have access to several subgroups of youth known to be at elevated risk for suicide. We briefly review relevant specialized risk processes related to three clinical subgroups: sexual and gender minority youth (S/GM), neurodiverse youth, and youth with chronic medical conditions.

LGBTQ Youth

As mentioned earlier, S/GM youth report higher levels of SI and SA relative to their heterosexual peers (Horwitz et al., 2021; Johns et al., 2020), with some studies indicating that S/GM youth may have an earlier age of onset of suicidal thinking and behavior, more attempts, and greater desire to die during an attempt relative to heterosexual peers (Fox et al., 2018). In an ED sample of over 6,000 youth ages 12 to 17 (Horwitz et al., 2021), 20% of whom identified as a sexual minority (SM), history of depression, bullying victimization, and sexual abuse emerged as the most significant risk factors for suicidal thinking and behaviors, with parent–family connectedness and positive affect the most significant protective factors against SI and SA. A subgroup of bisexual youth reported the highest levels of suicidal thinking and behavior, more risk factors, and fewer protective factors relative to other SM youth in this sample (Horwitz et al., 2021). In a study of 1,635 transgender or gender-nonconforming 9th- and 11th-grade students (e.g., ages 14–15 and 16–17) in Minnesota public schools, over half of the sample reported engaging in some type of self-harm, with 18% reporting NSSI in addition to a SA (Taliaferro et al., 2019). Factors that distinguished transgender youth who engaged in NSSI and reported a suicide attempt from those engaging in NSSI only were a mental health diagnosis, parent–family connectedness, relationship violence, history of physical or sexual abuse, lower grades, perceptions of school safety, and running away from home—with strongest effects for parent connectedness and school safety. Studies suggest that S/GM youth demonstrate similar patterns to those reviewed previously in terms of risk associated with psychopathology, interpersonal violence, and abuse. The Minority Stress Model (Meyer, 2003) suggests that being a S/GM may confer an increased burden of risk due to experiences of discrimination, rejection, stigma, having to conceal one's identity, or internalized homo- or transphobia. The role of the family as either a protective or risk factor in S/GM youth is also critical. The Family Acceptance Project (Ryan et al., 2010) is an intervention designed specifically to enhance parent support for and acceptance of LGBTQ youth to enhance their health and outcomes.

Neurodiverse Youth

Although neurodiverse youth, and especially youth with autism, have been shown to have elevated risk for suicide (Howe et al., 2020), tailored screening or assessment strategies are lacking for this population, with clinicians reporting a lack of training and need for additional guidance and clinical protocols (Cervantes et al., 2023). Risk factors for suicidal thinking and behavior among youth with autism are similar to those in the general population, including psychiatric comorbidities such as depression, anxiety, peer victimization/rejection, and adverse childhood experiences (O'Halloran et al., 2022). A unique challenge in interpreting the meager literature on suicide screening and risk assessment in neurodiverse youth is a lack of clarity about whether positive screens are due to higher incidence of suicide-related risk or to issues related to a unique interpretation of screening questions, cognitive impairments, or due to the practice of using parents as informants about suicide risk rather than youth themselves (Rybczynski et al., 2022).

Children With Chronic Medical Illness

Chronic medical conditions have long been associated with suicide risk in older adults, yet relatively little work has examined this issue in youth. In a systematic review of relationships between chronic medical illness and youth suicide risk, the following health conditions had evidence of association with suicidal thinking or behavior: chronic pain (including migraine and headache), respiratory diseases including asthma, cystic fibrosis, allergic diseases, epilepsy, diabetes, and cancer (Iannucci & Nierenberg, 2022). Across different health conditions, the authors documented a pattern whereby youth experiencing suicidal thinking and behavior were also experiencing comorbid depression. The mechanisms by which medical illness conveys suicide risk remain unclear, with factors varying by condition. For example, the severity of pain and its related impairment was associated with suicide risk in chronic pain patients, while nonadherence to medical regimens was associated with suicide risk in youth with diabetes (Iannucci & Nierenberg, 2022).

Across these subgroups likely to be encountered in health care settings, the need for additional developmental science is clear, along with the need to delve deeper into the mechanisms by which factors such as neurodiversity, health conditions, or being a sexual or gender minority may convey risk for suicide. It is incumbent on clinicians to be aware of both the limitations of current science along with the need to screen and assess for risk in these vulnerable subgroups of youth.

PREVENTION AND INTERVENTION: THE ROLE OF MEDICAL/BEHAVIORAL HEALTH PROVIDERS

A comprehensive approach to suicide prevention includes a continuum of strategies ranging from primary and indicated prevention to treatment, crisis management, and supports for bereaved individuals. We begin with strategies that can be used by pediatric psychologists and developmental-behavioral or primary care physicians in health care settings, turning to primary prevention and community-based, public health approaches. As this section suggests, everyone can play a role in preventing suicide, regardless of setting or discipline.

Screening

The importance of screening for suicide risk is predicated on data showing that many youth at elevated risk go unrecognized unless asked directly (Arango et al., 2021). Screening can be implemented in health care (primary care, emergency department, and subspecialty clinics), behavioral health settings (psychology, developmental-behavioral, and psychiatry clinics), and community settings (schools, juvenile justice, and child welfare) to identify youth in need of support. Given findings that 37.9% of youth suicide decedents had seen a health care provider in the month prior to their death by suicide (Ahmedani et al., 2014), and studies demonstrating that universal screening identifies individuals at risk for suicide who are not presenting with suicide-related complaints (King, Grupp-Phelan, et al., 2019), screening in health care settings is recommended by the National Strategy for Suicide Prevention (U.S. Surgeon General & National Action Alliance for Suicide Prevention, 2012), The Joint Commission (2019), and Zero Suicide Institute (n.d.-b). The American Academy of Pediatrics (2022), in concert with the American Foundation for Suicide Prevention, recommends universal screening for all youth ages 12 and older and indicated screening for ages 8 and older presenting with a behavioral health complaint. The Blueprint to Prevent Youth Suicide (American Academy of Pediatrics, 2022) provides step-by-step guidance, including the use of an evidence-based screening tool and standard workflows that detail which responses warrant a more thorough risk assessment, brief interventions, and referral. In any setting, screening must be paired with staff training, policies on communication and documentation, and an adequate referral network to ensure that youth who screen positive receive a risk assessment and are connected to helping resources.

Several evidence-based tools are available for youth suicide risk screening, including the Columbia Suicide Severity Rating Scale (C-SSRS; Posner et al., 2011), the Ask Suicide Screening Questions (ASQ; Horowitz et al., 2012), and the Computerized Adaptive Screen for Suicidal Youth (CASSY; King, Brent, et al., 2021). Each of these tools has shown predictive validity for one or more suicide-related outcomes, yet all screening tools are challenged by less-than-perfect accuracy and false positives (see Arango et al., 2021, for a review). Screening tools also have differing strengths in terms of availability, cost, and the amount of information provided. The ASQ and C-SSRS are publicly available online with training guidelines and suggested triage or response algorithms, whereas the CASSY requires the integration of a software program and use of a computer notebook. The CASSY's unique strengths are that it is a dimensional screen that provides information on the probability of a suicide attempt and enables settings to establish their own threshold for sensitivity versus specificity (as higher sensitivity is associated with more false positives), based on setting priorities and capacity for follow-up.

Risk Assessment

Once a youth has been identified as being at elevated risk for suicide, a comprehensive risk assessment should be conducted that is informed by the clinician's knowledge of risk and protective factors, warning signs, and a nuanced understanding of the youth's experiences and environmental contexts. A calm, compassionate, and collaborative stance is indicated (King et al., 2013), yet many clinicians report minimal training and low self-efficacy around suicide risk assessment (Schmitz et al., 2012), highlighting the need for continuing education and behavioral health consultation in emergency departments, primary care, subspecialty behavioral health care, and schools.

Responses to elevated risk: Brief interventions. Brief interventions are designed to promote safety and increase support during times of increased risk and can be used in a variety of settings by multidisciplinary providers including pediatric psychologists, developmental-behavioral pediatricians, primary care physicians, and others, bridging the gap between risk identification and recovery-oriented treatment. Brief interventions can support youth at many levels of acuity and include safety planning, lethal means counseling, and enhancing support and monitoring.

Safety planning. Safety planning has replaced no-harm contracts as a best-practice intervention in the context of elevated suicide risk (Stanley & Brown, 2012). In contrast to a no-harm contract, which simply asks a patient not to engage in self-harm until the next appointment, a safety plan is a step-by-step written guide that is collaboratively developed by a clinician and a patient and focuses on what patients can do to keep themselves safe. The most widely used safety plan (Stanley & Brown, 2012) includes the identification of triggers for suicidal thoughts, behaviors, or emotional distress as well as coping strategies, social support, professional crisis supports to call in an emergency, steps to make the environment safe, and reasons for living. As a suicidal crisis is typically time-limited, safety planning aims to prevent the individual from acting on suicidal thoughts until the suicidal crisis dissipates. There is significant evidence for the benefit of safety planning in adults (Stanley & Brown, 2012) and evidence that engaging parents (Asarnow et al., 2011) and supporting their self-efficacy (Ewell Foster et al., 2022) may be key components to safety planning with youth. The SAFETY-Acute Intervention (SAFETY-A; Zullo et al., 2020) is a family-oriented cognitive behavior intervention previously known as the Family Intervention for Suicide Prevention (Asarnow et al., 2011). SAFETY-A emphasizes youth and family strengths, identification of youth emotional reactions, and development of a safety plan. It also includes follow-ups that have been associated with improved treatment linkage. This type of collaborative approach is also emphasized by Czyz and colleagues (2019) in a motivational interviewing-enhanced safety planning intervention. In an open trial, youth with suicidal ideation or behavior reported improvements in their confidence to keep themselves safe, in addition to reductions in self-harm urges. Arango and colleagues (2021) review the benefits of incorporating technology into the safety planning process with youth.

Lethal means counseling. With many suicide attempt survivors reporting that only minutes elapsed between their decision and their attempt, reducing access to highly lethal means is a potentially life-saving brief intervention (Barber et al., 2022). Free, publicly available training in Counseling on Access to Lethal Means (CALM) is available via the Zero Suicide Institute (n.d.-a). Conversations about making the environment safe should include reducing access to firearms and reducing access to other potentially lethal methods of suicide such as medications and sharp objects. Among adults, assessment of lethal means has been associated with a 75% reduction in SA (Boggs et al., 2020), and among youth, means-restriction education in the ED has been shown to result in parent-reported safety improvements in the home setting 2 weeks later (Ewell Foster et al., 2022).

Enhancing support and monitoring. Given the well-documented relation between social connectedness and youth risk for suicide attempts (King, Grupp-Phelan, et al., 2019), interpersonal strategies designed to enhance support are indicated. In a clinical setting, these strategies may be incorporated into safety planning but may require additional communication with the school, parents' employers, or extended family to enhance emotional support, reduce stress (e.g., provide extensions on academic assignments), and increase the monitoring or supervision of youth. Follow-up caring contacts are a recommended strategy based on an early study of caring letters sent post hospital discharge, which demonstrated an impact on suicide mortality in adults (Motto, 1976). Subsequent studies have examined caring contacts as a continuity of care strategy to support treatment linkage (Asarnow et al., 2011), family education, or to prompt use of safety plans (Czyz et al., 2020). The Youth-Nominated Support Team intervention (YST; King, Arango, et al., 2019; King et al., 2009) exemplifies a social support strategy for adolescents with suicide risk by building an informed network of supportive adults who learn about the youth's mental health challenges, treatment plan, and suicide warning signs and about how to support the youth and their treatment adherence and positive choices. Support team members meet individually with the youth and YST staff check in with the support team adults weekly to provide resources and to address questions and concerns (King et al., 2009). In a rigorous randomized, controlled trial (RCT) of YST with a sample of 448 youth, adolescents in the YST + TAU (Treatment-As-Usual) group reported a more rapid reduction in SI and engaged in significantly more mental health and substance abuse treatment (King, Arango, et al., 2019; King et al., 2009). Mortality outcomes 11 to 14 years later revealed 13 deaths in the TAU group and 2 deaths in the YST + TAU group (hazard ratio: 6.62, $p < 0.01$). The low end of the confidence interval indicated 50% higher mortality in the TAU group. Although in need of replication, YST highlights one feasible and promising approach to increasing interpersonal connectedness for youth at risk for suicide.

TREATMENT

Currently, only one well-validated psychosocial treatment for youth suicide risk (*Dialectical Behavior Therapy With Suicidal Adolescents*; Miller et al., 2007) has demonstrated an impact on suicidal thoughts or behaviors across two separate RCTs (Substance Abuse and Mental Health Services Administration [SAMHSA], 2020). Five additional interventions are considered promising based on evidence from at least one RCT (SAMHSA, 2020): attachment-based family therapy (Diamond et al., 2010), multisystemic therapy (Henggeler et al., 1986), Safe Alternatives for Teens and Youth (SAFETY; Asarnow et al., 2015), integrated cognitive behavior therapy (Esposito-Smythers et al., 2011), and the Youth-Nominated Support Team (King, Arango, et al., 2019), which is an adjunctive intervention. Common elements among promising psychosocial interventions include a cognitive or behavioral framework that focuses on building emotion regulation and coping skills; a family component; and a distinct focus on suicidal thoughts, behaviors, and safety (SAMHSA, 2020). Psychopharmacology also plays a role in the treatment of youth at risk for suicide. Although beyond the scope of this chapter, a review of U.S. Food and Drug Administration–approved medications for youth is found in SAMHSA's guide to effective treatment for youth suicide (SAMHSA, 2020).

Risk Formulation and Crisis Management

One role of pediatric psychologists and developmental-behavioral pediatricians in concert with other mental health professionals may be to determine the acuity of a youth's risk to make determinations regarding need for emergency evaluation or hospitalization. A review of data regarding warning signs and precipitating events for suicide may be helpful in formulating the level of risk.

Warning signs. Warning signs are signals of acute or imminent risk. A consensus list of youth suicide warning signs, based on clinical experience and the limited research evidence available, includes (a) talking about or making plans for suicide; (b) expressing hopelessness about the future; (c) displaying severe or overwhelming psychic pain or distress; and (d) showing worrisome behavioral cues or marked changes in behavior such as social withdrawal, sleep changes, anger that seems out of context, or increased agitation or irritability (https://www.youthsuicidewarningsigns.org/).

Precipitating events. Suicide is rarely caused by a single factor but rather an accumulation of risks interacting with a precipitating event. NVDRS data from youth aged 5 to 11 years suggest that common precipitating factors for suicide in young children are family conflict and recent disciplinary action (Ruch et al., 2021); among youth aged 10 to 17 years, suicides are most often precipitated by family relationship (32%) and school problems (26%); and among youth aged 18 to 24 years, suicides are precipitated by intimate partner conflicts (33%) and substance abuse problems (21%; Ertl et al., 2020). Awareness of these common precipitants is key to risk formulation and decision-making in clinical settings. Given these data, providers in pediatric and behavioral health settings should inquire about stressors in family relationships, school difficulties, experiences of violence, and substance abuse difficulties. Health care providers should also assess for protective factors such as family and school connectedness.

Crisis supports. When there is concern for imminent risk, crisis services may include the brief interventions reviewed previously as well as evaluation in an ED, an inpatient psychiatric stay, or use of community-based crisis services. Although many youth first access mental health services in the ED setting (Grupp-Phelan et al., 2007), most EDs have limited behavioral health staff, resulting in variability in evidence-based risk assessment and care as well as lengthy boarding times. Despite widespread use, evidence for the benefit of psychiatric hospitalization on health outcomes is equivocal, with some former patients reporting benefits (e.g., brief respite from stress, mobilization of family support, or assistance with treatment linkage) but others reporting distressing experiences, including loss of autonomy and negative financial, academic, or social repercussions (Ward-Ciesielski & Rizvi, 2021). It is critical for clinicians to ensure that the more restrictive option of hospitalization is indicated and for youth and families to have reasonable expectations about the role of a hospital stay for safety and stabilization as opposed to recovery (Ward-Ciesielski & Rizvi, 2021).

The National Suicide Prevention Lifeline, a network of crisis centers available 24 hours a day by phone and, in some areas, via text messaging, offers a trained, supportive connection during a crisis. Given consistent findings regarding the benefit to callers (Hoffberg et al., 2020), enhancing awareness of the Lifeline is a goal of the National Strategy for Suicide Prevention. Exemplifying its impact, in the month following the release of hip-hop artist Logic's song titled "1-800-273-8255," the Lifeline received an additional 9,915 calls, a call volume increase of almost 7% with a reduction of 245 suicides that month, relative to expected rates (Niederkrotenthaler et al., 2021). In July 2022, the Lifeline transitioned to a three-digit number, 988, to improve ease of access. Other crisis response services include the Crisis Textline available at 741-741 and the Trevor Project for LGBTQ youth. A publication of the National Action Alliance for Suicide Prevention, titled *Crisis Now* (National Action Alliance for Suicide Prevention, 2016), provides a model for enhanced community-based crisis services that do not rely on EDs and inpatient hospitalizations, but rather peer support and respite services.

PRIMARY PREVENTION, HEALTH PROMOTION, AND INDICATED PREVENTION STRATEGIES

Primary prevention of suicide risk focuses on the promotion of protective factors such as emotion regulation, coping, problem-solving skills, and enhanced family functioning (Wyman, 2014). Often referred to as "upstream" prevention (Wyman, 2014), such strategies could be delivered in health care settings with trained subspecialty providers (e.g., developmental-behavioral pediatrics or pediatric psychology or psychiatry settings) or in community settings such as schools, reaching large numbers of youth, and target risk factors common to multiple adverse outcomes (e.g., suicide, substance abuse, violence).

Early Childhood/School-Aged Prevention Strategies

One example of a primary prevention approach is The Good Behavior Game (GBG; Kellam et al., 2008), a school-based positive behavioral support intervention for first- and second-grade classrooms (children ages 6–8 years) that was designed to reduce disruptive behavior, enhance self-regulation, and promote instructional time. Males randomized to the GBG displayed lower rates of substance use and violent behavior at ages 19–21 (Kellam et al., 2008); both males and females in the original GBG cohort displayed reduced rates of SI relative to control youth at ages 20–24 (Wilcox et al., 2008), with promising, but less definitive impacts of the GBG on SA.

Middle Childhood/Early Adolescent Prevention Strategies

Parenting interventions have also demonstrated a positive impact on SI and SA. The Family Check-Up (FCU; Connell et al., 2016) is a tiered intervention for parents of middle school youth targeting behavior management, family communication, and parental monitoring. In a long-term follow-up, youth whose families were randomized to FCU and engaged in the intervention had lower rates of SI/SA in young adulthood relative to those in a control condition. Interventions with youth having early markers of suicide risk have also been associated with positive outcomes. As one example, LET's Connect, a community mentorship program for urban youth who were at risk for suicide due to low social connectedness or peer victimization, was associated with modest improvements in social connectedness, self-esteem, and depression at 16-month follow-up (King, Gipson, et al., 2021). Interventions offered universally or early on for youth with emerging risk factors, prior to the onset of suicidal behavior, may have the potential to alter developmental trajectories and prevent the emergence of suicidal behavior.

Public Health Approaches to Prevention

A public health approach to reducing suicide also includes a focus on systems and societal-level risk reduction strategies. These may include training community gatekeepers, media messaging, health care system improvements, policy, and postvention strategies.

Community recognition and response to risk: Gatekeeper training. A key component of a comprehensive approach to suicide prevention are strategies to increase recognition of individuals at risk. In addition to screening, training concerned community members or gatekeepers shows promise as a prevention strategy.

Gatekeeper trainings educate community members regarding how to identify, respond, and refer individuals at risk for suicide to helping resources. "Gatekeepers" may be teachers, juvenile justice or child welfare staff, clergy, coaches, or anyone who could encounter a high-risk individual. When part of a larger prevention strategy, gatekeeper training has been shown to reduce suicide mortality rates for up to 2 years postimplementation (Godoy Garraza et al., 2019). Across different curricula, studies have consistently found that participants gain knowledge, improve their attitudes about suicide prevention, and increase their self-efficacy to intervene (e.g., Kuhlman et al., 2017) with some studies suggesting that trained participants go on to identify and refer more individuals to care (Ewell Foster et al., 2017; Kuhlman et al., 2017). A list of evidence-based gatekeeper trainings is available at the Suicide Prevention Resource Center (https://sprc.org/)

Safe and effective messaging. Decades of research have demonstrated links between exposure to suicide and increased community suicide deaths, otherwise known as contagion (Gould & Lake, 2013). To combat contagion, guidelines for safe and effective prevention messaging (National Action Alliance for Suicide Prevention, 2019) and responsible media reporting (Reporting on Suicide/SAVE, 2024) have been developed, which include refraining from glamorizing or providing details about the death while using the opportunity to educate, reduce stigma, instill hope, and provide resources such as the National Suicide Prevention Lifeline (988). Highlighting the potential danger of unsafe media portrayals, a time-series analysis of CDC suicide mortality data (Niederkrotenthaler et al., 2019) was conducted before and after the release of *13 Reasons Why*, a Netflix drama series that graphically depicted a female high school student's suicide (Gomez et al., 2017–2020). Consistent with media-related contagion, there were an additional 66 suicides among teen males and 37 among teen females in the months following the show's release, relative to the prior year, with no excess deaths in groups who were not the series' target audience (Niederkrotenthaler et al., 2019). Moreover, in a study of youth seeking psychiatric emergency services following the show's release, Hong et al. (2019) found that over half of youth surveyed felt that watching the show increased their risk for suicide to some extent. The Hong et al. (2019) study also highlighted the differential impact that media may have on youth who are already at elevated risk, as youth with higher levels of SI and more severe depressive symptoms were more likely to experience negative affect after watching the show.

Health care system improvements. As one example of a public health focus on improving community infrastructure, the Zero Suicide Institute (n.d.-c) aims to reform the way individuals at risk for suicide are cared for in health care settings, leading organizations through an implementation strategy designed to improve clinical care through leadership engagement, workforce training, improved screening and patient engagement practices, use of evidence-based treatments, ensuring continuity of care, and using data-driven quality improvement. The impact of the Zero Suicide Institute model is currently under investigation in several multisite trials, with an initial study in one health care system showing a 75% reduction in suicide rates from 89/100,000 at baseline to 22/100,000 at 4-year follow-up (Coffey, 2007).

Public policy. Public policy also has a role to play in a public health approach to suicide prevention, with reductions in access to lethal means as one example (Johnson & Coyne-Beasley, 2009). Naturalistic studies document a significant impact on suicide mortality when environmental interventions such as barriers or fencing are erected that prevent access to locations (bridges, tall buildings, railroad tracks) used in suicide attempts or deaths. Similarly, international suicide rates have been reduced by altering pesticide availability and by reducing concentrations of carbon monoxide in household gas (Johnson & Coyne-Beasley, 2009). In the United States, firearms policies, such as Extreme Risk Protection Orders (ERPOs), are available in 19 states and are being investigated as a suicide prevention strategy. In the United States, the Dickey Amendment, which restricted federal funds to study firearm-related injury and death, curtailed research from 1996 until 2020, when congressional funds resumed to study the role of firearms in public health.

Community postvention support. Postvention is defined as "activities developed by, with, or for suicide survivors, in order to facilitate recovery after suicide, and to prevent adverse outcomes including suicidal behavior" (Andriessen et al., 2019, p. 2). Across the lifespan, individuals bereaved by suicide are at elevated risk for their own psychopathology and suicide (Pitman et al., 2014), and surveys suggest that one suicide death can impact up to 135 family and community members (Cerel et al., 2019) with grief that is unique to suicide loss. Postvention services vary by community but may include trained first responders and victims' advocates who support on the scene, suicide bereavement support groups, and response protocols designed to reduce contagion. Recommended postvention guidelines are available at the National Action Alliance for Suicide Prevention (National Action Alliance for Suicide Prevention Survivors of Suicide Loss Task Force, 2015). Clinician survivor resources are available through the American Foundation for Suicide Prevention (https://afsp.org/ive-lost-someone) and the American Association of Suicidology (https://suicidology.org/).

EMERGING RESEARCH AND CLINICAL DIRECTIONS AND CHALLENGES: IMPLICATIONS FOR DEVELOPMENTAL SCIENCE, DEVELOPMENTAL-BEHAVIORAL PEDIATRICS, AND PEDIATRIC PSYCHOLOGY

Youth suicide risk is multifactorial and complex, emerging from a range of developmental trajectories. Moreover, the recommended multifaceted public health approach to suicide prevention includes strategies ranging from primary prevention to intervention, crisis management, and postvention. As such, there is a myriad of meaningful research directions aimed at furthering our understanding of youth suicide risk and developing and evaluating effective prevention strategies. This section highlights several broad research directions that could meaningfully inform youth suicide prevention.

In the realm of primary prevention, an interdisciplinary research approach is recommended that focuses on the prevention of child maltreatment and interpersonal violence—well-established risk factors for suicidal behavior and suicide—as well as the promotion of safe environments for all children and adolescents (King et al., 2018; Stone et al., 2017). A developmental science framework can help identify the multilevel ecological contexts associated with suicide risk, which can help guide the development of prevention and intervention strategies. Primary prevention moves beyond a narrow focus on preventing "close in time" suicide-related outcomes to consider how to reduce the development of suicide risk (e.g., child maltreatment), how to maximize resilience by improving children's socioemotional coping skills, and how to minimize environmental risk. Implementation of such upstream strategies (by subspecialists in developmental-behavioral pediatrics, pediatric psychology, or child psychiatry) can alter developmental trajectories and reduce suicide risk factors by early adulthood (Wilcox et al., 2008). As examples, further research could address how to most effectively support parents to reduce child maltreatment and how to most effectively support the safe storage of firearms, which are implicated in large numbers of adolescent suicides. Although such research is challenged by the need for well-powered and long-term prospective trials to demonstrate impacts on intermediary targets and suicide-related outcomes, these types of strategies have the potential to reduce suicide-related outcomes as well as a broad range of other adverse outcomes.

Further research is recommended on the development and implementation of selective prevention strategies designed for subgroups of youth with one or more suicide risk factors (e.g., youth in juvenile detention, youth with early-onset depressive disorders, youth with chronic health conditions, sexual/gender minority youth, neurodiverse youth). Taking a developmental science or developmental psychopathology perspective, which considers transactional influences on risk and protective factors across time (Oppenheimer et al., 2022), such research could examine strategies specifically tailored for a particular subgroup—for example, youth using substances to cope with depression. This targeted approach can help inform the optimal developmental timing and setting for each strategy (King, 1998), making use of tailored variables that increase the likelihood of effectiveness, or considering the use of sequential, multiple assignment, and randomized trials (Pistorello et al., 2018). An important research consideration will be to address the potential heterogeneity of effects across demographic and cultural subgroups, which will require large studies that sample diverse populations of youth and incorporate broad community stakeholder input.

Finally, further research is needed to improve systems of care for youth at risk who seek mental health services. Few evidence-based interventions exist, and they have only modest positive effects (SAMHSA, 2020). Research focused on improving understanding and recognition of youth transitions to higher levels of suicide risk may enable the design of more effective adaptive interventions. As an example, an improved understanding of the transition from ideation to action (Klonsky & May, 2015) may enable the development of a timely intervention for youth with suicidal ideation. In addition, the integration of innovative technology-based interventions, including accessible online platforms and cell phone mobile health approaches, has the potential to improve the fidelity of intervention delivery and intervention scalability, reducing disparities in care. Research is just beginning to examine the potential effectiveness of supportive messages, tips for coping strategies, and the provision of resources via website links. Finally, as screening and intervention strategies are brought together into systems of care, it will also be important to address the disparities in mental health service utilization across cultural subgroups of youth at risk of suicide (King et al., 2020). There is still much to learn about how to meet the needs of youth and families from diverse cultural backgrounds. Broad stakeholder input is needed to identify effective strategies for treatment engagement and retention.

CONCLUSION

As a leading cause of death for youth in the United States and globally, the prevention of suicide is an urgent priority. A comprehensive, multidisciplinary approach to prevention is indicated, and as this broad review suggests, *everyone* can play a role in professional or community settings as clinicians, researchers, or caring adult gatekeepers to develop, enhance, implement, evaluate, or disseminate effective suicide prevention practices. Developmental and clinical scientists have an important role to play in improving our understanding of suicide risk and protective factors, and in developing and evaluating more effective prevention and intervention strategies. Child-serving professionals, such as pediatric psychologists, child clinical psychologists, and developmental-behavioral and primary care pediatricians, have a key opportunity, via screening and compassionate and informed risk assessment coupled with brief interventions to interrupt the developmental trajectory of risk, supporting youth and families to obtain needed resources prior to the onset of suicidal behavior.

RESOURCES

Suicide Prevention: General Resources

- **National Strategy for Suicide Prevention**
  U.S. Department of Health and Human Services (HHS) Office of the Surgeon General and National Action Alliance for Suicide Prevention. (2012). *2012 national strategy for suicide prevention: Goals and objectives for action.* U.S. Department of Health and Human Services. https://www.ncbi.nlm.nih.gov/books/NBK109917/pdf/Bookshelf_NBK109917.pdf

- **Preventing Suicide: A technical package of policies, programs, and practice**
  https://stacks.cdc.gov/view/cdc/44275

- **Suicide Prevention Resource Center**
  https://sprc.org

- **Zero Suicide Institute**
  https://zerosuicide.edc.org

Clinical Resources: Screening and Intervention

- **Columbia Suicide Severity Rating Scale**
  https://cssrs.columbia.edu

- **Ask Suicide Screening Questions**
  https://www.nimh.nih.gov/research/research-conducted-at-nimh/asq-toolkit-materials

- **Safety Planning**
  https://suicidesafetyplan.com

- **CALM: Counseling on Access to Lethal Means**
  https://sprc.org/resources-programs/calm

- **Substance Abuse and Mental Health Services Administration guide to treatment**
  https://store.samhsa.gov/product/Treatment-for-Suicidal-Ideation-Self-harm-and-Suicide-Attempts-Among-Youth/PEP20-06-01-002

Support Following a Loss

American Foundation for Suicide Prevention, Living With Suicide Loss

https://afsp.org/ive-lost-someone

References

Ahmedani, B. K., Simon, G. E., Stewart, C., Beck, A., Waitzfelder, B. E., Rossom, R., Lynch, F., Owen-Smith, A., Hunkeler, E. M., Whiteside, U., Operskalski, B. H., Coffey, M. J., & Solberg, L. I. (2014). Health care contacts in the year before suicide death. *Journal of General Internal Medicine, 29*(6), 870–877. https://doi.org/10.1007/s11606-014-2767-3

American Academy of Pediatrics. (2022). *Suicide: Blueprint for youth suicide prevention.* https://www.aap.org/en/patient-care/blueprint-for-youth-suicide-prevention/

Andriessen, K., Krysinska, K., Kõlves, K., & Reavley, N. (2019). Suicide postvention service models and guidelines 2014–2019: A systematic review. *Frontiers in Psychology, 10,* 2677. https://doi.org/10.3389/fpsyg.2019.02677

Arango, A., Gipson, P. Y., Votta, J. G., & King, C. A. (2021). Saving lives: Recognizing and intervening with youth at risk for suicide. *Annual Review of Clinical Psychology, 17*(1), 259–284. https://doi.org/10.1146/annurev-clinpsy-081219-103740

Asarnow, J. R., Baraff, L. J., Berk, M., Grob, C. S., Devich-Navarro, M., Suddath, R., Piacentini, J. C., Rotheram-Borus, M. J., Cohen, D., & Tang, L. (2011). An emergency department intervention for linking pediatric suicidal patients to follow-up mental health treatment. *Psychiatric Services, 62*(11), 1303–1309. https://doi.org/10.1176/ps.62.11.pss6211_1303

Asarnow, J. R., Berk, M., Hughes, J. L., & Anderson, N. L. (2015). The SAFETY Program: A treatment-development trial of a cognitive-behavioral family treatment for adolescent suicide attempters. *Journal of Clinical Child and Adolescent Psychology, 44*(1), 194–203. https://doi.org/10.1080/15374416.2014.940624

Barber, C., Azrael, D., Miller, M., & Hemenway, D. (2022). Who owned the gun in firearm suicides of men, women, and youth in five US states? *Preventive Medicine, 164,* 107066. https://doi.org/10.1016/j.ypmed.2022.107066

Blair, J. M., Fowler, K. A., Jack, S. P., & Crosby, A. E. (2016). The national violent death reporting system: Overview and future directions. *Injury Prevention, 22*(Suppl. 1), i6–i11. https://doi.org/10.1136/injuryprev-2015-041819

Boggs, J. M., Beck, A., Ritzwoller, D. P., Battaglia, C., Anderson, H. D., & Lindrooth, R. C. (2020). A quasi-experimental analysis of lethal means assessment and risk for subsequent suicide attempts and deaths. *Journal of General Internal Medicine, 35*(6), 1709–1714. https://doi.org/10.1007/s11606-020-05641-4

Breton, J.-J., Labelle, R., Berthiaume, C., Royer, C., St-Georges, M., Ricard, D., Abadie, P., Gérardin, P., Cohen, D., & Guilé, J.-M. (2015). Protective factors against depression and suicidal behaviour in adolescence. *Canadian Journal of Psychiatry, 60*(2, Suppl. 1), S5–S15.

Bruckner, T. A., Singh, P., Yoon, J., Chakravarthy, B., & Snowden, L. R. (2020). African American/White disparities in psychiatric emergencies among youth following rapid expansion of Federally Qualified Health Centers. *Health Services Research, 55*(1), 26–34. https://doi.org/10.1111/1475-6773.13237

Castellví, P., Miranda-Mendizábal, A., Parés-Badell, O., Almenara, J., Alonso, I., Blasco, M. J., Cebrià, A., Gabilondo, A., Gili, M., Lagares, C., Piqueras, J. A., Roca, M., Rodríguez-Marín, J., Rodríguez-Jimenez, T., Soto-Sanz, V., & Alonso, J. (2017). Exposure to violence, a risk for suicide in youths and young adults. A meta-analysis of longitudinal studies. *Acta Psychiatrica Scandinavica, 135*(3), 195–211. https://doi.org/10.1111/acps.12679

Centers for Disease Control and Prevention. (2020). Youth Risk Behavior Surveillance—United States, 2019. *Morbidity and Mortality Weekly Report, 69*(1). https://www.cdc.gov/healthyyouth/data/yrbs/pdf/2019/su6901-H.pdf

Centers for Disease Control and Prevention National Center for Health Statistics. (2021). *Underlying cause of death 1999–2020: Multiple cause of death files, 1999–2020, as compiled from data provided by the 57 vital statistics jurisdictions through the Vital Statistics Cooperative Program.* CDC WONDER Online Database [Data set]. Retrieved January 20, 2022, from https://wonder.cdc.gov/ucd-icd10.html

Centers for Disease Control and Prevention, National Center for Injury Prevention and Control. (2020). *WISQARS: Web-based Injury Statistics Query and Reporting System.* U.S. Department of Health & Human Services. Retrieved March 20, 2022, from https://wisqars.cdc.gov/

Cerel, J., Brown, M. M., Maple, M., Singleton, M., van de Venne, J., Moore, M., & Flaherty, C. (2019). How many people are exposed to suicide? Not six. *Suicide and Life-Threatening Behavior, 49*(2), 529–534. https://doi.org/10.1111/sltb.12450

Cervantes, P. E., Li, A., Sullivan, K. A., Seag, D. E., Baroni, A., & Horwitz, S. M. (2023). Assessing and managing suicide risk in autistic youth: Findings from a clinician survey in a pediatric psychiatric emergency setting. *Journal of Autism and Developmental Disorders, 53*(5), 1755–1763. https://doi.org/10.1007/s10803-022-05448-8

Cha, C. B., Franz, P. J. M., Guzmán, E. M., Glenn, C. R., Kleiman, E. M., & Nock, M. K. (2018). Annual Research Review: Suicide among youth—Epidemiology, (potential) etiology, and treatment. *Journal of Child Psychology and Psychiatry, 59*(4), 460–482. https://doi.org/10.1111/jcpp.12831

Chu, C., Buchman-Schmitt, J. M., Stanley, I. H., Hom, M. A., Tucker, R. P., Hagan, C. R., Rogers, M. L., Podlogar, M. C., Chiurliza, B., Ringer, F. B., Michaels, M. S., Patros, C. H. G., & Joiner, T. E. (2017). The interpersonal theory of suicide: A systematic review and meta-analysis of a decade of cross-national research. *Psychological Bulletin*, *143*(12), 1313–1345. https://doi.org/10.1037/bul0000123

Cipriano, A., Cella, S., & Cotrufo, P. (2017). Nonsuicidal self-injury: A systematic review. *Frontiers in Psychology*, *8*, 1946. https://doi.org/10.3389/fpsyg.2017.01946

Coffey, C. E. (2007). Building a system of perfect depression care in behavioral health. *Joint Commission Journal on Quality and Patient Safety*, *33*(4), 193–199. https://doi.org/10.1016/S1553-7250(07)33022-5

Congressional Black Caucus (CBC) Emergency Task Force on Black Youth Suicide and Mental Health. (2019). *Ring the alarm: The crisis of Black youth suicide in America*. https://nbjc.org/wp-content/uploads/2020/11/Ring-the-Alarm-TASKFORCE-REPORT.pdf

Connell, A. M., McKillop, H. N., & Dishion, T. J. (2016). Long-term effects of the family check-up in early adolescence on risk of suicide in early adulthood. *Suicide and Life-Threatening Behavior*, *46*(Suppl. 1), S15–S22. https://doi.org/10.1111/sltb.12254

Conner, A., Azrael, D., & Miller, M. (2019). Suicide case-fatality rates in the United States, 2007 to 2014: A nationwide population-based study. *Annals of Internal Medicine*, *171*(12), 885–895. https://doi.org/10.7326/M19-1324

Crosby, A., Ortega, L., & Melanson, C. (2011). *Self-directed violence surveillance; uniform definitions and recommended data elements*. https://stacks.cdc.gov/view/cdc/11997

Czyz, E. K., Arango, A., Healy, N., King, C. A., & Walton, M. (2020). Augmenting safety planning with text messaging support for adolescents at elevated suicide risk: Development and acceptability study. *JMIR Mental Health*, *7*(5), e17345. https://doi.org/10.2196/preprints.17345

Czyz, E. K., King, C. A., & Biermann, B. J. (2019). Motivational interviewing-enhanced safety planning for adolescents at high suicide risk: A pilot randomized controlled trial. *Journal of Clinical Child and Adolescent Psychology*, *48*(2), 250–262. https://doi.org/10.1080/15374416.2018.1496442

Diamond, G., Kodish, T., Ewing, E. S. K., Hunt, Q. A., & Russon, J. M. (2022). Family processes: Risk, protective and treatment factors for youth at risk for suicide. *Aggression and Violent Behavior*, *64*, 101586. https://doi.org/10.1016/j.avb.2021.101586

Diamond, G. S., Wintersteen, M. B., Brown, G. K., Diamond, G. M., Gallop, R., Shelef, K., & Levy, S. (2010). Attachment-based family therapy for adolescents with suicidal ideation: A randomized controlled trial. *Journal of the American Academy of Child & Adolescent Psychiatry*, *49*(2), 122–131. https://doi.org/10.1016/j.jaac.2009.11.002

Ehlman, D. C., Yard, E., Stone, D. M., Jones, C. M., & Mack, K. A. (2022). Changes in suicide rates—United States, 2019 and 2020. *MMWR Morbidity and Mortality Weekly Report*, *71*(8), 306–312. https://doi.org/10.15585/mmwr.mm7108a5

Ertl, A., Crosby, A. E., & Blair, J. M. (2020). Youth suicide: An opportunity for prevention. *Journal of the American Academy of Child & Adolescent Psychiatry*, *59*(9), 1019–1021. https://doi.org/10.1016/j.jaac.2020.01.017

Esposito-Smythers, C., Spirito, A., Kahler, C. W., Hunt, J., & Monti, P. (2011). Treatment of co-occurring substance abuse and suicidality among adolescents: A randomized trial. *Journal of Consulting and Clinical Psychology*, *79*(6), 728–739. https://doi.org/10.1037/a0026074

Ewell Foster, C., Magness, C., Czyz, E., Kahsay, E., Martindale, J., Hong, V., Baker, E., Cavataio, I., Colombini, G., Kettley, J., Smith, P. K., & King, C. (2022). Predictors of parent behavioral engagement in youth suicide discharge recommendations: Implications for family-centered crisis interventions. *Child Psychiatry and Human Development*, *53*, 1240–1251. https://doi.org/10.1007/s10578-021-01176-9

Ewell Foster, C. J., Burnside, A. N., Smith, P. K., Kramer, A. C., Wills, A., & King, C. A. (2017). Identification, response, and referral of suicidal youth following applied suicide intervention skills training. *Suicide and Life-Threatening Behavior*, *47*(3), 297–308. https://doi.org/10.1111/sltb.12272

Fox, K. R., Hooley, J. M., Smith, D. M. Y., Ribeiro, J. D., Huang, X., Nock, M. K., & Franklin, J. C. (2018). Self-injurious thoughts and behaviors may be more common and severe among people identifying as a sexual minority. *Behavior Therapy*, *49*(5), 768–780. https://doi.org/10.1016/j.beth.2017.11.009

Geulayov, G., Gunnell, D., Holmen, T. L., & Metcalfe, C. (2012). The association of parental fatal and non-fatal suicidal behaviour with offspring suicidal behaviour and depression: A systematic review and meta-analysis. *Psychological Medicine*, *42*(8), 1567–1580. https://doi.org/10.1017/S0033291711002753

Godoy Garraza, L., Kuiper, N., Goldston, D., McKeon, R., & Walrath, C. (2019). Long-term impact of the Garrett Lee Smith Youth Suicide Prevention Program on youth suicide mortality, 2006–2015. *Journal of Child Psychology and Psychiatry*, *60*(10), 1142–1147. https://doi.org/10.1111/jcpp.13058

Goldstein, E. V., Prater, L. C., & Wickizer, T. M. (2022). Preventing adolescent and young adult suicide: Do states with greater mental health treatment capacity have lower suicide rates? *Journal of Adolescent Health, 70*(1), 83–90. https://doi.org/10.1016/j.jadohealth.2021.06.020

Gomez, S., Matyka, M., Son, D., McCarthy, T., Gorman Wettels, J., Golin, S., Sugar, M., Teefey, M., & Laiblin, K. (Executive Producers). (2017–2020). *13 reasons why* [TV series]. Netflix. https://www.netflix.com/title/80117470

Goodday, S. M., Shuldiner, J., Bondy, S., & Rhodes, A. E. (2019). Exposure to parental psychopathology and offspring's risk of suicide-related thoughts and behaviours: A systematic review. *Epidemiology and Psychiatric Sciences, 28*(2), 179–190. https://doi.org/10.1017/S2045796017000397

Gould, M. S., & Lake, A. M. (2013, February 6). The contagion of suicidal behavior. In D. M. Patel, M. A. Simon, & R. M. Taylor (Eds). *Contagion of violence: Workshop summary* (pp. 68–78). National Academies Press. https://www.ncbi.nlm.nih.gov/books/NBK207262/

Green, A. E., Taliaferro, L. A., & Price, M. N. (2021). Understanding risk and protective factors to improve well-being and prevent suicide among LGBTQ Youth. In R. Miranda & E. L. Jeglic (Eds.), *Handbook of youth suicide prevention* (pp. 177–194). Springer. https://doi.org/10.1007/978-3-030-82465-5_11

Grupp-Phelan, J., Harman, J. S., & Kelleher, K. J. (2007). Trends in mental health and chronic condition visits by children presenting for care at U.S. emergency departments. *Public Health Reports, 122*(1), 55–61. https://doi.org/10.1177/003335490712200108

Hatzenbuehler, M. L. (2011). The social environment and suicide attempts in lesbian, gay, and bisexual youth. *Pediatrics, 127*(5), 896–903. https://doi.org/10.1542/peds.2010-3020

Henggeler, S. W., Rodick, J. D., Borduin, C. M., Hanson, C. L., Watson, S. M., & Urey, J. R. (1986). Multisystemic treatment of juvenile offenders: Effects on adolescent behavior and family interaction. *Developmental Psychology, 22*(1), 132–141. https://doi.org/10.1037/0012-1649.22.1.132

Hoffberg, A. S., Stearns-Yoder, K. A., & Brenner, L. A. (2020). The effectiveness of crisis line services: A systematic review. *Frontiers in Public Health, 7*, 399. https://doi.org/10.3389/fpubh.2019.00399

Hong, V., Ewell Foster, C. J., Magness, C. S., McGuire, T. C., Smith, P. K., & King, C. A. (2019). *13 Reasons Why*: Viewing patterns and perceived impact among youths at risk of suicide. *Psychiatric Services, 70*(2), 107–114. https://doi.org/10.1176/appi.ps.201800384

Horowitz, L. M., Bridge, J. A., Teach, S. J., Ballard, E., Klima, J., Rosenstein, D. L., Wharff, E. A., Ginnis, K., Cannon, E., Joshi, P., & Pao, M. (2012). Ask Suicide-Screening Questions (ASQ): A brief instrument for the pediatric emergency department. *Archives of Pediatrics & Adolescent Medicine, 166*(12), 1170–1176. https://doi.org/10.1001/archpediatrics.2012.1276

Horwitz, A. G., Czyz, E. K., & King, C. A. (2015). Predicting future suicide attempts among adolescent and emerging adult psychiatric emergency patients. *Journal of Clinical Child and Adolescent Psychology, 44*(5), 751–761. https://doi.org/10.1080/15374416.2014.910789

Horwitz, A. G., Grupp-Phelan, J., Brent, D., Barney, B. J., Casper, T. C., Berona, J., Chernick, L. S., Shenoi, R., Cwik, M., King, C. A., & the Pediatric Emergency Care Applied Research Network. (2021). Risk and protective factors for suicide among sexual minority youth seeking emergency medical services. *Journal of Affective Disorders, 279*, 274–281. https://doi.org/10.1016/j.jad.2020.10.015

Howe, S. J., Hewitt, K., Baraskewich, J., Cassidy, S., & McMorris, C. A. (2020). Suicidality among children and youth with and without autism spectrum disorder: A systematic review of existing risk assessment tools. *Journal of Autism and Developmental Disorders, 50*(10), 3462–3476. https://doi.org/10.1007/s10803-020-04394-7

Hughes, K., Bellis, M. A., Hardcastle, K. A., Sethi, D., Butchart, A., Mikton, C., Jones, L., & Dunne, M. P. (2017). The effect of multiple adverse childhood experiences on health: A systematic review and meta-analysis. *The Lancet Public Health, 2*(8), e356–e366. https://doi.org/10.1016/S2468-2667(17)30118-4

Iannucci, J., & Nierenberg, B. (2022). Suicide and suicidality in children and adolescents with chronic illness: A systematic review. *Aggression and Violent Behavior, 64*, 101581. https://doi.org/10.1016/j.avb.2021.101581

Ivey-Stephenson, A. Z., Crosby, A. E., Jack, S. P. D., Haileyesus, T., & Kresnow-Sedacca, M. J. (2017). Suicide trends among and within urbanization levels by sex, race/ethnicity, age group, and mechanism of death—United States, 2001–2015. *MMWR Morbidity and Mortality Weekly Report Surveillance Summaries, 66*(18), 1–16. https://doi.org/10.15585/mmwr.ss6618a1

Ivey-Stephenson, A. Z., Demissie, Z., Crosby, A. E., Stone, D. M., Gaylor, E., Wilkins, N., Lowry, R., & Brown, M. (2020). Suicidal ideation and behaviors among high school students—Youth Risk Behavior Survey, United States, 2019. *MMWR Supplements, 69*(1), 47–55. https://doi.org/10.15585/mmwr.su6901a6

Johns, M. M., Lowry, R., Haderxhanaj, L. T., Rasberry, C. N., Robin, L., Scales, L., Stone, D., & Suarez, N. A. (2020). Trends in violence victimization and suicide risk by sexual identity among high school students—Youth Risk Behavior Survey, United States, 2015–2019. *MMWR Supplements, 69*(1), 19–27. https://doi.org/10.15585/mmwr.su6901a3

Johnson, R. M., & Coyne-Beasley, T. (2009). Lethal means reduction: What have we learned? *Current Opinion in Pediatrics, 21*(5), 635–640. https://doi.org/10.1097/MOP.0b013e32833057d0

Joiner, T. E., Jeon, M. E., Lieberman, A., Janakiraman, R., Duffy, M. E., Gai, A. R., & Dougherty, S. P. (2021). On prediction, refutation, and explanatory reach: A consideration of the interpersonal theory of suicidal behavior. *Preventive Medicine, 152*(Pt. 1), 106453. https://doi.org/10.1016/j.ypmed.2021.106453

The Joint Commission. (2019, November 20). *R³ report: Requirement, rationale, reference.* Issue 18. https://www.jointcommission.org/-/media/tjc/documents/standards/r3-reports/r3_18_suicide_prevention_hap_bhc_cah_11_4_19_final1.pdf

Kellam, S. G., Brown, C. H., Poduska, J. M., Ialongo, N. S., Wang, W., Toyinbo, P., Petras, H., Ford, C., Windham, A., & Wilcox, H. C. (2008). Effects of a universal classroom behavior management program in first and second grades on young adult behavioral, psychiatric, and social outcomes. *Drug and Alcohol Dependence, 95*(Suppl. 1), S5–S28. https://doi.org/10.1016/j.drugalcdep.2008.01.004

Kim, Y. J., Moon, S. S., Kim, Y. K., & Boyas, J. (2020). Protective factors of suicide: Religiosity and parental monitoring. *Children and Youth Services Review, 114,* 105073. https://doi.org/10.1016/j.childyouth.2020.105073

King, C. A. (1998). Suicide across the life span: Pathways to prevention. *Suicide and Life-Threatening Behavior, 28*(4), 328–337. https://doi.org/10.1111/j.1943-278X.1998.tb00969.x

King, C. A., Arango, A., & Ewell Foster, C. (2018). Emerging trends in adolescent suicide prevention research. *Current Opinion in Psychology, 22,* 89–94. https://doi.org/10.1016/j.copsyc.2017.08.037

King, C. A., Arango, A., Kramer, A., Busby, D., Czyz, E., Foster, C. E., Gillespie, B. W., & the YST Study Team. (2019). Association of the Youth-Nominated Support Team intervention for suicidal adolescents with 11- to 14-year mortality outcomes: Secondary analysis of a randomized clinical trial. *JAMA Psychiatry, 76*(5), 492–498. https://doi.org/10.1001/jamapsychiatry.2018.4358

King, C. A., Brent, D., Grupp-Phelan, J., Casper, T. C., Dean, J. M., Chernick, L. S., Fein, J. A., Mahabee-Gittens, E. M., Patel, S. J., Mistry, R. D., Duffy, S., Melzer-Lange, M., Rogers, A., Cohen, D. M., Keller, A., Shenoi, R., Hickey, R. W., Rea, M., Cwik, M., . . . Gibbons, R. (2021). Prospective development and validation of the computerized adaptive screen for suicidal youth. *JAMA Psychiatry, 78*(5), 540–549. https://doi.org/10.1001/jamapsychiatry.2020.4576

King, C. A., Brent, D., Grupp-Phelan, J., Shenoi, R., Page, K., Mahabee-Gittens, E. M., Chernick, L. S., Melzer-Lange, M., Rea, M., McGuire, T. C., Littlefield, A., Casper, T. C., & the Pediatric Emergency Care Applied Research Network (PECARN). (2020). Five profiles of adolescents at elevated risk for suicide attempts: Differences in mental health service use. *Journal of the American Academy of Child & Adolescent Psychiatry, 59*(9), 1058–1068.e5. https://doi.org/10.1016/j.jaac.2019.10.015

King, C. A., Foster, C. E., & Rogalski, K. M. (2013). *Teen suicide risk: A practitioner guide to screening, assessment, and management.* Guilford Press.

King, C. A., Gipson, P. Y., Arango, A., Lernihan, D., Clark, M., Ewell Foster, C., Caldwell, C., Ghaziuddin, N., & Stone, D. (2021). LET's CONNECT community mentorship program for adolescents with peer social problems: A randomized intervention trial. *American Journal of Community Psychology, 68*(3–4), 310–322. https://doi.org/10.1002/ajcp.12528

King, C. A., Grupp-Phelan, J., Brent, D., Dean, J. M., Webb, M., Bridge, J. A., Spirito, A., Chernick, L. S., Mahabee-Gittens, E. M., Mistry, R. D., Rea, M., Keller, A., Rogers, A., Shenoi, R., Cwik, M., Busby, D. R., Casper, T. C., & the Pediatric Emergency Care Applied Research Network. (2019). Predicting 3-month risk for adolescent suicide attempts among pediatric emergency department patients. *Journal of Child Psychology and Psychiatry, 60*(10), 1055–1064. https://doi.org/10.1111/jcpp.13087

King, C. A., Klaus, N., Kramer, A., Venkataraman, S., Quinlan, P., & Gillespie, B. (2009). The Youth-Nominated Support Team-Version II for suicidal adolescents: A randomized controlled intervention trial. *Journal of Consulting and Clinical Psychology, 77*(5), 880–893. https://doi.org/10.1037/a0016552

Klonsky, E. D., & May, A. M. (2015). The three-step theory (3ST): A new theory of suicide rooted in the "ideation-to-action" framework. *International Journal of Cognitive Therapy, 8*(2), 114–129. https://doi.org/10.1521/ijct.2015.8.2.114

Kuhlman, S. T. W., Walch, S. E., Bauer, K. N., & Glenn, A. D. (2017). Intention to enact and enactment of gatekeeper behaviors for suicide prevention: An application of the theory of planned behavior. *Prevention Science, 18*(6), 704–715. https://doi.org/10.1007/s11121-017-0786-0

Marttunen, M. J., Aro, H. M., Henriksson, M. M., & Lönnqvist, J. K. (1991). Mental disorders in adolescent suicide: *DSM-III-R* axes I and II diagnoses in suicides among 13- to 19-year-olds in Finland. *Archives of General Psychiatry, 48*(9), 834–839. https://doi.org/10.1001/archpsyc.1991.01810330058009

McKean, A. J. S., Pabbati, C. P., Geske, J. R., & Bostwick, J. M. (2018). Rethinking lethality in youth suicide attempts: First suicide attempt outcomes in youth ages 10 to 24. *Journal of the American Academy of Child & Adolescent Psychiatry, 57*(10), 786–791. https://doi.org/10.1016/j.jaac.2018.04.021

Meyer, I. H. (2003). Prejudice, social stress, and mental health in lesbian, gay, and bisexual populations: Conceptual issues and research evidence. *Psychological Bulletin, 129*(5), 674–697. https://doi.org/10.1037/0033-2909.129.5.674

Miller, A. L., Rathus, J. H., & Linehan, M. M. (2007). *Dialectical behavior therapy with suicidal adolescents*. Guilford Press.

Motto, J. A. (1976). Suicide prevention for high-risk persons who refuse treatment. *Suicide and Life-Threatening Behavior, 6*(4), 223–230. https://doi.org/10.1111/j.1943-278X.1976.tb00880.x

National Action Alliance for Suicide Prevention. (2016). *Crisis now: Transforming services is within our reach*. https://theactionalliance.org/resource/crisis-now-transforming-services-within-our-reach

National Action Alliance for Suicide Prevention. (2019). *Framework for successful messaging*. https://suicidepreventionmessaging.org/

National Action Alliance for Suicide Prevention Survivors of Suicide Loss Task Force. (2015). *Responding to grief, trauma, and distress after a suicide: U.S. national guidelines*. https://theactionalliance.org/resource/responding-grief-trauma-and-distress-after-suicide-us-national-guidelines

Niederkrotenthaler, T., Stack, S., Till, B., Sinyor, M., Pirkis, J., Garcia, D., Rockett, I. R. H., & Tran, U. S. (2019). Association of increased youth suicides in the United States with the release of *13 Reasons Why*. *JAMA Psychiatry, 76*(9), 933–940. https://doi.org/10.1001/jamapsychiatry.2019.0922

Niederkrotenthaler, T., Tran, U. S., Gould, M., Sinyor, M., Sumner, S., Strauss, M. J., Voracek, M., Till, B., Murphy, S., Gonzalez, F., Spittal, M. J., & Draper, J. (2021). Association of Logic's hip hop song "1-800-273-8255" with Lifeline calls and suicides in the United States: Interrupted time series analysis. *BMJ: British Medical Journal, 375*, e067726. https://doi.org/10.1136/bmj-2021-067726

Nock, M. K., Green, J. G., Hwang, I., McLaughlin, K. A., Sampson, N. A., Zaslavsky, A. M., & Kessler, R. C. (2013). Prevalence, correlates, and treatment of lifetime suicidal behavior among adolescents: Results from the National Comorbidity Survey Replication Adolescent Supplement. *JAMA Psychiatry, 70*(3), 300–310. https://doi.org/10.1001/2013.jamapsychiatry.55

Nock, M. K., Joiner, T. E., Jr., Gordon, K. H., Lloyd-Richardson, E., & Prinstein, M. J. (2006). Non-suicidal self-injury among adolescents: Diagnostic correlates and relation to suicide attempts. *Psychiatry Research, 144*(1), 65–72. https://doi.org/10.1016/j.psychres.2006.05.010

O'Halloran, L., Coey, P., & Wilson, C. (2022). Suicidality in autistic youth: A systematic review and meta-analysis. *Clinical Psychology Review, 93*, 102144. https://doi.org/10.1016/j.cpr.2022.102144

Oppenheimer, C. W., Glenn, C. R., & Miller, A. B. (2022). Future directions in suicide and self-injury revisited: Integrating a developmental psychopathology perspective. *Journal of Clinical Child and Adolescent Psychology, 51*(2), 242–260. https://doi.org/10.1080/15374416.2022.2051526

Padmanathan, P., Biddle, L., Hall, K., Scowcroft, E., Nielsen, E., & Knipe, D. (2019). Language use and suicide: An online cross-sectional survey. *PLOS ONE, 14*(6), e0217473. https://doi.org/10.1371/journal.pone.0217473

Palmer, L., Prindle, J., & Putnam-Hornstein, E. (2021). A population-based examination of suicide and child protection system involvement. *Journal of Adolescent Health, 69*(3), 465–469. https://doi.org/10.1016/j.jadohealth.2021.02.006

Pistorello, J., Jobes, D. A., Compton, S. N., Locey, N. S., Walloch, J. C., Gallop, R., Au, J. S., Noose, S. K., Young, M., Johnson, J., Dickens, Y., Chatham, P., Jeffcoat, T., Dalto, G., & Goswami, S. (2018). Developing adaptive treatment strategies to address suicidal risk in college students: A pilot sequential, multiple assignment, randomized trial (SMART). *Archives of Suicide Research, 22*(4), 644–664. https://doi.org/10.1080/13811118.2017.1392915

Pitman, A., Osborn, D., King, M., & Erlangsen, A. (2014). Effects of suicide bereavement on mental health and suicide risk. *The Lancet Psychiatry, 1*(1), 86–94. https://doi.org/10.1016/S2215-0366(14)70224-X

Posner, K., Brown, G. K., Stanley, B., Brent, D. A., Yershova, K. V., Oquendo, M. A., Currier, G. W., Melvin, G. A., Greenhill, L., Shen, S., & Mann, J. J. (2011). The Columbia-Suicide Severity Rating Scale: Initial validity and internal consistency findings from three multisite studies with adolescents and adults. *The American Journal of Psychiatry, 168*(12), 1266–1277. https://doi.org/10.1176/appi.ajp.2011.10111704

Reinherz, H. Z., Tanner, J. L., Berger, S. R., Beardslee, W. R., & Fitzmaurice, G. M. (2006). Adolescent suicidal ideation as predictive of psychopathology, suicidal behavior, and compromised functioning at age 30. *The American Journal of Psychiatry*, *163*(7), 1226–1232. https://doi.org/10.1176/ajp.2006.163.7.1226

Reporting on Suicide/SAVE. (2024). *Best practices and recommendations for reporting on suicide.* https://reportingonsuicide.org

Ruch, D. A., Heck, K. M., Sheftall, A. H., Fontanella, C. A., Stevens, J., Zhu, M., Horowitz, L. M., Campo, J. V., & Bridge, J. A. (2021). Characteristics and precipitating circumstances of suicide among children aged 5 to 11 years in the United States, 2013–2017. *JAMA Network Open*, *4*(7), e2115683. https://doi.org/10.1001/jamanetworkopen.2021.15683

Ruch, D. A., Sheftall, A. H., Schlagbaum, P., Rausch, J., Campo, J. V., & Bridge, J. A. (2019). Trends in suicide among youth aged 10 to 19 years in the United States, 1975 to 2016. *JAMA Network Open*, *2*(5), e193886. https://doi.org/10.1001/jamanetworkopen.2019.3886

Ryan, C., Russell, S. T., Huebner, D., Diaz, R., & Sanchez, J. (2010). Family acceptance in adolescence and the health of LGBT young adults. *Journal of Child and Adolescent Psychiatric Nursing*, *23*(4), 205–213. https://doi.org/10.1111/j.1744-6171.2010.00246.x

Rybczynski, S., Ryan, T. C., Wilcox, H. C., Van Eck, K., Cwik, M., Vasa, R. A., Findling, R. L., Slifer, K., Kleiner, D., & Lipkin, P. H. (2022). Suicide risk screening in pediatric outpatient neurodevelopmental disabilities clinics. *Journal of Developmental and Behavioral Pediatrics*, *43*(4), 181–187. https://doi.org/10.1097/DBP.0000000000001026

Schmitz, W. M., Jr., Allen, M. H., Feldman, B. N., Gutin, N. J., Jahn, D. R., Kleespies, P. M., Quinnett, P., & Simpson, S. (2012). Preventing suicide through improved training in suicide risk assessment and care: An American Association of Suicidology Task Force report addressing serious gaps in U.S. mental health training. *Suicide and Life-Threatening Behavior*, *42*(3), 292–304. https://doi.org/10.1111/j.1943-278X.2012.00090.x

Stanley, B., & Brown, G. K. (2012). Safety planning intervention: A brief intervention to mitigate suicide risk. *Cognitive and Behavioral Practice*, *19*(2), 256–264. https://doi.org/10.1016/j.cbpra.2011.01.001

Stone, D. M., Holland, K. M., Bartholow, B. N., Crosby, A. E., Davis, S. P., & Wilkins, N. (2017). *Preventing suicide: A technical package of policies, programs, and practice.* National Center for Injury Prevention and Control, Centers for Disease Control and Prevention. https://doi.org/10.15620/cdc.44275

Substance Abuse and Mental Health Services Administration (SAMHSA). (2020). *Treatment for suicidal ideation, self-harm, and suicide attempts among youth* (SAMHSA publication no. PEP20-06-01-002).

Taliaferro, L. A., McMorris, B. J., Rider, G. N., & Eisenberg, M. E. (2019). Risk and protective factors for self-harm in a population-based sample of transgender youth. *Archives of Suicide Research*, *23*(2), 203–221. https://doi.org/10.1080/13811118.2018.1430639

U.S. Surgeon General, & National Action Alliance for Suicide Prevention. (2012). *2012 national strategy for suicide prevention: Goals and objectives for action.* https://theactionalliance.org/our-strategy/national-strategy-suicide-prevention

Ward-Ciesielski, E. F., & Rizvi, S. L. (2021). The potential iatrogenic effects of psychiatric hospitalization for suicidal behavior: A critical review and recommendations for research. *Clinical Psychology: Science and Practice*, *28*(1), 60–71. https://doi.org/10.1111/cpsp.12332

Wilcox, H. C., Kellam, S. G., Brown, C. H., Poduska, J. M., Ialongo, N. S., Wang, W., & Anthony, J. C. (2008). The impact of two universal randomized first- and second-grade classroom interventions on young adult suicide ideation and attempts. *Drug and Alcohol Dependence*, *95*(Suppl. 1), S60–S73. https://doi.org/10.1016/j.drugalcdep.2008.01.005

World Health Organization. (2021). *Suicide worldwide in 2019: Global health estimates.* https://www.who.int/publications/i/item/9789240026643

Wyman, P. A. (2014). Developmental approach to prevent adolescent suicides: Research pathways to effective upstream preventive interventions. *American Journal of Preventive Medicine*, *47*(3, Suppl. 2), S251–S256. https://doi.org/10.1016/j.amepre.2014.05.039

Zero Suicide. (n.d.-a). *Counseling on access to lethal means.* Education Development Center. Retrieved February 14, 2025, from https://zerosuicide.edc.org/resources/resource-database/counseling-access-lethal-means-calm

Zero Suicide. (n.d.-b). *Screening.* Education Development Center. Retrieved February 14, 2025, from https://zerosuicide.edc.org/toolkit/identify-screening-and-assessment/screening#

Zero Suicide. (n.d.-c). *Zero suicide* [Homepage]. Education Development Center. Retrieved February 14, 2025, from https://zerosuicide.edc.org/

Zullo, L., Meza, J., Rolon-Arroyo, B., Vargas, S., Venables, C., Miranda, J., & Asarnow, J. R. (2020). Enhancing safety: Acute and short-term treatment strategies for youths presenting with suicidality and self-harm. *The Behavior Therapist*, *43*(8), 300–305.

Part IV

MULTIDISCIPLINARY ASSESSMENTS, INTERVENTIONS, AND TREATMENTS TO FOSTER CHILD HEALTH AND WELL-BEING

PART IV

CHAPTER 25

DEVELOPMENTAL ASSESSMENT OF INFANTS AND TODDLERS: CONCEPTS, PSYCHOMETRIC ISSUES, AND RELATED BRAIN DEVELOPMENT

Glen P. Aylward

This chapter reviews conceptual and pragmatic issues in the assessment of infants and toddlers. The first topic involves determining who needs developmental assessment and why. The ultimate goals of assessment—identifying risk and protective factors—and the difference between a delay and deficit or disorder are then addressed. The relationship between early brain development and developmental assessment is explored using the neuroenvironmental synthesis model (Aylward, 2020a). Prediction and factors that affect prediction, developmental domains, foci of assessment at different ages, milestones, and psychometric and testing issues, and the role of pediatric psychologists and developmental-behavioral pediatricians in developmental assessment of young children are also addressed.

Two obvious questions are: who should be assessed developmentally, and why is this assessment necessary? Children at established risk (e.g., genetic disorders), medical/biological risk (e.g., born extremely preterm or with hypoxic-ischemic encephalopathy), or environmental risk (e.g., poverty, lack of stimulation), who are often followed by pediatric psychologists and developmental-behavioral pediatricians, are prime candidates for assessment. Infants and toddlers who have none of the aforementioned risks, but who have been identified as having possible developmental delays via surveillance or screening by their primary care physician, also require developmental assessment. This assessment could be broad-based or it could be domain-specific and may be administered by allied specialists such as occupational therapists, physical therapists, or speech/language pathologists, in addition to developmental-behavioral pediatricians and pediatric psychologists. The assessment is necessary in order to identify the child's strengths and weaknesses and to intervene as early as possible.

Maturational theory emphasizes that development in infancy and toddlerhood proceeds in a predictable, "preprogrammed" fashion. However, this programming can be affected by various internal and external factors that influence the velocity, quality, and ultimate level of developmental change (Aylward, 2020a). Development is dynamic and proceeds in a cephalo-caudal and proximo-distal manner and moves from general to more specific acquisitions. It is against this dynamic backdrop that developmental-behavioral pediatricians, pediatric psychologists, and allied health professionals such as occupational and physical therapists, and speech/language specialists, are tasked with identification of problems in development. Each specialist may be called upon to perform assessments for different purposes, but all share the common issues involved with assessing infants and toddlers.

The ultimate goals of developmental assessment are to identify or verify a delay or disorder and address the problem by directing the child for additional medical evaluations to determine a potential etiology contributing to the delay and referring the family to services (e.g., private development therapies and early intervention services) to maximize a child's potential. The process of developmental assessment also helps to identify risk and protective factors in both the child and the environment that may positively or negatively affect the course of development (Wolraich et al., 1996). Risk factors increase the child's vulnerability to problematic developmental outcomes, while protective factors decrease this vulnerability. Identification of negative risk factors can also lead to efforts to ameliorate them. Early identification and intervention have been shown to improve outcomes for the 1 in 6 children who have developmental delays (Landa, 2018; Lipkin et al., 2020; Shonkoff & Hauser-Cram, 1987). Unfortunately, less than 25% of children with delays receive Early Intervention services before age 3 (Rosenberg et al., 2013).

DEFINITIONS: DELAY VERSUS A DISORDER OR DEFICIT

The primary reason for developmental assessment is to identify deviations in development that may be indicative of a delay or deficit (Bayley & Aylward, 2019a). A *delay* occurs when the child demonstrates the proper developmental sequence of a skill, but the pace and completeness of the acquisition are slower than in peers. Mastery of the developmental acquisition is lacking, but the infant shows components of emerging abilities that are assumed to eventually lead to mastery. However, delay implies 'catch-up' and cannot be used indefinitely. An infant who displays at least some components of a skill differs from the child in whom there is a total absence of these elements. In fact, this was the underlying reason for the adoption of the polytomous (3-level) scoring scheme on tests such as the Bayley-4 (Bayley & Aylward, 2019a). Mastery of an acquisition, emerging skills, or absence of age-appropriate behavior are scored differentially. A dichotomous scoring scheme would miss this distinction, essentially combining infants with emerging skills and those who show no proficiency whatsoever, with both not receiving any credit for the item. An example is midline, hand-to-hand transfer of objects. The child who can consistently transfer a small block or a ring from one hand to the other would be considered to have mastery; one who could transfer the ring (perhaps inconsistently) but not the block shows emerging proficiency, while the child who does not transfer at all may have a potential deficit in this area.

A *deficit* or a *disorder* is more long-lasting, and although the terms are often used interchangeably, the former indicates a deficiency or failing in development while the latter is a disruption in typical development. They both reflect atypical development. As such, the infant usually does not display any components of the developmental acquisition that is assessed, and the probability of mastering the skill in the future is low because this situation most likely reflects an impairment. The presence of abnormalities or "red flags" (such as persistence of primitive reflexes) are indicative of a disorder as well.

The following possibilities are offered as ways to differentiate a delay from a disorder/deficit:

- *Serial assessment.* Following a child longitudinally helps to determine whether there is continued developmental growth but on a slower trajectory, or if a plateau or decline is evident. A baseline needs to be established, and subsequent assessment results can be compared to previous levels of performance. If there continues to be progress, the likelihood of a delay is greater than the probability of a disorder or deficit. Subtest scaled scores, composite standard scores, or individual growth scores (used where there are minimal increments in development that would not change scaled scores, as on the Bayley-4) could be used for this purpose. Examiners should also evaluate changes within as well as between domains. Therefore, the course of development is best captured through change over time versus measurement at a single time point. This supports longitudinal monitoring.

- *Severity of the problematic skills.* A domain score that is 1 standard deviation (*SD*) below the mean may indicate either a delay or a disorder; scores that are −2 *SD* or more suggest a disorder. Related to severity is the number of domains that are below average: the more developmental domains that are 1 or more *SD* below the normative mean, the greater the likelihood that an underlying disorder exists. This is particularly true if cognitive and language domains are significantly below average. In this case, the likelihood of later intellectual disability is increased.
- *Red flags.* If the child displays so-called "red flags"—findings that are abnormal at any age, such as hyper- or hypotonicity, cortical thumbing, strong persistence of primitive reflexes, poor eye contact, absence of language, or unusual movements—a disorder is more likely than a delay (see Aylward, 1995, 2020a; Bayley & Aylward, 2019b). Observational skills are critical in detecting red flags and involve qualitative analyses that include patterns of developmental concerns and the *functional significance* of the aberrant finding. For example, if tight heel cords or brisk deep tendon reflexes are present but ambulation is not affected, these findings are considered to be of minimal functional importance.
- *Patterns of findings.* Whether specific positive findings are isolated or more generalized also helps to clarify the delay versus disorder question. Isolated findings raise caution but are not necessarily indicative of a disorder. However, if there are multiple indicators, such as increased tightness in axial tone, brisk deep tendon reflexes, and an inability to take steps with support at age 12 to 14 months, the pattern suggests a stronger likelihood of a disorder. The optimality concept is helpful as well (Aylward, 1995). This approach does not emphasize the accumulation of risk factors, but rather factors that are more likely to predict positive outcomes. For example, the likelihood of a disorder is reduced if the infant is able to perform test tasks that require higher-order processing, because this would indicate intact neural networks.

An Alternative Scheme

Accardo and colleagues (2008) have described the concepts of delay, dissociation, and deviance as a means to categorize and explain the developmental performance of infants and toddlers. A *delay* is defined in a similar fashion as was outlined previously, again allowing for the broad variation in normality. A delay can occur in one or more areas, but it is not intrinsically abnormal. A *dissociation* refers to a difference between two "streams" of development, with one being more delayed than the other. Marked differences between receptive and expressive language or verbal versus visual processing are examples. A disconnect between given milestones also are dissociations; examples include a child having a 100-word vocabulary but no two-word combinations, or an infant who can crawl (i.e., locomote "commando style," with the abdomen on the ground) but not sit without support. A dissociation has a high likelihood of evolving into a disorder. Finally, *deviance* involves the appearance of an indicator that is abnormal at any age (e.g., cortical thumb, scissoring in the downwards parachute, avoidance of eye contact, extremely poor self-regulation skills) and corresponds to a disorder.

RELATIONSHIP BETWEEN EARLY BRAIN DEVELOPMENT AND ASSESSMENT

Neuroenvironmental Synthesis Model

The neuroenvironmental synthesis model (Aylward, 2020a) provides a neurodevelopmental basis for infant assessment. In this integrated approach, external biological and environmental factors work together to affect the course of internal brain development (Shonkoff, 2016). Brain changes are then assumed to produce increasingly sophisticated behaviors that can be assessed with more complex developmental test items. Essentially, infant and toddler's central nervous system undergo biological maturation in conjunction with structural and functional changes that occur in response to experiences or injury. These influences affect the creation of synaptic connections and the formation of neural circuits necessary for increasingly complex behaviors that can be assessed (Aylward, 2020a)—or, conversely, the influences can interfere with these circuits. Biological components include brain growth and developmental plasticity, as well as epigenetic modifications (particularly methylation and microRNAs). It should be noted that brain development includes both additions (creation of new connections) as well as deletions (i.e., pruning or apoptosis). Under the environment umbrella are (a) physical exposures such as tobacco, bisphenol A, lead, prenatal substance and alcohol exposure, and other toxicants; (b) experiences such as the neonatal intensive care unit (NICU) environment that overwhelm the developing central nervous system; (c) social transactions including early adversity, low socioeconomic status (SES), poor social support, and cumulative allostatic load; and (d) poor nutrition. Via epigenetics, these factors can affect the underlying architecture of the infant's brain by altering gene expression.

Neuronal plasticity refers to structural and functional changes in neuronal circuits that are in response to experiences. Two types of circuits are important during infancy and toddlerhood and are relevant to infant assessment: (a) experience-expectant, innate, prewired circuits; and (b) experience-dependent circuits that are developed and modified by learning and memory formation (Greenough et al., 1987; Kolb et al., 2017). Synapses are the fundamental units of neuronal circuits, and synaptic plasticity involves the addition or removal of synapses (Fu & Zuo, 2011). The former circuits are innate and prewired but need environmental input to become functional—otherwise, without this input, they will be eliminated. This is evident in language, where input over time determines the child's ability to discriminate sounds specific to a language they have been exposed to better than sounds from unfamiliar languages. The second group of circuits, experience-dependent synapses, are developed and modified by environmental experiences and account for memory and learning (Greenough & Chang, 1989; Kolb et al., 2017). New learning involves the development of synaptic networks that are dynamic and become more complex over time. That is why assessment tasks also become more complex as the infant ages. Early intervention efforts will enhance the development of experience-dependent synapses and produce change over time.

Timing is critical, and certain brain areas are more or less responsive to environmental influences depending on age. The vulnerability or adaptability of the child's brain is dependent on critical and sensitive periods or windows defined as times when neuronal connections are highly susceptible to experience-expectant and experience-dependent modifications (Kolb et al., 2017).

There is also the potential for disruption or injury to affect brain development. For example, being born extremely preterm also interferes with the last wave of early brain development that includes proliferation, migration, and the intactness of the subplate neuronal layer. This transient structure experiences maximal thickness between 22 and 36 weeks' gestation and serves early placeholding functions for corticothalamic interconnections (Kiss et al., 2014). The end result of this disruption is decreased maturation and complexity of cortical circuitry. There is a resulting mixture of diffuse white and gray matter lesions that are presumed to be responsible for subtle neurodevelopmental problems later on (i.e., high prevalence/low severity dysfunctions; Albertine, 2012). There is evidence that higher-order complex cognitive skills develop later and involve longer, more geographically distant connections between neurons over white matter pathways (Willett, 2018). As a result, they are more susceptible to disruption or injury. Developmental assessment needs to be able to detect precursors of these potential deficits earlier, but we are not there yet.

Neuroanatomically, more complex neural circuits rely on earlier, simple neural assemblies. This variability of experiences, the functional levels in each of the five developmental domains (i.e., cognitive, language, motor, adaptive, and social-emotional), and interactions with the environment, make each child unique.

We now know that both cognitive and motor areas of the brain can be activated by a similar task. Damage to the motor circuits may be our first clue of increased risk of cognitive compromise, due in part to underlying neural connections and parallel circuits; damage to the tracts involved in motor function can also extend to cognitive circuits that may not be recruited into action until later in development (Volpe, 2009). This is sometimes referred to as a silent period.

Major, multiple changes in brain architecture and interconnections enable the expansion of the infant and toddler's behavioral repertoire. This, in turn, is assumed to correspond to the complexity of test tasks that can be administered to assess advances in development. This more complex function depends on integrated neural networks that are located in different areas of the brain.

The formation and elimination of synaptic structures happen rapidly in subpopulations of cortical neurons during sensorimotor learning experiences (Fu & Zuo, 2011). This synaptic proliferation and pruning phenomenon is referred to as *developmental plasticity* and differs from injury-induced plasticity. Behavioral and developmental acquisitions grossly parallel brain development as both begin with simple components and become more complex with increasing age.

To summarize, integrated neural circuits are extracted from a pool of less specific, basic neural groupings. These general, experience-dependent circuits are augmented or eliminated by the child's experiences, becoming more complex over time due to the increasing sophistication of these circuits that facilitate learning and memory. Environmental input is therefore critical to the infant and toddler's brain development (Aylward, 2020a). Higher-order integrated functional units are more complex and geographically distant—these factors make them more susceptible to disruption and insult (Keunen et al., 2017) the effects of which may not be apparent early on. There are changes within neural networks as well as between networks. The complexity of developmental assessment test items parallels these anatomic changes. Development involves the acquisition of new skills that are the result of maturation, experiential learning, and an array of emotional, social, and cultural environmental factors.

PREDICTION

There are contemporary (i.e., where the child is developmentally at the time of testing) as well as future (i.e., what level of development can be expected at later ages) dimensions inherent in developmental assessment. Associated with the primary goal of identification is the issue of prediction, which is often not specifically stated but is implied. Data obtained from these assessments are also routinely employed as outcome measures to determine the effects of certain medical/biological conditions (e.g., extreme prematurity) or innovative medical procedures (e.g., prenatal steroids, total body cooling).

The underlying assumption is that this early measure of development will also be predictive of later cognitive, language, motor functioning, or even academic functioning. Unfortunately, this is often not the case. This situation places developmental-behavioral pediatricians or pediatric psychologists in a quandary regarding whether to raise an early alarm to caregivers or provide reassurance, because lack of attainment of a skill could be due to the skill being emergent, latent, delayed, deficient, or disordered (Marks et al., 2008).

Numerous factors affect prediction, and these include:

- The ages at which the initial and end point measurements occur (due to plateaus and gradients)

- The time span between the assessment and outcome
- The developmental domain that is being considered
- The Flynn effect (Flynn, 1999) and other psychometric issues, including the "observational effect"
- How prediction is defined and the focus of later outcome
- The positive or negative influences of the environment
- The impact of early intervention or similar services
- Continuing effects of medical/biological issues

Ages of Initial and End Point Measurements

Development is dynamic and does not advance at the same rate equally in all domains or even within domains. Therefore, if the initial measure is taken at a time of rapid change, stability is compromised because of a high degree of variability. Conversely, if the initial or later outcome measures are assessed when development is at a plateau or there is a lull in progression, there might be better prediction at that point, but not necessarily when there is a resurgence of developmental change. The age of the infant at the initial assessment will also have an impact on prediction, because in the earlier age ranges, tests will contain a restricted repertoire of canalized, sensorimotor items, the predictive utility of which is limited.

Time Between Early Assessment and Outcome

The general rule of thumb is the closer two measurements are in time, the greater the correlation and, hence, the predictability is better. For example, if two measures are taken at 12 and 24 months, there might be a strong correlation, but the question remains just how predictive the 24-month assessment data is with regard to later, school-age function. A more stable level of cognitive and developmental function can be obtained at school age, and this is the recommended end point in predictive studies.

The Developmental Domain Being Considered

Motor function appears to be more "self-righting" than other domains, perhaps because it is canalized. However, as mentioned earlier, motor problems could also be a biomarker, with the cause for the motor problem also indirectly having an impact on neighboring systems that later turn out to be "cognitive" (Volpe, 2009). In contrast, compromised language function is more heavily dependent on environmental influences (Radesky et al., 2016), particularly low SES environments.

The Flynn Effect

Poor prediction has also been attributed to the Flynn effect (Flynn, 1999), where mean developmental test scores increase by 0.3 to 0.5 points per year or 3 to 5 points per decade. It is questionable whether this phenomenon is as applicable to infants and toddlers as it is to older children (Trahan et al., 2014); in fact, there is some contemporary evidence that the Flynn effect has weakened or even reversed (Bratsberg & Rogeberg, 2018). A review article on the "infant Flynn effect" revealed the mean increase in the Bayley developmental quotient was 3.4 points for the cognitive scale and 2.49 points for the motor scale (Lynn, 2009). A similar increase was found with the Griffiths Mental Developmental Scales-Revised (2.45 points). In addition, the observational effect means that familiarity with testing itself can change scores (Marks et al., 2008). Training to task (i.e., using test tasks to help a child with delays improve their skills during intervention) also inflates scores.

How Prediction Is Defined

There are various ways to define prediction. These include sensitivity (copositivity) and specificity (conegativity), odds ratios, correlations, and whether data are viewed as categorical or continuous. Outcomes also vary depending on whether the focus is on individual scale scores or composite scores. There are also combinations of outcomes that are used to place a young child in categories. For example, in the Neonatal Research Network, severe neurodevelopmental disabilities (NDDs) are defined as a Bayley-III motor or cognitive score < 70, cerebral palsy (GMFCS score of ≥3), bilateral sensory deficits (hearing, vision), or some combination. Moderate NDDs include cognitive or motor indexes between 70 and 85, mild cerebral palsy, or sensory deficits that can be corrected. Some clinicians use a combined score, while others use scores obtained for each domain of function. Adaptive functioning and quality of life measures are becoming more frequently used (Kilbride et al., 2018). Of note is the fact that the most frequent qualifier for NDDs are low cognitive scores. As a result, the group of children who manifest severe NDDs is very heterogeneous, having different deficits or combinations of disabilities (Cohen & Houtrow, 2019).

Environmental Effects: Considerations From Developmental Science

Environmental effects can be process/proximal (e.g., mother-infant interactions, amount of stimulation provided in the home, siblings) or status/distal (e.g., neighborhood, SES, poverty). As mentioned earlier, environmental factors have an impact on epigenetics (Aylward, 2020a). Either individually or cumulatively, these will undoubtedly have an impact on prediction.

There is also evidence that children raised in poverty have differences in brain size, such as smaller hippocampus and frontal and temporal lobes than peers who are not raised in poverty. These negative changes are related to poorer cognitive and academic performance as the child ages. "Toxic stress" due to continued exposure to poverty will produce more negative changes, underscoring the continued vulnerability of the developing brain and further disrupting prediction (Hair et al., 2015).

Environmental factors that influence development also change in terms of the magnitude of their effects depending on the age of the infant. Proximal or process factors are more influential over the first few years, while distal or status factors have a stronger impact as the child ages.

Effects of Early Intervention

Oftentimes, results of the initial evaluation qualify an infant for early intervention services that typically will be provided between the first assessment and later outcome determination. This intervention is geared to address the problematic developmental areas regardless of whether the cause is a delay or a disorder. Prediction will then be altered if the interventions are successful, underscoring the adaptability of the child's brain. Intervention may be less influential if the degree of deficit is more severe and causes a ceiling effect.

Continuing Effects of Medical/ Biological Issues

Medical/biological issues are typically found in infants who have had pre-, peri-, or postnatal trauma or illness. This would be evident in an infant who is born extremely preterm (<28 weeks gestation), for example, and whose respiratory distress syndrome evolved into bronchopulmonary dysplasia necessitating supplementary oxygen. This situation would subject the infant to frequent bouts of mild hypoxia that could have deleterious effects on brain development (Laptook, 2016). Similarly, a child with significant feeding problems may not have adequate intake of certain nutrients necessary for adequate growth and brain development. Extended stays in the NICU limit the infant's interactions with the environment and expose the central nervous system to sensory stimuli that may be overwhelming. This experience also impedes learning and exploration. Dealing with these and other limiting medical issues taxes the child's physiologic balance. This state also interferes with development, particularly in early to mid-infancy, causing lower early developmental scores that may improve with age and resolution of the physical problem. Again, prediction will be disrupted.

Similarly, the issue of when to discontinue correction for prematurity could affect prediction, particularly at younger ages where differences between corrected and uncorrected scores are greatest (Aylward, 2020b; Wilson-Ching et al., 2014). For example, if correction were used at 2 years and then discontinued at age 3, the impact could be greater than if it were discontinued at 5 or 6 years, particularly if the child fell in the upper end of the typical 3-month normative age band at the time of outcome. Moreover, the younger the gestational age at birth, the greater the need for correction, even to age 3 (Aylward, 2020b).

For both cognitive and motor domains, prediction is stronger if the child's scores fall in the very low (70–79) or extremely low (<70) range due to a limited ceiling effect. Conversely, if the initial scores fall in the high average (110–119), exceptional (120–129), or very exceptional range (>129), the likelihood of at least average later functioning is high, barring trauma or marked negative changes in the environment. There also might be some decline due to the statistical phenomenon of "regression toward the mean." The most unstable test performance (corresponding to the poorest levels of prediction) is found in infants and toddlers with mild to moderate problems (low average to borderline scores)—exactly the children we need to identify early.

DEVELOPMENTAL DOMAINS

Five domains of development are of interest to developmental-behavioral pediatricians, psychologists, and developmental scientists: *cognitive*, *language* (expressive, receptive, articulation), *motor* (gross and fine), *adaptive*, and *personal-social*. Developmental domains are unique but also interrelated. For example, motor skills enable the infant to explore the environment and manipulate objects—this leads to learning, which in turn facilitates cognitive development. Essentially, the infant moves from a "learning to manipulate" to a "manipulating to learn" mode. In addition, the development of more complex skills is dependent on the earlier foundational development of basic skills, drawn from different domains (C. P. Johnson & Blasco, 1997). Complicating developmental assessment is the possibility that a deficit or disorder in one domain such as gross motor may negatively affect parallel development in one or more other domains such as cognitive. It is also possible that skills contained in the cognitive domain could actually be normal, but the interference caused by the disorder in the motor development stream prevents the expression of true cognitive potential.

FOCUS OF ASSESSMENT AT DIFFERENT AGES

When administering developmental tests, assessment follows the evolving neurologic → motor → sensorimotor → cognitive sequence of increasingly complex developmental functions (Aylward, 2009, 2020a). Early on, developmental assessment primarily involves traditional neurologic exam items (e.g., tone, asymmetries, deep tendon reflexes). Next is the emergence of maturational, primitive reflexes (e.g., asymmetric tonic neck reflex, Moro, palmar grasp) and their subsequent disappearance by approximately 6 months of age due to the cerebral cortex inhibiting lower brain centers. These primitive reflexes are replaced by protective postural reactions (e.g., downward and forward parachute responses) from 4 months onwards. Later gross and fine motor skills that involve voluntary, purposeful movements allow for further development of cognition through interaction with the environment. There is debate as to the most optimal ages for assessment, particularly in follow-up programs. It is suggested that the key ages for developmental assessment correspond to the appearance and stability of major developmental acquisitions. Therefore at 6 months (corrected age in the case of those born preterm), there is emphasis on tone, primitive reflexes, and sensory functions such as hearing and vision. At 12 to 15 months, motor development is emphasized, while at 24 months, language is the focus. Cognitive abilities can be more thoroughly assessed at 36 months.

MILESTONES

Milestones in terms of cognitive, language, and motor development are typically used in developmental surveillance, screening, and to a lesser degree assessment, to gauge if the child's developmental progress falls in the "normal" range. These indicators are based primarily on maturational theory. However, there are differences in the ages used to determine when the lack of achieving a milestone is considered worrisome (Sheldrick et al., 2019). Many milestones are not evidence-based and 50%, 75%, and 90% success rates for milestones have been endorsed as "normal." Milestones vary by the population that is tested, environmental factors, normal variability in rates of development, and the specific domain from which the milestone is drawn. Of note is the fact that Bayley originally used a 50% mean score and a range of 5% and 95% success rate when presenting age estimates of successful item completion in her test manual (Bayley, 1969). The success rate issue is significant because, for example, if a 50% pass rate is selected as the mean milestone age, fully half of the children would fall below that cutoff age. Moreover, parents would be unjustifiably worried if the child was in the lower 50%, even though the child's performance might actually be normal. The U.S. Centers for Disease Control and Prevention (CDC) established the first set of milestones in 2004, and both the CDC (2018) and Bright Futures (Council on Children With Disabilities et al., 2006) report milestones based on ages that "most children pass." However, in both cases, it is not clear what "most" means (Sheldrick et al., 2019).

More recently, evidence-informed milestones for developmental surveillance (Zubler et al., 2022) at 15 and 30 months were based on a cutoff of 75%. The sequence of documenting development goes from surveillance to screening to assessment. While all infants and toddlers should be subject to continuous surveillance and periodic screening, not all children will receive a developmental assessment. If preliminary screening or dialogue between the parents and primary care physician (surveillance) raises concerns, then targeted screening using a validated screening instrument is the next step. If the results of the screening are indicative of delays, the third tier that involves assessment is warranted. Therefore, developmental-behavioral pediatricians, pediatric psychologists, and pediatric rehabilitation specialists have a third-tier role, because the primary care physician should routinely perform the surveillance and initial screening of the child's developmental status. This framework underscores the multidisciplinary approach involved in evaluating development in infants and toddlers.

The method of determination of item difficulty affects the age range given to milestones. Item sequences can be gauged by Conventional Test Theory (CTT), where the difficulty is age-based because some items are primarily for younger ages, and others for older age groups. Conversely, Item Response Theory (IRT) evaluates item difficulty across all ages. Item characteristic curves (ICCs) describe the probability of each response to each milestone as a function of developmental age (Sheldrick & Perrin, 2013; Sheldrick et al., 2019). Inferential norming is also employed in the development of assessment norms. The mean, SD, skewness, and kurtosis of scores are conditioned on age. Use of this model produces norms by age range and the normative age is the midpoint age of the range.

The current recommendation is to use a 75% pass rate as indicative of the age "normal" children would pass a given item (Zubler et al., 2022). It should be noted that the pass rate for a milestone has an impact on false-positive and false-negative rates. The 75% cutoff should decrease false positives and prevent unwarranted concerns in caregivers.

Developmental Quotients

Milestones often are used to produce a developmental quotient (DQ). The DQ is computed as the child's developmental age (determined to a significant degree by milestones) divided by the chronological age × 100. Although convenient, this computation depends on the numerator, which is based on the accuracy and content of the test used. Therefore, ratio DQs are not the best metric because (a) ratios are not comparable across ages, (b) the standard deviation does not remain constant, (c) resulting confidence intervals vary greatly, and (d) the velocity of developmental change is not consistent across ages.

Age Equivalents/Percent Delay

Age equivalents are frequently used in developmental assessment and are popular with caregivers.

Age equivalents are also a critical component of the computation of "percent delay." They refer to the age at which an infant's obtained raw score is comparable to what is considered average. A 12-month-old infant who is functioning at a 6-month level demonstrates a 50% delay; a 24-month-old functioning at an 18-month level has a 25% delay. Care must be taken to explain to parents that it is the proportion or ratio that is important for future comparisons, not the number of months. More specifically, the 12-month-old who scores at a 6-month level will not necessarily be at a 30-month level at the chronologic age of 36 months. Instead, there is a higher probability that the infant would fall around an 18-month level. Moreover, a 12-month-old who is functioning at a 6-month age equivalent is qualitatively different than a typical 6-month-old. The percent delay concept is widely used to determine eligibility for intervention services (e.g., a 30% delay in a specific domain). This practice assumes a degree of preciseness in developmental assessment that does not exist. Use of metrics such as standard deviations, percentiles, *t*-scores, or *z*-scores is a much better option.

PSYCHOMETRIC CONCERNS AND TEST ISSUES

Reference Standards

Even the most frequently used infant assessment instruments are not truly "gold standards." Instead, they should be considered "reference standards" because of the many factors that affect testing and the lack of absolute-value cutoffs (Aylward, 2009). That said, *sensitivity* is the proportion of children with a delay that are identified by the test. This could arguably be considered co-positivity in that both the reference standard and the test under consideration are in agreement that a problem exists. *Specificity* indicates the proportion of children who are normal and identified as normal by the test. Specificity would be more accurately deemed as co-negativity, namely, both measures are in agreement on the absence of a problem. Acceptable sensitivity and specificity values should be 0.70 or greater (Šimundić, 2009).

Children who have a developmental delay but are not identified are considered false negatives, while those who display typical development but are called delayed are false positives. The positive predictive value (PPV) refers to the proportion of children with a positive test result who actually are delayed; the negative predictive value (NPV) refers to the proportion of children with a negative test who do not have delays. In low-prevalence populations, sensitivity and specificity may be better measures for assessing developmental problems.

The ultimate goal of developmental assessment is to identify true positives while simultaneously limiting false negatives. False negatives in young children are more worrisome because interventions that address the child's delay or disorder would not occur as early as possible to optimize outcomes.

Reliability/Validity

Simply stated, no test is perfect. Successful test usage requires that the examiner understand both the test's strengths and weaknesses. Moreover, tests, per se, are not valid or invalid; validity depends on how the test is employed and interpreted. With infants and young children, validity is primarily established in two ways: (a) by comparing test results with other established tests (e.g., compare one version of a test to another), or (b) by evaluating how matched normative groups would differ from clinical samples (Aylward & Zhu, 2019). A developmental test should assess the important aspects of development and, at the same time, not be overly inclusive. The test should measure skills indicative of normal development but not reflect an attempt to be all-encompassing. Essentially a balance between theoretic and pragmatic considerations is necessary. While test items should be correlated with each other (assessed with split half reliability and alpha values), they should not be overly redundant. There simply is no reason to test the same skill two or three times. This makes the test too lengthy and limits the inclusion of potentially important items that tap other abilities. What the item is truly measuring should be clear. Many developmental tests have steep item gradients where a small change in the raw score would result in large changes in the scaled scores. This situation would cause test scores to be highly variable and have a major, negative impact on age equivalents.

Validity indicates whether a test measures what it claims to measure (i.e., whether the items are representative of the developmental domain that is under consideration). In developmental assessment, content validity and construct validity are critical issues and involve the test items covering the appropriate range of development. The test must also be reliable or consistent in measurement. *Reliability* includes internal consistency (i.e., all aspects of the test are measuring a cohesive construct), as well as test–retest reliability (i.e., the same score would be obtained if the test was readministered).

Test items that are strongly *canalized* are prominent at early ages on developmental tests. Canalization is conceptualized to involve prewired neural circuits present at birth that facilitate simple behaviors (Aylward, 2009, 2020a). These behaviors are primarily sensorimotor (e.g., smiling, reaching, babbling), self-righting, and less vulnerable to negative influences such as being born prematurely or having hypoxic-ischemic encephalopathy. Canalized behaviors tend to be buffered so that negative influences do not cause a major developmental disruption (M. H. Johnson et al., 2015). Because infant tests are heavily loaded with canalized behaviors early on, to the exclusion of items tapping higher-order cognitive skills, our ability to estimate the young child's true current and subsequent cognitive capacity (particularly the latter), is limited.

Another content issue involves *experiential bias* (Aylward, 2020a), where either familiarity or lack of experience with test items might give a false reading on the child's true abilities and cognitive capacity. Familiarization with test tasks such as form boards or pegboards would artificially benefit the toddler's actual test performance while a lack of experiences with these or other more common items (e.g., scissors) place the child at a disadvantage. Therefore, in addition to tasks that the infant or toddler potentially could have been exposed to, novel tasks should also be included in the developmental assessment that require a mix of acquired skills, learning, and problem solving.

Because of a limited behavioral repertoire at very young ages, it is difficult to identify and administer test items that may be more indicative of higher-order abilities. Moreover, tasks that do not appear linked to each other may actually be associated. Precursors to higher-order cognitive function include early skills such as habituation, awareness of surroundings, and object permanency; these behaviors are thought to reflect later critical functions of attention, inhibition, working memory and ability to shift (Aylward et al., 2022).

COMPONENTS OF DEVELOPMENTAL ASSESSMENT

Developmental assessment consists of four primary components: (a) observation, (b) administration of items, (c) caregiver report and participation, and (d) history and physical examination.

Observation

Bayley's (1969) statement that "[t]he order of presentation should be adapted to the responsiveness of the child and he/she may be scored for an ability manifested at any time during the observation period . . ." (p. 26) reflects an emphasis on the value of clinical observation in developmental assessment that still is true today. Keen observational skills necessitate that the clinician, regardless of specialty, has had much hands-on experience in assessment. Observations include the child's physical features, temperament, activity level, awareness of surroundings, interest and manipulation of objects, communication style and self-regulatory abilities; such observations can be made at any point in the evaluation, including the waiting room, hallway to the clinic, or as the child exits the examination room. Observation should be a critical tool for all disciplines performing developmental assessments.

Observations are particularly critical when testing infants or toddlers who have specific disabilities that require adjustments to the testing procedures in order to circumvent the effects the disability (e.g., motor, visual, hearing) might have on test performance. The negative effect of a disability on testing is magnified when the child is then compared to standardized norms derived from peers who are not disabled. Qualitative descriptions of what adaptations were used during testing are also helpful in designing subsequent interventions.

Because our ability to evaluate infants and toddlers with disabilities is more difficult in comparison to testing children without disabilities, developmental-behavioral pediatricians and pediatric psychologists have to be more flexible in the administration and scoring of items. The degree of flexibility and altered procedures potentially could be problematic, however. The terms *accommodations* and *modifications* are often used interchangeably to describe adaptations or adjustments to developmental testing. However, these terms are actually quite different: accommodations are acceptable or permissible changes in materials or procedures employed during testing, the purpose being to increase the validity of the test data and to obtain a more accurate estimation of the child's abilities that might be obscured using standard procedures. Conversely, a modification is a change in the content and presentation of an item and the actual construct being measured. Modifications should be avoided because comparison to normative test data is invalid (Aylward, 2020a). It also is assumed that the use of accommodations would not give the nondisabled child an advantage.

Administration of Test Items

The second component of the developmental assessment is the administration of actual test items. This provides qualitative and quantitative information obtained under structured, standardized situations. In so doing, examiners can evaluate the child's learning abilities, problem solving, cognitive flexibility, and attention—all precursors to higher-order cognitive function. Item administration also affords the opportunity to see how rapidly a child catches on to the task at hand and the ability to understand and follow directions. Evaluation of these abilities is critical in developmental assessment.

Linear and Nonlinear Formats

There are two types of administration schemes that are followed in developmental assessment: *linear* and *nonlinear* formats. With linear administration, the first item administered is based on chronologic age, a basal is established and items are administered sequentially until a ceiling is reached. Because linear assessments are standardized in this manner, if the procedures are not followed exactly, the data are considered invalid. While linear procedures ensure that all appropriate items are administered, administration is kept strictly in line with standardization procedures. Standard scores are provided but this approach is more applicable to older children. This is because linear administration mandates a rigid test administration style that can interfere with rapport-building, increase refusals, and lead to invalid test results in young children who tend to have their own testing agenda (Lane & Aylward, 2020).

Nonlinear administration still maintains many of the same requirements as linear scoring. However, it is more flexible in terms of administration sequence, allowing items and subtests to be administered in an order that best suits the child. The examiner can also group similar items that use the same test materials such as cubes or form boards to enhance the flow of testing. Nonlinear administration takes less time, is more flexible, and is conducive to scoring observational items noted at any time during the test session, versus when they come up in a prescribed, sequential order. It also allows the child to select items of interest first, enhancing cooperation and the production of a valid score. The computerized Q-Global format of Bayley-4 is an example of the nonlinear format. This again argues for the need for examiners having had practical experience, versus simply reading the test manual. It is assumed that accommodations would not give the nondisabled child an advantage.

Caregiver Report and Participation

The third component, information provided by caregivers, is extremely useful in assessing a child's development. Caregivers have a better understanding of the infant's strengths and weaknesses because of day-to-day contact in familiar surroundings. Caregiver report reduces testing time and fatigue, and it also minimizes missing information that might render the assessment incomplete or invalid. Nonetheless, total reliance on caregiver reports is not recommended in developmental assessment, although this procedure may be acceptable for initial screening purposes. It should be an adjunct to test administration. Test items that involve expressive language or motor development have a higher likelihood of refusal in infants and toddlers, making it difficult to determine if the child has mastery of the skill or not. Moreover, uncooperative behavior on the part of the child has been considered an indication of later risk and it is arguable as to what to do with items that are refused (i.e., should they be scored as failed or not; Wocadlo & Rieger, 2000). This is a particular problem on tests that have a low number of items. In addition to clarifying whether the refusal may be due to difficulty with the task, caregiver report also allows for verification of behavior that was ambiguous or not observed during the actual session. Many items that are complex, but very useful in determination of higher cognitive processes, tend to be difficult to elicit in standard testing situations. Examples include representational play (e.g., making believe an object is something else) and imaginary play (e.g., the child uses imaginary objects; Aylward, 2020a). These items, presumed to be indicative of higher-order functioning and underlying integrated neural networks, have a much greater likelihood of occurring in a familiar environment than in a clinic setting. In fact, these two items are now scored only by caregiver report on the Bayley-4.

Including caregivers in the testing process is also helpful in reducing anxiety in the parent and, reciprocally, in the child. Some caregivers may be overzealous and try to coach the child; they need to be discouraged from doing so in a calm, reassuring manner. Once again, this differs from testing older children, where parents are not present. Caregiver report and participation allow for a more "naturalistic" or "authentic" assessment whose proponents are critical of standardized, norm-referenced assessments because they perceive the testing as too artificial, not linked to intervention, and failing to tap the child's true potential (Macy et al., 2015).

There are a small number of caregivers who, for a variety of reasons, may exaggerate the child's abilities to make the infant look more "normal." Conversely, caregivers who are dealing with cumulative stress or mental health issues such as depression may report a more unfavorable view of their child's development. However, the majority of parents are quite accurate in their perception of their child's abilities (Aylward & Verhulst, 2008).

History and Physical Examination

The fourth component of developmental testing is the history and physical examination. The history can be taken by psychologists or developmental-behavioral pediatricians; the physical exam is performed by the developmental-behavioral pediatrician, although all disciplines can recognize dysmorphic features. Often, behavioral phenotypes are found with genetic or neurodevelopmental disorders, such as children with Down syndrome having problems with abstract language and scoring higher on tests in infancy than at later ages. In addition, children with certain medical histories may be at increased risk for later, associated problems, as in the case of children born at extremely premature gestational ages having an increased incidence of visual perceptual problems and later high prevalence/low severity dysfunctions such as lower IQ, attention deficit/hyperactivity disorder, executive dysfunction, and problems in academics (Aylward, 2002, 2005). Similarly, the child who sustains a Grade 3 or 4 intraventricular hemorrhage is at risk for motor problems (e.g., a developmental coordination disorder) or cerebral palsy. The family history is also helpful in the case of language disorders, genetic disorders, or intellectual disabilities. The infant's birth history, neonatal course, birth weight, and gestational age at birth should be considered. While some of these learning and neurodevelopmental problems cannot be diagnosed until later ages, the practitioner should pay particular attention to the emergence of particular areas of potential difficulty, many of which can be detected in the physical examination and history.

Homotypic and Heterotypic Behaviors

Some underlying developmental skills can be considered "homotypic" meaning that an early skill or acquisition has an obvious connection with a later behavior and appears to measure the same concept (e.g., attention). However due in part to the limited behavioral repertoires in infants, we are often faced with "heterotypic" behaviors where the links between the early manifestations of a skill and later abilities are not obvious and seem unrelated. Stated differently, there often is apparent discontinuity between the early manifestations of a skill and its later appearance.

For example, recently, Lowe et al. (2020) reported that early working memory at 18 to 22 months, measured with three test items ("finds hidden object," "finds hidden object reversed," and "finds hidden object visual displacement"), was a significant predictor of later verbal and processing skills at 6 to 7 years, but not executive function. There was also a sex difference, favoring girls. Kraybill et al. (2019) found a longitudinal association between infant attention at 5 months and 3-year executive function measures, suggesting that infant attention is an early marker of executive function (shorter look duration and higher shift rates indicating more efficient information processing and better attention). These findings raise caution that the selection of tasks assumed to measure a particular ability may have an effect on our assumptions regarding possible associations between early constructs; also, heterotypic associations make it difficult to predict specific outcomes. Additional studies like those mentioned above will enhance our knowledge of the relationships between early behaviors and later higher-order functions.

FUTURE DIRECTIONS

Advances in neuroimaging such as functional MRI, diffusion-weighted imagery, and positron emission tomography (Duerden et al., 2013), may be combined with developmental testing in the future in select cases, although there are practical issues, as well as procedural and technical difficulties, and the need for sedation. Such techniques could verify which circuits are involved in developmental tasks and provide additional information regarding developmental brain plasticity. Identification of critical items, that, if passed, would be indicative of intact neurocognitive networks, is another area that should be investigated. This is compatible with the optimality concept (Aylward, 1995) mentioned previously, where emphasis is placed on items that are passed, versus those that are failed. The more optimal responses a child receives, the greater the probability of normal functioning.

CONCLUSION

Early assessment provides a stronger associative linkage between test results and medical/biological factors or treatments. However, there is a limit as to what can be assessed early on. At later ages, more subtle issues may become apparent, but the degree of potential relationships is muddled because of the effects of the environment. The boundaries of normal and abnormal functioning are less clear in infants and toddlers than in older children, due to the dynamic backdrop of continuous developmental change. Therefore, we must often rely on an observational combination of pathognomic signs and patterns of performance (Aylward, 1997). In the past, functions were linked to test items in a posthoc fashion, versus defining a function proactively and devising a task to measure it. The latter approach is necessary if we are to move forward in developmental assessment. In addition, qualitative information must be translated into more objective, quantifiable data, because observation is a critical tool in the evaluation of infants and toddlers. This requires a delicate balance between rigid, linear test administration procedures and more flexible nonlinear administration—while at the same time maintaining standardized procedures so that the data are valid. Ultimately, the purpose of the assessment will determine the type and breadth of the evaluation instrument that is used.

Developmental assessment during infancy and toddlerhood needs to be administered by clinicians to enhance the validity of the findings. Developmental-behavioral pediatricians, pediatric psychologists, and allied health professionals who possess an understanding of central nervous system development and the relationship between developmental plasticity and the emergence of indicators of cognitive function should administer developmental testing. In fact, the so-called "infant specialist" should have a variety of interdisciplinary experiences and background knowledge that includes aspects of pediatrics (and normal development), pediatric neurology, genetics, psychology, and developmental-behavioral pediatrics.

RESOURCES

Developmental Milestones

- Ages and Stages. (2024). *Developmental milestone articles.*

  https://agesandstages.com/developmental-milestones-articles/

- American Academy of Pediatrics. (2024). *Bright futures guidelines and pocket guide* (4th ed.).

  https://downloads.aap.org/AAP/PDF/Bright%20Futures/BF4_POCKETGUIDE.pdf

- BrightFutures.org. (n.d.). *Promoting healthy mental development: Infant development checklist.* Georgetown University.

  https://www.brightfutures.org/development/infancy/checklist.html

- Centers for Disease Control and Prevention. *CDC's developmental milestones.*

  https://www.cdc.gov/ncbddd/actearly/milestones/index.html

- Child Mind Institute. (2023). *Complete guide to developmental milestones.*

  https://childmind.org/guide/parents-guide-to-developmental-milestones/

- Healthy Children.org, from the American Academy of Pediatrics

  https://www.healthychildren.org/

- Zubler, J. M., Wiggins, L. D., Macias, M. M., Whitaker, T. M., Shaw, J. S., Squires, J. K., Pajek, J. A., Wolff, R. B., Slaughter, K. S., Broughton, A. S., Gerndt, K. L., Mlodoch, B. J., & Lipkin, P. H. (2022). Evidence-informed milestones for developmental surveillance tools. *Pediatrics, 149*(3), e2021052138. https://doi.org/10.1542/peds.2021-052138

References

Accardo, P. J., Accardo, J., & Capute, A. J. (2008). A neurodevelopmental perspective on the continuum of developmental disabilities. In P. J. Accardo (Ed.), *Capute and Accardo's neurodevelopmental disabilities in infancy and childhood* (3rd ed., pp. 3–23). Paul H. Brookes.

Albertine, K. H. (2012). Brain injury in chronically ventilated preterm neonates: Collateral damage related to ventilation strategy. *Clinics in Perinatology, 39*(3), 727–740. https://doi.org/10.1016/j.clp.2012.06.017

Aylward, G. P. (1995). *Bayley infant neurodevelopmental screener manual.* The Psychological Corporation.

Aylward, G. P. (1997). *Infant and early childhood neuropsychology.* Plenum. https://doi.org/10.1007/978-1-4615-5927-6

Aylward, G. P. (2002). Cognitive and neuropsychological outcomes: More than IQ scores. *Mental Retardation and Developmental Disabilities Research Reviews, 8*(4), 234–240. https://doi.org/10.1002/mrdd.10043

Aylward, G. P. (2005). Neurodevelopmental outcomes of infants born prematurely. *Journal of Developmental and Behavioral Pediatrics, 26*(6), 427–440. https://doi.org/10.1097/00004703-200512000-00008

Aylward, G. P. (2009). Developmental screening and assessment: What are we thinking? *Journal of Developmental and Behavioral Pediatrics, 30*(2), 169–173. https://doi.org/10.1097/DBP.0b013e31819f1c3e

Aylward, G. P. (2020a). *Bayley 4: Clinical use and interpretation.* Academic Press.

Aylward, G. P. (2020b). Is it correct to correct for prematurity? Theoretic analysis of the Bayley-4 normative data. *Journal of Developmental and Behavioral Pediatrics, 41*(2), 128–133. https://doi.org/10.1097/DBP.0000000000000739

Aylward, G. P., Taylor, H. G. Anderson, P. J., & Vannier, L. C. (2022). Assessment of executive function in infants and toddlers: A potential role of the Bayley-4. *Journal of Developmental and Behavioral Pediatrics, 43*(7), e431–e441. https://doi.org/10.1097/DBP.0000000000001072

Aylward, G. P., & Verhulst, S. J. (2008). Comparison of caretaker report and hands-on neurodevelopmental screening in high-risk infants. *Developmental Neuropsychology, 33*(2), 124–136. https://doi.org/10.1080/87565640701884220

Aylward, G. P., & Zhu, J. J. (2019). *The Bayley scales: Clarification for clinicians and researchers.* NCS Pearson.

Bayley, N. (1969). *The Bayley scales of infant development.* The Psychological Corporation.

Bayley, N., & Aylward, G. P. (2019a). *Bayley scales of infant and toddler development: Administration manual* (4th ed.). NCS Pearson.

Bayley, N., & Aylward, G. P. (2019b). *Bayley scales of infant and toddler development: Technical manual* (4th ed.). NCS Pearson.

Bratsberg, B., & Rogeberg, O. (2018). Flynn effect and its reversal are both environmentally caused. *Proceedings of the National Academy of Sciences of the United States of America, 115*(26), 6674–6678. https://doi.org/10.1073/pnas.1718793115

Centers for Disease Control and Prevention. (2018). *CDC's developmental milestones.* https://www.cdc.gov/ncbddd/actearly/milestones/index.html

Cohen, E., & Houtrow, A. (2019). Disability is not delay: Precision communication about intellectual disability. *The Journal of Pediatrics, 207,* 241–243. https://doi.org/10.1016/j.jpeds.2018.12.040

Council on Children With Disabilities, Section on Developmental Behavioral Pediatrics, Bright Futures Steering Committee, & Medical Home Initiatives for Children With Special Needs Project Advisory Committee. (2006). Identifying infants and young children with developmental disorders in the medical home: An algorithm for developmental surveillance and screening. *Pediatrics, 118*(1), 405–420. https://doi.org/10.1542/peds.2006-1231

Duerden, E. G., Taylor, M. J., & Miller, S. P. (2013). Brain development in infants born preterm: Looking beyond injury. *Seminars in Pediatric Neurology, 20*(2), 65–74. https://doi.org/10.1016/j.spen.2013.06.007

Flynn, J. R. (1999). Searching for justice: The discovery of IQ gains over time. *American Psychologist, 54*(1), 5–20. https://doi.org/10.1037/0003-066X.54.1.5

Fu, M., & Zuo, Y. (2011). Experience-dependent structural plasticity in the cortex. *Trends in Neurosciences, 34*(4), 177–187. https://doi.org/10.1016/j.tins.2011.02.001

Greenough, W. T., Black, J. E., & Wallace, C. S. (1987). Experience and brain development. *Child Development, 58*(3), 539–559. https://doi.org/10.2307/1130197

Greenough, W. T., & Chang, F. F. (1989). Plasticity of synapse structure and pattern in the cerebral cortex. In S. Peters & E. G. Jones (Eds.), *Cerebral cortex* (Vol. 7, pp. 391–440). Plenum Press.

Hair, N. L., Hanson, J. L., Wolfe, B. L., & Pollak, S. D. (2015). Association of child poverty, brain development, and academic achievement. *JAMA Pediatrics, 169*(9), 822–829. https://doi.org/10.1001/jamapediatrics.2015.1475

Johnson, C. P., & Blasco, P. A. (1997). Infant growth and development. *Pediatrics in Review, 18*(7), 224–242. https://doi.org/10.1542/pir.18-7-224

Johnson, M. H., Jones, E. J., & Gliga, T. (2015). Brain adaptation and alternative developmental trajectories. *Development and Psychopathology, 27*(2), 425–442. https://doi.org/10.1017/S0954579415000073

Keunen, K., Benders, M. J., Leemans, A., Fieret-Van Stam, P. C., Scholtens, L. H., Viergever, M. A., Kahn, R. S., Groenendaal, F., de Vries, L. S., & van den Heuvel, M. P. (2017). White matter maturation in the neonatal brain is predictive of school age cognitive capacities in children born very preterm. *Developmental Medicine & Child Neurology, 59*(9), 939–946. https://doi.org/10.1111/dmcn.13487

Kilbride, H. W., Aylward, G. P., & Carter, B. (2018). What are we measuring as outcome? Looking beyond neurodevelopmental impairment. *Clinics in Perinatology, 45*(3), 467–484. https://doi.org/10.1016/j.clp.2018.05.008

Kiss, J. Z., Vasung, L., & Petrenko, V. (2014). Process of cortical network formation and impact of early brain damage. *Current Opinion in Neurology, 27*(2), 133–141. https://doi.org/10.1097/WCO.0000000000000068

Kolb, B., Harker, A., & Gibb, R. (2017). Principles of plasticity in the developing brain. *Developmental Medicine & Child Neurology, 59*(12), 1218–1223. https://doi.org/10.1111/dmcn.13546

Kraybill, J. H., Kim-Spoon, J., & Bell, M. A. (2019). Infant attention and age 3 executive function.

The Yale Journal of Biology and Medicine, 92(1), 3–11.

Landa, R. J. (2018). Efficacy of early interventions for infants and young children with, and at risk for, autism spectrum disorders. *International Review of Psychiatry, 30*(1), 25–39. https://doi.org/10.1080/09540261.2018.1432574

Lane, A. C., & Aylward, G. P. (2020). The Bayley-4 on Q-global. In G. P. Aylward (Ed.), *Bayley-4: Clinical use and interpretation* (pp. 113–135). Academic Press. https://doi.org/10.1016/B978-0-12-817754-9.00012-X

Laptook, A. R. (2016). Birth asphyxia and hypoxic-ischemic brain injury in the preterm infant. *Clinics in perinatology, 43*(3), 529–545. https://doi.org/10.1016/j.clp.2016.04.010

Li, P., Legault, J., & Litcofsky, K. A. (2014). Neuroplasticity as a function of second language learning: Anatomical changes in the human brain. *Cortex, 58*, 301–324. https://doi.org/10.1016/j.cortex.2014.05.001

Lipkin, P. H., Macias, M. M., & Council on Children With Disabilities, Section on Developmental and Behavioral Pediatrics. (2020). Promoting optimal development: Identifying infants and young children with developmental disorders through developmental surveillance and screening. *Pediatrics, 145*(1), e20193449. https://doi.org/10.1542/peds.2019-3449

Lowe, J., Bann, C. M., Fuller, J., Vohr, B. R., Hintz, S. R., Das, A., Higgins, R. D., Watterberg, K. L., & the SUPPORT Study Group of the Eunice Kennedy Shriver National Institute of Child Health and Human Development Neonatal Research Network. (2020). Early working memory is a significant predictor of verbal and processing skills at 6–7 years in children born extremely preterm. *Early Human Development, 147*, 105083. https://doi.org/10.1016/j.earlhumdev.2020.105083

Lynn, R. (2009). What has caused the Flynn effect? Secular increases in the developmental quotients of infants. *Intelligence, 37*(1), 16–24. https://doi.org/10.1016/j.intell.2008.07.008

Macy, M., Bagnato, S. J., Macy, R. S., & Salaway, J. (2015). Conventional tests and testing for early identification eligibility. *Infants & Young Children, 28*(2), 182–204. https://doi.org/10.1097/IYC.0000000000000032

Marks, K., Glascoe, F. P., Aylward, G. P., Shevell, M. I., Lipkin, P. H., & Squires, J. K. (2008). The thorny nature of predictive validity studies on screening tests for developmental-behavioral problems. *Pediatrics, 122*(4), 866–868. https://doi.org/10.1542/peds.2007-3142

Radesky, J. S., Carta, J., & Bair-Merritt, M. (2016). The 30 million word gap: Relevance for pediatrics. *JAMA Pediatrics, 170*(9), 825–826. https://doi.org/10.1001/jamapediatrics.2016.1486

Rosenberg, S. A., Robinson, C. C., Shaw, E. F., & Ellison, M. C. (2013). Part C early intervention for infants and toddlers: Percentage eligible versus served. *Pediatrics, 131*(1), 38–46. https://doi.org/10.1542/peds.2012-1662

Sheldrick, R. C., & Perrin, E. C. (2013). Evidence-based milestones for surveillance of cognitive, language, and motor development. *Academic Pediatrics, 13*(6), 577–586. https://doi.org/10.1016/j.acap.2013.07.001

Sheldrick, R. C., Schlichting, L. E., Berger, B., Clyne, A., Ni, P., Perrin, E. C., & Vivier, P. M. (2019). Establishing new norms for developmental milestones. *Pediatrics, 144*(6), e20190374. https://doi.org/10.1542/peds.2019-0374

Shonkoff, J. P. (2016). Capitalizing on advances in science to reduce the health consequences of early childhood adversity. *JAMA Pediatrics, 170*(10), 1003–1007. https://doi.org/10.1001/jamapediatrics.2016.1559

Shonkoff, J. P., & Hauser-Cram, P. (1987). Early intervention for disabled infants and their families: A quantitative analysis. *Pediatrics, 80*(5), 650–658. https://doi.org/10.1542/peds.80.5.650

Šimundić, A. M. (2009). Measures of diagnostic accuracy: Basic definitions. *EJIFCC: The Electronic Journal of the International Federation of Clinical Chemistry and Laboratory Medicine, 19*(4), 203–211.

Straathof, E. J. M., Heineman, K. R., Hamer, E. G., & Hadders-Algra, M. (2021). Patterns of atypical muscle tone in the general infant population—Prevalence and associations with perinatal risk and neurodevelopmental status. *Early Human Development, 152*, 105276. https://doi.org/10.1016/j.earlhumdev.2020.105276

Trahan, L. H., Stuebing, K. K., Fletcher, J. M., & Hiscock, M. (2014). The Flynn effect: A meta-analysis. *Psychological Bulletin, 140*(5), 1332–1360. https://doi.org/10.1037/a0037173

Volpe, J. J. (2009). Brain injury in premature infants: A complex amalgam of destructive and developmental disturbances. *The Lancet Neurology, 8*(1), 110–124. https://doi.org/10.1016/S1474-4422(08)70294-1

Willett, S. (2018). Developmental care in the nursery. In H. Needelman & B. J. Jackson (Eds.), *Follow-up for NICU graduates. Promoting positive developmental and behavioral outcome for at-risk infants* (pp. 15–58). Springer. https://doi.org/10.1007/978-3-319-73275-6_2

Wilson-Ching, M., Pascoe, L., Doyle, L. W., & Anderson, P. J. (2014). Effects of correcting for prematurity on cognitive test scores in childhood. *Journal of Paediatrics and Child Health*, *50*(3), 182–188. https://doi.org/10.1111/jpc.12475

Wocadlo, C., & Rieger, I. (2000). Very preterm children who do not cooperate with assessments at three years of age: Skill differences at five years. *Journal of Developmental and Behavioral Pediatrics*, *21*(2), 107–113. https://doi.org/10.1097/00004703-200004000-00004

Wolraich, M. L., Felice, M. E., & Drotar, D. (1996). *The classification of child and adolescent mental diagnoses in primary care* (DSM-PC). American Academy of Pediatrics.

Zubler, J. M., Wiggins, L. D., Macias, M. M., Whitaker, T. M., Shaw, J. S., Squires, J. K., Pajek, J. A., Wolf, R. B., Slaughter, K. S., Broughton, A. S., Gerndt, K. L., Mlodoch, B. J., & Lipkin, P. H. (2022). Evidence-informed milestones for developmental surveillance tools. *Pediatrics*, *149*(3), 1–29. https://doi.org/10.1542/peds.2021-052138

CHAPTER 26

LEARNING, COGNITION, AND INTELLECTUAL AND LEARNING DISORDERS—EVALUATION AND MANAGEMENT IN PEDIATRIC SETTINGS

Danielle N. Shapiro and Jennifer C. Gidley Larson

Intellectual disability (ID) and specific learning disorders (SLDs) constitute significant public health problems. Because these conditions are generally diagnosed in childhood, have broad implications for multiple aspects of individuals' functioning across the lifespan, and benefit from an interdisciplinary approach combining educational, psychological, medical, and developmental perspectives, professionals interested in development must be familiar with these disorders. This chapter aims to provide a broad background in the conceptualization, diagnosis, course, assessment, and treatment of ID and SLD.

Specifically, the chapter will cover the following areas:

- Historical overview of the constructs of intellect and learning
- The current definitions and diagnostic criteria for ID and SLD
- The epidemiology of ID and SLD
- Determinants of risk and resilience for ID and SLD
- Assessment of intellect and learning
- Intervention in clinical practice, including the role of pediatricians, developmental-behavioral pediatricians, and neuropsychologists
- Resources for professionals and families

HISTORICAL OVERVIEW OF INTELLECTUAL DISABILITY

Historically, individuals with learning and cognitive differences—particularly those with moderate to severe ID—were explicitly marginalized and separated from society, sometimes in institutional settings with unhealthy, unsafe, and understimulating conditions. In the late 19th and early 20th centuries, increased scientific interest in disorders of cognition coupled with educational initiatives targeting people with diverse educational needs prompted greater delineation of patterns of intellectual difficulties (Sattler, 2001). More specifically, at the request of the French government, Alfred Binet, Victor Henri, and Theodore Simon developed the 1905 Binet-Simon Scales to measure higher-order mental processes, which would later be recognized as the first intelligence test. Tests proliferated in other areas of Europe and in the United States in the years that followed. While there were regional differences in the approach to measuring intellect and learning, the principles underlying intellectual assessment were consistent and emphasized the following underlying functions: sensation, attention, perception, association, and memory (Sattler, 2001). In 1916, Terman published the Stanford Revision

https://doi.org/10.1037/0000414-026
APA Handbook of Pediatric Psychology, Developmental-Behavioral Pediatrics, and Developmental Science: Vol. 2. Pediatric Psychology and Developmental-Behavioral Pediatrics: Clinical Applications of Developmental Science, P. E. Shah and M. H. Bornstein (Editors-in-Chief)
Copyright © 2025 by the American Psychological Association. All rights reserved.

and Extension of the Binet-Simon Scale, which featured standardization by age and introduced the intelligence quotient (IQ). In the late 1930s, the Wechsler-Bellevue Intelligence Scale, Form 1, was published and, after several iterations and modifications, it eventually transitioned into what is more commonly known as the Wechsler Scales of Intelligence. The Wechsler scales remain some of the most widely used tests of intelligence for children and adults today (see Danforth et al., 2010; Sattler, 2001; Wechsler, 1981). With the development of these tools, the construct of a clinically significant impairment in cognition emerged.

Conceptualizations of ID have evolved over time. Impairment in intellect has had numerous labels, many of which either contemporaneously had, or evolved to have, a pejorative meaning, including such terms as *feeblemindedness*, *moron*, *idiot*, *imbecile*, *mentally deficient* or *slow*, *mentally challenged*, and *mental retardation* (Schalock et al., 2007). Mental retardation was the predominant term used throughout much of the 20th century. However, due to persisting stigma and its pejorative use, combined with the impact of the disability movement and shift to a socioecological concept of disability (i.e., the fit of the person within their context/environment), the term "intellectual disability" emerged in the early 21st century (Schalock, 2011). *Intellectual disability* is the diagnostic term used in the fifth edition of the *Diagnostic and Statistical Manual of Mental Disorders* (*DSM-5*; American Psychiatric Association, 2013), which is the most recent version of this diagnostic manual. Notably, the World Health Organization's (2019) *International Classification of Diseases* (*ICD*) proposed that "mental retardation" be replaced with "disorder of intellectual development" in the recently updated 11th revision (*ICD-11*; initially released in 2019 and most recently updated in 2024; see Zigic et al., 2023). The term *cognitive impairment* is frequently used interchangeably with ID; however, cognitive impairment is not a diagnostic term and reflects more broad-based impairments in cognitive processes including, but not limited to, attention, visuospatial skills, memory, executive functions, and processing speed. For example, an individual with traumatic brain injury or stroke may have cognitive impairments, but not necessarily meet criteria for ID.

Conceptually, the construct of mental retardation (hereafter, intellectual disability) was originally derived from a discrepancy between one's chronological age and mental age on intelligence tests, literally reflecting slowed or "retarded" mental growth (Schalock, 2011; Wehmeyer et al., 2008). This construct failed to appreciate the relation between a person's functional capacity and his/her environmental context (what is referred to as a socioecological framework). In the 1950s, the medical field shifted from emphasizing only intellectual/mental functioning to include social competency/adjustment, adaptability to the environment, management of daily life skills, learning, and maturation. These factors were eventually operationalized under the construct of "adaptive behaviors/adaptive functioning" (Schalock, 2011). In 1959 Heber introduced the "dual-criterion approach," which conceptualized ID as the combination of impaired intellectual functioning and impaired adaptive functioning and included an age-of-onset criterion (Heber, 1959; Tassé et al., 2012). This approach emphasizes a multidimensional understanding of human functioning and is the foundation of the current diagnosis of ID, which shifts the emphasis from a "defect," internal to a person (i.e., mental retardation), to an incongruence between a person's capacity and the demands of their environment.

HISTORICAL OVERVIEW OF SPECIFIC LEARNING DISORDER

Complementary to these developments in our general understanding of intellectual functioning, and as testing became more sophisticated in the late 19th century, there was a shift from recognition of general deficits in cognition to identification of more specific deficits in functioning, including in domain-specific learning. For example, in 1877 Adolf Kussmaul described a patient as being unable to read in the context of intact intellectual and perceptual skills (Matteson & Kluge, 2003). Shortly thereafter, the term "dyslexia" was coined by Rudolf Berlin to describe reading difficulties associated with a neurological basis despite intact visual acuity and language skills (Anderson & Meier-Hedde, 2001; Kirby, 2020). The broader early construct of what later came to be called SLD emerged out of research on institutionalized children with perinatal brain injury in the 1930s and 1940s in which a distinction was made between those who had more general mental impairment and those with specific learning difficulties in the absence of general impairment. In 1960, Samuel Kirk introduced the term "learning disabilities" to describe children who had difficulties in the development of language, speech, reading, and communication skills but without primary sensory impairment or generalized cognitive impairment (Danforth et al., 2010). Recognition of the construct of learning disabilities by parents and educators gained momentum in the 1960's and 1970's, and eventually, the definition was broadened to recognize specific impairments in reading, math, and written expression.

As recognition of learning disabilities continued to gain momentum in the 1970s, advocacy efforts emerged resulting in protections for individuals with disabilities and special education services for children. First, Congress passed the Rehabilitation Act of 1973 (public law 93-112), Section 504 of which states that individuals with disabilities cannot be excluded from, or subjected to discrimination within, any program receiving federal financing, including public schools. Shortly thereafter, the Education for All Handicapped Children Act of 1975 was passed, which ensured a free, appropriate public education (FAPE) for all students, protection for students with disabilities and their families, and financial assistance to states to provide these services. This law has been amended numerous times, and in its 1990 reauthorization it was renamed the Individuals With Disabilities Education Act (IDEA; IDEA, 2024; Yell et al., 2017). Since its most recent reauthorization in 2004, the IDEA has continued to be revised, most recently in 2017 (IDEA, 2024). It is enforced by the U.S. Department of Education, Office of Special Education, and currently upholds and protects the rights of infants through young adults with disabilities, guaranteeing FAPE in the least restrictive environment through access to early intervention services, evaluation, goal attainment monitoring, and transition planning. At this time, 14.1% of youth ages 3 to 21 receive services under IDEA (National Center for Education Statistics, 2023).

DEFINITIONS: INTELLECTUAL DISABILITY

Intellectual disability as currently conceptualized involves two basic elements: low intellectual ability, as measured on standardized tests, and low adaptive functioning. *Adaptive functioning* is defined as the collection of learned skills that enable people to function in their everyday environment as expected based on their age and cultural context. Factor analyses have consistently identified four adaptive factors/domains: (a) *motor/physical competence*, including basic fine and gross motor skills; (b) *conceptual skills*, including functional academics and communication; (c) *social skills*, including interpersonal social communication, social problem solving, and empathy; and (d) *practical skills*, including community use, home living, and activities of daily living such as bathing, grooming, transferring, and so on. Motor/physical competence is considered a relevant factor only in young children (i.e., under 9 years old; see Schalock, 1999; Tassé et al., 2012). Together this collection of skills allows an individual to function adequately within their expected environments including, home, work, school, community, and social context.

The *DSM-5* (American Psychiatric Association, 2013) categorizes ID as a neurodevelopmental disorder beginning in childhood, meaning that impairment should be present prior to age 18, though recent literature highlighting continued brain development into the early 20s has suggested that it may be more appropriate to extend the diagnostic period to age 22 (Giedd et al., 1999; Schalock et al., 2021). Because by definition symptoms of ID emerge in childhood, ID is often diagnosed in children who have previously been identified as delayed. While there is no lower age limit at which ID can be diagnosed, it is often conceptualized as an evolution of the diagnosis of global developmental delay (GDD), which is a diagnostic term reserved for children under 5. GDD is diagnosed in young children who are unable to undergo systematic assessment of functioning due to their age but who do not meet expected developmental milestones across several areas of developmental functioning (e.g., language, motor, or social development).

In addition to onset occurring during the developmental period, a diagnosis of ID requires impairment in both intellectual functioning and adaptive functioning domains. More specifically, intellectual functioning (i.e., IQ) must be at least two standard deviations below the population mean, including a margin for measurement error (i.e., a standard score on a standardized test of 70 ± 5). Likewise, adaptive functioning as reported by informant(s) or the individual (as they are able) must also be at least two standard deviations below the mean when compared to others of similar age and sociocultural background. There must also be sufficient impairment to require ongoing support for the person to function adequately across environments. To meet diagnostic criteria, impairments in adaptive functioning can be in any one of the four domains described previously or in multiple domains. Importantly, ID is distinguishable from other disorders affecting cognition and adaptive functioning because ID is characterized within the context of development rather than as loss of an acquired skill—for example, loss of cognitive function due to dementia or injury. ID does co-occur with other medical and mental health diagnoses including, but not limited to, genetic disorders (see Table 26.1), preterm birth and birth-related complications (e.g., hypoxic-ischemic encephalopathy, cerebral palsy), epilepsy, and autism spectrum disorder (ASD), as well as anxiety and attention deficit/hyperactivity disorder (ADHD; Oeseburg et al., 2011; Schieve et al., 2016). In the *DSM-5*, ID is specified by severity level (i.e., mild, moderate, severe) that reflects the level of supports required due to adaptive functioning needs (see the *DSM-5*, pp. 33–36, for diagnostic criteria [American Psychiatric Association, 2013]).

DEFINITIONS: SPECIFIC LEARNING DISORDERS

Like ID, in the *DSM-5* specific learning disorders (SLDs) are categorized as neurodevelopmental disorders. Importantly, children must have had exposure to an opportunity to develop core academic skills before an SLD can be diagnosed. Therefore, while risk factors for SLD may be

TABLE 26.1

Common Genetic Disorders Associated With Intellectual Disability (ID)

Disorder	Percentage of known ID cases	Base rate in population of live births
Chromosomal aberrations	15%–20%	
Down syndrome (trisomy 21)		1/700
Edwards syndrome (trisomy 18)		1/2,000–6,000
DiGeorge syndrome (22q11 deletion)		1/4,000
X-linked syndromes	10% in males	
Fragile X syndrome		1/4,000 males and 1/8,000 females
Single gene mutations	Unknown	
Prader-Willi syndrome		1/10,000–30,000
Angelman syndrome		1/15,000

identified earlier in development, as outlined below, these disorders should not be diagnosed until a child is school-age. The current diagnostic criteria for SLD include (a) difficulty in at least one core academic area (i.e., reading, spelling, written expression, or math), (b) academic attainment that is below age expectations, (c) learning problems start during the school-age years, and (d) learning problems are not better explained by another condition such as ID. Of note, while an SLD presentation should not be better explained by another condition such as ID, SLD is at times diagnosed in children with ID or another comorbid condition if there is a clear, additional pattern of learning difficulty not fully explained by broader deficits.

Models to Diagnose SLDs

Several key models are used to diagnose SLDs: the low achievement model, the aptitude achievement discrepancy model, and the response to intervention model.

Low achievement model. The *DSM-5* uses a low achievement model to determine the diagnosis of SLDs. In this model, "clinically significant" deficits (definitions of which vary in the literature but generally range from one to two standard deviations below the mean) in academic skills alone are sufficient to render a diagnosis, assuming the lack of a more parsimonious explanation for the deficit, such as inadequate exposure or ID. The low achievement model has the strongest empirical support and best discriminant validity of the current models of SLD. Discriminant validity refers to the degree to which a construct is unrelated to conceptually different constructs. For example, learners with SLDs designated by low achievement differ in patterns of strength and weakness in neurocognitive profiles, patterns of heritability, and neural correlates. However, alternative ways of conceptualizing SLD are common, particularly in school settings (see the response to intervention model).

Aptitude achievement discrepancy model. In the aptitude achievement discrepancy model, a statistically significant discrepancy between scores on measures of verbal or visual-perceptual abilities, and academic testing in the same domain, indicates the presence of a learning disorder. For example, a child with average-range verbal IQ and impaired reading aptitude might be classified as having an SLD in reading. This model has high face validity (i.e., would appear to be valid on the surface), as it stems from the historical conceptualization of SLD as impacting individuals who "should" be able to learn given their cognitive abilities but are unable to do so. However, the aptitude achievement discrepancy model has not held up under empirical scrutiny. Validity studies have highlighted that there is, at most, a very small observable difference on key metrics, such as prognosis, among students with low reading scores who do or do not have a discrepancy with IQ (Fletcher et al., 2005). Similar studies in other academic domains, such as math, have arrived at similar conclusions.

Response to intervention model. Response to intervention (RTI) models are common in the school setting and rely on serial curriculum-based assessments to establish a failure to respond to typical instructional techniques (termed "appropriate instruction") among students with SLD. This model has the advantage of a longitudinal framework, which can account for a student's developmental trajectory, and has been demonstrated to have strong reliability and validity. However, this model is difficult to apply in a clinical setting given the frequent need for follow-up; in school settings, problems arise around how to define "appropriate instruction" and how to differentiate an inadequate versus adequate response to intervention.

Domains of Impairment for SLDs

There are three recognized SLDs—in the domains of reading, written expression/spelling, and mathematics. These are further subdivided. SLD in reading can occur at the level of the word (i.e., dyslexia) or the text (i.e., fluency or reading comprehension). SLD in math includes computational difficulties (i.e., dyscalculia; such as difficulty with arithmetic) and difficulties with problem solving or story problems. SLD in written expression can manifest as problems with transcription or handwriting (i.e., dysgraphia), spelling, or generation of text.

SLD in reading. SLD in reading is the most common SLD, affecting up to 15% of school-age children (Altarac & Saroha, 2007). SLD in reading has two main presentations, with problems occurring at the level of the word or the text. Word-level reading problems, namely dyslexia, are phonologically based and are more commonly diagnosed in younger school-age children (typically by third grade). Essential to word-level reading is an appreciation of the sounds, or phonemes, that make up words. This broad skill can be broken down into multiple subskills including phonemic awareness (identification of phonemes), phonological processing (efficiently hearing, recalling, and reproducing speech sounds), and phonetic decoding (pulling phonemes out of words). The term dyslexia is often colloquially used to describe letter reversals but can include multiple aspects of foundational reading skills including phonemic awareness, phonetic decoding, and/or rapid letter naming. Together, phonological awareness and rapid naming of letters are hypothesized to be the strongest predictors of reading attainment in the early elementary years, and a "double deficit" in these domains is indicative of risk for SLD in reading (Wolf & Bowers, 1999).

Older children are more often diagnosed with a text-level reading learning disability, namely reading fluency or comprehension. These difficulties may evolve from dyslexia and/or may be associated with underlying deficits in vocabulary, listening comprehension, or attention and executive functions. Reading comprehension, in particular, is a complex skill involving phonological (individual sounds) as well as morphological (words) processing, attention, memory, organization, and problem solving or inference. In other words, the reader not only must process linguistic elements of the text but must also sustain attention throughout a passage, organize and accurately recall previously learned context, and distill meaning from individual passages and the text as a whole. Perhaps in part due to these complexities, about 41% of students with SLD in reading have *late-emerging reading disorder*, defined as emerging after the third grade in students who have no previous history of dyslexia (Leach et al., 2003).

SLD in mathematics. SLD in mathematics includes two broad subtypes: dyscalculia (poor computational skills or reduced knowledge of math facts) and math reasoning problems (issues with logic-based problem solving or story problems). SLD in mathematics is often associated with an underlying deficit in phonological decoding and is therefore commonly comorbid with SLD in reading. Attainment in mathematics has also been linked with working memory, attention, basic numeracy concepts (e.g., concepts of quantity or size), and visual-spatial skills, although these associations are generally weaker than those observed in the dyslexia literature.

SLD in written expression. SLD in written expression may be characterized by deficits in transcription (dysgraphia), spelling, mechanics, and/or text generation. Dysgraphia is defined as impairments in legible, automatic letter writing and typically results from fine motor impairment. Dysgraphia may contribute to reduced text generation, as writing is often laborious, but it is phenotypically distinct from writing problems based in language deficits. Deficits in spelling are often associated with a primary deficit in phonological processing and are commonly comorbid with SLD in reading. Individuals with SLD in written expression may also struggle with the organization and generation of text, including poor mechanics (grammar, punctuation), organization, or clarity. Problems generating the content of the text are commonly associated with underlying language or executive impairments.

EPIDEMIOLOGY AND PREVALENCE

Epidemiology of Intellectual Disability

Worldwide, the prevalence of ID is about 1% to 3%, although low- and middle-income countries have prevalence rates almost two times that of high-income countries (Maulik et al., 2011). Of those classified with ID, approximately 85% have mild cases, 10% moderate, 3% to 4% severe, and 1% to 2% have profound impairment (Harris, 2006). There is a greater prevalence of ID in older school-aged children and adolescents than in younger children, and a 1.5 times greater prevalence of ID in males than in females across all age groups (Harris, 2006; Maulik et al., 2011), likely reflecting gender differences in genetic risk factors. In the literature, ID is associated with other sociodemographic factors, including population setting, access to services, socioeconomic status (SES), and maternal characteristics such as maternal diabetes during pregnancy, pregnancy hypertension, infection, placenta previa, and antepartum hemorrhage, as well as study factors such as sampling strategy or diagnostic tool used (Harris, 2006; Langridge et al., 2013; Maulik et al., 2011).

Within the United States, similar rates of ID were reported in a National Health Interview Survey conducted between 2014 and 2016 with an overall prevalence rate of 1.3% to 1.6% for boys and 0.9% for girls. The prevalence of an ID diagnosis does not differ significantly by ethnicity (Zablotsky et al., 2017).

Epidemiology of Learning Disorders

Worldwide, learning disorders impact millions of children, although prevalence estimates across countries vary widely (Al-Yagon et al., 2013). These disparities most likely reflect differences in criteria but also potentially reflect differences in education and other socioeconomic factors. Using data from the National Survey of Children's Health, the lifetime prevalence of learning disorder diagnosis among children in the United States is nearly 10% (Altarac & Saroha, 2007). Within the United States, prevalence was higher among boys, children in poverty, and children of parents with a high school education or less (Altarac & Saroha, 2007).

Depending on the definition applied in individual studies, reading disorders affect 5% to 10% of the population (Siegel, 2006). Gender differences have been identified in risk for SLD in reading, but these differences appear to be small and are unlikely to be clinically significant. For example, one epidemiological study found a small gender difference in the number of elementary-age children diagnosed with dyslexia, a difference largely explained by a substantial referral bias for boys (Shaywitz et al., 1992).

Similar problems around inclusion criteria impact studies aimed at identifying the prevalence of learning disorders in written expression and mathematics. Depending on the model used, SLD in written expression has been found to impact 8% to 15% of students (Lyon, 1996). A prospective study of elementary school students ($N = 2,241$) found that 5.7% of students met the criteria for SLD in mathematics on standardized tests (Morsanyi et al., 2018). The literature has not found a consistent or significant gender difference in risk for SLD in mathematics, although SLD in mathematics has been found to be more common in children with language difficulties or social-emotional concerns, such as ADHD or autism (Morsanyi et al., 2018).

RISK AND RESILIENCE IN INTELLECTUAL DISABILITY

Etiology is unknown for nearly half of the identified cases of ID. When etiology is known, risk can be differentiated broadly into genetic and nongenetic factors.

Genetic and Nongenetic Risk Factors for Intellectual Disability

Genetic factors linked to ID are thought to account for 30% to 50% of known ID cases (L. Kaufman et al., 2010). Research on human genetics over the past decade has identified around 750 genes linked to ID, which include chromosomal aberrations (e.g., aneuploidies), single-gene mutations (e.g., Fragile X, Prader-Willi; see Table 26.1), as well as inherited genetic traits (L. Kaufman et al., 2010; Kochinke et al., 2016). Although the heritability of ID among families was historically thought to be high, research on mixed nonconsanguineous families has found that 75% of genetic causes of ID are *de novo* or suspected *de novo* (Järvelä et al., 2021). This pattern is even more pronounced for cases of severe ID (see Reichenberg et al., 2016).

Nongenetic causes of ID are thought to fall into the following categories: prenatal, perinatal, and postnatal. A meta-analysis identified the following prenatal risk factors for ID: advanced maternal age, African American maternal ethnicity, low maternal education, third or more parity (i.e., previously delivered fetus), maternal alcohol/tobacco use during pregnancy, and maternal pre-existing health conditions, including diabetes, hypertension, and asthma (Huang et al., 2016). Perinatal and neonatal risk factors include birth injury, such as hypoxic-ischemic encephalopathy, preterm birth, and postterm birth, although the latter has shown a weaker correlation with cognitive outcome (Heuvelman et al., 2018). Postnatal causes and risk factors include infection, systemic illness, exposure to toxins, neurometabolic processes, and acquired or traumatic brain injury.

Ecological/Sociodemographic Risk Factors Associated With Intellectual Disability

Sociodemographic factors, although not a direct cause of ID, are correlated with the diagnosis of ID and can exacerbate ID presentation or borderline ID symptoms. Sociodemographic factors include social and emotional deprivation (i.e., inadequate or inconsistent interpersonal attachments), early home environment (i.e., stimulation deficiency), low parent education, SES, and malnutrition (Cicek et al., 2020). These factors seem to be most associated with less severe forms of ID and reflect environmental risks and determinants that can contribute to less-than-optimal brain development, likely through poorer access to resources and interventions. Research also indicates that individuals with ID have an increased risk of experiencing adversity during their lifetime. When they occur during childhood, adverse experiences have been found to be a better predictor of poor physical health and illness, and increased psychiatric, emotional, and conduct problems in those with ID when compared to those without ID (Scheffers et al., 2020).

Life expectancy among individuals with mild ID is similar to that of typically developing peers; however, those with moderate to severe ID have 16.5% to 75% higher rates of chronic physical and mental health conditions, leading to lower life expectancy (Cicek et al., 2020). Individuals with ID also have a disproportionate rate of comorbid psychiatric illness (Einfeld et al., 2011).

Ecological/Sociocultural Factors Associated With Resilience in Intellectual Disability

While the literature on resiliency in ID is relatively new and sparse, individuals with ID who have access to educational, social, and mental health services may experience improved outcomes including higher functional independence and well-being (Crnic et al., 2017). Scheffers et al. (2020) identified internal (i.e., autonomy, self-acceptance, and physical health) and external (i.e., supportive social network and daily activities) sources of resilience in individuals with ID, many of which are modifiable and may serve as points of intervention to improve quality of life in individuals with ID. Importantly, children are part of a dynamic family system, and parents of children with ID report higher levels of stress than do parents of typically developing children. Early intervention, including parent training and support for positive parent coping, can promote family well-being and more positive outcomes in children with ID (Crnic et al., 2017).

RISK AND RESILIENCE IN SPECIFIC LEARNING DISORDERS

Etiology of SLDs is multifactorial and includes genetic, developmental, and environmental factors.

Genetic and Nongenetic Risk Factors for Specific Learning Disorders

Twin and family studies suggest that reading disorders are moderately heritable. A meta-analysis of studies on familial patterns of risk for SLD found a 34% to 53% prevalence among children with an affected first-degree relative, depending on the threshold used for diagnosis (Snowling & Melby-Lervåg, 2016). Meta-analyses of twin studies have found that upwards of 50% of the variance in reading achievement is attributable to genetics (Grigorenko, 2005). The research literature on the genetics of SLD in mathematics and written expression is smaller but has also suggested that heritability is a significant risk factor (Fletcher & Grigorenko, 2017). As has been found in studies on other neurodevelopmental disorders, such as ADHD and ASD, the impact of genetics on academic achievement is more pronounced among individuals with more severe SLD symptoms (Fletcher & Grigorenko, 2017). Learning disorders are also more common in children with certain genetic disorders (see Table 26.2).

Most studies examining the neuropathology of SLDs have focused on reading. Functional neuroimaging studies have identified a network of regions in the left hemisphere that appears to develop in response to exposure to printed text and has been associated with achievement in reading (Fletcher & Grigorenko, 2017). This network links a ventral stream (occipital and posterior temporal lobes; associated with visual processing of written text), dorsal stream (temporal and temporal-parietal regions; involved with lexicon and word meaning), and the inferior frontal lobe (Fletcher & Grigorenko, 2017). This network has been linked with risk for dyslexia in both English and non-English speakers, such as Italian speakers who, because of the orthographic features of the Italian language, are generally thought to be at lower risk for SLD in reading (Paulesu et al., 2001). Even preverbal infants with a genetic risk for SLD in reading have been found to have differences in functional magnetic resonance imaging studies, as well as behavioral differences such as requiring longer to categorize speech sounds (Lyytinen et al., 2003).

Diffusion tensor imaging research has identified white matter tracts that appear to be of particular relevance to number sense and math abilities. Among individuals with SLDs in math, white matter abnormalities have been observed in the inferior parietal and temporal lobes (Matejko & Ansari, 2015). Very little imaging research has been focused on written expression, specifically, although neural substrates are thought to overlap with other language-based skills including reading.

General cognitive abilities (e.g., IQ) are by definition not associated with SLD, but certain developmental and cognitive factors may confer risk for SLD. Children who have other neurodevelopmental diagnoses, such as language delay and ADHD, are at an increased risk for SLDs, as indicated by a higher comorbidity among these conditions than would be expected from the base rates of the conditions alone (Willcutt & Pennington, 2000). Overlap between SLDs and other conditions points to a shared underlying set of risks (Fletcher & Grigorenko, 2017). For example, underlying deficits in processing speed and working memory contribute to symptoms of ADHD and SLD and may help to account for the high comorbidity between these conditions (Willcutt & Pennington, 2000). Among children with ADHD, treatment for ADHD symptoms may reduce the risk of developing an SLD and, in children with comorbid ADHD and SLD, treatment of ADHD may improve academic performance. For example, methylphenidate therapy has been linked with improved reading scores in a clinical trial of children with comorbid ADHD and SLD in reading (Keulers et al., 2007). A meta-analysis revealed that treatment with methylphenidate was associated with small but consistent improvements in math and reading fluency (Kortekaas-Rijlaarsdam et al., 2019).

Similarly, treatment of developmental speech and language disorders in the toddler and preschool years may decrease the risk for SLD in reading in elementary school. As outlined below, prior to the school-age period, it is not possible to assess specific domains of learning in a valid and

TABLE 26.2

Genetic Disorders Associated With Specific Learning Disorder (SLD) Profiles

Disorder	Common SLD profile
Neurofibromatosis Type 1	SLD in reading, mathematics, and/or written expression
Williams syndrome	SLD in mathematics
22q11.2 deletion syndrome	SLD in mathematics
Klinefelter syndrome	SLD in reading
Turner syndrome	SLD in mathematics

reliable way, and therefore children are not diagnosed with SLD prior to school entry. However, young children may be identified as being at an increased risk for SLD based on family history of learning disorders or speech and language impairments, which have been linked to later difficulties in reading acquisition (Gallagher et al., 2000). Early articulation, expressive language, and letter knowledge predict reading outcomes and may be especially important targets for preventing SLDs among at-risk children (Gallagher et al., 2000).

Ecological and Sociodemographic Risk Factors Associated With Specific Learning Disorders

Environmental factors also predict risk for diagnosis of an SLD. In a large, epidemiological sample, poverty, as well as multiple other markers of SES such as parents' education, family structure (one-parent household), and presence of a smoker in the home, were associated with an increased risk for an SLD (Altarac & Saroha, 2007). A link was also found between risk for SLD and parenting style. For example, parents who reported higher aggravation and reduced tendency to discuss conflicts calmly were more likely to have children with an SLD. These associations raise the question of the extent to which SLDs, and low academic attainment in general, reflect differences in underlying cognitive factors versus differences in exposure and opportunity for learning. They also suggest avenues for promoting resilience against SLD, such as parent training and programs to address food and housing insecurity (Bigelow, 2006).

As is true for ID, individuals with SLD are at an increased risk for psychological, behavioral, and social problems. Children with SLD have increased rates of mood/anxiety disorders, conduct problems, and are more likely to be the targets and perpetrators of bullying (Alexander-Passe, 2008; Turunen et al., 2021). These comorbidities reflect the psychological toll of learning problems and the importance of identifying and pursuing modifiable pathways to resilience. Helping children to understand and contextualize their learning difficulties, effective educational intervention, and promotion of family and individual coping are all important strategies to reduce the educational and psychological impact of SLDs. The earlier the better for these interventions (Fricke et al., 2013), highlighting the importance of identifying potential risks as early as possible and ideally prior to the start of formal education.

ASSESSMENT OF INTELLECT AND ACADEMIC ATTAINMENT

The Role of General Pediatricians and Developmental-Behavioral Pediatricians

General pediatricians survey and screen development throughout infancy and childhood during planned well-child visits, which are an excellent opportunity for early identification of developmental deviations (Lipkin et al., 2020). Starting at age 4 or 5, well-child visits include questions about learning and academic performance and should ideally include feedback from child care providers and/or teachers (Lipkin et al., 2020). Health care providers may suspect a learning or cognitive concern when parents report that their child has one or more of the following challenges: difficulty with learning, either in general or in a specific area; unexplained low academic attainment despite intervention and/or repeated practice or exposure; or unexplained or sudden behavioral or emotional problems at school. When a specific learning disorder or ID is suspected, a formal evaluation is the first step toward clarifying the diagnosis and potential interventions. For children with uncomplicated SLD or ID, such as when there is not a suspected comorbid ADHD or underlying medical process that would complicate interpretation or impact diagnosis (e.g., epilepsy, brain injury, etc.), a school-based evaluation will typically provide a good assessment of intellectual and learning abilities and needs.

For children with learning difficulties and a suspected dual diagnosis (e.g., when there is a suspected comorbid ADHD, ASD, or underlying medical process that would complicate interpretation or impact diagnosis), a referral to a developmental-behavioral pediatrician may be helpful in the evaluation process. Developmental-behavioral pediatricians may also serve as a resource for families to help contextualize psychoeducational testing results performed through the school system within a child's broader medical and behavioral history. They can also help to facilitate referrals for further evaluation or to appropriate therapies. Relatedly, developmental-behavioral pediatricians can help evaluate for the medical comorbidities associated with ID and SLD and make appropriate referrals to other subspecialists as indicated.

The Role of the School System in the Evaluation of Intellectual and Academic Attainment

Parents can request through their child's school that their children be evaluated for an individualized education program (IEP), which will typically include a formal assessment of learning and identification of a need for special education support. IEPs are provided through IDEA. As an alternative to an IEP, schools may also offer to provide services through a 504 plan (as provided by Section 504 of the Rehabilitation Act of 1973). Both IEP's and 504 plans provide accommodations and support to students with disabilities, though 504 plans adopt a looser definition of disabilities and, in line with the objectives of the Rehabilitation Act of 1973, aim to reduce discrimination against people with disabilities. As such, while IEPs provide special education services to ensure FAPE, 504 plans aim to remove barriers for students with disabilities. In other words, students do not receive special education under 504 plans. All public schools, including public charters, are required by federal law to be compliant with IDEA and Section 504 of the Rehabilitation Act of 1973 and therefore provide IEPs and 504 plans as necessary. Unlike students in public schools, students whose parents decide to place them in private schools or homeschool them are not entitled to FAPE, although certain services such as therapies may be available through nonpublic service learning plans. To request an evaluation for an IEP or 504 plan, parents can generally contact the counselor or special education coordinator at their child's school or, alternatively, directly contact the intermediate school district. School staff will then talk parents through the IEP evaluation, determination, and if warranted, implementation processes.

The Role of Neuropsychologists in the Evaluation of Intellectual and Academic Attainment

A medical neuropsychological evaluation may be justified if school testing is inconclusive or there are additional suspected contributing factors relevant to cognitive concerns, including medical or behavioral comorbidities. A medical neuropsychological evaluation is informed by an appreciation for brain-behavior relationships and can provide broader contextual and diagnostic information. These evaluations are completed by a clinical neuropsychologist, typically outside of the school setting.

Whether psychoeducational or neuropsychological, evaluation of intellect and learning includes a few basic components: intellect, adaptive functioning, and academic achievement. Common instruments used to evaluate these domains are described in Table 26.3. Tests have relative strengths and weaknesses that make them more or less appropriate in a given situation. In general, a strong instrument will have established normative data, including demographic properties matching the child being tested, good sensitivity (the test's ability to accurately identify positive cases) and specificity (the test's ability to accurately identify negative cases) for the population of interest, and demonstrated reliability and validity. Examiners should have specific training in test administration and interpretation and conduct tests in a standardized setting using standardized procedures as described in manuals accompanying the tests.

Each of the measures described in Table 26.3 is comprised of multiple subtests that in turn comprise index scores that then comprise a composite score. Subtests and index scores aim to measure different aspects of the underlying dimension, such as intellect. Generally speaking,

TABLE 26.3

Common Intellectual, Academic Achievement, and Adaptive Measures

Domain	Instrument	Current edition	Age range	Format
Intellect	Wechsler Preschool and Primary Scale of Intelligence (Wechsler, 2012)	Fourth	2:6–7:7	Direct measure
	Wechsler Intelligence Scale for Children (Wechsler, 2014)	Fifth	6:0–16:11	Direct measure
	Wechsler Adult Intelligence Scale (Wechsler, 2008)	Fourth	16:0–90:11	Direct measure
	Differential Ability Scales (Elliott, 2007)	Second	2:6–17:11	Direct measure
	Woodcock Johnson Tests of Cognitive Abilities (Schrank et al., 2014)	Fourth	2:0–90+	Direct measure
	Stanford-Binet Intelligence Scales (Roid & Pomplun, 2012)	Fifth	2:0–85+	Direct measure
	Leiter International Performance Scale (Roid & Miller, 2013)	Third	3:0–75+	Direct measure
	Test of Nonverbal Intelligence (Brown et al., 2010)	Fourth	6:0–89:11	Direct measure
Academic achievement	Wechsler Individual Achievement Test (Wechsler, 2009)	Third	4:0–50:11	Direct measure
	Kaufman Test of Individual Achievement (A. S. Kaufman & Kaufman, 2014)	Third	4:6–25:11	Direct measure
	Woodcock Johnson Tests of Achievement (Schrank et al., 2014)	Fourth	2:0–90+	Direct measure
	Wide Range Achievement Test (Wilkinson & Robertson, 2017)	Fifth	5:0–94:11	Direct measure
	Bracken Basic Concept Scale (Bracken, 2006)	Third	3:0–6:11	Direct measure
Adaptive functioning	Adaptive Behavior Assessment System (Harrison & Oakland, 2015)	Third	Birth–89:11	Parent/informant/self report
	Vineland Adaptive Behavior Scales (Sparrow et al., 2016)	Third	Birth–89:11	Parent/informant report; interview

Note. Ages are expressed as youngest year:month through oldest year:month.

intellectual tests examine multiple aspects of problem solving such as verbal reasoning, fluid (novel, nonverbal) problem solving, and/or visual-spatial problem solving. Some intellectual tests examine other domains that are highly correlated with general intellect, such as speed of processing, working memory, attention, or aspects of memory.

Psychometric research has indicated that for children, and particularly young children, differentiation between these multiple aspects of problem solving can be somewhat artificial (Watkins & Beaujean, 2014). Reliability of intellectual testing and the nuance with which aspects of cognition can be assessed increase with age. More specifically, neurodevelopmental assessment (birth through 3.5 years) using developmental measures (most commonly the Bayley Scales of Infant Development; Bayley & Aylward, 2019), has been shown to have variable predictive validity for school-aged cognitive abilities, with greater predictive validity in clinical samples (e.g., children with a history of preterm birth) or children with moderate to severe deficits (Bode et al., 2014; Månsson et al., 2019). Likewise, longitudinal research has shown that IQ obtained during the preschool years (i.e., 4 years of age) was moderately correlated ($r = .36$ and $.59$) with IQ at 6 and 7 years respectively. Scores obtained at 7 years of age were a more stable predictor of later IQ ($r = .79$) and those obtained later in elementary school had the greatest predictive validity of IQ at age 23 (Schneider et al., 2014). As is true of early developmental assessments, IQ scores obtained in the preschool period are most stable and predictive in those at the lower end of the IQ distribution (Schneider et al., 2014).

Assessment of adaptive functioning, which is necessary for a diagnosis of ID, is often parent-reported (either via survey or interview) and examines children's independence across conceptual, social, practical, and/or motor domains. Notably, adaptive functioning is a better predictor of functional outcomes in adults with neurodevelopmental disabilities than IQ (Woolf et al., 2010).

While relatively global indicators of reasoning can be assessed during infancy and toddler years, preacademic skills and academic achievement are not usually assessed until at least preschool age because these skills require exposure to develop. Screeners of school readiness assess preacademic skills including mastery of colors and basic shapes, as well as basic alphabetic or numeracy skills, which can identify children who are at risk for learning problems in the preschool period. Assessment of academic achievement typically begins in kindergarten and assesses major domains such as reading, mathematics, and written expression. Assessments may break these domains down further, including evaluating aspects of phonics, reading comprehension, and/or reading fluency, math computation, math fluency, applied math skills, and spelling and the mechanics of writing. Research indicates that in typically developing kindergarteners, the best predictors for SLD in mathematics at grades 2 and 3 include deficits in any or all of the following: reading numbers, number constancy, magnitude judgments of numbers (i.e., is 7 more/less than 3), and mental addition of 1 digit numbers (Mazzocco & Thompson, 2005). Consistent with the "double deficit" model described above, research indicates that for typically developing kindergarteners, the best predictors of reading performance (though not necessarily risk for SLD in reading) at grades 1 and 2 include the following: letter naming, letter sound knowledge, naming speed, and phonological awareness (Schatschneider et al., 2004).

In interpreting and applying psychoeducational or neuropsychological reports, it is important to attend to certain, key information. We recommend first reviewing behavioral observations and validity sections, paying attention to factors that may interfere with interpretation (e.g., inadequate effort, behavioral problems, situational variables that interfered with standard administration, etc.). After establishing that scores are valid, reliance on the psychologist's interpretation if available will generally take into account the psychometric properties of the tests and give a good indication of whether scores are clinically meaningful. A high level of caution is recommended when interpreting scores in the absence of this context.

INTERVENTION IN CLINICAL PRACTICE

A new ID or SLD diagnosis can be overwhelming and scary, and helping families to label and process emotions associated with a diagnosis can facilitate engagement in, and improvement from, interventions. In general, families benefit from concrete next steps and hope. Fortunately, there is good reason to be optimistic. There are multiple, effective interventions for SLD. ID cannot be remediated to the same extent as SLD, but multiple efficacious interventions exist to minimize the behavioral and functional impact of ID.

Interventions Targeting Intellectual Disability

No universally accepted standardized intervention protocol or practice guidelines currently exist for clinical management of ID. There is consensus that the goals of intervention for people with ID should aim to (a) lessen the effects of the disability on day-to-day functioning by optimizing environmental supports and building on skills/strengths of the individual; and (b) prevent or limit further deterioration of functioning, for example, by treating an underlying health condition, if known. Interventions should be put in place as early as possible and should be sustained throughout development, changing as needed to meet the child at their developmental level. For example, supports may focus on developing foundational academic skills in early childhood and later shift to the development of vocational and daily living skills as the child develops.

Whenever possible, intervention should be evidence-based; however, the literature on the clinical effectiveness of treatments and interventions for individuals with ID is limited (see Bhaumik et al., 2011). Individuals with ID often have broad-based deficits, and intervention is often multifaceted. Early intervention may include speech, occupational, or physical therapies. Hearing and vision services may also be important, as a large portion of individuals with moderate to severe ID have comorbid sensory impairment (van den Broek et al., 2006). Access to learning and cognitive assessment and special education services during early childhood can be beneficial for children with ID and are supported under IDEA. A wide range of supports and services may be available through an IEP, ranging from a contained special education environment, paraprofessional support, and therapies (speech, occupational, physical, or behavioral) to supplementary supports like curriculum modifications, extended time, or a reduced homework burden.

Interventions targeting behavior and socioemotional needs are also critical for children and adolescents with ID and typically include family-centered intervention, social skills support and training, and behavioral intervention techniques. For example, the principles of applied behavior analysis (ABA) including token economies have been demonstrated to have clinical utility for individuals with ID (Matson & Boisjoli, 2009). Consultation with a dietitian or feeding specialist can address associated malnutrition, oral aversion, or failure to thrive.

As a child transitions into adolescence, intervention should target functional living, vocational skills, and coordination with adult service agencies. IDEA mandates that transition planning from school to postschool environments be included in an IEP prior to the student turning 16 (IDEA, 2004). As an initial step, there should be a discussion among the student, family, and school personnel to determine which high school track (i.e., high school diploma vs. certificate of completion/alternative certificate) best supports the needs and postsecondary goals of the student. A high school diploma requires that the student meet the state/district standards for high school graduation, while a certificate of completion is an alternative that can be provided to indicate any number of accomplishments, including attendance/completion, achievement, or meeting modified graduation requirements and is given at the discretion of the local districts, but is not a diploma. To be eligible for the certificate track, the student must be receiving services through an IEP. With a certificate of completion, students are eligible to continue to receive special education services after completion of high school through the age of 21 in most states, with a few states extending up through age 25. According to the National Center for Education Statistics (2022), in the 2019–2020 school year, of those served under IDEA who were ages 14–21, about 76% exited with a diploma, 10% exited school with a certificate of completion, 13% dropped out, and 1% aged out of services. Of those individuals with an ID designation on their IEP (8.6% of all IEPs), about 49% exited with a diploma, 34% exited school with a certificate of completion, 11% dropped out, and 5% aged out of services.

Although the IDEA mandate is that transition planning be in place by age 16, research has shown that in "early transition" states where transition services are provided by age 14, individuals with ID were more likely to be employed than peers residing in "late transition" states where transition services are provided by age 16 (Cimera et al., 2017). As such, schools and providers should encourage transition planning in middle school, ideally around age 12, to promote optimal outcomes for individuals with ID (Cooley et al., 2011). In addition to early transition planning, research indicates the following best practices for promoting a successful transition from school to postschool environments: (a) active student, family, and school involvement in transition planning processes; (b) individualized transition plans; (c) vocational educational experiences or opportunities in high school; (d) implementation of a functional curriculum that builds skills for independent living (typically through a certificate of completion program); (e) education inclusion; and (f) intra-agency collaboration (i.e., adult service agencies, community agencies, and local businesses; Park & Bouck, 2018; Povenmire-Kirk et al., 2015; Shogren & Plotner, 2012).

Planning for transition into adulthood should also provide support for parents/caregivers, particularly as they navigate issues like guardianship, conservatorship, and/or power of attorney to ensure that their child/ward has an appropriate level of support and protection based on their functional needs when they turn 18 (see Pivalizza, 2021).

Interventions Targeting Specific Learning Disorder

The idea that SLD can be treated as a clinical problem using a structured therapy has roots in the work of Samuel Orton, who in 1925 first described an intervention for children who struggled to read and were labeled by teachers as "dull, subnormal, or failing or retarded in school work" (Orton, 1925). Since that time, a wide range of interventions has become available, many of which have been systematically studied in large clinical trials. Encouragingly, this body of research has found that interventions contribute to clinically significant improvements in learning, which do not seem to be systematically mitigated by factors such ethnicity, SES, or intellectual ability (Morris et al., 2012).

Across all SLDs, more intensive intervention programs have been found to be more effective. For SLD in reading, and regardless of the level of the reading difficulty, interventions that are explicit, structured, and focused on a specific strategy rather than being "discovery-based" have been found to be the most efficacious, as have interventions that combine multiple strategies into a comprehensive approach toward reading instruction. A meta-analysis conducted by the National Reading Panel found that word-level reading disorders and spelling impairments respond to specific and targeted instruction in phonemic awareness (Eunice Kennedy Shriver National Institute of Child Health and Human Development, 2000). Interventions targeting phonemic awareness take a variety of forms but typically involve repeated and scaffolded instruction, and games for practice, that help learners to more fluently combine and decode phonemes.

The meta-analysis also identified that fluency was improved with techniques that promoted guided practice and speeded reading. The NRP's meta-analysis did not identify a specific approach to address comprehension difficulties but rather indicated that a combination of multiple text-comprehension teaching techniques is most helpful for students with SLD impacting reading comprehension.

Implications for Multidisciplinary Practice

Individuals with SLD and ID benefit from a multidisciplinary, coordinated approach toward assessment and intervention. Professionals in pediatric psychology, developmental-behavioral pediatrics, and developmental science play a critical role in the identification, assessment, and treatment of people with ID and SLD. Given the importance of early identification and intervention, it is especially important for professionals who work with children to know when to refer for educational or neuropsychological assessment. Screening tools, such as the Ages and Stages Questionnaire (Squires & Bricker, 2009), as well as a thorough clinical interview about developmental and academic history can help to determine next steps.

Behavioral and developmental experts then play a critical role in management of symptoms such as attention deficits, coping difficulties, behavioral problems, or social skill concerns that impact functional outcomes and quality of life. As described above, people with SLD and ID area at an increased risk for a mental health conditions such as depression, anxiety, and substance abuse (Alexander-Passe, 2008; Capozzi et al., 2008; Einfeld et al., 2011). Managing behavioral problems and psychological symptoms not only improves coping and adjustment more broadly, but also allows individuals with ID and SLD to take full advantage of educational, vocational, and adaptive interventions.

CONCLUSION

Early identification and intervention are crucial to set the trajectory and maximize the potential for future growth in people with ID or SLD and therefore should be top priorities for providers. Continued monitoring through academic and medical settings and referral for further evaluation as warranted are also key to optimizing development because as children grow, deficits may pose new and unique challenges. With careful, multidisciplinary management including helping children and families to understand and process their emotions related to their children's learning and cognitive differences, children can and generally do learn to manage these differences, leading lives that are rich, happy, and fulfilled.

RESOURCES

Most states have state-funded and/or private organizations aimed at providing support to people with learning disorders or intellectual disabilities (IDs). A selection of the numerous national organizations and government resources are provided here. Families may find support through these resources or through groups organized on social media or other websites.

- American Association on Intellectual and Developmental Disabilities:

  https://www.aaidd.org

  Professional organization for people who work with people with ID with educational and advocacy resources.

- The Arc:

  https://thearc.org

  The Arc has chapters throughout the country and works directly with adults with intellectual disabilities to provide supports that increase independence.

- Center for Parent Information and Resources:

  https://www.parentcenterhub.org

  Repository of webinars, literature, and live events for parents of youth with disabilities.

- National Reading Panel (NRP) Report:

  https://www.nichd.nih.gov/sites/default/files/publications/pubs/nrp/Documents/report.pdf

  Commissioned in 1997 by the federal government, the NRP summarized the literature on reading disorders and interventions.

- Think College:

  https://thinkcollege.net

  National organization dedicated to improve access to higher education options for individuals with ID.

- U.S. Department of Education Individuals With Disabilities Education Act website:

  https://sites.ed.gov/idea

  Information about special education for parents and educators.

- What Works Clearinghouse:

  https://ies.ed.gov/ncee/wwc

  Reviews the scientific literature on academic interventions to help educators and parents make evidence-based decisions.

- Wright's Law:

  https://www.wrightslaw.com/advoc

  Advice for parents on advocating for individualized education programs.

References

Al-Yagon, M., Cavendish, W., Cornoldi, C., Fawcett, A. J., Grünke, M., Hung, L. Y., Jiménez, J. E., Karande, S., van Kraayenoord, C. E., Lucangeli, D., Margalit, M., Montague, M., Sholapurwala, R., Sideridis, G., Tressoldi, P. E., & Vio, C. (2013). The proposed changes for *DSM-5* for SLD and ADHD: International perspectives—Australia, Germany, Greece, India, Israel, Italy, Spain, Taiwan, United Kingdom, and United States. *Journal of Learning Disabilities, 46*(1), 58–72. https://doi.org/10.1177/0022219412464353

Alexander-Passe, N. (2008). The sources and manifestations of stress amongst school-aged dyslexics, compared with sibling controls. *Dyslexia, 14*(4), 291–313. https://doi.org/10.1002/dys.351

Altarac, M., & Saroha, E. (2007). Lifetime prevalence of learning disability among US children. *Pediatrics, 119*(Suppl. 1), S77–S83. https://doi.org/10.1542/peds.2006-2089L

American Psychiatric Association. (2013). *Diagnostic and statistical manual of mental disorders* (5th ed.). https://doi.org/10.1176/appi.books.9780890425596

Anderson, P. L., & Meier-Hedde, R. (2001). Early case reports of dyslexia in the United States and Europe. *Journal of Learning Disabilities, 34*(1), 9–21. https://doi.org/10.1177/002221940103400102

Bayley, N., & Aylward, G. P. (2019). *Bayley scales of infant and toddler development* (4th ed.). NCS Pearson.

Bhaumik, S., Gangadharan, S., Hiremath, A., & Russell, P. S. (2011). Psychological treatments in intellectual disability: The challenges of building a good evidence base. *The British Journal of Psychiatry, 198*(6), 428–430. https://doi.org/10.1192/bjp.bp.110.085084

Bigelow, B. J. (2006). There's an elephant in the room: The impact of early poverty and neglect on intelligence and common learning disorders in children, adolescents, and their parents. *Developmental Disabilities Bulletin, 34*, 177–215.

Bode, M. M., D'Eugenio, D. B., Mettelman, B. B., & Gross, S. J. (2014). Predictive validity of the Bayley, Third Edition at 2 years for intelligence quotient at 4 years in preterm infants. *Journal of Developmental & Behavioral Pediatrics, 35*(9), 570–575. https://doi.org/10.1097/DBP.0000000000000110

Bracken, B. (2006). *Bracken basic concept scale, third edition: Receptive*. PsychTESTS. Pearson.

Brown, L., Sherbenou, R. J., & Johnsen, S. K. (2010). *Test of Nonverbal Intelligence (TONI-4)*. Pro-Ed.

Capozzi, F., Casini, M. P., Romani, M., De Gennaro, L., Nicolais, G., & Solano, L. (2008). Psychiatric comorbidity in learning disorder: Analysis of family variables. *Child Psychiatry and Human Development, 39*(1), 101–110. https://doi.org/10.1007/s10578-007-0074-5

Cicek, A. U., Sari, S. A., & Isik, C. M. (2020). Sociodemographic characteristics, risk factors, and prevalence of comorbidity among children and adolescents with intellectual disability: A cross-sectional study. *Journal of Mental Health Research in Intellectual Disabilities, 13*(2), 66–85. https://doi.org/10.1080/19315864.2020.1727590

Cimera, R. E., Burgess, S., & Bedesem, P. L. (2017). Does providing transition services by age 14 produce better vocational outcomes for students with intellectual disability? *Research and Practice for Persons With Severe Disabilities, 39*(1), 47–54. https://doi.org/10.1177/1540796914534633

Cooley, W. C., Sagerman, P. J., American Academy of Pediatrics, American Academy of Family Physicians, American College of Physicians, & Transitions Clinical Report Authoring Group. (2011). Supporting the health care transition from adolescence to adulthood in the medical home. *Pediatrics, 128*(1), 182–200. https://doi.org/10.1542/peds.2011-0969

Crnic, K. A., Neece, C. L., McIntyre, L. L., Blacher, J., & Baker, B. L. (2017). Intellectual disability and developmental risk: Promoting intervention to improve child and family well-being. *Child Development, 88*(2), 436–445. https://doi.org/10.1111/cdev.12740

Danforth, S., Slocum, L., & Dunkle, J. (2010). Turning the educability narrative: Samuel A. Kirk at the intersection of learning disability and "mental retardation." *Intellectual and Developmental Disabilities, 48*(3), 180–194. https://doi.org/10.1352/1944-7558-48.3.180

Education for All Handicapped Children Act, Pub. L. No. 94-142, 89 Stat. 773 (1975).

Einfeld, S. L., Ellis, L. A., & Emerson, E. (2011). Comorbidity of intellectual disability and mental disorder in children and adolescents: A systematic review. *Journal of Intellectual and Developmental Disability, 36*(2), 137–143. https://doi.org/10.1080/13668250.2011.572548

Elliott, C. D. (2007). *Differential ability scales* (2nd ed.). The Psychological Corporation.

Eunice Kennedy Shriver National Institute of Child Health and Human Development (NICHD). (2000). *Report of the National Reading Panel: Teaching children to read: An evidence-based assessment of the scientific research literature on reading and its implications for reading instruction*. NIH Publication No. 00-4754. U.S. Government Printing Office. https://www.nichd.nih.gov/publications/pubs/nrp/findings

Fletcher, J. M., Denton, C., & Francis, D. J. (2005). Validity of alternative approaches for the identification of learning disabilities: Operationalizing unexpected underachievement. *Journal of Learning Disabilities, 38*(6), 545–552. https://doi.org/10.1177/00222194050380061101

Fletcher, J. M., & Grigorenko, E. L. (2017). Neuropsychology of learning disabilities: The past and the future. *Journal of the International Neuropsychological Society, 23*(9–10), 930–940. https://doi.org/10.1017/S1355617717001084

Fricke, S., Bowyer-Crane, C., Haley, A. J., Hulme, C., & Snowling, M. J. (2013). Efficacy of language intervention in the early years. *Journal of Child Psychology and Psychiatry, 54*(3), 280–290. https://doi.org/10.1111/jcpp.12010

Gallagher, A., Frith, U., & Snowling, M. J. (2000). Precursors of literacy delay among children at genetic risk of dyslexia. *Journal of Child Psychology and Psychiatry, 41*(2), 203–213. https://doi.org/10.1111/1469-7610.00601

Giedd, J. N., Blumenthal, J., Jeffries, N. O., Castellanos, F. X., Liu, H., Zijdenbos, A., Paus, T., Evans, A. C., & Rapoport, J. L. (1999). Brain development during childhood and adolescence: A longitudinal MRI study. *Nature Neuroscience, 2*(10), 861–863. https://doi.org/10.1038/13158

Grigorenko, E. L. (2005). A conservative meta-analysis of linkage and linkage-association studies of developmental dyslexia. *Scientific Studies of Reading, 9*(3), 285–316. https://doi.org/10.1207/s1532799xssr0903_6

Harris, J. C. (2006). *Intellectual disability: Understanding its development, causes, classification, evaluation, and treatment*. Oxford University Press.

Harrison, P. L., & Oakland, T. (2015). *Adaptive behavior assessment system* (3rd ed.). Western Psychological Services.

Heber, R. (1959). A manual on terminology and classification in mental retardation. *American Journal of Mental Deficiency, 64*(2, Suppl. 64), 1–111.

Heuvelman, H., Abel, K., Wicks, S., Gardner, R., Johnstone, E., Lee, B., Magnusson, C., Dalman, C., & Rai, D. (2018). Gestational age at birth and risk of intellectual disability without a common genetic cause. *European Journal of Epidemiology, 33*(7), 667–678. https://doi.org/10.1007/s10654-017-0340-1

Huang, J., Zhu, T., Qu, Y., & Mu, D. (2016). Prenatal, perinatal and neonatal risk factors for intellectual disability: A systemic review and meta-analysis. *PLOS ONE, 11*(4), e0153655. https://doi.org/10.1371/journal.pone.0153655

Individuals With Disabilities Education Act (IDEA). (2024). *A history of the Individuals With Disabilities Education Act*. U.S. Department of Education. https://sites.ed.gov/idea/IDEA-History

Individuals With Disabilities Education Improvement Act, 20 U.S.C. §§ 1400-1482 (2004).

Järvelä, I., Määttä, T., Acharya, A., Leppälä, J., Jhangiani, S. N., Arvio, M., Siren, A., Kankuri-Tammilehto, M., Kokkonen, H., Palomäki, M., Varilo, T., Fang, M., Hadley, T. D., Jolly, A., Linnankivi, T., Paetau, R., Saarela, A., Kälviäinen, R., Olme, J., . . . Schrauwen, I. (2021). Exome sequencing reveals predominantly de novo variants in disorders with intellectual disability (ID) in the founder population of Finland. *Human Genetics, 140*(7), 1011–1029. https://doi.org/10.1007/s00439-021-02268-1

Kaufman, A. S., & Kaufman, N. L. (2014). *Kaufman test of educational achievement* (3rd ed.). NCS Pearson.

Kaufman, L., Ayub, M., & Vincent, J. B. (2010). The genetic basis of non-syndromic intellectual disability: A review. *Journal of Neurodevelopmental Disorders, 2*(4), 182–209. https://doi.org/10.1007/s11689-010-9055-2

Keulers, E. H., Hendriksen, J. G., Feron, F. J., Wassenberg, R., Wuisman-Frerker, M. G., Jolles, J., & Vles, J. S. (2007). Methylphenidate improves reading performance in children with attention deficit hyperactivity disorder and comorbid dyslexia: An unblinded clinical trial. *European Journal of Paediatric Neurology, 11*(1), 21–28. https://doi.org/10.1016/j.ejpn.2006.10.002

Kirby, P. (2020). Dyslexia debated, then and now: A historical perspective on the dyslexia debate. *Oxford Review of Education, 46*(4), 472–486. https://doi.org/10.1080/03054985.2020.1747418

Kochinke, K., Zweier, C., Nijhof, B., Fenckova, M., Cizek, P., Honti, F., Keerthikumar, S., Oortveld, M. A., Kleefstra, T., Kramer, J. M., Webber, C., Huynen, M. A., & Schenck, A. (2016). Systematic phenomics analysis deconvolutes genes mutated in intellectual disability into biologically coherent modules. *American Journal of Human Genetics, 98*(1), 149–164. https://doi.org/10.1016/j.ajhg.2015.11.024

Kortekaas-Rijlaarsdam, A. F., Luman, M., Sonuga-Barke, E., & Oosterlaan, J. (2019). Does methylphenidate improve academic performance? A systematic review and meta-analysis. *European Child & Adolescent Psychiatry, 28*(2), 155–164. https://doi.org/10.1007/s00787-018-1106-3

Langridge, A. T., Glasson, E. J., Nassar, N., Jacoby, P., Pennell, C., Hagan, R., Bourke, J., Leonard, H., & Stanley, F. J. (2013). Maternal conditions and perinatal characteristics associated with autism spectrum disorder and intellectual disability. *PLOS ONE, 8*(1), e50963. https://doi.org/10.1371/journal.pone.0050963

Leach, J. M., Scarborough, H. S., & Rescorla, L. (2003). Late-emerging learning disabilities. *Journal of Educational Psychology, 95*(2), 211–224. https://doi.org/10.1037/0022-0663.95.2.211

Lipkin, P. H., Macias, M. M., Norwood, K. W., Jr., Brei, T. J., Davidson, L. F., Davis, B. E., Ellerbeck, K. A., Houtrow, A. J., Hyman, S. L., Kuo, D. Z., Noritz, G. H., Yin, L., Murphy, N. A., Levy, S. E., Weitzman, C. C., Bauer, N. S., Childers, D. O., Jr., Levine, J. M., Peralta-Carcelen, A. M., . . . the Council on Children With Disabilities, Section on

Developmental and Behavioral Pediatrics. (2020). Promoting optimal development: Identifying infants and young children with developmental disorders through developmental surveillance and screening. *Pediatrics, 145*(1), e20193449. https://doi.org/10.1542/peds.2019-3449

Lyon, G. R. (1996). Learning disabilities. *The Future of Children, 6*(1), 54–76. https://doi.org/10.2307/1602494

Lyytinen, H., Leppänen, P. H. T., Richardson, U., & Guttorm, T. K. (2003). Brain functions and speech perception in infants at risk for dyslexia. In V. Csépe (Ed.), *Dyslexia: Different brain, different behavior* (pp. 113–152). Springer. https://doi.org/10.1007/978-1-4615-0139-8_4

Månsson, J., Stjernqvist, K., Serenius, F., Ådén, U., & Källén, K. (2019). Agreement between Bayley-III measurements and WISC-IV measurements in typically developing children. *Journal of Psychoeducational Assessment, 37*(5), 603–616. https://doi.org/10.1177/0734282918781431

Matejko, A. A., & Ansari, D. (2015). Drawing connections between white matter and numerical and mathematical cognition: A literature review. *Neuroscience and Biobehavioral Reviews, 48*, 35–52. https://doi.org/10.1016/j.neubiorev.2014.11.006

Matson, J. L., & Boisjoli, J. A. (2009). The token economy for children with intellectual disability and/or autism: A review. *Research in Developmental Disabilities, 30*(2), 240–248. https://doi.org/10.1016/j.ridd.2008.04.001

Matteson, E. L., & Kluge, F. J. (2003). Think clearly, be sincere, act calmly: Adolf Kussmaul (February 22, 1822–May 28, 1902) and his relevance to medicine in the 21st century. *Current Opinion in Rheumatology, 15*(1), 29–34. https://doi.org/10.1097/00002281-200301000-00006

Maulik, P. K., Mascarenhas, M. N., Mathers, C. D., Dua, T., & Saxena, S. (2011). Prevalence of intellectual disability: A meta-analysis of population-based studies. *Research in Developmental Disabilities, 32*(2), 419–436. https://doi.org/10.1016/j.ridd.2010.12.018

Mazzocco, M. M., & Thompson, R. E. (2005). Kindergarten predictors of math learning disability. *Learning Disabilities Research & Practice, 20*(3), 142–155. https://doi.org/10.1111/j.1540-5826.2005.00129.x

Morris, R. D., Lovett, M. W., Wolf, M., Sevcik, R. A., Steinbach, K. A., Frijters, J. C., & Shapiro, M. B. (2012). Multiple-component remediation for developmental reading disabilities: IQ, socioeconomic status, and race as factors in remedial outcome. *Journal of Learning Disabilities, 45*(2), 99–127. https://doi.org/10.1177/0022219409355472

Morsanyi, K., van Bers, B. M. C. W., McCormack, T., & McGourty, J. (2018). The prevalence of specific learning disorder in mathematics and comorbidity with other developmental disorders in primary school-age children. *British Journal of Psychology, 109*(4), 917–940. https://doi.org/10.1111/bjop.12322

National Center for Education Statistics. (2022). *Students with disabilities*. U.S. Department of Education, Institute of Education Sciences. Retrieved June 12, 2024, from https://nces.ed.gov/programs/coe/indicator/cgg

National Center for Education Statistics. (2023). *Fast facts: Students with disabilities*. U.S. Department of Education, Institute of Education Sciences. https://nces.ed.gov/fastfacts/display.asp?id=64

Oeseburg, B., Dijkstra, G. J., Groothoff, J. W., Reijneveld, S. A., & Jansen, D. E. (2011). Prevalence of chronic health conditions in children with intellectual disability: A systematic literature review. *Intellectual and Developmental Disabilities, 49*(2), 59–85. https://doi.org/10.1352/1934-9556-49.2.59

Orton, S. T. (1925). "Word blindness" in school children. *Archives of Neurology and Psychiatry, 14*(5), 581–615. https://doi.org/10.1001/archneurpsyc.1925.02200170002001

Park, J., & Bouck, E. (2018). In-school service predictors of employment for individuals with intellectual disability. *Research in Developmental Disabilities, 77*, 68–75. https://doi.org/10.1016/j.ridd.2018.03.014

Paulesu, E., Démonet, J. F., Fazio, F., McCrory, E., Chanoine, V., Brunswick, N., Cappa, S. F., Cossu, G., Habib, M., Frith, C. D., & Frith, U. (2001). Dyslexia: Cultural diversity and biological unity. *Science, 291*(5511), 2165–2167. https://doi.org/10.1126/science.1057179

Pivalizza, P. (2021). *Intellectual disability (ID) in children: Management, outcomes, and prevention*. UpToDate. Retrieved April 25, 2024, from https://www.uptodate.com/contents/intellectual-disability-id-in-children-clinical-features-evaluation-and-diagnosis

Povenmire-Kirk, T., Diegelmann, K., Crump, K., Schnorr, C., Test, D., Flowers, C., & Aspel, N. (2015). Implementing CIRCLES: A new model for interagency collaboration in transition planning. *Journal of Vocational Rehabilitation, 42*(1), 51–65. https://doi.org/10.3233/JVR-140723

Rehabilitation Act of 1973. Public Law 93-112, 29 U.S.C. §701 et seq. (1973).

Reichenberg, A., Cederlöf, M., McMillan, A., Trzaskowski, M., Kapra, O., Fruchter, E., Ginat, K., Davidson, M., Weiser, M., Larsson, H., Plomin, R., & Lichtenstein, P. (2016). Discontinuity in the genetic and environmental causes of the intellectual disability spectrum. *Proceedings of the National Academy of Sciences of the United States of America*, 113(4), 1098–1103. https://doi.org/10.1073/pnas.1508093112

Roid, G. H., & Miller, L. J. (2013). *Leiter international performance scale*. Torrence WPS.

Roid, G. H., & Pomplun, M. (2012). *The Stanford-Binet intelligence scales* (5th ed.). Riverside Publishing Company.

Sattler, J. M. (2001). *Assessment of children: Cognitive applications* (4th ed.). Jerome M. Sattler Publishers.

Schalock, R. L. (1999). The merging of adaptive behavior and intelligence: Implications for the field of mental retardation. In R. L. Schalock (Ed.), *Adaptive behavior and its measurement: Implications for the field of mental retardation* (pp. 43–59). American Association on Mental Retardation.

Schalock, R. L. (2011). The evolving understanding of the construct of intellectual disability. *Journal of Intellectual and Developmental Disability*, 36(4), 223–233. https://doi.org/10.3109/13668250.2011.624087

Schalock, R. L., Luckasson, R., & Tassé, M. J. (2021). An overview of *Intellectual Disability: Definition, Diagnosis, Classification, and Systems of Supports* (12th ed.). *American Journal on Intellectual and Developmental Disabilities*, 126(6), 439–442. https://doi.org/10.1352/1944-7558-126.6.439

Schalock, R. L., Luckasson, R. A., Shogren, K. A., Borthwick-Duffy, S., Bradley, V., Buntinx, W. H., Coulter, D. L., Craig, E. M., Gomez, S. C., Lachapelle, Y., Reeve, A., Snell, M. E., Spreat, S., Tassé, M. J., Thompson, J. R., Verdugo, M. A., Wehmeyer, M. L., & Yeager, M. H. (2007). The renaming of mental retardation: Understanding the change to the term intellectual disability. *Intellectual and Developmental Disabilities*, 45(2), 116–124. https://doi.org/10.1352/1934-9556(2007)45[116:TROMRU]2.0.CO;2

Schatschneider, C., Fletcher, J. M., Francis, D. J., Carlson, C. D., & Foorman, B. R. (2004). Kindergarten prediction of reading skills: A longitudinal comparative analysis. *Journal of Educational Psychology*, 96(2), 265–282. https://doi.org/10.1037/0022-0663.96.2.265

Scheffers, F., van Vugt, E., & Moonen, X. (2020). Resilience in the face of adversity in adults with an intellectual disability: A literature review. *Journal of Applied Research in Intellectual Disabilities*, 33(5), 828–838. https://doi.org/10.1111/jar.12720

Schieve, L. A., Tian, L. H., Rankin, K., Kogan, M. D., Yeargin-Allsopp, M., Visser, S., & Rosenberg, D. (2016). Population impact of preterm birth and low birth weight on developmental disabilities in US children. *Annals of Epidemiology*, 26(4), 267–274. https://doi.org/10.1016/j.annepidem.2016.02.012

Schneider, W., Niklas, F., & Schmiedeler, S. (2014). Intellectual development from early childhood to early adulthood: The impact of early IQ differences on stability and change over time. *Learning and Individual Differences*, 32, 156–162. https://doi.org/10.1016/j.lindif.2014.02.001

Schrank, F. A., McGrew, K., Mather, N., Wendling, B. J., & LaForte, E. (2014). *The Woodcock–Johnson IV: Tests of cognitive abilities, tests of oral language, tests of achievement*. Riverside Publishing Company.

Section 504 of the Rehabilitation Act of 1973, 34 C.F.R. Part 104. https://www2.ed.gov/policy/rights/reg/ocr/34cfr104.pdf

Shaywitz, S. E., Escobar, M. D., Shaywitz, B. A., Fletcher, J. M., & Makuch, R. (1992). Evidence that dyslexia may represent the lower tail of a normal distribution of reading ability. *The New England Journal of Medicine*, 326(3), 145–150. https://doi.org/10.1056/NEJM199201163260301

Shogren, K. A., & Plotner, A. J. (2012). Transition planning for students with intellectual disability, autism, or other disabilities: Data from the National Longitudinal Transition Study-2. *Intellectual and Developmental Disabilities*, 50(1), 16–30. https://doi.org/10.1352/1934-9556-50.1.16

Siegel, L. S. (2006). Perspectives on dyslexia. *Paediatrics & Child Health*, 11(9), 581–587. https://doi.org/10.1093/pch/11.9.581

Snowling, M. J., & Melby-Lervåg, M. (2016). Oral language deficits in familial dyslexia: A meta-analysis and review. *Psychological Bulletin*, 142(5), 498–545. https://doi.org/10.1037/bul0000037

Sparrow, S., Saulnier, C., Cicchetti, D., & Doll, E. (2016). *Vineland-3: Vineland adaptive behavior scales* (3rd ed.). Pearson Assessments.

Squires, J., & Bricker, D. (2009). *Ages & Stages Questionnaires®, Third Edition (ASQ®-3): A parent-completed child monitoring system*. Paul H. Brookes Publishing Co.

Tassé, M. J., Schalock, R. L., Balboni, G., Bersani, H., Jr., Borthwick-Duffy, S. A., Spreat, S., Thissen, D., Widaman, K. F., & Zhang, D. (2012). The construct of adaptive behavior: Its conceptualization, measurement, and use in the field of intellectual disability. *American Journal on Intellectual and Developmental Disabilities*, 117(4), 291–303. https://doi.org/10.1352/1944-7558-117.4.291

Turunen, T., Poskiparta, E., Salmivalli, C., Niemi, P., & Lerkkanen, M. K. (2021). Longitudinal associations between poor reading skills, bullying and victimization across the transition from elementary to middle school. *PLOS ONE, 16*(3), e0249112. https://doi.org/10.1371/journal.pone.0249112

van den Broek, E. G., Janssen, C. G., van Ramshorst, T., & Deen, L. (2006). Visual impairments in people with severe and profound multiple disabilities: An inventory of visual functioning. *Journal of Intellectual Disability Research, 50*(6), 470–475. https://doi.org/10.1111/j.1365-2788.2006.00804.x

Watkins, M. W., & Beaujean, A. A. (2014). Bifactor structure of the Wechsler Preschool and Primary Scale of Intelligence—Fourth Edition. *School Psychology Quarterly, 29*(1), 52–63. https://doi.org/10.1037/spq0000038

Wechsler, D. (1981). The psychometric tradition: Developing the Wechsler Adult Intelligence Scale. *Contemporary Educational Psychology, 6*(2), 82–85. https://doi.org/10.1016/0361-476X(81)90035-7

Wechsler, D. (2008). *WAIS-IV administration and scoring manual*. Psychological Corporation.

Wechsler, D. (2009). *Wechsler individual achievement test* (3rd ed.). Psychological Corporation.

Wechsler, D. (2012). *WPPSI-IV: Wechsler preschool and primary scale of intelligence*. Pearson, Psychological Corporation.

Wechsler, D. (2014). *WISC-V: Technical and interpretive manual*. Pearson.

Wehmeyer, M. L., Buntinx, W. H., Lachapelle, Y., Luckasson, R. A., Schalock, R. L., Verdugo, M. A., Borthwick-Duffy, S., Bradley, V., Craig, E. M., Coulter, D. L., Gomez, S. C., Reeve, A., Shogren, K. A., Snell, M. E., Spreat, S., Tassé, M. J., Thompson, J. R., & Yeager, M. H. (2008). The intellectual disability construct and its relation to human functioning. *Intellectual and Developmental Disabilities, 46*(4), 311–318. https://doi.org/10.1352/1934-9556(2008)46[311:TIDCAI]2.0.CO;2

Wilkinson, G. S., & Robertson, G. J. (2017). *Wide range achievement test* (5th ed.). Pearson.

Willcutt, E. G., & Pennington, B. F. (2000). Comorbidity of reading disability and attention-deficit/hyperactivity disorder: Differences by gender and subtype. *Journal of Learning Disabilities, 33*(2), 179–191. https://doi.org/10.1177/002221940003300206

Wolf, M., & Bowers, P. (1999). The double-deficit hypothesis for the developmental dyslexias. *Journal of Educational Psychology, 91*(3), 415–438. https://doi.org/10.1037/0022-0663.91.3.415

Woolf, S., Woolf, C. M., & Oakland, T. (2010). Adaptive behavior among adults with intellectual disabilities and its relationship to community independence. *Intellectual and Developmental Disabilities, 48*(3), 209–215. https://doi.org/10.1352/1944-7558-48.3.209

World Health Organization. (2019). *International classification of diseases* (11th ed.). https://icd.who.int/

Yell, M. L., Katsiyannis, A., & Bradley, M. R. (2017). The Individuals With Disabilities Education Act: The evolution of special education law. In J. Kauffman, D. Hallahan, & P. Pullen (Eds.), *Handbook of special education* (pp. 53–68). Routledge. https://doi.org/10.4324/9781315517698-7

Zablotsky, B., Black, L. I., & Blumberg, S. J. (2017). Estimated prevalence of children with diagnosed developmental disabilities in the United States, 2014–2016. *NCHS Data Brief, 291*, 1–8.

Zigic, N., Pajevic, I., Hasanovic, M., Avdibegovic, E., Aljukic, N., & Hodzic, V. (2023). Neurodevelopmental disorders in ICD-11 classification. *European Psychiatry, 66*(Suppl. 1), S737. https://doi.org/10.1192/j.eurpsy.2023.1547If

CHAPTER 27

PSYCHOLOGICAL CONSULTATION IN INPATIENT PEDIATRIC MEDICAL SETTINGS

Cassie N. Ross and Kristin A. Kullgren

Pediatric psychology consultation-liaison is the primary method of psychological service delivery in the pediatric hospital setting. The main components of this practice are *consultation,* capturing the direct provision of evidence-based psychological services at the request of the referring medical team, and *liaison,* representing indirect systems-level activities that occur as part of the psychologist's integration in the medical system or team (Kullgren & Carter, 2020). Consultation activities may include a request by the oncology team to evaluate a child and family coping with a new cancer diagnosis, behavioral recommendations to a nurse when a child's aggression interferes with postsurgical care, or a brief developmental assessment to determine if a toddler with a long hospitalization has characteristics of autism spectrum disorder (ASD). Liaison activities may include leading a multidisciplinary hospital-wide trauma-informed care committee, participating in cardiac developmental rounds, advocating at the state legislature for insurance coverage, or creating educational modules for pediatric residents on socioecological factors impacting child adjustment to hospitalization.

This chapter will focus on pediatric psychology consultation-liaison to promote child wellness and optimal development during a hospitalization while acknowledging that there are many opportunities for liaison work to achieve these goals. This chapter will start with an introduction to the foundation of pediatric psychology consultation-liaison including how it differs from traditional psychological practice and theoretical models, drawn from developmental science, that provide an integrated risk and resilience systems perspective. A brief consideration of health inequities and developmental stages that impact hospitalized youth will follow. The chapter will end with discussion of the consultation process and considerations for evaluation and intervention in pediatric psychology consultation-liaison (see the Resources box for practice resources).

INPATIENT PEDIATRIC PSYCHOLOGY CONSULTATION-LIAISON VERSUS TRADITIONAL PSYCHOLOGICAL PRACTICE

Kullgren and Carter (2020) describe the differences between the practice of pediatric psychology consultation-liaison and traditional psychotherapy including

- focus of intervention (individual/family, medical team, and/or medical system),
- source of the referral (medical team, protocol, or clinical pathway),
- responsibility for the patient (referring physician),

- timing (often same day, depending on access to patient, or as concerns arise),
- target of intervention (focused, solution oriented),
- treatment length (short term; most often one or two sessions),
- integration (highly integrated into setting), and
- liaison work (integrated into practice).

The practice of the pediatric consultation-liaison psychologist varies based on composition of the team (including psychologists, psychiatrists, social workers, nurses, developmental-behavioral pediatricians, and board-certified behavioral analysts), assignment location (whole hospital or specific unit [e.g., neonatal intensive care unit]), specific population (e.g., oncology), and scope of practice (boundaries between psychology and other services, evaluation vs. standardized assessment vs. intervention). Pediatric consultation-liaison psychologists need a flexible skill set specific to the consultant role while integrating core pediatric psychology competencies into consultation-liaison practice (Kullgren & Carter, 2020):

- foundational knowledge of biopsychosocial factors and child development, psychological functioning, and health or illness;
- effective use of current research in practice;
- professionalism in all contexts including patient care, training and education, and multidisciplinary work;
- effective communication skills tailored to the specific needs of the audience and rapport building;
- clinical skills in evidence-based practice, assessment, intervention, and consultation; and
- teaching, supervision, professional leadership, and advocacy skills.

The rationale for integrated pediatric psychology consultation-liaison support is grounded in risk of comorbid psychiatric concerns in youth with chronic medical conditions that can contribute to poor health outcomes, increased vulnerability to exacerbation of mental health concerns from the medical setting/potential trauma, and higher health care utilization (Zima et al., 2016). International research found a significant relationship between psychiatric diagnoses and physical illness, with an increased likelihood of developing physical illness associated with the diagnosis of more than one psychiatric condition (Scott et al., 2016). Youth with comorbid psychiatric and medical issues typically have more complex mental health diagnoses, higher health care costs, and more complicated health outcomes than youth who do not (Steiner et al., 1993).

In children, the chronic illness experience may disrupt important aspects of development resulting in overdependence on caregiver(s), difficulties in separation from parents, reduced peer socialization, reduced adolescent experimentation, and disrupted identity development. In addition to developmental disturbances, youth with chronic medical conditions often have complex biopsychosocial predisposing and predictive vulnerabilities to the development of comorbid psychiatric concerns such as physiological changes related to their medical condition, high rates of peer victimization, family stressors, and social determinants of health (Brady et al., 2021). Early involvement by a pediatric consultation-liaison psychologist may result in shortened hospital stays, highlighting the vital role of these providers (Bowling et al., 2021, Bowling & Bearman, 2023). Finally, integrated psychology supports the medical team's care of patients and families with complex developmental and biopsychosocial needs.

THEORETICAL MODELS AND ECOLOGICAL CONTEXTS RELEVANT TO PEDIATRIC PSYCHOLOGY CONSULTATION-LIAISON

Theoretical models of practice can provide a foundation for both the novice and seasoned pediatric consultation-liaison psychologists as well as for multidisciplinary providers who aim for holistic systems-level evaluations of their patients. As the role of a pediatric consultation-liaison psychologist tends to focus on interdisciplinary patient care, the models that are widely used as a basis for practice are integrative including ecological contexts as they relate to patient functioning (Carter et al., 2020). The integrated comprehensive consultation-liaison model (ICCLM; see Figure 27.1; Carter et al., 2017) provides a visual framework integrating three major biopsychosocial models utilized in pediatric psychological consultation-liaison practice—bioecological systems theory (BST), the pediatric psychosocial preventative health model (PPPHM), and the seven C's of consultation-liaison—to provide a robust and thorough theoretical foundation. The ICCLM illustrates the breadth of pediatric psychology consultation-liaison services as spanning various levels of systems through evaluation and intervention to optimize pediatric health and well-being.

Bioecological Systems Theory

Bronfenbrenner's bioecological systems theory (1979) evaluates the relationships between and impact of complex systems on a child's development including the individual child, microsystem (e.g., family, peers, school, medical providers), mesosystem (interactions between members of the microsystem), exosystem (neighborhood, social services, legal system), macrosystem (cultural and societal values and norms), and chronosystem (time). Pediatric psychology consultation-liaison utilizes BST to evaluate aspects of risk and resilience within each system as well as the impact of the interactions between systems on the child and family (Carter et al., 2020). This evaluation then informs interventions focused on bolstering aspects of resilience and

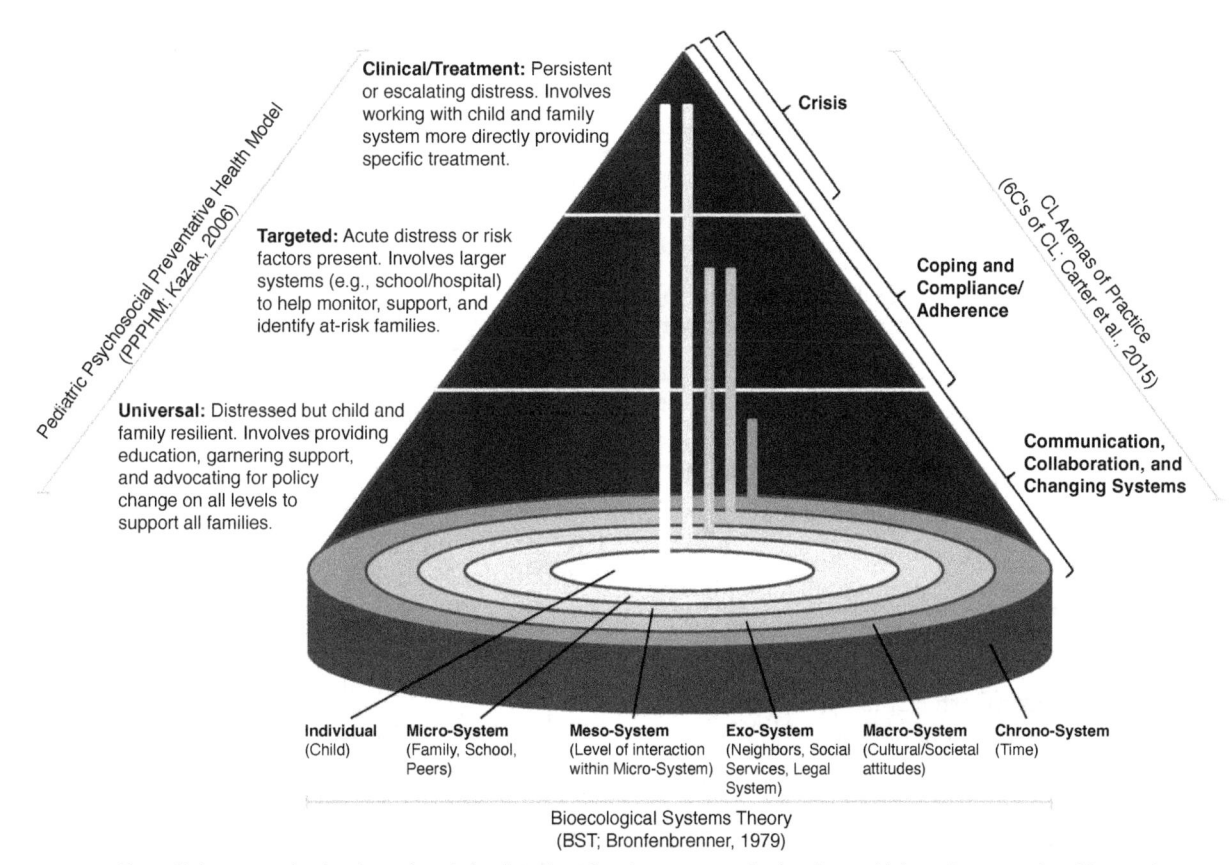

Note: Columns projecting from the circles into the triangle represent the levels at which each system is addressed. For example, the Individual system (child) is targeted at all three treatment/care levels while the Macrosystem is involved primarily at the Universal level.

FIGURE 27.1. Integrated comprehensive consultation-liaison (CL) model. From "Inpatient Pediatric Consultation–Liaison," by B. D. Carter, W. G. Kronenberger, E. L. Scott, K. A. Kullgren, C. Piazza-Waggoner, and C. E. Brady, in M. C. Roberts and R. G. Steele (Eds.), *Handbook of Pediatric Psychology* (5th ed., p. 108), 2017, Guilford Press. Copyright 2017 by Guilford Press. Reprinted with permission.

targeting areas of risk to improve functioning within and between systems. A strength of BST is the wide lens of systems that impact health, but it lacks a theoretical base to guide intervention. Therefore, it is common for practitioners to utilize multiple theoretical models to inform their practice.

Pediatric Psychosocial Preventative Health Model

The PPPHM provides a targeted public health and risk and resilience model provides a targeted public health and risk and resilience model guiding intervention for families with chronically ill children (Kazak, 2006). It targets three levels of risk- and resilience-focused evaluations to inform intervention. The universal level recognizes resilience in most children and families while identifying systematic risk factors, barriers, bias, and health care inequities as opportunities for change. An example would be a pediatric consultation-liaison psychologist leading an initiative on developmentally informed pain management across the hospital.

The targeted level of the PPPHM includes patients and families identified as at risk for poor health outcomes. The pediatric consultant-liaison psychologist contributes to evaluation via risk screening to inform interventions for family-specific education and brief focused interventions for improving health behaviors (Carter et al., 2020; Kazak, 2006). This may include screening post-surgical patients and providing a single-session brief intervention on pain coping strategies. Finally, the clinical/treatment level includes patients and families who require more intensive or direct mental health care (Carter et al., 2020; Kazak, 2006). A child with severe pain and depressed mood following a traumatic injury would require clinical intervention by a pediatric consultation-liaison psychologist to address the impact of these symptoms on the child's recovery.

Indications for consultation: The seven C's of pediatric psychology consultation-liaison. Although BST and the PPPHM provide a strong theoretical foundation for evaluation and intervention, further specifications are required for pediatric psychology consultation-liaison. Therefore, practitioners utilize the seven C's of consultation—crisis, coping, compliance/adherence, communication, collaboration, changing systems, and championing/advocacy—as a model for practice-specific roles and responsibilities that can be integrated with these other models (Carter et al., 2017). Pediatric consultation-liaison psychologists are often called upon for evaluation and intervention for acute crises such as coping with new onset medical illnesses/injuries and psychiatric emergencies (Carter et al., 2020). For example, they might consult with a teen who has a new cancer diagnosis and is expressing suicidal thoughts.

Evaluation of and intervention around coping with illness is one of the more common consultation requests for pediatric consultation-liaison psychologists, particularly for adolescents (Kullgren et al., 2018). These providers take a strength-based approach by identifying existing coping strategies and then providing evidence-based coping skills to help patients and families through hospitalization and illness. Compliance/adherence is also a common challenge in the pediatric population, creating risk for poor health outcomes (Rapoff, 2010). Pediatric consultation-liaison psychologists are trained in evaluating biopsychosocial barriers to adherence, problem solving to remove or reduce these barriers, and addressing additional systemic barriers toward optimal adherence to care recommendations (Carter et al., 2020). For example, when consulted to evaluate a child with cystic fibrosis admitted due to worsening lung functioning, a pediatric consultation-liaison psychologist would assess family knowledge about the regimen and beliefs around treatment efficacy, determine if child emotional or behavioral factors are interfering, assess the family's response, and consider whether systemic factors are impacting care (e.g., access to medications, insurance status).

When a child is hospitalized, the various multidisciplinary providers, family members, and community supports involved can create communication challenges. In this case the pediatric consultant-liaison psychologist can work to promote effective communication between disciplines, for example, by consulting with the child's outpatient developmental-behavioral pediatrician to better understand the child's behavioral and developmental needs impacting their inpatient care (Carter et al., 2020). Similarly, the goal of the pediatric consultation-liaison psychologist is to increase collaboration among direct care providers, collaborate with multidisciplinary providers on patient care and quality improvement efforts, and conduct research regarding the integration of behavioral health into medicine. Scheduling a team meeting with outpatient providers to discuss discharge planning is an example of this collaborative role. Looking to the larger system, pediatric consultation-liaison psychologists are uniquely positioned to champion advocacy efforts focused on prevention, accessibility of care, and integration of behavioral health via changes in the larger systems. The roles and responsibilities of these providers can range from individual patient needs to larger national and sometimes international systems in which patients and families live.

Integrated comprehensive consultation-liaison model in practice. Using the ICCLM in practice, the pediatric consultation-liaison psychologist assumes a role in evaluation and intervention that varies depending on whether the needs are at the systemic level, for prevention, targeting at risk-populations, or addressing the needs of those with clinical levels of disease or psychiatric needs (Carter et al., 2020). To illustrate with a case example, a pediatric consultation-liaison psychologist may utilize the ICCLM when consulted for adherence concerns for a child with Type 1 diabetes admitted in diabetic ketoacidosis. First, evaluation of BST domains will determine resilience and risk factors that impact multiple levels of systems. At the individual level, the pediatric consultation-liaison psychologist would consider the individual child's developmental and cognitive ability to engage in their care and emotional and behavioral factors that could impact compliance/adherence. Microsystem inquiry would explore interactive bidirectional factors between the child and family, peer, and school settings that either support or hinder adherence. Understanding the interactions between the child's microsystems, such as between the school and outpatient endocrine clinic (mesosystem), can help identify additional opportunities to address risk and build resilience. The larger context of the child's world, represented in the child's exosystem, can provide awareness of social and community influences on the child and family, such as neighborhood violence, which can inform the family's illness experience. Finally, social determinants of health within the child's macrosystem that could impact adherence, such as socioeconomic status, poverty, and ethnicity, would be assessed (see the "Consideration of Health Inequities" section later in this chapter).

From the PPPHM perspective, the pediatric consultation-liaison psychologist would determine the level of intervention needed (clinical/treatment level) and then develop interventions that target each BST system. For example, this might include:

- utilizing the seven C's of pediatric psychology consultation-liaison to bolster resilience factors of motivation (BST: individual system; seven C's: compliance/adherence),
- improving adherence by conducting behavioral interventions for needle phobia (BST: individual system; seven C's: crisis),
- providing parent management training and requesting additional school services (BST: microsystem; seven C's: communication),
- increasing communication between school and medical providers regarding treatment at school (BST: mesosystem; seven C's: collaboration), and/or
- advocating for additional community social services (BST: exosystem; seven C's: changing systems).

Taken together, the ICCLM's integration of BST, the PPPHM, and the seven C's provides a strong theoretical base for the practice of pediatric psychology consultation-liaison.

Consideration of health inequities. When models of care are considered, it is important to highlight the importance of health inequities in youth. Health inequities among diverse populations impact all facets of health and access to quality care (McKay & Parente, 2019). Underserved and oppressed populations are more likely to be hospitalized, have longer admissions, require more invasive interventions and be readmitted, have complications, or die in the hospital. Systemic bias and discrimination increase risk for mental health concerns that further impact long-term health and hospitalization experiences (Bardach et al., 2014). Patients from diverse backgrounds have a variety of norms and perceptions of illness, pain, and psychological distress to be considered. Guidelines for multicultural clinical practice have shifted from a knowledge-based competency paradigm to a focus on cultural humility, encouraging provider self-reflection, recognition of limits of knowledge, and curiosity about the complexities of a family's identity and values (Patallo, 2019). Pediatric consultation-liaison psychologists play a significant role with underserved populations by providing mental health services guided by cultural humility to reduce distress and trauma related to hospitalization. By facilitating communication between families and medical providers, these providers can encourage and support family engagement, shared decision making, and effective communication. They can work to educate multidisciplinary providers about family cultural values, support understanding and acceptance of treatment recommendations, identify potential barriers due to inequities, and increase awareness about impact of implicit or explicit bias on care. They are uniquely suited to advocate for positive change through educational, departmental, institutional, state, and national initiatives focused on diversity, equity, inclusion, and justice.

Consideration of developmental factors across the childhood lifespan. Developmental factors play a key role in the child's coping with illness and hospitalization. Pediatric consultation-liaison psychologists see patients throughout their development from newborns to young adults and must consider the foundations of developmental science in case conceptualization and treatment. Distress related to illness and hospitalization occurs throughout the lifespan, but younger children, particularly those with biological or developmental ages between 6 months and 6 years, are at higher risk for acute distress and posttraumatic stress symptoms (Perrin & Shipman, 2009). Children with developmental disorders have increased vulnerability to both comorbid medical and mental health conditions and diminished access to high-quality specialized health care (Cheak-Zamora & Thullen, 2017).

Illness and hospitalization are often difficult for young children or youth with developmental disorders due to the external locus of control, disrupted routine, social communication requirements with providers, sensory sensitivity, limited coping skills, and potentially limited understanding of medical care/diagnoses (Straus et al., 2019). A thorough assessment of the role of developmental level, communication skills, preferences, and behavioral/emotional functioning can help to direct patient-focused interventions (Noeder & Davis, 2020). Therefore, pediatric consultation-liaison psychologists commonly consult with developmental-behavioral pediatricians to provide a united developmental conceptualization and treatment recommendations for the hospital admission and postdischarge care. Together these providers play a vital role in implementing developmentally informed interventions that are rooted in developmental science (e.g., consistent care team, routine, reduced stimulation, use of concrete language, informing before doing), coping skill development, and supporting coordination of outpatient services. Interventions should be developed in collaboration with the patient's caregiver, emphasizing environmental modifications such as reducing room stimulation by limiting the number of providers, providing recommendations for nurses or other medical providers on developmental and trauma-informed care practices, and developing behavior plans to ensure consistency in provider and parent responses to behaviors (Noeder & Davis, 2020).

THE CONSULTATION PROCESS

Consultation processes differ depending on the structure and resources of the health system. Typically, a physician, nurse practitioner, or other member of the primary medical team will initiate the consult order. The pediatric consultation-liaison psychologist will then conduct an evaluation, provide recommendations to multidisciplinary providers, support discharge planning and care coordination, and provide evidence-based intervention to the patient and family.

Evaluation

Pediatric consultation-liaison psychologists collaborate with the referring providers, relevant medical specialists (e.g., developmental-behavioral pediatricians), the patient, and family to clarify the referral question and develop consultation goals that are specific, measurable, attainable, relevant, and timely (SMART; Doran, 1981). Collateral information is obtained from the medical record, community supports (e.g., school counselor, teacher, spiritual leader), and outpatient health care providers (e.g., primary care provider, developmental-behavioral pediatrician, mental health provider, physical therapist). The pediatric consultation-liaison psychologist then conducts a targeted comprehensive biopsychosocial evaluation via an interview with the family and patient. Standardized assessment measures may be used to evaluate specific domains of concern (see the Resources box). Please see Albright et al. (2020) for a detailed list of assessment measures commonly utilized in pediatric psychology consultation-liaison. The data collected from multiple sources are organized to develop a case conceptualization and treatment recommendations to be communicated to the patient, family, and medical team.

Treatment Recommendations/Discharge Planning/Care Coordination

In addition to direct psychological intervention, discussed later in this chapter, pediatric consultation-liaison psychologists provide collaborative care to support treatment goals. They may recommend and participate in team conferences and/or family care conferences with the goal of improving communication and care coordination across different systems for a patient with complex biopsychosocial needs. They can cotreat with other providers (e.g., developmental-behavioral pediatricians, physical therapists, occupational therapists, child life specialists, psychiatrists) by joining a session to evaluate and provide intervention recommendations to improve a child's participation. They can provide direct intervention or recommendations when broader exosystem factors are impacting the child's health. For example, pediatric consultation-liaison psychologists often provide accommodation or evaluation recommendations to the child's school; provide education and training to parents; relay events of admission and treatment recommendations to the patient's outpatient mental health provider; and/or consult with child protective services, foster care agencies, or other exosystem entities. Due to the often time-limited nature of these services, a key role psychologists play is disposition planning as part of the discharge process (e.g., inpatient psychiatric admission, intensive outpatient program, individual or family psychotherapy, applied behavior analysis therapy).

Evidence-Based Interventions

Pediatric consultation-liaison psychologists utilize evidence-based interventions that are customized and adapted to be accessible to the patient and family in the hospital setting while prioritizing the SMART goals of consultation (Doran, 1981). This section provides an overview of commonly used evidence-based interventions; condition-specific interventions will be addressed in the section that follows.

Motivational interviewing. Motivational interviewing is an evidence-based, patient-centered, directive treatment modality originally developed to treat substance abuse concerns, with efficacy in various domains of behavior change, particularly adherence concerns (Lundahl et al., 2019; Miller & Rollnick, 1991). Pediatric consultation-liaison psychologists utilize motivational interviewing to evaluate aspects of risk and resilience including a patient's values and goals, level of ambivalence toward behavior change, and barriers to behavior change (Miller & Rollnick, 1991). The evaluation informs interventions such as education, highlighting discrepancies between values and behaviors, evoking reasons for change, and problem solving (Erickson et al., 2005; Miller & Rollnick, 1991). Although motivational interviewing is a valuable tool for a variety of patients needing improved motivation for behavior change, the variability in patient ages, developmental level, and consultation concerns requires a similarly vast repertoire of treatment modalities.

Cognitive behavior therapy. Cognitive behavior therapy (CBT) is a highly researched psychological treatment modality that has demonstrated efficacy in treating a broad range of mental health concerns throughout the lifespan (Hofmann et al., 2012). Beck (1970/2016) and Ellis (1962) described the theoretical basis of CBT as maladaptive cognitions are the foundation of psychological distress and behavioral problems, and these maladaptive cognitions can be changed via therapeutic intervention (psychoeducation, reframing maladaptive cognitions, problem solving, relaxation/coping skill development). Whereas traditional outpatient CBT relies on structured protocols, the short-term and unpredictable nature of the inpatient medical setting requires pediatric consultation-liaison psychologists to conduct focused modified CBT interventions to meet SMART goals.

Acceptance and commitment therapy. Acceptance and commitment therapy (ACT) is considered a third-wave of CBT that includes the functional and contextual phenomena of psychological inflexibility/flexibility as domains of risk and resilience (Hayes et al., 2006). For patients with symptoms of depression or anxiety, patients who are struggling with their identity, or patients with a chronic illness, pediatric consultation-liaison psychologists may utilize the lens of ACT during evaluation to guide interventions that bolster resiliency in psychological flexibility and utilize mindfulness and cognitive interventions to improve one's ability to be present in the moment (Hayes et al., 2006). Acceptance and commitment therapy may be more appropriate for patients with internalizing concerns or those whose externalizing concerns do not pose harm to themself or others.

Dialectical behavior therapy. Dialectical behavior therapy (DBT), also a third-wave of CBT, was originally developed for the treatment of borderline personality disorder and posits that emotional and behavioral dysregulation are due to the complex interplay between biology and the individual within multilevel systems (Linehan et al., 1991). Dialectic behavior therapy has been adapted to treat pediatric populations experiencing emotional and behavioral dysregulation, non-suicidal self-injury, suicidal behaviors, and eating disorders. Evaluation includes the function of behaviors within and between systems, triggers and warning signs of behaviors, and existing coping or self-soothing skills. Common interventions include interdisciplinary behavior plans to prevent and respond to problematic or dangerous behaviors, education of system members (family, schools, medical teams), and building coping/self-soothing behaviors. Along with motivational interviewing, CBT, and ACT, DBT is among the most common evidence-based treatment modalities utilized by pediatric consultation-liaison psychologists, although interventions must be tailored based upon the referral question and the complexities of the hospital setting.

EVALUATION AND EVIDENCE-BASED INTERVENTION CONSIDERATIONS FOR COMMON REFERRAL CONCERNS

This section will briefly describe common physical health, adaptation, and mental health concerns seen by pediatric consultation-liaison psychologists. This is an introduction to common evaluation and intervention strategies with the understanding that general pediatric psychological competencies are modified to support hospitalized youth.

Common Physical Health Conditions

Historically, there has been an illusionary division between physical and mental health as separate conditions. As medicine and psychological sciences have advanced, it has become evident that physical and mental health are inseparable (Sinyor et al., 2019). The integration of pediatric consultation-liaison psychologist into medical system allows for holistic care.

Feeding disorders. Pediatric consultation-liaison psychologists are often consulted to assess the complex psychosocial contributors to weight loss or poor growth due to poor oral intake. When a child is admitted with poor oral intake, the broad differential diagnoses include medical conditions, functional gastrointestinal conditions, eating disorders, avoidant/restrictive food intake disorder (ARFID), and other psychiatric diagnoses impacting eating (e.g., major depression, psychosis anxiety).

Chapter 23 of this volume of the handbook is dedicated to the topic of eating disorders, but in this chapter we will focus on ARFID, which results from lack of interest in food, aversion based on sensory aspects of food, and/or fear of aversive consequences of eating (i.e., pain, nausea), leading to nutritional deficiency, need for supplemental nutrition, and impairment in psychosocial functioning (American Psychiatric Association, 2013). This disorder presents throughout development, often starting in infancy and young childhood, and is more common in youth with ASD, attention deficit/hyperactivity disorder, intellectual disabilities, picky eating history, anxiety, and/or history of medical conditions impacting feeding (Andersen et al., 2020). Inpatient management involves a coordinated interdisciplinary effort often including pediatric hospitalists, developmental-behavioral pediatricians, adolescent medicine specialists, psychiatrists, psychologists, social workers, occupational therapists/speech-language pathologists (SLP), and/or child life specialists (Andersen et al., 2020; Tsang et al., 2020). For youth with ARFID, the appropriateness of inpatient feeding treatment prior to the initiation of refeeding must be considered given the risk of further reinforcement of food aversion and avoidance (see Table 27.1; Andersen et al., 2020). Many children require enteral feeding due to persistent food refusal, severe malnutrition, or contraindications for behavioral refeeding (Andersen et al., 2020). Pediatric consultation-liaison psychologists play an important role in management utilizing bioecological contexts, providing psychoeducation, supporting coping skills development, increasing distress tolerance/emotional regulation, and providing other cognitive behavior techniques focused on awareness, cognitive distortions, cognitive restructuring, and disposition planning (Tsang et al., 2020).

Pain. Pain is a common experience of children and youth admitted to the hospital and may be

TABLE 27.1

Considerations for Inpatient Refeeding for Patients With ARFID

Considerations	Recommendations
Length of admission	Create realistic goals for anticipated length of admission
Comorbid medical concerns	Contraindicated for patients with current medical concerns causing pain and nausea due to likelihood of worsening aversion
	Aspiration or oral motor deficits
Acuity of feeding concerns	Acute feeding problems without comorbid medical issues causing pain or nausea: ■ Brief interventions focused on short term goals of acceptance of supplemental nutrition, preferred foods, and reducing anxiety surrounding intake ■ Referral to outpatient feeding specialist Chronic or severe feeding problems: ■ Not suitable for brief behavioral refeeding interventions and may require nasogastric tube feeding during hospital admission. Behavioral intervention may be appropriate for long admissions ■ Referral to multidisciplinary feeding program for intensive outpatient treatment

Note. ARFID = avoidant/restrictive food intake disorder. Data from Andersen et al. (2020).

chronic (e.g., migraine), acute (e.g., postsurgical), or an acute exacerbation of a chronic pain condition (e.g., sickle cell vaso-occlusive crisis). The role of the pediatric consultation-liaison psychologist is to understand the contributing biopsychosocial factors (child factors, family factors, medical conditions, pain history, treatment plan, organizational context; MacKenzie et al., 2020) and the impact of pain on functioning to develop brief targeted interventions to support pain coping during hospitalization. CBT has a strong evidence base for treating chronic pain; modifications for the inpatient setting may be necessary due to the limited time for intervention (Foxen-Craft et al., 2020). Using a structured brief intervention such as the ABCD mnemonic (activity, breathing, counter-stimulation, distraction) can be a successful starting point for pain intervention. To encourage activity, the pediatric consultation-liaison psychologist may work with medical providers, physical therapists/occupational therapists, the family, and the patient to set goals for movement and time out of bed. Diaphragmatic breathing can be supported utilizing videos or phone apps to help pace breathing. Counter-stimulation includes sensory coping using heat, ice, aromatherapy, and massage, for example. Finally, distraction includes engaging in pleasant activities that keep the mind off the pain. For youth with chronic pain, outpatient referral to a pain management therapist may be recommended.

Gastrointestinal symptoms: Functional nausea and vomiting. Gastrointestinal symptoms are a common concern for hospital admission and pose a complicated diagnostic challenge. Symptoms may be related to an acute self-resolving illness, organic disease, functional symptoms (functional vomiting disorders, rumination, functional abdominal pain disorder, functional defecation disorders), or formal eating or feeding disorder (Maddux et al., 2020; Rome Foundation, 2016).

The following discussion focuses on treatment of patients with functional gastrointestinal symptoms. Prior to formal treatment of functional conditions, it is necessary to determine if factors such as malnutrition, dehydration, constipation, or other modifiable sources of discomfort are well managed (Maddux et al., 2020). It is common for pediatric consultation-liaison psychologists to consult with outpatient developmental-behavioral pediatricians to aid in conceptualization and treatment planning, particularly for youth with chronic constipation or other elimination disorders. Observation of oral intake is necessary to support differential diagnosis and to evaluate for additional factors that may contribute to nausea and vomiting, followed by direct feedback to the patient, family, and medical team regarding diagnosis and treatment recommendations. The initial stage of intervention includes increasing the child's and family's awareness of contributing biopsychosocial factors as well as the use of coping skills such as diaphragmatic breathing, which can be supported by biofeedback. Treatment then transitions to a gradual food exposure plan. Setting realistic expectations for the treatment team, patients, and families is essential as resolution of symptoms is often time consuming and challenging due to ongoing and aversive symptoms.

Somatic symptom and related disorders. Somatic symptom and related disorders (SSRD) are characterized by physical symptoms accompanied by excessive thoughts, feelings, and behaviors about the symptoms that cause significant impairment and distress and cannot be explained by a medical condition (American Psychiatric Association, 2013). These diagnoses can co-occur with a known medical condition, with symptoms that are amplified or inconsistent with the known medical cause. They are a common consultation concern when there is concern about psychological factors affecting the medical presentation and/or the medical evaluation is not consistent with a medical cause (Williams et al., 2020). Pediatric consultation-liaison psychologists will conduct a thorough evaluation of the bio-ecological context of the patient's presentation with specific attention to environmental response to symptoms that may inadvertently reinforce the symptoms, patient/parent distress, functional impact, and degree of control over symptoms. The primary intervention is the communication of the SSRD diagnosis and conceptualization, which, if accepted by the family, will lay the groundwork for outpatient intervention. Secondary interventions include supporting the medical team and family around a common language for the symptoms, creation of a symptom response plan, and supporting discharge planning. Finally, pediatric consultation-liaison psychologists may introduce coping strategies as a bridge to outpatient intervention and develop a therapeutic alliance that will increase family acceptance of outpatient interventions (Weiss et al., 2021).

Pretransplant or surgical evaluations. Pediatric consultation-liaison psychologists may be involved in pretransplant (solid organ, bone marrow, hematopoietic stem cell) or presurgical evaluations to determine psychosocial risk and protective factors and provide recommendations for interventions or resources throughout the transplantation process (Cousino et al., 2020). Evaluation includes clinical interviews and assessment measures (see the Resources box) focusing on the following factors:

- history of treatment adherence;
- barriers to adherence or potential challenges (i.e., pill swallowing, needle phobia, history of delirium);
- history of hospitalization and surgery;
- patient and family knowledge of current condition and the planned procedure;
- developmentally appropriate responsibility of care;
- cognitive or developmental functioning; and
- patient or family history of mental illness, trauma history, coping skills, and social support.

Data are integrated, and the pediatric consultation-liaison psychologist provides feedback to the patient, family, and multidisciplinary team regarding the strengths-based conceptualization and concrete recommendations for immediate interventions, additional service needs (e.g., neuropsychological assessment, outpatient psychotherapy, school accommodations), and resources to address potential risk factors (Cousino et al., 2020).

COMMON CONCERNS OF ADAPTATION ADDRESSED THROUGH PEDIATRIC PSYCHOLOGY CONSULTATION-LIAISON

Hospitalization is very disruptive to children and their families, requiring children and families to quickly adapt to the loss of control due to the hospital environment (Cammarata et al., 2020). It is common for children and families to experience complex psychological reactions (distress, difficulty complying with cares or interacting with providers) which may impact functioning and the ability to participate in medical care (National Child Traumatic Stress Network, 2014; Rennick et al., 2014).

Coping With Illness and Hospitalization

Pediatric consultation-liaison psychologists use a strength-based approach to provide education about common emotional reactions to illness and hospitalization and developmentally appropriate coping skills (see Table 27.2). CBT is tailored to a patient's specific needs including recognition and restructuring of maladaptive cognitions (e.g., anticipatory anxiety, catastrophizing, avoidance, emotional reaction toward help seeking) and increasing perceived control over modifiable factors (e.g., effective communication of needs and wants, care preferences, self-care, adherence; Marsac et al., 2016). To reduce distress and further trauma related to illness and/or hospitalization, pediatric cognitive-liaison psychologists collaborate with multidisciplinary teams to provide holistic trauma-informed care for the patient and family.

Behaviors That Interfere With Care

Verbal or physical aggression, self-harm, attempts to unsafely leave the room or hospital, and/or care refusal are more likely among patients with acute psychiatric concerns, developmental disorders, mental status changes, and/or medical

TABLE 27.2
General Coping Recommendations

Parent/child domain	Interventions
Parent	
Communication	Acknowledge distress and encourage emotional expression; developmentally appropriate education
Comfort	Bring comfort/familiar items from home
Planning	Have plans for visits and transitions; create daily visual schedule for child
Child	
Relaxation tools	Diaphragmatic breathing, imagery, hypnosis, mindfulness, muscle relaxation, grounding techniques
Distraction	Engagement in pleasant activities; referrals to child life, music therapy, art therapy, pet therapy
Living tools	Sleep hygiene strategies, nutrition and hydration strategies, behavioral activation, routines and structure
Sensory tools	Weighted blankets, massage, stress balls, Play Doh, kinetic sand, fidgets, slime, cold water or ice on hands or face, heating pads, warm showers/bath, yoga or other physical practice, aromatherapy
Cognitive tools	Emotion identification, processing, and expression. Identifying relationships among thoughts, feelings, and behaviors; cognitive distortions; cognitive reframing. Problem solving. Goal setting.

trauma or other adverse life experiences (Gerson et al., 2019). Management of these behaviors in the hospital can be challenging and complex, requiring interdisciplinary teamwork and coordination with the child's primary medical team, other potential inpatient consultants, and outpatient providers (i.e., developmental-behavioral pediatricians, board-certified behavior analysts, applied behavior analysts, psychiatrists, psychotherapists). Pediatric consultation-liaison psychologists gather information regarding behaviors, biopsychosocial factors, antecedents/triggers, consequences/responses, and behavioral de-escalation techniques (e.g., keeping calm; simple, concrete, and empathetic communication style; redirection; use of coping skills, preferred activities, selective attention) and collaborate with psychiatrists and other medical providers on instructions regarding psychotropic medication use or restraints should behavioral techniques fail (Gerson et al., 2019). As many medical providers have not received formal training in behavioral de-escalation, pediatric consultation-liaison psychologists often provide education and direction to staff in preparation or response to a child's escalation.

Neonatal Intensive Care

Parents whose babies are admitted to the neonatal intensive care unit (NICU) commonly experience significant emotional distress including grief, stress, depression, anxiety, and posttraumatic stress (Hoge & Shaw, 2021; Hynan et al., 2015). Because parental mental health concerns impact both acute and long-term infant outcomes, there is a movement for universal screening of parental mental health (see the Resources box) as well as increasing the presence of psychosocial staffing within NICUs (Hynan et al., 2015). Pediatric consultation-liaison psychologists may provide services to parents of babies in NICU. Areas of intervention include supporting and developing the parent–infant narrative to improve parent–infant interaction and coregulation; parent coping skill development; and CBT to support effective communication, information retention, decision-making, and accessing outpatient mental health treatment (Hoge & Shaw, 2021).

Medical Traumatic Stress

The integrative model of pediatric medical traumatic stress defines changes in health status due to acute or chronic illness or injury; hospitalization; and painful, invasive, and scary medical care, tests, and/or procedures as potentially traumatic events for both pediatric patients and their family members (National Child Traumatic Stress Network, 2014; see also Chapter 4, this volume). Adverse or traumatic experiences are significantly related to long-term consequences for both physical and mental health (Oh et al., 2018). Evaluation, recognition, and intervention focused on historical, ongoing, or current traumatic or adverse experiences are integral to optimal care of hospitalized youth and their families. Pediatric consultation-liaison psychologists can identify traumatic reactions and mitigate or prevent worsening symptoms via trauma-informed intervention focused on identifying stressful aspects of medical care that are potentially modifiable; providing psychoeducation; engaging the patient and family in problem solving or coping skill development; and offering targeted CBT, such as thought recognition and restructuring, relaxation techniques, and graded exposure in which the child faces their smallest fears while working their way up to their largest. They provide education to multidisciplinary staff regarding culturally sensitive, trauma-informed, family-focused care practices (see Table 27.3), recommendations for medical management of pain as appropriate, and involvement of additional support staff such as child life, social work, or spiritual care. These interventions can reduce a patient's traumatic reaction, decrease distress, and support active coping while also minimizing vicarious trauma and burnout of medical providers (Marsac et al., 2016).

TABLE 27.3

Trauma-Informed Care Recommendations

Domain	Intervention
Control	Provide patient with as much control as possible. Patient should: ■ Understand and have a say in what is about to happen. ■ Have some control over pain management.
Knowledge	Use words and ideas patients can understand. Assess understanding of diagnosis or procedure via teach-back method. Clarify misconceptions.
Parents	Encourage parent presence and support of child's emotional expression and coping. Encourage parental basic self-care. Provide resources to support parental coping via support system and hospital staff.
Resources	Utilize psychosocial resources (e.g., social work, interpreter services) to mitigate impact on child traumatic stress by addressing challenges with housing, finances, insurance, language barriers, immigration, care of other children, and so on.

Note. Data from Lerwick (2016).

Medical Regimen Nonadherence

Pediatric consultation-liaison psychologists are consulted for concerns about adherence to medical recommendations such as medications, diet, fluid intake, physical activity, attending appointments, completion of other medical care (e.g., blood glucose checks, airway clearance, self-catheterization). Adherence to medical advice is strongly linked to health outcomes and health care utilization, but due to numerous biopsychosocial and systemic barriers, an estimated 50% of pediatric patients struggle with adherence (Rapoff, 2010). Evaluation of nonadherence requires clinical finesse due to the potential sensitivity of the topic. By utilizing a nonjudgmental, normalizing, motivational interview style, the pediatric consultation-liaison psychologists can shift the focus to a united goal of improving health. This can occur via targeted evaluation of side effects, impact on quality of life, barriers to adherence, and potential solutions, which can be supplemented by adherence assessment measures (see the Resources box). As barriers to adherence are often complex and span ecological systems, concerns may not resolve in the brief time available during the patient's hospital stay (Ramsey & Holbein, 2020). Therefore, pediatric consultation-liaison psychologists can identify barriers, provide basic adherence interventions (Table 27.4), and offer referrals to outpatient therapy after discharge.

Loss and End of Life

In collaboration with medical teams and other providers specializing in palliative and spiritual care, pediatric consultation-liaison psychologists commonly support patients and families in coping with loss, end of life, and bereavement. They provide education, normalize and encourage emotional expression surrounding grief and bereavement, and offer CBT for emotional or behavioral concerns, as well as interventions focused on symptom management (Cousino et al., 2020). Intervention may include supporting parents in having open and honest communication with their child surrounding prognosis and end of life. Every family has different preferences, and

TABLE 27.4
Adherence Barriers and Consultation-Liaison Interventions

Level domain	Intervention
Individual	
Cognitive functioning	Referral for neuropsychological evaluation; memory aids: alarms, tracking tools, and so on
Knowledge or perceived benefits	Developmentally and cognitively appropriate value-driven education
Psychological barriers	Referral for outpatient therapy; evaluate health beliefs, incentives or rewards, problem solving
Family	
Knowledge and care responsibility	Education, problem solving
Support, resources, logistics	Referral to social work
Stress or mental health concerns	Referral to outpatient therapy, social work, or behavioral systems therapy
Medications	
Taste	Mix with pleasant tastes, try preferred food/drink before or after, switch to pills from liquid
Pill swallowing and needle phobia	Behavioral pill swallowing intervention, graded exposure, referral to outpatient therapy
Side effects	Consult with medical providers regarding concerns
Regimen complexity	Work with medical providers for simplifying regimen, problem solving, creating daily schedule

Note. Adapted from "Treatment Adherence Within Consultation-Liaison Services," by R. R. Ramsey and C. E. Holbein, in B. D. Carter and K. A. Kullgren (Eds.), *Clinical Handbook of Psychological Consultation in Pediatric Medical Settings* (pp. 432–433), 2020, Springer International Publishing (https://doi.org/10.1007/978-3-030-35598-2_32). Copyright 2020 by Springer Nature. Adapted with permission.

pediatric consultation-liaison psychologists can provide guidance and education on developmentally appropriate ways to discuss end of life; use tools to understand patient wishes (i.e., *My Wishes* [Aging With Dignity, 2018], *Voicing My Choices* [see Zadeh et al., 2015], also see the Resources box); facilitate discussions among patient, family, and/or medical team; and provide guidance to the medical team regarding the patient's and family's wishes and values for the child's end-of-life care (Flowers et al., 2020). They may also provide support to the grieving medical team.

Common Mental Health Concerns

In terms of common psychiatric diagnoses, Bowling et al. (2021) reported that trauma- and stressor-related disorders, depression, and anxiety are the primary diagnoses treated by pediatric consultation-liaison psychologists. Developmental stage can impact common referral concerns, with younger children more often referred for anxiety or feeding concerns and adolescents referred for evaluation and treatment of depression, pain, other somatic complaints, and maladjustment (Kullgren et al., 2018). Considerations for these common concerns will be described in the following paragraphs.

Depression and anxiety. Pediatric patients with acute or chronic illness or injury are at higher risk for depression and anxiety, which may further disease burden, impact treatment engagement, and reduce overall health and well-being (Kline-Simon et al., 2016). Pediatric consultation-liaison psychologists support patients and families in identifying sources of anxiety or low mood, engaging in problem solving, creating coping plans, teaching relaxation techniques, scheduling worry time, and offering anxiety/phobia-targeted interventions as well as environmental interventions to reduce modifiable sources of distress. A common initial intervention includes utilizing behavioral activation through participation in pleasant activities with family members or multidisciplinary team members like child life specialists, participation in physical therapy and/or occupational therapy, and encouragement to complete activities of daily living and physical activity despite limitations due to medical status (Martin & Oliver, 2019). Pediatric consultation-liaison psychologists provide strength-based interventions to build on resilience factors as well as more formal CBT (i.e., identifying cognitive distortions, thought challenging, restructuring; Thabrew et al., 2018).

Psychiatric emergencies and crisis intervention. The prevalence of suicidality in youth continues to rise worldwide, especially in the face of the mental health crisis exacerbated by the COVID-19 pandemic (Yard et al., 2021). There is a movement toward universal risk screening of pediatric patients 10 years and older in the emergency department or early in hospital admission (Brahmbhatt et al., 2019; King et al., 2021; also see the Resources box). Pediatric consultation-liaison psychologists may evaluate patients specifically for concerns related to suicidal/homicidal ideation as well as conduct universal risk assessments. They then integrate data collected from the patient and collateral resources to determine the patient's acute level of risk and guide decision making with regard to the next steps. They conduct safety education and planning with the patient and family, provide crisis resources, inform the primary care physician and/or current mental health provider of risk, initiate immediate safety precautions (often including bedside staff for direct supervision, limitations to patient privacy, and removal of potentially dangerous items), and disposition planning (individual psychotherapy, intensive outpatient programs, inpatient psychiatric care; Brahmbhatt et al., 2019; Pettit et al., 2018).

Mental status changes. Changes in a child's mental status can be due to a broad range of medical or psychiatric concerns that require multidisciplinary evaluation to determine etiology and treatment. In pediatric patients, delirium is the most common explanation for a change in mental status due to medical causes including infection; trauma; metabolic conditions; or substance ingestion, intoxication, or withdrawal (Patti & Gupta, 2021). The first-line treatment for delirium is medical management of the underlying medical cause, and symptom course/severity can be evaluated with evidence-based measures (Silver et al., 2015; also see the Resources box). Psychotropic medications can help reduce agitation when paired with environmental interventions (verbal reassurance and redirection, access to familiar objects/pictures from home, lighting during the day to reinforce day and night cycles, easily readable date and time to reorient the patient, a calm environment with limited number of providers as appropriate). If a judicious medical workup has been completed, is generally reassuring, and symptoms are inconsistent with a known medical condition, psychiatric causes for a change in mental status can be evaluated. These may include psychosis, catatonia, severe depression, and SSRD. Pediatric consultation-liaison psychologists develop behavior plans to provide the patient with consistent behavioral expectations and support medical staff with the goal of reducing the need for chemical or physical restraints.

CONCLUSION

Pediatric psychology consultation-liaison practice is an exciting field with a range of opportunities to impact patient care and medical systems. In addition to direct patient care, a significant role for pediatric consultation-liaison psychologist is interdisciplinary (liaison with developmental-behavioral pediatricians, medical specialists, nurses, and others) with additional collaborations to inform systemic changes to support the health and well-being of patients and families. Modification of core pediatric psychology competencies can lead to significant positive impact in the health outcomes of hospitalized children and youth.

RESOURCES

Commonly Used Pediatric Psychology Consultation-Liaison Assessment Measures by Areas of Concern

Adherence

- Adolescent/Parent Medication Barriers Scale. Evaluates barriers to adherence for parents and children (Simons & Blount, 2007).
- Medical Adherence Measure. Evaluates medical knowledge and treatment adherence in children and parents (Zelikovsky & Schast, 2008).

ARFID

Gastrointestinal and Gastroesophageal Reflux Scale for Infants and Toddlers. Evaluates gastrointestinal distress and reflux (via parent report) in children younger than 2 years (Pados et al., 2021).

Transplant

- Pediatric Transplant Rating Instrument. Evaluates psychosocial risk factors for pretransplant candidates via parent and child report (Fung & Shaw, 2008).
- PedsQL Transplant Module. Evaluates health-related quality of life in pediatric patients, aged 5–18 years, with transplant (Weissberg-Benchell et al., 2010).

Mental Status

- Mini-Mental State Pediatric Examination. This tool screens for higher mental function and mental status in children 4–18 years (Ouvrier et al., 1993).
- School-Years Screening Test for the Evaluation of Mental Status. This tool, for children aged 5–17 years, can be used to assess suspected cognitive problems and mental status change (Ouvrier et al., 1999).

Delirium

Cornell Assessment for Pediatric Delirium. This observational screener is used to detect delirium in pediatric patients from neonates through 21 years (Silver et al., 2015).

Risk Assessment

- Columbia Suicide Severity Rating Scale. Evaluates suicide risk via interview in young people aged 11–18 years (Posner et al., 2011).
- Ask Suicide-Screening Questions. This screening tool can be used to assess suicide risk, via interview, in children and young people ages 8–24 years (Horowitz et al., 2012).

Pediatric Psychology Consultation-Liaison Practice Resources

Adherence

https://www.e-lfh.org.uk/programmes/kidzmed/

Coping With Hospitalization and Illness

- https://www.childrenshospital.org/patient-resources/you-arrive/your-visit/my-hospital-story
- https://copingclub.com/tools/k
- https://kidshealth.org/en/kids/hospital.html

End of Life

- https://www.bioethics.northwestern.edu/programs/epec/
- https://www.nhpco.org/
- https://fivewishes.org/

Feeding Disorders

https://www.feedingmatters.org

Neonatal Intensive Care Unit

Shaw, R. J., & Horowitz, S. (2021). *Treatment of psychological distress in parents of premature infants: PTSD in the ICU*. American Psychiatric Association Publishing.

Pain

- https://aci.health.nsw.gov.au/chronic-pain/painbytes
- https://www.thecomfortability.com/
- https://www.zoffness.com/resources/
- Coakley, R. (2016). *When your child hurts: Effective strategies to comfort, reduce stress, and break the cycle of chronic pain*. Yale University Press.
- Culbert, C. (2007). *Be the boss of your pain: Self-care for kids*. Free Spirit Publishing.

- Miles, B. S. (2006). *Imagine a rainbow: A child's guide for soothing pain*. Magination Press.
- Palmero, T., & Law, E. (2015). *Managing your child's chronic pain*. Oxford University Press.
- Zoffness, R. (2019). *The chronic pain and illness workbook for teens: CBT and mindfulness-based practices to turn the volume down on pain*. New Harbinger.

Somatic Symptom and Related Disorders

- https://keltymentalhealth.ca/somatization
- https://www.neurosymptoms.org/
- https://nonepilepticseizures.com/
- https://childmind.org/guide/somatic-symptom-disorder/
- https://fndhope.org

Traumatic Stress

- https://www.nctsn.org/
- https://www.aftertheinjury.org/
- https://umhs-adolescenthealth.org/wp-content/uploads/2022/02/trauma-informed-care-starter-guide-official.pdf
- https://www.healthcaretoolbox.org/

References

Aging With Dignity. (2018). *My wishes*. https://store.fivewishes.org/ShopLocal/en/p/MW-MASTER-000/my-wishes

Albright, D., Bruni, T., & Kronenberger, W. (2020). Assessment in pediatric psychology consultation-liaison. In B. D. Carter & K. A. Kullgren (Eds.), *Clinical handbook of psychological consultation in pediatric medical settings* (pp. 125–136). Springer. https://doi.org/10.1007/978-3-030-35598-2_11

American Psychiatric Association. (2013). *Diagnostic and statistical manual of mental disorders* (5th ed.). https://doi.org/10.1176/appi.books.9780890425596

Andersen, M. N., Dempster, R., Garbacz, L. L., Sayers, L., Shepard, H., Drayton, A., & Knight, R. M. (2020). Pediatric feeding disorders. In B. D. Carter & K. A. Kullgren (Eds.), *Clinical handbook of psychological consultation in pediatric medical settings* (pp. 227–238). Springer. https://doi.org/10.1007/978-3-030-35598-2_18

Bardach, N. S., Coker, T. R., Zima, B. T., Murphy, J. M., Knapp, P., Richardson, L. P., Edwall, G., & Mangione-Smith, R. (2014). Common and costly hospitalizations for pediatric mental health disorders. *Pediatrics*, *133*(4), 602–609. https://doi.org/10.1542/peds.2013-3165

Beck, A. T. (2016). Cognitive therapy: Nature and relation to behavior therapy—Republished article. *Behavior therapy*, *47*(6), 776–784. https://doi.org/10.1016/j.beth.2016.11.003 (Original work published 1970)

Bowling, A. A., Bearman, S. K., Wang, W., Guzman, L. A., & Daleiden, E. (2021). Pediatric consultation-liaison: Patient characteristics and considerations for training in evidence-based practices. *Journal of Clinical Psychology in Medical Settings*, *28*(3), 529–542. https://doi.org/10.1007/s10880-020-09738-0

Bowling, A. A., & Bearman, S. K. (2023). Pediatric consultation-liaison: Relationship between time to initial consult and length of hospitalization. *Clinical Practice in Pediatric Psychology*, *11*(3), 274–279. https://doi.org/10.1037/cpp0000446

Brady, A. M., Deighton, J., & Stansfeld, S. (2021). Chronic illness in childhood and early adolescence: A longitudinal exploration of co-occurring mental illness. *Development and Psychopathology*, *33*(3), 885–898. https://doi.org/10.1017/S0954579420000206

Brahmbhatt, K., Kurtz, B. P., Afzal, K. I., Giles, L. L., Kowal, E. D., Johnson, K. P., Lanzillo, E., Pao, M., Plioplys, S., Horowitz, L. M., & the PaCC Workgroup. (2019). Suicide risk screening in pediatric hospitals: Clinical pathways to address a global health crisis. *Psychosomatics*, *60*(1), 1–9. https://doi.org/10.1016/j.psym.2018.09.003

Bronfenbrenner, U. (1979). *The ecology of human development: Experiments by nature and design*. Harvard University Press. https://doi.org/10.2307/j.ctv26071r6

Cammarata, C., Bujoreanu, S., & Wohlheiter, K. (2020). Hospitalization and its impact: Stressors associated with inpatient hospitalization for the child and family. In B. D. Carter & K. A. Kullgren (Eds.), *Clinical handbook of psychological consultation in pediatric medical settings* (pp. 37–49). Springer. https://doi.org/10.1007/978-3-030-35598-2_4

Carter, B. D., Kronenberger, W. G., Scott, E. L., Kullgren, K. A., Piazza-Waggoner, C., & Brady, C. E. (2017). Inpatient pediatric consultation–liaison. In M. C. Roberts & R. G. Steele (Eds.), *Handbook of pediatric psychology* (5th ed., pp. 105–117). Guilford Press.

Carter, B. D., Tsang, K. K., Brady, C. E., & Kullgren, K. A. (2020). Pediatric consultation-liaison: Models and roles in pediatric psychology.

In B. D. Carter & K. A. Kullgren (Eds.), *Clinical handbook of psychological consultation in pediatric medical settings* (pp. 11–24). Springer. https://doi.org/10.1007/978-3-030-35598-2_2

Cheak-Zamora, N. C., & Thullen, M. (2017). Disparities in quality and access to care for children with developmental disabilities and multiple health conditions. *Maternal and Child Health Journal, 21*(1), 36–44. https://doi.org/10.1007/s10995-016-2091-0

Cousino, M. K., Rea, K. E., & Fredericks, E. M. (2020). Psychological consultation in pediatric solid organ transplantation. In B. D. Carter & K. A. Kullgren (Eds.), *Clinical handbook of psychological consultation in pediatric medical settings* (pp. 355–371). Springer. https://doi.org/10.1007/978-3-030-35598-2_27

Doran, G. T. (1981). There's a SMART way to write management's goals and objectives. *Management Review, 70*(11), 35–36.

Ellis, A. (1962). *Reason and emotion in psychotherapy*. Lyle Stuart.

Erickson, S. J., Gerstle, M., & Feldstein, S. W. (2005). Brief interventions and motivational interviewing with children, adolescents, and their parents in pediatric health care settings: A review. *Archives of Pediatrics & Adolescent Medicine, 159*(12), 1173–1180. https://doi.org/10.1001/archpedi.159.12.1173

Flowers, S. R., Hildenbrand, A. K., & Hansen-Moore, J. A. (2020). Pediatric oncology. In B. D. Carter & K. A. Kullgren (Eds.), *Clinical handbook of psychological consultation in pediatric medical settings* (pp. 295–314). Springer. https://doi.org/10.1007/978-3-030-35598-2_23

Foxen-Craft, E., Williams, A. E., & Scott, E. L. (2020). The problem of pain: Chronic pain. In B. D. Carter & K. A. Kullgren (Eds.), *Clinical handbook of psychological consultation in pediatric medical settings* (pp. 155–167). Springer. https://doi.org/10.1007/978-3-030-35598-2_13

Fung, E., & Shaw, R. J. (2008). Pediatric Transplant Rating Instrument—A scale for the pretransplant psychiatric evaluation of pediatric organ transplant recipients. *Pediatric Transplantation, 12*(1), 57–66. https://doi.org/10.1111/j.1399-3046.2007.00785.x

Gerson, R., Malas, N., Feuer, V., Silver, G. H., Prasad, R., & Mroczkowski, M. M. (2019). Best Practices for Evaluation and Treatment of Agitated Children and Adolescents (BETA) in the emergency department: Consensus statement of the American Association for Emergency Psychiatry. *The Western Journal of Emergency Medicine, 20*(2), 409–418. https://doi.org/10.5811/westjem.2019.1.41344

Hayes, S. C., Luoma, J. B., Bond, F. W., Masuda, A., & Lillis, J. (2006). Acceptance and commitment therapy: Model, processes and outcomes. *Behaviour Research and Therapy, 44*(1), 1–25. https://doi.org/10.1016/j.brat.2005.06.006

Hofmann, S. G., Asnaani, A., Vonk, I. J. J., Sawyer, A. T., & Fang, A. (2012). The efficacy of cognitive behavioral therapy: A review of meta-analyses. *Cognitive Therapy and Research, 36*(5), 427–440. https://doi.org/10.1007/s10608-012-9476-1

Hoge, M. K., & Shaw, R. J. (2021). Best practice guidelines on parental mental health in the neonatal intensive care unit: The importance and impact on infant health and developmental outcomes. *Early Human Development, 154*, 105277. https://doi.org/10.1016/j.earlhumdev.2020.105277

Horowitz, L. M., Bridge, J. A., Teach, S. J., Ballard, E., Klima, J., Rosenstein, D. L., Wharff, E. A., Ginnis, K., Cannon, E., Joshi, P., & Pao, M. (2012). Ask Suicide-Screening Questions (ASQ): A brief instrument for the pediatric emergency department. *Archives of Pediatrics & Adolescent Medicine, 166*(12), 1170–1176. https://doi.org/10.1001/archpediatrics.2012.1276

Hynan, M. T., Steinberg, Z., Baker, L., Cicco, R., Geller, P. A., Lassen, S., Milford, C., Mounts, K. O., Patterson, C., Saxton, S., Segre, L., & Stuebe, A. (2015). Recommendations for mental health professionals in the NICU. *Journal of Perinatology, 35*(Suppl. 1), S14–S18. https://doi.org/10.1038/jp.2015.144

Kazak, A. E. (2006). Pediatric psychosocial preventative health model (PPPHM): Research, practice, and collaboration in pediatric family systems medicine. *Families, Systems, & Health, 24*(4), 381–395. https://doi.org/10.1037/1091-7527.24.4.381

King, C. A., Brent, D., Grupp-Phelan, J., Casper, T. C., Dean, J. M., Chernick, L. S., Fein, J. A., Mahabee-Gittens, E. M., Patel, S. J., Mistry, R. D., Duffy, S., Melzer-Lange, M., Rogers, A., Cohen, D. M., Keller, A., Shenoi, R., Hickey, R. W., Rea, M., Cwik, M., . . . Gibbons, R. (2021). Prospective development and validation of the Computerized Adaptive Screen for Suicidal Youth. *JAMA Psychiatry, 78*(5), 540–549. https://doi.org/10.1001/jamapsychiatry.2020.4576

Kline-Simon, A. H., Weisner, C., & Sterling, S. (2016). Point prevalence of co-occurring behavioral health conditions and associated chronic disease burden among adolescents. *Journal of the American Academy of Child & Adolescent Psychiatry, 55*(5), 408–414. https://doi.org/10.1016/j.jaac.2016.02.008

Kullgren, K. A., & Carter, B. D. (2020). Introduction to the *Clinical Handbook of Psychological*

Consultation in Pediatric Medical Settings. In B. D. Carter & K. A. Kullgren (Eds.), *Clinical handbook of psychological consultation in pediatric medical settings* (pp. 3–9). Springer. https://doi.org/10.1007/978-3-030-35598-2_1

Kullgren, K. A., Sullivan, S. K., & Bravender, T. (2018). Understanding the unique needs of hospitalized adolescents and young adults referred for psychology consults. *Clinical Pediatrics, 57*(11), 1286–1293. https://doi.org/10.1177/0009922818774339

Lerwick, J. L. (2016). Minimizing pediatric healthcare-induced anxiety and trauma. *World Journal of Clinical Pediatrics, 5*(2), 143–150. https://doi.org/10.5409/wjcp.v5.i2.143

Linehan, M. M., Armstrong, H. E., Suarez, A., Allmon, D., & Heard, H. L. (1991). Cognitive-behavioral treatment of chronically parasuicidal borderline patients. *Archives of General Psychiatry, 48*(12), 1060–1064. https://doi.org/10.1001/archpsyc.1991.01810360024003

Lundahl, B., Droubay, B. A., Burke, B., Butters, R. P., Nelford, K., Hardy, C., Keovongsa, K., & Bowles, M. (2019). Motivational interviewing adherence tools: A scoping review investigating content validity. *Patient Education and Counseling, 102*(12), 2145–2155. https://doi.org/10.1016/j.pec.2019.07.003

MacKenzie, N. E., Tutelman, P. R., & Chambers, C. T. (2020). The problem of pain: Acute pain and procedures. In B. D. Carter & K. A. Kullgren (Eds.), *Clinical handbook of psychological consultation in pediatric medical settings* (pp. 139–153). Springer. https://doi.org/10.1007/978-3-030-35598-2_12

Maddux, M. H., Deacy, A. D., & Colombo, J. M. (2020). Organic gastrointestinal disorders. In B. D. Carter & K. A. Kullgren (Eds.), *Clinical handbook of psychological consultation in pediatric medical settings* (pp. 195–210). Springer. https://doi.org/10.1007/978-3-030-35598-2_16

Marsac, M. L., Kassam-Adams, N., Hildenbrand, A. K., Nicholls, E., Winston, F. K., Leff, S. S., & Fein, J. (2016). Implementing a trauma-informed approach in pediatric health care networks. *JAMA Pediatrics, 170*(1), 70–77. https://doi.org/10.1001/jamapediatrics.2015.2206

Martin, F., & Oliver, T. (2019). Behavioral activation for children and adolescents: A systematic review of progress and promise. *European Child & Adolescent Psychiatry, 28*(4), 427–441. https://doi.org/10.1007/s00787-018-1126-z

McKay, S., & Parente, V. (2019). Health disparities in the hospitalized child. *Hospital Pediatrics, 9*(5), 317–325. https://doi.org/10.1542/hpeds.2018-0223

Miller, W., & Rollnick, S. (1991). *Motivational interviewing: Preparing people to change addictive behavior*. Guilford Press.

National Child Traumatic Stress Network. (2014). *Pediatric medical traumatic stress toolkit for health care providers*. https://www.nctsn.org/resources/pediatric-medical-traumatic-stress-toolkit-health-care-providers

Noeder, M. M., & Davis, A. L. (2020). Developmental considerations in consultation-liaison psychology. In B. D. Carter & K. A. Kullgren (Eds.), *Clinical handbook of psychological consultation in pediatric medical settings* (pp. 375–385). Springer. https://doi.org/10.1007/978-3-030-35598-2_28

Oh, D. L., Jerman, P., Silvério Marques, S., Koita, K., Purewal Boparai, S. K., Burke Harris, N., & Bucci, M. (2018). Systematic review of pediatric health outcomes associated with childhood adversity. *BMC Pediatrics, 18*(1), 83. https://doi.org/10.1186/s12887-018-1037-7

Ouvrier, R., Hendy, J., Bornholt, L., & Black, F. H. (1999). SYSTEMS: School-Years Screening Test for the Evaluation of Mental Status. *Journal of Child Neurology, 14*(12), 772–780. https://doi.org/10.1177/088307389901401202

Ouvrier, R. A., Goldsmith, R. F., Ouvrier, S., & Williams, I. C. (1993). The value of the Mini-Mental State Examination in childhood: A preliminary study. *Journal of Child Neurology, 8*(2), 145–148. https://doi.org/10.1177/088307389300800206

Pados, B. F., Repsha, C., & Hill, R. R. (2021). The Gastrointestinal and Gastroesophageal Reflux (GIGER) Scale for infants and toddlers. *Global Pediatric Health, 8*. https://doi.org/10.1177/2333794X211033130

Patallo, B. J. (2019). The multicultural guidelines in practice: Cultural humility in clinical training and supervision. *Training and Education in Professional Psychology, 13*(3), 227–232. https://doi.org/10.1037/tep0000253

Patti, L., & Gupta, M. (2021). *Change in mental status*. StatPearls Publishing. https://www.ncbi.nlm.nih.gov/books/NBK441973/

Perrin, E. C., & Shipman, D. (2009). Hospitalization, surgery, and medical and dental procedures. In W. B. Carey, A. C. Crocker, W. L. Coleman, E. R. Elias, & H. M. Feldman (Eds.), *Developmental-behavioral pediatrics* (4th ed., pp. 329–336). W. B. Saunders. https://doi.org/10.1016/B978-1-4160-3370-7.00033-X

Pettit, J. W., Buitron, V., & Green, K. L. (2018). Assessment and management of suicide risk in children and adolescents. *Cognitive and Behavioral Practice*, 25(4), 460–472. https://doi.org/10.1016/j.cbpra.2018.04.001

Posner, K., Brown, G. K., Stanley, B., Brent, D. A., Yershova, K. V., Oquendo, M. A., Currier, G. W., Melvin, G. A., Greenhill, L., Shen, S., & Mann, J. J. (2011). The Columbia-Suicide Severity Rating Scale: Initial validity and internal consistency findings from three multisite studies with adolescents and adults. *The American Journal of Psychiatry*, 168(12), 1266–1277. https://doi.org/10.1176/appi.ajp.2011.10111704

Ramsey, R. R., & Holbein, C. E. (2020). Treatment adherence within consultation-liaison services. In B. D. Carter & K. A. Kullgren (Eds.), *Clinical handbook of psychological consultation in pediatric medical settings* (pp. 425–438). Springer. https://doi.org/10.1007/978-3-030-35598-2_32

Rapoff, M. A. (2010). *Adherence to pediatric medical regimens*. Springer. https://doi.org/10.1007/978-1-4419-0570-3

Rennick, J. E., Dougherty, G., Chambers, C., Stremler, R., Childerhose, J. E., Stack, D. M., Harrison, D., Campbell-Yeo, M., Dryden-Palmer, K., Zhang, X., & Hutchison, J. (2014). Children's psychological and behavioral responses following pediatric intensive care unit hospitalization: The caring intensively study. *BMC Pediatrics*, 14(1), 276. https://doi.org/10.1186/1471-2431-14-276

Rome Foundation. (2016). *Appendix A: Rome IV diagnostic criteria for functional gastrointestinal disorders* [Webpage]. https://theromefoundation.org/rome-iv/rome-iv-criteria/

Scott, K. M., Lim, C., Al-Hamzawi, A., Alonso, J., Bruffaerts, R., Caldas-de-Almeida, J. M., Florescu, S., de Girolamo, G., Hu, C., de Jonge, P., Kawakami, N., Medina-Mora, M. E., Moskalewicz, J., Navarro-Mateu, F., O'Neill, S., Piazza, M., Posada-Villa, J., Torres, Y., & Kessler, R. C. (2016). Association of mental disorders with subsequent chronic physical conditions: World mental health surveys from 17 countries. *JAMA Psychiatry*, 73(2), 150–158. https://doi.org/10.1001/jamapsychiatry.2015.2688

Silver, G., Kearney, J., Traube, C., & Hertzig, M. (2015). Delirium screening anchored in child development: The Cornell Assessment for Pediatric Delirium. *Palliative & Supportive Care*, 13(4), 1005–1011. https://doi.org/10.1017/S1478951514000947

Simons, L. E., & Blount, R. L. (2007). Identifying barriers to medication adherence in adolescent transplant recipients. *Journal of Pediatric Psychology*, 32(7), 831–844. https://doi.org/10.1093/jpepsy/jsm030

Sinyor, M., Goldstein, B. I., & Schaffer, A. (2019). Bridging the mental-physical divide in health care. *CMAJ: Canadian Medical Association Journal/journal de l'Association medicale canadienne*, 191(26), E722–E723. https://doi.org/10.1503/cmaj.190709

Steiner, H., Fritz, G. K., Mrazek, D., Gonzales, J., & Jensen, P. (1993). Pediatric and psychiatric comorbidity. Part I: The future of consultation-liaison psychiatry. *Psychosomatics*, 34(2), 107–111. https://doi.org/10.1016/S0033-3182(93)71899-X

Straus, J., Coburn, S., Maskell, S., Pappagianopoulos, J., & Cantrell, K. (2019). Medical encounters for youth with autism spectrum disorder: A comprehensive review of environmental considerations and interventions. *Clinical Medicine Insights: Pediatrics*, 13. https://doi.org/10.1177/1179556519842816

Thabrew, H., Stasiak, K., Hetrick, S. E., Donkin, L., Huss, J. H., Highlander, A., Wong, S., & Merry, S. N. (2018). Psychological therapies for anxiety and depression in children and adolescents with long-term physical conditions. *Cochrane Database of Systematic Reviews*, 2018(12), CD012488. https://doi.org/10.1002/14651858.CD012488.pub2

Tsang, K. K., Hayes, L. C., & Cammarata, C. (2020). Eating disorders and avoidant/restrictive food intake disorder. In B. D. Carter & K. A. Kullgren (Eds.), *Clinical handbook of psychological consultation in pediatric medical settings* (pp. 211–226). Springer. https://doi.org/10.1007/978-3-030-35598-2_17

Weiss, K. E., Steinman, K. J., Kodish, I., Sim, L., Yurs, S., Steggall, C., & Fobian, A. D. (2021). Functional neurological symptom disorder in children and adolescents within medical settings. *Journal of Clinical Psychology in Medical Settings*, 28(1), 90–101. https://doi.org/10.1007/s10880-020-09736-2

Weissberg-Benchell, J., Zielinski, T. E., Rodgers, S., Greenley, R. N., Askenazi, D., Goldstein, S. L., Fredericks, E. M., McDiarmid, S., Williams, L., Limbers, C. A., Tuzinkiewicz, K., Lerret, S., Alonso, E. M., & Varni, J. W. (2010). Pediatric health-related quality of life: Feasibility, reliability and validity of the PedsQL transplant module. *American Journal of Transplantation*, 10(7), 1677–1685. https://doi.org/10.1111/j.1600-6143.2010.03149.x

Williams, S. E., Zahka, N. E., & Kullgren, K. A. (2020). Somatic symptom and related disorders.

In B. D. Carter & K. A. Kullgren (Eds.), *Clinical handbook of psychological consultation in pediatric medical settings* (pp. 169–181). Springer. https://doi.org/10.1007/978-3-030-35598-2_14

Yard, E., Radhakrishnan, L., Ballesteros, M. F., Sheppard, M., Gates, A., Stein, Z., Hartnett, K., Kite-Powell, A., Rodgers, L., Adjemian, J., Ehlman, D. C., Holland, K., Idaikkadar, N., Ivey-Stephenson, A., Martinez, P., Law, R., & Stone, D. M. (2021). Emergency department visits for suspected suicide attempts among persons aged 12–25 years before and during the COVID-19 pandemic—United States, January 2019–May 2021. *MMWR: Morbidity and Mortality Weekly Report, 70*(24), 888–894. https://doi.org/10.15585/mmwr.mm7024e1

Zadeh, S., Pao, M., & Wiener, L. (2015). Opening end-of-life discussion: How to introduce Voicing My CHOiCES™, an advance care planning guide for adolescents and young adults. *Palliative and Supportive Care, 13*(3), 591–599. https://doi.org/10.1017/S1478951514000054

Zelikovsky, N., & Schast, A. P. (2008). Eliciting accurate reports of adherence in a clinical interview: Development of the Medical Adherence Measure. *Pediatric Nursing, 34*(2), 141–146.

Zima, B. T., Rodean, J., Hall, M., Bardach, N. S., Coker, T. R., & Berry, J. G. (2016). Psychiatric disorders and trends in resource use in pediatric hospitals. *Pediatrics, 138*(5), e20160909. https://doi.org/10.1542/peds.2016-0909

CHAPTER 28

INTEGRATED BEHAVIORAL HEALTH IN PEDIATRIC HEALTH CARE SETTINGS

Blake M. Lancaster, Hannah L. Ham, Alexandra Neenan, Eleah Sunde, Sharnita D. Harris, Luke K. Turnier, Richard Birnbaum, and Alexandros Maragakis

Integrating behavioral health providers into primary care is a model of primary care designed to provide health care that addresses both the mind and the body—the whole person—in the primary care setting. It is virtually impossible for a pediatrician to address all of the potential physical and behavioral issues that children present within the primary care setting. Embedding a behavioral health provider in the primary care context provides the opportunity for patients to receive collaborative physical and behavioral health care in one setting. Although the notion of embedding a psychologist in primary care seems to be relatively simple, a variety of issues need to be considered and addressed to accomplish this modest goal. These issues include but are not limited to specialized training required for the behavioral health provider to function effectively as an integrated provider in primary care, scope of practice, authorizations and billing considerations, and assessment and treatment models.

This chapter begins with an overview of integrated behavioral health (IBH) and how it evolved in partnership with pediatric primary care to address a critical gap in mental health care. The chapter will consider the ecological contexts (informed by developmental science) relevant to IBH models and will present models of screening, assessment, and treatment in primary care. We will highlight how IBH can help address disparities and inequities in health care delivery and discuss practical considerations for implementing IBH models of care (training, education, reimbursement). We will discuss ethical considerations in IBH models, including issues of privacy and information sharing, and we will describe how IBH models of care can integrate with other behavioral health systems of care, including developmental-behavioral pediatrics, to address behavioral health needs of children.

ADDRESSING IDENTIFIED HEALTH NEEDS AND SERVICE GAPS THROUGH INTEGRATED BEHAVIORAL HEALTH SERVICES

Most children who experience a mental health issue will not receive any form of behavioral health treatment (Godoy et al., 2017). Current research shows that 35% of youth will experience a diagnosable mental disorder by age 15 and that prevalence of a diagnosable mental disorder will increase to 50% by age 18 (Caspi et al., 2020). Among adolescents diagnosed with a mental health disorder, fewer than half (45%) receive some form of service (Costello et al., 2014). In contrast, more than 90% of children in the United States receive primary care services (Stein et al., 2008).

Despite reported discomfort and lack of behavioral health training, primary care pediatricians have been labeled as the de facto behavioral health care providers because they deliver approximately 80% of behavioral health services for children (Leslie et al., 2006; Norquist & Regier, 1996). Pediatricians make up the majority of behavioral health providers in the United States. However, 65% of primary care pediatricians reported a lack of training in the treatment of children and adolescents with mental health problems, 40% reported lacking confidence in their ability to recognize these problems, and more than 50% reported lacking confidence in their ability to treat mental health concerns (Lancaster et al., 2019; McMillan et al., 2017). Although primary care pediatricians report some comfort with identifying mental health issues compared with managing treatment, a majority report significant barriers to identifying outpatient treatment providers (Bettencourt et al., 2021).

When primary care pediatricians refer patients to outpatient service, the literature shows the rate of attendance at first visit ranges from near zero (Wildman & Langkamp, 2012) to less than 50% (Kelleher et al., 2006). The lack of follow-through to outpatient service, as a result of long wait-lists or a dearth of providers, often results in patients returning to their primary care pediatrician for continuing/repeated treatment of behavioral health problems (Hine et al., 2017). When patients are successful in obtaining behavioral health services outside of the primary care office, challenges with effective collaboration of care can undermine effective treatment (Kolko & Perrin, 2014). Difficulties with obtaining an appropriate referral, in addition to challenges with treatment collaboration, potentially increase the likelihood that primary care pediatricians will rely more heavily on medication management of behavioral health issues (e.g., attention-deficit/hyperactivity disorder [ADHD]), although evidence-based behavioral health intervention is recommended as the first-line intervention (Pelham Jr. et al., 2016).

The mismatch between pediatrician expertise and the increase in behavioral health issues has created a demand for behavioral health services in primary care. Difficulties with obtaining referrals for behavioral health treatment, in addition to a shortage of behavioral health providers (Mongelli et al., 2020). Challenges and opportunities to meet the mental health needs of underserved and disenfranchised populations in the United States (Mongelli et al., 2020) have increased this demand for integrated behavioral health care across the United States (Asarnow et al., 2017). Integrating behavioral health services into primary care, where most children receive their health care, increases access to these services by 66% to 95% (Kolko et al., 2010; Lieberman et al., 2006), with an 85% rate of attendance for the first visit (Valleley et al., 2020). It also reduces the burden on primary care providers who are frequently tasked with addressing behavioral health concerns (Riley et al., 2019). Increased behavioral health screening in primary care and training for pediatricians provide a myriad of benefits including increased collaboration of care with behavioral health specialists (Godoy et al., 2017), improved identification of behavior health concerns, and establishment of evidence-based treatment plans for patients with reported mental health concerns (Bitsko et al., 2016). Integrating behavioral health into the primary care setting has notable benefits including the potential to increase access and more efficiently address both physical- and mental-health-related concerns among pediatric patients (Campo et al., 2015).

INTEGRATING BEHAVIORAL HEALTH INTO PEDIATRIC PRIMARY CARE

Pediatricians signaled openness to integrating behavioral health providers into primary care as early as the 1960s. At the annual conference of the American Academy of Pediatrics in 1964, J. L. Wilson suggested that, due to the frequency with which behavioral health issues present in primary care, groups of primary care pediatricians should hire psychologists to address children's and adolescents' mental health issues. Welcomed by pediatricians who were providing up to 80% of the mental health care for children in the United States while being largely untrained in behavioral health assessment and treatment, Wilson's proposal set the stage for the emergence of integrated behavioral health clinics (Sharp et al., 1992).

Despite the long-standing enthusiasm for the IBH model, only about 15% of pediatric primary care clinics had a behavioral health provider as of 2009 (Guevara et al., 2009). A variety of barriers contributed to the modest growth of integrated models in pediatric primary care. These barriers related to the lack of a specialized behavioral health workforce and logistical concerns including clinic space and legal, insurance, and professional guild issues. Some of the professional guild issues stemmed from psychological guilds that were initially resistant to collaborating with physicians in the medical field (Allen et al., 1993; Friman, 2010). There were concerns that the discipline would lose professional independence and become reliant on and/or absorbed by the physicians' guild. Other guild issues centered on psychologists' ability to function within a medical setting, adjusting to performance measures in medical settings, and concerns about the professional hierarchy. Ultimately, most of these logistical and guild issues have been resolved, but they are in constant flux and often need to be addressed in each instance of collaboration between psychologists and physicians in order to establish an integrated behavioral health clinic.

The purpose of IBH is to embed behavioral health providers in primary care clinics to provide coordinated/collaborative care with physicians and thereby ensure that patients receive health care services addressing both the mind and body. Integrated behavioral health providers are trained to assess and treat the wide variety of behavioral health issues that present in primary care. Figure 28.1 provides a breakdown of common reasons for referral to IBH services (Bruni et al., 2016).

Historically, the majority of behavioral health problems that present in primary care have revolved around mild to moderate externalizing behavioral problems (e.g., oppositional defiant disorder and ADHD; Schuhmann et al., 1996). Although these issues still represent roughly half of referrals to IBH providers, the relative prevalence of referrals for internalizing symptoms (e.g., anxiety, depression) has increased from

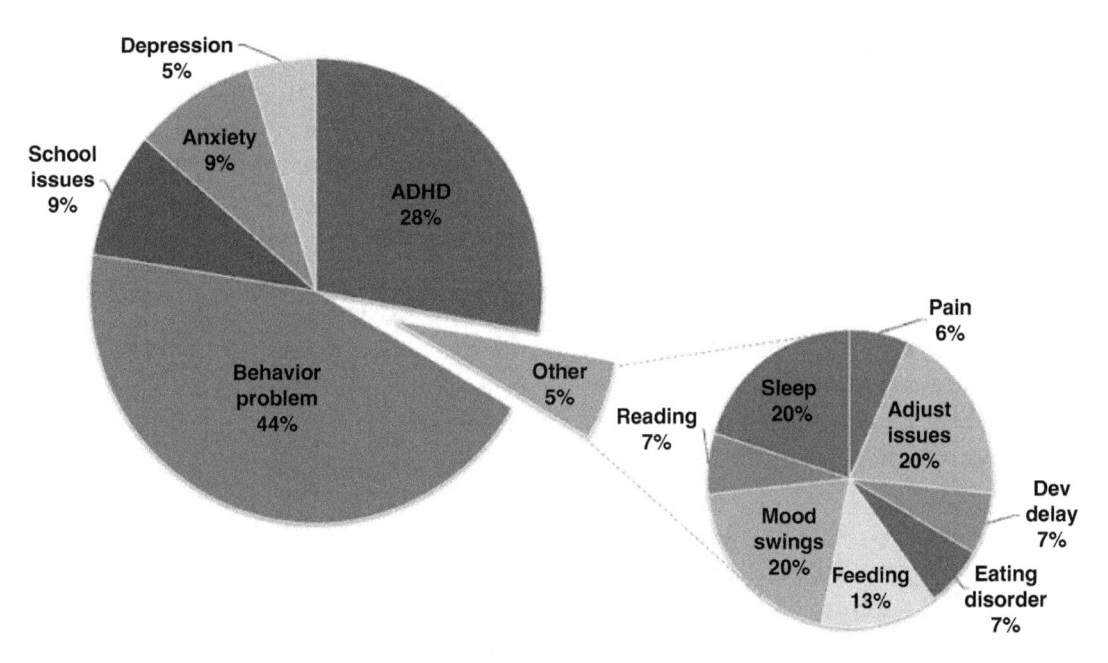

FIGURE 28.1. Common reasons for referral to integrated behavioral health services. Dev = developmental. From *Applied Behavior Analysis in Pediatric Primary Care: Bringing Applied Behavior Analysis to Scale* [Poster presentation], by T. P. Bruni and B. M. Lancaster, 45th Annual Convention of Applied Behavior Analysis International, Chicago, IL, United States, 2019. Copyright 2019 by T. P. Bruni and B. M. Lancaster. Reprinted with permission.

roughly 20% to 30% in the context of the COVID-19 pandemic (Chakawa et al., 2021). Concerns with health behaviors such as toileting, sleeping, and eating issues represent an additional smaller portion of IBH referrals (Talmi et al., 2016; Valleley et al., 2020). An IBH provider needs to be trained in a developmental context to be able to assess the severity of the presenting behavioral health issues and to titrate treatment based on developmental context. Additionally, IBH providers need to be able to identify the severity of the presenting issue and refer to providers such as a developmental-behavioral pediatrician (e.g., for autism, complex/high-intensity ADHD) or a pediatric psychologist (e.g., for pain, sleep, encopresis). To conduct these activities effectively, it is widely considered essential that IBH providers maintain a physical presence in the primary care clinic, although there are several models for integrating a behavioral health provider into primary care.

INTEGRATED CARE MODELS

Models of IBH service delivery (Heath et al., 2013; Peek & the National Integration Academy Council, 2013) differ in the way that providers coordinate and collaborate on behavioral health services. The phrase "integrated behavioral health" is ambiguous and requires a more specific description of how evidenced-based behavioral health services are implemented in a modular, time-limited, goal-focused manner in different settings. This vagueness in terminology and lack of a standard universally agreed upon structure to describe model differences presents challenges for researchers and policy makers attempting to compare model effects, such as those relating to operating costs and patient outcomes (Berwick et al., 2008)

Heath et al. (2013) developed a standard six-level framework specifying how behavioral health services are integrated within primary care. It consists of three core classifications—coordinated, colocated, and integrated care models—categorizing the lowest to the highest forms of integration. Each classification has two levels that indicate the extent of collaboration. Heath and colleagues characterized *collaboration* in their framework as the way in which health care providers in clinics work together and *integration* as the way in which services are implemented and clinics are operated.

Coordinated Care

The core features of coordinated care reflect the lowest degree of communication and integration between behavioral health and primary care providers. Coordinated care is sporadic and occurs only when there is a distinct need. Level 1, minimal collaboration, involves infrequent contact, with providers operating in different environments and systems. Level 2, basic collaboration at a distance, involves a logistic relationship similar to that in level 1, with more frequent but still intermittent communication based on necessity.

Colocated Care

The core characteristic of colocated care is that behavioral health and primary care providers are housed in the same facility. Level 3, basic collaboration on-site, involves more regular communication between providers (facilitated by their physical presence in the office) but still includes maintaining distinct systems. Level 4, close collaboration with some system integration, can include sharing of some administrative functions, such as scheduling and use of electronic medical records. Colocation facilitates better communication between providers but does not ensure formal integration.

Integrated Care

Integrated care necessitates modifications in how primary care and behavioral health providers deliver services. Level 5, close collaboration approaching an integrated practice, involves behavioral health and primary care providers working together to devise system-level solutions. This means that a change in service delivery has begun but is not complete. Level 6, collaboration in a transformed/merged practice, represents a fully integrated system of primary care and behavioral health for every patient.

There are also models that describe a focus on providing behavioral health services to specific patient populations. For example, the collaborative care model is designed for patients with more chronic mental illnesses and often involves collaboration among primary care providers, care managers, and a consulting psychiatrist (American Psychiatric Association & the Academy of Psychosomatic Medicine, 2016). In contrast, the primary care behavioral health model is focused on a larger proportion of patients with behavioral health needs within a primary care clinic (Reiter et al., 2018). This model includes a behavioral health generalist (e.g., psychologist or social worker) working in conjunction with primary care providers to provide more consultative short-term evidence-based treatments with patients until symptoms have appropriately improved.

Research is currently limited regarding comparative outcomes among the different care models (Stancin, 2016). Nonetheless, Yonek and colleagues (2020) found that, regardless of the different behavioral health models, the most effective features were population-based care, measurement-based care, and evidence-based behavioral health service. Unfortunately, multiple barriers exist that impede behavioral health integration in organizations.

Barriers to implementing behavioral health into primary care include existing health care policies and reimbursement regulations, organizational structures, inefficiency, financial resources, and workforce reluctance and training (Gerrity et al., 2014; Grazier et al., 2016; Miller et al., 2013). Research by Grazier et al. (2016) identified various ways these barriers to integration can be effectively surmounted:

- by focusing on under-resourced and at-risk populations,
- by using a data-centered approach to assess and address both system strengths and gaps in care,
- by forming partnerships with community organizations to better manage the broad range of patient needs,
- by gaining support from prominent community stakeholders,
- by developing an organizational team-focused solution including provider teams and administrators as well as patients and their families, and
- by maintaining and generating diverse funding mechanisms.

BENEFITS OF INTEGRATING BEHAVIORAL HEALTH INTO PRIMARY CARE

Most families present to their primary care pediatrician with behavioral health concerns; IBH care offers these families accessible behavioral health care services within the patient's medical home. From the perspective of the patient and family, working with a behavioral health professional who works directly with the child's trusted pediatrician within the same building can increase accessibility of services and comfort and reduce stigma associated with disclosing mental health concerns (Stancin & Perrin, 2014). It also allows for interdisciplinary communication and coordinated physical and behavioral health care for patients. Additionally, patients experience reduced costs because integrated behavioral health care can minimize unnecessary repeat medical visits (Valleley et al., 2004) and medical inpatient services (Highland et al., 2020).

Integrating behavioral health care into primary care also benefits primary care physicians. In a health care setting in which they are being asked to do increasingly more, physicians experience time (Cooper et al., 2006; Meadows et al., 2011) and reimbursement barriers (Connor et al., 2006; deGruy, 1997; Meadows et al., 2011) when addressing behavioral health concerns. The average 20 minutes required for pediatricians to address behavioral health concerns exceeds the typical 12- to 15-minute time allotment per patient, which can have adverse effects on physician efficiency and workflow. Pediatricians are also reimbursed at a significantly lower rate per minute than behavioral health providers for the treatment of behavioral health concerns (Meadows et al., 2011). Integrated behavioral health providers are able to provide more minutes of service to patients while also receiving mental health reimbursement for service provision. The idea that IBH results in increased productivity and improved workflow is known as the "physician leveraging effect" (Cummings et al., 2009) by which pediatricians spend more time on medical concerns and primary prevention efforts and less time addressing time-intensive behavior problems (Chaffee, 2008). Physicians report satisfaction with IBH services (Hine et al., 2017).

ECOLOGICAL CONTEXTS RELEVANT TO IBH: CONSIDERATIONS FROM DEVELOPMENTAL SCIENCE

The IBH model has shown potential for addressing behavioral health disparities, reducing symptoms across diagnoses, and is appropriate across development. Behavioral health disparities have been well documented among communities of color. Black/African Americans and Latin Americans are less likely to access behavioral health treatment (Agency for Healthcare Research and Quality, 2015). However, integrating a psychologist in primary care has led to favorable outcomes for Black/African Americans and Latin Americans, including significant reductions in symptoms and improvements in functioning, satisfaction with behavioral health services, and a strong therapeutic alliance (Bridges et al., 2014; O'Loughlin et al., 2019; Pickford et al., 2021). Spanish-speaking patients have also demonstrated a strong therapeutic alliance with integrated behavioral health providers, even when an interpreter was used (Villalobos et al., 2016), which suggests that having trained interpreters within primary care is essential for increasing access to services for patients with limited English proficiency. Moreover, providers will want to consider the impact of ethnicity and culture when providing care. More specifically, it is critical for behavioral health care providers to be aware of unconscious biases influencing diagnosis and treatment. One study found that, at their initial IBH appointment, Latin Americans are significantly less likely to receive a psychiatric diagnosis than non-Latin Americans (Bridges et al., 2014). Disparities in diagnosis and treatment can be reduced by providers remaining vigilant and checking their own biases through ongoing professional development focused on identifying and addressing implicit biases (Lelutiu-Weinberger et al., 2023; Zestcott et al., 2016).

Additionally, IBH models (i.e., colocated and fully integrated) are ideal for addressing externalizing and internalizing problems commonly seen in childhood, such as oppositional defiant behavior, ADHD, anxiety, and depression (Moore et al., 2018; Weersing et al., 2017) through evidenced-based treatment strategies including cognitive behavior therapy, behavior therapy, and parent management training. Careful consideration must be given to the appropriateness of treating trauma within primary care given time limits and high patient volume. Evidence supports the feasibility and acceptability of screening for trauma in primary care and providing preventative services for infants screening positive for adverse childhood experiences (Kia-Keating et al., 2019). Although ongoing trauma treatment for posttraumatic stress disorder, reactive attachment disorder, acute stress disorder, disinhibited social engagement disorder, and grief and loss may not be the best fit for the scope of IBH, behavioral health providers can offer preliminary recommendations (e.g., relaxation strategies, behavior activation) and connect families to appropriate community providers.

SCREENING, ASSESSMENT, TREATMENT, AND INTERVENTIONS IN CLINICAL PRACTICE

Patients with behavioral health concerns frequently present first to their primary care pediatrician, necessitating a process for identifying and referring patients to behavioral services even in IBH settings (Njoroge et al., 2016). Children's behavioral health concerns frequently go unaddressed, particularly when they are mild enough to be amenable to brief solution-focused interventions (Kolko & Perrin, 2014). Given limited time to address children's health needs in the primary care setting, relying on non-formalized or idiosyncratic processes for identification of behavioral health concerns by physician or parent risks that these difficulties will go unnoticed.

Screening and Referral Processes

Universal, proactive, systematic screening that accurately captures children's difficulties can provide a more robust approach to determining which children need IBH services. Such screening requires systems-level changes to allow for additional time spent administering and scoring screening measures. To successfully implement screening procedures, buy-in from members of the medical team who would be delivering screening measures is essential (Godoy et al., 2017). Similarly, identifying appropriate opportunities for parents to complete screening measures (e.g., at check-in, online prior to the appointment) is necessary to ensure uptake. Systematic screening procedures for common behavioral health concerns should be implemented using tools that take no more than 5 to 10 minutes for patients or caregivers to complete. Appropriate screening measures for IBH settings can be easily scored and interpreted by medical professionals, who can then determine whether a child's concerns should be addressed by a behavioral health clinician (BHC; Maruish, 2018). Referral to IBH may occur alongside referral to allied services, such as developmental-behavioral pediatrics or child psychiatry for additional diagnostic evaluation or medication management of behavioral health issues (Godoy et al., 2017). Table 28.1 provides a list of screening measures that are appropriate for primary care.

Purpose of IBH Interventions

The purpose of IBH is to provide and coordinate behavioral health care across the entire population of a primary care clinic, including patients with a full range of behavioral health concerns. In early childhood, these may include tantrum behaviors or toileting difficulties; older children may exhibit mood or anxiety concerns. Many patients in primary care settings may not seek out behavioral health services, or they may only have subclinical concerns (Kolko & Perrin, 2014; Robinson & Reiter, 2016). Serving these patients in the familiar setting of the primary care practice allows BHCs to increase overall access while

TABLE 28.1

Sample Screening Measures Appropriate for Integrated Behavioral Health Settings

Name of assessment	Brief description	Number of items	Respondent	Psychometrics
Pediatric Symptom Checklist (Gardner et al., 1999)	Measures externalizing, internalizing, and attention problems in children ages 4–17; Spanish version available (Piqueras et al., 2021)	17	Parent	80% sensitivity for detecting externalizing disorders and depression; 68% sensitivity for detecting anxiety (Gardner et al., 2007)
Patient Health Questionnaire (Kroenke et al., 2001)	Measures depression symptoms and subjective distress in individuals ages 13 and older	9	Self	Scores ≥11 demonstrate 89% sensitivity and 77% specificity for identifying major depressive disorder in adolescents (Richardson et al., 2010)
Generalized Anxiety Disorder Scale (Spitzer et al., 2006)	Measures generalized anxiety symptoms and subjective distress in individuals ages 12 and older	7	Self	Scores ≥11 demonstrate 97% sensitivity and 100% specificity for identifying generalized anxiety disorder (Mossman et al., 2017)
Ages and Stages Questionnaires (3rd ed.; Squires & Bricker, 2009)	Series of questionnaires that assesses social, motor, and language development from ages 2 to 66 months; versions available in several languages (Singh et al., 2017)	30	Parent	Test–retest reliability of 92%, sensitivity of 87% and specificity of 96% for detecting significant developmental concerns (Singh et al., 2017)

meeting the needs of a large number of patients (Robinson & Reiter, 2016). Unlike traditional psychotherapy, IBH interventions serve to facilitate improvement only in a circumscribed behavior or small set of behaviors (e.g., sleep onset, toileting, tantrums, noncompliance; see Table 28.2). As with primary care more broadly, specialty concerns (i.e., significant functional impairment, safety concerns) typically warrant outside referrals.

A stepped care approach is a model that utilizes the least intensive approach that can be reasonably expected to benefit the patient and escalates to a higher levels of care only when needed (Snipes et al., 2015). This model can be employed to most efficiently utilize limited resources among the medical team. For example, the BHC may create handouts or brochures that the pediatrician can provide to patients with mild and circumscribed concerns without needing to involve the BHC directly in each case. For patients with mild to moderate concerns, the BHC may meet with the patient once or several times to facilitate psychoeducational or brief behavioral interventions in either an individual or group format. Many evidence-based behavioral interventions, such as parent–child interaction therapy and Coping Cat, have been adapted for use in primary care settings (Kolko & Perrin, 2014). As with traditional psychotherapy, IBH interventions should produce measurable improvements in the patient's functioning as evidenced by decreased frequency, length, or severity of problem behavior and improvements in functioning. However, due to the time constraints inherent to IBH, interventions that require weekly sessions or full-length therapy sessions are not feasible (Kolko & Perrin, 2014).

TABLE 28.2

List of Common Integrated Behavioral Health Interventions

Name of intervention	Brief description of intervention	Resource
Motivational interviewing	Collaborative style of interviewing and engagement to foster patients' commitment to health behavior change	Erickson et al., 2005 (https://jamanetwork.com/journals/jamapediatrics/fullarticle/486200)
Parent management behavioral training	Parent training that fosters skills in positive communication, positive reinforcement, structure, and discipline	https://www.cdc.gov/adhd/treatment/behavior-therapy.html
Brief cognitive behavior therapy	Individualized approach to address distorted cognitions and physiological activation through skill-based techniques	Friedberg & Paternostro, 2019 (https://doi.org/10.1007/978-3-030-21683-2_7)
P.R.I.D.E. skills	Child-directed interaction to teach caregivers skills in praise, reflection, imitation, describing children's behavior, enjoyment in interaction	Parent–child interaction therapy (PCIT), n.d. (https://www.parentchildinteractiontherapy.com/pcit-child-directed-interaction)
Special playtime	Scheduled, consistent 1:1 play time with parents and children to foster positive parenting interactions	Centers for Disease Control and Prevention, 2019 (https://www.cdc.gov/parenting-toddlers/communication/special-playtime.html?CDC_AAref_Val=https://www.cdc.gov/parents/essentials/toddlersandpreschoolers/communication/specialplaytime.html)
Emotion regulation strategies		
Zones of regulation	Occupational therapy strategies to foster self-regulation	The Zones of Regulation, 2023 (https://zonesofregulation.com/)
Mindfulness techniques/mind–body therapies in children and youth	A review of evidence-based mind–body techniques to promote self-regulation including biofeedback, hypnosis, guided imagery, meditation and mindfulness	American Academy of Pediatrics Section on Integrative Medicine, 2016 (https://publications.aap.org/pediatrics/article/138/3/e20161896/52650/Mind-Body-Therapies-in-Children-and-Youth)

Addressing Risk and Significant Concerns

Because IBH clinicians see a high volume of patients with a limited amount of time to spend with each, not all presenting concerns can be comprehensively managed with the resources available in a primary care setting. Patients who demonstrate risk for suicide or other dangerous behavior may require more intensive services from a community therapist or psychiatrist, if not emergency psychiatric care. Still, psychologists working in IBH settings should be prepared to screen and intervene for high-risk concerns with the same degree of care as would be provided in more traditional psychotherapy settings. According to Section 2.02 of the American Psychological Association's (2017) *Ethical Principles of Psychologists and Code of Conduct*, even in a setting where it is not typical to work with high-risk individuals, psychologists should at least provide emergency services. In the case of high-risk suicidal ideation, IBH providers should conduct screenings that are brief but thorough, assessing current suicidal behaviors such as planning or acquiring means, attempt history, and protective factors (Bryan et al., 2009). When imminent risk is present, providers should ensure that patients are referred to emergency services and coordinate with the primary care pediatrician to facilitate follow-through on referrals to specialty mental health care.

INCREASING EQUITY IN POPULATIONS WITH LIMITED ACCESS TO CARE

Pediatric primary care providers who serve children in rural areas, as well as those who serve children from racial and ethnic minority groups, are less likely to have access to a geographically proximal behavioral health provider (Vander Wielen et al., 2015). Thus, integrating behavioral health services into primary care clinics offers a key opportunity to increase service access to historically excluded groups. From a practical standpoint, IBH can increase access to care by allowing families to receive services in the same physical location where children see their pediatricians (Kolko & Perrin, 2014). Telehealth formats, such as videoconference and phone appointments, further increase accessibility, particularly for children with complex medical conditions (Milne Wenderlich & Herendeen, 2021). However, integration of behavioral health providers within primary care settings is not sufficient to ensure that disparities are addressed (Arora et al., 2017). Integration is more likely to be successful at increasing equity if BHCs have strong relationships with trusted primary care pediatricians, develop culturally relevant interventions that leverage community resources, and proactively attend to potential concerns about stigma and previous negative experiences with mental health care services. These issues are particularly relevant given recent data documenting racial disparities in IBH utilization, with Black children notably at risk for lower IBH utilization in the context of the COVID-19 pandemic (Chakawa et al., 2021; Walters et al., 2021). Further research is needed to leverage the potential of IBH for reducing behavioral health disparities.

PAYMENT, REIMBURSEMENT, AND INSURANCE ISSUES

As the field of IBH has grown, a variety of sustainable financial models has emerged. Unsustainable business models have been a barrier to the development and growth of the field, as many behavioral health providers have depended on grant funding to support salaries and administrative support. Integrated behavioral health initiatives that rely too heavily on grant or other external funding tend to have a predetermined shelf life, and the program is discontinued after the funding period expires. When an IBH program is discontinued, physicians, families, and behavioral health providers experience significant behavioral health access issues, leaving them in a more challenging situation than before IBH was introduced to primary care.

Several sustainable financial models can prevent an IBH program from expiring. Behavioral health providers who obtain licensure can bill standard current procedural terminology codes for the provision of behavioral health services in primary care if services meet the threshold for a billable encounter (i.e., 16 minutes or longer). A licensed psychologist, for example, can bill standard CPT codes for conducting new patient visits and individual/family therapy sessions. These standard fee-for-service models provide a pathway for behavioral health providers to receive reimbursement for their efforts and build an IBH program within primary care clinics. However, individual insurance companies may vary with regard to reimbursement practices and procedures so that follow-through for reimbursement is not guaranteed. Behavioral health providers can partner with the primary care administration to garner authorization, submit bills, and receive reimbursement for services, or they can contract with an outside billing agency to conduct these tasks in an effective manner.

The standard fee-for-service model potentially presents the simplest method to develop and sustain an IBH initiative. Some new CPT codes have been proposed to allow more collaborative care between physicians and behavioral health providers. These fee-for-performance models consist of larger bundled payments to the entire primary care clinic and provide an incentive for clinics to achieve better health outcomes for patients (with behavioral health being a significant factor in children's overall health). In some cases, a primary care clinic will pay the behavioral health provider's salary with the increased revenue that pediatricians realize from the increased efficiency they achieve when relieved of addressing behavioral health concerns. Behavioral health providers are encouraged to explore business models before partnering with a primary care clinic, and the financial sustainability of an IBH program should be reviewed often to ensure consistent access to behavioral health services for the children and families receiving services.

EDUCATION

There is a severe shortage of psychologists in the United States. The American Psychological Association (2018) estimated that a 27% increase in the number of available psychologists will be needed by 2030 to address unmet mental health needs. Given the increased demand for integrated behavioral health care, psychologists with specialized training in identifying and treating behavioral disorders within integrated care settings are needed to optimize access to evidence-based behavioral health services.

Despite the ubiquity of behavioral concerns in primary care, few graduate programs offer training in primary care prior to internship, and fewer than 100 accredited internships offer training in integrated primary care (Blount & Miller, 2009). Many graduate health psychology programs prepare students for research and practice in medical settings that differ substantially from primary care in terms of the culture, pace, and wide range of treatment needs that present. Generalist training is insufficient to prepare clinicians to function effectively within primary care settings; therefore, innovations in training and education are necessary to address the workforce shortage within pediatric integrated primary care.

Integrated behavioral health psychologists working within pediatric primary care require unique competencies and skills (McDaniel et al., 2014). They must have training in and exposure to building and integrating behavioral health services into a pediatric primary care setting (Dobmeyer et al., 2003). This training involves developing successful partnerships with medical providers to achieve the common goals of providing preventive care, managing health conditions, and improving the medical and behavioral health outcomes of pediatric patients (Dobmeyer et al., 2003; Jackson et al., 2012; McDaniel et al., 2014). It utilizes valid and reliable screening measures to identify patients in need of behavioral health consultations or interventions (Jackson et al., 2012; McDaniel et al., 2014; Palermo et al., 2014). Additionally, the training focuses on developing a consistent and reliable referral system and engaging in concise, meaningful, and respectful conversations with all members of the interdisciplinary team.

Knowledge about child and adolescent development is a core competency that permeates assessment, intervention, and consultation services within pediatric IBH. The psychologist should utilize the biopsychosocial model to conceptualize cases and assess risk and protective factors that promote resilience within pediatric populations (Jackson et al., 2012; McDaniel et al., 2014). Notably, the psychologist should have the skills to utilize assessment results to promote eligibility for meaningful interventions through school systems via 504 plans or individualized education plans (Jackson et al., 2012). Integrated behavioral health psychologists must be knowledgeable of common behavioral health concerns that occur during child and adolescent development (e.g., feeding, toileting, sleep, behavior, school issues, attention, anxiety, depression), as well as competent in brief, problem-focused, evidence-based interventions that may be indicated to treat the identified concern. Proficiency in parent-mediated intervention is often required to promote positive outcomes for pediatric populations. When planning treatment and care coordination, the pediatric IBH psychologist should consider time constraints, level of integration in primary care, and resources available and mindfully select interventions that can be supported and monitored by other members of the interdisciplinary team (McDaniel et al., 2014). Furthermore, when coordinating care, IBH psychologists should understand the role and interactions of other providers serving youth, such as pediatricians, educators, and community-based providers (McDaniel et al., 2014). Additional competencies that are critical for provision of pediatric IBH services include:

- knowledge of ethical and legal requirements unique to the treatment of youth in primary care (Daly et al., 2011; Jackson et al., 2012),
- understanding of guidelines within the health care organization and national/state health care policy that affect the behavioral health care of pediatric populations,
- experience in advocacy initiatives and training of stakeholders within the institution and broader health care system (McDaniel et al., 2014),
- knowledge of how to conduct research and quality improvement initiatives in primary care to address pediatric problems while minimizing risk to vulnerable populations (Jackson et al., 2012; Palermo et al., 2014),

- experience in the supervision and teaching of other health professionals and future IBH psychologists (Mancini et al., 2019; McDaniel et al., 2014), and
- recognition of the importance of self-assessment and self-care for the behavioral health provider.

Given the unique competencies required of BHCs, the supervision and training model for these practitioners should differ from generalist training models. One well-established model of supervision that is designed to meet these training needs within the fast-paced context of a primary care visit is the patient ask recommend see evaluate (PARSE) model, which aims to mirror the physicians' medical training model (Mancini et al., 2019). In this approach, the trainee succinctly presents relevant details about the *patient* to the supervisor, the supervisor *asks* clarifying and Socratic method questions to facilitate the trainee's case conceptualization, the supervisor and trainee develop *recommendation(s)* for the visit, the supervisor and trainee the patient, and finally the supervisor *evaluates* the trainee and provides feedback on performance. The trainee receives live supervision during patient visits in addition to weekly hour-long individual and group supervision that is more common in traditional psychotherapy settings.

ETHICAL CONSIDERATIONS

The IBH model is designed to serve the behavioral health needs of all patients in a primary care clinic, including screening for high-risk behaviors.

Considerations for Patients Who Need Intensive Treatment

A small proportion of patients with identified behavioral health concerns, such as those with severe mental illness or those who are at high risk of harm to themselves or others, would be better addressed in placements that can provide a higher level of care. In these instances, the BHC has an ethical obligation to guide the patient toward effective treatment through a community referral to prevent a disruption in services (see standard 3.12, Interruption of Psychological

Services; American Psychological Association, 2017). However, patient follow-through on such referrals is often low (Davis et al., 2016; Hacker et al., 2014), and even for individuals who do pursue the referral, extensive wait-lists can present an additional barrier to access services (American Public Health Association, 2016). Thus, simply providing a patient with a referral to more intensive or specialized services is insufficient, as it does not necessarily mean that the patient will receive adequate care (Runyan et al., 2013).

Behavioral health clinicians must instead adopt an active role as case managers in the referral process (see Maragakis et al., 2018). Providing a brief consultation with the patient regarding referral options (Davis et al., 2016) and checking in with the patient throughout the referral process via telephone (Cucciare et al., 2015) are both strategies that increase the likelihood of the patient accessing outside services. Behavioral health clinicians may also coordinate with local mental health professionals to reserve space for referrals or provide emergency prescriptions to prevent a delay in services due to wait-lists. Finally, patients may benefit from problem solving around practical barriers to accessing treatment, including identifying community resources (e.g., transportation, child care).

When immediate referral to specialty services is not possible, the BHC must balance adherence to the IBH model, which prioritizes immediate availability of the clinician for brief treatment of a large volume of patients, with the obligation to support individuals who need but cannot immediately access longer term or intensive care. Even if the IBH model is not the ideal fit, the BHC may best serve such patients by providing treatment in the interim until the patient can receive appropriate care within the community. Such an approach accords with the American Psychological Association's *Ethical Principles of Psychologists and Code of Conduct* (2017, Standard 2.02), which states that psychologists may provide emergency services for individuals for whom other mental health services are unavailable to ensure that they have access to some care.

Considerations for Evidence-Based Practice

According to the American Psychological Association's ethical principles and code of conduct, clinicians have an ethical obligation to deliver interventions that are "based upon established scientific and professional knowledge of the discipline" (American Psychological Association, 2017, Standard 2.04). Current practice guidelines recommend integrating scientific knowledge into clinical care through the use of evidence-based practices (American Psychological Association Presidential Task Force, 2006). In support of this goal, the American Psychological Association has moved to endorsing manualized empirically supported treatments (ESTs) for a variety of psychological disorders to aid clinicians in identifying interventions that are supported within the scientific literature (Tolin et al., 2015). However, as noted by Maragakis et al. (2018), full manualized ESTs are not generally feasible within the brief treatment model of IBH (Shepardson et al., 2016). Instead, interventions in IBH are often abbreviated versions of manualized treatments that have empirical support (e.g., Berkovits et al., 2010; Shepardson et al., 2016), although there is currently little empirical evidence for the effectiveness of this briefer treatment model (Kolko & Perrin, 2014).

These limitations necessitate a different conceptualization of what it means to engage in evidence-based practice within an IBH setting compared with a more traditional outpatient setting. Maragakis et al. (2018) suggested that, rather than consider adherence to ESTs as the marker of engaging in evidence-based practice, IBH clinicians should instead consider evidence-based principles. That is, clinicians should identify the underlying theory, principles, mechanisms of change, and contextual variables (Baucom & Boeding, 2013; Follette & Beitz, 2003; Hofmann, 2013) that make interventions (including ESTs) effective and deliver those components in an efficient manner. Clinicians then base their interventions on a conceptual understanding of psychological principles that are grounded within the broader scientific literature and can better tailor them to fit the context of the patient and the IBH model. This approach requires that such mechanisms of change have been identified within the literature, yet the field is still far from understanding why and how evidence-based therapies lead to change (Kazdin, 2009).

Engaging in data-based decision making means that clinicians use interventions that have a basis in the scientific literature and that they evaluate whether the intervention results in improvement for a specific patient. Monitoring a patient's response to treatment and the performance of the IBH system are important quality improvement practices in an IBH setting that can contribute to knowledge within the field regarding the effectiveness of the IBH model and directly inform clinical care (see Maragakis & O'Donohue, 2016).

Considerations for Patient Privacy and Information Sharing

The IBH model is meant to facilitate collaboration between providers. All members of the care team (e.g., primary care pediatricians, BHCs, medical specialists) must have access to all patient data, including therapy progress notes, to coordinate care (Snipes et al., 2015). Access generally occurs within a shared electronic medical record. This process differs from that of other behavioral health models in which the patient's session notes are kept separate from their medical record and are not released to other providers without explicit written permission from the client (i.e., a release of information). Given this difference, it is critical that patients understand that the BHC will share relevant information with the patient's primary care pediatrician and vice versa. Such informed consent is consistent with the American Psychological Association's ethics principles and code of conduct (2017, Standards 3.10, 9.03, and 10.01), which require patients to be informed of the limits of confidentiality in the process of consent for medical treatment or in the context of a "warm handoff" to a behavioral health provider.

IMPLICATIONS FOR DEVELOPMENTAL-BEHAVIORAL PEDIATRICIANS, DEVELOPMENTAL SCIENTISTS, AND OTHER PEDIATRIC PSYCHOLOGISTS NOT WORKING IN PRIMARY CARE

The presentation of behavioral health concerns in primary care settings varies, and the severity of these concerns exists on a continuum from mild/moderate to severe. Integrated primary care models are designed to address population health issues. That is, the overarching purpose of integrated care models is to improve access to evidence-based treatment for the most commonly presenting behavioral health issues in the setting in which parents most commonly raise these concerns: the primary care setting. As mentioned earlier, behavioral health concerns are among the commonly presenting concerns in the primary care setting. These issues are also the most time consuming for primary care pediatricians to address and the ones they feel most uncomfortable and least trained to address. The vast majority of behavioral health issues that present in primary care are mild to moderate and can be treated in the course of a few sessions with an integrated behavioral health specialist. Efficient and effective treatment of behavioral health in primary care achieves the goal of treating both the mind and body of pediatric patients: the whole child.

More severe behavioral health issues that present in primary care may require referrals to the services of a specialized child psychologist, a developmental-behavioral pediatrician, or a child psychiatrist. Children should be referred to these more specialized services when the presenting problem is too severe or when an extended course of treatment in primary care fails to meet treatment goals. In the end, the IBH model closely mimics the medical primary care model, in which primary care pediatricians address mild to moderate presenting problems and refer for specialized care when necessary. This IBH model serves as part of a continuum of care in which population health is largely addressed in the medical home and more significant presenting problems are addressed by more specialized services.

When an IBH system is running smoothly, access to behavioral health services is improved and most medical and behavioral issues can be addressed effectively and efficiently. Currently, many behavioral health issues go untreated in traditional primary care, which significantly impairs the efficiency of care in these settings. Too many behavioral health issues are currently being referred for specialty services, resulting in long waitlists and contributing to the majority of behavioral health issues being untreated. Ultimately, integrating behavioral health into primary care allows the majority of behavioral health concerns to be efficiently addressed in the medical home and minimizes the number of referrals to specialized care, thus reserving specialized services for patients experiencing more complex and severe presenting problems.

CONCLUSION

The emergence of the IBH field stems from an ever-increasing demand for behavioral health services in the pediatric setting. Over the next decade, this service sector is projected to be among the leading growth sectors, with growth estimated at roughly 14% (Health Resources and Services Administration, 2016). Although more research is needed to fully understand the barriers to accessing behavioral health services, integrating behavioral health providers into pediatric primary care appears to be one of the most effective methods of increasing access to behavioral health services for children. The IBH model reduces mental health stigma, helps overcome insurance barriers, allows for collaborative care between behavioral health providers and physicians, and significantly increases follow-through for children referred for behavioral health services (Kolko et al., 2010; Lieberman et al., 2006; Valleley et al., 2020). Training programs also appear to have finally "gotten the memo," as a consistent number of specially trained behavioral health providers are graduating into the workforce with the skills necessary to integrate their services into primary care (although more programs are always needed). Behavioral health providers interested in working in the primary care setting should seek the proper training and reach out to pediatrician groups.

RESOURCES

Anxiety

Chorpita B. F., Weisz J. R. (2009). *MATCH-ADC: Modular approach to therapy for children with anxiety, depression, trauma, or conduct problems.* PracticeWise.

Lebowitz, E. R., & Omer, H. (2013). *Treating childhood and adolescent anxiety: A guide for caregivers.* Wiley.

March, J. S., & Mulle, K. (1998). *OCD in children and adolescents: A cognitive-behavioral treatment manual.* Guilford Press.

Attention-Deficit/Hyperactivity Disorder

Barkley, R. A. (2022). *Treating ADHD in children and adolescents.* Guilford Press.

Volpe, R. J., & Fabiano, G. A. (2013). *Daily behavior report cards: An evidence-based system of assessment and intervention.* Guilford Press.

Behavior Management

Barkley, R. A. (2013). *Defiant children: A clinician's manual for assessment and parent training.* Guilford Press.

Barkley, R. A., & Robin, A. L. (2014). *Defiant teens: A clinician's manual for assessment and family intervention.* Guilford Press.

Hembree-Kigin, T. L., & McNeil, C. B. (2013). *Parent–child interaction therapy.* Springer Science & Business Media.

Depression

Craighead, L. W. E., Craighead, W., Kazdin, A. E., & Mahoney, M. J. (1994). *Cognitive and behavioral interventions: An empirical approach to mental health problems.* Allyn & Bacon.

Hertfordshire Partnership University NHS Foundation Trust. (2016). *Cognitive behavioural therapy (CBT) skills workbook*. https://www.hpft.nhs.uk/media/1655/wellbeing-team-cbt-workshop-booklet-2016.pdf

Little, S. G., & Akin-Little, A. (Eds.). (2019). *Behavioral interventions in schools: Evidence-based positive strategies* (2nd ed.). American Psychological Association. https://doi.org/10.1037/0000126-000

Meltzer, L. J., & McLaughlin Crabtree, V. (2015). *Pediatric sleep problems: A clinician's guide to behavioral interventions*. American Psychological Association. https://doi.org/10.1037/14645-000

Rosselló, J., & Bernal, G. (2007). *Treatment manual for cognitive behavior therapy for depression: Adaptation for Puerto Rican adolescents*. University of Puerto Rico. https://i4health.paloaltou.edu/downloads/CBT_adolescents_individual_manual_eng.pdf (PDF, 2MB)

Evidence-Based Treatments

Curry, J. F., Wells, K. C., Brent, D. A., Clarke, G. N., Rohde, P., Albano, A. M., Reinecke, M. A., Benazon, N., & March, J. S. (2005). *Treatment for adolescents with depression study (TADS) cognitive behavior therapy manual: Introduction, rationale, and adolescent sessions*. Duke University Medical Center. https://aaronkrasner.com/wp-content/uploads/2017/10/TADS_CBT.pdf

Davis, J. P., Palitz, S. A., Knepley, M., & Kendall, P. C. (2019). Cognitive-behavioral therapy with youth. In K. S. Dobson, & D. J. A. Dozois (Eds.), *Handbook of cognitive-behavioral therapies* (4th ed., pp. 349–382). Guilford Press.

Ehrenreich-May, J., Kennedy, S. M., Sherman, J. A., Bilek, E. L., Buzzella, B. A., Bennett, S. M., & Barlow, D. H. (2017). *Unified protocols for transdiagnostic treatment of emotional disorders in children and adolescents: Therapist guide*. Oxford University Press.

Palmiter, D. J., Jr. (2016). *Practicing cognitive behavioral therapy with children and adolescents: A guide for students and early career professionals*. Springer.

Feeding

Williams, K. E., & Seiverling, L. J. (2018). *Broccoli boot camp: Basic training for parents of selective eaters*. Woodbine House.

Parenting

Christophersen, E. R., & Mortweet, S. L. (2003). *Parenting that works: Building skills that last a lifetime*. American Psychological Association.

Christophersen, E. R., & VanScoyoc, S. M. (2013). *Treatments that work with children: Empirically supported strategies for managing childhood problems*. American Psychological Association. https://doi.org/10.1037/14137-000

Forgatch, M. S., & Patterson, G. R. (1989). *Parents and adolescents living together. Part 2: Family problem solving*. Castalia Publishing.

Forgatch, M. S., & Patterson, G. R. (2010). Parent Management Training—Oregon Model: An intervention for antisocial behavior in children and adolescents. In J. R. Weisz & A. E. Kazdin (Eds.), *Evidence-based psychotherapies for children and adolescents* (2nd ed., pp. 159–177). Guilford Press.

Webster-Stratton, C. (2000). *The Incredible Years training series*. U.S. Department of Justice.

Toileting

Azrin, N., & Foxx, R. M. (2019). *Toilet training in less than a day*. Gallery Books.

References

Agency for Healthcare Research and Quality. (2015). *2014 national healthcare quality & disparities report* (Publication No. 15-0007). https://www.ahrq.gov/sites/default/files/wysiwyg/research/findings/nhqrdr/nhqdr14/2014nhqdr.pdf

Allen, K. D., Barone, V. J., & Kuhn, B. R. (1993). A behavioral prescription for promoting applied behavior analysis within pediatrics. *Journal of Applied Behavior Analysis, 26*(4), 493–502. https://doi.org/10.1901/jaba.1993.26-493

American Academy of Pediatrics Section on Integrative Medicine. (2016). Mind–body therapies in children and youth. *Pediatrics, 138*(3), e20161896. https://doi.org/10.1542/peds.2016-1896

American Psychiatric Association & the Academy of Psychosomatic Medicine. (2016). *Dissemination of integrated care within adult primary care settings: The collaborative care model*. https://www.psychiatry.org/File%20Library/Psychiatrists/Practice/Professional-Topics/Integrated-Care/APA-APM-Dissemination-Integrated-Care-Report.pdf

American Psychological Association. (2017). *Ethical principles of psychologists and code of conduct* (2002, amended effective June 1, 2010, and January 1, 2017). https://www.apa.org/ethics/code/index.aspx

American Psychological Association. (2018). *APA fact sheet series on psychologist supply and demand projections 2015-2030: Unmet need*. https://www.apa.org/workforce/publications/supply-demand/unmet-need.pdf

American Psychological Association Presidential Task Force on Evidence-Based Practice. (2006). Evidence-based practice in psychology. *American Psychologist*, 61(4), 271–285. https://doi.org/10.1037/0003-066X.61.4.271

American Public Health Association. (2016). *Removing barriers to mental health services for veterans* [Policy no. 201411]. https://www.apha.org/policies-and-advocacy/public-health-policy-statements/policy-database/2015/01/28/14/51/removing-barriers-to-mental-health-services-for-veterans

Arora, P. G., Godoy, L., & Hodgkinson, S. (2017). Serving the underserved: Cultural considerations in behavioral health integration in pediatric primary care. *Professional Psychology: Research and Practice*, 48(3), 139–148. https://doi.org/10.1037/pro0000131

Asarnow, J. R., Kolko, D. J., Miranda, J., & Kazak, A. E. (2017). The pediatric patient-centered medical home: Innovative models for improving behavioral health. *American Psychologist*, 72(1), 13–27. https://doi.org/10.1037/a0040411

Baucom, D. H., & Boeding, S. (2013). The role of theory and research in the practice of cognitive-behavioral couple therapy: If you build it, they will come. *Behavior Therapy*, 44(4), 592–602. https://doi.org/10.1016/j.beth.2012.12.004

Berkovits, M. D., O'Brien, K. A., Carter, C. G., & Eyberg, S. M. (2010). Early identification and intervention for behavior problems in primary care: A comparison of two abbreviated versions of parent-child interaction therapy. *Behavior Therapy*, 41(3), 375–387. https://doi.org/10.1016/j.beth.2009.11.002

Berwick, D. M., Nolan, T. W., & Whittington, J. (2008). The triple aim: Care, health, and cost. *Health Affairs*, 27(3), 759–769. https://doi.org/10.1377/hlthaff.27.3.759

Bettencourt, A. F., Ferro, R. A., Williams, J.-L. L., Khan, K. N., Platt, R. E., Sweeney, S., & Coble, K. (2021). Pediatric primary care provider comfort with mental health practices: A needs assessment of regions with shortages of treatment access. *Academic Psychiatry*, 45(4), 429–434. https://doi.org/10.1007/s40596-021-01434-x

Bitsko, R. H., Holbrook, J. R., Robinson, L. R., Kaminski, J. W., Ghandour, R., Smith, C., & Peacock, G. (2016). Health care, family, and community factors associated with mental, behavioral, and developmental disorders in early childhood—United States, 2011–2012. *MMWR: Morbidity and Mortality Weekly Report*, 65(9), 221–226. https://doi.org/10.15585/mmwr.mm6509a1

Blount, F. A., & Miller, B. F. (2009). Addressing the workforce crisis in integrated primary care. *Journal of Clinical Psychology in Medical Settings*, 16(1), 113–119. https://doi.org/10.1007/s10880-008-9142-7

Bridges, A. J., Andrews, A. R., III, Villalobos, B. T., Pastrana, F. A., Cavell, T. A., & Gomez, D. (2014). Does integrated behavioral health care reduce mental health disparities for Latinos? Initial findings. *Journal of Latina/o Psychology*, 2(1), 37–53. https://doi.org/10.1037/lat0000009

Bruni, T. P., Lancaster, B. M., & Cook, A. (2016, May 27–31). *The application of applied behavior analysis within integrated behavioral health care* [Poster presentation]. Annual Meeting of the Association for Applied Behavior Analysis, Chicago, IL, United States.

Bryan, C. J., Corso, K. A., Neal-Walden, T. A., & Rudd, M. D. (2009). Managing suicide risk in primary care: Practice recommendations for behavioral health consultants. *Professional Psychology: Research and Practice*, 40(2), 148–155. https://doi.org/10.1037/a0011141

Campo, J. V., Bridge, J. A., & Fontanella, C. A. (2015). Access to mental health services: Implementing an integrated solution. *JAMA Pediatrics*, 169(4), 299–300. https://doi.org/10.1001/jamapediatrics.2014.3558

Caspi, A., Houts, R. M., Ambler, A., Danese, A., Elliott, M. L., Hariri, A., Harrington, H., Hogan, S. Poulton, R., Ramrakha, S., Reuben, A., Richmond-Rakerd, L., Sugden, K., Wertz, J., Williams, B. S., & Moffitt, T. E. (2020). Longitudinal assessment of mental health disorders and comorbidities across 4 decades among participants in the Dunedin birth cohort study. *JAMA Network Open*, 3(4), e203221. https://doi.org/10.1001/jamanetworkopen.2020.3221

Centers for Disease Control and Prevention. (2019). *Tips for special playtime*. Retrieved January 30, 2025, from https://www.cdc.gov/parenting-toddlers/communication/special-playtime.html

Chaffee, B. (2008). Financial models for integrated behavioral health care. In W. T. O'Donohue & L. James (Eds.), *The primary care toolkit* (pp. 19–30). Springer. https://doi.org/10.1007/978-0-387-78971-2_3

Chakawa, A., Belzer, L. T., Perez-Crawford, T., & Yeh, H. W. (2021). COVID-19, telehealth, and pediatric integrated primary care: Disparities in service use. *Journal of Pediatric Psychology, 46*(9), 1063–1075. https://doi.org/10.1093/jpepsy/jsab077

Connor, D. F., McLaughlin, T. J., Jeffers-Terry, M., O'Brien, W. H., Stille, C. J., Young, L. M., & Antonelli, R. C. (2006). Targeted child psychiatric services: A new model of pediatric primary clinician—Child psychiatry collaborative care. *Clinical Pediatrics, 45*(5), 423–434. https://doi.org/10.1177/0009922806289617

Cooper, S., Valleley, R. J., Polaha, J., Begeny, J., & Evans, J. H. (2006). Running out of time: Physician management of behavioral health concerns in rural pediatric primary care. *Pediatrics, 118*(1), e132–e138. https://doi.org/10.1542/peds.2005-2612

Costello, E. J., He, J. P., Sampson, N. A., Kessler, R. C., & Merikangas, K. R. (2014). Services for adolescents with psychiatric disorders: 12-month data from the National Comorbidity Survey-Adolescent. *Psychiatric Services, 65*(3), 359–366. https://doi.org/10.1176/appi.ps.201100518

Cucciare, M. A., Coleman, E. A., & Timko, C. (2015). A conceptual model to facilitate transitions from primary care to specialty substance use disorder care: A review of the literature. *Primary Health Care Research and Development, 16*(5), 492–505. https://doi.org/10.1017/S1463423614000164

Cummings, N. A., O'Donohue, W. T., & Cummings, J. L. (2009). The financial dimension of integrated behavioral/primary care. *Journal of Clinical Psychology in Medical Settings, 16*(1), 31–39. https://doi.org/10.1007/s10880-008-9139-2

Daly, E. J., III, Doll, B., Schulte, A. C., & Fenning, P. (2011). The competencies initiative in American professional psychology: Implications for school psychology preparation. *Psychology in the Schools, 48*(9), 872–886. https://doi.org/10.1002/pits.20603

Davis, M. J., Moore, K. M., Meyers, K., Mathews, J., & Zerth, E. O. (2016). Engagement in mental health treatment following primary care mental health integration contact. *Psychological Services, 13*(4), 333–340. https://doi.org/10.1037/ser0000089

deGruy, F. V. (1997). Mental healthcare in the primary care setting: A paradigm problem. *Families, Systems, & Health, 15*(1), 3–26. https://doi.org/10.1037/h0089802

Dobmeyer, A. C., Rowan, A. B., Etherage, J. R., & Wilson, R. J. (2003). Training psychology interns in primary behavioral health care. *Professional Psychology: Research and Practice, 34*(6), 586–594. https://doi.org/10.1037/0735-7028.34.6.586

Erickson, S. J., Gerstle, M., & Feldstein, S. W. (2005). Brief interventions and motivational interviewing with children, adolescents, and their parents in pediatric health care settings: A review. *Archives of Pediatric and Adolescent Medicine, 159*(12), 1173–1180. https://doi.org/10.1001/archpedi.159.12.1173

Follette, W. C., & Beitz, K. (2003). Adding a more rigorous scientific agenda to the empirically supported treatment movement. *Behavior Modification, 27*(3), 369–386. https://doi.org/10.1177/0145445503027003006

Friedberg, R. D., & Paternostro, J. K. (2019). Cognitive behavioral therapy with youth: Essential foundations and elementary practices. In R. D. Friedberg & J. K. Paternostro (Eds.), *Handbook of cognitive behavioral therapy for pediatric medical conditions* (pp. 87–101). Springer. https://doi.org/10.1007/978-3-030-21683-2_7

Friman, P. C. (2010). Come on in, the water is fine: Achieving mainstream relevance through integration with primary medical care. *The Behavior Analyst, 33*(1), 19–36. https://doi.org/10.1007/BF03392201

Gardner, W., Lucas, A., Kolko, D. J., & Campo, J. V. (2007). Comparison of the PSC-17 and alternative mental health screens in an at-risk primary care sample. *Journal of the American Academy of Child & Adolescent Psychiatry, 46*(5), 611–618. https://doi.org/10.1097/chi.0b013e318032384b

Gardner, W., Murphy, M., Childs, G., Kelleher, K., Pagano, M., Jellinek, M., McInerny, T. K., Wasserman, R. C., Nutting, P., & Chiappetta, L. (1999). The PSC-17: A brief pediatric symptom checklist including psychosocial problem subscales. A report from PROS and ASPN. *Ambulatory Child Health, 5*(3), 225–236.

Gerrity, M., Zoller, E., Pinson, N., Pettinari, C., & King, V. (2014). *Integrating primary care into behavioral health settings: What works for individuals with serious mental illness.* Milbank Memorial Fund. https://www.milbank.org/wp-content/uploads/2016/04/Integrating-Primary-Care-Report.pdf

Godoy, L., Long, M., Marschall, D., Hodgkinson, S., Bokor, B., Rhodes, H., Crumpton, H., Weissman, M., & Beers, L. (2017). Behavioral health integration in health care settings: Lessons learned from a pediatric hospital primary care system. *Journal of Clinical Psychology in Medical Settings, 24*(3–4), 245–258. https://doi.org/10.1007/s10880-017-9509-8

Grazier, K. L., Smiley, M. L., & Bondalapati, K. S. (2016). Overcoming barriers to integrating behavioral health and primary care services. *Journal of Primary Care & Community Health, 7*(4), 242–248. https://doi.org/10.1177/2150131916656455

Guevara, J. P., Greenbaum, P. E., Shera, D., Bauer, L., & Schwarz, D. F. (2009). Survey of mental health consultation and referral among primary care pediatricians. *Academic Pediatrics, 9*(2), 123–127. https://doi.org/10.1016/j.acap.2008.12.008

Hacker, K., Arsenault, L., Franco, I., Shaligram, D., Sidor, M., Olfson, M., & Goldstein, J. (2014). Referral and follow-up after mental health screening in commercially insured adolescents. *Journal of Adolescent Health, 55*(1), 17–23. https://doi.org/10.1016/j.jadohealth.2013.12.012

Health Resources and Services Administration. (2016). *National projections of supply and demand for selected behavioral health practitioners: 2013–2025.* U.S. Department of Health and Human Services. https://bhw.hrsa.gov/sites/default/files/bureau-health-workforce/data-research/behavioral-health-2013-2025.pdf

Heath, B., Wise Romero, P., & Reynolds, K. (2013). *A standard framework for levels of integrated healthcare.* SAMHSA-HRSA Center for Integrated Health Solutions. https://www.hrsa.gov/behavioral-health/standard-framework-levels-integrated-healthcare

Highland, J., Nikolajski, C., Kogan, J., Ji, Y., Kukla, M., & Schuster, J. (2020). Impact of behavioral health homes on cost and utilization outcomes. *Psychiatric Services, 71*(8), 796–802. https://doi.org/10.1176/appi.ps.201900141

Hine, J. F., Grennan, A. Q., Menousek, K. M., Robertson, G., Valleley, R. J., & Evans, J. H. (2017). Physician satisfaction with integrated behavioral health in pediatric primary care: Consistency across rural and urban settings. *Journal of Primary Care & Community Health, 8*(2), 89–93. https://doi.org/10.1177/2150131916668115

Hofmann, S. G. (2013). Bridging the theory-practice gap by getting even bolder with the Boulder model. *Behavior Therapy, 44*(4), 603–608. https://doi.org/10.1016/j.beth.2013.04.006

Jackson, Y., Wu, Y. P., Aylward, B. S., & Roberts, M. C. (2012). Application of the competency cube model to clinical child psychology. *Professional Psychology: Research and Practice, 43*(5), 432–441. https://doi.org/10.1037/a0030007

Kazdin, A. E. (2009). Understanding how and why psychotherapy leads to change. *Psychotherapy Research, 19*(4–5), 418–428. https://doi.org/10.1080/10503300802448899

Kelleher, K. J., Campo, J. V., & Gardner, W. P. (2006). Management of pediatric mental disorders in primary care: Where are we now and where are we going? *Current Opinion in Pediatrics, 18*(6), 649–653. https://doi.org/10.1097/MOP.0b013e3280106a76

Kia-Keating, M., Barnett, M. L., Liu, S. R., Sims, G. M., & Ruth, A. B. (2019). Trauma-responsive care in a pediatric setting: Feasibility and acceptability of screening for adverse childhood experiences. *American Journal of Community Psychology, 64*(3–4), 286–297. https://doi.org/10.1002/ajcp.12366

Kolko, D. J., Campo, J. V., Kelleher, K., & Cheng, Y. (2010). Improving access to care and clinical outcome for pediatric behavioral problems: A randomized trial of a nurse-administered intervention in primary care. *Journal of Developmental and Behavioral Pediatrics, 31*(5), 393–404. https://doi.org/10.1097/DBP.0b013e3181dff307

Kolko, D. J., & Perrin, E. (2014). The integration of behavioral health interventions in children's health care: Services, science, and suggestions. *Journal of Clinical Child and Adolescent Psychology, 43*(2), 216–228. https://doi.org/10.1080/15374416.2013.862804

Kroenke, K., Spitzer, R. L., & Williams, J. B. W. (2001). The PHQ-9: Validity of a brief depression severity measure. *Journal of General Internal Medicine, 16*(9), 606–613. https://doi.org/10.1046/j.1525-1497.2001.016009606.x

Lancaster, B., Cook, A., Bruni, T., Sturza, J., Sevecke, J., Ham, H., Knight, R., Hoffses, K., Wickham, C. A., & Orringer, K. A. (2019). Comparing primary care pediatricians' perceptions of clinics with and without integrated behavioral health. *Primary Health Care Research and Development, 20*, e63. https://doi.org/10.1017/S1463423618000579

Lelutiu-Weinberger, C., Clark, K. A., & Pachankis, J. E. (2023). Mental health provider training to improve LGBTQ competence and reduce implicit and explicit bias: A randomized controlled trial of online and in-person delivery. *Psychology of Sexual Orientation and Gender Diversity.* https://doi.org/10.1037/sgd0000560

Leslie, L. K., Stallone, K. A., Weckerly, J., McDaniel, A. L., & Monn, A. (2006). Implementing ADHD guidelines in primary care: Does one size fit all? *Journal of Health Care for the Poor and Underserved, 17*(2), 302–327. https://doi.org/10.1353/hpu.2006.0064

Lieberman, A., Adalist-Estrin, A., Erinle, O., & Sloan, N. (2006). On-site mental health care: A route to improving access to mental health services in an inner-city, adolescent medicine clinic. *Child: Care, Health and Development, 32*(4), 407–413. https://doi.org/10.1111/j.1365-2214.2006.00620.x

Mancini, K., Wicoff, M., & Stancin, T. (2019). Clinical supervision in integrated pediatric primary care: The PARSE model in action. *Training and Education in Professional Psychology, 13*(4), 316–322. https://doi.org/10.1037/tep0000238

Maragakis, A., Lindeman, S., & Nolan, J. (2018). Evidence based and intensity specific services in the integrated care setting: Ethical considerations for a developing field. *Behavior Analysis: Research and Practice, 18*(4), 425–435. https://doi.org/10.1037/bar0000127

Maragakis, A., & O'Donohue, W. (2016). Creating a quality improvement system for an integrated care (IC) program: The why, what, and how to measure. In W. O'Donohue & A. Maragakis (Eds.), *Quality improvement in behavioral health* (pp. 207–227). Springer. https://doi.org/10.1007/978-3-319-26209-3_14

Maruish, M. E. (2018). Selection of psychological measures and associated administration, scoring, and reporting technology for use in pediatric primary care settings. In M. E. Maruish (Ed.), *Handbook of pediatric psychological screening and assessment in primary care* (pp. 71–92). Routledge. https://doi.org/10.4324/9781315193199

McDaniel, S. H., Grus, C. L., Cubic, B. A., Hunter, C. L., Kearney, L. K., Schuman, C. C., Karel, M. J., Kessler, R. S., Larkin, K. T., McCutcheon, S., Miller, B. F., Nash, J., Qualls, S. H., Connolly, K. S., Stancin, T., Stanton, A. L., Sturm, L. A., & Johnson, S. B. (2014). Competencies for psychology practice in primary care. *American Psychologist, 69*(4), 409–429. https://doi.org/10.1037/a0036072

McMillan, J. A., Land, M., Jr., & Leslie, L. K. (2017). Pediatric residency education and the behavioral and mental health crisis: A call to action. *Pediatrics, 139*(1), e20162141. https://doi.org/10.1542/peds.2016-2141

Meadows, T., Valleley, R., Haack, M. K., Thorson, R., & Evans, J. (2011). Physician "costs" in providing behavioral health in primary care. *Clinical Pediatrics, 50*(5), 447–455. https://doi.org/10.1177/0009922810390676

Miller, B. F., Talen, M. R., & Patel, K. K. (2013). Advancing integrated behavioral health and primary care: The critical importance of behavioral health in health care policy. In M. R. Talen & A. Burke Valeras (Eds.), *Integrated behavioral health in primary care: Evaluating the evidence, identifying the essentials* (pp. 53–62). Springer. https://doi.org/10.1007/978-1-4614-6889-9_4

Milne Wenderlich, A., & Herendeen, N. (2021). Telehealth in pediatric primary care. *Current Problems in Pediatric and Adolescent Health Care, 51*(1), 100951. https://doi.org/10.1016/j.cppeds.2021.100951

Mongelli, F., Georgakopoulos, P., & Pato, M. T. (2020). Challenges and opportunities to meet the mental health needs of underserved and disenfranchised populations in the United States. *Focus, 18*(1), 16–24.

Moore, J. A., Karch, K., Sherina, V., Guiffre, A., Jee, S., & Garfunkel, L. C. (2018). Practice procedures in models of primary care collaboration for children with ADHD. *Families, Systems, & Health, 36*(1), 73–86. https://doi.org/10.1037/fsh0000314

Mossman, S. A., Luft, M. J., Schroeder, H. K., Varney, S. T., Fleck, D. E., Barzman, D. H., Gilman, R., DelBello, M. P., & Strawn, J. R. (2017). The Generalized Anxiety Disorder 7-item scale in adolescents with generalized anxiety disorder: Signal detection and validation. *Annals of Clinical Psychiatry, 29*(4), 227–234A. https://www.ncbi.nlm.nih.gov/pmc/articles/PMC5765270/pdf/nihms929209.pdf

Njoroge, W. F. M., Hostutler, C. A., Schwartz, B. S., & Mautone, J. A. (2016). Integrated behavioral health in pediatric primary care. *Current Psychiatry Reports, 18*(12), 106. https://doi.org/10.1007/s11920-016-0745-7

Norquist, G. S., & Regier, D. A. (1996). The epidemiology of psychiatric disorders and the de facto mental health care system. *Annual Review of Medicine, 47*, 473–479. https://doi.org/10.1146/annurev.med.47.1.473

O'Loughlin, K., Donovan, E. K., Radcliff, Z., Ryan, M., & Rybarczyk, B. (2019). Using integrated behavioral healthcare to address behavioral health disparities in underserved populations. *Translational Issues in Psychological Science, 5*(4), 374–389. https://doi.org/10.1037/tps0000213

Palermo, T. M., Janicke, D. M., Beals-Erickson, S. E., & Fritz, A. M. (2014). Training and competencies in pediatric psychology. In M. C. Roberts & R. G. Steele (Eds.), *The handbook of pediatric psychology* (5th ed., pp. 55–66). Guilford Press.

Parent Child Interaction Therapy (PCIT). (n.d.). *Child Directed Interaction (CDI) phase of parent child interaction therapy*. Retrieved December 6, 2024, from https://www.parentchildinteractiontherapy.com/pcit-child-directed-interaction

Peek, C. J., & The National Integration Academy Council. (2013). *Lexicon for behavioral health and primary care integration: Concepts and definitions developed by expert consensus* [AHRQ Publication No. 13-IP001-EF]. Agency for Healthcare Research and Quality. https://integrationacademy.ahrq.gov/sites/default/files/2020-06/Lexicon.pdf

Pelham, W. E., Jr., Fabiano, G. A., Waxmonsky, J. G., Greiner, A. R., Gnagy, E. M., Pelham, W. E., III, Coxe, S., Verley, J., Bhatia, I., Hart, K., Karch, K., Konijnendijk, E., Tresco, C., Nahum-Shani, I., & Murphy, S. A. (2016). Treatment sequencing for childhood ADHD: A multiple-randomization study of adaptive medication and behavioral interventions. *Journal of Clinical Child & Adolescent Psychology, 45*(4), 396–415.

Pickford, D. Y., Hill, T. L., Arora, P. G., & Baker, C. N. (2021). Prevention of conduct problems in integrated pediatric primary care. In W. O'Donohue & M. Zimmermann (Eds.), *Handbook of evidence-based prevention of behavioral disorders in integrated care* (pp. 193–220). Springer. https://doi.org/10.1007/978-3-030-83469-2_9

Piqueras, J. A., Vidal-Arenas, V., Falcó, R., Moreno-Amador, B., Marzo, J. C., Holcomb, J. M., & Murphy, M. (2021). Short form of the Pediatric Symptom Checklist–Youth Self-Report (PSC-17-Y): Spanish validation study. *Journal of Medical Internet Research*, 23(12), e31127. https://doi.org/10.2196/31127

Reiter, J. T., Dobmeyer, A. C., & Hunter, C. L. (2018). The primary care behavioral health (PCBH) model: An overview and operational definition. *Journal of Clinical Psychology in Medical Settings*, 25(2), 109–126. https://doi.org/10.1007/s10880-017-9531-x

Richardson, L. P., McCauley, E., Grossman, D. C., McCarty, C. A., Richards, J., Russo, J. E., Rockhill, C., & Katon, W. (2010). Evaluation of the Patient Health Questionnaire-9 Item for detecting major depression among adolescents. *Pediatrics*, 126(6), 1117–1123. https://doi.org/10.1542/peds.2010-0852

Riley, A. R., Paternostro, J. K., Walker, B. L., & Wagner, D. V. (2019). The impact of behavioral health consultations on medical encounter duration in pediatric primary care: A retrospective match-controlled study. *Families, Systems, & Health*, 37(2), 162. https://doi.org/10.1037/fsh0000406

Robinson, P. J., & Reiter, J. T. (2016). *Behavioral consultation and primary care: A guide to integrating services*. Springer. https://doi.org/10.1007/978-3-319-13954-8

Runyan, C., Robinson, P., & Gould, D. A. (2013). Ethical issues facing providers in collaborative primary care settings: Do current guidelines suffice to guide the future of team based primary care? *Families, Systems, & Health*, 31(1), 1–8. https://doi.org/10.1037/a0031895

Schuhmann, E., Durning, P., Eyberg, S. M., & Boggs, S. R. (1996). Screening for conduct problem behavior in pediatric settings using the Eyberg Child Behavior Inventory. *Ambulatory Child Health*, 2, 35–41.

Sharp, L., Pantell, R. H., Murphy, L. O., & Lewis, C. C. (1992). Psychosocial problems during child health supervision visits: Eliciting, then what? *Pediatrics*, 89(4), 619–623. https://doi.org/10.1542/peds.89.4.619

Shepardson, R. L., Funderburk, J. S., & Weisberg, R. B. (2016). Adapting evidence-based, cognitive-behavioral interventions for anxiety for use with adults in integrated primary care settings. *Families, Systems, & Health*, 34(2), 114–127. https://doi.org/10.1037/fsh0000175

Singh, A., Yeh, C. J., & Boone Blanchard, S. (2017). Ages and Stages Questionnaire: A global screening scale [English edition]. *Boletín Médico del Hospital Infantil de México*, 74(1), 5–12. https://doi.org/10.1016/j.bmhimx.2016.07.008

Snipes, C., Maragakis, A., & O'Donohue, W. (2015). Team-based stepped care in integrated delivery settings. *Family Medicine and Community Health*, 3(1), 39–46. https://doi.org/10.15212/FMCH.2015.0101

Spitzer, R. L., Kroenke, K., Williams, J. B. W., & Löwe, B. (2006). A brief measure for assessing generalized anxiety disorder: The GAD-7. *Archives of Internal Medicine*, 166(10), 1092–1097. https://doi.org/10.1001/archinte.166.10.1092

Squires, J., & Bricker, D. (2009). *Ages and Stages Questionnaires (ASQ-3; 3rd ed.): A parent-completed child monitoring system*. Paul Brookes Publishing Company. https://products.brookespublishing.com/Ages-Stages-Questionnaires-Third-Edition-ASQ-3-P569.aspx

Stancin, T. (2016). Commentary: Integrated pediatric primary care: Moving from why to how. *Journal of Pediatric Psychology*, 41(10), 1161–1164. https://doi.org/10.1093/jpepsy/jsw074

Stancin, T., & Perrin, E. C. (2014). Psychologists and pediatricians: Opportunities for collaboration in primary care. *American Psychologist*, 69(4), 332–343. https://doi.org/10.1037/a0036046

Stein, R. E. K., Horwitz, S. M., Storfer-Isser, A., Heneghan, A., Olson, L., & Hoagwood, K. E. (2008). Do pediatricians think they are responsible for identification and management of child mental health problems? Results of the AAP periodic survey. *Ambulatory Pediatrics*, 8(1), 11–17. https://doi.org/10.1016/j.ambp.2007.10.006

Talmi, A., Muther, E. F., Margolis, K., Buchholz, M., Asherin, R., & Bunik, M. (2016). The scope of behavioral health integration in a pediatric primary care setting. *Journal of Pediatric Psychology*, 41(10), 1120–1132. https://doi.org/10.1093/jpepsy/jsw065

Tolin, D. F., McKay, D., Forman, E. M., Klonsky, E. D., & Thombs, B. D. (2015). Empirically supported treatment: Recommendations for a new model. *Clinical Psychology: Science and Practice*, 22(4), 317–338. https://doi.org/10.1111/cpsp.12122

Valleley, R. J., Meadows, T. J., Burt, J., Menousek, K., Hembree, K., Evans, J., Gathje, R., Kupzyk, K., Sevecke, J. R., & Lancaster, B. (2020). Demonstrating the impact of colocated behavioral health in pediatric primary care. *Clinical Practice in Pediatric*

Psychology, 8(1), 13–24. https://doi.org/10.1037/cpp0000284

Valleley, R. J., Polaha, J., & Evans, J. (2004). The impact of behavioral healthcare services on medical utilization for children with externalizing disorders in a rural community. *Journal of Rural Community Psychology, e*7. https://works.bepress.com/jodi-polaha/8/

Vander Wielen, L. M., Gilchrist, E. C., Nowels, M. A., Petterson, S. M., Rust, G., & Miller, B. F. (2015). Not near enough: Racial and ethnic disparities in access to nearby behavioral health care and primary care. *Journal of Health Care for the Poor and Underserved, 26*(3), 1032–1047. https://doi.org/10.1353/hpu.2015.0083

Villalobos, B. T., Bridges, A. J., Anastasia, E. A., Ojeda, C. A., Hernandez Rodriguez, J. H., & Gomez, D. (2016). Effects of language concordance and interpreter use on therapeutic alliance in Spanish-speaking integrated behavioral health care patients. *Psychological Services, 13*(1), 49–59. https://doi.org/10.1037/ser0000051

Walters, J., Johnson, T., DeBlasio, D., Klein, M., Sikora, K., Reilly, K., Hutzel-Dunham, E., White, C., Xu, Y., & Burkhardt, M. C. (2021). Integration and impact of telemedicine in underserved pediatric primary care. *Clinical Pediatrics, 60*(11–12), 452–458. https://doi.org/10.1177/00099228211039621

Weersing, V. R., Brent, D. A., Rozenman, M. S., Gonzalez, A., Jeffreys, M., Dickerson, J. F., Lynch, F. L., Porta, G., & Iyengar, S. (2017). Brief behavioral therapy for pediatric anxiety and depression in primary care: A randomized clinical trial. *JAMA Psychiatry, 74*(6), 571–578. https://doi.org/10.1001/jamapsychiatry.2017.0429

Wildman, B. G., & Langkamp, D. L. (2012). Impact of location and availability of behavioral health services for children. *Journal of Clinical Psychology in Medical Settings, 19*(4), 393–400. https://doi.org/10.1007/s10880-012-9324-1

Yonek, J., Lee, C. M., Harrison, A., Mangurian, C., & Tolou-Shams, M. (2020). Key components of effective pediatric integrated behavioral health care models: A systematic review. *JAMA Pediatrics, 174*(5), 487–498. https://doi.org/10.1001/jamapediatrics.2020.0023

Zestcott, C. A., Blair, I. V., & Stone, J. (2016). Examining the presence, consequences, and reduction of implicit bias in health care: A narrative review. *Group Processes & Intergroup Relations, 19*(4), 528–542. https://doi.org/10.1177/1368430216642029

The Zones of Regulation. (2023). *A simple approach to developing self-regulation* [Homepage]. Retrieved December 6, 2024, from https://zonesofregulation.com

CHAPTER 29

RELATIONSHIP-FOCUSED INTERVENTIONS AND PSYCHOTHERAPY: APPLICATIONS FOR CHILD AND ADOLESCENT HEALTH AND BEHAVIOR

Megan M. Julian, Fiona K. Miller, and Jerrica Pitzen

Relationships are a foundational component of human development. From forming emotional connections to learning about the world to basic survival, humans depend on the relationships they have with others. The relationship that is arguably most important to development is that between caregiver and child. The benefits of early, secure, and nurturing relationships extend beyond the immediacy of trusting another individual to meet one's physical or emotional needs or provide regulation during periods of distress. Rather, the skills acquired in infancy and early childhood build a foundation that extends into the future, promoting wellness and protecting against adversity, with the potential for these skills to be passed from one generation to the next. Caregivers too benefit from the relationship they have with their child, from the shared joy experienced during play to the pride of witnessing their child meet a new developmental milestone.

The capacity to develop and grow these kinds of strong connections with caregivers, friends, or other important figures has been enveloped under the term of "relational health" (FrameWorks Institute, 2020), which is recognized as an increasingly important contributor to well-being beyond the infant and early childhood period. If practitioners seek to prevent poor health outcomes, understanding the caregiver–child relationship is the most beneficial area on which to focus their efforts. Child health practitioners are uniquely positioned to support the relational health of the child as they see nearly every infant through well-child and other visits. The practitioner's office is one of the first environments in which the caregiver–child relationship can be observed and intervention can occur (Willis & Eddy, 2022). Child health practitioners can support the relational health of their patients and caregivers in several ways that will be discussed further in this chapter. To promote relational health, the first steps a practitioner can take are to understand the importance of relationships to development, to consider the various contextual factors impacting relationships, and to make a conscious effort to model positivity and support in their own relationships with families.

This chapter discusses the origins of relational health and the theoretical framework on which it is based, including a focus on attachment theory and risk and resilience factors grounded in developmental psychopathology. Relational health will be considered in the context of disorders and mental health conditions that can benefit from relationally focused interventions. The chapter provides an overview of evidence-based relationship-focused assessment methods and treatments beginning in infancy and early childhood and extending into school age and adolescence. It concludes with strategies for applying relationally focused interventions with special clinical populations, such as children with chronic illness, served by clinical psychologists, pediatric psychologists, and developmental-behavioral pediatricians. It presents future considerations and resources for practitioners interested in applying relational health to their work with children and families.

RELATIONAL HEALTH ACROSS DEVELOPMENT

The renowned psychoanalyst and pediatrician Donald Winnicott (1960) famously said, "There is no such thing as an infant" (p. 587). There is always an infant *and* someone to care for and nurture them. Infants are born into the world deeply intertwined in a relationship with their caregiver(s) that is essential to their survival and development. Impairment of this first caregiving relationship can have significant and lasting consequences, and therefore relationally focused psychotherapeutic treatment during infancy and early childhood can be critical.

Willis and Eddy (2022) defined early relational health (ERH) as "a foundational, culturally embedded and developing set of positive, responsive, and reciprocal interactions from birth that nurture and build emotional connections between caregivers, infants, and young children and result in emerging confidence, competence, and emotional well-being for all" (p. 364). The concept of ERH is rooted in attachment and infant mental health (IMH), which focuses on the importance of the caregiver–child relationship and the use of interventions specifically targeted at improving the quality of that relationship. Early relational health seeks to promote child well-being through a broader understanding of the contextual factors that impact families, parents' capacities to engage in caregiving, and other social determinants of health.

Although many characteristics of ERH may be considered culturally universal, such as mutual engagement between the caregiver and child, little research has empirically examined how ERH may look similar or different across cultures (Charlot-Swilley et al., 2022). Given the significance of culture to family interactions, practitioners interested in ERH should not only be mindful of the current dearth of research around culture and ERH, but they should also recognize how their own culture and implicit biases, as well as the historical and structural racism within the larger health care system, may contribute to their perceptions of what a healthy caregiving relationship should look like.

What might ERH look like within a caregiver–child dyad? One key observable characteristic is mutuality or responsivity in interactions, for example, seeing a caregiver respond to an infant's smile by making eye contact and smiling back or commenting on a child's story by repeating back details. These types of serve-and-return interactions, with the child using their skills to initiate an interaction and the caregiver noticing and responding in kind, are a snapshot of the relational health between a caregiver and child. As the child grows and methods of interacting with caregivers evolve over time, these reciprocal interactions act as building blocks in the foundation of future healthy relationships.

In fact, the centrality of relational health to an individual's well-being continues throughout middle childhood and adolescence. With development, the child is afforded new opportunities to form progressively complex, contingent, and reciprocal relationships with peers, novel adults, and broader communities. As relational health moves beyond the primacy of the parent–child relationship, a child's psychological health is enhanced through mutual and enduring emotional connections with others (Bronfenbrenner, 1975). To self-regulate and function effectively across these broader developmental systems, children continue to require senses of safety, security, and support to explore and effectively participate in a larger world as they strive for increased autonomy and still maintain a deep connection to their roots.

Growth-fostering relationships continue to be critical to well-being throughout development as the components of relational health shift with age (Liang et al., 2010). By young adulthood, relational health is broadly conceptualized and assessed as the quality of interpersonal interactions that may nurture growth and be mutually empathic and empowering to individuals (Liang et al., 2002, 2017; Liang & West, 2011). Developing measures to assess relational health beyond infancy has been a focus of more recent work. To assess broader relational health in late adolescent and young adult women, for example, the Relational Health Indices (RHI) were developed to examine engagement, authenticity, and empowerment/zest across relationships with different relational partners, including mentors, peers, and community members (Liang et al., 2002). Findings indicated that strong community relationships are associated with lower levels of depression in young women and increased authenticity, mutual engagement, empowerment, and conflict tolerance in LGBTQ youth (Gamarel et al., 2014; Lund et al., 2014).

Mentoring relationships may be protective in that they are associated with increased well-being (i.e., interpersonal relationship skills, knowledge of culture, knowledge of healthy relationships) in Indigenous youth (Crooks et al., 2017) and with increased self-esteem in affluent adolescent girls during early and mid-adolescence (Liang et al., 2016). Mentoring relationships are also associated with lower levels of depression and stress and increased life satisfaction in youth transitioning out of foster care systems (Munson & McMillen, 2009). Together these findings suggest a range of applicability of relational health across diverse populations throughout development.

Poor relational health, as indicated by an absence of safe, stable, and nurturing relationships (SSNRs), in combination with childhood adversity and/or toxic stress, can lead to biological changes, such as methylation, increases in brain activity, or hypersensitivity to certain cues, with negative impacts on child health and behavior outcomes, educational achievement, and later economic productivity (Garner et al., 2021). However, the presence of SSNRs together with mild instances of childhood adversity may promote positive stress responses, leading to greater resilience. Additionally, children with mental, social, or behavioral health problems in families with greater relational health demonstrated greater capacities to engage consistently in self-regulation, which was associated with greater school performance (Bethell et al., 2022). Similarly, positive connections with caregivers in the context of early adversity may protect against poor mental health in adulthood (Bethell, Jones, et al., 2019).

As a key driver of developmental health across the lifespan, relational health has long been a central focus of early intervention. Clinicians working within a biopsychosocial framework prioritize early relational health and the child–parent relationship as both a target of and vehicle for early intervention. In doing so, they actively attend to the historical, ecological, and developmental factors that create vulnerability or promote resilience within a relational dyad and subsequently identify ports of entry for intervention (e.g., see child–parent psychotherapy [CPP], described later in this chapter).

Given the importance of relational health, interventions have been developed to improve the quality of caregiver–child relationships, particularly in infancy and early childhood, although relationship-focused interventions are also salient for the school-aged child and adolescent. Relational health is both a contributor to and a viable intervention target for a multitude of problems including internalizing problems, externalizing problems, trauma responses, and developmental concerns.

THEORETICAL FRAMEWORK

Early relationships play an important role in the young child's development and have been a focus of many theories of child development.

Attachment Theory

The framework of attachment theory originated from developmental science and centered on the ethological and biobehavioral advantages of attachment figures before the theory transformed into a deeper understanding of how secure attachments with caregivers improve the quality of the relationship and contribute to a child's emotional regulation. As Bowlby (1988) wrote, attachment relationships serve to protect children from harm and promote their survival, and caregivers provide other benefits such as helping a child learn about the environment and teaching their child how to self-regulate and interact with other people.

A child will utilize different attachment behaviors that make up what is called the attachment behavioral system. During times of distress or fear, infants develop a set of attachment behaviors through trial and error to determine what will be most effective at gaining the attention and support of specific caregivers during specific situations (Cassidy, 2016). Once the child establishes contact with the caregiver, the caregiver responds reassuringly, and a sense of safety has been reestablished, the attachment behavioral system disengages. The way in which a caregiver responds to a child's attachment behaviors plays an important role in the security or insecurity of the attachment relationship. Caregivers who respond promptly and appropriately often establish secure attachment, whereas inconsistent or inappropriate responses can lead to attachment insecurity.

Classifications of attachment insecurity, identified by Ainsworth's Strange Situation Procedure (Ainsworth et al., 1978) and later expanded upon by Main and Solomon (1990), include avoidant, ambivalent, and disorganized/disoriented. An infant with an avoidant attachment classification displays little or no affect during separations from a caregiver and appears to avoid the caregiver during reunion. A child with an ambivalent classification displays visible distress during separations, has a difficult time regulating during reunions, and may vacillate between anger and passivity (Solomon & George, 2016). Lastly, Main and Solomon's (1990) disorganized/disoriented classification was added to consider the infant who displays unusual or contradictory behaviors during separations and reunions, such as freezing/stilling, seeming fearful of their caregiver, or not appearing to use any clear attachment strategy. Strong research support exists demonstrating relations between attachment insecurity and later externalizing (e.g., Aguilar et al., 2000; Fearon & Belsky, 2011; Keller et al., 2005) and internalizing problems (e.g., Colonnesi et al., 2011; Lyons-Ruth et al., 1997).

A child's experiences form the basis of representations (known as internal working models) regarding their caregivers, themselves, and the broader environment (Bowlby, 1969/1982). Bowlby suggested that internal working models help the child anticipate and plan for future events and that the child relies on these models to know which attachment behavior to utilize with specific caregivers or attachment figures. The child then carries their internal working models into future relationships with friends and other caregivers, interpreting the behaviors of others through a perspective that has developed over time. However, these models and lenses are often continuously revised as the child develops and has more and varied experiences to consider (Cassidy, 2016).

A child's attachment with their caregivers continues to play an important role in later childhood development, but the child's world expands to include relationships with other individuals, such as friends, teachers, and other important figures. The caregiver and child become more adept at reading each other's cues, which results in a smoother, more coordinated process of engaging and subsequently disengaging from the attachment behavioral system (Brumariu, 2015). Additionally, the emphasis of this system shifts from requiring the caregiver to be in proximity of the child to help regulate to the child finding comfort in knowing the caregiver is available if needed. Likewise, the child's ability to regulate without relying on the caregiver grows, and the attachment behavioral system is activated less frequently as the child becomes more autonomous.

Risk and Resilience in Relational Health

The importance of relationships has also been highlighted in theories of atypical development, such as developmental psychopathology, which is relevant to pediatric psychology and developmental-behavioral pediatrics. According to this view, relationships can serve as either risk or protective factors in the development of psychopathology in childhood. Extremes in the caregiving relationship, such as abuse and neglect, have been shown to contribute to childhood psychopathology, but less severe instances of poor parent–child relationship quality may also contribute to behavioral or emotional dysfunction. Insecure attachment relationships have the potential to lead to over-dependence or under-dependence on caregivers, and a child who has experienced maltreatment in caregiving relationships can demonstrate unusual or distorted attachment behaviors in an effort to have their needs met (Sroufe, 1990). On the other hand, based on their own experiences of caregiving, mental health, or other factors, a parent may find their child's cues so distressing that they engage in caregiving behaviors such as shutting down when a child is distressed or increasing distance between themselves and their child (George & Solomon, 2008). As a child's emotional regulation capacities often depend on caregivers responding calmly, sensitively, and consistently during times of distress, a child's ability to regulate is diminished if they feel unable to signal their distress or their caregiver struggles to respond to those signals.

Theories of developmental psychopathology also consider the role of adaptation—that psychopathology results when circumstances occur that require the child to continually adapt, leading the child increasingly farther away from typical development (Sroufe et al., 1999). The child actively engages in behaviors and seeks out experiences that support continuity in adaptation. Therefore, a child with a history of being rejected by caregivers may become so accustomed to that response that they may engage in potentially maladaptive behaviors in order to experience rejection by other individuals, including later in life. Additionally, a child may perceive and interpret new events in a manner that corresponds to and reinforces their relational history.

Biological Factors in Early Relationships

Caregiving relationships have also been considered in the context of gene-environment interactions. Some genotypes have been shown to predispose a child to adversity and/or psychopathology, but secure attachment relationships may serve to protect against genetic risk factors being determinative (Calkins et al., 2013). More broadly, positive caregiving behaviors may buffer the risk of certain alleles such as the A1 polymorphism of DRD2 (Propper et al., 2008) and the short polymorphism of DRD4 (Propper et al., 2007), whereas negative caregiving behaviors interact with genes that have been associated with childhood psychopathology, including L-DRD4 (Bakermans-Kranenburg & van IJzendoorn, 2006) and MAOA (Vanyukov et al., 2007). Gene-environment interactions specifically in the context of early parent–child relationships predict a child's later self-regulatory capacities (Kochanska et al., 2009), noncompliance (Sulik et al., 2012), and externalizing symptoms (DiLalla et al., 2009). Research examining biological mediators of the relation between parenting and child development has shown that early parenting relationships and behaviors are related to hypothalamic–pituitary–adrenal axis functioning in the child. Research shows greater infant cortisol recovery following a stressful event when caregivers displayed more sensitive or engaged behavior (Albers et al., 2008; Blair et al., 2008) and greater increases in cortisol when fathers engaged in more negative behavior (Mills-Koonce et al., 2011). The relation between maternal stress and infant stress reactivity (as measured by cortisol) is buffered by mothers' sensitive caregiving (Nazzari et al., 2022). Therefore, early parent–child relationships marked by warmth and sensitivity appear to play important roles in promoting positive social-emotional development and protecting against preexisting genetic risk factors for psychopathology.

Parental Mentalization

Parental mentalization has been theorized as an additional mechanism by which the caregiving relationship protects against childhood psychopathology. Sharp and Fonagy (2008) viewed mentalization as a form of "meeting of minds" between the caregiver and child, in that mentalizing involves a coordinated and intentional sharing of emotional states between the two. Through parents' capacity to recognize and accurately interpret their child's thoughts and feelings, a form of mentalizing known as parental reflective functioning (Slade, 2005), a child's own mentalizing abilities develop, which as proposed by Sharp and Fonagy (2008) leads to the development of emotional regulation. A child who lacks the ability to consider their own and others' mental states may demonstrate maladaptive patterns in self-regulation, leading to psychopathology. Parents with greater reflective functioning tend to use more sensitive and fewer problematic parenting behaviors than less reflective parents (e.g., Möller et al., 2017; Rosenblum et al., 2008; Smaling et al., 2016; Stacks et al., 2014). In support of Sharp and Fonagy (2008), various forms of parental mentalization, including reflective functioning and mind-mindedness, are associated with greater emotion regulation (Heron-Delaney et al., 2016; Senehi et al., 2018; Smaling et al., 2017) and fewer internalizing and externalizing disorders in children (Ensink et al., 2017; Hughes et al., 2017; Meins et al., 2013). Many relationally focused interventions aim to increase a parent's mentalizing or reflective capacity (see the Intervention for At-Risk Dyads: Strong Roots and the Infant Mental Health Home Visiting sections later in this chapter).

Although much research has examined how specific parenting behaviors such as insensitivity, harshness, warmth, or responsiveness and/or biological stress responses contribute to child outcomes at a certain point in time, it is important to understand how multiple parent–child interactions over months and years impact the child. Developmental cascades consider the cumulative nature of a child's interactions on development (Masten & Cicchetti, 2012). For example, for a child exposed to repeated instances of poor parental mental health leading to more negative caregiving and increased cortisol reactivity, the number of these events and their frequency work together to lead to potential developmental concerns or psychopathology. On the other hand, repeated experiences of positive caregiving, even in light of stressors, have the potential to predict developmental progress that continues throughout a child's development.

Importantly, influences between children and their caregivers are bidirectional. A child's characteristics or behavior may elicit certain parenting behavior, and parenting behavior in turn elicits certain child behavior, allowing for change in one relational partner to result in change in the other and in their relationship (Sameroff, 2009). When considering treatment from a developmental cascades perspective, early intervention should focus on increasing behaviors associated with positive cascades or decreasing behaviors associated with negative cascades (Cicchetti & Gunnar, 2008; Masten & Cicchetti, 2010).

RELATIONSHIP DISTURBANCES AND DISORDERS

Across the fifth edition of the *Diagnostic and Statistical Manual of Mental Disorders* (American Psychiatric Association, 2013), the parent–child relationship is either explicitly or implicitly identified as an important part of diagnosis and/or treatment across a myriad of disorders. For example, in some disorders, a child's symptoms may be expressed in the context of their relationship with their caregivers. A child with separation anxiety may fear the loss of a caregiving relationship so much that they struggle to appropriately separate during brief or routine events. Those with selective mutism may have such high levels of anxiety that they require the presence of caregivers in social settings to speak on their behalf. For a child with a trauma-related disorder, the caregiver is often involved in the traumatic event either as a witness, a victim, or the perpetrator. A child with experiences of abuse or neglect may have perceptions of the event that are likely shaped by their relationship with their caregiver and the belief that this individual is supposed to keep them safe from harm (Lieberman et al., 2015). As a result, the child may blame themselves for their trauma, augmenting their symptom presentation and negatively impacting their sense of self. A child who has experienced the most disrupted or deprived caregiving during infancy or early childhood may present with symptoms of reactive attachment disorder or disinhibited social engagement, disorders characterized by difficulties forming attachment relationships and distorted or inappropriate attachment behavior (American Psychiatric Association, 2013).

For special clinical populations, such as a child with intellectual disabilities or neurodevelopmental disorders, relationships with family members and friends play an important role in determining the degree to which their social functioning is impacted by their disorder. Likewise, the quality of a child's social communication with family members and friends is important to consider when making a diagnosis of autism spectrum disorder. Other diagnoses or symptom presentations may not explicitly relate to the caregiver–child relationship; however, relational issues are often present and can both impact and be impacted by the child's presenting concerns. Therefore, interventions with children often require engaging the caregiver in treatment as well as targeted work to improve aspects of the relationship impacted by the disorder or traumatic experience and to develop skills to change those aspects of the relationship that may be promoting maladaptive behavior.

Relational health is grounded in tenets from attachment theory and neurodevelopment and recognizes the importance of developing interventions to mitigate the effects of toxic stress on the caregiver–child relationship (Garner et al., 2021). Relationally focused interventions (RFI) consider the ecological factors that contribute to vulnerabilities across relationships and development, including parent and child experiences, and seek to identify opportunities to engage families in treatment through the development of a strong therapeutic alliance. Engagement, an element central to relationally focused practice, can be utilized across disciplines with those who work with children and families, including but not limited to primary care physicians, developmental-behavioral pediatricians, and psychologists.

THE RELATIONAL PERSPECTIVE IN ACTION

Given their centrality in development, relationships have been the focus of therapeutic assessment and interventions. Relational work is not bound to a particular discipline, but rather can be applied by any practitioner who has been trained in relational techniques—psychologists, social workers, or pediatricians, among others. Similarly, relational work can take place in a wide variety of clinical settings, ranging from a brief pediatric visit to a more in-depth psychological evaluation. Relational work is unique in that the focus is not a specific individual but rather what happens between individuals. Most commonly, relational work focuses on the caregiver–child relationship. Although the deepest body of work pertains to relationally oriented assessment and intervention in infancy and early childhood, elements of the relational perspective are also found in interventions with older children and adolescents.

Relationally Oriented Assessment

Relationally focused assessment is defined by a focus on what happens between people rather than within an individual. Clinical observation and clinical interview questions are at the core of relationally oriented assessment, as most formal measures consider one individual's perspective rather than what happens between individuals. Because the relationship is the target of relational work, relational assessment attends closely to both verbal and nonverbal communication between members of the dyad or family. Facial expressions, eye contact, body posture, and other nonverbal cues can shed light on an individual's internal experience, even in the absence of verbal cues. Relationally focused clinicians aim to be acutely attuned to the internal experience of both members of the dyad to understand each member's unique contributions to and experiences of the relationship. Specifically, each member of the dyad's thoughts, feelings, representations, and reflections are relevant to their subjective experience of the relationship and will influence observable behaviors that each individual exhibits in interaction with the another.

Table 29.1 offers some ideas of how clinicians can tune in to the relationship between a caregiver and child to better support the family's functioning. The goal of relational assessment is typically a relationally informed conceptualization of the problem rather than a specific score on a measure.

Although it is common for a clinician when getting to know a family to form an opinion about which member of the dyad is the problem, relational assessment aims to get beyond this dichotomy and instead see and understand the perspective of both members of the dyad. Relational assessment goes beyond a simple list of symptoms exhibited by an individual and focuses instead on the ways that caregivers and children interact with one another and how these interactions relate to the presenting problem. For instance, when the child is upset, does the caregiver escalate their affect or share their calmness with the child? Does the dyad have moments of joy or pleasure together? These positive interactions serve as the foundation for resilience and are particularly vital for families experiencing stress or behavioral challenges.

Clinical observations suggesting that there is relational dysfunction guide recommendations about treatment. For instance, for a child with attention-deficit/hyperactivity disorder (ADHD)

TABLE 29.1

Relationship Assessment: Notice, Ask, Reflect

Notice
- Body positioning (eye contact, turned toward/away from each other)?
- Emotional attunement (do they appear to be aware of and to understand each other's emotional experience)?
- Do they delight in one another?
- If both are verbal, do they rely on each other to share information or create a joint narrative when describing an event?
- How does the caregiver respond when the child is upset or has a challenging behavior? With empathy? Resentment? Helplessness?
- What does it feel like for you, the clinician, to be in the room with this dyad/family? Is there tension? Warmth? Distance?

Ask
- How do you help your child soothe when they are upset?
- How does your child soothe on their own? With you? And with others?
- What is going on when your child soothes easily? What might be happening when your child has difficulty soothing?
- How can you tell what your child is thinking or feeling?
- What do you like to do together?
- Tell me three words or phrases to describe your relationship with your child/parent. Give an example/memory for each one.
- Tell me about your support system.
- What is your greatest challenge in parenting? Greatest joy?

Reflect
- Reflective statements and questions can help a dyad to shift in their understanding of one another or their understanding of the problem. For example:
    - "What do you think [child] was feeling when [challenging event/behavior happened]?"
    - "What did you [caregiver] feel when [challenging event/behavior happened]?"
    - "I wonder if that reminded you [caregiver or child] of [another experience, potentially a traumatic experience]."
    - "I can see how much you [caregiver] care about [child] and how important it is to you that [child feels better, child stays out of trouble, child is not showing distress, child gets good grades, and so forth]."
    - "I noticed that [child] brightened/leaned into you [or other positive response] when you [positive parenting behavior]. How do you think your child felt when you did that?"
    - "I can see that you are important to each other. I wonder how your child is able to show you that you are important to him/her. In what ways is your child important to you?"

who gets adequate support from and is regulated by their parents, coaching in executive functioning strategies and/or medication may be a sufficient treatment plan. However, for a child with ADHD who becomes more dysregulated by their parents when upset, these strategies are likely to be inadequate. In this case, a relational approach, such as parent–child dyadic psychotherapy, may be a necessary supplement to standard ADHD treatment.

Relationally Focused Intervention

Relationally focused intervention can take place within relationally focused psychotherapy, but it can also be implemented in smaller pieces within a pediatric visit or other brief clinical encounters. The goal of relationally focused intervention is to support the caregiver–child relationship and to enhance the dyad's ability to understand each other and co-regulate. A relationally focused clinician will make comments and observations that aim to make each member of the dyad's internal experiences more apparent with the goal of helping them better understand their own and the other's experience in the relationship (see Table 29.1). Ultimately, as relational patterns emerge (i.e., escalating one another's emotions in times of distress), a relationally focused clinician helps each member of the dyad to reduce their reactivity to the other.

For example, in a pediatric visit, a mother may appear frustrated, angry, and resentful as she describes her son's impulsive and aggressive behaviors. A relationally focused clinician may empathize with the mother while also acknowledging the son's experience and perspective: "I can tell that this is hard to talk about. I can tell that you really value your friendships, and something really upsetting must have happened for you to hit your classmate." As each member of the dyad feels valued and understood by the clinician, they are likely to also feel more regulated in one another's presence. As members notice, reflect, and practice new ways of being together, the relationship can gradually shift from one that escalates distress to one that promotes a feeling of security.

Central to relational interventions is a focus on regulation and co-regulation. Because a feeling of safety is critical in relationships, relationally focused clinicians are attentive to how each member of the dyad is regulating and acts to support their regulation. As young children require the assistance of their caregivers to regulate, clinicians actively support caregivers in co-regulating with their young children (i.e., by coaching parents in strategies to regulate themselves, in strategies for them to use with their children). Clinicians balance the needs of both members of the dyad and ensure that each is able to experience regulation in their relationship. The experience of regulation builds security and trust in the relationship and increases the dyad's capacity to continue to feel safe and connected.

As consistency, reliability, and accessibility are qualities that are critical to a well-functioning relationship, relationally focused clinicians aim to exemplify these qualities in their interaction with the dyad and support the dyad in exemplifying these qualities as well. When dysregulation is experienced in a relationship, a relationally focused clinician attends to the relational processes that contribute to or escalate dysregulation. By considering the history and subjective experience of each member of the dyad, a clinician can reveal processes that contribute to relational dysfunction (e.g., help a caregiver to see the role of their trauma in shaping their interpretation of their child's behavior) and help both members of the dyad achieve regulation and a feeling of safety.

Interactions in relationships are typically deeply rooted and are driven by a plethora of earlier experiences in relationships. In turn, interventions that target observable behaviors may provide a temporary improvement in relational functioning, but fail to create lasting change. Relational interventions target the roots of our behaviors in relationships by considering how these behaviors developed and the purposes that they serve in relationships. Ultimately, this focus is meant to create more lasting and impactful change in relational functioning. In fact, research suggests that interventions designed to enhance relationships also are broadly associated with improved cortisol regulation (Slopen et al., 2014). Further, even among children who have experienced adversity, family resilience and connection are associated with a variety of positive developmental outcomes including children's ability to regulate their emotions, demonstration of persistence, and interest and curiosity in learning new things (Bethell, Gombojav, et al., 2019).

Relationships are a central force in our lives, and connection with those we care about can be a powerful motivator of behavior. In turn, improving the quality of relationships is typically a highly desired and meaningful treatment goal that can motivate participation in treatment. Just as relational clinicians are attuned to the quality of a dyad's relationship, they are also attuned to the quality of their own relationship with the dyad. A strong therapeutic relationship between the provider and the dyad can help the dyad to feel more connected to the provider and reduce the likelihood of premature dropout from treatment. In considering clinical environments that support relational health, it may be useful to attend to the ways in which providers and staff can attend to each other and to their patients. Creating warm, consistent, and predictable work spaces and carving out time for reflective supervision among staff may ultimately foster stronger relationships among patients, staff, and providers and more broadly in relationships outside the therapeutic practice.

Addressing Ecological Contexts in Relational Work

The relational perspective is unique in its attention to how each individual's historical experiences impact their subjective experience in the current relationship. For example, for a young child who experienced early separation related to foster care or adoption, a clinician and caregiver may observe and think together about how the child experiences other more routine separations from caregivers. For parents, their own history of trauma, stress, separations, and loss is critical to understanding the way that they experience their current relationships, including their relationship with their children. A mother who experienced domestic violence, for instance, may experience reminders of those traumatic experiences when her young child shows developmentally normative aggression. Helping a parent to understand the ways that their own history can impact their thoughts, feelings, and representations in their relationship with their child is important and perhaps necessary to shift relational patterns and ultimately increase satisfaction in the relationship for both partners.

A relational perspective also places attention on factors that occur outside of the focal dyad and how those factors can influence the functioning of the dyad. For instance, factors like employment, community violence, support services, and culture are all likely to affect an individual's functioning. Those contextual factors also influence the way an individual interacts with others and in turn the individual's relationships. For example, a parent experiencing high levels of stress due to community violence or financial insecurity may become irritable and respond to his or her child with less sensitivity. The child in turn may have more difficulty regulating emotions and show less synchronous interactions with their parents.

Effects of sociohistorical influences, including ethnicity and socioeconomic status, can play out in relationships as well. For instance, a young African American boy showing age-typical aggressive behavior may elicit a strong response from a parent due to their understanding of systemic racism and the ways that U.S. society criminalizes African American men and boys. A relationally focused intervention attends to these distal and proximal factors, and by revealing various factors that influence how people exist in relationships, it can help dyads to shift into healthier ways of being together.

Relationally Focused Interventions in Infancy and Early Childhood

There are several intervention programs that are designed to support caregiver–child relationships during infancy and early childhood. These programs range from universal prevention programs, designed to screen and support dyads at all levels of functioning, to more intensive intervention programs designed to support dyads with clinical levels of risk. Although the therapy programs described in the following paragraphs are conducted primarily by psychologists or social workers with specialized training in the specific intervention, other providers, such as pediatricians, play an important role in identifying patients who would be a good fit for these programs and providing a warm handoff to ensure their enrollment and connection with a therapy provider.

Universal prevention: Early relational health screen and early relational health conversations. Pediatric care typically involves routine screening for a variety of medical and developmental conditions and risks. Developmental, behavioral, and social delays are very common, with as many as one in four children between birth and 5 years old at moderate to high risk for such problems (Child & Adolescent Health Measurement Initiative, 2012). Given the centrality of relationships to young children's development and well-being, the Early Relational Health Screen (ERHS) was developed as a universal strategy to support early relational health in infancy and toddlerhood (ages 4 to 24 months) that quickly identifies caregiver–child dyads who may require additional support and clinical intervention (Willis et al., 2022). It can be administered by any provider who has been trained in its use; most often, given the limited time that a pediatrician can spend with a family, it is completed by a social worker or other clinician at a pediatric clinic. It includes both a screening component and a promotion component. The screening component involves a brief parent–child interaction that is video recorded, observed, and coded by a trained clinician (or non-clinician) to assess a number of dyadic relational qualities (e.g., mutual enjoyment, mutual pacing). The promotion component involves review of the video with the caregiver and a conversation about early relational health that is designed to promote caregivers' observations and reflective skills. Caregivers are asked questions including

- What was this experience like for you? For your child?
- Was there anything that bothered or surprised you?
- What do you think was your child's sweetest or favorite moment?
- Do you have any concerns or questions about the relationship you and your child have with one another?

Through this conversation, caregivers are supported in reflecting on their relationship with their child and practice observing aspects of their interaction that might otherwise go unnoticed. Caregivers thereby enhance their ability to understand their own mental states as well as those of their child, which are known to relate to the child's attachment security (Shai & Meins, 2018). Interactions are rated on a set of qualities that vary by age, with some applied to all ages (e.g., mutual engagement, pacing) and others only to older ages (e.g., shared goals/objectives, mutual response to a challenge, shared pretend play). The ERHS is unique in that it is a truly relational approach; it is driven not by caregiver behavior or child behavior but instead by what happens between caregivers and children.

The ERHS has been implemented in settings including pediatric primary care, infant mental health home visiting (IMH-HV), and research studies, but empirical research is so far limited (Willis & Eddy, 2022). Preliminary findings suggest that it is feasible to utilize this approach in pediatric primary care settings (Willis et al., 2022). In-the-moment ratings are consistent with ratings made from a video recording and align well with other established measures of caregiver–child relationships (e.g., the National Institute of Child Health and Human Development's Dyadic Mutuality scale; Rosenblum et al., 2022). Mothers who are depressed have lower ratings on the ERHS (Rosenblum et al., 2022), suggesting that the ERHS may be a helpful tool to identify dyads with relational health challenges related to maternal mental health. Given the ERHS's ability to screen and identify families who may need more comprehensive support services, as well as to support all dyads through brief relational health conversations, it should be considered a promising practice for universal prevention and promotion of relational health.

An alternative to the ERHS, the Early Relational Health-Conversations (ERH-C) model was developed following experiences of African American families using the ERHS and was designed to minimize potential implicit biases within health care settings (Charlot-Swilley et al., 2022). This model is grounded using an Afrocentric worldview and prioritizes the voices of nondominant cultures. The ERH-C model considers all members of the family who interact with a child and gives space for families to tell their own stories. As in the ERHS, interactions between parent and child are recorded and watched by the family and the ERH-C facilitator. The family and facilitator then discuss strengths observed during the interaction and engage in broader conversations around family values and hopes.

Eight components of ERH-C were developed to guide conversations between families and facilitators: preparing and entering, accessing, pausing and co-creating, storytelling, witnessing, mutual reflection, claiming, and mutual insight (Charlot-Swilley et al., 2022). These components and their prompts are designed to prepare the facilitator to have safe, nonjudgmental conversations with families while also recognizing areas in which families may benefit from additional support. Unlike ERHS, the ERH-C model does not provide ratings but rather allows for a qualitative approach to understanding ERH within families. Facilitators are expected to receive reflective supervision and consultation in order to best utilize ERH-C in their practice. Further research is needed to better understand methods of applying ERH-C in pediatric or other health care settings, but practitioners may find ERH-C to be a useful measure of connecting with and understanding the early relational health of families, particularly those from marginalized populations.

Intervention for at-risk dyads: Strong Roots. For dyads that have been identified as having risk factors for poor relational health, intervention may be appropriate. Whether risk arises from caregiver mental health, sociodemographic factors, trauma, or problems related to child development, intervention programs that bolster caregiver–child relationships can promote resilience and reduce the likelihood of ongoing risk. The Strong Roots programs are one example of a brief intervention program designed for dyads experiencing risk. These programs are a set of group-based interventions to support mothers (Mom Power; Muzik et al., 2016), fathers (Fraternity of Fathers), military families (Strong Military Families; Rosenblum et al., 2015), and teachers (Hearts and Minds on Babies; Barron et al., 2020) in developing safe, strong, and positive relationships for young children, families, and communities. These programs are designed for families from pregnancy through child age 6 and have a curriculum based on attachment theory, trauma theory, and social learning theory. Strong Roots programs are designed to be led by mental health clinicians (i.e., social workers, psychologists, counselors) who have been trained in the model. The program uses a metaphor of a tree to illustrate a caregiver's role in being both a secure base for exploration (branching out) and a safe haven in times of connection (building roots). Caregivers and group leaders discuss how to understand often confusing child behavior and how to co-regulate with their child and meet their child's needs for both exploration and connection. In a child-directed play group that is concurrent with the parent group child team members carefully observe and assess their developmental functioning, and children and caregivers practice safe and predictable separation and reunion routines. Group sessions also have a focus on promoting self-care through evidence-based strategies such as mindfulness and guided imagery. Group discussions allow caregivers to reflect on the ways that their current parenting—including their values, behaviors, and emotions—is a product of the caregiving that they experienced when they were children themselves. Strong Roots programs typically include individual check-in sessions for each participant to assess their current needs and connect them to any additional support services that may be indicated.

Strong Roots programs are widely available in Michigan and can be found in nine other states, with additional expansion ongoing. Mom Power has been subject to an open trial and a randomized controlled trial (RCT), which found that participation in Mom Power is associated with improved maternal mental health, reduced parenting stress, and widening social support (Muzik et al., 2015, 2016; Rosenblum, Muzik et al., 2017). Mothers who participated in Mom Power were more likely to have a "balanced" representational style (i.e., reflections that are characterized by warmth and acceptance of the child, associated with attachment security) and improved reflective functioning (Rosenblum, Lawler et al., 2017). Brain imaging suggested that these mothers have more activation in brain circuits associated with parental empathy (Swain et al., 2016, 2017). Similarly, Strong Military Families has been associated with improved reflective functioning and representations as well as improved positive affect in caregiver–child interactions (Julian, Muzik, Kees, Valenstein, Dexter, et al., 2018; Julian, Muzik, Kees, Valenstein, & Rosenblum, 2018). The Strong Roots programs utilize strategies that support relational health from both the caregiver's and child's individual perspectives but also through supported dyadic interactions. Participation in Strong Roots programs is associated with meaningful changes in factors that underlie relational health, such as reflective capacity, mental health, and social support.

Additional relationally focused interventions appropriate for dyads experiencing risk include Circle of Security (Huber et al., 2015) and Attachment and BioBehavioral Catch-up (Bernard et al., 2012).

Interventions for dyads requiring ongoing clinical support. Although brief interventions are appropriate for many families, more intensive intervention may be necessary for those experiencing more significant symptoms and risks.

Infant mental health home visiting. In the early 1970s, the field of IMH began to emerge, led by the understanding that a nurturing caregiver–child relationship lies at the center of an infant's well-being (Weatherston et al., 2020). The IMH model was one of the first true relational interventions; it has been the root of numerous other early childhood relational interventions that are practiced widely in the United States and around the world, including CPP (Lieberman & Van Horn, 2004, 2008) and Child FIRST (Lowell et al., 2011). Components of the intervention (e.g., video review) are utilized in a wide variety of relational intervention approaches.

IMH-HV is a home-based parent–child intervention model in which a trained clinician (typically a masters-level mental health provider, such as a licensed social worker) supports caregiver–child dyads from pregnancy into early childhood through weekly therapy in the family's home (Weatherston et al., 2020). Families are referred to IMH-HV for a variety of reasons, including maternal mental health concerns, child behavior or development concerns, or social or demographic risk factors (e.g., teenage parenthood, domestic violence, family stress). This intervention is unique in its attention to families' needs at multiple levels; it supports parents in material ways (i.e., provision of concrete support, connection to other needed services), attends to and supports family systems, and provides infant–parent psychotherapy to more directly support early relational health. Infant–parent psychotherapy supports the infant–parent relationship through observation and interpretation of infants' and parents' behavior and emotions and facilitation of their co-regulation. Clinicians are trained to support caregivers' development of reflective functioning and frequently discuss with parents the ways in which their own history in relationships shows up in their interactions with and responses to their own children. The focus of IMH-HV on meeting families' material needs is reflective of its recognition that factors outside of the focal dyad (e.g., connection to needed services, lack of material resources) impact the infant–parent relationship and that sensitive and responsive caregiving is much more challenging for families whose basic needs are not met. Clinicians also provide developmental guidance and work to bolster a family's social support system and connection to needed services, often going so far as to accompany families to medical or social service appointments and sign them up for needed services (e.g., Supplemental Nutrition Program for Women, Infants, and Children).

The Michigan model of IMH-HV has been subject to a RCT as well as studies examining its effects as it is currently practiced in the community (Lawler et al., 2017; Rosenblum et al., 2020). Those who were referred to IMH-HV services by Michigan's Baby Court (i.e., children served by the child welfare system) showed improvements in parental responsiveness, positive affect, and reflective functioning over the course of IMH-HV treatment (Stacks et al., 2019). A randomized controlled trial found that more IMH-HV sessions were associated with increased maternal sensitivity. Participation in video review—a strategy in which parents and clinicians reflect together on video-recorded observations of the parent's interaction with the child—was associated with improved maternal sensitivity, over and above the effect of number of sessions (Rosenblum et al., 2020). IMH-HV services are associated with improvements in child expressive language, positive affect, and enthusiasm (Stacks et al., 2020).

Although maternal adverse childhood experiences are negatively associated with child language competence, this association was eliminated among mother–child dyads who were randomized to receive IMH-HV treatment, suggesting that IMH-HV can mitigate the intergenerational transmission of risk (Riggs et al., 2022). Maternal adverse childhood experiences are associated with maternal posttraumatic stress disorder symptoms, and in turn with more toddler emotional problems; however, even among mothers with mild to moderate posttraumatic stress disorder symptoms, participation in IMH-HV is linked to improved toddler social-emotional well-being over the course of treatment (Ribaudo et al., 2022). In brief, IMH-HV treatment is associated with improvements in both parental and child functioning in domains that relate to the way parents and children interact with one another.

Child–parent psychotherapy. CPP is a trauma-focused relational psychotherapy that is conducted by mental health clinicians (e.g., psychologists, social workers) who have been trained in the model. As with other psychotherapy models, pediatricians and other providers play an important role in identifying families that could be a good fit for this work and making a referral to this treatment. More specifically, CPP is a dyadic psychotherapy model for children under 6 years of age who have experienced trauma and have behavioral or emotional challenges (Lieberman & Van Horn, 2004). One of the foundational pieces of CPP is the understanding that the caregiver–child relationship is central to the dyad's recovery from trauma and resolution of behavioral and emotional challenges.

CPP begins with a foundational phase, during which information is gathered about both the child's and the caregiver's trauma history, and the clinician and caregiver explore both how the child's symptoms may be connected to their experience of trauma and how the caregiver's history impacts the way they experience and respond to their child. The core intervention phase of treatment then begins by presenting a play-based narrative about the trauma to the child, along with acknowledgment of the impact of the trauma on their emotions and behavior and an explanation of how treatment will help. As the core intervention phase continues, treatment is centered around play-based developmental-relational psychotherapy, in which the clinician is deeply attuned to the emotions and behaviors of each member of the dyad. During play, the clinician makes comments to help the dyad notice something (e.g., how a child's memory of an event might be showing up in play), to shift their understanding of something (e.g., an emotional reaction by caregiver or child as a response to a trauma reminder), or to provide developmental guidance (e.g., understanding of a behavior as developmentally normative, sharing strategies that may help a young child regulate emotions). Throughout treatment, safety is a core theme. The clinician helps the caregiver to ensure that the dyad experiences both psychological and physical safety, that the dyad's material needs are met (e.g., safe housing, access to needed services), and that the dyad is able to experience the difference between then (i.e., the trauma) and now (i.e., safety). On average, a course of CPP lasts about a year or more, with weekly sessions.

Several RCTs have been completed to evaluate the effect of CPP on participating dyads. This intervention is associated with improvements in child behavior problems and child trauma symptoms and with reductions in mothers' general distress and avoidant symptoms (Lieberman et al., 2005, Weiner et al., 2009). These effects have been documented to last at least 6 months beyond the end of treatment (Ghosh Ippen et al., 2011). Some studies have examined how CPP is related to caregiver–child interaction. One such RCT found that, for anxiously attached Latin American infants, those who participated in CPP had lower avoidance, resistance, and anger when interacting with their mothers; their mothers in turn showed greater empathy and enhanced interactions with their children (Lieberman et al., 1991). Some studies have reported outcomes related to attachment security. For example, two RCTs found that CPP is associated with increased rates of secure attachment, but rates of secure attachment may not differ between CPP and a psychoeducational parenting intervention (Cicchetti et al., 1999, 2006). Young children who have participated in CPP may also enjoy improved representations of themselves and of their caregivers and healthier relationship expectations (Toth et al., 2002). Notably, the change to secure attachment mediates the effect of CPP on both maternal warmth and child problem behavior (Guild et al., 2021).

Relationally Focused Interventions for School-Aged Children

There are more efficacious relationship-focused interventions designed to promote relational health in early life than there are for any other developmental period. That is, fewer intervention programs for middle childhood and adolescence target what is happening in the transactions between or among members of a relational system in real time. However, relational components form the foundation of evidence-based Parent Management Training (PMT) programs designed to reduce disruptive, noncompliant, and oppositional behavior in children, in which providers work on activities that increase the frequency of positive parent–child interactions.

For example, under the supervision of an interventionist, parents participating in parent–child interaction therapy (PCIT), begin by learning PRIDE (i.e., **p**raise, **r**eflection, **i**mitation, **d**escription, **e**njoyment) skills (Eyberg & Funderburk, 2011; Niec, 2018). The Incredible Years Parenting Program (Webster-Stratton & Bywater, 2019) also begins by teaching parents how to enrich interactions with their children through child-centered play and by learning to deliver praise effectively. Activities focus on teaching parents how to follow their child's lead, pace play, increase their ability to read and be sensitive to their children's cues, praise their children's ideas and creativity, and encourage imaginative play. Parents are also taught to encourage problem solving and to attend to children during special time dedicated to play. Specific strategies for delivering effective praise are reviewed. They help parents to catch children being "good" (not "perfect") and to offer labeled praise that is authentic, specific, immediate, contingent on behavior, positive, enthusiastic, and combined with affection (Webster-Stratton, 2000; Webster-Stratton & Bywater, 2019). Both parent training and relational health interventions encourage caregivers to observe, attend to, and reflect on child behaviors and experiences and to increase their awareness and responsiveness to child cues. In relational interventions, caregivers work with both members of the dyad jointly in real time while holding in mind and reflecting upon the unique aspects of the dyad's relational history.

Relationally Focused Interventions in Adolescence

Evidence supporting relationship-focused interventions in youth is emerging in several areas, including work with adolescent girls who are incarcerated (Lenz et al., 2012) and therapeutic work with girls participating in inpatient treatment for chemical dependency (Vandermause, Fougere, et al., 2018; Vandermause, Roberts, et al., 2018), as well as in recommendations for treatment with adolescent survivors of sexual abuse (Haiyasoso & Schuermann, 2018). There is also empirical support for Attachment Based Family Therapy (ABFT; Diamond, 2014; Diamond et al., 2019), which is a relationship-focused intervention for families whose teens show depression and suicidality (Diamond, 2014). This intervention targets what is happening between teens and their caregivers. In doing so, clinicians aim to restore safety and security in relationships between parents and their teens, with the goal of establishing or restoring adolescents' confidence in relying on their caregivers for support, especially during times of stress and psychiatric crisis (Diamond, 2014; Diamond et al., 2019).

Rooted in both attachment theory and family therapy, ABFT is a component-based 12- to 16-week (or longer) therapy that aims to reduce youth suicidality and depression through five modules or components:

1. a *relational reframe*, which shifts how family members view or make attributions about the problem, generate potential solutions, and encourage members to agree to participate in family therapy;
2. an *adolescent alliance*, which focuses on understanding the adolescent's thoughts, feelings, and experiences of the attachment relationship so that the relationship becomes valued and the adolescent develops an openness to renegotiating the relationship;
3. a *parent alliance*, which addresses parents' working model of their teen and explores how they conceive of parenting to increase their motivation (especially after experiencing the stress of rearing a teen with suicidality) and promote an increase in supportive parenting behavior;
4. *attachment repair*, in which relational partners engage in corrective attachment episodes and providers work with caregivers and teens conjointly to shift interactions, thereby increasing the likelihood that teens will seek support from caregivers when distressed and in return experience parental validation, comfort, and help around problem solving; and
5. *promoting autonomy*, the last phase of ABFT, in which parents support their teens in managing typical developmental tasks faced by many adolescents (i.e., navigating academics, driving a car, part-time employment), as well as symptoms of depression (Diamond, 2014; Diamond et al., 2019).

Participation in ABFT is associated with lower rates of suicide and depression in youth than treatment-as-usual or wait-list controls (Diamond et al., 2002; Ewing et al., 2018). Reductions in depression and suicidal ideation are similar to those found for suicidal youth participating in comparable supportive treatments (Diamond et al., 2019). The therapeutic focus on relational work during sessions enables dyads to practice different ways of relating to each other, which is especially important given associations among adolescent depression, suicide risk, and poor family functioning. The relational work involving corrective attachment episodes in ABFT is a mechanism through which change occurs in cases with positive outcomes (Tsvieli et al., 2021). The relational focus of ABFT may also be particularly helpful for hard to reach adolescents who have "failed" previous interventions, lost prior hard-earned gains, or not benefited from prior treatments for depression and suicidality, including individual therapy (Ewing et al., 2018).

RELATIONALLY FOCUSED INTERVENTIONS IN CLINICAL POPULATIONS WHERE RELATIONAL HEALTH IS AT RISK: RELEVANCE FOR PEDIATRIC PSYCHOLOGY AND DEVELOPMENTAL-BEHAVIORAL PEDIATRICS

Beyond early childhood, the development of relationship-focused interventions and relationship-focused treatment environments may be especially useful for providers working with populations at risk for poor relational health across the lifespan (e.g., clinical and pediatric psychologists and developmental-behavioral pediatricians). Relational health in individuals and families impacted by neurodevelopmental disorders, including autism spectrum disorder and other chronic health conditions (e.g., asthma, cancer, cystic fibrosis, diabetes, epilepsy, allergies, juvenile arthritis) may be particularly vulnerable. Treatment for core symptoms of chronic conditions often necessitates intense, complex, multifaceted interdisciplinary care over long periods of time, placing relational health at risk. Infants and children, for example, may be medically or physically fragile, hospitalized, and separated at times from their primary caregivers. Their behavior may be less predictable, and cues about their needs may be less readable, making sensitive contingent caregiving and predictable, sustained, pleasurable, reciprocal interactions more difficult (Fraiberg, 1971; Goldberg, 1977; Hallett et al., 2021). Therefore, relational partners may be more likely to disengage over time as they are involved in multiple systems of medical, therapeutic, and educational care.

Some caregivers may see their role expand to that of a parent–therapist, delivering and evaluating specialized curricula or therapeutic activities. In contrast, others may become increasingly dependent on professionals or experts for children to achieve significant developmental milestones (Affleck et al., 1982; Bishop & Lord, 2023; Bronfenbrenner, 1975). Relational health may suffer as caregivers are at increased risk for parental over-involvement or under-involvement, burnout, and withdrawal. Further challenges may arise as opportunities for interactions that support the development of joint and independent emotional and behavioral regulation are limited while dyads focus on interventions treating developmental and/or medical symptoms.

Although it has not yet been researched or applied in these populations, the Strong Roots framework is also appropriate for care targeting relational health in populations with chronic conditions. The process of branching out, connecting with, and exploring broader systems (e.g., day care, school, extracurricular activities) with different caregivers and diverse relational partners (e.g., peers, teaches coaches, mentors) while maintaining roots in primary relationships may be comparatively more difficult and fraught with unexpected challenges for children with chronic conditions. Increased understanding, empathy, sensitivity, as well as larger toolkits and specific strategies, may be necessary to establish, foster, and sustain relational health with developmentally and medically impacted children and youth.

Independent of or in addition to treating the core symptoms of chronic conditions, a relationally focused provider will conceptualize relational health as a unique and specific target worthy of intentional assessment and intervention, which may also require ongoing monitoring or check-ins across developmental transition periods. Expanding on Winnicott's observation that there is no such thing as an infant, but that there is always an "infant and . . .," a relationally focused provider will formally assess and treat, as necessary, the relational components of the patient–caregiver system throughout childhood and adolescence. Despite the challenges inherent in managed care, relationally focused clinics or primary care offices function as a "holding environment" throughout childhood by investing in support structures that foster positive interactions with office staff and intentionally screen and/or promote relational health at each pediatric visit. In these environments, providers have time to intentionally check in on familial, peer, and community relationships; on parent–child perceptions of their experience of reciprocity in those relationships; and on what "on the ground" engagement looks like as children and youth branch out to broader relationships and communities. Understanding how children can engage in, access, and participate in broader relationships drives questions about more specific interventions for relational health.

Historically, relationally focused providers have valued mindfulness in themselves as they reflect on their own role in their relationship to patients with chronic conditions (Affleck et al., 1982). They practice and model reflective functioning and encourage that practice as part of their desire to support the emotional quality of their relationship with their patients and their patients' relationships with each other (Frosch et al., 2021). Given that reflective functioning has been identified as a potential mechanism for increasing sensitivity in social interactions, a relationally focused provider will hold in mind the potential thoughts, feelings, and intentions of the relational partners within a system. The provider becomes an informed and active member of the decision-making treatment team rather than a dispenser of advice that may or may not be followed. In doing so, the provider is conceptualizing the broader system of relational health (e.g., with co-parents, parenting partners, grandparents, therapists), exploring the types of interventions that may be accessible and feasible with the treatment team, and addressing relational health needs in addition to treatment needs associated with specific medical, neurodevelopmental, or behavioral phenotypes. Particular attention is paid to interactions that enhance safety, stability, and growth fostering interactions when the dyad is together by observing the form of interaction, by exploring unstated assumptions of either partner, by making the implicit explicit, and by querying opportunities for relational enhancement and joy beyond preset roles.

Within autism spectrum disorder, for example, a relationally focused provider may consider the child's challenging behavior (i.e., protesting, hitting, yelling) and the function of that behavior (e.g., preventing change; escaping social demands; accessing attention, tangible rewards, or sensory experiences) as well as the meaning of that behavior within the context of the relationships in which it is observed. A relationally focused provider will observe and ask both members of the relational dyad about the meaning of that behavior, thereby making the implicit explicit while targeting what is happening in real time between members of the dyad. Over time, the relational provider will reflect on strengths and challenges or opportunities for growth available within a relational dyad with the goal of promoting increased attunement, positivity, and engagement.

In addition to therapeutic interventions aimed at treating core symptoms of autism spectrum disorder, a relationally focused provider will assess, reflect on, and practice therapeutic activities that characterize growth-fostering relationships to improve quality of life. Providers will examine the developmental and relational histories of all parties, reflect on the meaning and understanding of each other's behaviors, and integrate those findings into therapeutic activities. They will strive to facilitate increases in mutuality, reciprocity, and contingent responsiveness among relational partners, beginning with where a given relationship and phenotypic presentation resides. In doing so, providers may offer concrete support and help with resource acquisition (i.e., access to a board-certified behavior analyst/therapist) while separately working with dyads to increase connection, safety, and feelings of security to promote relational health. For example, they may spend time intentionally helping caregivers distinguish perceptions and attributions about behaviors from phenotypic symptoms to help each party coregulate, deescalate, and engage in sustained interactions together (Frosch et al., 2021; Goldberg, 1977; Lieberman et al., 2005). The potential for RFI extends into middle childhood, adolescence, and young adulthood, offering significant promise for improving the daily quality of life in family systems impacted by chronic conditions.

CONCLUSION

Relational health is a key factor in well-being throughout the lifespan, and relationship-focused interventions have a distinguished foundation rooted in both developmental and clinical science. These interventions are efficacious in promoting relational quality and in reducing distress, including symptoms related to depression, suicidality, trauma, and emotional and behavioral problems. They are also associated with increased parent sensitivity, positive mood, reflective functioning, and attachment security. In altering relationships, relationship-focused interventions can create resilience that mitigates the impact of historical and current life stress while promoting a more positive self-sustaining developmental trajectory. The demonstrated efficacy of these interventions across a range of clinical populations, diagnostic groups, and relational branches suggests that they are a powerful if underutilized methodology. They are well-established, evidence-based approaches for use during the early childhood years; however, they may also be particularly useful in improving relational health, if not core symptoms, in older children and adolescents presenting with chronic and pervasive lifelong developmental disorders such as neurodevelopmental disorders, autism spectrum disorder, and chronic illness. These conditions, in conjunction with the developmental processes involved in branching out, maintaining connections, and finding security, cause intense, enduring, and novel distress in relational systems, which present shifting challenges and evolving targets for intervention (Hayes & Watson, 2013; Hollocks et al., 2021). Conceptualizing, measuring, and intervening in relational health across development are evolving foci, with numbers of facets that require both more intense and more extensive research. Chief among these is the development of reliable and valid measurement tools that can be used effectively in clinical environments and across different relational partners, clinical populations, and developmental periods. Further work specifying relational health as a unique assessment and intervention target across the lifespan is needed. Elements of relational health should be clearly defined for a given intervention, focusing on the development of growth-fostering relationships that are joyful, safe, mutually supportive, contingent, accessible, and reciprocal, with the potential for including diverse relational partners.

Developing new relationship-focused interventions to create or enhance sustained reciprocal, contingent, and growth-fostering relationships across development is a goal worthy of intervention efforts that extend well beyond the infant and preschool period. Further research is essential to probe and validate interventions with multiple populations and to identify the active components of efficacious interventions to extend the benefits of increasing relational health, for its own sake, and for its potential value for improving quality of life in a range of more pervasive and entrenched developmental difficulties.

RESOURCES

Early Relational Health

- Early Relational Health Screen

    https://www.allianceaimh.org/early-relational-health-screen

- Playlist of a series of conversations about early relational health by leaders in the field

    https://www.youtube.com/playlist?list=PL-oK-jkL0HeWl7PjNESa_QsSN7UdWJFci

- Short summaries and videos demonstrating early relational health principles in pediatric settings

    https://www.aap.org/en/patient-care/early-childhood/early-relational-health/

Relationally Focused Interventions

- Child Parent Psychotherapy

    https://childparentpsychotherapy.com/

- Infant Mental Health Home Visiting

    https://www.allianceaimh.org/infant-mental-health-home-visiting

- Strong Roots

    https://zerotothrive.org/strong-roots/

Practical Recommendations for Health Care Providers on Supporting Relational Health

- An initiative around promoting social-emotional development in pediatric settings

    https://cssp.org/our-work/project/pediatrics-supporting-parents/

- Frosch, C. A., Schoppe-Sullivan, S. J., & O'Banion, D. D. (2021). Parenting and child development: A relational health perspective. *American Journal of Lifestyle Medicine, 15*(1), 45–59. https://doi.org/10.1177/1559827619849028
- Garner, A., Yogman, M., & Committee on Psychosocial Aspects of Child and Family Health, Section on Developmental and Behavioral Pediatrics, Council on Early Childhood. (2021). Preventing childhood toxic stress: Partnering with families and communities to promote relational health. *Pediatrics, 148*(2), e2021052582. https://doi.org/10.1542/peds.2021-052582

References

Affleck, G., McGrade, B. J., McQueeney, M., & Allen, D. (1982). Promise of relationship-focused early intervention in developmental disabilities. *The Journal of Special Education, 16*(4), 413–430. https://doi.org/10.1177/002246698201600405

Aguilar, B., Sroufe, L. A., Egeland, B., & Carlson, E. (2000). Distinguishing the early-onset/persistent and adolescence-onset antisocial behavior types: From birth to 16 years. *Development and Psychopathology, 12*(2), 109–132. https://doi.org/10.1017/S0954579400002017

Ainsworth, M. D. S., Blehar, M. C., Waters, E., & Wall, S. (1978). *Patterns of attachment: A psychological study of the strange situation.* Erlbaum.

Albers, E. M., Riksen-Walraven, J. M., Sweep, F. C., & de Weerth, C. (2008). Maternal behavior predicts infant cortisol recovery from a mild everyday stressor. *Journal of Child Psychology and Psychiatry, 49*(1), 97–103. https://doi.org/10.1111/j.1469-7610.2007.01818.x

American Psychiatric Association. (2013). *Diagnostic and statistical manual of mental disorders* (5th ed.). https://doi.org/10.1176/appi.books.9780890425596

Bakermans-Kranenburg, M. J., & van IJzendoorn, M. H. (2006). Gene-environment interaction of the dopamine D4 receptor (DRD4) and observed maternal insensitivity predicting externalizing behavior in preschoolers. *Developmental Psychobiology, 48*(5), 406–409. https://doi.org/10.1002/dev.20152

Barron, C., Washington, B., Powell, S., Bell, S., & Stacks, A. M. (2020). A relationship-based approach to professional development in the early childhood education setting: The role of relationships in collaboration and implementation. *Zero to Three Journal, 41*(1), 5–11.

Bernard, K., Dozier, M., Bick, J., Lewis-Morrarty, E., Lindhiem, O., & Carlson, E. A. (2012). Enhancing attachment organization among maltreated children: Results of a randomized clinical trial. *Child Development, 83*(2), 623–636. https://doi.org/10.1111/j.1467-8624.2011.01712.x

Bethell, C., Jones, J., Gombojav, N., Linkenbach, J., & Sege, R. (2019). Positive childhood experiences and adult mental and relational health in a statewide sample: Associations across adverse childhood experiences levels. *JAMA Pediatrics, 173*(11), e193007. https://doi.org/10.1001/jamapediatrics.2019.3007

Bethell, C. D., Garner, A. S., Gombojav, N., Blackwell, C., Heller, L., & Mendelson, T. (2022). Social and relational health risks and common mental health problems among US children: The mitigating role of family resilience and connection to promote positive socioemotional and school-related outcomes. *Child and Adolescent Psychiatric Clinics of North America, 31*(1), 45–70. https://doi.org/10.1016/j.chc.2021.08.001

Bethell, C. D., Gombojav, N., & Whitaker, R. C. (2019). Family resilience and connection promote flourishing among US children, even amid adversity. *Health Affairs, 38*(5), 729–737. https://doi.org/10.1377/hlthaff.2018.05425

Bishop, S. L., & Lord, C. (2023). Commentary: Best practices and processes for assessment of autism spectrum disorder—The intended role of standardized diagnostic instruments. *Journal of Child Psychology and Psychiatry, 64*(5), 834–838.

Blair, C., Granger, D. A., Kivlighan, K. T., Mills-Koonce, R., Willoughby, M., Greenberg, M. T., Hibel, L. C., Fortunato, C. K., & the Family Life Project Investigators. (2008). Maternal and child contributions to cortisol response to emotional arousal in young children from low-income, rural communities. *Developmental Psychology, 44*(4), 1095–1109. https://doi.org/10.1037/0012-1649.44.4.1095

Bowlby, J. (1982). *Attachment and loss: Vol. 1. Attachment.* Basic Books. (Original work published 1969)

Bowlby, J. (1988). *A secure base.* Basic Books.

Bronfenbrenner, U. (1975). Is early intervention effective? In M. Guttentag & E. Streuning (Eds.), *Handbook of evaluation research* (Vol. 2, pp. 519–603). Sage.

Brumariu, L. E. (2015). Parent–child attachment and emotion regulation. *New Directions for Child and Adolescent Development, 2015*(148), 31–45. https://doi.org/10.1002/cad.20098

Calkins, S. D., Propper, C., & Mills-Koonce, W. R. (2013). A biopsychosocial perspective on parenting and developmental psychopathology. *Development and Psychopathology*, 25(4, Pt. 2), 1399–1414. https://doi.org/10.1017/S0954579413000680

Cassidy, J. (2016). The nature of the child's ties. In J. Cassidy & P. R. Shaver (Eds.), *Handbook of attachment: Theory, research, and clinical applications* (3rd ed., pp. 3–24). Guilford Press.

Charlot-Swilley, D., Condon, M.-C., & Rahman, T. (2022). At the feet of storytellers: Implications for practicing early relational health conversations. *Infant Mental Health Journal*, 43(3), 373–389. https://doi.org/10.1002/imhj.21981

Child and Adolescent Health Measurement Initiative (CAHMI). (2012). *National Survey of Children's Health*. https://childhealthdata.org/learn/NSCH

Cicchetti, D., & Gunnar, M. R. (2008). Integrating biological measures into the design and evaluation of preventive interventions. *Development and Psychopathology*, 20(3), 737–743. https://doi.org/10.1017/S0954579408000357

Cicchetti, D., Rogosch, F. A., & Toth, S. L. (2006). Fostering secure attachment in infants in maltreating families through preventive interventions. *Development and Psychopathology*, 18(3), 623–649.

Cicchetti, D., Toth, S. L., & Rogosch, F. A. (1999). The efficacy of toddler–parent psychotherapy to increase attachment security in offspring of depressed mothers. *Attachment & Human Development*, 1(1), 34–66. https://doi.org/10.1080/14616739900134021

Colonnesi, C., Draijer, E. M., Stams, G. J. J. M., Van der Bruggen, C. O., Bögels, S. M., & Noom, M. J. (2011). The relation between insecure attachment and child anxiety: A meta-analytic review. *Journal of Clinical Child and Adolescent Psychology*, 40(4), 630–645. https://doi.org/10.1080/15374416.2011.581623

Crooks, C. V., Exner-Cortens, D., Burm, S., Lapointe, A., & Chiodo, D. (2017). Two years of relationship-focused mentoring for First Nations, Métis, and Inuit adolescents: Promoting positive mental health. *The Journal of Primary Prevention*, 38(1–2), 87–104. https://doi.org/10.1007/s10935-016-0457-0

Diamond, G. M. (2014). Attachment-based family therapy interventions. *Psychotherapy*, 51(1), 15–19. https://doi.org/10.1037/a0032689

Diamond, G. S., Kobak, R. R., Krauthamer Ewing, E. S., Levy, S. A., Herres, J. L., Russon, J. M., & Gallop, R. J. (2019). A randomized controlled trial: Attachment-based family and nondirective supportive treatments for youth who are suicidal. *Journal of the American Academy of Child & Adolescent Psychiatry*, 58(7), 721–731. https://doi.org/10.1016/j.jaac.2018.10.006

Diamond, G. S., Reis, B. F., Diamond, G. M., Siqueland, L., & Isaacs, L. (2002). Attachment-based family therapy for depressed adolescents: A treatment development study. *Journal of the American Academy of Child & Adolescent Psychiatry*, 41(10), 1190–1196. https://doi.org/10.1097/00004583-200210000-00008

DiLalla, L. F., Elam, K. K., & Smolen, A. (2009). Genetic and gene-environment interaction effects on preschoolers' social behaviors. *Developmental Psychobiology*, 51(6), 451–464. https://doi.org/10.1002/dev.20384

Ensink, K., Bégin, M., Normandin, L., & Fonagy, P. (2017). Parental reflective functioning as a moderator of child internalizing difficulties in the context of child sexual abuse. *Psychiatry Research*, 257, 361–366. https://doi.org/10.1016/j.psychres.2017.07.051

Ewing, E. S. K., Levy, S., Scott, S. A., & Diamond, G. S. (2018). Attachment-based family therapy for adolescent depression and suicide risk. In H. Steele & M. Steele (Eds.), *Handbook of attachment-based interventions* (pp. 401–418). Guilford Press.

Eyberg, S., & Funderburk, B. W. (2011). *Parent–child interaction therapy*. PCIT International.

Fraiberg, S. (1971). Intervention in infancy: A program for blind infants. *Journal of the American Academy of Child Psychiatry*, 10(3), 381–405. https://doi.org/10.1016/S0002-7138(09)61746-5

FrameWorks Institute. (2020). *Building relationships: Framing early relational health*. Center for the Study of Social Policy. https://cssp.org/resource/building-relationships-framing-early-relational-health/

Frosch, C. A., Schoppe-Sullivan, S. J., & O'Banion, D. D. (2021). Parenting and child development: A relational health perspective. *American Journal of Lifestyle Medicine*, 15(1), 45–59. https://doi.org/10.1177/1559827619849028

Fearon, R. M. P., & Belsky, J. (2011). Infant–mother attachment and the growth of externalizing problems across the primary-school years. *Journal of Child Psychology and Psychiatry*, 52(7), 782–791. https://doi.org/10.1111/j.1469-7610.2010.02350.x

Gamarel, K. E., Garrett-Walker, J. J., Rivera, L., & Golub, S. A. (2014). Identity safety and relational health in youth spaces: A needs assessment with LGBTQ youth of color. *Journal of LGBT Youth*, 11(3), 289–315. https://doi.org/10.1080/19361653.2013.879464

Garner, A., Yogman, M., & Committee on Psychosocial Aspects of Child and Family Health, Section on Developmental and Behavioral Pediatrics,

Council on Early Childhood. (2021). Preventing childhood toxic stress: Partnering with families and communities to promote relational health. *Pediatrics, 148*(2), e2021052582. https://doi.org/10.1542/peds.2021-052582

George, C., & Solomon, J. (2008). The caregiving system: A behavioral systems approach to parenting. In J. Cassidy & P. R. Shaver (Eds.), *Handbook of attachment: Theory, research, and clinical applications* (2nd ed., 833–856). Guilford Press.

Ghosh Ippen, C., Harris, W. W., Van Horn, P., & Lieberman, A. F. (2011). Traumatic and stressful events in early childhood: Can treatment help those at highest risk? *Child Abuse and Neglect, 35*(7), 504–513. https://doi.org/10.1016/j.chiabu.2011.03.009

Goldberg, S. (1977). Social competence in infancy: A model of parent-infant interaction. *Merrill-Palmer Quarterly, 23*(3), 163–177.

Guild, D. J., Alto, M. E., Handley, E. D., Rogosch, F., Cicchetti, D., & Toth, S. L. (2021). Attachment and affect between mothers with depression and their children: Longitudinal outcomes of child parent psychotherapy. *Research on Child and Adolescent Psychopathology, 49*, 563–577.

Hallett, V., Mueller, J., Breese, L., Hollett, M., Beresford, B., Irvine, A., Pickles, A., Slonims, V., Scott, S., & Simonoff, E. (2021). Introducing 'Predictive Parenting': A feasibility study of a new group parenting intervention targeting emotional and behavioral difficulties in children with autism spectrum disorder. *Journal of Autism and Developmental Disorders, 51*, 323–333. https://doi.org/10.1007/s10803-020-04442-2

Haiyasoso, M., & Schuermann, H. (2018). Application of relational-cultural theory with adolescent sexual abuse survivors. *Journal of Child and Adolescent Counseling, 4*(2), 164–177. https://doi.org/10.1080/23727810.2017.1381933

Hayes, S. A., & Watson, S. L. (2013). The impact of parenting stress: A meta-analysis of studies comparing the experience of parenting stress in parents of children with and without autism spectrum disorder. *Journal of Autism and Developmental Disorders, 43*(3), 629–642. https://doi.org/10.1007/s10803-012-1604-y

Heron-Delaney, M., Kenardy, J. A., Brown, E. A., Jardine, C., Bogossian, F., Neuman, L., de Dassel, T., & Pritchard, M. (2016). Early maternal reflective functioning and infant emotional regulation in a preterm infant sample at 6 months corrected age. *Journal of Pediatric Psychology, 41*(8), 906–914. https://doi.org/10.1093/jpepsy/jsv169

Hollocks, M. J., Meiser-Stedman, R., Kent, R., Lukito, S., Briskman, J., Stringer, D., Lord, C., Pickles, A., Baird, G., Charman, T., & Simonoff, E. (2021). The association of adverse life events and parental mental health with emotional and behavioral outcomes in young adults with autism spectrum disorder. *Autism Research, 14*(8), 1724–1735. https://doi.org/10.1002/aur.2548

Hughes, C., Aldercotte, A., & Foley, S. (2017). Maternal mind-mindedness provides a buffer for pre-adolescents at risk for disruptive behavior. *Journal of Abnormal Child Psychology, 45*(2), 225–235. https://doi.org/10.1007/s10802-016-0165-5

Huber, A., McMahon, C. A., & Sweller, N. (2015). Efficacy of the 20-week Circle of Security intervention: Changes in caregiver reflective functioning, representations, and child attachment in an Australian clinical sample. *Infant Mental Health Journal, 36*(6), 556–574. https://doi.org/10.1002/imhj.21540

Julian, M. M., Muzik, M., Kees, M., Valenstein, M., Dexter, C., & Rosenblum, K. L. (2018). Intervention effects on reflectivity explain change in positive parenting in military families with young children. *Journal of Family Psychology, 32*(6), 804–815. https://doi.org/10.1037/fam0000431

Julian, M. M., Muzik, M., Kees, M., Valenstein, M., & Rosenblum, K. L. (2018). Strong Military Families intervention enhances parenting reflectivity and representations in families with young children. *Infant Mental Health Journal, 39*(1), 106–118. https://doi.org/10.1002/imhj.21690

Keller, T. E., Spieker, S. J., & Gilchrist, L. (2005). Patterns of risk and trajectories of preschool problem behaviors: A person-oriented analysis of attachment in context. *Development and Psychopathology, 17*(2), 349–384. https://doi.org/10.1017/S0954579405050170

Kochanska, G., Philibert, R. A., & Barry, R. A. (2009). Interplay of genes and early mother–child relationship in the development of self-regulation from toddler to preschool age. *Journal of Child Psychology and Psychiatry, 50*(11), 1331–1338. https://doi.org/10.1111/j.1469-7610.2008.02050.x

Lawler, J. M., Rosenblum, K. L., Muzik, M., Ludtke, M., Weatherston, D. J., & Tableman, B. (2017). A collaborative process for evaluating infant mental health home visiting in Michigan. *Psychiatric Services, 68*(6), 535–538. https://doi.org/10.1176/appi.ps.201700047

Lenz, A. S., Speciale, M., & Aguilar, J. V. (2012). Relational-cultural therapy intervention with incarcerated adolescents: A single-case effectiveness design. *Counseling Outcome Research and Evaluation, 3*(1), 17–29. https://doi.org/10.1177/2150137811435233

Liang, B., Lund, T. J., Mousseau, A. M. D., & Spencer, R. (2016). The mediating role of engagement in mentoring relationships and self-esteem among affluent adolescent girls. *Psychology in the Schools*, *53*(8), 848–860. https://doi.org/10.1002/pits.21949

Liang, B., Tracy, A., Taylor, C. A., Williams, L. M., Jordan, J. V., & Miller, J. B. (2002). The Relational Health Indices: A study of women's relationships. *Psychology of Women Quarterly*, *26*(1), 25–35. https://doi.org/10.1111/1471-6402.00040

Liang, B., Tracy, A. J., Kenny, M. E., Brogan, D., & Gatha, R. (2010). The Relational Health Indices for Youth: An examination of reliability and validity aspects. *Measurement and Evaluation in Counseling & Development*, *42*(4), 255–274. https://doi.org/10.1177/0748175609354596

Liang, B., & West, J. (2011). Relational health, alexithymia, and psychological distress in college women: Testing a mediator model. *American Journal of Orthopsychiatry*, *81*(2), 246–254. https://doi.org/10.1111/j.1939-0025.2011.01093.x

Liang, B., White, A., Mousseau, A. M. D., Hasse, A., Knight, L., Berado, D., & Lund, T. J. (2017). The four P's of purpose among college bound students: People, propensity, passion, prosocial benefits. *The Journal of Positive Psychology*, *12*(3), 281–294. https://doi.org/10.1080/17439760.2016.1225118

Lieberman, A. F., Ghosh Ippen, C., & Van Horn, P. (2015). *Don't hit my mommy! A manual for child-parent psychotherapy with young children exposed to violence and other trauma*. Zero to Three.

Lieberman, A. F., & Van Horn, P. (2004). *Don't hit my mommy: A manual for child parent psychotherapy with young witnesses of family violence*. Zero to Three.

Lieberman, A. F., & Van Horn, P. (2008). *Psychotherapy with infants and young children: Repairing the effects of stress and trauma on early attachment*. Guilford Press.

Lieberman, A. F., Van Horn, P., & Ippen, C. G. (2005). Toward evidence-based treatment: Child-parent psychotherapy with preschoolers exposed to marital violence. *Journal of the American Academy of Child & Adolescent Psychiatry*, *44*(12), 1241–1248. https://doi.org/10.1097/01.chi.0000181047.59702.58

Lieberman, A. F., Weston, D. R., & Pawl, J. H. (1991). Preventive intervention and outcome with anxiously attached dyads. *Child Development*, *62*(1), 199. https://doi.org/10.2307/1130715

Lowell, D. I., Carter, A. S., Godoy, L., Paulicin, B., & Briggs-Gowan, M. J. (2011). A randomized controlled trial of Child FIRST: A comprehensive home-based intervention translating research into early childhood practice. *Child Development*, *82*(1), 193–208. https://doi.org/10.1111/j.1467-8624.2010.01550.x

Lund, T. J., Chan, P., & Liang, B. (2014). Depression and relational health in Asian American and European American college women. *Psychology in the Schools*, *51*(5), 493–505. https://doi.org/10.1002/pits.21758

Lyons-Ruth, K., Easterbrooks, M. A., & Cibelli, C. D. (1997). Infant attachment strategies, infant mental lag, and maternal depressive symptoms: Predictors of internalizing and externalizing problems at age 7. *Developmental Psychology*, *33*(4), 681–692. https://doi.org/10.1037/0012-1649.33.4.681

Main, M., & Solomon, J. (1990). Procedures for identifying infants as disorganized/disoriented during the Ainsworth Strange Situation. In M. T. Greenberg, D. Cicchetti, & E. M. Cummings (Eds.), *Attachment in the preschool years* (pp. 121–160). University of Chicago Press.

Masten, A. S., & Cicchetti, D. (2010). Developmental cascades. *Development and Psychopathology*, *22*(3), 491–495. https://doi.org/10.1017/S0954579410000222

Masten, A. S., & Cicchetti, D. (2012). Risk and resilience in development and psychopathology: The legacy of Norman Garmezy. *Development and Psychopathology*, *24*(2), 333–334. https://doi.org/10.1017/S0954579412000016

Meins, E., Centifanti, L. C. M., Fernyhough, C., & Fishburn, S. (2013). Maternal mind-mindedness and children's behavioral difficulties: Mitigating the impact of low socioeconomic status. *Journal of Abnormal Child Psychology*, *41*(4), 543–553. https://doi.org/10.1007/s10802-012-9699-3

Mills-Koonce, W. R., Garrett-Peters, P., Barnett, M., Granger, D. A., Blair, C., Cox, M. J., & the Family Life Project Key Investigators. (2011). Father contributions to cortisol responses in infancy and toddlerhood. *Developmental Psychology*, *47*(2), 388–395. https://doi.org/10.1037/a0021066

Möller, C., Odersjö, C., Pilesjö, F., Terpening, K., Österberg, M., & Holmqvist, R. (2017). Reflective functioning, limit setting, and emotional availability in mother–child dyads. *Parenting: Science and Practice*, *17*(4), 225–241. https://doi.org/10.1080/15295192.2017.1369311

Munson, M. R., & McMillen, J. C. (2009). Natural mentoring and psychosocial outcomes among older youth transitioning from foster care. *Children and Youth Services Review*, *31*(1), 104–111. https://doi.org/10.1016/j.childyouth.2008.06.003

Muzik, M., Rosenblum, K. L., Alfafara, E. A., Schuster, M. M., Miller, N. M., Waddell, R. M., & Kohler, E. S. (2015). Mom Power: Preliminary outcomes of a group intervention to improve mental health and parenting among high-risk mothers. *Archives of Women's Mental Health*, *18*(3), 507–521. https://doi.org/10.1007/s00737-014-0490-z

Muzik, M., Rosenblum, K. L., Schuster, M. M., Kohler, E. S., Alfafara, E. A., & Miller, N. M. (2016). A mental health and parenting intervention for adolescent and young adult mothers and their infants. *Journal of Depression and Anxiety*, *5*(3), 233. https://web.archive.org/web/20190225150052id_/

Nazzari, S., Fearon, P., Rice, F., Molteni, M., & Frigerio, A. (2022). Maternal caregiving moderates the impact of antenatal maternal cortisol on infant stress regulation. *Journal of Child Psychology and Psychiatry*, *63*(8), 871–880. https://doi.org/10.1111/jcpp.13532

Niec, L. N. (Ed.). (2018). *Handbook of parent–child interaction therapy: Innovations and applications for research and practice*. Springer. https://doi.org/10.1007/978-3-319-97698-3

Propper, C., Moore, G. A., Mills-Koonce, W. R., Halpern, C. T., Hill-Soderlund, A. L., Calkins, S. D., Carbone, M. A., & Cox, M. (2008). Gene-environment contributions to the development of infant vagal reactivity: The interaction of dopamine and maternal sensitivity. *Child Development*, *79*(5), 1377–1394. https://doi.org/10.1111/j.1467-8624.2008.01194.x

Propper, C., Willoughby, M., Halpern, C. T., Carbone, M. A., & Cox, M. (2007). Parenting quality, DRD4, and the prediction of externalizing and internalizing behaviors in early childhood. *Developmental Psychobiology*, *49*(6), 619–632. https://doi.org/10.1002/dev.20249

Ribaudo, J., Lawler, J. M., Jester, J. M., Riggs, J., Erickson, N. L., Stacks, A. M., Brophy-Herb, H., Muzik, M., & Rosenblum, K. L. (2022). Maternal history of adverse experiences and posttraumatic stress disorder symptoms impact toddlers' early socioemotional wellbeing: The benefits of Infant Mental Health-Home Visiting. *Frontiers in Psychology*, *12*, 792989. https://doi.org/10.3389/fpsyg.2021.792989

Riggs, J. L., Rosenblum, K. L., Muzik, M., Jester, J., Freeman, S., Huth-Bocks, A., Waddell, R., Alfafara, E., Miller, A., Lawler, J., Erickson, N., Weatherston, D., Shah, P., Brophy-Herb, H., & Michigan Collaborative for Infant Mental Health Research. (2022). Infant mental health home visiting mitigates impact of maternal adverse childhood experiences on toddler language competence: A randomized controlled trial. *Journal of Developmental & Behavioral Pediatrics*, *43*(4), e227–e236. https://doi.org/10.1097/dbp.0000000000001020

Rosenblum, K. L., Lawler, J. M., Alfafara, E., Miller, N., Schuster, M., & Muzik, M. (2017). Improving maternal representations in high-risk mothers: A randomized, controlled trial of the Mom Power parenting intervention. *Child Psychiatry & Human Development*. https://doi.org/10.1007/s10578-017-0757-5

Rosenblum, K. L., McDonough, S. C., Sameroff, A. J., & Muzik, M. (2008). Reflection in thought and action: Maternal parenting reflectivity predicts mind-minded comments and interactive behavior. *Infant Mental Health Journal*, *29*(4), 362–376. https://doi.org/10.1002/imhj.20184

Rosenblum, K. L., Muzik, M., Jester, J. M., Huth-Bocks, A., Erickson, N., Ludtke, M., Weatherston, D., Brophy-Herb, H., Tableman, B., Alfafara, E., & Waddell, R. (2020). Community-delivered infant–parent psychotherapy improves maternal sensitive caregiving: Evaluation of the Michigan model of infant mental health home visiting. *Infant Mental Health Journal*, *41*(2), 178–190. https://doi.org/10.1002/imhj.21840

Rosenblum, K. L., Muzik, M., Morelen, D. M., Alfafara, E. A., Miller, N. M., Waddell, R. M., Schuster, M. M., & Ribaudo, J. (2017). A community-based randomized controlled trial of Mom Power parenting intervention for mothers with interpersonal trauma histories and their young children. *Archives of Women's Mental Health*, *20*(5), 673–686. https://doi.org/10.1007/s00737-017-0734-9

Rosenblum, K. L., Muzik, M., Waddell, R. M., Thompson, S., Rosenberg, L., Masini, G., & Smith, K. (2015). Strong Military Families: A multifamily group approach to strengthening family resilience. *Zero to Three*, (November), 8–14. https://zerotothrive.org/wp-content/uploads/2020/02/Strong-Military-Families_A-Multifamily-Group-Approach-to-Strengthening-Family-Resilience_Rosenblum-et-al_2015.pdf

Rosenblum, K. L., Riggs, J., Freeman, S., Shah, P. E., Muzik, M., & Michigan Collaborative for Infant Mental Health Research. (2022). In-the-moment ratings on the Early Relational Health Screen: A pilot study of application in home visiting and primary care. *Infant Mental Health Journal*, *43*(3), 410–423. https://doi.org/10.1002/imhj.21978

Sameroff, A. (2009). The transactional model. In A. Sameroff (Ed.), *The transactional model of development: How children and contexts shape each other* (pp. 3–21). American Psychological Association. https://doi.org/10.1037/11877-001

Senehi, N., Brophy-Herb, H. E., & Vallotton, C. D. (2018). Effects of maternal mentalization-related parenting on toddlers' self-regulation. *Early Childhood Research Quarterly*, *44*, 1–14. https://doi.org/10.1016/j.ecresq.2018.02.001

Shai, D., & Meins, E. (2018). Parental embodied mentalizing and its relation to mind-mindedness, sensitivity, and attachment security. *Infancy, 23*(6), 857–872. https://doi.org/10.1111/infa.12244

Sharp, C., & Fonagy, P. (2008). The parent's capacity to treat the child as a psychological agent: Constructs, measures and implications for developmental psychopathology. *Social Development, 17*(3), 737–754. https://doi.org/10.1111/j.1467-9507.2007.00457.x

Slade, A. (2005). Parental reflective functioning: An introduction. *Attachment & Human Development, 7*(3), 269–281. https://doi.org/10.1080/14616730500245906

Slopen, N., McLaughlin, K. A., & Shonkoff, J. P. (2014). Interventions to improve cortisol regulation in children: A systematic review. *Pediatrics, 133*(2), 312–326. https://doi.org/10.1542/peds.2013-1632

Smaling, H. J. A., Huijbregts, S. C. J., Suurland, J., van der Heijden, K. B., Mesman, J., van Goozen, S. H. M., & Swaab, H. (2016). Prenatal reflective functioning and accumulated risk as predictors of maternal interactive behavior during free play, the still-face paradigm, and two teaching tasks. *Infancy, 21*(6), 766–784. https://doi.org/10.1111/infa.12137

Smaling, H. J. A., Huijbregts, S. C. J., van der Heijden, K. B., Hay, D. F., van Goozen, S. H. M., & Swaab, H. (2017). Prenatal reflective functioning and development of aggression in infancy: The roles of maternal intrusiveness and sensitivity. *Journal of Abnormal Child Psychology, 45*(2), 237–248. https://doi.org/10.1007/s10802-016-0177-1

Solomon, J., & George, C. (2016). The measurement of attachment security and related constructs in infancy and early childhood. In J. Cassidy & P. R. Shaver (Eds.), *Handbook of attachment: Theory, research, and clinical applications* (3rd ed., pp. 366–396). Guilford Press.

Sroufe, L. A. (1990). Considering normal and abnormal together: The essence of developmental psychopathology. *Development and Psychopathology, 2*(4), 335–347. https://doi.org/10.1017/S0954579400005769

Sroufe, L. A., Carlson, E. A., Levy, A. K., & Egeland, B. (1999). Implications of attachment theory for developmental psychopathology. *Development and Psychopathology, 11*(1), 1–13. https://doi.org/10.1017/S0954579499001923

Stacks, A. M., Barron, C. C., & Wong, K. (2019). Infant mental health home visiting in the context of an infant–toddler court team: Changes in parental responsiveness and reflective functioning. *Infant Mental Health Journal, 40*(4), 523–540. https://doi.org/10.1002/imhj.21785

Stacks, A. M., Muzik, M., Wong, K., Beeghly, M., Huth-Bocks, A., Irwin, J. L., & Rosenblum, K. L. (2014). Maternal reflective functioning among mothers with childhood maltreatment histories: Links to sensitive parenting and infant attachment security. *Attachment & Human Development, 16*(5), 515–533. https://doi.org/10.1080/14616734.2014.935452

Stacks, A. M., Wong, K., Barron, C., & Ryznar, T. (2020). Permanency and well-being outcomes for maltreated infants: Pilot results from an infant-toddler court team. *Child Abuse and Neglect, 101*(January), 104332. https://doi.org/10.1016/j.chiabu.2019.104332

Sulik, M. J., Eisenberg, N., Lemery-Chalfant, K., Spinrad, T. L., Silva, K. M., Eggum, N. D., Betkowski, J. A., Kupfer, A., Smith, C. L., Gaertner, B., Stover, D. A., & Verrelli, B. C. (2012). Interactions between serotonin transporter gene haplotypes and quality of mothers' parenting predict the development of children's noncompliance. *Developmental Psychology, 48*(3), 740–754. https://doi.org/10.1037/a0025938

Swain, J. E., Ho, S. S., Rosenblum, K. L., Morelen, D., Dayton, C. J., & Muzik, M. (2017). Parent–child intervention decreases stress and increases maternal brain activity and connectivity during own baby-cry: An exploratory study. *Development and Psychopathology, 29*(02), 535–553. https://doi.org/10.1017/S0954579417000165

Swain, J. E., Ho, S. S., Rosenblum, K. L., Morelen, D. M., & Muzik, M. (2016). Emotion processing and psychopathological risk in the parental brain: Psychosocial intervention increases activity and decreases stress. *Journal of the American Academy of Child & Adolescent Psychiatry, 55*(10), S320–S321. https://doi.org/10.1016/j.jaac.2016.07.350

Toth, S. L., Maughan, A., Manly, J. T., Spagnola, M., & Cicchetti, D. (2002). The relative efficacy of two interventions in altering maltreated preschool children's representational models: Implications for attachment theory. *Development and Psychopathology, 14*(04), 877–908. https://doi.org/10.1017/S095457940200411X

Tsvieli, N., Lifshitz, C., & Diamond, G. M. (2021). Corrective attachment episodes in attachment-based family therapy: The power of enactment. *Psychotherapy Research, 32*(2), 209–222. https://doi.org/10.1080/10503307.2021.1913295

Vandermause, R., Fougere, M., Liu, Y. H., & Odom-Maryon, T. (2018). Relational health and recovery: Adolescent girls in chemical dependency treatment. *Journal of Addictions Nursing, 29*(1), 4–12. https://doi.org/10.1097/JAN.0000000000000207

Vandermause, R., Roberts, M., & Odom-Maryon, T. (2018). Relational health in transitions: Female adolescents in chemical dependency treatment. *Substance Use & Misuse, 53*(8), 1353–1360. https://doi.org/10.1080/10826084.2017.1408655

Vanyukov, M. M., Maher, B. S., Devlin, B., Kirillova, G. P., Kirisci, L., Yu, L. M., & Ferrell, R. E. (2007). The MAOA promoter polymorphism, disruptive behavior disorders, and early onset substance use disorder: Gene-environment interaction. *Psychiatric Genetics, 17*(6), 323–332. https://doi.org/10.1097/YPG.0b013e32811f6691

Weatherston, D. J., Ribaudo, J., & the Michigan Collaborative for Infant Mental Health Research. (2020). The Michigan infant mental health home visiting model. *Infant Mental Health Journal, 41*(2), 166–177. https://doi.org/10.1002/imhj.21838

Webster-Stratton, C. (2000). *The Incredible Years training series*. U.S. Department of Justice.

Webster-Stratton, C., & Bywater, T. (2019). The Incredible Years® series: An internationally evidenced multimodal approach to enhancing child outcomes. In B. H. Fiese, M. Celano, K. Deater-Deckard, E. N. Jouriles, & M. A. Whisman (Eds.), *APA handbook of contemporary family psychology: Family therapy and training* (pp. 343–359). American Psychological Association. https://doi.org/10.1037/0000101-021

Weiner, D. A., Schneider, A., & Lyons, J. S. (2009). Evidence-based treatments for trauma among culturally diverse foster care youth: Treatment retention and outcomes. *Children and Youth Services Review, 31*(11), 1199–1205. https://doi.org/10.1016/j.childyouth.2009.08.013

Willis, D. W., Condon, M. C., Moe, V., Munson, L., Smith, L., & Eddy, J. M. (2022). The context and development of the early relational health screen. *Infant Mental Health Journal, 43*(3), 493–506. https://doi.org/10.1002/imhj.21986

Willis, D. W., & Eddy, J. M. (2022). Early relational health: Innovations in child health for promotion, screening, and research. *Infant Mental Health Journal, 43*(3), 361–372. https://doi.org/10.1002/imhj.21980

Winnicott, D. W. (1960). The theory of the parent-infant relationship. *International Journal of Psychoanalysis, 41*(6), 585–595.

Index

A page number in italics in the index refers to an entry that appears in a table, figure, or exhibit. Items in italics indicate the name of a publication or website. Individuals referred to or discussed in the text are also included in the index.

ABA. *See* Applied behavior analysis–based interventions
ABA therapy, 152
ABFT. *See* Attachment Based Family Therapy
Abusive head trauma, 197
Academic achievement
    assessment of, 624–627
    cancer impact on, 240–241
    epilepsy and, 195
    obesity and, 349
    pulmonary disorders and, 268
    SB and, 189–190
    SCD and, 219–220
    sleep and, 452–453
    TBI and, 199
Academic/school functioning, PMTS impacts on, 81
Acceptance, of chronic health condition diagnosis, 7–8
Acceptance and commitment therapy (ACT), 86
    consultation process and, 644
Accidents, PMTS and, 78
Acculturation, 87
ACEs. *See* Adverse childhood experiences
Achenbach System of Empirically Based Assessment (ASEBA), 220
Acquired capability, 576
Acrocyanosis, 559
ACT. *See* Acceptance and commitment therapy
Actigraphy, 454–455
Active coping attempts, 223
Activity processes, 498

Acute lymphoblastic leukemia, 241
Acute medical care phase, 76
Acute myeloid leukemia (AML), 247
Acute pain, 49–50
    SCD and, 217–218
Acute stress disorder, 72, 80
    pain and, 74
    peritraumatic dissociation and, 74
ADA. *See* Americans with Disabilities Act
Adaptation
    congenital medical conditions and, 176–177
    to diabetes, 307
    family processes associated with, 7–14
    pediatric psychology consultation-liaison and common concerns of, 647–651
    T1D and, 312
Adaptive functioning, 617
    assessment of, 627
Adenotonsillectomy, 460–461
ADHD. *See* Attention-deficit/hyperactivity disorder
ADHD Rating Scale-5, 502
ADHD Rating Scale-IV Preschool Version, 503
Adherence, 27
    assessment of, 33–36
    asthma and, 265–266
    cancer care and, 239–240
    CF and, 266
    community-level factors, 33
    defining, 28–29
    epilepsy and, 196

    family-level factors, 32–33
    future research directions, 39
    implications for pediatrics and developmental science, 38–39
    individual and public health outcomes and, 29–30
    interventions, 36–38, 266–267
    passive adherence coping, 223
    pediatric psychology consultation-liaison and, 649, *650*
    prevalence and clinical cut points, 29
    SB and, 191
    SCD and, 223–224
    self-management and, 28, 30–33
    socioecological determinants of, 31–33
    T1D and, 308–309
    T2D and, 321
    taxonomy of, 28
    theory and contextual determinants of, 30–33
ADI-R. *See* Autism Diagnostic Interview-Revised
Adjunctive pharmacologic therapy, 60
Adolescence
    ADHD evaluation in, 504
    ADHD outcomes in, 501
    ASD development and, 370, 371
    CHD and parent and family functioning during, 291
    CHD and psychosocial concerns in, 288–289
    developmental stage of, 131
    RFIs in, 695–696

Adolescence *(continued)*
  SI and SA in, 577
  sleep–wake patterns in, 448
  suicide prevention strategies, 585
  T2D management in, 321
  VI in, 432
Adolescent Sleep Wake Scale, 57, 454
ADOS-2. *See* Autism Diagnostic Interview-Revised
Adult health care
  epilepsy and transition to, 196
  SB and transition to, 191
  SCD and transition to, 226–227
  TBI and transition to, 200–201
Advance care planning, 106
Adverse childhood experiences (ACEs), 346
  internalizing and externalizing problems and, 531
  maternal, 694
  suicide risk factors, 578–579
Affective disorders, chronic pain and, 52
Affordable Care Act (2010), 100
Age equivalents, 605–606
Agency for Healthcare Research and Quality (AHRQ), 295
Agender, 129
Ages and Stages Questionnaire, 629
AHA. *See* American Heart Association
AHI. *See* Apnea-hypopnea index
AHRQ. *See* Agency for Healthcare Research and Quality
Airway obstruction, 458
Alagille syndrome, 285
Alcohol, suicide risk factors and, 578
Allergies, structural racism and, 261
Allostatic load, 320
Allow natural death orders (AND orders), 99
Alpha 2 adrenergic receptor agonists, 60, 86
Alpha agonists, 510, 540
Amenorrhea, 559
American Academy of Pediatrics, 283–284, 287, 295, 660
  ASD screening recommendations, 377
  Down syndrome screening guidelines, 147
  neonatal follow-up guidelines from, 407
  obesity screening guidelines, 350
  OSA guidelines, 460
  palliative care guidelines, 100

  on screening for internalizing and externalizing problems, 534
  suicide risk screening recommendation, 581
American Academy of Sleep Medicine, 454
American Heart Association (AHA), 283, 287
American Psychiatric Association, screening tools, 534
American Society of Hematology (ASH), 224
Americans With Disabilities Act (ADA), 435
AML. *See* Acute myeloid leukemia
Amphetamine, 509, 511
AN. *See* Anorexia nervosa
Analgesia, racial disparities in use of, 53
AND orders. *See* Allow natural death orders
Anemia. *See also* Sickle cell anemia
  hemolytic, 214
Anorexia nervosa (AN), 551, 555, 558
  categories of, 552–553
  CBT-ED for, 562–563
  diagnostic components, 552
  epidemiology of, 554
  FBT for, 561–562
  medical complications of, 559
  medication management of, 563
  neurobiology of, 557
  psychiatric complications of, 560
ANSD. *See* Auditory neuropathy spectrum disorder
Antihistamines, 468
Antipsychotics, 372
Anxiety, 523
  ADHD and, 506–507
  cancer and, 242
  CBT for, 539
  chronic pain and, 52
  continuity in, 526
  costs of, 527
  disorders of, 532–533
  insomnia and, 457
  obesity and, 349
  pediatric psychology consultation-liaison and, 650
  preterm birth and caregiver symptoms of, 400
  PTMS and, 81
  PTSS and, 73
  social support and, 400
  22q and, 146

Apnea-hypopnea index (AHI), 460
Appearance concerns, 170–171
Applied behavior analysis– (ABA-) based interventions, 379–380, 628
Aptitude achievement discrepancy model, 619
ARFID. *See* Avoidant/restrictive food intake disorder
Aripiprazole, 152, 383
Armodafinil, 466
ASD. *See* Autism spectrum disorder
ASEBA. *See* Achenbach System of Empirically Based Assessment
ASH. *See* American Society of Hematology
Ask Suicide Screening Questions (ASQ), 581
Assessment. *See also* Developmental assessment
  of adaptive functioning, 627
  CHD and, 294–295
  of chronic pain, 56–58
  congenital medical conditions and, 176
  of DHH children, 427
  gender-affirmative, 128
  IBH and, 664–667
  of ID, 624–627
  of incontinence disorders, 486–487, 487
  of intellect and academic attainment, 624–627
  of internalizing and externalizing disorders, 534–536, 535
  of multisensory impairment, 434–435
  obesity and, 349–350
  of pain interference, 57–58
  for PMTS, 80
  relationally oriented, 687–689, 688
  SB, 192
  serial, 598–599
  T1D and, 314–315
  T2D and, 321–322
  of treatment adherence, 33–36
  for VI, 433–434
Assistive devices, for hearing impairment, 429
Asthma, 8, 12, 27, 87, 255
  academic and social functioning impacts, 268
  adherence and, 265–266
  background and significance for, 256

708

clinical guidelines and standards of care, 262–263
coping and, 269–271
ecological contexts and outcomes from, 265
ecological factors, 258–259
emotional well-being and, 267
mental health and, 260, 267
pathophysiology of, 258
PMTS and, 77
prevalence and public health impacts, 256
social determinants of health and health equity and, 260, 262
social support and, 267, 271
socioeconomic risk factors and, 259
symptom management, 263
Atomoxetine, 383, 509–510, 539
At-risk dyads, interventions for, 692–693
Attachment
caregivers and, 684
preterm birth and, 401–402
Attachment and BioBehavioral Catch-up, 693
Attachment Based Family Therapy (ABFT), 696
Attachment theory, 684
Attention-deficit/hyperactivity disorder (ADHD)
ASD and, 370, 382
cancer care and, 246
CHD and, 298
comorbidities of, 505–507
defining, 498
developmental science foundations for care for, 497–498
diagnosis of, 502–507
domain-specific presentations in, 498
Down syndrome and, 148
dual pathway model of, 498–499
eating disorders and, 561
epidemiology and risk factors, 500–501
externalizing problems and, 533–534
FXS and, 151–152, 155
gender and, 526
ID and, 624
incontinence disorders and, 483
interventions for, 507–511
natural history of, 501
outcomes, 501
physical examination and observation elements, 504–505
preschool and, 503

preterm birth and, 397
prognostic factors for, 501–502
SCD and, 225
SLDs and, 623
sleep and, 453
sleep disorders and, 466–467
sociodemographic considerations in diagnosis, 505
T1D and, 312
treatment adherence and, 27, 32, 33
treatment of, 507–513
22q and, 146
Attention problems, preterm birth and, 397
Attention processes, 497–498
Attention regulation, 508
Attributions, identifying internalizing and externalizing problems and, 527–528
Audiology, 428–429
Audiometry, 425
Auditory brainstem implantation, 429
Auditory evoked potentials, 425
Auditory neuropathy spectrum disorder (ANSD), 422, 423
Autism Diagnostic Interview-Revised (ADI-R), 377, 379
Autism Diagnostic Observation Schedule, Second Edition (ADOS-2), 377, 379
Autism Speaks, 376
Autism spectrum disorder (ASD), 143, 365, 637
ADHD and, 506
behavioral interventions in, 379–381
CAM and, 382
cancer care and, 246
caregiver well-being and, 375–376
cultural considerations and health equity and, 376
developmental emergence of, 369–370
developmental trajectories, 372
diagnostic evaluation, 377, 379
Down syndrome and, 148
economic considerations, 376
EF and, 373
epidemiology, 370–371
etiology and neurobiology of, 370–371
family systems approach, 375–376
FXS and, 150–151, 154
gender diversity and, 370
guardianship in, 375
heterogeneity in, 367
incontinence disorders and, 483

internalizing and externalizing problems and, 530
medications in, 382, 383–384
outcomes, 371–375
peer relationships and bullying and, 372–373
personal agency and self-determination and, 373–374
postsecondary education and vocational outcomes, 374–375
preschool and development of, 369–370
preterm birth and, 396–397
psychoeducation and, 382, 385
residential and adult day programs, 375
RFI and, 698
screening and diagnosis of, 376–379, 378
services through IDEA, 381
signs and symptoms of, 367–370
sleep disorders and, 467
social cognition and, 367
social skills interventions, 381–382
transition services and services cliff, 374
treatments and interventions, 379–385
22q and, 146
VI and, 432
Autonomy, development of, 5
Autopsy, 106
Avoidant coping, 312
Avoidant/restrictive food intake disorder (ARFID), 553, 555, 557, 562–563, 645, *645*

Bariatric surgery, 323
BASC. *See* Behavioral Assessment System for Children
BASC-3. *See* Behavior Assessment System for Children, Third Edition
Bath Adolescent Pain Questionnaire, 57
BCVA. *See* Best-corrected visual acuity
BEARS sleep screening tool, 453, *454*
Beck Depression Inventory, 57
BED. *See* Binge eating disorder
Bedtime fading, 457
Bedwetting, 480, 489
Behavioral Assessment System for Children (BASC), 534
Behavioral classroom management, 508
Behavioral comorbidities
OSA and, 459–460
screening for, 57
22q and, 146

Behavioral functioning
  ADHD outcomes and, 501
  hearing impairment and, 427–428
  VI and, 434
Behavioral health. *See also* Integrated behavioral health
  benefits of integrating into primary care, 663–664
  health disparities, 664
  integrating into pediatric primary care, 660–662
Behavioral insomnia of childhood, 455–457
Behavioral interventions
  in ASD, 379–381
  hearing impairment and, 429
Behavioral screening
  for incontinence disorders, 486–487
  T1D and, 314–315
Behavioral sleep disorders, 455–458
Behavior Assessment System for Children, Third Edition (BASC-3), 220, 503
Benzodiazepines, 539
Bereavement care, 97
  communication and, 105–106
  goal-directed partnerships and, 105–106
  supporting families in, 103–106
Berlin, Rudolf, 617
Best-corrected visual acuity (BCVA), 430
Bifidobacteria, 345
Billing codes, for chronic pain, 50
Binet, Alfred, 615
Binet-Simon Scale, 616
Binge eating disorder (BED), 553–555, 557, 559, 560, 562–564
Bioassays, 34
Bioecological systems theory (BST), 639–640
Biofeedback, 489
  EEG, 509
Biomarkers, ASD and, 371
Biometric data, 36
Biopsychosocial development, contexts shaping, 6–7
Biopsychosocial models
  asthma and, 262
  of chronic pain, 55–56
  of continence development, 477
  of incontinence, 482
  obesity and, 344
Birth defects, 163
Blindness, 430

Blueprint to Prevent Youth Suicide, 581
BMI. *See* Body mass index
Body dysphoria, 129–130, 136
Body image
  CL/P and, 170–171
  DSD and, 174
  gender dysphoria and, 174
Body mass index (BMI), 342, 343, 348, 350
  CF and, 259
  genetics and, 345
Bone marrow transplantation, 78
Brain growth, ASD and, 371
Brain tumors, 241
Brief Adherence Rating Scale, 34
Brief Infant Sleep Questionnaire, 454
Bright Futures, 605
Bronchiolitis, 87
Bronchodilators, 263, 264
Bruch, Hilda, 552
BST. *See* Bioecological systems theory
Bulimia nervosa, 553–555, 558, 563
  neurobiology of, 557
  psychiatric complications of, 560
Bullying, 5
  ASD and, 372–373
  T1D and, 313
Bupropion, 563
Burns, PMTS and, 78–79

CAH. *See* Congenital adrenal hyperplasia
CALM. *See* Counseling on Access to Lethal Means
CAM. *See* Complementary and alternative medicine
Canalization, 607
Cancer, 27
  acute and late effects, 238–239
  adaptive outcomes, 243–245
  caregiver distress and, 243
  coping and, 244–245
  defining, 235
  developmental-behavioral care and, 241
  diagnosis, treatment, and survival, 236–237
  epidemiology, 236–237
  etiology, prevalence, and incidence, 236
  follow-up and transition care, 239
  HRQoL and, 240, 243–244
  models of care, 245–246
  multidisciplinary care and, 246
  physical appearance impacts, 241

PMTS and, 78
  psychosocial outcomes, 240–243
  resilience and growth and, 244
  self-management and adherence, 239–240
  stigma and, 241
  talking about, 102
Cancer disparities, 236–237
Cannabidiol (CBD), 146, 153
Care, behaviors that interfere with, 647–648
Care ambassadors, 316
Care coordination
  CHD and, 294–295
  consultation process and, 643
  defining, 295
  IBH and, 669
Caregiver distress
  cancer and, 243
  incontinence and, 485–486
Caregiver parenting stress, preterm birth and, 399–400
Caregiver report and participation, 608–609
Caregivers
  attachment and, 684
  PMTS impacts on, 82
  preterm birth impacts on, 393
  relationships and, 681
Caregiver well-being, 375–376
Caregiving factors, internalizing and externalizing problems and, 530–531
Caring contacts, 583
Cascades theory, 365
CASSY. *See* Computerized Adaptive Screen for Suicidal Youth
Cataplexy, 465–467
Catastrophizing, parental, 9
Catechol-O-methyl-transferase (COMT), 150
Cayler cardiofacial syndrome, 144, *144*
CBCL. *See* Child Behavior Checklist
CBD. *See* Cannabidiol
CBFLI. *See* Comprehensive behavioral family lifestyle interventions
CBT. *See* Cognitive behavior therapy
CBT-ED. *See* Cognitive behavior therapy for eating disorders
CBT-I. *See* Cognitive behavior therapy for insomnia
CDC. *See* Centers for Disease Control and Prevention
CDS. *See* Cognitive disengagement syndrome

Celebrations of life, 106–107
Centers for Disease Control and Prevention (CDC), 60, 342, 376
  on developmental milestones, 605
  hearing screening guidelines, 428
  mild TBI management guidelines, 201
  1-3-6 Early Hearing Detection and Intervention goal, 428
Central disorders of hypersomnolence, 465
Central nervous system (CNS)
  cancers of, 240
  cancer treatments impacting, 240
  etiologies for abnormalities of, 285–286, 286
  SCD complications in, 218
Central sensitization, 55
Cerebral blood flow, SCA and, 214
Cerebral palsy (CP), 396
Cerebral (cortical) visual impairment (CVI), 430
CF. *See* Cystic fibrosis
CFTR modulators, 264
CGM. *See* Continuous glucose monitoring
CHARGE, 285
CHD. *See* Congenital heart disease
Chiari II malformation, 188
Child Activity Limitations Interview, 57
Child Behavior Checklist (CBCL), 6, 503, 534
Child behavior problems, chronic health conditions and, 5–6
Child coping strategies, resilience and, 6
Child end-of-life care, 99
Child FIRST, 693
Childhood deaths, epidemiology of, 97–98
Child–parent psychotherapy (CPP), 85, 693, 694–695
Child Protective Services (CPS), 579
Child psychology
  chronic health condition clinical implications for, 17–18
  pediatrics collaboration with, 3
Children's Depression Rating Scale-Revised, 221
Children's Sleep Habits Questionnaire, 454
Child Trauma Screening Questionnaire, 80
Chromosomal microarray (CMA), 143, 150

Chromosome 21, 147
Chromosome 22q11.2 deletion syndrome (22q), 143, 154, 155, 285
  future treatments, 146–147
  management and intervention, 146
  medical, developmental, and behavioral phenotype, 145–146
  names associated with, *150*
  overview, prevalence, and genetics, 144–145
Chronically suboptimal metabolic control, 317–318
Chronic anemia, 213
Chronic health conditions, 3
  behavior problems and, 5–6
  beliefs about causes of, 8
  challenges faced by children and adolescents with, 4–5
  clinical implications, 17–18
  collaborative care and, 311
  consequences and parent perceptions of child vulnerability, 8–9
  controllability and self-efficacy, 10
  developmental considerations, 5
  developmental issues and, 10
  disruptions from, 638
  emotional functioning and, 221, 267
  family and parenting influences on coping with, 6–14
  family communication, 12–13
  family ecological contexts and, 7
  family history and, 53
  family monitoring and shared decision making, 13–14
  family processes associated with adaptation to, 7–14
  family stress and coping, 11–12
  health outcomes in children with, 5–6
  life expectancy and, 98
  methodological critique and future research directions, 16–17
  obesity and, 343
  pain from, 50
  parental attitudes and beliefs and, 7–10
  parental minimizing and dispositional optimism, 9
  parenting and family functioning and adaptation to, 14–18
  parent modeling, 10–11

  PMTS and, 77–78
  quality of life and, 5
  social activities and, 5
  suicide prevention and, 580–581
  treatment adherence and, 32
  treatment of, 8
Chronic pain, 4, 646
  assessment of, 56–58
  behavioral comorbidity screening, 57
  billing codes for, 50
  biopsychosocial models of, 55–56
  common types of, 50–51
  conceptual models of, 55–56
  COVID-19 pandemic and, 61
  defining and classifying, 49–51
  ecological and contextual factors in, 52–55
  epidemiology and economic impact of, 51–52
  individual factors in, 52–53
  parental attitudes and beliefs and, 7–8
  parent and family factors in, 53–54
  psychological therapies for, 59
  resilience factors for adjustment in, 56
  SCD and, 213, 217–218
  treatment of, 58–61
  underlying health conditions and, 50
Chronotherapy, 464
Circadian rhythm disorders, 464–465
Circadian rhythms, 447–448
Circle of Security, 693
Citalopram, *384*, 539
Cleft lip and/or palate (CL/P), 163
  body image and appearance concerns, 170–171
  care for, 165
  clinical implications of management of, 174–177
  education and support for, 175
  family and adjustment to, 169–170
  overview, 164
  peer relationships and, 169–170
  psychosocial adjustment, 168–170
  psychosocial assessment and intervention in, 176
  psychosocial screening in, 175–176
  research gaps and future directions in care for, 177
  risk and resilience factors, 167
  stigma and, 166
  treatment adherence and, 176–177
Clonazepam, *468*

Clonidine, 86, 152, *383*, *468*, 510
CL/P. *See* Cleft lip and/or palate
CMA. *See* Chromosomal microarray
CMV. *See* Cytomegalovirus
CNS. *See* Central nervous system
Cochlear implants, 428, 429
Cogmed, 241
Cognitive behavior therapy (CBT), 155
   chronic pain and, 646
   consultation process and, 644
   internalizing and externalizing disorders and, 538–540
   physical therapy combination with, 58–59
   PMTS interventions and, 85
   SCD and, 218
   T1D and, 315
Cognitive behavior therapy for eating disorders (CBT-ED), 562–563
Cognitive behavior therapy for insomnia (CBT-I), 457–458
Cognitive development
   DHH children and, 423–424
   VI and, 431
Cognitive disengagement syndrome (CDS), 499–500
Cognitive functioning
   ASD and, 372
   cancer impact on, 240–241
   CL/P and, 169
   DSD and, 172–173
   preterm birth and, 396
   SCD and, 218–219
   T1D and, 313
Cognitive impairment, defining, 616
Cognitive training interventions, 508
Collaborative care, T1D and, 311
Colocated care, 662
Color of Autism Foundation, 376
Columbia Suicide Severity Rating Scale (C-SSRS), 581
Combined behavioral and medication therapy, in ADHD, 511
Communication
   death, dying, and bereavement and, 105–106
   DHH children and, 424
   DSD and, 171–172
   family, 12–13
   social, 367
Community
   internalizing and externalizing problems and, 531
   suicide risk factors, 578–579
   treatment adherence and, 33

Complementary and alternative medicine (CAM), 59–60
   ASD and, 382
Complete androgen insensitivity syndrome, 174
Complete gonadal dysgenesis, 174
Complex CHD, 283
   neurodevelopmental risks, 284
Complicated mild TBI, 197
Comprehensive behavioral family lifestyle interventions (CBFLI), 352
Computerized Adaptive Screen for Suicidal Youth (CASSY), 581
COMT. *See* Catechol-O-methyl-transferase
Conceptual skills, 617
Concerta, 146
Concussion, 197
Conductive hearing loss, 422
Confusion arousal, *461*, 461–462
Congenital adrenal hyperplasia (CAH), 164, 174
Congenital differences, 163
Congenital hearing loss, 422
Congenital heart disease (CHD), 283
   assessment and care coordination and, 294–295
   ecological contexts and outcomes in, 289–295
   epidemiology and risk factors, 284
   health disparities and outcomes in, 292–294
   medical home and multidisciplinary care roles, 295
   neurodevelopmental risk in, 284–289, *285*
   parents and outcomes, 289–292
   practice considerations for, 289
   predicting developmental outcomes, 287–288
   predicting psychosocial outcomes, 289
   psychosocial outcomes, 288
   resilience and intervention, 296–298
   social determinants of health and, 292–293
Congenital medical conditions
   clinical implications of management of, 174–177
   education and support for, 175
   frameworks for risk and resilience in, 167
   psychosocial assessment and intervention in, 176

   psychosocial screening in, 175–176
   research gaps and future directions in care for, 177
   stigma and, 165–167
   treatment adherence and, 176–177
Conners Early Childhood Rating Scale, 503
Conners Rating Scale, 502
Constipation, 478, 482
Consultation, 637
   indications for, 640–641
   process of, 643–644
Continence, 477
   development of, 478–480
Continuous glucose monitoring (CGM), 315
Control-based model of coping, 223, 244
Controller medications, 263
Conventional Test Theory (CTT), 605
Coordinated care, 662
COPE. *See* Creating Opportunities for Parent Empowerment
Coping
   active attempts, 223
   avoidant, 312
   cancer and, 244–245
   control-based model of, 223
   family, 11–12
   general recommendations for, *648*
   with illness and hospitalization, 647
   medical mistrust as, 28
   pulmonary disorders and, 269–271
   resilience and strategies of, 6
   SCD and, 222–223
   socialization of strategies for, 11
   T1D and, 312
Coping Cat, 666
Corticosteroids, 263, 264
   OSA management and, 461
Counseling on Access to Lethal Means (CALM), 582
COVID-19 pandemic, 49
   CF care and, 265
   chronic pain and, 61
   mental health crisis and, 651
   obesity and, 341
   PTSD symptoms and, 79
   social anxiety and, 532
   telehealth and, 86
CP. *See* Cerebral palsy
CPP. *See* Child–parent psychotherapy
CPS. *See* Child Protective Services
Creating Opportunities for Parent Empowerment (COPE), 85

Crisis intervention, pediatric psychology consultation-liaison and, 650–651
Crisis supports, 584
Crisis Textline, 584
Critical periods, 600
Crizanlizumab, 215
Cross-gender identifications, 126
C-SSRS. *See* Columbia Suicide Severity Rating Scale
CTT. *See* Conventional Test Theory
Culture
　health disparities and, 16
　internalizing and externalizing problems and, 526
　PMTS and, 86–87
CVI. *See* Cerebral (cortical) visual impairment
CVI Range assessment, 433
Cyproheptadine, *468*
Cystic fibrosis (CF), 12, 216, 255
　academic and social functioning impacts, 268
　adherence and, 266
　background and significance for, 256–257
　clinical guidelines and standards of care, 263
　coping and, 269–271
　diabetes and, 264
　ecological contexts and outcomes from, 265
　ecological factors, 259
　mental health and emotional well-being and, 267
　pathophysiology of, 258
　prevalence and public health impacts, 256–257
　screening for, 262, 263
　social determinants of health and health equity and, 262
　social support and, 267, 271
　symptom management, 263–264
Cytomegalovirus (CMV), 423

Daily report cards, 508
DB. *See* Deaf-Blindness
DBDs. *See* Disruptive behavior disorders
DBT. *See* Dialectical behavior therapy
Deaf, 422
Deaf and hard of hearing (DHH)
　emotional and behavioral functioning and, 427–428
　management and interventions in, 428–430
　medical evaluation of, 427
　outcomes, 423–425
Deaf-Blindness (DB), 434–435
Death and dying
　communication and, 105–106
　developmental considerations in, 101–102
　family system and, 102–103
　goal-directed partnerships and, 105–106
　lifespan considerations, 98–99
　methodological considerations in research, 108
　risk and resilience factors and, 104–105
　rituals after, 106–107
　supporting families through, 103–106
　talking about, 102
Decision making, shared, 13–14
Default mode network (DMN), 498
D-E-F Framework, 84
Deficit, 598–599
Delay, 598–599
Delay aversion, 498
Delayed-onset hearing loss, 422
Delayed sleep–wake phase disorder (DSWPD), 464–465
Demi-boy, 129
Demi-girl, 129
Depression, 523
　ADHD and, 506–507
　cancer and, 242
　CBT for, 539
　chronic pain and, 52
　continuity in, 526
　maternal, 400
　obesity and, 349
　pediatric psychology consultation-liaison and, 650
　preterm birth and caregiver symptoms of, 400
　PTMS and, 81
　T1D and, 311–312
　T2D and, 319
Depressive disorders, 533
Desmopressin, 488, 489
Development
　ADHD diagnosis and, 503–504
　ADHD treatment and, 511–513
　ASD and trajectories of, 372
　authentic gender self emergence in, 130–131
　body image and, 170–171
　CHD and neural, 285–289
　CHD interventions and, 297–298
　chronic health conditions and, 5
　chronic pain and, 52–55
　of continence, 478–480
　death and dying and, 101–102
　delay *versus* disorder or deficit in, 598–599
　domains of, 604
　family factors in, 15–16
　gender identity as milestone of, 124
　internalizing and externalizing problems and status of, 530
　milestones in, 604–606
　pediatric sleep and, 448, *449*
　PMTS and, 74
　relational health across, 682–683
　stigma and, 166–167
　suicidal thinking and behavior and, 577
　22q and, 145–146
Developmental assessment, 597
　components of, 607–610
　definitions for, 598–599
　focus at different ages of, 604
　future directions in, 610
　neuroenvironmental synthesis model and, 599–601
　prediction and, 601–604
　psychometric concerns and test issues, 606–607
Developmental behavioral pediatrics
　ADHD and, 502–513
　chronic pain and, 60–61
　DHH children and, 428
　diabetes and role of, 323–324
　IBH implications for, 671–672
　intellect assessment and, 624–625
　RFI relevance for, 696–698
　SCD and, 225
　sleep disorder implications for, 469
Developmental cascade models, 32
Developmental delay, 143
Developmental Origins of Health and Disease hypothesis (DOHAD), 344
Developmental plasticity, 601
Developmental quotients, 605
Developmental science, treatment adherence implications for, 38–39
Developmental stage, of adolescence, 131
Deviance, 599

Index

Dextroamphetamine, 509, 511
DHH. *See* Deaf and hard of hearing
Diabetes, 12. *See also* Type 1 diabetes; Type 2 diabetes
  adaptation to, 307
  CF and, 264
  clinical practice recommendations, 323–324
  future research directions, 324
  Type 1, 4, 27
Diabetes Distress Scale, 321
Diabetes Management Summary Score, 322
Diabetic ketoacidosis (DKA), 308, 312, 313, 317
Diagnosis, acceptance of, 7–8
Diagnostic and Statistical Manual of Mental Disorders, 5th edition (*DSM-5*)
  on ADHD, 498, 500, 502–504
  ASD diagnostic criteria in, 367
  on depression, 506
  on eating disorders, 552, 552–553
  on elimination disorders, 480, *480*
  on externalizing problems, 533
  gender dysphoria in, 125, 138
  on generalized anxiety disorder, 506
  on ID, 616, 617–618
  on insomnia, 455
  on internalizing and externalizing problems, 524
  models for SLDs, 619
  on parent–child relationship, 686
  PMTS screening and assessment and, 80
  on stress disorders, 72
Dialectical behavior therapy (DBT), consultation process and, 644
Diaper rashes, 482
Dickey Amendment, 586
Differences of sex development (DSD), 163
  body image and appearance concerns, 174
  care for, 165
  clinical implications of management of, 174–177
  communication and, 171–172
  education and support for, 175
  family and adjustment to, 173
  overview, 164
  peer relationships and, 173–174
  prenatal care and, 171
  psychosocial adjustment, 171–174
  psychosocial assessment and intervention in, 176
  psychosocial screening in, 175–176
  research gaps and future directions in care for, 177
  risk and resilience factors, 167
  stigma and, 166, 171
  treatment adherence and, 176–177
DiGeorge syndrome, 150, 285
Digital health interventions, 37–38
Digital interventions, 317
Diphenhydramine, *468*
Discharge planning, 643
Discomfort, sources of, 4
Discrete trial training (DTT), 380
Disorder, 598–599
Disordered eating, T2D and, 320
Dispositional optimism, parental, 9
Disruption, factors in, 4
Disruptive behavior disorders (DBDs), ADHD and, 507
Dissociation, 599
  peritraumatic, 74
Distress, 642
Divalproex, 540
Diversity
  epilepsy and, 194–195
  SB and, 189
  TBI and, 198–199
DKA. *See* Diabetic ketoacidosis
DMN. *See* Default mode network
DNR orders. *See* Do-not-resuscitate orders
DOHAD. *See* Developmental Origins of Health and Disease hypothesis
Do-not-resuscitate orders (DNR orders), 99
Double deficit model, 627
Down syndrome (DS), 143, 147–149, 154, 155, 236, 285
  OSA and, 459
Doxepin, *468*
DS. *See* Down syndrome
DSD. *See* Differences of sex development
DSM-5. *See Diagnostic and Statistical Manual of Mental Disorders*, 5th edition
DSWPD. *See* Delayed sleep–wake phase disorder
DTT. *See* Discrete trial training
Duloxetine, 539
Dyscalculia, 620
Dysgraphia, 620
Dyslexia, 617, 620
Dyslipidemia, 319
Dyspepsia, functional, 51

Early brain development, 597
Early intervention, CHD and, 294–295
Early literacy supports, hearing impairment and, 430
Early relational health (ERH), 682
Early Relational Health-Conversations (ERH-C), 692
Early Relational Health Screen (ERHS), 691–692
Early Start Denver Model (ESDM), 152, 380
Eating disorders, 646
  appropriate level of care for, 560–565
  clinical presentations of, 557–558
  defining, 551
  epidemiology of, 554
  etiology and maintaining mechanisms, 554–555
  historical overview for, 551–552
  impacts of, 556–557
  major types of, 552–554
  medical complications of, *558*, 558–560
  neurobiology of, 557
  psychiatric complications of, 560
  risk factors, 555–556
  T1D and, 312
  T2D and, 320
  treatment outcomes and prevention, 564–565
Ecological contexts
  CHD outcomes and, 289–295
  family, 7
  IBH and, 664
  ID and, 622
  obesity and, 343–344
  pulmonary disorder outcomes and, 264–265
  relational work and, 690
  SLDs and, 624
  suicide and, 587
  T1D and, 309–311
  T2D and, 318–320
Ecological momentary assessment (EMA), 35
Ecological Systems Theory, 215–216
Economic hardship, health disparities and, 15–16
EDI. *See* Emotional development interaction
EDS. *See* Excessive daytime sleepiness
Education
  ASD and, 374–375
  congenital medical condition management and, 175

epilepsy and, 195
IBH and, 668–669
internalizing and externalizing problems and, 531
obesity interventions in, 353
postsecondary, 374–375
preterm birth impacts on, 396
SB and, 189–190
TBI and, 199
Education of All Handicapped Children Act (1975), 617
EEG biofeedback, 509
EF. *See* Executive function
Electronic monitors, 35
Elimination disorders, 477
definitions for, *480*, 480–481
epidemiology of, 481–482
intervention for, 487–488
outcome measures, 490–491
theoretical models of, 482
Elimination log, 486
EMA. *See* Ecological momentary assessment
EMDR. *See* Eye movement desensitization and reprocessing
Emotional development interaction (EDI), 538–539
Emotional distress, parent, 53
Emotional functioning
cancer impacts on, 242–243
chronic health conditions and, 221, 267
CL/P and, 168–169
DSD and, 172–173
hearing impairment and, 427–428
obesity and, 348–349
preterm birth and, 397
pulmonary disorders and, 267
SCD and, 221
VI and, 434
Empirically supported treatments (ESTs), 670
Enacted stigma, 166
Encopresis, 480, 481, *481*
Endocrine Society Clinical Practice Guideline, 134
End-of-life care, 97
of children, 99
ecological contexts relevant to, 101–103
of infants in NICU, 98–99
methodological considerations in research, 108
models of, 99–101

pediatric psychology consultation-liaison and, 649–650
Enuresis, 480, *480*, 481–482, 488
ADHD and, 483
Environmental conditions
ADHD and, 500–501
ASD and, 370
brain development and, 600
development prediction and, 603
eating disorders and, 556
Environmental tobacco smoke, 260
Epigenetics, 345, 600
Epilepsy, 187
clinical intervention and research recommendations, 197
clinical management, 196
clinical presentation and developmental course, 194
diversity and equity and, 194–195
epidemiology, 194
etiology and prognosis, 194
outcomes, 195
risk and resilience factors, 195–196
self-management and adherence, 196
types of, 194
EpiTRAQ, 196
Equity
epilepsy and, 194–195
IBH and, 667
SB and, 189
TBI and, 198–199
ERH. *See* Early relational health
ERH-C. *See* Early Relational Health-Conversations
ERHS. *See* Early Relational Health Screen
ERPOs. *See* Extreme Risk Prevention Orders
Escitalopram, *384*, 539
ESDM. *See* Early Start Denver Model
ESPA-COMP. *See* European Society for Patient Adherence, Compliance and Persistence
ESTs. *See* Empirically supported treatments
Ethics, IBH and, 669–671
Ethnicity
ADHD and, 500, 505, 512
obesity differences and, 343
preterm birth and, 394–395
race, 255, 259, 264, 341, 394–395, 469, *576*
European Society for Patient Adherence, Compliance and Persistence (ESPA-COMP), 28

Ewing sarcoma, 236
Excessive daytime sleepiness (EDS), 450, *450*, 454
narcolepsy and, 465–466
Excess weight
ASD and, 372
defining and diagnosing, 342–343
Executive function (EF), 367
ADHD and, 498
ASD and, 373
Experiential bias, 607
Exposure therapy, 539
Externalizing disorders, 523, 525
classification of, 524–525
clinical presentations of, 533–534
epidemiology and societal costs of, 525–527
IBH models and, 664
identification of, 527–528
risk and protective factors, 528–531
screening and clinical assessment of, 534–536
treatment and intervention, 536, *537*, *538*, 539–540
External locus of control, 642
Extinction/rapid withdrawal, 456
Extreme Risk Prevention Orders (ERPOs), 586
Eye movement desensitization and reprocessing (EMDR), 539

Families
adaptation and processes in, 7–14
as agent of change interventions, 352–353
ASD and, 375–376
CHD outcomes and, 289–292
chronic health condition adaptation and functioning of, *14*, 14–18
chronic health conditions and, 3
CL/P adjustment and, 169–170
communication, 12–13
coping with chronic health conditions and, 6–14
death and dying and, 102–103
DSD adjustment and, 173
ecological contexts, 7
epilepsy and, 195
grief interventions for, 107–108
health disparities and, 15–16
ICU hospitalization impacts on, 79
incontinence and stress on, 485–486
monitoring, 13–14
obesity and functioning of, 347–348

Families *(continued)*
   palliative care implementation and, 101
   PMTS impacts on functioning of, 83
   preterm birth impacts on, 393
   preterm birth outcomes and, 402
   SB and, 190
   stress and coping, 11–12
   suicide risk factors, 578–579
   supporting through death, dying, and bereavement, 103–106
   T1D and, 309, 314, 316
   T2D and, 318–319, 322
   TBI and, 199–200
   treatment adherence factors, 32–33
Family and Medical Leave Act, 107
Family-based treatment (FBT), 561–562
Family Check-Up (FCU), 585
Family-level interventions, 36–37
Family Nurture Intervention, 404
Family systems-illness model, 365
FAPD. *See* Functional abdominal pain disorders
FAPE. *See* Free, appropriate public education
FBT. *See* Family-based treatment
FCU. *See* Family Check-Up
FDA. *See* Food and Drug Administration
Fear avoidance model, 55
Fecal incontinence, 481, *481*, 482
   interventions, 489–490
Federal nutrition programs, 353–354
Feeding disorders, 645
Fee-for-service models, 668
Felt stigma, 166
Fibromyalgia, 51
Firearms, suicide and, 575, 586
FISH. *See* Fluorescence in-situ hybridization
504 plans, 625
Fluorescence in-situ hybridization (FISH), 150
Fluoxetine, *384*, 539, 563
Fluvoxamine, *384*, 539
Flynn effect, 602
Focal onset seizures, 194
Food and Drug Administration (FDA), 215, 463
   ADHD medications and, 509, 512
Food supplements, ADHD treatment and, 511
Fragile X syndrome (FXS), 143, 530
   autism and, 150–151, 154
   diagnosis and management, 154
   molecular overview and disorders of, 150
   outcomes in childhood, 151–152
   treatment, 152–154
Free, appropriate public education (FAPE), 617, 625
Friendships, ASD and, 373
Full Scale IQ (FSIQ), 218–220
Functional abdominal pain disorders (FAPD), 51
Functional Disability Inventory, 57
Functional dyspepsia, 51
Functional nausea and vomiting, 646
Functional significance, 599
Funerals, 106–107
FXS. *See* Fragile X syndrome

Gabapentin, 469
Gabapentinoids, 60
GAD. *See* Generalized anxiety disorder
GAM. *See* Gender Affirmative Model
Gastrointestinal symptoms, 646
Gatekeeper training, 585
GBG. *See* The Good Behavior Game
GCS. *See* Glasgow Coma Scale
GDD. *See* Global developmental delay
Gender, 123
   ADHD and, 512
   developmental emergence of authentic self, 130–131
   eating disorders and, 555
   explorations of, 131
   internalizing and externalizing problems and, 526
   obesity differences and, 343
   self-realization of, 128
   suicide and, 574–575
   theoretical models of, 124–125
Gender-affirmative assessment, 128
Gender Affirmative Model (GAM), 123
   evolution of, 124–125
   relevance of, 131–138
   stages in, 126
Gender diversity
   anticipatory guidance and considerations, 138–139
   ASD and, 370
   awareness of, 131
   clinical evaluation of, 133–136
   clinical intervention guidelines for, 136–138
   clinical management of, 132–133
   profiles and trajectories in children of, 126–130
   study findings on, 131–138
Gender dysphoria, 127, 130–132, 136, 138–139
   ASD and, 370
   body image and, 174
   epidemiology of, in childhood, 125–126
Gender expressions, 123, 124, 127
   clinical intervention guidelines and, 137–138
   exploring outside binary boxes, 129–130
Gender fluid, 129–131
Gender health, 123, 138–139
Gender identity, 123, 124
   awareness of, 127
   clinical intervention guidelines and, 138
   cross-gender identifications, 126
   early awareness of, 136–137
   exploring outside binary boxes, 129–130
Gender Identity Disorder (GID), 125
Gender literacy, 132–133
Gender minority stress, 139
Gender pathology, 124
Genderqueer, 129
Gender resilience, 138–139
Gender reveal parties, 171
Gender stress, 138–139
Generalized anxiety disorder (GAD), 533
   ADHD and, 506
Generalized onset seizures, 194
Generalized tonic-clonic seizures (GTCS), 194
Gene therapy, SCD and, 215
Genetic disorders
   cancer risk and, 236
   CHD and, 285
   ID and, 618, *618*
   SLDs and, 623, *623*
Genetics
   ADHD and, 500
   ASD and, 370
   early relationships and, 685
   eating disorders and, 555
   ID and, 621–622
   internalizing and externalizing problems and, 528
   obesity and, 345
   SLDs and, 622–624
Genetic syndromes, multidisciplinary care for children with, 154–155
Genetic workups, 143
GID. *See* Gender Identity Disorder

Glasgow Coma Scale (GCS), 197, 198
Global developmental delay (GDD), 618
Glycemic control, 314, 317, 319, 321, 322
Glymphatic system, 447
Goal-directed partnerships, death, dying, and bereavement and, 105–106
The Golden Cage (Bruch), 552
The Good Behavior Game (GBG), 584–585
Graduated extinction/withdrawal, 456
Grief, 103
    interventions for families and providers, 107–108
    parental, 104
Growth charts, 350
Growth-fostering relationships, 683
Growth hormone deficiency, 145
GTCS. *See* Generalized tonic-clonic seizures
Guanfacine, 86, 152, *383*, *468*, 510, 511
Guardianship, 375
Gull, William, 552
Gut microbiome, 345

Hard of hearing, 422, 423
HbA1c. *See* Hemoglobin A1c
HbS. *See* Hemoglobin S
Headaches
    migraines, 51
    primary, 51
    tension-type, 51
Health behaviors
    household chaos and, 347
    sleep and, 452
Health care
    access to, 15–16
    chronic pain and utilization and costs of, 52
    disparities in, 15
    treatment adherence factors, 33
Health Care Toolbox (website), 84
Health disparities
    behavioral health, 664
    cancer and, 236–237
    CHD outcomes and, 292–294
    chronic pain and, 54–55
    family factors in, 15–16
    obesity and, 343–344
    preterm birth and, 396
    suicide risk factors, 579
    T2D and, 318

Health equity
    ASD and, 376
    IBH and, 667
    PPPHM and, 642
    pulmonary disorders and, 259–262
    T1D and, 308–309
    T2D and, 318
Health Equity Framework, 216
Health insurance
    cancer care and, 237
    IBH and, 667–668
Health outcomes, 3
    adherence and, 29–30
    chronic health conditions and, 5–6
    PMTS impacts on, 81
Health-related quality of life (HRQoL), 189, 190
    cancer and, 240, 243–244
    incontinence and, 484
    preterm birth and, 397
    SCD and, 224
Hearing aids, 428
Hearing impairment
    assistive devices for, 429
    behavioral interventions and, 429
    causes and clinical features of, 422
    early literacy supports and, 430
    emotional and behavioral functioning and, 427–428
    epidemiology of, 422–423
    etiology, 423
    management and interventions in, 428–430
    medical evaluation of, 427
    neurobiology, 423
    outcomes, 423–425
    psychotherapy and, 429
    screening for, 425, 427
    terminology for, 422
Heart disease, 283
Hematopoietic stem cell transplantation, 215
Hemoglobin A1c (HbA1c), 308, 312, 314, 318, 323
Hemoglobin S (HbS), 214, 215, 217, 219
Hemolytic anemia, 214
Henri, Victor, 615
Heterotypic behaviors, 610
History, in developmental assessment, 609–610
Homotypic behaviors, 610
Hospice care, 100
HOTV letter charts, 433
Household chaos, health behaviors and, 347

HPA axis. *See* Hypothalamic–pituitary–adrenal axis
HRQoL. *See* Health-related quality of life
Human-centered principles, 38
Hydroxyurea, 215
Hydroxyzine, *468*
Hyperglycemia, 320
Hypersomnia, 465
Hypertension, obesity and, 343
Hyperthyroidism, 145
Hypnogogic/hypnopompic hallucinations, 465
Hypoglycemia, 310, 316, 317
Hypogonadism, 559
Hypothalamic–pituitary–adrenal axis (HPA axis), 345–347, 526
Hypoxic-ischemic encephalopathy, 622

IASP. *See* International Association for the Study of Pain
IBD. *See* Inflammatory bowel disease
IBH. *See* Integrated behavioral health
IBS. *See* Irritable bowel syndrome
ICCLM. *See* Integrated comprehensive consultation-liaison model
ICCs. *See* Item characteristic curves
ICD-11. *See International Classification of Diseases*, 11th revision
ICSs. *See* Inhaled corticosteroids
ICU hospitalization
    family system impacts on, 79
    palliative care and, 100
ID. *See* Intellectual disability
IDEA. *See* Individuals With Disabilities Education Act
Identity
    development of, 5
    gender, 123, 124, 129–130
    transgender, 126
Identity *vs.* Role Confusion, 131
IEPs. *See* Individualized Education Plans
iManage, 38
IMH. *See* Infant mental health
IMH-HV. *See* Infant mental health home visiting
Immunological disparities, structural racism and, *261*
Impairment Rating Scale, 502
Implicit bias, identifying internalizing and externalizing problems and, 527–528
Impulse control processes, 498

717

Incontinence
　assessment of disorders of, 486–487, 487
　definitions of disorders of, *480*, 480–481
　epidemiology of disorders of, 481–482
　fecal, 481, *481*, 482, 489–490
　impact and outcomes of disorders of, 484–486
　intervention for, 487–490
　medical risk factors for, 483–484, *484*
　neurodevelopmental disorders and, 478
　outcome measures, 490–491
　risk and comorbidities in disorders of, 482–484
　urinary, *480*, 480–481, 489
Incredible Years Parenting Program, 695
Incredible Years Series, 540
Individualized Education Plans (IEPs), 435, 625
　ASD and, 381
　504 plans, 625
　genetic disorders and, 155
Individuals With Disabilities Education Act (2004) (IDEA), 294, 435, 617, 625, 628
　ASD services through, 381
Infancy
　ASD development and, 369
　RFIs in, 690–695
Infant end-of-life care, 98–99
Infant mental health (IMH), 682
Infant mental health home visiting (IMH-HV), 691, 693–694
Inflammatory bowel disease (IBD), 50, 57, 58
Information sharing considerations, 671
Ingestible sensor systems, 35–36
Inhaled corticosteroids (ICSs), 263
Insomnia
　behavioral, of childhood, 455–457
　primary, psychophysiologic, or learned, 457–458
　secondary, 464
Insulin, 308–309, 312, 314, 320
Insulin resistance, 319
Integrated behavioral health (IBH), 16
　addressing identified health needs and service gaps through, 659–660
　barriers to implementing, 663

benefits of, 663–664
ecological contexts, 664
education for, 668–669
ethical considerations in, 669–671
evidence-based practice and, 670–671
increasing equity and, 667
introduction of, 660–661
payment, reimbursement, and insurance issues, 667–668
purpose of, 661
screening, assessment, treatment, and interventions in clinical practice of, 664–667, *665*, *666*
Integrated care
　models of, 662–663
　T1D and, 311
Integrated comprehensive consultation-liaison model (ICCLM), 639, *639*, 641
Integrative medicine, 59–60
Integrative Trajectory Model, 75, 75–77, 85
Intellect, assessment of, 624–627
Intellectual disability (ID), 143
　ADHD and, 506
　ASD and, 371
　assessment of, 624–627
　conceptualizations of, 616
　definitions for, 617–618
　diagnosis of, 618
　epidemiology of, 620–621
　genetic disorders in, 618, *618*
　historical overview, 615–616
　interventions, 627–629
　preterm birth and, 396
　PTSD and, 74
　relationships and, 687
　risk factors for, 621–622
Intelligence quotient (IQ), 616
Intensive Training Program (ITP), 36
Interactive behaviors, preterm birth and, 400–401
Interdisciplinary pediatric pain clinics, 60–61
Intergenerational trauma, PMTS and, 87
Internalizing disorders, 349, 523, *525*
　ADHD and, 506–507
　classification of, 524–525
　clinical presentations of, 532–533
　epidemiology and societal costs of, 525–527
　IBH models and, 664
　identification of, 527–528

risk and protective factors, 528–531
screening and clinical assessment of, 534–536
treatment and intervention, 536, *537*, *538*, 538–539
International 22q11.2 Deletion Syndrome Consortium, 145
International Association for the Study of Pain (IASP), 49, 50
International Children's Continence Society, 480, *480*, 490
International Classification of Diseases, 11th revision (*ICD-11*), 50
　on ID, 616
　on internalizing and externalizing problems, 524
International Society for Pediatric and Adolescent Diabetes (ISPAD), 310, 321, 323
Interpersonal Theory of Suicide (IPTS), 575–576
Interventions
　for ADHD, 507–511
　adherence, 36–38, 266–267
　for at-risk dyads, 692–693
　for CHD, 296–298
　cognitive training, 508
　in consultation process, 643–644
　development prediction and, 603
　for DHH children, 428–430
　digital, 317
　digital health, 37–38
　early intervention programs, 294–295
　family-level, 36–37
　grief, 107–108
　IBH and, 664–667, *666*
　for incontinence disorders, 487–490
　for internalizing and externalizing disorders, 536, *537*, *538*, 538–540
　lifestyle, 322
　in multisensory impairment, 435
　multisystemic, 37
　patient-level, 36
　peer group, 317, 322, 323
　relationally focused, 689–690
　safety planning, 582
　social skills, 381–382
　T1D and, 315–318
　T2D and, 322–323
　in VI, 434
IPTS. *See* Interpersonal Theory of Suicide

IQ. *See* Intelligence quotient
Iron, 511
    RLS and, 463
Irritable bowel syndrome (IBS), 51
IRT. *See* Item Response Theory
ISPAD. *See* International Society for Pediatric and Adolescent Diabetes
Item characteristic curves (ICCs), 605
Item Response Theory (IRT), 605
ITP. *See* Intensive Training Program

Jacobsen deletion, 285
JIA. *See* Juvenile idiopathic arthritis
Joint Committee on Infant Hearing, 428
Juvenile idiopathic arthritis (JIA), 50, 57, 58

K6. *See* Kessler distress score
Kangaroo care, 403
Kessler distress score (K6), 321
Kirk, Samuel, 617
Klinefelter syndrome, 172
Kussmaul, Adolf, 616

Language
    ASD and, 372
    DHH children development and, 423–424
    health disparities and, 16
    suicide stigma and, 574
    VI and, 431
Language delay, SLDs and, 623
Late-emerging reading disorder, 620
Late preterm infants (LPIs), 397
Learned insomnia, 457–458
Learning disabilities, 617
Learning disorders. *See also* Specific learning disorders
    ADHD and, 506
    epidemiology of, 621
Learning outcomes, preterm birth and, 396
Least restrictive environment (LRE), 381
LEA symbols, 433
Leiter International Performance Scale, Third Edition, 427
Lethal means counseling. *See* Counseling on Access to Lethal Means
Leukemias, 236
    acute lymphoblastic, 241
Level 1 Cross-Cutting Symptoms Measures, 534

LGBTQ youth
    suicide prevention, 579–580
    suicide risk and, 575
    suicide risk factors, 579
L-glutamine, 215
Liaison activities, 637
Life course models, 55–56
Life-limiting conditions, 98
    deaths from, 99
    siblings and, 103
Lifestyle factors, T2D and, 319
Lifestyle interventions, 322
Lifestyle modifications, ADHD and, 511
Light exposure, 464
Limit-setting sleep problems, 456
Linear formats, 608
Lipomeningocele SB, 188
Lisdexamfetamine, 564
LOC. *See* Loss of consciousness
Locus of control, 642
logMar chart, 430, 433
Loss, pediatric psychology consultation-liaison and, 649–650
Loss of consciousness (LOC), 198
Low achievement model, 619
Low vision, 430
LPIs. *See* Late preterm infants
LRE. *See* Least restrictive environment
Lymphomas, 236

Magnesium, 511
Malaria, 214
Malnutrition, 558–559
Maltreatment, ADHD and, 507
Marginalized populations, suicide risk factors, 579
Maternal depression, 400
Mathematics, SLD in, 620
Maturational theory, 597
M-CHAT-R/F. *See* Modified Checklist for Autism in Toddlers, Revised With Follow-Up
Media-related contagion, 585–586
Medicaid, CF and, 259
Medical Adherence Measure, 34
Medical complexity, 98
Medical-legal partnerships (MLPs), 259
Medical mistrust, 28
Medical regimen nonadherence, 649
Medical risk factors
    ADHD and, 501
    for incontinence, 483–484, *484*
    T2D and, 319

Medical system factors
    T1D and, 310–311
    T2D and, 319
Medical traumatic stress, 648–649
Medication Adherence Rating Scale, 34
Medication Adherence Self-report Inventory, 34
Medications
    ADHD management with, 509–510, 512
    ASD management and, 382, *383–384*
    eating disorder management and, 563–564
    palliative care and, 101
    PMTS and, 86
    sleep disorder management with, 467, *468, 469*
Melanoma, 236
Melatonin, 372, 382, *384*, 448, 464, *468, 469*
Memorials, 106–107
Meningocele SB, 188
Mental health
    asthma and, 260
    bladder or bowel problem risks and, 483
    parental, NICU screening for, 405–407, *406*
    pediatric psychology consultation-liaison and common concerns of, 650–651
    sleep and, 452
    suicide risk factors, 578, 579
Mentalization, 686
Mental retardation. *See* Intellectual disability
Mental status, changes in, 651
Mentoring relationships, 683
Metabolic syndrome, ASD and, 372
Metformin, 153, 322, 382
Methylphenidate, *383*, 509, 511
Metyrosine, 146
Microbiome, 345
Microdeletion syndromes, 143, 150
Migraines, 51
Mild TBI, 197
    clinical management, 201
    clinical presentation and developmental course, 198
    outcomes, 199
    risk and resilience factors, 200
Mindfulness-based CBT, 539
Mindfulness-based stress reduction, 539
Mind wandering, 499, 500
Minimizing, parental, 9

Minocycline, 153
Minority Stress Model, 580
MIS-C. *See* Multisystem inflammatory syndrome
MLPs. *See* Medical-legal partnerships
Mobile medicine, 16
Modafinil, 466
Modeling, parent, 10–11
Modified Checklist for Autism in Toddlers, Revised With Follow-Up (M-CHAT-R/F), 377
Mom Power, 693
Monocular blindness, 430
Mood disorders
　ADHD and, 506–507
　chronic pain and, 52
Mosaicism, 147
Motivational interviewing, 643–644
Motor development, VI and, 431
Motor/physical competence, 617
MSEL. *See* Mullen Scales of Early Learning
MSLT. *See* Multiple sleep latency test
Mullen Scales of Early Learning (MSEL), 153
Multidimensional Anxiety Scale for Children, 534
Multi-inflammatory syndrome, 341
Multiple sleep latency test (MSLT), 454
Multisensory impairment, 434–435
Multisystemic interventions, adherence, 37
Multisystemic therapy, 37
Multisystem inflammatory syndrome (MIS-C), 79, 341
Musculoskeletal and joint pain, 51
Myelomeningocele SB, 188, 192

N-acetyl-cysteine, *383*
Narcolepsy, 465–467
National Action Alliance for Suicide Prevention, 584, 586
National Child Traumatic Stress Network (NCTSN), 84
National Health Examination Survey (NHANES), 342
National Institutes of Health, 216
National Reading Panel, 629
National School Lunch Program, 353
National Strategy for Suicide Prevention, 573, 577, 581
National Suicide Prevention Lifeline, 584, 585
National Violent Death Reporting System (NVDRS), 574, 584

Naturalistic developmental behavioral interventions (NDBIs), 380
NCTSN. *See* National Child Traumatic Stress Network
NDBIs. *See* Naturalistic developmental behavioral interventions
NDDs. *See* Neurodevelopmental disabilities
Neighborhoods, obesity and, 348
Neonatal follow-up programs, 407–408
Neonatal intensive care unit (NICU), 73, 74, 398–400
　developmental surveillance and longitudinal monitoring after discharge from, 407–408
　discharge planning and transition to home from, 407
　end-of-life care in, 98–99
　family system impacts of, 79
　interventions to facilitate family bonding in, 403–404
　mental health and psychological support in, 404–407
　neuroprotective approaches, 403
　parental mental health screening in, 405–407, *406*
　pediatric psychology consultation-liaison and, 648
Neonatal mortality, 395–396
Nervous system disorders, 187
Neural tube, 188
Neurobiology
　ASD and, 370–371
　of hearing impairment, 423
　of sleep, 446–448
　of visual impairment, 430
Neuroblastoma, 236
Neurocognitive functioning
　T1D and, 313
　T2D and, 319–320
Neurodevelopmental and neurosensory disabilities
　preterm birth and, 396
　relationships and, 687
Neurodevelopmental disabilities (NDDs), 602–603
Neurodevelopmental disorders
　ADHD and, 500
　incontinence and, 483
　toilet training and, 482
Neurodiverse youth, suicide prevention and, 580
Neuroenvironmental synthesis model, 599–601
Neurofeedback, 509

Neuronal plasticity, 600
Neurosensory disorders
　assessment and management of, 425, *426*
　equity and inclusion and rights and advocacy for, 435
　future research directions, 436
　prognostic factors for, 421
Newborn Individualized Developmental Care and Assessment Program (NIDCAP), 298, 403–404
New Forrest Program, 540
NHANES. *See* National Health Examination Survey
NICH. *See* Novel Interventions in Children's Healthcare
NICU. *See* Neonatal intensive care unit
NIDCAP. *See* Newborn Individualized Developmental Care and Assessment Program
Nightmares, 461, 461–462
Night wakings, 455–457
Nocturnal seizures, 461, *461*
No-harm contracts, 582
Nonbinary, 129
Nonheterosexuality, ASD and, 370
Nonlinear formats, 608
Nonsuicidal self-injury (NSSI), 574, 578, 580
Norepinephrine reuptake inhibitors, 509–510
Novel Interventions in Children's Healthcare (NICH), 37
NRC-1, 146
NSSI. *See* Nonsuicidal self-injury
NVDRS. *See* National Violent Death Reporting System

OAE. *See* Otoacoustic emissions
OAHI. *See* Obstructive AHI
Obesity, 319, 341
　ASD and, 372
　biological factors in, 345–346
　defining and diagnosing, 342–343
　ecological contexts and social determinants of health and, 343–344
　health disparities and, 343–344
　outcomes, 348–349
　pediatrician's role, 351–352
　pediatric psychologist's role, 352
　prevalence of pediatric, 343
　psychological factors, 346–347
　risk and resilience factors, 345–348
　school-based interventions, 353

screening and assessment of, 349–350
social factors, 347–348
staged approach to treatment, 351
stigma and, 346
stress and, 345, 346–347
theoretical models of, 344–345
trauma and, 346–347
treatment and interventions in clinical practice, 350–354
Objective diagnostic testing, ADHD evaluation and, 505
Objective measures
technology-supported, 35–36
of treatment adherence, 34–36
Observation, 607–608
Observational effect, 602
Obstructive AHI (OAHI), 460
Obstructive sleep apnea (OSA), 319
defining, 458
etiology, 458–459
evaluation of, 460
pathophysiology and clinical symptoms, 459
treatment, 460–461
Occulta SB, 188
ODD. *See* Oppositional defiant disorder
OI. *See* Orthopedic injury
Olanzapine, 563
Omega-3 supplements, 511
1-3-6 Early Hearing Detection and Intervention goal, 428
Ongoing care phase, 76
Opioids, 60
Opitz G/BBB, 150
Oppositional defiant disorder (ODD), 370, 533, 540
Organ donation, 106
Organizational skills training, 508
Orthopedic injury (OI), 199–200
Orton, Samuel, 629
OSA. *See* Obstructive sleep apnea
OSFEDs. *See* Other specified feeding and eating disorders
Osteosarcoma, 236
Other specified feeding and eating disorders (OSFEDs), 554
Otoacoustic emissions (OAE), 425
Otolaryngology, 428–429
Overprotectiveness, 8–9, 18
Oxybutynin, 489

Pain. *See also* Chronic pain
acute, 49–50, 217–218
acute stress disorder and, 74
chronic, 213, 646
classification of, 49–51
consultation-liaison considerations and, 645–646
parental attitudes and beliefs and chronic, 7–8
parental grief, 104
PMTS and management of, 84
recurrent, 50–51
underlying health conditions and, 50
Pain catastrophizing, 217
Pain interference, assessment of, 57–58
Palliative care, 97, 100–101
methodological considerations in research, 108
PAP. *See* Positive airway pressure
Parasomnias, *461*, 461–462
Parental attitudes and beliefs
acceptance of diagnosis and, 7–8
catastrophizing, 9
causes and, 8
chronic health condition adaptation and, 7–10
chronic pain and, 53–54
controllability and self-efficacy, 10
developmental issues and, 10
minimizing and dispositional optimism, 9
perceptions of child vulnerability, 8–9
psychological flexibility, 9
treatment and, 8
uncertainty tolerance, 9–10
Parental distress
emotional, 53
PMTS and level of, 73–74
Parental grief, 104
Parental mentalization, 686
Parental stress and adjustment, T1D and, 310
Parent–child interaction therapy (PCIT), 539–540, 666, 695
Parenting
ADHD and, 502
CHD outcomes and, 290
chronic health condition adaptation and, *14*, 14–18
coping with chronic health conditions and, 6–14
family stress and coping, 11–12
food-specific, 347
mentalization and, 686
preterm birth and transition to, 398–402
self-management and, 13

Parent management training (PMT), 539–540, 695
Parent Management Training: the Oregon Model, 540
Parent-mediated therapies, 380
Parent modeling, 10–11
Parents
CHD and mental health of, 289–292
child death impact on, 102–103
incontinence disorders and, 483
PMTS impacts on, 82
psychosocial adaptation to CL/P diagnosis, 168
psychosocial adaptation to DSD diagnosis, 171–172
T1D interventions and, 318
Paroxetine, 539
PARSE. *See* Patient ask recommend see evaluate model
Partial arousal parasomnias, 462
Passive adherence coping, 223
PAT. *See* Psychosocial Assessment Tool
Patient ask recommend see evaluate model (PARSE), 669
Patient Health Questionnaire-9, 57
Patient Health Questionnaire-Adolescents, 534
Patient-level interventions, adherence, 36
Patient privacy, 671
Patient Reported Outcomes Measurement Information System (PROMIS), 57
PCIT. *See* Parent–child interaction therapy
Pediatric Emotional Distress Scale, 80
Pediatric ICU (PICU), 74
family system impacts of, 79
parent well-being impacts of, 82
PMTS interventions and, 85
Pediatric medical traumatic stress (PMTS), 71
chronic diseases and, 77–78
clinical conditions associated with, 77–80
conceptual frameworks for, 75–77
defining, symptoms, and epidemiology of, 72
impacts on well-being of, 80–83
Integrative Trajectory Model of, *75*, 75–77, 85
interventions, 83–87
medications and, 86
pain management and, 84

Pediatric medical traumatic stress (PMTS) *(continued)*
  posttraumatic growth and resilience following, 83
  risk and protective factors in, 73–75, 76
  screening and assessment for, 80
  trajectories of, 76–77
  trauma nature and risk for development of, 72–73
Pediatric Medical Traumatic Stress Toolkit for Health Care Providers, 84
Pediatric palliative care, 97
Pediatric psychology consultation, 637
Pediatric psychology consultation-liaison
  adaptation concerns and, 647–651
  consultation process, 643–644
  evaluation and evidence-based intervention considerations in, 644–647
  theoretical models and ecological contexts for, 638–642
  traditional psychological practice difference from, 637–638
Pediatric Psychosocial Preventative Health Model (PPPHM), 84, 245–246, 639, 640–642
Pediatric Quality of Life Inventory, 57–58, 322
Pediatrics
  child psychology collaboration with, 3
  genetic syndromes and, 154
  treatment adherence implications for, 38–39
Pediatric Self-Management Model, 240
Pediatric Sleep Questionnaire, 454
Peer group interventions, 317, 322, 323
Peer relationships
  ASD and, 372–373
  CL/P adjustment and, 169–170
  DHH children and, 424
  DSD adjustment and, 173–174
  epilepsy and, 195
  SB and, 190
  SCD and, 220–221
  TBI and, 199–200
PEERS. *See* Program for the Education and Enrichment of Relational Skills

Peers, obesity and, 348
Peer victimization, 348–349
Perceived burdensomeness, 576
Percent delay, 605–606
Perinatal mental health professionals (PMHPs), 404–405
Periodic limb movement disorder (PLMD), 462–463
Periodic limb movements (PLMs), 462–463
Peripheral sensitization, 55
Peritrauma phase, 76
Peritraumatic dissociation, 74
Persisters, 126, 127
Personal agency, ASD and, 373–374
PFTs. *See* Pulmonary function testing
Phobias, 533
PHQ-9, 321
Physical examination, in developmental assessment, 609–610
Physical health
  ASD and, 371–372
  internalizing and externalizing problems and, 530
  pediatric psychology consultation-liaison and considerations, 645–647
  sleep and, 452
Physical therapy, chronic pain and, 58–59
Pica, 553
PICU. *See* Pediatric ICU
Pill counts, 34–35
Placental dysfunction, 285
PLMD. *See* Periodic limb movement disorder
PLMs. *See* Periodic limb movements
PMHPs. *See* Perinatal mental health professionals
PMT. *See* Parent management training
PMTS. *See* Pediatric medical traumatic stress
Polycystic ovary syndrome, 319
Polyethylene glycol, 488
Polysomnography (PSG), 454, 460
Positive airway pressure (PAP), 461
Postconcussive syndrome, 198, 201
Posttraumatic amnesia (PTA), 198
Posttraumatic growth (PTG), 83, 87
Posttraumatic stress disorder (PTSD), 72
  childbirth and, 398–399
  COVID-related disruptions and, 79
  health outcomes and, 81
  intellectual disability and, 74

  peritraumatic dissociation and, 74
  psychological functioning and, 81
  quality of life and, 81–82
  SCD and, 77
  screening and assessment for, 80
Posttraumatic stress symptoms (PTSS), 72, 80
  cancer and, 242
  caregivers and, 243
  factors in development of, 73–75
  preterm birth and, 398–399
  PTE subjective experience and, 73
Posttraumatic stress syndrome (PTSS), 6
Postvention services, 586
Potential traumatic event (PTE), 71
  subjective experience of, 73
Poverty, SLDs and, 624
PPPHM. *See* Pediatric Psychosocial Preventative Health Model
Practical skills, 617
Premutation disorders, 150–155
Prenatal care, DSD and, 171
Prenatal context, internalizing and externalizing problems and, 528–529
Prenatal infections, hearing loss from, 423
Prescription refill measures, 35
Preterm birth, 393
  ASD and, 396–397
  attachment and, 401–402
  biopsychosocial antecedents and risks with, 394–395
  caregiver parenting stress and, 399–400
  clinical care for, 402–404
  consequences of, 395–398
  defining and, 394
  developmental surveillance and longitudinal monitoring after, 407–408
  family-level factors in, 402
  future research directions, 408
  interactive behaviors and, 400–401
  outcomes, 402
  posttraumatic stress and, 398–399
  prevalence, 394
  risk factors in, 394
  social determinants of health and, 394–395
Pretransplant or surgical evaluations, 647
Prevention Plus, 351
PRIDE skills, 695

Primary care pediatricians
    benefits of integrating behavioral health with, 663–664
    integrating behavioral health with, 660–662
    referrals from, 660, 661
Primary headache, 51
Primary insomnia, 457–458
Primary pain disorder, 50–51
Problem-solving therapy (PST), 12
Process C, 447
PRODH. See Proline dehydrogenase
Program for the Education and Enrichment of Relational Skills (PEERS), 382
Proline dehydrogenase (PRODH), 144–145
PROMIS. See Patient Reported Outcomes Measurement Information System
PROMIS Pediatric Anxiety, 57
PROMIS Pediatric Pain Interference Scale, 57
PROMIS Pediatric Sleep Disturbances survey, 454
PROMIS Pediatric Sleep-Related Impairments survey, 454
PROMIS Sleep Disturbance Scale, 57
Propranolol, 86
Protogay children, 128–129
Providers, grief interventions for, 107–108
PSG. See Polysomnography
PST. See Problem-solving therapy
Psychiatric comorbidities, 22q and, 146
Psychiatric conditions, ASD and, 371
Psychiatric emergencies, 650–651
Psychoeducation
    ASD and, 382, 385
    CBT and, 538
    for internalizing and externalizing problems, 536
Psychological flexibility, parental, 9
Psychological functioning, PMTS impacts on, 81
Psychophysiologic insomnia, 457–458
Psychosis
    ADHD evaluation and, 504
    22q and, 144, 146
Psychosocial Assessment Tool (PAT), 80, 246
Psychosocial functioning
    CL/P and, 170–171
    DSD and, 174

Psychosocial screening
    T1D and, 314–315
    T2D and, 321–322
Psychosocial Standards of Care for Childhood Cancer, 245, 245
Psychosocial support, 267
Psychotherapy
    in ASD, 380–381
    hearing impairment and, 429
PTA. See Posttraumatic amnesia
PTE. See Potential traumatic event
PTEN hamartoma tumor syndrome, 236
PTG. See Posttraumatic growth
PTSD. See Posttraumatic stress disorder
PTSS. See Posttraumatic stress symptoms; Posttraumatic stress syndrome
Public health
    adherence and outcomes in, 29–30
    suicide prevention strategies, 585–586
Public policy, suicide prevention and, 586
Pulmonary disorders, 255
    academic and social functioning impacts, 268
    caregiver and family functioning and, 268–269
    clinical implications across developmental stages, 265–269
    coping and, 269–271
    ecological contexts and outcomes from, 264–265
    mental health and emotional well-being and, 267
    social determinants of health and health equity and, 259–262
    social support and, 267, 271
Pulmonary function testing (PFTs), 256, 266
Pure tone and speech audiometry, 425

QoL. See Quality of life
Quality of death, 99–100
    impacts on family and, 103
Quality of life (QoL)
    ASD and, 372
    CHD and, 292, 297
    chronic health conditions and, 5
    DHH children, 424–425
    epilepsy and, 195–196
    incontinence and, 484, 490
    obesity and, 349
    PMTS impacts on, 81–82
    SB and, 189, 191

    screening for, 57–58
    T2D and, 320
    TBI and, 199
    VI and, 432

Race
    ADHD and, 500, 505, 512
    analgesia use disparities and, 53
    behavioral health disparities and, 664
    CHD outcomes and, 292–294
    ethnicity, 255, 259, 264, 341, 394–395, 469, 576
    IBH and, 667
    identifying internalizing and externalizing problems and, 527–528
    obesity differences and, 343
    preterm birth and, 394–395
    T1D and, 308
    T2D and, 318
    technology-supported adherence measures and, 36
    treatment adherence factors and, 31
Racial bias
    relational work and, 690
    SCD and, 217, 221–224
Radio frequency identification tags, 36
Reading, SLD in, 620, 629
Reading comprehension, 620
Recurrent pain, common types of, 50–51
Red flags, 599
Reference standards, 606
Rehabilitation Act, 435, 617, 625
Reimbursement, IBH and, 667–668
Relational health, 681, 687
    across development, 682–683
    ecological contexts and, 690
    risk and resilience in, 685
    theoretical framework for, 683–686
Relationally focused interventions (RFI), 687, 689
    in adolescence, 695–696
    in clinical populations at risk, 696–698
    in infancy and early childhood, 690–695
    for school-aged children, 695
Relationally oriented assessment, 687–689, 688
Relationships, 681
    biological factors in early, 685
    disturbances and disorders in, 686–687
    growth-fostering, 683
    mentoring, 683
    safe, stable, and nurturing, 683

Reliability, 606–607
Reliever medications, 263
Remotely delivered psychological therapies, 59
REM sleep, 447
Residential and adult day programs, 375
Resilience
    bereavement and, 104–105
    cancer and, 244
    CHD and, 296–298
    child coping strategies and, 6
    chronic pain adjustment and, 56
    congenital conditions and, 167
    defining, 269, 296
    in DHH children, 425
    epilepsy and, 195–196
    ID and, 622
    internalizing and externalizing problems and, 528–531
    obesity and, 345–348
    promoting, 269–271, 270
    pulmonary disorders and, 268–269
    relational health and, 685
    SB and, 190–191
    SCD and, 224
    T1D and, 314
    T2D and, 320
    TBI and, 200
    VI and, 432–433
Response to intervention model (RTI), 619
Restless leg syndrome (RLS), 462–463
Restricted and repetitive behaviors (RRBs), 367, 372
Retinoblastoma, 236
Retinopathy, of prematurity, 396
Revised Children's Manifest Anxiety Scale, 534
RFI. *See* Relationally focused interventions
Risk factors
    in ADHD, 500–501
    cancer and, 236–237
    CHD and, 284, 288
    congenital conditions and, 167
    epilepsy and, 195–196
    internalizing and externalizing problems and, 528–531
    obesity, 345–348
    preterm birth and, 394
    pulmonary disorders and, 268–269
    relational health and, 685
    SB and, 190
    in suicide, 577–579

T1D and, 313–314
T2D and, 320
TBI and, 200
Risperidone, 146, 152, *383*
RLS. *See* Restless leg syndrome
RRBs. *See* Restricted and repetitive behaviors
RTI. *See* Response to intervention model
Rumination disorder, 553–554

SA. *See* Suicide attempt
SAD. *See* Separation anxiety disorder
Safe, stable, and nurturing relationships (SSNRs), 683
Safe Alternatives for Teens and Youth (SAFETY), 583
SAFETY-Acute Intervention, 582
Safety plans, 582
SAMHSA. *See* Substance Abuse and Mental Health Services Administration
S. aureus, 345
SB. *See* Spina bifida
SCA. *See* Sickle cell anemia
Scanning devices, 434
SCD. *See* Sickle cell disease; Social (pragmatic) communication disorder
Schizophrenia
    PRODH and, 145
    22q and, 146
School age
    ADHD and, 503–504
    ASD development and, 370
School-based interventions, 353
School environment, obesity and, 348
School functioning
    cancer impact on, 240–241
    CHD and, 287
    CL/P and, 169
    DSD and, 172–173
    SCD and, 219–220
SCIs. *See* Silent cerebral infarcts
SCQ. *See* Social Communication Questionnaire
Screen for Child Anxiety and Related Emotional Disorders, 57, 534
Screening
    for ASD, 376–377, *378*
    for CF, 262, 263
    congenital medical conditions and psychosocial, 175–176
    hearing, 425, 427
    IBH and, 664–667, *665*
    in incontinence disorders, 486–487

for internalizing and externalizing disorders, 534–536
obesity and, 349–350
for parental mental health concerns, in NICU, 405–407, *406*
for PMTS, 80
sleep, 453–454
for social determinants of health, 293
for suicide risk, 581
T1D and, 314–315
for VI, 433
Screening Tool for Early Predictors of PTSD, 80
Screen reading software, 434
Screen time, obesity and, 347–348
SDB. *See* Sleep-disordered breathing
SDBP. *See* Society for Developmental and Behavioral Pediatrics
SDBP Complex ADHD guidelines, 511, 512
Secondary control coping, 244
Secondary insomnia, 464
Seizures
    ASD and, 371
    nocturnal, 461, *461*
Selective histamine receptor antagonists, *468*
Selective mutism, 532
Selective serotonin reuptake inhibitors (SSRIs), 60, 152, 155, 539, 563
Self-care, ADHD and, 501
Self-determination, ASD and, 373–374
Self-efficacy
    parental, 10
    T1D coping and, 314
    T2D and, 320
    treatment adherence and, 31
Self-esteem, obesity and, 349
Self-management
    adherence and, 28, 32
    cancer care and, 239–240
    epilepsy and, 196
    parental involvement and, 13
    SB and, 191
    SCD and, 222
Self-regulation, 346
Self-report scales, for chronic pain, 57
Self-soothing, sleep and, 456
Sensitive periods, 423, 600
Sensitivity, 606
Sensorineural hearing loss, 422
Sensory impairment, 421
    equity and inclusion and rights and advocacy, 435
    future research directions, 436

Sensory input, 421
Sensory processing impairment, incontinence disorders and, 483
Separation anxiety disorder (SAD), 532
Serial assessment, 598–599
Serotonin and norepinephrine reuptake inhibitors, 60
Sertraline, 86, 153, *384*, 539
Service gaps, 659–660
Services cliff, 374
SES. *See* Socioeconomic status
Sex-chromosome aneuploidies, 172
Sex designated at birth, 126
Sex formation, 127
Sex roles, socialization of, 124
Sexual abuse, incontinence disorders and, 483
Sexuality, socialization and, 128
Shared decision making, 13–14
SI. *See* Suicidal ideation
Siblings
    ASD and, 376
    child death impact on, 103
    PMTS impacts on, 82
Sickle cell anemia (SCA), 213
Sickle cell disease (SCD), 31, 50
    academic, emotional, and psychosocial morbidities associated with, 219–221
    adherence and, 223–224
    coping and, 222–223
    epidemiology, 214–215
    lifelong management and transition to adult care, 226–227
    medical morbidities associated with, 216–219
    multidisciplinary care and assessment, 224–227
    pain in, 213, 217–218
    pathophysiology, 214
    PMTS and, 77–78
    predictors of health outcomes and disparities, 215–216
    prevalence and incidence, 214
    racial bias and stigma and, 221–224
    resilience and health-related quality of life and, 224
    self-management and, 222–224
    survival and mortality, 215
    treatment, 215
Silent cerebral infarcts (SCIs), 213
Simon, Theodore, 615
Six Cs model, 344
Skills acquisition, 477
SLDs. *See* Specific learning disorders

Sleep
    diagnostic tools for, 454–455
    neurobiology and regulation of, 446–448
    normative developmental patterns of pediatric, 448, *449*
    principles of healthy habits of, *450*
    regulation of, *447*, 447–448
    scope and public health significance of, 446
    stages of, 446–447
Sleep diaries, 454
Sleep-disordered breathing (SDB), 458–461
Sleep disorders
    behavioral, 455–458
    clinical assessment of, 453–455
    conceptual framework of, *450*, 450–451
    consequences associated with, 452–453
    medical comorbidities and considerations in evaluation of, 466–467
    movement disorders, 462–463
    pharmacological management of, 467, *468*, 469
    prevalence, 451
Sleep disturbances, 445
    ASD and, 372
    chronic pain and, 52–53
    screening for, 57
Sleep-onset association disorders, 455
Sleep terrors, *461*, 461–462
Sleep–wake patterns, 464–465
Sleepwalking, *461*, 461–462
Slow-wave sleep (SWS), 446–447
SMART. *See* Social-ecological model of young adult readiness for transition
Smart glasses, 434
Smoking, asthma and, 260
Social activities, chronic conditions and, 5
Social anxiety disorder, 532–533
Social assessment, of DHH children, 427
Social cognition, 367
Social communication, 367
Social (pragmatic) communication disorder (SCD), 367
Social Communication Questionnaire (SCQ), 377
Social competence, DHH children and, 424
Social context, chronic pain and, 54–55

Social determinants of health
    CHD and, 292–293
    chronic pain and, 54–55
    defining, 259
    obesity and, 343–344
    preterm birth and, 394–395
    pulmonary disorders and, 259–262
    screening for, 293
    suicide risk factors, 579
Social development
    DHH children, 424
    VI and, 431–432
Social-ecological model of young adult readiness for transition (SMART), 239
Social exclusion, 5
Social factors
    obesity and, 347–348
    T1D and, 310
Social functioning
    cancer impacts on, 241–242
    obesity and, 348–349
    pulmonary disorders and, 268
    SCD and, 220–221
Social isolation, 271
Socialization
    continence development and, 477
    of coping strategies, 11
    sex role, 124
    sexuality and, 128
Social jet lag, 448
Social perspective taking, development of, 5
Social Responsiveness Scale-Second Edition (SRS-2), 377
Social skills, 617
Social skills interventions (SSI), 381–382, 508
Social support, 267, 271
    anxiety and, 400
    suicide interventions, 582–583
    T1D and, 309, 310
Social transition, 127, 132–133, 135–137
Society for Developmental and Behavioral Pediatrics (SDBP), 511
Sociodemographic factors
    ADHD diagnosis and, 505
    ADHD treatment and, 511–513
    ID and, 622
    PMTS development and, 74
    SB and, 189
    SLDs and, 624
    T1D and, 314
    T2D and, 318

Socioecological contexts
  determinants of adherence, 31–33
  SCD and, 216
  treatment adherence and, 28–29
Socioeconomic risk factors
  asthma and, 259
  SLDs and, 624
Socioeconomic status (SES)
  ADHD and, 500, 502
  cancer disparities and, 236, 237
  CF and, 259
  CHD outcomes and, 292–294
  obesity and, 344
  preterm birth and, 401
  SB and, 189
  T1D and, 308
Sodium oxybate, 466, 467
Somatic symptom and related disorders (SSRD), 646–647
Somnambulism. *See* Sleepwalking
Special Supplemental Nutrition Program for Women, Infants, and Children (WIC), 353
Specificity, 606
Specific learning disorders (SLDs), 615
  definitions for, 618–620
  domains of impairment, 619–620
  epidemiology of, 621
  historical overview for, 616–617
  interventions, 629
  models for diagnosing, 619
  risk factors for, 622–624
Specific phobias, 533
Speech and language pathology, 429
Spence Children's Anxiety Scale, 534
Spina bifida (SB), 187
  clinical management, 191–193
  clinical presentation and developmental course, 189
  clinical recommendations, 193
  diversity and equity and, 189
  epidemiology of, 188
  etiology and prognosis for, 188–189
  future research, 193–194
  medical and psychological assessments, 192
  outcomes, 189–191
  self-management and adherence in, 191
  transition to adult health care, 191
  types of, 188
SRS-2. *See* Social Responsiveness Scale-Second Edition

SSI. *See* Social skills interventions
SSNRs. *See* Safe, stable, and nurturing relationships
SSRD. *See* Somatic symptom and related disorders
SSRIs. *See* Selective serotonin reuptake inhibitors
Standards of Care, Version 7 (WPATH), 136
Standards of Care, Version 8 (WPATH), 133–136
Stanford Revision and Extension of the Binet-Simon Scale, 615–616
Starvation, 556–557
State-Trait Anxiety Inventory for Children, 534
Stem cell transplants, psychological impacts on siblings, 82
Stepped care approach, 666
Stigma
  cancer and, 241
  congenital medical conditions and, 165–167
  development and related factors, 166–167
  DSD and, 171
  enacted, 166
  felt, 166
  obesity and, 346
  SCD and, 221–224
  T1D and, 313
Stimulant medications, 509, 540
Stool softeners, 488
Stool withholding behaviors, 482
Strange Situation Procedure, 684
Strengths and Difficulties Questionnaire, 168
Stress
  family, 11–12
  gender, 138–139
  gender minority, 139
  health disparities and, 16
  incontinence and, 485–486
  medical traumatic, 648–649
  obesity and, 345–347
  preterm birth and caregiver parenting, 399–400
  T1D and, 312
  toxic, 603
Strong Military Families, 692, 693
Strong Roots, 692–693, 697
Structural racism
  allergies and immunological disparities and, 261
  cancer disparities and, 236

  defining, 259–260
  preterm birth and, 396
Subjective assessment measures, of treatment adherence, 33–34
Substance Abuse and Mental Health Services Administration (SAMHSA), 583
Sudden unexpected death in epilepsy (SUDEP), 194
Suicidal ideation (SI), 574, 576, 577
  risk factors, 578
Suicidal thinking and behavior, 577
Suicide, 524, 573
  definitions and terminology for, 574
  emerging research and clinical directions, 587–588
  epidemiology and prevalence, 574–575
  means of, 575
  media-related contagion and, 585–586
  precipitating events, 584
  prevention and intervention, 581–583
  prevention in special clinical populations, 579–581
  prevention strategies, 584–586
  risk and protective factors, 577–579
  safety planning interventions, 582
  theories of, 575–577
  treatment, 583–584
Suicide attempt (SA), 574, 576, 577, 580
  risk factors, 578
Surviving Cancer Competently Intervention Program, 85
Sweat testing, for CF, 263
SWS. *See* Slow-wave sleep

T1D. *See* Type 1 diabetes
T2D. *See* Type 2 diabetes
Task-unrelated thought, 499
TBI. *See* Traumatic brain injury
T-box transcription factor-1 (TBX-1), 145
Teacher's Report Form, 503
Telehealth, 86
  ASD and, 376
Telemedicine, 16
  pill counts and, 35
Tension-type headaches, 51
Tetrahydrocannabinol (THC), 153
Text-level reading learning disabilities, 620
TF-CBT. *See* Trauma-focused CBT

GREYSCALE

BIN TRAVELER FORM

Cut By Meriane #6 Qty 10 Date 02/3

Scanned By Elieny Mendoza Qty 10 Date 02/19/26

Scanned Batch ID's

Notes/Exception